CAUSE	RATE
Rheumatic fever and chronic rheumatic heart disease	6.1
Congenital anomalies	5.9
Birth injury, difficult labor, and hypoxia	5.4
Nephritis and nephrosis	4.1
Septicemia	3.6
Hypertensive heart disease	3.2
Hernia and intestinal obstruction	2.6
Peptic ulcer	2.5
Hypertension	2.5
Influenza	1.9
Anemia	1.5
Hypertensive heart and renal disease	1.5
Infections of kidney	1.4
Avitaminosis	1.3
Cholelithiasis, cholecystitis, and cholangitis	1.3
Tuberculosis	1.0
Asthma	0.9
Meningitis	0.7
Acute bronchitis and bronchiolitis	0.3
Cerebral embolism	0.3
Appendicitis	0.3
Angina pectoris	0.1
Complications of pregnancy, childbirth	0.1

From the National Center for Health Statistics, *Vital Statistics Report,* Vol. 29, No. 6, September 17, 1980.

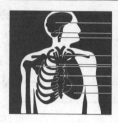

PROFESSIONAL GUIDE TO
DISEASES™

INTERMED COMMUNICATIONS, INC.
SPRINGHOUSE, PENNSYLVANIA

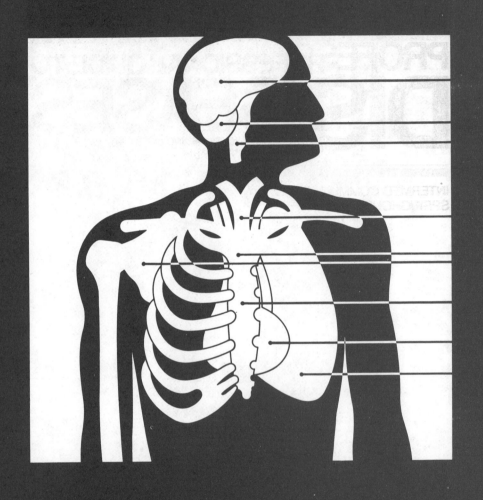

PROFESSIONAL GUIDE TO
DISEASES™

INTERMED COMMUNICATIONS, INC.
SPRINGHOUSE, PENNSYLVANIA

INTERMED COMMUNICATIONS BOOKS

Library of Congress Cataloging in Publication Data
Main entry under title:

Professional guide to diseases.

 Bibliography: p.
 Includes index.
 1. Medicine—Handbooks, manuals, etc.   2. Diseases—Handbooks, manuals, etc.   3. Nursing—Handbooks, manuals, etc.   I. Intermed Communications, inc.
 [DNLM: 1. Disease.   2. Health.   3. Medicine. WB 100 P962]
 RT65.P69   616   81-19996
 ISBN 0-916730-36-0   AACR2

Editorial and production staff

Senior Editor: Thomas Leibrandt

Associate Editors: Lisa Z. Cohen, Martin DiCarlantonio

Assistant Editors: Laura Albert, Brenda Moyer, William Kelly

Clinical Editors: Joanne Patzek DaCunha, RN; Susan M. Glover, RN, BSN; Lenora Haston, RN, MSN; Patrice Nasielski, RN

Clinical Pharmacy Editor: Larry Gever, PharmD

Production Coordinator: Patricia A. Hamilton

Copy Editors: Linda S. Hewlings, Barbara Hodgson, Jo Lennon

Designer: Kathaleen Motak Singel

Art Production Manager: Wilbur D. Davidson

Art Assistants: Diane Fox, Christopher Laird, Sandra Simms, Bob Walsh, Joan Walsh, Ron Yablon

Illustrators: Robert Jackson, Thomas Lewis, Cynthia Mason, Bud Yingling

Typography Manager: David C. Kosten

Typography Assistants: Nancy Merz Ballner, Ethel Halle, Diane Paluba

Production Manager: Robert L. Dean

Editorial Assistants: Maree DeRosa, Helen O'Connor Smith

Indexer: Grinstead/Feik Indexers

Researcher: Vonda Heller

Staff for this edition

Editors: Alan M. Rubin, Richard Samuel West

Assistant Editor: Dario F. Bernardini

Clinical Editor: Barbara McVan, RN

Copy Editor: Karen E. Loudon

Editorial Staff Assistants: Evelyn M. James, Cynthia A. Lotz

Special thanks to the following, no longer on the staff, who assisted in preparation of this volume: Susan Callaway, Katherine W. Carey, Bernard Haas, John Isely, Mary R. McCole, RN, BSN, Joan P. McNamara, RN, Genevieve O'Hara, Elaine Schott-Jones, Sara M. Sumner, RN.

Contents

1 Immune Disorders

2 Genetic Disorders

3 Mental and Emotional Disorders

4 Trauma

5 Neoplasms

6 Infection

7 Respiratory Disorders

Appendices and Index

A Note To Readers

The clinical procedures described and recommended in this publication are based on research and consultation with medical and nursing authorities. To the best of our knowledge, these procedures reflect currently accepted clinical practice; nevertheless, they can't be considered absolute and universal recommendations. For individual application, treatment recommendations must be considered in light of the patient's clinical condition and, before administration of new or infrequently used drugs, in light of latest package-insert information. The authors and the publisher disclaim responsibility for any adverse effects resulting directly or indirectly from the suggested procedures, from any undetected errors, or from the reader's misunderstanding of the text.

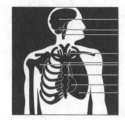

Advisory Board

At the time of original publication, these advisors, clinical consultants, and contributors held the following positions.

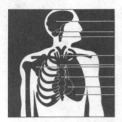

Clinical Consultants

Barbara Kupfer Alonso, RN, BSN, Nurse Clinician, High-Risk Obstetrics, Prentice Women's Hospital and Maternity Center of Northwestern Memorial Hospital, Chicago, Ill.

Charold L. Baer, RN, PhD, Professor and Chairperson, Department of Medical-Surgical Nursing, University of Oregon Health Sciences Center School of Nursing, Portland.

Edmund Martin Barbour, MD, Vice-Chief of Gastroenterology, Harper Hospital, Detroit, Mich.; Assistant Professor of Medicine, Wayne State University, Detroit.

Henry D. Berkowitz, MD, Associate Professor of Surgery; Assistant Chief of Vascular Service; Director, Peripheral Vascular Laboratory, Hospital of the University of Pennsylvania, Philadelphia.

William F. Bruther, MD, Chief of Ophthalmology, Anne Arundel General Hospital, Annapolis, Md.

Barbara R. Burroughs, RN, MSN, Pediatric Nurse Clinical Specialist and Education Coordinator, Philadelphia Regional Chronic Pulmonary Disease Program, Children's Hospital of Philadelphia (Pa.).

Monica Wolcott Choi, RN, MSN, Nurse Specialist, Health Care for Women, Penn Urban Health Maintenance Program, Philadelphia, Pa.

Susan Corbett, RN, Dermatology Nurse, Skin and Cancer Hospital and Mycosis Fungoides Center of Temple University, Philadelphia, Pa.

Robert L. Cox, MD, Clinical Infectious Diseases Consultant, Rose Medical Center, Porter Memorial Hospital, Denver, Colo.

Irene Cullin, RN, BSN, Coordinator of Nursing Education, Massachusetts Eye and Ear Infirmary, Boston.

Scott Decker, MD, Chief of Resident Training, James-Lawrence Kernan Hospital, Baltimore, Md.

Richard Depp, MD, Associate Professor and Head, Maternal-Fetal Medicine, Department of Obstetrics and Gynecology, Northwest University Medical School, Chicago, Ill.; Director of Obstetrics, Prentice Women's Hospital and Maternity Center of Northwestern Memorial Hospital, Chicago.

Toby R. Engel, MD, Professor of Medicine, Medical College of Pennsylvania, Philadelphia.

Lee Gigliotti, RN, MSN, Nursing Coordinator, University of Pennsylvania Cancer Center, and Assistant Clinical Professor of Nursing, University of Pennsylvania, Philadelphia.

Rodolfo I. Godinez, MD, PhD, Assistant Professor of Anesthesiology, Children's Hospital of Philadelphia (Pa.) and University of Pennsylvania Medical School, Philadelphia.

Pamela Miller Gotch, RN, MSN, Clinical Nurse Specialist, St. Luke's Hospital, Milwaukee, Wis.

Mitchell M. Jacobson, MD, Associate Clinical Professor of Medicine, Medical College of Wisconsin, and University of Wisconsin Medical School, Milwaukee.

Sheila M. Jenkins, RN, BSN, Instructor, Nursing of Children, Bridgeport (Conn.) Hospital School of Nursing.

Mildred L. Kistenmacher, MD, Associate Professor, Temple University, Philadelphia, Pa.; Chief of Clinical Genetics, St. Christopher's Hospital for Children, Philadelphia.

Elaine Kohler, MD, Associate Professor of Pediatrics, Medical College of Wisconsin, Milwaukee; Chief of Metabolic Division, Milwaukee (Wis.) Children's Hospital.

John Laszlo, MD, Professor of Medicine, Director of Clinical Programs, Duke University Comprehensive Cancer Center, Durham, N.C.

Herbert A. Luscombe, MD, Professor and Chairman, Department of Dermatology, Jefferson Medical College, Thomas Jefferson University, Philadelphia, Pa.

Evan G. McLeod, MD, Associate Attending Physician, Michael Reese Hospital and Medical Center, Chicago, Ill.; Assistant Professor of Medicine, University of Chicago School of Medicine.

Lorna MacNutt, RN, BSN, Nursing Education Instructor, Massachusetts Eye and Ear Infirmary, Boston.

Kenneth J. Mamot, RN, Infection Control Nurse, Genesee Hospital, Rochester, N.Y.

Celine Marsden, RN, MN, CCRN, Lecturer, University of California at Los Angeles School of Nursing.

William D. Minard, MD, Obstetrician-Gynecologist, Lansdale (Pa.) Medical Group.

Brenda M. Nevidjon, RN, MSN, Head Nurse, Inpatient Cancer Research Unit, Duke University Medical Center, Durham, N.C.

Barbara Ellen Norwitz, RN, BS, Pediatric Nurse Practitioner, Johns Hopkins Hospital, Baltimore, Md.

Patricia A. O'Brien, RN, MSN, Clinical Specialist, Orthopedics, Thomas Jefferson University Hospital, Philadelphia, Pa.

Eileen Egan Pannese, RN, BSN, MS, Coordinator, Advanced Placement Program, and Instructor, Bridgeport (Conn.) Hospital School of Nursing.

R. Parameswaran, MD, Director of CCU, Staff Cardiologist, and Clinical Associate Professor of Medicine, Albert Einstein Medical Center, Northern Division, Philadelphia, Pa.

Shaukat M. Qureshi, MD, FRCSEd, Urology Resident, Thomas Jefferson University Hospital, Philadelphia, Pa.

Kathleen Redelman, RN, BS, Clinical Specialist and Research Nurse, Division of Neurosurgery, Indiana University Medical School, Indianapolis.

Max L. Ronis, MD, Professor and Chairman, Department of Otorhinology, Temple University School of Medicine, Philadelphia, Pa.

Thomas J. Rosko, MD, Emergency Physician, Doylestown (Pa.) Hospital.

Sarah Sanford, RN, Critical Care Coordinator, Overlake Memorial Hospital, Bellevue, Wash.

Gregory Sarna, MD, Assistant Professor of Medicine, Division of Hematology/Oncology, University of California at Los Angeles Center for the Health Sciences.

Linda Patti Sarna, RN, MN, Visiting Lecturer, Graduate Oncology Program, University of California at Los Angeles School of Nursing.

Irene F. Schepartz, RN, MSN, Assistant Professor, Mental Health, Psychologic Nursing, Medical College of Georgia School of Nursing, Athens.

Allan Schwartz, MD, Professor of Medicine, Hahnemann Hospital Medical School, Philadelphia, Pa.

Joan Kelley Simoneau, RN, MICN, CCRN, Director, Nursing Practice and Education, Prime-care Corp., Marina Del Rey, Calif.

Susan E. Sweny, RN, Gastrointestinal Nurse Coordinator, Mount Auburn Hospital, Cambridge, Mass.

Madeline Musante Wake, RN, MSN, Director, Continuing Education in Nursing, Marquette University, Milwaukee, Wis.

Martin Weisburg, MD, Assistant Professor of Obstetrics and Gynecology, and Psychology, Thomas Jefferson University, Philadelphia, Pa.

Barbara Whitney, RN, MS, Executive Director, Sex Information and Education Council of the U.S. (SIECUS), New York, N.Y.

John K. Wiley, MD, Chief of Neurosurgery, Miami Valley Hospital, Dayton, Ohio; Assistant Professor of Surgery, Wright State University, Dayton.

Camille Gorman Woodward, RN, RRT, CCRN, BS, Instructor, Department of Anesthesiology, Northwestern University Medical School, Chicago, Ill.; Nurse Clinician, Department of Respiratory Therapy, Northwestern Memorial Hospital, Chicago.

Warren Jay Zalut, MD, Psychiatric Consultant, Assistant in Psychiatry, Presbyterian-University of Pennsylvania Medical Center, Philadelphia.

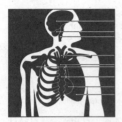

Contributors

Virginia P. Arcangelo, RN, MSN, Staff, Thomas Jefferson University Hospital, Philadelphia, Pa.

Cynthia L. Ashe, RN, Oncology Nurse Clinician, Duke University Medical Center, Durham, N.C.

Charold L. Baer, RN, PhD, Professor and Chairperson, Department of Medical-Surgical Nursing, University of Oregon Health Sciences Center School of Nursing, Portland.

Katherine Green Baker, RN, MN, Clinical Nurse Specialist, University of California at Los Angeles Center for the Health Sciences.

Judy Beniak, RN, BSN, Community Program Specialist, Comprehensive Epilepsy Program, University of Minnesota, Minneapolis.

Jo Anne Bennett, RN, CCRN, MA, Assistant Executive Director, Maternal-Child Care Services, Metropolitan Hospital Center, New York, N.Y.

Patricia M. Bennett, RN, BSN, Instructor, Shepard Gill School, Massachusetts General Hospital, Boston.

Margaret Hamilton Birney, RN, MSN, Instructor, University of Delaware College of Nursing, Newark.

Phyllis Bitner, RN, Oncology Coordinator, Medical College of Pennsylvania, Philadelphia.

Heather Boyd-Monk, RN, BSN, Educational Coordinator, Wills Eye Hospital, Philadelphia, Pa.

Hirotaka Katsumata Brailey, RN, Student, Southern Missionary College, Collegedale, Tenn.

Christine S. Breu, RN, MN, Cardiovascular Clinical Specialist, University of California at Los Angeles Hospital and Clinics.

Susan A. Budassi, RN, MSN, MICN, Clinical Specialist, Department of Emergency Medicine, Dr. David M. Brotman Memorial Hospital, Culver City, Calif.; Assistant Professor of Clinical Nursing, University of California at Los Angeles School of Nursing.

Judith Suter Burkholder, RN, MSN, Nurse Practitioner—Dermatology, Yale-New Haven Hospital, New Haven Conn.

Barbara R. Burroughs, RN, MSN, Pediatric Nurse, Clinical Specialist and Education Coordinator, Philadelphia Regional Chronic Pulmonary Disease Program, Children's Hospital of Philadelphia (Pa.).

Priscilla A. Butts, RN, MSN, Former Assistant Director of Nursing, Women and Children Care Program, Thomas Jefferson University Hospital, Philadelphia, Pa.

Mary P. Cadogan, RN, MN, Instructor, Community Health Nursing, Yale University School of Nursing, New Haven, Conn.; Family Nurse Practitioner, Hill Health Center, New Haven.

Constance C. Cooper, RN, Supervisor, Gastroenterology, Allegheny General Hospital, Pittsburgh, Pa.

Susan Corbett, RN, Dermatology Nurse, Skin and Cancer Hospital and Mycosis Fungoides Center of Temple University, Philadelphia, Pa.

H. Patricia Culp, RN, Rehabilitation Nursing Coordinator, James M. Jackson Memorial Hospital, Miami, Fla.

Joanne Patzek DaCunha, RN, Clinical Editor, Nurse's Reference Library, Intermed Communications, Inc., Springhouse, Pa.

T. Forcht Dagi, MD, Senior Neurosurgical Resident, Massachusetts General Hospital, Boston.

Janet S. D'Agostino, RN, MSN, Pulmonary Clinician, St. Elizabeth's Hospital of Boston, Brighton, Mass.

Joanne D'Agostino, RN, BA, MSN, Rehabilitation Clinical Leader, Massachusetts General Hospital, Boston.

Helen L. Davis, RN, Neonatal Nurse Clinician, Intensive Care Nursery, Thomas Jefferson University Hospital, Philadelphia, Pa.

Joan B. Davis, RN, CCRN, Critical Care Instructor, Pacific Northwest Inservice Specialists, Seattle, Wash.

Andrea L. Devoti, RN, BSN, Head Nurse, Elliot Neurological Center, Pennsylvania Hospital, Philadelphia.

Stella R. Doherty, RN, BSEd, MSN, Nursing Services Consultant for Tuberculosis, Pennsylvania Department of Health, Bureau of Epidemiology and Disease Prevention, Harrisburg.

Judy Donlen, RN, Neonatal Nursing Instructor, St. Christopher's Hospital for Children, Philadelphia, Pa.

Kathleen A. Dracup, RN, MN, CCRN, Research Fellow, Department of Medicine/Cardiology, University of California at Los Angeles.

Diane Dressler, RN, MSN, Clinical Nurse Specialist, St. Luke's Hospital, Milwaukee, Wis.

Colleen Jane Dunwoody, RN, BA, Head Nurse, Orthopedics, Presbyterian-University Hospital, Pittsburgh, Pa.

Jeanne Dupont, RN, Head Nurse, Emergency Department, Massachusetts Eye and Ear Infirmary, Boston.

Marjorie M. Eichler, RN, Staff, Dermatology Department, Yale University Health Services Center, New Haven, Conn.

Mary Ellen Florence, RN, MSN, Marital and Sex Counselor and Therapist, University of Pennsylvania, Philadelphia.

Kathleen T. Flynn, RN, MS, Assistant Professor, Medical-Surgical Nursing Program, Yale University School of Nursing, New Haven, Conn.

Bernadette M. Forget, RN, MSN, Clinical Nurse Specialist, Dermatology Department, Yale University School of Medicine, New Haven, Conn.

Nora L. Freeze, RN, MSN, Clinical Instructor, Helene Fuld School of Nursing, West Jersey Hospital, Camden, N.J.

Carolyn P. Fritz, RN, Nurse Manager, Emergency Department, Presbyterian-University of Pennsylvania Medical Center, Philadelphia.

Sally Santmyer Gammon, RN, MS, Medical/Pulmonary Clinical Nurse Specialist, St. Mary's Hospital, Richmond, Va.

Catherine D. Garofano, RN, BS, Clinical Nurse in Endocrinology and Metabolism, and Senior Instructor in Medicine, Hahnemann Medical College and Hospital, Philadelphia, Pa.

Anna Gawlinski, RN, MSN, Cardiovascular Clinical Nurse Specialist, University of California at Los Angeles Hospital.

Susan M. Glover, RN, BSN, Clinical Coordinator, Nurse's Reference Library, Intermed Communications, Inc., Springhouse, Pa.

Carol Ann Gramse, RN, MA, Assistant Director, Education and Training, Pilgrim Psychiatric Center, West Brentwood, N.Y.

Sherry Pawlak Greifzu, RN, Staff, American Oncologic Hospital, Philadelphia, Pa.

Donna H. Groh, RN, BSN, Head Nurse, Pediatric ICU, Children's Hospital of Philadelphia (Pa.)

Rebecca G. Hathaway, RN, MSN, Assistant Director of Nursing, Critical Care Division, University of California at Los Angeles Hospital, Clinics, and Center for the Health Sciences; Assistant Clinical Professor of Nursing, University of California at Los Angeles School of Nursing.

Laura Lucia Hayman, RN, MSN, Associate Professor, University of Pennsylvania School of Nursing, Philadelphia.

Eddie R. Hedrick, BS, MT (ASCP), Epidemiologist, Morristown (N.J.) Memorial Hospital.

Patricia Turk Horvath, RN, MSN, Assistant Professor, Cardiovascular-Thoracic Nursing, Medical-Surgical Nursing Program, Yale University School of Nursing, New Haven, Conn.

Mary Louise H. Jones, RN, BSN, Head Nurse, Obstetrics Department, Florida Hospital, Orlando.

Joyce L. Kee, RN, MSN, Assistant Professor, University of Delaware College of Nursing, Newark.

Margaret A. Keen, RN, MSN, Nurse Clinician, Health Care of Women, Albert Einstein Medical Center, Southern Division, Philadelphia, Pa.

Patricia Lockhart Kelley, RN, MS, Clinical Specialist/Clinical Educator in Neurology, James M. Jackson Memorial Hospital, Miami, Fla.

Karen Kennedy, RN, BSN, Staff, Emergency Room, Winter Park (Fla.) Memorial Hospital.

Joan E. Kenny, RN, Urology Nurse, Pennsylvania Hospital, Philadelphia.

Ruth S. Kitson, RN, Head Nurse, Thoracic Surgery-Respiratory Diseases, Toronto Western Hospital, Ont.

Mary E. LaBove, RN, MSN, Medical-Surgical Clinical Specialist, Our Lady of Lourdes Hospital, Camden, N.J.

Mary Ann Lafferty, PhD, Assistant Professor, University of Pennsylvania School of Nursing, Philadelphia.

Cheryl Ann Gross Lane, RN, Oncology Nurse Specialist, Bowman Gray School of Medicine of Wake Forest University, Winston-Salem, N.C.

Linda Lass-Schuhmacher, RN, MEd, Instructor, Shepard-Gill School of Practical Nursing of the Massachusetts General Hospital, Boston.

Rhea D. Lemerman, RN, BS, MEd, Instructor, Nursing Research and Development, James M. Jackson Memorial Hospital, Miami, Fla.

Blanche M. Lenard, RN, Nurse Epidemiologist, Crozer-Chester Medical Center, Chester, Pa.

Dorrett N. Linton, RN, Staff, Pennsylvania Hospital, Philadelphia.

Gail D'Onofrio Long, RN, MS, Clinical Specialist, Medical ICU/CCU, University Hospital, Boston, Mass.

Pamela Peters Long, RN, BSN, Oncology Nurse Clinician, Memorial Medical Center, Savannah, Ga.

Donna Orrill McCarthy, RN, MSN, Assistant Professor, Marquette University College of Nursing, Milwaukee, Wis.

Mary R. McCole, RN, BSN, Head Nurse, CCU, Albert Einstein Medical Center, Northern Division, Philadelphia, Pa.

Edwina A. McConnell, RN, MS, Clinical Director, Surgical Nursing, Madison (Wis.) General Hospital.

Joan P. McNamara, RN, Former Chemotherapy Nurse, Abington (Pa.) Memorial Hospital.

Shirley Heaton Marshburn, RN, Supervisor, Emergency Department, Winter Park (Fla.) Memorial Hospital.

Linda L. Martin, RN, MSN, Clinical Nurse Specialist—Pulmonary, University of Virginia Medical Center, Charlottesville.

Celestine B. Mason, RN, BSN, MA, Assistant Professor, Pacific Lutheran University School of Nursing, Tacoma, Wash.

Vivian Meehan, RN, Nursing Supervisor, Highland Park (Ill.) Hospital.

Rita V. Miller, RN, BA, Nurse Manager, Presbyterian-University of Pennsylvania Medical Center, Philadelphia.

M. Leslie Mitman, RN, BSN, Staff, Thomas Jefferson University Hospital, Philadelphia, Pa.

Karen Moore, RN, MSN, Coordinator of Quality Assurance for Nursing, Hospital of the University of Pennsylvania, Philadelphia.

Elaine Helen Niggemann, RN, MS, Student, University of Arizona College of Medicine, Tucson.

Mary Beth Pais, RN, BSN, Clinical Instructor, Orthopedics, Presbyterian-University Hospital, Pittsburgh, Pa.

A. June Partyka, RN, ET, Rehabilitation Nurse Coordinator, Ostomy Therapist, St. Francis Medical Center, Trenton, N.J.

Linda Pelczynski, RN, MSN, Neurologic Clinical Specialist, Carney Hospital, Boston, Mass.

Chris Perkins, RN, MN, Associate Professor of Nursing, Southern Missionary College, Collegedale, Tenn.

Patricia Hogan Pincus, RN, BS, Assistant Nursing Practice Coordinator, University of Rochester (N.Y.) Medical Center.

Rosemary Carol Polomano, RN, MSN, Oncology Clinical Specialist, Hospital of the University of Pennsylvania, Philadelphia.

Kathryn Preston, RN, MS, Instructor, University of Delaware College of Nursing, Newark.

Katherine S. Puls, RN, CNM, MS, Nurse-Midwife, Illinois Masonic Medical Center, Chicago.

Jo-Ellen Quinlan, RN, MSN, Gastrointestinal Nurse Clinician, Department of Gastroenterology, Children's Hospital Medical Center, Boston, Mass.

Roger L. Ready, RN, Nurse Endoscopist, Mayo Clinic, Rochester, Minn.

Mary Kay Rhoads, RN, BSN, CCRN, Clinical Instructor, Medical ICU, Duke University Medical Center, Durham, N.C.

Hazel V. Rice, RN, MS, EdS, Coordinator, Southern Missionary College, Orlando, Fla.

Marilyn A. Roderick, RN, BSN, Infection Control Consultant, Stanford, Calif.

Lisa Sehrt Rodriguez, RN, BSN, Nurse Clinician—Education, Ochsner Foundation Hospital, New Orleans, La.

Mary E. Ropka, RN, MSN, Clinical Nurse Specialist, Yale-New Haven Hospital, New Haven, Conn.

Minnie B. Rose, RN, BSN, MEd, Clinical Director, Nurse's Reference Library, Intermed Communications, Inc., Springhouse, Pa.

Pamela M. Rowe, RN, BSN, MEd, Clinical Instructor, Memorial Sloan-Kettering Cancer Center, New York, N.Y.

Sarah A. Ryan, RN, Infection Control Nurse, Crozer-Chester Medical Center, Chester, Pa.

Linda Patti Sarna, RN, MN, Visiting Lecturer, Graduate Oncology Program, University of California at Los Angeles School of Nursing.

Marilyn R. Shahan, RN, MS, Communicable Disease Nursing Consultant, Denver (Colo.) Visiting Nurse Service.

Frances W. "Billie" Sills, RN, MSN, Director of Nursing, Ortho-Rehab-Neuro Services, James M. Jackson Memorial Hospital, Miami, Fla.

Christine McNamee Smith, RN, BSN, Nurse Clinician, Thomas Jefferson University Hospital, Philadelphia, Pa.

Janis B. Smith, RN, BSN, Staff Education Instructor, Pediatric ICU, Children's Hospital of Philadelphia (Pa.).

Mary Lillian (Lilleé) Smith, RN, MSN, Assistant Director, Maternal/Child Health, Burlington County Memorial Hospital, Mount Holly, N.J.

June L. Stark, RN, Critical Care Instructor, Tufts-New England Medical Center, Boston, Mass.

Deborah Steiner, RN, Staff, Gastroenterology Laboratory, St. Francis General Hospital, Pittsburgh, Pa.

Janice G. Stewart, RN, MSN, Respiratory Clinical Nurse Specialist, Thomas Jefferson University Hospital, Philadelphia, Pa.

Nancy S. Storz, RD, MS, Assistant Professor, University of Pennsylvania School of Nursing, Philadelphia.

Sara M. Sumner, RN, Supervisor, Critical Care, Sacred Heart General Hospital, Chester, Pa.

Mona R. Sutnick, RD, MS, Clinical Associate, University of Pennsylvania School of Dental Medicine, Philadelphia.

Maureen K. Toal, RN, BSN, Staff, Jackson Clinic, Temple University Hospital, Philadelphia, Pa.

Mary Mishler Vogel, RN, MSN, Renal Clinical Specialist, Thomas Jefferson University Hospital, Philadelphia, Pa.

Nancy Wade, RN, BS, Clinical Education Coordinator, Neurosurgery, James M. Jackson Memorial Hospital, Miami, Fla.

Peggy L. Wagner, RN, MSN, Cardiovascular Clinical Nurse Specialist, St. Michael Hospital, Milwaukee, Wis.

Madeline Musante Wake, RN, MSN, Director of Continuing Education in Nursing and Assistant Professor, Marquette University, Milwaukee, Wis.

Connie Walleck, RN, CNRN, Nurse Clinician II, Neurosurgery, University of Maryland Hospital, Baltimore.

Charlene R. Wandel, RN, MN, Head Nurse, Orthopedic and Arthritis Rehabilitation Unit, Presbyterian-University Hospital, Pittsburgh, Pa.

Joanne Schlosser Ware, RN, Staff, Indian River Kidney Center, Stuart, Fla.

Marilee J. Warner, RN, BSN, Nurse Clinician, Pediatrics, Thomas Jefferson University Hospital, Philadelphia, Pa.

Juanita Watson, RN, MSN, Assistant Professor of Nursing, College of Allied Health Services, Thomas Jefferson University, Philadelphia, Pa.

Rosalyn Jones Watts, RN, MSN, Assistant Professor of Nursing, University of Pennsylvania School of Nursing, Philadelphia.

Terri E. Weaver, RN, MSN, Pulmonary Clinician Nurse Specialist, Hospital of the University of Pennsylvania, Philadelphia.

Erma L. Webb, RN, MS, Assistant Professor of Nursing, Southern Missionary College, Collegedale, Tenn.

Joanne F. White, RN, MNEd, Assistant Dean, School of Nursing; and Coordinator, Continuing Education, Duquesne University, Pittsburgh, Pa.

Barbara A. Wojtkiewicz, RN, BSN, Adult Nurse Practitioner, Martha Eliot Health Center, Boston, Mass.

Hilary Wood, RN, Clinical Nurse Specialist, Medical Oncology, North Carolina Memorial Hospital, Chapel Hill.

Gayle Ziegler, RN, Rheumatology Nurse Clinician, Research Assistant II, University of Pittsburgh (Pa.) School of Medicine.

Mary Frazier Zimmerman, RN, MS, Acting Clinical Director, Medical Nursing, Madison (Wis.) General Hospital.

Foreword

IN NO AREA OF HUMAN ENDEAVOR is it as critically important as in the practice of medicine that all members of the profession consistently seek and maintain excellence. Continuity and maximum effectiveness of patient management cannot be achieved without two things: up-to-date medical knowledge, experience, and technology, and the commitment of all health-care team members to understand and cope with the pathophysiology of a variety of conditions. Moreover, all members of the health-care team must not only comprehend and fulfill their responsibilities to the patient, but they must recognize their obligation to integrate their individual efforts, expertise, and services with those of their colleagues.

Remaining abreast with the myriad advances being made in medicine today is virtually impossible. But each of us who shares the responsibility for patient care *must* command at least a working knowledge of current concepts and a state-of-the-art knowledge of the more important and common conditions we confront everyday.

The scope and organization of PROFESSIONAL GUIDE TO DISEASES make this volume uniquely capable of providing the essential elements of more than 600 disease processes in a comprehensive and coordinated, yet concise and ready manner. Students, trainees, and practitioners in all areas and at all levels of the health-care profession will appreciate how current clinical information and relevant aspects of treatment are summarized in each entry.

The book is divided into two major sections. Section I (Chapters 1-6) deals with disorders such as genetic abnormalities and trauma that affect the whole body. Section II (Chapters 7-21) describes conditions such as respiratory, gastrointestinal, and neurologic disorders that primarily affect a specific body system.

Beginning with the *Introduction* that summarizes general considerations and normal anatomy and physiology, each chapter reviews normal functions before considering the abnormal. There follows a concise definition of the disease, often including incidence and prognosis, a brief summary of *Causes* and, when appropriate, pathophysiology. Next, a *Signs and Symptoms* section details the disease's expected clinical effects, and a *Diagnosis* section summarizes various clinical findings and special tests that suggest, confirm, or support the presence of the disease. Tests that unequivocally confirm a diagnosis are graphically highlighted. The *Treatment* section describes commonly accepted forms of therapy, including surgery, and summarizes possible complications together with any ominous changes that signal onset of rapid and life-threatening deterioration in the patient's condition. Finally, the section on *Additional Considerations* lists relevant information concerning customary care in the hospital and at home.

When appropriate, each entry also includes helpful information that a patient can use, including rehabilitation and prevention techniques. Charts, anatomic drawings, and illustrations clarify and amplify the text; carefully selected marginal notes isolate and emphasize useful supplementary information.

I'm delighted to have this opportunity to introduce this most valuable addition to your professional library. I am confident that you'll find it most useful in helping you provide the best possible care for your patients.

—STANLEY J. DUDRICK, MD, FACS
Professor of Surgery
The University of Texas Medical School at Houston
St. Luke's Episcopal Hospital and Texas Children's Hospital
Houston, Texas

Overview

Disease: The twilight process

Definitions of health and disease are easy to come by, but hard to live with. In most cases, they're concrete statements drawn from highly fluid abstractions—private beliefs and prejudices, religion and folklore—and only occasionally from rational thought and scientific evidence.

Not too long ago, health was understood to be simply the absence of disease—a definition we now realize is unrealistic. Even more utopian is the concept that health is a state of absolute physical, mental, and social well-being. Recent proof of the long-term gestation of chronic disease renders one part of this notion obsolete, and if health depended on perfect mental and social equanimity, it would be an even rarer commodity than it already is.

The fact is that health and disease are parallel dimensions in the life of every human being, overlapping and intermingling in such a way as to defy precise definition.

Consider the individual who's fully recovered from a myocardial infarction. He takes no medication, observes only minimal restrictions in his diet and daily activities, appears perfectly healthy in every respect—yet he does have heart disease. Do you interrupt this man in the middle of a red-hot tennis game to tell him he's sick? Or is he again healthy?

A hemophiliac may strike most of us as being far from healthy. But what it means to be healthy and what it means to be sick are concepts so colored by one's personal perceptions that many who are physically or mentally impaired—if they're able to function in what, for them, is a normal manner—may consider themselves in perfect health. And who can argue with them?

Disease, in other words, is often a twilight process—born in obscurity, nurtured in darkness, capable of flagrant and awful destruction, but just as likely to lapse into remission—during which the individual is neither totally healthy nor totally sick. As nurses, we must take this less starry-eyed view of the disease process into account, recognize the myriad factors that can cause the process to begin, and above all, strive to prevent it from ever getting started in the first place.

Environment: The inescapable factor

A thoroughly pragmatic examination of health and disease begins by considering human beings in relation to environment. Human interaction with environment starts at conception and continues throughout life until the very moment of death, clearly influencing health and disease in many ways. To simplify matters, we'll distinguish between internal and external environmental factors, noting, however, that no part of a person's

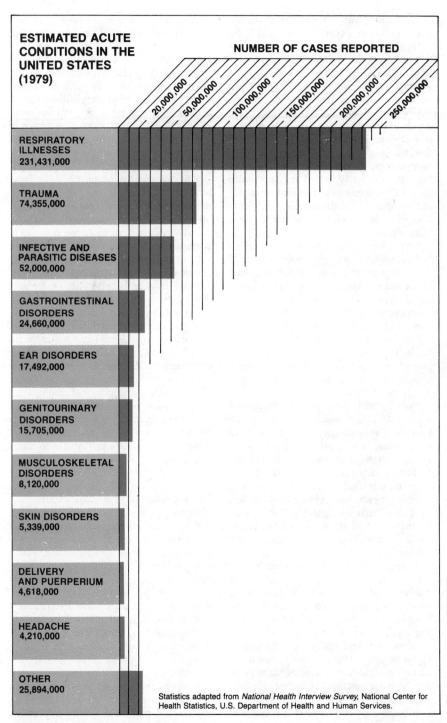

ESTIMATED ACUTE CONDITIONS IN THE UNITED STATES (1979)

NUMBER OF CASES REPORTED

20,000,000
50,000,000
100,000,000
150,000,000
200,000,000
250,000,000

RESPIRATORY ILLNESSES
231,431,000

TRAUMA
74,355,000

INFECTIVE AND PARASITIC DISEASES
52,000,000

GASTROINTESTINAL DISORDERS
24,660,000

EAR DISORDERS
17,492,000

GENITOURINARY DISORDERS
15,705,000

MUSCULOSKELETAL DISORDERS
8,120,000

SKIN DISORDERS
5,339,000

DELIVERY AND PUERPERIUM
4,618,000

HEADACHE
4,210,000

OTHER
25,894,000

Statistics adapted from *National Health Interview Survey,* National Center for Health Statistics, U.S. Department of Health and Human Services.

environment can be strictly divorced from any other aspect.

Genetic endowment, familial tendency, and personal predisposition appear to be the primary determinants of *internal environment*. The line between genetic endowment and familial tendency is fine but real. Scientific proof firmly supports the existence of genetic defects, such as muscular dystrophy, Down's syndrome, and many forms of mental retardation, while theories of familial tendency stand on less solid ground. Nevertheless, familial tendency can be defined as the apparent inclination of family members to acquire the same disease.

By personal predisposition, we mean certain physical and psychological traits that seem to characterize the majority of persons with a particular disease. Men with Type A behavior patterns (success-oriented, hard-driving), for example, are said to run a greater risk of having myocardial infarctions than those with Type B patterns (placid, easygoing). A link may also exist between personality and somatic disorders such as ulcers and colitis.

Only recently have the destructive effects of *external environment* on health become frighteningly clear. Pure food, clean water, and fresh air are treasures to be cherished in our highly mobile, heavily industrialized society. At one time the burning environmental issue of the day was sewage treatment versus septic tanks. Now we must find safer ways to dispose of all sorts of deadly environmental debris—gases, chemicals, and nuclear waste.

Today, entire populations may develop eye problems, hearing disorders, lung diseases, or cancer simply because of where they live or work. Occupational diseases caused by handling or breathing coal, asbestos, or wheat dust and various chemical sprays are becoming commonplace. Unfortunately, not all of us can escape such hazards by altering our life-styles or moving to healthier environments. The well-to-do may find it feasible, but poverty traps countless others—coal-mining families, migrant workers and their children—forcing them to live under perilous conditions.

Food poisoning could once be traced rather easily to bacterial contamination during preparation or storage. Today, the widespread use of preservatives in commercially prepared foods raises more complex health questions. How much of a chemical preservative is it safe to use? How can we monitor the long-term effects of preservatives?

The scarcity of scientific data from human populations hampers researchers and restricts our role in this area. Many of us feel unqualified to evaluate the available information; we hesitate to suggest limits to those seeking advice. All too often we ourselves are trying to decide whether to stop using hair dryers, to start buying bread with no preservatives, or to give up sugar.

Knowledge of genetic aberrations, family history, personal inclination, and the impact of external environment on health allows us to screen patients more effectively for disease. Our role can only broaden as we perfect our skills in history-taking and physical assessment, as we become more sensitive to the need for providing emotional support, and as we learn more about cue syndromes— unique clusters of signs and symptoms indicative of specific disease states—and the disease process in general.

Pathogenesis: The imperfect science

Pathogenesis—the process of tracing the history of a disease from its inception— is hardly a simple matter. Many intermediate factors that contribute to disease never come to light. Elevated blood cholesterol, hypertension, and cigarette smoking, for example, are the primary risk factors in heart disease, according to the American Heart Association. Yet these same factors don't figure at all in more than half the cases of coronary artery disease.

In short, pathogenesis is an imperfect science, which makes our role in screening and referral all the more important.

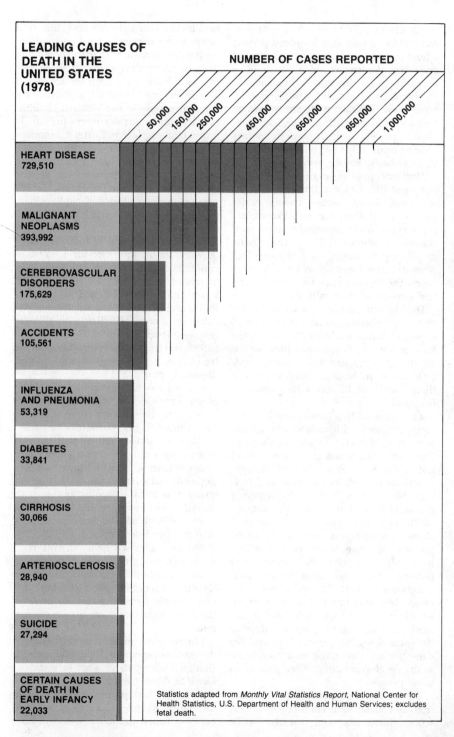

LEADING CAUSES OF DEATH IN THE UNITED STATES (1978)

NUMBER OF CASES REPORTED

50,000 — 150,000 — 250,000 — 450,000 — 650,000 — 850,000 — 1,000,000

HEART DISEASE
729,510

MALIGNANT NEOPLASMS
393,992

CEREBROVASCULAR DISORDERS
175,629

ACCIDENTS
105,561

INFLUENZA AND PNEUMONIA
53,319

DIABETES
33,841

CIRRHOSIS
30,066

ARTERIOSCLEROSIS
28,940

SUICIDE
27,294

CERTAIN CAUSES OF DEATH IN EARLY INFANCY
22,033

Statistics adapted from *Monthly Vital Statistics Report,* National Center for Health Statistics, U.S. Department of Health and Human Services; excludes fetal death.

Disease usually begins in one of two ways: either a pathogen invades a person whose resistance to that particular pathogen has decreased, as a result of a breakdown in the body's homeostatic mechanisms, the integrity of the skin or other body organs, or the entire reticuloendothelial system; or a person, perhaps in perfect health, comes in contact with an unusually toxic pathogen (rabies virus or heavy smoke, for example).

Multisystem diseases occur, of course, but most illnesses are limited in scope and time. Renal disease, treated early, can be controlled; the cardiovascular, pulmonary, and endocrine systems may remain unimpaired for years. Pneumonia, appendicitis, and acute infectious diseases last only so long. In most cases, the disease runs its course; signs and symptoms eventually abate.

During our initial contact with patients, we should define the scope and expected duration of their illnesses, since for most people these factors indicate the gravity of a disease. Our patients will be anxious and troubled until we answer their questions in terms they can understand.

Pathogens such as viruses and bacteria represent readily identifiable *physiologic stressors,* directly linked to disease. However, other kinds of stressors—loud noise, for example—affect physiologic functions as well as attitudes and feelings. Noise above 70 decibels triggers a predictable response from the sympathetic nervous system. Cardiac rate changes, respirations increase, and blood pressure may rise, but the point at which loud noise can consistently raise blood pressure and sustain hypertension until symptoms of heart disease appear is not clear. Research has linked noise exposure to elevated blood cholesterol in animals, but we can't say for certain that the same thing happens in humans. We can only say that noise may contribute to the development of cardiac disease in some people.

The same is true of *psychological stress* and its concomitant emotions of anger, worry, bitterness, and anxiety. While health-care professionals find it hard to define stress precisely, most people have no trouble recognizing it in their daily lives. So many things can cause it—loss of a job, disaffection for a spouse, death of a loved one, financial problems. We say that people in the Western civilization live under greater stress than their more contemplative Eastern counterparts, that city folks pursue a more stressful existence than their country cousins. We often evaluate one another by our ability to "handle" stress, naively prizing the appearance of being at harmony with the world and oneself despite adversity.

The energy needed to maintain such outward calm, to create the illusion of coping successfully with life in the eyes of others, may exact a heavy toll. We know that stressful physical, psychologic, and symbolic stimuli can—separately or in concert—elicit a physiologic response from the body.

Such a response, however, cannot safely be elicited indefinitely; at some point, disease begins.

In most cases, we can identify physiologic stressors and weaken their effect by altering the patient's environment or by attenuating his reaction to the stressor. We may advise a patient with cardiac disease, for example, to find a new house or apartment so he won't have to climb flights of stairs. In addition, we may instruct him to take medication, such as digitalis, to strengthen his heart's contractions. Both approaches represent viable nursing interventions.

But how can we help patients cope with psychological stress? Providing sound health information, taking the time to teach patients the facts about this more subtle form of stress, is perhaps the most important contribution we can make.

Moreover, we must learn to emphasize the positive aspects of dealing with stress. Don't tell your patient what he stands to *lose* if he doesn't learn to cope with stress intelligently and maturely; tell him what he stands to *gain* if he does learn to cope—a fuller and more bountiful life.

Health expectations: The new emphasis

Today, the public is more aware than ever of our responsibilities in health care. High schools and colleges offer comprehensive courses on health; the media present informative programs and detailed articles on modern medicine. Diet and nutrition, physical fitness, the causes of cardiac disease are but a few of the subjects with which the layman has become intimately familiar.

The rapid growth of technology has forced all of us to think about health in its broadest sense. Prevention has become every bit as important as treatment, if not more so. Today, people don't want a good doctor—or a good nurse—so much as they want to avoid getting sick in the first place.

This change in the public's perception of health and disease has created disturbing repercussions throughout the health-care system in the United States. Interest has shifted so dramatically from sickness to "wellness," from medical cure to healthful living, that we can no longer ignore a corresponding shift in society's expectations of its members entrusted with health care.

This provocative new emphasis underlies the philosophy behind health maintenance organizations (HMOs), proliferating group cooperatives which hold that health and well-being are better served through education and prevention than through reactionary attempts to treat disease. HMOs encourage consumers to participate in the formulation of health policy by serving on committees, boards, and the like.

Because these organizations are regulated by the Department of Health and Human Services, the extent of our participation is subject to guidelines. But as a matter of practice, we enjoy great flexibility in their day-to-day functioning. If the stated goal of HMOs—to provide quality health care at the lowest possible cost—is to be realized, we must play a more active role in the future.

The hard fact is that socioeconomic status, a measure of affluence, often determines the amount and quality of health care that people seek for themselves and their families in the United States. The poor visit a doctor only when symptoms become acute. A migrant worker explained his reason for not seeing a doctor: "I wasn't bleeding anywhere and I didn't even have a temperature." This man was experiencing constant but subdued pain, which was later attributed to cancer.

Our responsibility to the public has never been greater, nor has it ever been under more intense scrutiny. Our expanded role in the health-care system calls for advanced knowledge of health and disease, and the ambiguous relationship between the two. We can no longer rely on "basic training" to see us through, because in most cases, that training did not cover the in-depth anatomy, physiology, and pharmacology required for today's responsibilities. Nor did it offer sufficient understanding of vital skills, such as auscultation, palpation, percussion, and inspection; these, too, must be learned and perfected. Recognition of cue syndromes is just being introduced into nursing curricula but is sure to become important.

Fortunately, most of us want to acquire the knowledge and skills necessary to serve our patients in the most effective way. Understanding health and disease in the context of both internal and external environments is one step toward this goal. Shifting the focus of our care from merely treating disease to advocating healthful living is another direction in which we must begin to move.

With these goals firmly in mind, and with proper dedication and discipline, we can act as indispensable catalysts to far-reaching change.

—FRANCES J. STORLIE, RN, PHD

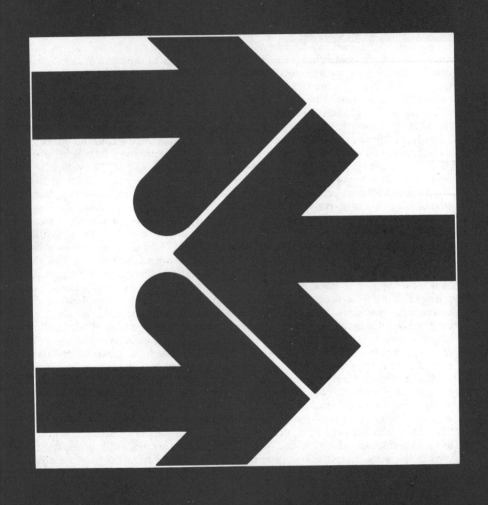

1 Immune Disorders

Immune Disorders

Introduction

Immunity describes the body's defense system against microorganisms or malignancy. Briefly stated, an immune response is the body's production of antibodies and the resulting protection (immunity) to exposure (invasion) by an antigen (foreign substance). In a hypersensitive (allergic) response, the body abnormally produces antibodies in response to an antigen (allergen). Usually, the antigen is made up of or attached to a protein molecule. It is this protein that provokes the immune response.

This response works through countless cells that operate through the reticuloendothelial system (thymus, lymphoid tissue, liver, spleen, and bone marrow). Each cell develops from stem cells originating from the fetal liver and, after birth, from the bone marrow. These stem cells produce all cells of the hematopoietic system which are lymphocytes (T cells if processed via the thymus, or B cells via bursa equivalent) or other leukocytes (granulocytes, monocytes), as well as erythrocytes, and platelets. Each lymphoid cell has a special immune system function assigned during embryonic life.

The immune system protects the body from invasion via three levels of defense: local barriers, inflammation, and a specific immune response. Local barriers provide chemical and mechanical defenses through the skin (natural oils), mucous membranes (cilia), and conjunctiva (tears). Then, inflammation sends polymorphonuclear leukocytes, or neutrophils, via the blood to the site of injury, where these phagocytes engulf the invading organism. If these first levels of defense fail or are inadequate, a specific immune response develops. This defensive response is possible because the immune system recognizes the carrier protein as a foreign substance, setting off a humoral or a cell-mediated response or both.

Humoral immunity is created by humoral antibodies (immunoglobulins), a heterogenous group of proteins, each specially modified to react with a particular antigen. Humoral immunity is most important in protecting against bacterial and viral reinfections. The major cells of this system are the B lymphocytes. When these immunoglobulin-coated cells recognize an intruder to the system, they stimulate antibody production (an antigen-antibody reaction), while the minor cells, T cells, assist in this reaction. Immunoglobulins are divided into five classes: IgM, IgG (gamma globulin), IgA, IgE, and IgD. The amount of each present at any given time depends on the challenging antigen, but all five classes are normally present during any antigenic challenge.

Antigen-antibody reactions activate the complement system, a mechanism for removing antigen from the body. The complement system is a nonspecific series of ordered chemical reactions which amplify humoral immunity response. When the complement system, normally present in serum, is activated by antigen-antibody reactions, its discrete plasma proteins (C_1 to C_9) result in lysis of the antigen's cell wall and opsonization (tagging and identification) of the antigenic substance, enabling phagocytosis of the antigen. A special characteristic of a humoral response is rapid onset. A humoral response may start immediately after antigen contact or up to 48 hours later. The speed of humoral response is dramatized in anaphylactic reactions.

Cell-mediated (cellular) immunity

Cellular immunity is predominant at the tissue level and is most evident in a localized inflammatory response. Such immunity is highly effective against fungal

FIVE CLASSES OF IMMUNOGLOBULIN

• *IgM,* the immunoglobulin with the largest molecular structure, is the first antibody synthesized after antigenic challenge. Most often it is found within circulating fluids. It initiates increased production of IgG and the complement fixation process essential for a successful antibody response. This is the major functioning antibody in ABO incompatibilities.

• *IgG,* the dominant immunoglobulin in serum, is produced in response to bacterial, fungal, and viral invasion. It protects against both red and white cell antigens and crosses the placenta.

• *IgA* is found in all body secretions. Produced in the lymphoid tissues along mucosal surfaces, it combines with a protein (secretory piece) in the mucosa and is secreted onto the mucosal surfaces as a secretory antibody. IgA defends exposed body surfaces against invading microorganisms by recognizing them as foreign and probably initiating antigen-antibody reaction.

• *IgD* is found in minute amounts in serum tissues. Its specific function is unknown, though it is found in increased amounts during allergic reactions to milk, penicillin, insulin, and various toxins.

• *IgE* is probably responsive to IgA. It is concentrated mostly in lung, skin, and in mucous membrane tissue cells, and is the key antibody in allergic response. Contact between IgE and antigen causes the release of chemical mediators, resulting in Type I hypersensitivity reactions, which are characterized by flare and wheal. It also provides the first defense against environmental antigens.

and viral invasion and tumors, and is the primary reaction in organ transplant rejection.

Unlike humoral immunity, which depends mainly on B cells, cell-mediated, or cellular immunity, depends on T cells. T cells, stored in the spleen and the lymphatic system, are processed in the thymus. Unlike B cells, T cells carry little or no immunoglobulin on their surface and always maintain their lymphocyte structure. These cells fall into three distinct groups: circulating T cells (within circulating fluids), noncirculating T cells (including T cells that produce lymphokines and selectively migrate to inflammation sites), and memory T cells (which recognize antigens on repeated exposure).

When a memory T cell recognizes an antigen as foreign, it mobilizes tissue macrophages in the presence of the migratory inhibitory factor (MIF). Like complement reaction, MIF is actually a series of chemical reactions. Once activated, MIF transforms local macrophages into intense phagocytes and prevents macrophages from leaving the invasion site until they have destroyed the antigen.

Humoral and cell-mediated responses function interdependently. For example, although T cells' primary function is in a cell-mediated response, they can also activate a humoral response and rush previously formed circulating antibodies to the invasion site. Similarly, B cells can influence cell-mediated responses.

Natural or acquired immunity

Both humoral and cell-mediated immunity can be either natural or acquired. *Natural immunity*, genetically inherited resistance to specific infectious organisms, is constant for a species and cannot be transferred to another species. (For example, dogs are susceptible to distemper, but humans are immune to it.) Genetically inherited immunity of individuals, species, and races can be enhanced or reduced by diet, mental health, environment, virulence of invading organisms, and metabolism. *Acquired immunity* is individual resistance to antigens (infectious organisms) that may be developed actively or passively. Acquired immunity may be *natural* (when a person develops antibodies as a result of infection), *active artificial* (when antibodies follow inoculation with vaccine or toxoid), or *passive artificial* (after injection of immune serum).

TWO THEORIES OF ANTIBODY FORMATION

The first, the *instructive theory*, holds that each antigenic contact made during one's lifetime forms a new antibody. For example, when an immunoglobulin-coated B cell comes into contact with an antigen, it surveys it, and the B cell's RNA simultaneously undergoes changes that allow new cells to form antibodies against the antigen. This random process allows the reticuloendothelial system to instruct cells to produce antibody against any antigen at any time.

The second and more complex theory, the *specific, or clonal selective, theory* (clone cells transmit immunologic memory), holds that antibody patterns are established before or soon after birth. The thymus, located in the mediastinal cavity, changes bone marrow lymphocytes into T cells, each with the potential of producing antibody, even against self. The cells that could produce antibody against self are destroyed and removed via phagocytosis. The remaining cells mature with the fetus, leave the thymus, and seed the reticuloendothelial system. Each remaining cell can produce antibody against specific antigens. According to this theory, the body can recognize any antigen and increase antibody production specific to that antigen at any time. Once an antigenic challenge occurs, an immunologic template for the antibody formed is passed on to future cells. Within these theories, immunity is humoral or cell-mediated.

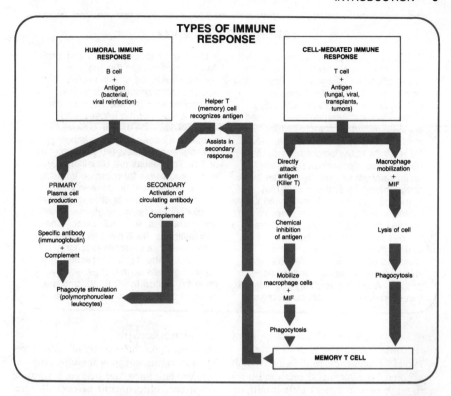

TYPES OF IMMUNE RESPONSE

The numerous vaccines and toxoids we use today are based on Pasteur's method of attenuating (weakening) disease organisms. An attenuated organism is recognized as an antigen once it enters the body but is too weak to cause severe disease. But it does provoke formation of circulating antibodies. Immunization with attenuated live organisms (example: Sabin's oral polio vaccine) offers most effective immunity.

Passive artificial immunity provides preformed antibodies against an organism. Because acquired preformed antibodies aren't actively produced by the recipient, they offer only transient immunity. For example, gamma globulin B contains antibodies that attack the invading antigens of hepatitis B, but its protective effect soon wears off. Infants have natural passive immunity, received through placental circulation. This immunity lasts from 3 to 6 months; then acquired immunization must begin.

Allergy: Immunity gone wrong ·

Allergy is a hypersensitive response to antigens (usually environmental) that are not intrinsically harmful. According to the National Institutes of Health, one out of every six Americans has a serious allergy.

Allergy reflects four kinds of hypersensitivity:
• Type I (atopy, anaphylaxis, urticaria, angioedema), in which IgE antibodies fixed to tissue mast cells react with antigen and trigger release of histamine and other chemotactic factors.
• Type II (drug reactions, transfusion reactions, erythroblastosis fetalis), in which IgG or IgM antibodies react with antigen on target cells (usually red blood cells) and activate complement, causing cell wall lysis in serum or tissues.
• Type III (serum sickness, systemic lupus erythematosus), in which IgG or IgM antibodies form complexes with antigen and complement, activating neutrophil

TESTING FOR ALLERGY

Successful treatment of an allergy always requires accurate identification of the offending allergen. The most common method of identification, skin testing, is best for persons with atopy or anaphylaxis. Allergens to be tested are determined by allergic history, medical history, environment, and diet. (At least 24 hours before testing, the person must discontinue using any antihistamines or hydroxyzine, as these drugs inhibit or diminish skin-test responses.) Several allergens can be tested safely at the same time. Within minutes of a positive skin test, histamine is released from the mast cells, causing vasodilation (erythema), localized edema from increased vascular permeability (wheal), and localized pruritus. A positive reaction to a skin test can even occur in distant target organs.

Cutaneous (prick/scratch) and intradermal injection are the two most common methods of skin testing. Cutaneous testing should be done first. The preferred sites are the inner aspect of the forearm or the upper back. For small children, the back is preferred, because it allows a large number of simultaneous tests (40 to 80 in rows of 10). The results are usually ready to be read within 20 minutes. Intradermal testing should be done following a scratch test with negative or unclear results. These tests are always done on the extremities. Although intracutaneous testing is much more accurate, it can lead to a systemic reaction. Because of the threat of reaction, the number of tests done simultaneously must be limited to 20 to 30, and the allergen tested may be more dilute.

chemotactic factors which cause local tissue inflammation and destruction.
• Type IV (contact dermatitis), in which sensitized T cells react directly with an antigen to produce local inflammation.

Allergies can be further described as immediate (antibody-mediated) or delayed (cell-mediated) reactions. In an immediate allergic reaction (types I, II, and III), allergens (antigens) stimulate production of specific antibodies that may circulate freely in the serum or may be attached to specific cells (sessile). Antigen-antibody reaction activates certain enzymes, creating an imbalance between these enzymes and their inhibitors. Simultaneously, certain pharmacologically active substances are released into the circulation (histamine, slow-reacting substances [SRS-A], bradykinin, acetylcholine, gamma globulin G, and leukotaxine).

Delayed reactions also stem from allergens but don't seem to need antibodies. Mediators differ with the allergen. The symptoms in a delayed allergic reaction depend on the specific mediator and on the extent of tissue damage resulting from the reaction.

Immunotherapy

Depending on the severity of allergic response, treatment may include drugs to relieve symptoms and decrease immune response, elimination of the allergen from the environment, or immunotherapy (hyposensitization).

Immunotherapy is based on the assumption that *low* doses of an offending allergen will bind with IgG to prevent an allergic reaction by inhibiting the effect of IgE and stimulating formation of blocking antibody (IgG). The more a person is exposed to offending allergens, the more blocking antibody he forms. Blocking antibody binds to the circulating antigen, decreasing or eliminating the allergic response seemingly by creating immunologic tolerance toward the antigen.

Immunotherapy begins with low doses of an allergen, gradually increasing as the patient's tolerance to it grows. It can be perennial (throughout the year) or preseasonal (beginning 3 to 6 months before the season starts). The starting dose is very small but is gradually increased to a point at which systemic reaction or severe local reaction is absent.

Treatment usually continues until the patient has been reasonably free of allergic symptoms for 2 to 5 years.

Four theories of autoimmunity

In allergy, the immune system is overly sensitive to foreign substance; in autoimmunity, the immune system cannot distinguish between self and foreign substance—probably because of some change in the function of cellular or humoral immune system components.

Several theories attempt to explain the autoimmune reaction.

1. The *forbidden clone theory* is based on the clonal evolution theory (at birth, all cells that might react against self have been eliminated from the system, leaving only cells which will react against foreign substance). This theory maintains that certain of these cells that can react against self (clone cells) persist latent until some stimulus—a viral infection or some metabolic change—activates these hidden clone cells. If the viral stimulus is structurally similar to a body cell, the immune response against it also destroys body tissues. The normal cells of the immune system attack only the virus, while the clone cells attack the body tissues.

2. The *sequestered antigens theory* holds that certain levels of antigen exposure and contact between immunogenic cells and body cells are needed to maintain immunologic tolerance. Because of their isolation from blood and lymphatic circulation, certain sequestered antigens (in brain tissues, eye lenses, and spermatozoa) have no contact with the immune system. After tissue damage, these sequestered antigens may be exposed to immune system cells. An autoimmune response may follow if sequestered antigens are not recognized as self.

3. The theory that *T-lymphocytes* are the major immunocompetent cells in cellular immunity and regulator (helper and suppressor) cells in humoral response holds that during immune response, T cells help to maintain the level of B-cell response needed to completely eliminate the antigenic substance. Once the antigen has been eliminated, a second type of T cell suppresses the B cell and/or the helper T cell. Absence of this suppressor T cell leads to persistent immune response and to destruction of self. For example, when hapten that attaches to a body protein is recognized as foreign, self cells are destroyed. If suppressor T-cell activity is abnormal or absent, B- or T-cell activity may continue, even against body cells.

4. The *immune complex activity theory* holds that in a prolonged antigen-antibody reaction, antibody may not be produced rapidly enough, and complement may be depleted and smaller immune complexes (antigen-antibody) formed. Inadequate complement allows these complexes to settle in the inner lining of blood vessels, the basement membrane of the glomeruli, or other target organs, leading to destruction of self cells as well as of antigen.

Why these mechanisms occur in autoimmune disorders is still a mystery. We know that some microorganisms resemble body cells; beta-hemolytic streptococcus releases a toxin that closely resembles heart tissue. Why does this cause heart disease in some and have no effect on others? Are autoimmune disorders preventable? Are they genetically transmitted? We may eventually know these answers as research continues.

EARLY VACCINES

The discovery of acquired (artificial) immunity led to our present immunization programs. In 1798, Edward Jenner realized that persons who survived smallpox did not get the disease again, even after reexposure. Jenner also discovered vaccines by taking pus from a cow infected with cowpox (cowpox in cows is equivalent to smallpox in humans) and injecting it into humans, to create a mild form of smallpox.

One hundred years later, Louis Pasteur clarified Jenner's work. He discovered that cultured serum taken from a recovered patient produced acquired immunity when given to a healthy person.

ALLERGY

Allergic Asthma

Allergic asthma is a chronic reactive airway disorder that produces episodic, reversible airway obstruction via bronchospasms, which narrow the bronchioles, with increased mucus secretion and mucosal edema. Its symptoms range from mild wheezing and dyspnea to life-threatening respiratory failure. Symptoms of bronchial airway obstruction may or may not persist between acute episodes.

Causes and incidence

This common condition (9,000,000 cases in the U.S. alone) begins in children under age 10 in 50% of all cases, and in such children affects twice as many boys as girls. In another third, asthma begins before age 30—though it can strike at any age—but by age 30, distribution is even between men and women. Underlining the significance of hereditary predisposition, about one third of all asthmatics share the disease with at least one member of their immediate family, and three fourths of the children with two asthmatic parents also have asthma.

Asthma may result from sensitivity to specific external allergens (extrinsic) or from internal, nonallergenic factors (intrinsic). Extrinsic allergens cause approximately 50% of all cases of asthma. Such allergens include pollen, animal dander, house dust (fungal spores), kapok or feather pillows, some foods, or any other sensitizing substance. Most *extrinsic asthma* (atopic asthma) begins in children and is usually accompanied by other manifestations of atopy (Type I—IgE-mediated allergy), such as eczema and allergic rhinitis. *Intrinsic asthma* (nonatopic asthma) is triggered by a severe respiratory infection (usually in adults) and may result from hypersensitivity to the specific bacteria. Irritants, emotional stress, fatigue, endocrine changes, temperature and humidity changes, and exposure to noxious fumes may aggravate intrinsic asthma attacks. In many asthmatics, especially children, intrinsic and extrinsic asthma coexist.

What actually causes the fundamental reaction in asthma is still unclear, but many suspect that bronchoconstriction results from a malfunctioning autonomic reflex mechanism which decreases chemical inhibition, and allows asthma reaction mediators (histamine, SRS-A, and eosinophil chemotactic factor) to rise.

Signs and symptoms

An asthma attack may begin dramatically, with simultaneous onset of severe, multiple symptoms, or insidiously, with gradually increasing respiratory distress. Typically, the acute asthmatic attack causes sudden dyspnea; wheezing (most pronounced on expiration); tightness in the chest, with increasing difficulty during inspiration and expiration; and sometimes coughing, with thick, tenacious sputum that may be clear or yellow. The patient feels as if he is suffocating. During a severe attack, he may be unable to speak more than a few words without pausing for breath.

Such a patient usually shows these signs: tachypnea, though respiratory rate is frequently normal; audible wheezing, sometimes loud enough to hear across the room; obvious use of accessory respiration muscles; rapid pulse; profuse perspiration; hyperresonant lung fields; and diminished breath sounds with wheezes and rhonchi. Cyanosis, confusion, and lethargy may signal onset of status asthmaticus and respiratory failure.

Diagnosis

Laboratory studies in patients with asthma often show the following abnormalities:

• *CBC with differential:* increased eosinophil count, with possible neutropenia (suggesting an allergic cause).

• *Chest X-ray:* possible hyperinflation, with areas of focal atelectasis (mucus plugging).

• *Pulmonary function studies:* signs of airway obstructive disease (decreased flow rates and forced expiratory volume in 1 second [FEV_1]), low normal or decreased vital capacity, and increased total lung and residual capacity. However, pulmonary function studies are often normal between attacks. During an asthma attack, arterial blood gases show decreased O_2 saturation and PO_2 levels, and increased PCO_2 level and decreased pH, which return to normal soon after the attack.

• *History of familial allergy:* If the patient with asthma symptoms has no allergic history, he'll need skin testing for specific allergens and, later, inhalation bronchial challenge testing to evaluate the clinical significance of allergens identified by skin testing.

Before testing, other causes of airway obstruction and wheezing must be ruled out. In children, such causes include cystic fibrosis; aspiration; congenital anomaly; benign or malignant tumors of the bronchi, thyroid, thymus, or mediastinum; and acute viral bronchitis; in adults, obstructive pulmonary disease and congestive heart failure.

Treatment

The best treatment for asthma is prevention, by eliminating the allergens, irritants, or other provocative stimuli from the patient's environment. Usually, such stimuli can't be removed entirely, so desensitization to specific antigens can be helpful but isn't totally effective or persistent. In patients whose asthma is related to bronchial infections, treatment with antibiotics and vaccines during the winter may greatly decrease asthma symptoms, and occasionally, the doctor

BREATHING EXERCISES FOR CHILDREN AND ADULTS WITH ASTHMA

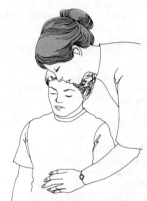

—A family member may promote diaphragmatic breathing by firmly putting her hand on the patient's abdomen, just below his ribs. His abdomen should swell as he inhales, and return to a relaxed position when he exhales.

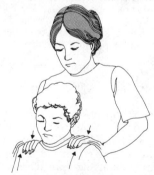

—To promote relaxation, she can put her hands on the patient's shoulders, as shown above, and ask him to push up against the pressure of her hands. The patient should relax at regular intervals.

—A young child can learn proper breathing techniques by trying to:
• inflate balloons.
• extinguish candles.
• blow Ping-Pong balls across a table.
• blow butterflies made from facial tissues across a table.

HOW TO TREAT STATUS ASTHMATICUS

Unless it is promptly and correctly treated, status asthmaticus may lead to fatal respiratory failure. The patient with increasingly severe asthma that's unresponsive to drug therapy (status asthmaticus) is usually admitted to the ICU for the following special medical and nursing care:
• frequent arterial blood gas measurements to assess respiratory status; particularly after ventilator therapy, a change in oxygen concentration, or $NaHCO_3$ administration (to correct or prevent metabolic acidosis)
• careful oxygen administration (the patient will be hypoxemic) and, if necessary, endotracheal intubation and mechanical ventilation (when the patient has an elevated PCO_2)
• administration of I.V. fluids according to the patient's clinical status and age (dehydration is likely because of inadequate fluid intake and increased insensible loss)
• administration of corticosteroids, epinephrine, and I.V. aminophylline (sedation must be used only with caution)
• frequent chest X-rays, taken routinely to assess the patient's condition.

may order vaccines for protection against bacteria.

Drug treatment for allergic asthma usually includes some form of bronchodilator and is more effective when begun soon after onset of symptoms. Drugs used include rapid-acting epinephrine, epinephrine in oil, which is not recommended for infants; terbutaline; metaproterenol; aminophylline or a combination of theophylline, ephedrine, and phenobarbital; oral bronchodilators; corticosteroids; or cromolyn sodium powder oral inhalant (only a preventive measure, not for use in an attack).

Additional considerations

During an acute attack:
• Immediate treatment is needed to maintain respiratory function and re-lieve bronchoconstriction, while allowing mucus plug expulsion. If the patient's specific allergens, irritants, or other precipitating factors are known, an asthmatic attack may be relieved simply by removing the offending stimulus.
• If the attack is induced by exercise, it may be controlled if the patient sits down, rests, and sips warm water. This helps slow breathing, promotes bronchodilation, and loosens secretions. (Before exercise, asthmatic children should use an oral bronchodilator for 30 to 60 minutes or an inhaled bronchodilator for 15 to 20 minutes.)
• The patient should be asked if he has a nebulizer and if he's used it. He should have access to an isoproterenol or isoetharine nebulizer at all times. But, he should take no more than two or three whiffs every 4 hours. If he needs the nebulizer again in less than 4 hours, he should call the doctor for further instruction. (Overuse of a nebulizer can progressively weaken the patient's response until the nebulizer has no effect at all. Extended overuse can even lead to cardiac arrest and death.)
• Loss of breath is terrifying, so the patient needs to be reassured and helped to relax. Then, he should be placed in a semi-Fowler's position, and encouraged to begin diaphragmatic breathing.
• A severe asthma attack unrelieved by epinephrine is a medical emergency. Special care must be taken to give epinephrine using the correct administration route, concentration, and dosage.
• Administering oxygen by nasal cannula at 2 liters per minute eases difficulty in breathing and increases arterial oxygen saturation. Later, oxygen should be adjusted according to the patient's vital functions and arterial blood gas measurements. (A high percentage of oxygen [over 40%] administered to a chronic asthma patient may stop his breathing.)
• The doctor will order drugs and I.V. fluids. He'll continue epinephrine, and administer aminophylline by I.V. bolus as a loading dose, followed by I.V. drip. (Elderly patients with hepatic or cardiac insufficiency are predisposed to ami-

nophylline toxicity.) The drip rate is monitored closely. An I.V. infusion pump may be used for greater accuracy. Simultaneously, a loading dose of corticosteroids can be given I.V. or I.M. I.V. fluids combat dehydration until the patient can tolerate oral fluids, which will help loosen secretions.

When the patient is ready, he'll be given expectorants to begin clearing bronchial passages of mucus and other debris collected during the acute attack. Isoproterenol will be administered at a dose of 0.25 to 0.5 ml diluted with 1.5 to 8.5 ml sterile saline solution at 4-hour intervals. Administration by an O_2-powered nebulizer minimizes the risk of associated decreases in arterial PO_2. (Delivery with intermittent positive pressure breathing should be avoided, because together they may increase airway resistance and the risk of pneumothorax and pneumomediastinum.)

During long-term care:
• The patient's drug regimen must be supervised. When he's using an aminophylline bronchodilator, his blood levels must be monitored, as oral absorption of aminophylline can be erratic. With long-term steroid therapy, cushingoid side effects are possible. Alternate-day dosage or use of an orally inhalable steroid, beclomethasone, may minimize these side effects. Because of their respiratory depressant effect, sedatives and narcotics are not recommended in *acute* asthmatic attacks.

To prevent recurring attacks:
• The patient should follow a leisurely morning routine. He should breathe deeply, cough up secretions accumulated overnight, and allow time for medication to work. He can best loosen secretions by coughing correctly—inhaling fully and gently, then bending over with arms crossed over the abdomen before coughing—and by drinking 3 quarts of liquid daily.
• The patient should avoid known allergens, irritating fumes of any kind, aerosol spray, smoke, and automobile exhaust. His family must understand the importance of their cooperation. If he can't avoid all irritants, he should at least limit them and amend his personal habits to include good posture and moderate exercise and to exclude smoking and overeating.

Allergic Rhinitis

Allergic rhinitis is a reaction to airborne (inhaled) allergens. Depending on the allergen, the resulting rhinitis and conjunctivitis may be seasonal (hay fever) or occur year round (perennial allergic rhinitis). Allergic rhinitis is the most common atopic allergic reaction, affecting over 20 million Americans. It's most prevalent in young children and adolescents but can occur in all age groups.

Causes
Hay fever reflects a heightened capacity, probably inherited, for becoming sensitized to an allergen. It is usually induced by windborne pollens: in spring by tree pollens (oak, elm, maple, alder, birch, cottonwood); in summer by grass pollens (sheep sorrel, English plantain); and in the fall by weed pollens (ragweed). Occasionally, between June and October, hay fever is induced by allergy to mold (fungal spores).

In perennial allergic rhinitis, inhalant allergens provoke antigen responses that produce recurring symptoms year round. The major perennial allergens are house dust, feather pillows, mold, cigarette smoke, upholstery, and animal danders. Seasonal pollen allergy may exacerbate symptoms of perennial rhinitis.

Signs and symptoms
In hay fever, the key symptoms are paroxysmal sneezing, profuse watery rhi-

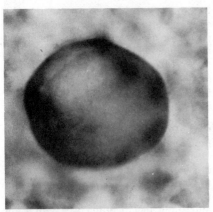

Photomicrograph of pollen grain in nasal smear. Hay fever is usually induced by windborne pollens: in spring, by tree pollens (oak, elm, maple, alder, birch, cottonwood); in summer, by grass pollens (sheep sorrel, English plantain); and in fall, by weed pollens (ragweed).

norrhea, nasal obstruction or congestion, and pruritus of the nose and eyes, sometimes accompanied by malaise and fever but usually by pale, irritated, edematous nasal mucosa; red and edematous eyelids and conjunctivae; excessive lacrimation; and headache or sinus pain. Some children complain of itching in the throat.

In perennial allergic rhinitis, conjunctivitis and other extranasal symptoms are rare, but chronic nasal obstruction is common and often extends to eustachian tube obstruction, particularly in children. In both conditions, dark circles appear under the patient's eyes ("allergic shiners") because of venous congestion in the maxillary sinuses. The severity of signs and symptoms may vary from year to year.

Untreated allergic rhinitis may lead to asthma; recurrent otitis media, with hearing loss; sinusitis; nasal or sinusal polyps; alveolar hypoventilation, with cor pulmonale; epistaxis; and orofacial dental deformities.

Diagnosis
Microscopic examination of sputum and nasal secretions reveals presence of large numbers of eosinophils. Blood chemistry shows normal or slightly elevated IgE; chest X-ray is normal. Firm diagnosis rests on the patient's personal and family history of allergies, and on physical findings during a symptomatic phase. Skin testing, paired with tested responses to environmental stimuli, can pinpoint the responsible allergens.

To distinguish between allergic rhinitis and other disorders of the nasal mucosa, these differences must be considered. In chronic vasomotor rhinitis, eye symptoms are absent, rhinorrhea is mucoid, and seasonal variation is absent. In infectious rhinitis (common cold), the nasal mucosa is beet red, nasal secretions contain polymorphonuclear exudate, and symptoms include fever and sore throat. In rhinitis medicamentosa, which results from excessive use of nasal sprays or drops, the only symptom is nasal drainage. In children, differential diagnosis should rule out a nasal foreign body.

Treatment and additional considerations
Treatment aims to control symptoms by eliminating the environmental antigen and by drug therapy and immunotherapy. Antihistamines effectively block histamine effects but commonly produce anticholinergic side effects (sedation, dry mouth, nausea, anorexia, vomiting, constipation, diarrhea, dizziness, blurred vision, insomnia, tinnitus, palpitations, headache, and nervousness). For severe and resistant flare-ups, short-term use of topical or systemic corticosteroids may be helpful.

The patient with allergic rhinitis must comply strictly with prescribed drug treatment regimens, because drug misuse can cause complications. He should be advised to report any change in symptoms to the doctor.

Long-term management includes immunotherapy, or desensitization with injections of extracted allergens, administered preseasonally, coseasonally, or perennially. Seasonal allergies require particularly close dosage regulation.

Before such injections, the patient's symptom status is assessed. For 30 minutes afterward, he's watched closely for adverse reactions, including anaphylaxis and severe localized erythema. In case of adverse reaction, epinephrine and emergency resuscitative equipment should be on hand. The patient should be instructed to call a doctor if a delayed reaction occurs.

Patients can reduce environmental exposure to airborne allergens in several ways: by sleeping with the windows closed, by avoiding the countryside during pollination seasons, by using air conditioning to filter allergens and keep down moisture and dust, and by being prepared for attacks after unavoidable exposure to animals (for instance, in other people's homes). Occasionally, in severe and resistant cases, patients may have to consider drastic changes in life style, such as relocation to a pollen-free area either seasonally or year round.

Anaphylaxis

Anaphylaxis is a dramatic, acute atopic reaction, marked by the sudden onset of rapidly progressive urticaria, respiratory distress, and vascular collapse, leading to systemic shock and, sometimes, death.

Causes and incidence
The source of anaphylactic reactions is ingestion of or other systemic exposure to sensitizing drugs or other substances. Such substances may include serums (usually horse serum), vaccines, allergen extracts, enzymes (L-asparaginase), hormones, penicillin and other antibiotics, sulfonamides, local anesthetics, salicylates, polysaccharides, procaine, diagnostic chemicals (sulfobromophthalein, sodium dehydrocholate, and radiographic contrast media), foods (legumes, nuts, berries, seafoods, and egg albumin), insect venom (honeybees, wasps, hornets, yellow jackets, fire ants, mosquitoes, and certain spiders), and rarely, ruptured hydatid cyst.

The single most common cause of anaphylaxis is penicillin, which induces anaphylaxis in 1 to 4 of every 10,000 patients treated with it. Penicillin is most likely to induce anaphylaxis after parenteral administration and in patients with a familial history of atopic allergy.

Anaphylaxis may occur after a single exposure to an antigen or after repeated exposures. However, the sooner the reaction occurs after exposure, the more likely it is to be severe.

Systemic anaphylaxis is similar to the atopic reaction in other allergic states, such as asthma. In anaphylaxis, the allergen enters the systemic circulation and sets up a humoral response. If this humoral response were carried out completely, the allergen would be removed from the system, as are bacteria. Instead, the allergen combines with IgE, provoking release of histamine from its mast cell stores. IgG or IgM enters into the reaction and activates the release of complement fractions, which also stimulate histamine release. This rise in histamine levels leads to vascular collapse.

At the same time, two other chemical mediators, bradykinin and SRS-A (slow-reactive substance of anaphylaxis), induce vascular collapse by stimulating contraction of certain groups of smooth muscles and by increasing vascular permeability. In turn, increased vascular permeability leads to decreased peripheral resistance and plasma leakage from the circulation to extravascular tissues (which lowers blood volume, causing hypotension, hypovolemic shock and cardiac dysfunction).

Signs and symptoms
Anaphylactic reaction produces sudden physical distress that occurs within sec-

PATIENT TEACHING AID

How to use an anaphylaxis kit

1. Contact doctor, if possible; then proceed with emergency kit.
2. Remove insect stinger if it's still there. Be careful not to imbed stinger farther into skin.
3. If you were stung on an arm or leg, apply tourniquet between sting and body. To tighten, pull end of one string.

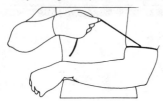

push plunger until it stops (0.3 ml). Do not force farther. Remove the needle, and replace the needle cover. A second injection of 0.3 ml remains in the syringe. H-S Epinephrine 1:1,000 syringe has graduations of 0.1 ml so that doses less than 0.3 ml can be measured for children: 6 to 12 years, 0.2 ml;

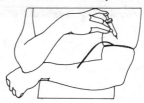

Release tourniquet every 10 minutes by pulling metal ring. If you were stung on the body, neck, or face, apply ice to the affected area.
4. Using an alcohol swab, cleanse a 4" (10 cm) area on your arm or thigh (above tourniquet).
5. Prepare prefilled syringe. First, remove needle cover. Then, expel air from syringe by holding syringe with needle pointing up and carefully pushing plunger.
6. Inject epinephrine. Insert whole needle straight down into cleansed skin area. When this is done, pull back on plunger. If blood enters syringe, the needle is in a blood vessel. Withdraw needle, and reinsert in another site. For adults, and children over 12 years,

2 to 6 years, 0.15 ml; infants to 2 years, 0.05 to 0.1 ml.
7. Chew and swallow Chlo-Amine (antihistamine) tablets. Adults, and children over 12 years should take four tablets; children 12 years or younger, two tablets.
8. Apply ice packs, if available.
9. Keep warm. Avoid exertion.
10. Prepare prefilled syringe for second injection. Turn rectangular plunger one quarter turn to right, to line up with rectangular slot in syringe. Do not depress plunger until ready for second injection.
11. Second injection: If no noticeable improvement in 10 minutes, repeat steps 4, 5, and 6.
12. See doctor as soon as possible.

onds or minutes (usually no later than 45 minutes, although an insect reaction may be delayed) after exposure to an allergen. Severity of the reaction is inversely related to the interval between exposure to the allergen and the onset of symptoms. Usually, the first symptoms include a feeling of impending doom or fright, weakness, sweating, sneezing, shortness of breath, nasal pruritus, urticaria, and angioedema, followed rapidly by symptoms in one or more target organs. Cardiovascular symptoms include hypotension, shock, and sometimes cardiac dysrhythmias (possible secondary ischemic EKG changes: flattening and inversion of T waves, S-T segment elevation or depression, and nodal rhythms). Respiratory symptoms can occur at any level in the respiratory tract and commonly include nasal mucosal edema, profuse watery rhinorrhea, itching, nasal congestion, and sudden sneezing attacks. Edema of the upper respiratory tract, resulting in hypopharyngeal and laryngeal obstruction (hoarseness, stridor, and dyspnea), is an early sign of acute respiratory failure, which can be fatal. Gastrointestinal and genitourinary symptoms include severe stomach cramps, nausea, diarrhea, and urinary urgency and incontinence.

Diagnosis
Anaphylaxis is characterized by the rapid onset of severe respiratory or cardiovascular symptoms after ingestion or injection of a drug, vaccine, diagnostic agent, or food, or after an insect sting. If these symptoms occur without a known allergic stimulus, other possible causes of shock (acute myocardial infarction, status asthmaticus, congestive heart failure) must be ruled out.

Treatment and additional considerations
Anaphylaxis is always an emergency. It requires an *immediate* injection of epinephrine 1:1,000 aqueous solution, 0.1 to 0.5 ml, repeated every 5 to 20 minutes, as necessary.

In the early stages of anaphylaxis, when the patient has not lost consciousness and is normotensive, epinephrine is given intramuscularly or subcutaneously, and moved into circulation faster by massaging the site of injection. In severe reactions, when the patient has lost consciousness and is hypotensive, epinephrine is given I.V.

The airway must be maintained and the patient observed for early signs of laryngeal edema (stridor, hoarseness, and dyspnea). Development of laryngeal edema will probably necessitate endotracheal tube insertion or a tracheotomy, and oxygen therapy.

In case of cardiac arrest, the patient is given cardiopulmonary resuscitation, including closed-chest heart massage, assisted ventilation, and sodium bicarbonate; other therapy is indicated by clinical response.

The patient must be watched closely for hypotension and shock, and circulatory volume is maintained with volume expanders (plasma, plasma expanders, saline, and albumin), as needed. Blood pressure is stabilized with the I.V. vasopressors norepinephrine and dopamine. Blood pressure, central venous pressure, and urinary output are monitored as a response index.

After the initial emergency, other medications may be ordered: subcutaneous epinephrine, longer-acting epinephrine, corticosteroids, and diphenhydramine I.V. for long-term management; and aminophylline I.V. over 10 to 20 minutes for bronchospasm. (Aminophylline is given cautiously, since rapid infusion may cause or aggravate severe hypotension.)

To prevent anaphylaxis, the patient must avoid exposure to known allergens. In food or drug allergy, the sensitized person must learn to avoid the offending food or drug in all its forms. With allergy to insect stings, he should avoid open fields and wooded areas during the insect season. In addition, he should carry an anaphylaxis kit (epinephrine, antihistamine, tourniquet) whenever he goes outdoors.

If a patient must receive a drug to which he is allergic, careful desensitization with gradually increasing doses of the antigen or advance administration of steroids will prevent a severe reaction. Of course, a person with a known allergic history should receive a drug with a high anaphylactic potential only after cautious pre-testing for sensitivity. The patient must be monitored closely during testing, and resuscitative equipment and epinephrine should be handy. When any patient needs a drug with a high anaphylactic potential (particularly parenteral drugs), he should receive each dose under close medical observation, again with resuscitative equipment and epinephrine handy.

Some diagnostic tests may produce anaphylaxis; for example, intravenous pyelogram (IVP), cardiac catheterization, and any angiography using radiographic contrast media.

Urticaria: Angioedema
(Hives)

Urticaria is an episodic, usually self-limited skin reaction that produces dermal wheals surrounded by an erythematous flare. Angioedema (angioneurotic edema) is a subcutaneous and dermal eruption that produces deeper, larger wheals, usually on the hands, feet, lips, and eyelids. When angioedema causes laryngeal edema, it can lead to asphyxiation and death. Urticaria and angioedema can occur simultaneously, but angioedema may last longer.

Causes and incidence

Urticaria and angioedema are common allergic reactions that may occur in 20% of the general population at some time or other. Their causes include allergy to drugs (cutaneous anaphylaxis), foods and insect stings, and occasionally, inhalant allergens (animal danders, flour, cosmetics) that provoke IgE-mediated response to protein allergens. However, certain drugs may cause urticaria without an IgE response. When urticaria and angioedema are part of an anaphylactic reaction, they almost always persist long after the systemic response has subsided. This is so because circulation to the skin is restored last after an allergic reaction, resulting in slow histamine reabsorption at the reaction site.

Nonallergic urticaria and angioedema are probably also related to histamine release by some still unknown mechanism. External physical stimulus, such as cold (usually in young adults),

heat, water, or sunlight, may also provoke urticaria and angioedema. *Dermographism* urticaria that develops after stroking or scratching the skin, occurs in as many as 20% of the population. Such urticaria develops with varying pressure, most often under tight clothing, and is aggravated by scratching.

Several conditions provoke urticaria via secondary IgE response: localized or secondary infection (respiratory infection), neoplastic disease (Hodgkin's lymphoma), connective tissue diseases (systemic lupus erythematosus), collagen vascular disease, and psychogenic disease. Physical or emotional stress may trigger the release of acetylcholine by nerve endings, which may induce cholinergic urticaria or angioedema. However, stress alone doesn't seem to cause urticaria or angioedema.

Hereditary angioedema results from an autosomal dominant trait—a hereditary deficiency of an alpha globulin, the normal inhibitor of C1 esterase (a component of the complement system). Such deficiency allows uninhibited C1 esterase release, resulting in the vascular changes common to angioedema.

HEREDITARY ANGIOEDEMA

Hereditary angioedema usually begins in childhood with recurrent subcutaneous or submucosal edema at regular intervals of weeks, months, or years, often following trauma. Urticarial lesions are usually not pruritic but may be mildly painful. Involvement of the GI tract may cause nausea, vomiting, and severe abdominal pain. Laryngeal angioedema may be fatal and carries an overall mortality rate as high as 50%.

Signs and symptoms

The characteristic features of urticaria are distinct, raised evanescent dermal wheals surrounded by an erythematous flare. These lesions may be as small as ½" to ¾" (1.3 to 1.9 cm) but may cover an entire body region with confluent flares. In cholinergic urticaria, the wheals may be tiny and blanched, surrounded by erythematous flares.

Angioedema characteristically produces nonpitted swelling of deep subcutaneous tissue, usually on the eyelids, lips, genitalia, and mucous membranes. These swellings don't usually itch but may burn and tingle. The clinical features of hereditary angioedema are slightly different. Such angioedema is unifocal, without urticarial pruritus but associated with recurrent, transient edema of skin and mucosa (especially of the respiratory tract).

Diagnosis

An accurate patient history can help determine the causes of hives. Such a history should include:

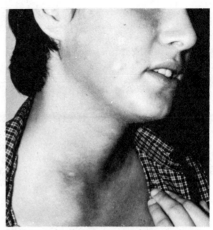

Distinct, raised evanescent dermal wheals surrounded by erythematous flare

• drug history, including over-the-counter preparations (vitamins, aspirin, antacids)

• frequently ingested foods (strawberries, milk products, fish)

• environmental influences (pet, carpet, clothing, soap, inhalants, cosmetics, hair dye, insect bites and stings)

• psychiatric climate (current stress, job situation, family role, patient's feelings).

Diagnosis also requires physical assessment to rule out similar conditions, and CBC, urinalysis, erythrocyte sedimentation rate (ESR), and chest X-ray to rule out inflammatory infections. Skin testing, an elimination diet, and a food diary (recording time and amount of food eaten, and circumstances) can pinpoint allergens that provoke urticaria and angioedema. The food diary may also suggest other allergies. For instance, a patient allergic to fish may also be allergic to iodine contrast materials.

Recurrent angioedema, without urticaria, points to hereditary angioedema. Decreased levels of C4 and C1 esterase inhibitor can confirm this diagnosis.

Treatment and additional considerations

Treatment aims to prevent or limit contact with triggering factors or, if this is impossible, to desensitize the patient to them and to relieve symptoms. Treatment for acute hereditary angioedema may require epinephrine, antihistamines,

corticosteroids (of limited value), danazol (new experimental treatment), and positive pressure breathing and tracheotomy to relieve respiratory obstruction resulting from laryngeal edema. Once the triggering stimulus has been removed, urticaria usually subsides in a few days, except for drug reactions, which may persist as long as the drug is in the bloodstream.

During desensitization, progressively larger doses of specific antigens (determined by skin testing) are injected intradermally. Diphenhydramine or some other antihistamine can ease itching and

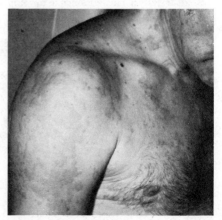

Confluent flares in urticaria

swelling with every kind of urticaria. Phenobarbital may help control urticaria traced to emotional stress. Patients receiving antihistamines or phenobarbital should be warned that they may experience drowsiness. Aspirins and corticosteroids are contraindicated in urticaria treatment.

Drug Hypersensitivity

An allergic reaction can occur after exposure to a drug by any route and can reflect any of four kinds of hypersensitivity: Type I, atopic reactions, including anaphylaxis; Type II, complement-dependent reactions; Type III, multisystem complement-dependent reactions; or Type IV, cell-mediated reactions. These account for roughly 10% of all adverse reactions to drugs.

Causes

The root cause of hypersensitivity is still unknown, but it may reflect genetic susceptibility. In any case, we do know *how* hypersensitivity works: a drug bonds with serum proteins (becomes immunogenic) and induces antibody formation. Thus, hypersensitivity reactions are most common after administration of natural proteins, such as animal serums, vaccines, biologicals, and allergen extracts. They also occur after exposure to sulfa drugs, penicillin, and penicillin-related drugs.

Drug hypersensitivity is potentially more severe after oral or parenteral administration, and is most likely to develop in patients with infection (probably because infection increases immune system activity). The tendency to develop hypersensitivity also depends on the nature of the drug, the degree and duration of exposure to it, the patient's age and sex, an atopic history, prior drug reactions, and underlying disease.

Type I reactions are particularly likely with systemically administered drugs (especially ACTH and insulin) and reflect the formation of IgE antibodies. Type II reactions, often due to blood group and Rh incompatibility, are complement-dependent and therefore involve IgG or IgM antibodies. In such reactions, plasma immunoglobulins recognize a drug as foreign and destroy it via certain blood cells, resulting in hemolytic anemia. Type III reactions, such as serum sickness, deposit immune complexes along the blood vessels and stimulate inflammation and cell wall damage. Type IV reactions, such as contact dermatitis and homograft rejection, are cell-

---

PENICILLIN WITH CAUTION

To prevent allergic response from penicillin or its derivatives (such as ampicillin or carbenicillin), the World Health Organization recommends the following actions:

• having an emergency kit available to treat allergic reactions.
• taking a detailed patient history, including history of penicillin allergy and other allergies. If the patient's a child younger than 3 months, his mother should be checked for penicillin allergy. Penicillin must never be given if the patient's ever had an allergic reaction to it, or (in the case of an infant) if his mother's ever had such a reaction.
• confirming suspected penicillin allergy with skin and immunologic tests *before* administration.
• informing the patient that he is going to receive penicillin before he takes the first dose.
• observing carefully for adverse effects for at least half an hour after administering penicillin or one of its derivatives.

mediated and follow topical application of antibiotics, local anesthetics, or additives (lanolin, paraben).

Signs and symptoms

The clinical features of drug hypersensitivity vary, ranging from mild local symptoms (pruritus, erythema, rash, edema) to severe systemic disorders (asthma, anemia, blood dyscrasia, or anaphylaxis). Type I symptoms usually include flushing, urticaria, coughing, anxiety, pruritus, erythema, rash, and edema and can escalate to anaphylaxis. In Type II, an erythematous rash (mainly on the trunk, upper arms, and legs) and blood dyscrasia usually develop after several days of drug treatment or even after treatment has stopped. However, infections may mask Type II symptoms. Similarly, in Type III, fever, malaise, and urticaria are likely soon after drug administration but may be delayed. In Type IV, syncope, hypotension, or contact dermatitis follow use of a local anesthetic (sometimes after 12 hours but usually after 24 to 72 hours). In all four types, the patient complains of unusual and severe malaise.

Diagnosis

Diagnosis depends primarily on the physical examination, and the patient's medical history (particularly regarding drug treatment) and blood count determination. Drug hypersensitivity should be suspected if the patient shows signs of allergy following two or more exposures to a drug. Since hypersensitivity develops after repeated drug exposures, the patient probably will not have an allergic reaction after only one exposure.

Specific tests for hypersensitivity include skin tests for IgE hypersensitivity, when the reaction follows drugs that are complete antigen compounds (serum, protein hormones, and penicillin), but such testing is ineffective for most drugs. Specific tests for Type II reactions include monitoring of platelets, hemoglobin, and hematocrit for hematologic changes, and in vitro agglutination tests for an antigen-antibody reaction. Another test, the radioallergosorbent test (RAST), detects the allergen by its ability to bind with a radioactive substance.

Treatment and additional considerations

At the first sign of a hypersensitivity reaction, the offending drug must be discontinued at once (unless doing so will endanger the patient's life). If the doctor isn't present, he must be notified immediately. Then, specific symptoms are treated as follows:
• For Type I reactions, antihistamines, epinephrine, or corticosteroids
• For severe Type II reactions, a blood transfusion for anemia and if platelet destruction is severe, evaluation of renal and hepatic function. In patients with platelet destruction, drugs that alter platelet function (aspirin) are contraindicated.

CLASSIFICATION OF PENICILLIN REACTIONS

STAGE	REACTION TIME	SIGNS AND SYMPTOMS
I. **Immediate** (most dangerous)	Within 30 minutes	Urticaria, systemic anaphylaxis
II. **Accelerated**	Within 2 to 72 hours	Pruritus, urticaria, wheezing, laryngeal edema, local inflammatory reactions
III. **Late** (most common: 80% to 90%)	After 72 hours (sometimes weeks later)	Morbilliform, urticarial, and erythematous eruptions; serum sickness; local inflammatory reactions

• For Type III reactions, corticosteroids and supportive measures, as needed (tranfusions, analgesics).

• For Type IV reactions, discontinuation of allergenic topical medication. However, localized symptoms, such as dermatitis, may persist for weeks to months afterward.

Special care must be taken to prevent a hypersensitive reaction. For instance, a meticulous history of the patient's drug, food, and environmental allergies must be taken before any drug regimen begins. A patient who has other allergies is also apt to develop drug hypersensitivity; and a patient who is allergic to one drug (such as penicillin) may develop cross-sensitivity to a related drug.

Patients should know how to recognize early signs of hypersensitivity (pruritis, erythema, rash, edema), and immediately report them. Often, early recognition of drug hypersensitivity and prompt discontinuation of the allergenic drug can mean the difference between a slight rash and fatal anaphylaxis.

Transfusion Reaction

A transfusion reaction is a cytotoxic reaction that accompanies or follows I.V. administration of blood or blood components. Its severity varies from mild (fever or chills) to severe (acute renal failure or complete vascular collapse and death) with the amount of blood transfused, the type of reaction, and the patient's general health.

Causes

A cytotoxic reaction to transfusion (Type II allergic) results when humoral antibodies react with antigenic cell components or haptens (antigens) that have become bound to cells. In a cytotoxic reaction, the antibody itself destroys the antigen without the intervention of phagocytic cells for cellular lysis. The subsequent release of toxic material, such as histamine, then produces systemic symptoms. Transfusion reactions can be hemolytic, caused by the administration of mismatched blood (occur immediately after transfusion is started in one out of every 5,000 patients, but are sometimes delayed, as in Rh incompatibility) or nonhemolytic, caused by patient sensitivity to infused components.

Hemolytic reactions fall into two groups:

• *Blood transfusions with serologically incompatible blood* lead to intravascular agglutination of red cells. The recipient's antibodies (IgG or IgM) attach themselves to the donated red cells, leading to the clumping and destruction of large numbers of cells.

• *Delayed extravascular hemolytic reactions due to Rh incompatibility* occur several days to 2 weeks after transfusion. They are usually less serious than serologically incompatible reactions. Rh reactions are most likely to occur in women sensitized to red blood cell antigens by prior pregnancy, or by unknown factors that may include bacterial or viral infection; and in persons who have had more than five transfusions.

Signs and symptoms

Immediate symptoms of transfusion reaction develop within a few minutes of the start of transfusions or hours after transfusions, and may include chills, fever, urticaria,, tachycardia, dyspnea, nausea, vomiting, tightness in the chest, chest and back pain, hypotension, bronchospasm, angioneurotic edema, anaphylaxis, shock, pulmonary edema, and congestive heart failure. In a surgical patient under anesthesia, these symptoms are masked, but blood oozes from mucous membranes or the incision site. If the patient develops shock, he does not respond to blood administration.

Delayed symptoms, such as anemia, usually occur within 2 weeks. Symptoms of malaria or serum hepatitis appear weeks or months after transfusion.

Diagnosis

Confirming a transfusion reaction requires proof of blood incompatibility and evidence of hemolysis, such as hemoglobinuria. When such a reaction is suspected, a blood sample is drawn; then, it's retyped and cross-matched with the donor's blood, and the patient's urine is checked for red cells. After a transfusion reaction, laboratory tests will show increased indirect bilirubin, decreased haptoglobin, increased serum hemoglobin, and hemoglobin in urine. Later, as the reaction progresses, tests may show disseminated intravascular coagulation (DIC)—thrombocytopenia, increased prothrombin time, decreased fibrinogen level—and acute tubular necrosis—increased serum BUN, and creatinine.

Treatment and additional considerations

At the first sign of a reaction, the transfusion must be stopped at once and a doctor summoned. To prevent hypovolemia, he'll probably substitute an infusion of normal saline solution for the blood transfusion. For adults, the infusion rate is between 150 and 300 ml per hour; for children, the infusion rate is calculated according to body weight.

Subsequent procedures include:

• inserting a Foley catheter and collecting midstream urine for cultures and sensitivity. A record of fluid intake and output is kept, and the patient is watched for hematuria, oliguria, and anuria.

• monitoring vital signs every 15 to 30 minutes.

• covering the patient with blankets to ease chills, and reassuring him.

• giving an I.V. antihypotensive drug and normal saline solution to combat shock; oxygen (by nasal cannula or venturi mask at low flow rates); epinephrine to treat dyspnea and wheezing; diphenhydramine to combat cellular histamine released from destroyed tissue; corticosteroids to reduce inflammation; and mannitol or furosemide to maintain urinary function.

• fully documenting the transfusion reaction on the patient's chart, noting length of transfusion, amount of blood absorbed, and how the patient reacted.

To prevent transfusion reaction, hospital policy on giving blood transfusions must be clear and rigorously enforced. Any health care professional administering a blood transfusion must make sure he has the right blood and the right patient before proceeding. With another health care professional, he should check and double-check the patient's name, his hospital identification number, ABO group, and Rh status. The blood must not be given if even a small discrepancy is discovered. Instead, the blood bank should be notified at once, and the blood

---

Rh SYSTEM

The Rh system contains more than 30 antibodies and antigens. Eighty-five percent of the world's population is Rh-positive, which means their red blood cells carry the D or Rh antigen. The remaining 15% of the population who are Rh-negative do not carry this antigen.

When Rh-negative persons receive Rh-positive blood for the first time, they become sensitized to the D antigen but show no immediate reaction to it. If they receive Rh-positive blood a second time, they then develop a massive hemolytic reaction. For example, an Rh-negative mother who delivers an Rh-positive baby is sensitized by the baby's Rh-positive blood. During her next Rh-positive pregnancy, her sensitized blood would cause a hemolytic reaction in fetal circulation. Thus, the Rh-negative mother should receive Rh_o (D) immune globulin, human I.M., within 72 hours after delivering an Rh-positive baby to prevent formation of antibodies against Rh-positive blood.

returned unopened.

To begin the transfusion, the health care professional should first make sure an 18G (or larger) needle or catheter is in place and functioning well; then connect the blood setup, and begin to slowly infuse blood. He'll closely watch the patient for any adverse reaction, which is most likely to occur within the first 15 minutes. Also, he'll monitor vital signs every 15 to 30 minutes during the entire transfusion.

He won't administer any drugs or fluids through the same I.V. while transfusing blood. However, if immediate drug administration is necessary, he'll stop the transfusion and flush the line with 10 to 20 ml normal saline solution. (Since dextrose solution causes hemolysis of blood cells, it must not be substituted for normal saline solution.) Then, he'll administer the medication, flush the line again, and resume the blood transfusion.

Most severe transfusion reactions occur with the use of whole blood. The use of blood components radically decreases the possibility of a reaction.

AUTOIMMUNITY

DiGeorge's Syndrome
(Congenital thymic hypoplasia or aplasia)

DiGeorge's syndrome is a disorder known typically by the partial or total absence of cellular immunity that results from a deficiency of T-lymphocytes. It characteristically produces life-threatening hypocalcemia that may be associated with cardiovascular and facial anomalies. Prognosis is excellent when fetal thymic transplant, correction of hypocalcemia, and repair of cardiac anomalies are possible.

Causes
DiGeorge's syndrome is probably caused by abnormal fetal development of the third and fourth pharyngeal pouches (12th week of gestation) that interferes with the formation of the thymus. As a result, the thymus is completely or partially absent and abnormally located, causing deficient cellular immunity.

ROLE OF THE THYMUS IN IMMUNE RESPONSE
Although the exact relationship between the thymus and the immunologic system remains unclear, possible thymic functions include:
• destruction of T cells that would have "mistaken" components of the human organism as foreign during the fetal stage. This establishes immunologic differentiation between self and nonself.
• development of lymphocytes in the thymic epithelium or mesenchymal cells.
• regulation of the humoral immune response through the interaction of B and T cells.

Signs and symptoms
Symptoms are usually obvious at birth or shortly thereafter. An infant with DiGeorge's syndrome may have low-set ears, notched ear pinnae, a fish-shaped mouth, an undersized jaw, and abnormally wide-set eyes (hypertelorism) with antimongoloid eyelid formation (downward slant). Cardiovascular abnormalities include great blood vessel anomalies (these may also develop soon after birth) and tetralogy of Fallot. The thymus may be absent or underdeveloped, and abnormally located. An infant with thymic hypoplasia (rather than aplasia) may

experience a spontaneous return of cellular immunity but can develop severe T cell deficiencies later in life, allowing exaggerated susceptibility to viral, fungal, or bacterial infections, which may be overwhelming. Typically, hypoparathyroidism, usually associated with DiGeorge's syndrome, causes tetany, hyperphosphoremia, and hypocalcemia. Hypocalcemia develops early and is both life-threatening and unusually resistant to treatment. It can lead to seizures, central nervous system damage, and early congestive heart failure.

Diagnosis

Immediate diagnosis is difficult unless the infant shows typical facial anomalies, normally the first clues to the disorder. Definitive diagnosis depends on successful treatment of hypocalcemia and other life-threatening birth defects during the first few weeks of life. Such diagnosis rests on proof of decreased or absent T-lymphocytes (sheep cell test, lymphopenia) and of an absent thymus (chest X-ray). Immunoglobulin assays are useless, because antibodies present are usually from maternal circulation.

Additional tests showing low serum calcium, elevated serum phosphorus, and missing parathyroid hormone confirm hypoparathyroidism.

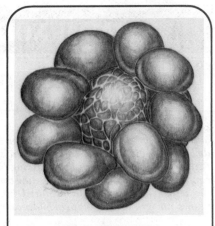

SHEEP CELL TEST

When human blood cells are mixed with sheep red blood cells, the sheep cells aggregate peripherally around human T-lymphocytes to form characteristic rosettes.

Treatment and additional considerations

Life-threatening hypocalcemia must be treated immediately, but it's unusually resistant and requires aggressive treatment; for example, with a rapid I.V. infusion of 10% solution of calcium gluconate. During such an infusion, heart rate must be monitored and the infusion watched carefully to avoid infiltration. Calcium supplements *must* be given with vitamin D, or sometimes also with parathyroid hormone, to ensure effective calcium utilization. After hypocalcemia is under control, fetal thymic transplant may restore normal cellular immune function. Cardiac anomalies require surgical repair when possible.

A patient with DiGeorge's syndrome also needs a low-phosphorous diet and careful preventive measures for infection. The mother of such an infant must be taught to watch for signs of infection and get it treated immediately; to keep the infant away from crowds or any other sources of infection; and to provide good hygiene and adequate nutrition and hydration.

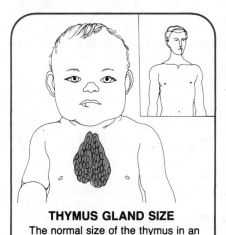

THYMUS GLAND SIZE

The normal size of the thymus in an infant and in an adult.

IMMUNODEFICIENCY

B Cell Deficiency
(Agammaglobulinemia or hypogammaglobulinemia)

B cell, or antibody-mediated, deficiencies interfere with effective humoral response and increase vulnerability to infection. Prognosis varies with the severity of the deficiency but is guarded. In X-linked infantile hypogammaglobulinemia (also called Bruton's or X-linked infantile agammaglobulinemia), infections such as encephalitis, hepatitis, or chronic lung disease may cause permanent organ damage and shorten the patient's life span. In acquired hypogammaglobulinemia, correct treatment allows normal life (including childbearing) and a normal life span.

Causes
X-linked infantile hypogammaglobulinemia, the most severe B cell deficiency, is a congenital X-linked disorder affecting males, in which all five immunologic classes (IgM, IgG, IgA, IgD, and IgE) are totally or partially absent. Circulating B cells (normally present in the lymph system and the blood) are absent, but T cells are usually normal. It usually appears in infants who are between 4 and 12 months old, when transplacental maternal immunoglobulins that provided immune response have been depleted.

The cause of acquired hypogammaglobulinemia isn't known, but genetic factors and stress may play a part. This disorder affects both males and females, and may occur at any age, but the usual age of onset is between 15 and 30 years. In acquired hypogammaglobulinemia, circulating B cells are present but dysfunctional, diminishing synthesis or release of immunoglobulin.

Signs and symptoms
Signs of X-linked infantile hypogammaglobulinemia include recurrent bacterial otitis media, dermatitis, meningitis, pneumonia, and bronchitis—usually caused by gram-positive organisms (pneumococci, meningococci, Staphylococcus aureus) and Hemophilus influenzae and other gram-negative bacteria. Purulent conjunctivitis, abnormal dental decay, retarded development, and rheumatoid-arthritis–like symptoms in large joints may also occur. Despite recurrent infections, lymphadenopathy and splenomegaly are usually absent.

In acquired hypogammaglobulinemia, pyogenic bacterial infections are also common, often accompanied by marked lymphadenopathy and splenomegaly. Generally, recurrent sinopulmonary infections, chronic bacterial conjunctivitis, and malabsorption (often associated with infestation by Giardia lamblia) are the first clues that something is wrong but at times may follow rheumatoid-arthritis–like symptoms with sterile effusions into large joints. Acquired hypogammaglobulinemia may also appear with neoplastic diseases, such as lymphoma, lymphatic leukemia, thymoma, and myeloma.

Diagnosis
For both these B cell deficiencies, diagnosis rests on clinical features, an accurate patient history (with particular attention to age of onset), family history (which may show severe infection as a common cause of death), and laboratory data. Diagnosis of X-linked infantile hypogammaglobulinemia may be especially difficult, since recurrent infections are common even in normal infants (many of whom don't start producing their own antibodies until between 18 and 20 months). Diagnosis must also rule out

cystic fibrosis and other congenital disorders that cause recurrent respiratory infections.

In X-linked infantile hypogammaglobulinemia and in acquired hypogammaglobulinemia, immunoelectrophoresis shows decreased IgM, IgA, and IgG globulins in the serum. However, in X-linked infantile hypogammaglobulinemia, diagnosis by this method isn't possible until the infant is 6 or 8 months old. But before then, a continual drop in these immunoglobulins suggests this disorder.

Antigenic stimulation confirms an inability to produce specific antibodies. In the most common test, diphtheria, pertussis, and tetanus (DPT) combined vaccine is injected in the thigh, followed by inguinal lymph node biopsy. In acquired hypogammaglobulinemia, this biopsy may show B cells but no plasma cells (B cells mature to form plasma cells as part of a normal immune response).

Treatment and additional considerations

B cell deficiencies can't be prevented or cured, but effective treatment can control infections, boost the patient's immune defenses and reduce rheumatoid-arthritis–like symptoms. For example, replacement of gamma globulin (beginning with a loading dose, followed by increasing monthly or more frequent doses until symptoms subside) can help maintain immune response.

• Since these injections are very painful, they're given deep into a large muscle mass, such as the gluteal or thigh muscles. The injection site is massaged well. If the doctor orders more than 1.5 ml, he'll divide the dose, and inject it into more than one site; for frequent injections, he'll rotate the injection sites.

• Because gamma globulin is composed primarily of IgG, the patient may also need fresh frozen plasma infusions (obtained from donors immunized to produce specific antibodies) to provide IgA and IgM. The doctor (or other health care professional) will double-check to make sure he has the right plasma for the patient, infuse it quickly, and observe for an allergic reaction (fever, urticaria, malaise).

• Prophylactic antibiotics aren't necessary, but antibiotics can control infections when they occur. To help prevent severe infection, patients should know how to recognize its early signs and avoid crowds and persons who have active infections.

• These patients must not be immunized with live virus vaccines, since serious illness, with neurologic damage, may result. Corticosteroids and other immunosuppressive drugs are contraindicated, as is splenectomy, because these further impair the patient's immune response.

• Parents of children with these disorders may need genetic counseling.

Severe Combined Immunodeficiency Disease (SCID)

In SCID, also called Swiss-type agammaglobulinemia, both T and B cell immunity are either completely absent or severely deficient, leading to extreme susceptibility to infection and severely shortened life span. Prognosis is poor. Most patients die from infection within a year after birth.

Causes

SCID exists in an X-linked recessive form (which occurs only in males) and an autosomal recessive form. Exactly how these genetic defects cause such severe immunodeficiency isn't known, but possibly it is due to the failure of the embryonic stem cell to differentiate into

T cells and B cells. The absence of these circulating lymphocytes results in a very small thymus. Certain enzyme deficiencies (such as adenosine deaminase deficiency) also are associated with SCID.

Signs and symptoms

An extreme susceptibility to infection becomes obvious in the infant with SCID by age 3 to 6 months, when maternal immunoglobulin stores are at least partly depleted. Commonly, such an infant fails to thrive and develops chronic otitis, sepsis, watery diarrhea (associated with *Salmonella* or *Escherichia coli*), recurrent pulmonary infections (usually caused by *Pseudomonas*, cytomegalovirus, or *Pneumocystis carinii*), and persistent oral candidiasis, with esophageal erosions and hoarseness, and common viral infections (measles, chickenpox) that are often fatal.

The infant infected with *P. carinii* may have a low-grade fever and a cough for months, while he uses maternal immunoglobulin to fight the infection. However, as soon as he uses up these immunoglobulin stores, the infection flares, producing full-blown symptoms: cyanosis; rapid respirations; and normal chest sounds, with an abnormal chest X-ray. Because of persistent maternal IgG, gram-negative infections don't usually appear until after the infant is 6 months old. Maternal antibodies are totally depleted within 1 year.

Diagnosis

Diagnosis is difficult, since most SCID infants die of overwhelming infection within a year after birth, and defective antibody-mediated (B cell) immunity is hard to detect before the child is 5 months old (at this time immunoglobulin levels should be 1% of normal). Before 5 months, even normal infants have very small amounts of serum immunoglobulins IgM and IgA. Normal IgG levels merely reflect maternal IgG. However, severely diminished or absent T cell and B cell immunity (less than 10% T cell rosettes and absent lymphocyte response); lymph node biopsy showing absence of lymphocytes,

plasma cells, and lymphoid follicles; and lack of skin reactivity to painting with dinitrochlorobenzene can confirm this diagnosis.

Treatment

Treatment aims to restore immune response and prevent infection. Histocompatible bone marrow transplant is the only satisfactory treatment available to correct immunodeficiency. Since bone marrow cells must be HL-A- (human leukocyte antigen) and MLC- (mixed leukocyte culture) matched, the most common donors are histocompatible siblings. However, bone marrow transplant may cause a graft-versus-host reaction, which increases vulnerability to infection and may be fatal.

Fetal thymus transplants are ineffective, since they restore only T cell (and not B cell) immunity. Some SCID infants have been rescued by being placed in a completely sterile, long-term environment. However, this treatment isn't effective if the child already has had recurring infections.

Additional considerations

Patient care is primarily supportive. Although an SCID infant must remain in strict protective isolation, he needs a stimulating atmosphere to promote normal growth and development. Parents should visit their child often, hold him, and bring him toys that can be sterilized easily. All procedures should be thoroughly explained to them. The child needs a normal day/night routine, and health care professionals responsible for his care should talk to the child as much as possible.

Since parents will have questions about the vulnerability of future offspring, they need genetic counseling. In addition, the child's parents and siblings need psychologic and spiritual support to help them cope with the child's inevitable long-term illness and early death. They may also need a social service referral for assistance in coping with the financial burden of the child's long-term hospitalization.

Chronic Mucocutaneous Candidiasis

Chronic mucocutaneous candidiasis is an uncommon form of candidiasis (moniliasis) that usually develops during the first year of life but occasionally may occur as late as the 20s. It's a persistent infection, affecting males and females, that may result from an inherited defect in the cell-mediated (T cell) immune system. (The humoral immune system, mediated by B cells, is intact and gives a normal antibody response to Candida albicans.) *In some patients, an autoimmune response affecting the endocrine system may induce various endocrinopathies.*

Despite chronic candidiasis, these patients rarely die of systemic infection. Instead, they usually die of hepatic or endocrine failure. Patients with Addison's disease, for example, may die suddenly and unexpectedly because of adrenal failure. So, prognosis for chronic mucocutaneous candidiasis depends on the severity of the associated endocrinopathy. Indeed, patients with associated endocrinopathy rarely live beyond their 30s.

Causes

Autoimmunity, with the thymus acting as an endocrine organ, may cause the defect in the cellular-mediated immune system and the associated endocrinopathy. This immune defect may then allow autoantibodies to develop against target organs. This disease's changeable nature depends on the start and severity of this destructive process.

Signs and symptoms

Chronic candidal infections can affect the skin, mucous membranes, nails, and vagina, usually causing large, circular lesions. These infections rarely produce systemic symptoms but in late stages may be associated with recurrent respiratory tract infections. Other associated conditions include severe viral infections that may precede the onset of endocrinopathy and, sometimes, hepatitis. Involvement of the mouth, nose, and palate may cause speech and eating difficulties.

Symptoms of endocrinopathy are peculiar to the organ involved. Tetany and hypocalcemia are most common and are associated with hypoparathyroidism. Addison's disease, hypothyroidism, diabetes, and pernicious anemia are also connected with chronic mucocutaneous candidiasis. Psychiatric disorders are likely because of disfigurement and multiple endocrine aberrations.

Diagnosis

Laboratory findings show a normal circulating T cell count, with normal immunologic response to antigens other than *Candida*, possibly with decreased circulating T cells. Most patients don't have delayed hypersensitivity skin tests to *Candida*, even during the infectious stage. Migration inhibiting factor (MIF) that indicates presence of activated T cells may not respond to *Candida*.

Nonimmunologic abnormalities result from endocrinopathy and may include hypocalcemia, abnormal hepatic function studies, hyperglycemia, iron deficiency, and abnormal vitamin B_{12} absorption (pernicious anemia). Diagnosis must rule out other immunodeficiency disorders associated with chronic *Candida* infection, especially DiGeorge's syndrome, ataxia-telangiectasia, and severe combined immunodeficiency disease (SCID), all of which produce severe immunologic defects. After diagnosis, the patient needs evaluation of adrenal, pituitary, thyroid, gonadal, pancreatic, and parathyroid functions, with careful follow-up. The disease is progressive, and most patients eventually develop endocrinopathy.

Treatment and additional considerations

Treatment aims to control infection but isn't always successful. Topical antifungal agents are often ineffective against chronic mucocutaneous candidiasis. Miconazole and nystatin are sometimes useful but ultimately fail to control this infection.

Systemic infections may not be fatal, but they're serious enough to warrant vigorous treatment. Amphotericin B is sometimes effective against systemic infection but is highly nephrotoxic, so the patient's renal function must be monitored closely. In severe cases, transfer factor from a *Candida*-positive donor with delayed sensitivity, with intravenous amphotericin B is most successful. Fetal thymus transplants are effective

with some patients, but immunotherapy doesn't prevent progressive development of endocrinopathies; these must be treated individually with hormone replacement. (Experimentally, injections of thymosin and levamisole have had some positive effect.) Oral or intramuscular iron replacement may also be necessary.

The patient should learn about progressive manifestations of the disease, expecially the importance of seeing an endocrinologist for regular checkups. Treatment may also include plastic surgery, when possible, and counseling to help the patient cope with his disfigurement.

Wiskott-Aldrich Syndrome

Wiskott-Aldrich syndrome is an X-linked recessive immunodeficiency disorder in which both B and T cell functions are defective. Its clinical features include thrombocytopenia, with severe bleeding; eczema; recurrent infection; and an increased risk of malignancy. Prognosis is poor. This syndrome causes early death (average life span is 4 years), usually from massive bleeding during infancy; later, from malignancy or severe infection.

Causes

Since Wiskott-Aldrich syndrome results from an X-linked recessive trait, it affects only males. Patients with this genetic defect are born with a normal thymus gland and normal plasma cells and lymphoid tissues, but as they get older, an acquired thymic system deficiency results in a decline in both B and T cell functions, compromised immunity, and vulnerability to infection. These patients also have a metabolic defect in platelet synthesis and produce only small, short-lived platelets and incompetent phagocytes (unable to process foreign antigens), resulting in abnormal immunoglobulin patterns.

Signs and symptoms

Characteristically, newborns with Wiskott-Aldrich syndrome develop bleeding, petechiae, and purpura, resulting from thrombocytopenia. As these infants get older, the bleeding subsides. But at about

1 year, eczema occurs, which becomes progressively more severe. Skin is easily infected because of scratching. They're also likely to develop recurrent systemic infections, such as chronic pneumonia, sinusitis, otitis media, herpes of the skin and eyes (which may cause keratitis and vision loss) with hepatosplenomegaly. Usually, pneumococci, meningococci, and *Hemophilus influenzae* are the infecting organisms. These infants are also highly vulnerable to malignancy, especially leukemia and lymphoma.

Diagnosis

The most important clue to diagnosis of Wiskott-Aldrich syndrome is thrombocytopenia (with a platelet count below 100,000/mm^3 and prolonged bleeding time) and bleeding disorders at birth. In such newborns, immunization with antigens, especially those containing polysaccharides (for example, bacterial capsular antigens), reveals an inability to produce antibodies; in older infants and toddlers, there is faulty antibody response to other antigens. Laboratory tests show elevated IgE and IgA levels, decreased IgM levels, normal IgG levels, low to absent isohemagglutinins, and (sometimes) shortened half-life of IgG, IgA, and albumin.

Treatment

Treatment of Wiskott-Aldrich syndrome aims to limit bleeding through the use of fresh, cross-matched platelet transfusions; to control infection with prophylactic antibiotics and, once bleeding problems are controlled, to supply passive immunity with gamma globulin injections; and to control eczema with topical corticosteroids. Systemic corticosteroids are contraindicated, since they further compromise immunity. An antipruritic may relieve itching.

Although still investigational, treatment with transfer factor has increased resistance to infection and has reduced eczema, splenomegaly, and bleeding tendencies in about half these patients. However, it may cause hemolytic anemia and nephrotic syndrome, and doesn't increase platelet production.

The parents of children with Wiskott-Aldrich syndrome need genetic counseling to answer their questions about the vulnerability of future offspring.

Additional considerations

Physical and psychologic support, and patient teaching can help these patients and their families cope with this disorder. A baseline platelet count should be established before platelet transfusions begin; then, the count should be checked often during therapy. Each platelet unit transfused should raise the count by 10,000/mm³.

• Parents must watch for signs of bleeding, such as bruising; painful, swollen joints; and tenderness in the trunk area. They should plan their child's activity levels so he can develop normally. While such a child must avoid contact sports, he can ride a bike (wearing protective football gear) and swim.

• Parents also must observe the child for signs of infection, such as fever, cold-like symptoms, or drainage and redness around any superficial wound, and clean all skin wounds carefully. Meticulous mouth and skin care, good nutrition, and adequate hydration are essential. Parents should avoid exposing the child to crowds or persons with active infections.

• As soon as the child is old enough, he should learn about his disease and his limitations.

Nezelof's Syndrome

Nezelof's syndrome is a primary immunodeficiency disease characterized by absent T cell function and deficient B cell function, with fairly normal immunoglobulin levels and little or no specific antibody production. The degree of B cell deficiency varies. Nezelof's syndrome causes early onset of recurrent, progressively severe, and eventually fatal infections.

Causes

The cause of Nezelof's syndrome is unknown. It may be a genetic disorder transmitted as an autosomal recessive trait, because it affects both male and female siblings. However, not all patients with Nezelof's syndrome have a positive family history, so alternative explanations are possible. For example, the syndrome could result from a stem cell deficiency that causes T cell and B cell deficiencies; it could result from an underdeveloped thymus gland that inhibits T-lymphocyte development; or, result from failure to produce or secrete thymic humoral factors, particularly thymosin.

Signs and symptoms

Clinical signs of Nezelof's syndrome may appear in infants or in toddlers up to 4 years, and usually include recurrent pneumonia, otitis media, chronic fungal infections, upper respiratory tract infections, hepatosplenomegaly, and diarrhea. Lymph nodes and tonsils may be absent or enlarged; a tendency toward malignancy is common. Eventually, infection may cause sepsis, which is the usual cause of death in patients with this disorder.

Diagnosis

Failure to thrive, poor eating habits, weight loss, and recurrent infections in children may all suggest Nezelof's syndrome. But definite diagnosis requires the following: evidence of defective B cell and T cell immunity (although the number of circulating B cells is normal), moderate to marked decrease in T cells, a deficiency or rise in one or more immunoglobulins, a nonreactive Schick test after DPT immunization, a reduced or absent antibody response after immunization with a specific antigen, missing thymus shadow on a chest X-ray, abnormal lymphoid structure of thymus dependent areas, and lymphopenia (decreased lymphocytes in the blood).

Treatment

Initial treatment is primarily supportive and includes aggressive use of antibiotics to fight infection, and monthly injections of gamma globulin or fresh frozen plasma infusions, especially if the patient can't produce specific antibodies.

Fetal thymus transplant can fully restore T cell immunity within weeks, but its effect is transient, necessitating repeated transplants. Both transfer factor therapy and repeated injections of thymosin are only partially effective in restoring T cell immunity. While histocompatible bone marrow transplants may restore immunity, they haven't been used enough to make a clear evaluation.

Additional considerations

To prepare a child for painful gamma globulin injections, a nurse or other health care professional may let the child give a doll an injection. Then, when the nurse gives the child a gamma globulin injection, she'll encourage the child to cry if he wants.

• To prevent tissue damage, gamma globulin is injected deep into a large muscle mass, and injection sites are rotated. Injection site rotation is documented carefully. If the child receives more than 1.5 ml gamma globulin at one time, the dose should be divided and injected into several injection sites.

• Parents need to watch for signs of infection in the child. They must keep the child away from crowds and persons with active infections.

Ataxia-telangiectasia

Inherited as an autosomal recessive disorder, ataxia-telangiectasia is characterized by progressively severe ataxia; telangiectasia, particularly of the face, earlobes, and conjunctivae; and chronic, recurrent sinopulmonary infections that may reflect both antibody-mediated (B cell) and cell-mediated (T cell) immune deficiencies. Initially, ataxia-telangiectasia was considered a neurologic disease, because its dominant sign is cerebellar ataxia. It's now known to have associated endocrine and vascular aspects. Ataxia usually appears within 2 years after birth but may develop as late as age 9. The degree of immunodeficiency determines the rate of deterioration. Some patients die within several years; others survive until their 30s. Severe abnormalities cause rapid clinical deterioration and premature death due to overwhelming sinopulmonary infection or malignancy.

Causes
In ataxia-telangiectasia, immunodeficiency stems from an underdeveloped (often seemingly embryonic) thymus, which probably results from defective fetal development of mesenchyme (connective tissue in the mesoderm). A tropic hormone deficiency may explain the involvement of the thymus and the endocrine organs.

Signs and symptoms
The earliest and most dominant symptoms are neurologic: slurred speech, irregular gait, continual and involuntary jerky (choreoathetoid) movements, nystagmus, and extrapyramidal symptoms (pseudoparkinsonism, motor restlessness, dystonias), and posterior column signs (unsteady gait, with forward leaning to maintain balance; decreased arm movements; and purposeless tremors). These signs of cerebellar ataxia usually develop by the time the infant begins to use his motor skills. The associated telangiectasia usually appears later and may not develop until age 9, appearing first as a vascular lesion on the sclera and later on the bridge or side of the nose, the ear, or the antecubital or popliteal areas. More than 50% of affected children develop recurrent or chronic respiratory infections because of IgA deficiency early in life, but some may be symptom-free for 10 years or more. These children are unusually vulnerable to lymphomas, particularly lymphosarcomas and lymphoreticular malignancies but may also develop leukemia, adenocarcinoma, dysgerminoma, or medulloblastoma. They may fail to develop secondary sex characteristics during puberty and eventually may become mentally retarded. Some patients show signs of progeria: premature graying, senile keratoses, and vitiligo.

Diagnosis
If a patient has the complete syndrome (ataxia, telangiectasia, and recurrent sinopulmonary infection), the diagnosis can be made on these clinical facts alone. However, the complete syndrome may not be apparent, and ataxia may be the only symptom for 6 years or longer. So, early diagnosis usually depends on immunity tests. A patient with ataxia-telangiectasia usually shows:
- selective absence of IgA (in 60% to 80%) or deficient IgA and IgE
- normal IgM and IgD levels
- absence of Hassall's corpuscles on examination of thymic tissue
- high serum levels of oncofetal proteins
- decreased T cells.

Other findings in these patients may include cutaneous anergy and delayed rejection of skin grafts; absent or underdeveloped ovaries; abnormal hepatic function tests; gonadal dysgenesis and testicular atrophy; and small, abnormal lymph node structure. Older patients have diminished excretion of 17-ketosteroids, associated with elevated follicle-stimulating hormone (FSH) levels. Pneumoencephalography reveals dilation of the ventricular system and diffuse cerebral atrophy.

Treatment and additional considerations
No treatment is yet available to stop progression of this disease. However, prophylactic use of broad-spectrum antibiotics does help control recurrent infections. To help prevent infections, parents are advised to keep the affected child away from crowds and persons with active infections, and are taught to recognize early signs of infection. They're also taught physical therapy and postural drainage techniques if their child has chronic bronchial infections. Proper nutrition and adequate hydration is important. Frozen plasma infusion can passively replace missing antibodies and may also help prevent infection. The effectiveness of other forms of immunotherapy—such as fetal thymus transplant, transfer factor, or histocompatible bone marrow transplant—is unproven.

Standard treatment for malignancies is inappropriate for patients with ataxia-telangiectasia. Because these patients are extremely sensitive to chemotherapy and radiation therapy, such treatments may cause severe and sometimes fatal reactions.

Parents of a child with ataxia-telangiectasia may have questions about the vulnerability of future offspring and may need genetic counseling. Some parents may also require psychologic therapy to help them cope with the child's long-term illness and inevitable early death.

IgA Deficiency
(Janeway Type 3 dysgammaglobulinemia)

Selective deficiency of IgA is the most common immunoglobulin deficiency, appearing in as many as 1 in 400 persons. IgA—the major immunoglobulin in human saliva, nasal and bronchial fluids, and intestinal secretions—guards against bacterial and viral reinfections. Consequently, IgA deficiency leads to chronic sinopulmonary infections, gastrointestinal diseases, and other disorders. Prognosis is good for patients who receive correct treatment, especially if they are free of associated disorders. Such patients have been known to survive to 70 years.

Causes
IgA deficiency seems to be linked to autosomal dominant or recessive inheritance. The presence of normal numbers of peripheral blood lymphocytes carrying IgA receptors and of normal amounts of other immunoglobulins suggests that B cells may not be secreting IgA. In an occasional patient, suppressor T cells appear to inhibit IgA. IgA deficiency also seems related to autoimmune disorders, since many patients with rheumatoid arthritis or systemic lupus erythematosus are also IgA-deficient.

Signs and symptoms
Some IgA-deficient patients have no symptoms, possibly because they have extra amounts of low-molecular-weight IgM, which take over IgA function and help maintain adequate immunologic defenses. Among those patients who do develop symptoms, chronic sinopulmonary infection is most common. Other effects are respiratory allergy, often triggered by infection; gastrointestinal tract diseases, such as celiac disease, ulcerative colitis, and regional enteritis; autoimmune diseases, such as rheumatoid arthritis, systemic lupus erythematosus, immuno-hemolytic anemia, and chronic hepatitis; and malignant tumors, such as squamous cell carcinoma of the lungs,

reticulum cell sarcoma, and thymoma. Age of onset varies. Some IgA-deficient children with recurrent respiratory disease and middle-ear inflammation may begin to synthesize IgA spontaneously as recurrent infections subside and their condition improves.

Diagnosis
Immunologic analyses of IgA-deficient patients show IgA levels below 5 mg/dl in serum. While IgA is usually absent from secretions in IgA-deficient patients, levels may be normal in rare cases. IgE is normal, while IgM may be normal or elevated in serum and secretions. Normally absent low-molecular–weight IgM (7S) may be present.

Tests may also indicate autoantibodies and antibodies against IgG (rheumatoid factor), IgM, and bovine milk. Cell-mediated immunity and secretory piece (the glycopeptide that transports IgA) are usually normal, and most circulating B cells appear normal. Some IgA-deficient patients have subnormal T cell interferon production, which may increase susceptibility to infection.

Treatment and additional considerations
Selective IgA deficiency has no known cure. Treatment aims to control symp-

toms of associated diseases, such as respiratory and gastrointestinal infections, and is generally the same as for a patient with normal IgA, with one exception: An IgA-deficient patient is not treated with gamma globulin, because sensitization may lead to anaphylaxis during future administration of blood products. If transfusion with blood products is necessary, the risk of adverse reaction can be minimized by using washed red blood cells, or can be avoided completely by crossmatching the patient's blood with that of an IgA-deficient donor. Since this is a lifelong disorder, the patient must learn to prevent infection, to recognize its early signs, and to seek treatment promptly.

Complement Abnormalities

Complement is a series of circulating enzymatic serum proteins with nine functional components, labeled C1 through C9. When the immunoglobulins IgG or IgM react with antigens as part of an immune response, they activate the complement system. Complement then combines with the antibody-antigen complex and undergoes a sequence of complicated reactions that amplify the immune response against the antigen. This complex process is called complement fixation.

Complement abnormalities are rare. The most common are C2 and C3 deficiencies and C5 familial dysfunction. Theoretically, any complement component may be deficient or dysfunctional, and many such disorders are under investigation. Complement deficiency or dysfunction may increase susceptibility to infection and also seems related to collagen vascular diseases. Complement abnormalities have been confirmed in a few patients with lupus erythematosus (and their relatives), in some with dermatomyositis, in one with scleroderma (and in his family), and in a few with gonococcal and meningococcal infections. Prognosis varies with the abnormality and the severity of associated diseases.

Causes

Primary complement deficiencies are probably inherited. Secondary deficiencies may follow complement-fixing (complement consuming) immunologic reactions (such as drug-induced serum sickness), acute streptococcal glomerulonephritis, and acute active systemic lupus erythematosus.

Signs and symptoms

C2 and C3 deficiencies and C5 familial dysfunction increase susceptibility to bacterial infection (which may involve several body systems simultaneously). C2 deficiency is also related to lupus erythematosus and chronic renal failure. C5 dysfunction, usually associated with normal C5 levels, is a familial defect in infants. C5 dysfunction causes failure to thrive, diarrhea, and seborrheic dermatitis.

Diagnosis

Diagnosis is difficult and requires careful interpretation of both clinical features and laboratory results, since no single test is definitive. Total serum complement levels (measured by complement fixation) may be low in complement deficiency but may be normal in dysfunction. Unfortunately, detection of specific complement components is expensive, complicated, and not widely available. But certain other clues strongly suggest complement abnormalities (see p. 34).

Treatment

Treatment replaces complement-fixing antibodies and controls infection and associated illnesses. Infection requires prompt antibiotic therapy and other appropriate treatment. Usually, fresh frozen plasma provides replacement antibodies, but bone marrow transplant

THEORIES OF COMPLEMENT FUNCTION

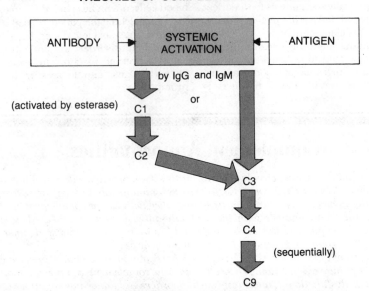

FACTORS OF IMMUNE RESPONSE ENHANCED BY THE COMPLEMENT SYSTEM:

C1 through C9, the active complement system components, don't react simultaneously after systemic activation by IgG and IgM. Instead, they proceed sequentially, usually starting with C1 and continuing to C9, but sometimes starting with C3. How do they enhance an immune response?

● In *lysis,* complement proteins digest portions of the antigen's cell membrane and destroy the cell.

● In *chemotaxis,* complement directs neutrophils (enzyme-loaded leukocytes) to the immune reaction site.

● *Anaphylatoxins* produced during complement fixation induce vascular permeability and dilation.

● In *opsonization,* complement proteins tag, or identify, antigens, rendering them particularly susceptible to *phagocytosis.*

● In *agglutination,* complement proteins alter antigenic surfaces, causing antigens to adhere to one another.

Complement components also limit antigen movement by causing local inflammation, and may neutralize viruses. Unfortunately, complement amplifies harmful immunologic reactions, such as hypersensitivity, as well as beneficial ones.

Clues to complement abnormalities:

● detection of complement and immunoglobulin in the walls of blood vessels in glomerulonephritis

● detection of complement components and IgG by immunofluorescent examination of glomerular tissues in glomerulonephritis

● EKG conduction abnormalities

● increased erythrocyte sedimentation rate

● pleocytosis in cerebrospinal fluid

● RBCs, RBC casts, and protein in urine.

---

or gamma globulin injections may augment such treatment. However, replacement therapy doesn't cure complement abnormalities, and beneficial effects are transient. Bone marrow transplant may be helpful but can cause a potentially fatal graft-versus-host reaction.

Additional considerations

Before plasma is infused, leukocytes are matched carefully for HL-A cell types to prevent a graft-versus-host (GVH) reaction and other harmful immunologic responses.

If the doctor orders gamma globulin injections, he'll monitor symptoms and laboratory results to assure precise dosage adjustment. Before the doctor gives a gamma globulin injection, he'll warn the patient that it will be painful. Then, he'll inject gamma globulin into a large muscle mass, which he'll massage thoroughly after the injection. If he injects more than 1.5 ml, he'll use more than one site; if he orders frequent doses, he'll rotate the injection sites.

After bone-marrow transplant, the patient is monitored closely for transfusion and GVH reaction. Such a patient should avoid crowds and persons with infections, and learn to recognize early signs of infection. In addition, he must use proper skin hygiene, and promptly treat even small wounds.

But when prevention fails, meticulous medical and nursing care can speed recovery and avoid complications. For example, renal infection requires careful monitoring of fluid intake and output, tests for serum electrolytes and acid-base balance, and observation for signs of renal failure. If changes in mental activity or signs of ataxia are noted, neurologic damage must be suspected.

Selected References

Arndt, K. MANUAL OF DERMATOLOGIC THERAPEUTICS: WITH ESSENTIALS OF DIAGNOSIS, 2nd ed. Boston: Little, Brown & Co., 1978.

Back, F., et. CLINICAL IMMUNOBIOLOGY, Vol. 4. New York: Academic Press, 1980.

Back, J., ed. IMMUNOLOGY. New York: John Wiley & Sons, 1978.

Bergsma, Daniel, ed. IMMUNODEFICIENCY IN MAN AND ANIMALS (Robert E. Krieger: 11:1). White Plains, N.Y.: National Foundation-March of Dimes, 1976.

Bigley, Nancy J. IMMUNOLOGIC FUNDAMENTALS, 2nd ed. Chicago: Year Book Medical Publishers, 1980.

Carpenter, Philip L. IMMUNOLOGY AND SEROLOGY, 3rd ed. Philadelphia: W.B. Saunders Co., 1975.

Dahl, Mark V. CLINICAL IMMUNODERMATOLOGY. Chicago: Year Book Medical Publishers, 1980.

Erslev, Allan J., and Thomas G. Gabuzda. PATHOPHYSIOLOGY OF BLOOD. Philadelphia: W.B. Saunders Co., 1975.

Freedman, Samuel O., and Phil Gold. CLINICAL IMMUNOLOGY, 2nd ed. New York: Harper & Row, 1976.

Fudenberg, Hugh, et al. BASIC AND CLINICAL IMMUNOLOGY, 2nd ed. Los Altos, Calif.: Lange Medical Pubns., 1978.

Gell, P., et al, eds. CLINICAL ASPECTS OF IMMUNOLOGY, 3rd ed. Philadelphia: J.B. Lippincott Co., 1975.

Johnson, F., ed. ALLERGY: IMMUNOLOGY AND TREATMENT. Miami: Symposia Specialists, 1980.

NURSE'S GUIDE TO DRUGS. Nursing80 Books, Springhouse, Pa.: Intermed Communications, Inc., 1980.

Patterson, Roy. ALLERGIC DISEASES: DIAGNOSIS AND MANAGEMENT. Philadelphia: J.B. Lippincott Co., 1972.

Rajka, E., and S. Korossy, eds. IMMUNOLOGICAL ASPECTS OF ALLERGY AND ALLERGIC DISEASES, Vol. 4. New York: Plenum Publishing Corp., 1977.

Safai, B., and R. Good, eds. IMMUNODERMATOLOGY (Comprehensive Immunology Series), Vol. 7. New York: Plenum Publishing Corp., 1980.

Stiehm, E. Richard, and Vincent A. Fulginiti. IMMUNOLOGIC DISORDERS IN INFANTS AND CHILDREN. Philadelphia: W.B. Saunders Co., 1973.

Vaughn, Victor C., and R. James McKay, eds. NELSON TEXTBOOK OF PEDIATRICS, 11th ed. Philadelphia: W.B. Saunders Co., 1980.

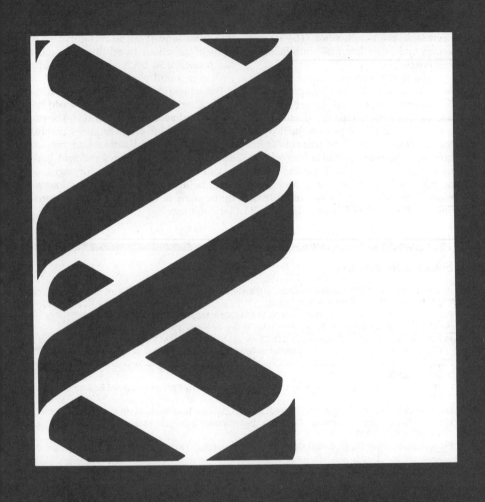

2 Genetic Disorders

Genetic Disorders

Introduction

Genetic diseases result from single gene (mendelian) substitutions, chromosome abnormalities, or multifactorial (polygenic) errors. Well over 2,000 such abnormalities have been identified in humans, ranging from mild differences (as in certain hemoglobin abnormalities) to fatal or overwhelmingly disabling conditions, such as Down's syndrome (trisomy 21). In the United States alone approximately 200,000 infants are born each year with an overt genetic abnormality. Such abnormalities account for up to 20% of all pediatric hospital admissions and at least 10% to 20% of all stillbirths and neonatal deaths.

Although genetic disorders are determined entirely by a person's genetic makeup, and as such are unchangeable throughout life, they can and do interact with environmental factors. For example, albinism (an inherited inability to generate the protective pigment melanin) greatly increases susceptibility to skin cancer after excessive exposure to sunlight.

Pedigree analysis

Genetics, the study of heredity, uses pedigree (family tree) analysis, karyotypic (chromosomal) analysis, and biochemical analysis of blood, urine, or body tissues to unravel the effects and patterns of inheritance. With the resulting increased understanding of heredity, genetic influences are likely to assume greater importance in health-care delivery as time goes by.

The essential ingredient of heredity is *DNA* (deoxyribonucleic acid), which makes up *genes* (basic units of hereditary material) that are arranged into threadlike organelles called *chromosomes*, in the cell nucleus. Together, these contribute to a person's genotype and phenotype (genetic and physical makeup). In humans, each body cell (except ova and sperm) has 46 chromosomes arranged in 23 pairs. One such pair is the sex chromosomes: females have a matched (homologous) pair of ·X chromosomes; males, an unmatched (heterologous) pair, an X and a Y. Thus, the normal human chromosome complement is 46,XX in females and 46,XY in males. The remaining 22 chromosome pairs (autosomes) are all homologous.

The position that the gene for a given trait occupies on a chromosome is called a *locus*. Different loci exist for hair color, blood group, and so on. The number and arrangement of the locus on homologous chromosomes are the same. A different form of the same gene that occupies a corresponding locus on a homologous chromosome is called an *allele* and determines alternative (and inheritable) forms of the same characteristic. Some alleles control normal trait variation, such as hair color; other defective alleles may cause a congenital defect or even induce abortion. Both heterologous (co-dominant) alleles may express their own effects, or one (the dominant allele) may be expressed and the other (the recessive) suppressed.

A mutation—a permanent inheritable change in a gene—may cause serious,

PATTERNS OF TRANSMISSION IN GENETIC DISORDERS

- **Autosomal recessive**
  Hartnup disease
  Xeroderma pigmentosum
  Congenital afibrinogenemia
  Congenital virilizing adrenal hyperplasia
  Fabry's disease
  Galactosemia
  Niemann Pick disease
  Retinitis pigmentosa
  Thalassemia
  Cystic fibrosis
  Tay-Sachs disease
  Cystinuria
  Cretinism
  Phenylketonuria
  Albinism
  Fanconi's syndrome
  Sickle cell anemia

- **Chromosomal**
  Turner's syndrome
  Trisomy 13
  Trisomy 18
  Down's syndrome (trisomy 21)
  Klinefelter's syndrome
  Hermaphroditism
  Cri du chat syndrome

- **Autosomal dominant**
  Achondroplastic dwarfism
  Colorectal polyposis
  Familial nonhemolytic jaundice
  Renal glycosuria
  Spherocytosis
  Pituitary diabetes insipidus
  Hyperlipidemias
  Neurofibromatosis
  Huntington's chorea
  Osteogenesis imperfecta
  Retinoblastoma
  Marfan's syndrome
  Hereditary hemorrhagic telangiectasia

- **X-linked**
  Some immunodeficiencies
  Pseudohypoparathyroidism
  G 6-PD deficiency
  Hemophilia
  Duchenne-type muscular dystrophy

- **Multifactorial**
  Rheumatoid arthritis
  Diabetes mellitus (some cases)
  Congenital heart anomalies
  Neural tube anomalies
  Mental retardation (some cases)
  Cleft lip/palate

DNA AND HOW IT WORKS

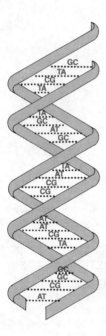

Deoxyribonucleic acid (DNA) is a polymer (macromolecule) made up of individual units called *nucleotides*. Each nucleotide is composed of the pentose (5-carbon) sugar deoxyribose and phosphate, plus two nitrogen-containing bases—a purine and a pyrimidine. These bases are paired by hydrogen bonds to form two coiled chains, known as a double helix. In DNA, the purines are adenine (A) and guanine (G); the pyrimidines, thymine (T) and cytosine (C) (see illustration).

DNA transmits its genetic code by acting as a template (pattern) for the synthesis of messenger ribonucleic acid (RNA). Messenger RNA, in turn, arranges amino acids in the correct sequence to build polypeptide chains, the basis for enzymes that control the cell's essential biochemical processes and other proteins.

even lethal defects, or it may be relatively benign. Teratogenic agents such as radiation, drugs, viruses, and synthetic chemicals may produce mutations (gene changes), but such changes may also occur spontaneously. Mutations can occur anywhere in the DNA chain of bases that transmit the genetic code.

Types of genetic defects
Genetic disorders occur in three different forms:
• *Mendelian* or *single-gene disorders* are inherited in clearly identifiable patterns.
• *Chromosomal aberrations or abnormalities* include structural defects within a chromosome, such as deletion and translocation, plus absence or addition of complete chromosomes.
• *Multifactorial (polygenic) disorders* reflect the interaction of at least two abnormal genes and environmental factors to produce a defect.

Single-gene disorders
Single-gene disorders are inherited through a single allelic gene form and, except for new mutations, usually follow mendelian rules of inheritance. They may be autosomal (result from defective genes on one of the 22 pairs of autosomes) or X-linked (result from a defective gene on the X chromosome). Autosomal defects are by far the most common genetic disorders; in fact, about 90% of *all* genetic defects result from such inheritance. Single-gene disorders may be further classified as dominant or recessive, depending on whether the defective gene is a dominant or a recessive allele.

Single-gene inheritance patterns
A dominant gene produces its effect even in heterozygotes (persons who also carry a normal gene for the same trait), since the dominant gene masks the effects of the normal paired gene. Because a person with an autosomal dominant disease is usually a heterozygote and carries a normal gene, his children have a 50% chance of inheriting the defective dominant gene and the disease (see page 43).

This probability remains the same for each and every pregnancy, since each pregnancy is a separate event. Unaffected persons (normal homozygotes) don't carry the gene and therefore can't transmit it to their children. Gender doesn't influence transmission of the abnormal autosomal dominant trait. Unless the defective dominant gene has arisen as a new mutation, every affected person has an affected parent, so autosomal dominant traits don't tend to skip generations.

Since a defective recessive gene can only produce a disorder in homozygotes (*autosomal recessive inheritance*) to inherit the recessive trait, offspring must receive one copy of the same defective gene from each parent. Since both parents must be heterozygous carriers, such autosomal recessive disorders are more common in children of consanguineous parents (blood relatives). Autosomal recessive disorders affect males and females equally.

In *X-linked recessive inheritance*, nearly all affected persons are male, since females inherit a dominant normal allelic gene that doesn't permit expression of the recessive trait. Females do, however, act as carriers for such traits. X-linked recessive disorders are never transmitted directly from father to son, since the father gives the son a Y chromosome, which can't carry the trait.

In *X-linked dominant inheritance*, which is rare, an affected male transmits the defective trait to all his daughters but none of his sons. His daughters, in turn, may pass on the trait (and the disorder) to their sons. Such inheritance also affects heterozygous females but to a lesser extent than males.

Genetic accidents

During germ cell formation by meiosis, failure of chromosomes to divide (*nondisjunction*) results in a germ cell that contains less or more than the normal 23 chromosomes. Usually, such abnormal germ cells fail to unite at conception, or if fertilization does take place, the embryo is aborted early. Experts believe

MITOSIS AND MEIOSIS

Old   New   New   Old

The body grows and replaces all dividing cells other than germ cells (sperm and ova) by *mitosis*. In mitosis, the cell's DNA exactly replicates itself and leads to the creation of a new daughter cell with the identical genetic makeup as the parent cell. Each new cell has a diploid number of chromosomes (in humans, 46).

Germ cells, however, form by *meiosis*. In meiosis, DNA first replicates. Then, through a complicated process, two cell divisions create four daughter cells (a sperm or ovum) from each parent cell, each of which has a haploid number of chromosomes (in humans, 23).

that up to 60% of spontaneous abortions at less than 90 days' gestation result from abnormal fetal chromosome number; offspring with grosser abnormalities are probably never even implanted. Absence of an autosomal chromosome is incompatible with life; but absence of a sex chromosome, as in Turner's syndrome (in which a female offspring receives only one X chromosome), is better tolerated. Presence of an extra chromosome (a trisomy), as in Down's syndrome, usually produces some combination of physical malformation and mental retardation.

Chromosomal disorders may also result from structural changes within chromosomes. For instance, in *deletion*, loss of part of a chromosome during cell division produces varying effects in the offspring, depending on the type and amount of genetic material lost. An example of a chromosomal disorder resulting from deletion is the cri du chat syndrome, in which part of the short arm of the number 5 chromosome is missing.

Another type of chromosome abnormality is *translocation*, in which part of a chromosome breaks off and attaches itself to another chromosome. If little or no genetic material is lost, the translocation is balanced (symmetrical), and the person is normal.

Another abnormality, *ring chromosomes*, results when a chromosome loses a section of genetic material from each end and the remaining stumps join together to form a ring. The effect of such a structural abnormality varies with the type of genetic material lost.

In *mosaicism*, a rare condition, abnormal chromosomal division in the *zygote* (the cell formed at conception by the union of the sperm and ova) results in two or more cell lines with different chromosomes. One cell line may be normal, the other abnormal, such as trisomy 21. The patient's phenotype depends on the percentage of normal cells, but usually he shows the effect of the abnormal cell line.

Multifactorial (polygenic) disorders are inherited abnormalities that result from the interaction of at least two inherited abnormal genes and environmental factors. They include common malformations such as neural tube abnormalities, cleft lip, and cleft palate, as well as disorders that might not become apparent until later in life. Such disorders don't follow the mendelian patterns of inheritance, but study of the frequency of specific birth defects within families suggests familial transmission. So far, however, exactly *how* multifactorial disorders result remains unclear.

Detecting genetic disorders

Although genetic disorders can't be cured, genetic testing and counseling can help prevent them and can help patients and their families deal with such disorders when they do develop. Genetic testing relies primarily on pedigree (family tree) analysis, karyotype (chromosomal) analysis, and biochemical analysis of blood, urine, or body tissues (including amniocentesis) to detect abnormal gene products. Newborn screening for inherited metabolic disorders such as phenylketonuria (PKU) has become standard, and prompt treatment of such disorders can avoid or minimize their results. Simple blood tests can detect carriers of recessive genes such as Tay-Sachs and sickle cell anemia. This gives a couple at risk the option of prenatal diagnosis (amniocentesis) to detect affected offspring. Recent developments, such as chromosomal banding (identifying areas on chromosomes responsible for specific abnormalities), have further helped unravel genetic mysteries. But even with such testing, certain genetic disorders remain undetectable until they produce irreversible clinical features. And unfortunately, we still have no way to look at a specific gene directly.

A *pedigree*, the study of a trait or a disease in the patient's family, helps determine the inheritance pattern of this trait or disease, including the probability of occurrence. The pedigree chart begins with the patient (index) and traces all living and remembered blood relatives in order of their birth, listing the following data:

INHERITANCE PATTERNS

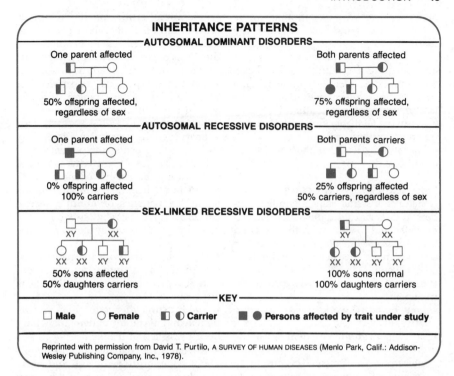

Reprinted with permission from David T. Purtilo, A SURVEY OF HUMAN DISEASES (Menlo Park, Calif.: Addison-Wesley Publishing Company, Inc., 1978).

- current age or age at death
- health status (including abortions, miscarriages, stillbirths, and their reasons; the site and nature of congenital anomalies; acquired heart lesions; primary site malignancies; and types of arthritis)
- relationships (if he's a twin or involved in a consanguineous marriage).

This information can be culled from the patient's memory, or from autopsy and pathology reports, and photographs. After gathering such information, the pedigree chart is viewed in relation to the clinical features of the suspected genetic disorder and appropriate laboratory tests. One such test is the *karyotype*. In a karyotype, blood cells drawn from the patient's vein are grown in a special culture until the stage of mitosis, when chromosomes are most easily seen with a microscope. Then the cells are broken open and stained to show specific bands on the chromosomes. Staining techniques can be varied to help identify each chromosome and the bands it contains.

Amniocentesis, needle aspiration of amniotic fluid following transabdominal puncture of the uterus under local anesthetic, can now detect over a hundred genetic disorders before birth by:
- karyotyping fetal chromosomes.
- culturing fetal cells in amniotic fluid to measure fetal enzymes or identify cell characteristics.
- analyzing alpha-fetoprotein (AFP). Usually, this procedure is done at 15 to 16 weeks' gestation.

Amniocentesis allows parents to choose elective abortion or prepare themselves during pregnancy for the birth of a child with a genetic disorder. It's recommended when:
- the mother is over age 35.
- a familial history of chromosomal abnormality, or translocations exists.
- a history of neural tube defect in a child of a previous birth or in a primary relative exists.
- the parents are known carriers of an

autosomal recessive disease that can be detected prenatally, such as Tay-Sachs disease.

In most other situations, the risks of amniocentesis (bleeding, fluid leakage, abortion, and infection) outweigh the benefits. Safer alternatives to amniocentesis now under investigation include:
• culturing fetal chorionic cells that desquamate into the cervical canal.
• karyotyping fetal lymphocytes in maternal blood.

How the family can cope

Genetic counseling helps a family to understand its risk for a particular genetic disorder and to cope with the disorder, if that risk becomes reality. Counseling sessions make it easier for the family to comprehend:
• medical facts (diagnosis, prognosis, treatment)
• how heredity works (risks to other relatives)
• options available to deal with the problem
• consequences of their decision.

Psychologic support to relieve stress and improve the patient's or parents' self-concept is as important as the correct information. Birth of a child with a genetic defect may provoke parental feelings of isolation, insecurity, and helplessness; strain marital relations; and initiate a period of shock and denial, followed by grief and mourning. After diagnosis of genetic disease, psychologic support can be provided in these ways:
• Helping the persons concerned deal with their initial shock, anger, or denial so that they will be ready to accept genetic counseling.
• Learning what services are offered by the counseling center the patient's been referred to so he'll know what to expect.
• Providing the genetic counselor with pertinent medical data and information about the patient's or family's special concerns, such as religious and social restraints, and about any family pressure and discord.
• Communicating with the patient and his family in an unhurried and non-technical manner, being sure all the facts are accurate.
• Making sure, after counseling, that the patient and his family understand what's been presented to them.
• Advising the patient and his family about community resources and agencies that are available to help them deal with genetic disorders.
• Helping them get in touch with the families of other patients with the same disorder.
• Coordinating the assistance of other members of the health-care team.
• Recognizing the parents' everyday stresses in caring for a child with a congenital defect, and allowing them to vent their feelings.

List of counseling services

The National Foundation of the March of Dimes publishes a list of genetic counseling services located throughout the United States. To obtain this list, write to the Professional Education Department, The National Foundation of the March of Dimes, 1275 Mamaroneck Ave., White Plains, NY 10605.

Local March of Dimes chapters can also provide information about local genetic counseling services and educational material about specific birth defects.

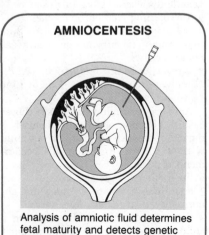

AMNIOCENTESIS

Analysis of amniotic fluid determines fetal maturity and detects genetic abnormalities.

AUTOSOMAL DOMINANT INHERITANCE

Neurofibromatosis

(Von Recklinghausen's Disease)

Neurofibromatosis is an inherited developmental disorder of the nervous system, muscles, bones, and skin that causes formation of multiple, pedunculated, soft tumors (neurofibromas), and café-au-lait spots. Approximately 100,000 Americans are known to have neurofibromatosis; in many other persons, this disorder is overlooked because symptoms are mild. Prognosis is usually good, though spinal or intracranial tumors or malignant changes in tumors can shorten life span.

Causes and incidence

Neurofibromatosis generally becomes apparent during childhood or adolescence but can occur at any stage of life. Sometimes progression stops as the patient matures. It's often associated with meningiomas, suprarenal medullary secreting tumors, spina bifida, meningocele, kyphoscoliosis, vascular and lymphatic nevi, and ocular and renal anomalies. In about half these patients, neurofibromatosis is transmitted as an autosomal dominant trait; in the remainder, it occurs as a new mutation. Persons with neurofibromatosis have a 50% risk that their offspring will have the same disease.

Signs and symptoms

Symptoms result from an overgrowth of mesodermal and ectodermal elements in the skin, central nervous system, and other organs. Such overgrowth produces multiple pedunculated nodules (neurofibromas) of varying sizes on the nerve trunks of extremities and on the nerves of head, neck, and body. Signs and symptoms vary according to the location and size of the tumors and include:
• neurologic impairment from intracranial, spinal, and orbital tumors—and in 10% of patients, seizures, blindness, deafness, mental deficiency.
• cutaneous lesions—six or more flat-pigmented or hyperpigmented skin areas (café-au-lait spots).

• skeletal involvement—scoliosis, severe kyphoscoliosis, and spina bifida.
• endocrine abnormalities.
• renal damage—hypertension.

Complications include congenital tibial pseudoarthrosis; cancer of the nerve sheath, or neurofibrosarcoma, which occurs in up to 8% of patients; and malignant changes in tumors themselves, present in up to 10% of patients.

Diagnosis

Diagnosis rests on characteristic clinical findings, especially neurofibromas and café-au-lait spots. X-rays showing a wid-

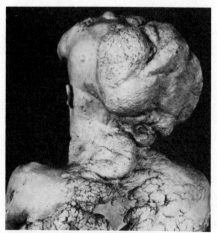

Severe neurofibromatosis—postmortem cast of the back of the head of John Merrick, "the Elephant Man."

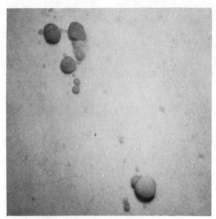

Multiple pedunculated nodules (neuro-fibromas) of varying sizes

ening internal auditory meatus and intervertebral foramen further support this diagnosis. Such diagnosis rarely requires a tumor biopsy.

Treatment

Treatment consists of surgical removal of intracerebral or intraspinal tumors, when possible; correction of kyphoscoliosis; and if necessary, cosmetic surgery for disfiguring or disabling growths.

Additional considerations

• Disfigurement may cause overwhelming social embarrassment and regression. To accept his condition, the patient must be accepted by others first.
• The patient should be encouraged to wear attractive clothing that covers unsightly nodules. He may be interested in obtaining special cosmetics to cover skin lesions.
• The patient will need genetic counseling regarding the 50% risk of transmitting this disorder to offspring. The National Neurofibromatosis Foundation, 340 E. 80th St., New York, NY 10021, can provide more information.

Osteogenesis Imperfecta

Osteogenesis imperfecta (brittle bones) is a hereditary disease of bones and connective tissue that causes skeletal fragility, thin skin, blue sclera, poor teeth, hypermobility of joints, and progressive deafness. This disease occurs in two forms. In the rare congenital form, fractures are present at birth. This form is usually fatal within the first few days or weeks of life. In the late-appearing form (osteogenesis imperfecta tarda), the child appears normal at birth but develops recurring fractures (mostly of the extremities) after the first year of life.

Causes

Congenital osteogenesis imperfecta results from autosomal recessive inheritance; osteogenesis imperfecta tarda, from autosomal dominant inheritance. Clinical signs can probably be attributed to defective osteoblastic activity and a defect of mesenchyma (embryonic connective tissue) and its derivatives (scleras, bones, and ligaments). Consequently, the reticulum fails to differentiate into mature collagen or causes abnormal collagen development, leading to immature and coarse bone formation. In addition, the disturbed formation of periosteum causes cortical bone thinning.

Signs and symptoms

Both congenital and delayed osteogenesis imperfecta produce bilaterally bulging skull, triangular-shaped head and face, prominent eyes, blue sclera, and protruding ears. One third of patients become deaf by ages 30 to 40 as a result of osteosclerosis and pressure on the auditory nerve. These disorders also cause thin, translucent skin; possible subcutaneous hemorrhages; and discolored (blue-gray or yellow-brown) teeth, which break easily and are cavity-prone because of dentin deficiency. Other signs and symptoms include poorly developed skeletal muscles (atrophy) and hypermobility of joints, from laxity of ligaments and capsule.

The hallmark of this disease, though, is fractures that occur with even slight trauma. In the congenital form, birth itself may cause fractures; other skeletal deformities reflect intrauterine fractures that healed in abnormal positions. In both forms, incomplete and relatively painless fractures after birth that receive no treatment can produce deformities from bones healing in poor alignment. The incidence of such fractures decreases after puberty.

Osteogenesis imperfecta tarda may also cause stunted growth from epiphyseal fractures, or short stature from deformities following fractures.

Diagnosis

Family history and characteristic features, such as blue sclera, establish this diagnosis. X-rays showing evidence of multiple old fractures and skeletal deformities, and skull X-ray showing wide sutures, with small, irregularly shaped islands of bone (wormian bones) between them supports the diagnosis. Serum calcium and serum phosphorus levels are within normal limits.

Treatment

The aim of treatment is to prevent deformities by traction, immobilization, or both; and to emphasize normal development and rehabilitation. Supportive treatment includes:

• checking the patient's circulatory, motor, and sensory abilities (frequent hearing tests).

• encouraging him to walk when possible (these children develop a fear of walking).

• teaching preventive measures. For example, the child must avoid contact sports or strenuous activity, or wear knee pads, helmets, or other protective devices when he does engage in these activities.

Additional considerations

• The parents and child must be taught how to recognize fractures and how to correctly splint a fracture.

• Parents should encourage their child to develop interests that don't require strenuous physical activity, and to develop his fine motor skills. These will help increase the child's sense of self-worth.

• Parents should make arrangements for tutoring throughout hospitalization and home care.

• The child must assume some responsibility for precautions during physical activity to help foster his independence.

• The child will need good nutrition to promote bone healing.

• The parents and child may need to be referred to the proper agency for genetic counseling.

Marfan's Syndrome

(Arachnodactyly)

Marfan's syndrome is a rare inherited, degenerative, generalized disease of the connective tissue that causes ocular, skeletal, and cardiovascular anomalies. It probably results from elastin and collagen abnormalities.

Death is usually attributed to cardiovascular complications and may occur anytime from early infancy to adulthood, depending on the severity of the symptoms. Marfan's syndrome affects males and females equally. Probably its most famous victim was Abraham Lincoln.

Causes

Marfan's syndrome is inherited as an autosomal dominant trait. In 85% of patients with this disease, family history confirms Marfan's syndrome in one parent as well. In the remaining 15%, a negative family history suggests fresh mutation, possibly because of advanced paternal age.

Signs and symptoms

Characteristically, the clinical effects of Marfan's syndrome are absent at birth and develop slowly over a period of years. These effects vary even among siblings.

The most common signs of this disorder are skeletal abnormalities, particularly excessively long tubular bones and an arm span exceeding the patient's height. Usually, the patient is taller than average for his family, with the upper half of his body shorter than average and the lower half, longer. His fingers are long and slender (spider fingers). Weakness of ligaments, tendons, and joint capsules results in joints that are loose, hyperextensible, and habitually dislocated. Excessive growth of the rib bones gives rise to chest deformities, such as pectus excavatum (funnel breast) and pigeon breast.

Eye problems are also common: 75% of patients have crystalline lens displacement (ectopia lentis), the ocular hallmark of Marfan's syndrome. Frequently, quivering of the iris with eye movement (iridodonesis) suggests this disorder. Most patients are severely myopic, many have retinal detachment, and some have glaucoma.

The most serious complications occur in the cardiovascular system and include weakness of the aortic media that leads to progressive dilation or dissecting aneurysm of the ascending aorta. Such dilation appears first in the coronary sinuses and is often preceded by aortic regurgitation. Less common cardiovascular complications include mitral regurgitation and endocarditis.

Other general symptoms and associated problems include sparsity of subcutaneous fat, frequent hernia, cystic lung disease, recurrent spontaneous pneumothorax, and scoliosis.

Diagnosis

Because no specific test confirms Marfan's syndrome, diagnosis rests on typical clinical features (particularly skeletal deformities *and* ectopia lentis) and a history of the disease in close relatives. Useful supplementary procedures, though not definitive for diagnosis, include X-rays for skeletal abnormalities and auscultation for abnormal heart sounds.

Treatment

Attempts to stop the degenerative process have met with little success. Therefore, treatment of Marfan's syndrome is basically symptomatic, such as surgical repair of aneurysms and of ocular deformities. In young patients with early dilation of the aorta, prompt treatment with propranolol can often decrease ventricular ejection and protect the aorta; extreme dilation requires surgical replacement of the aorta and the aortic valve. Steroids and sex hormones have been successful (especially in girls) in inducing precocious puberty and early epiphyseal closure to prevent abnormal adult height. Genetic counseling is important, particularly since pregnancy and resultant increased cardiovascular workload can produce aortic rupture.

Additional considerations

Aside from general health care, as required by the patient's condition, the patient and his family will need education concerning:
• the course of the disease and potential complications, such as lung disease or pneumothorax.
• the need for frequent checkups so the degenerative changes can be discovered and treated early.
• the importance of taking prescribed medication in the amount and on the schedule that the doctor has ordered.
• the benefits of hormonal therapy to induce early epiphyseal closure, thus preventing abnormal adult height (subject to doctor's recomendation).
• the need for the parents to have only realistic expectations of the child despite his height and looks, which make him appear older and more mature than he actually is.

AUTOSOMAL RECESSIVE INHERITANCE

Cystic Fibrosis
(Mucoviscidosis)

Cystic fibrosis is a generalized dysfunction of the exocrine glands, affecting multiple organ systems in varying degrees of severity. It's transmitted as an autosomal recessive trait and is the most common fatal genetic disease of Caucasian children. Cystic fibrosis is a chronic disease that severely shortens the patient's life span. About 50% of affected children die by age 16; of the rest, some survive to age 30.

Causes and incidence

Incidence of cystic fibrosis is highest (approximately 1 in 2,000 live births) in persons of central European ancestry. Incidence is lower in American Blacks (1 in 17,000 live births), American Indians, and persons of Asian ancestry. Frequency is equal in both sexes.

The underlying biochemical defect probably reflects an alteration in a protein or enzyme. In fact, cystic fibrosis accounts for almost all cases of pancreatic enzyme deficiency in children.

The immediate causes of symptoms in cystic fibrosis are increased viscosity of bronchial, pancreatic, and other mucous gland secretions, and consequent obstruction of glandular ducts.

Signs and symptoms

The clinical effects of cystic fibrosis may become apparent soon after birth or may take years to develop. They include major aberrations in sweat gland, respiratory, and gastrointestinal functions. Sweat gland dysfunction is the most consistent abnormality. Increased concentrations of sodium and chloride in the sweat lead to hyponatremia and hypochloremia, and can eventually induce fatal shock and arrhythmias, especially in hot weather, when sweating is profuse.

Respiratory symptoms reflect disabling obstructive changes in the lungs: wheezy respirations; a dry, nonproductive paroxysmal cough; dyspnea; and tachypnea. These changes stem from the accumulation of thick, tenacious secretions in the bronchioles and the alveoli, and eventually lead to severe atelectasis and emphysema. Consequently, children with cystic fibrosis typically display a barrel chest, cyanosis, and clubbing of the fingers and toes. They suffer recurring bronchitis and pneumonia, and may have associated nasal polyps and sinusitis. Pneumonia, emphysema, or atelectasis usually causes death.

The gastrointestinal effects of cystic fibrosis occur mainly in the intestines, pancreas, and liver. One of the earliest such symptoms is meconium ileus; the newborn with cystic fibrosis doesn't excrete meconium, a dark green mucilaginous material found in the intestine at birth. Therefore, he develops symptoms of intestinal obstruction, such as abdominal distention, vomiting, constipation, dehydration, and electrolyte imbalance. Eventually, obstruction of the pancreatic ducts and resulting deficiency of trypsin, amylase, and lipase prevent the conversion and absorption of fat and protein in the intestinal tract. The undigested food is then excreted in characteristically frequent, bulky, foul-smelling, and pale stools, with a high fat content. This malabsorption induces other abnormalities: poor weight gain, ravenous appetite, distended abdomen, thin extremities, and sallow skin with poor turgor. The inability to absorb fats produces deficiency of fat-soluble vitamins (A, D, E, and K), leading to clotting problems and retarded bone growth. A common complication in infants and children with such symptoms is rectal prolapse, secondary to malnutrition and wasting of perirectal supporting tissues.

In the pancreas, fibrotic tissue, multiple cysts, thick mucus, and eventually fat replace the acini (small, saclike swellings normally found in this gland), producing symptoms of pancreatic insufficiency: insufficient insulin production, abnormal glucose tolerance, and glycosuria. Biliary obstruction and fibrosis may prolong neonatal jaundice. In some patients, cirrhosis and portal hypertension may lead to esophageal varices, episodes of hematemesis, and occasionally, hepatomegaly.

Diagnosis

 The presence of elevated electrolyte (sodium and chloride) concentration in sweat in a patient with pulmonary disease or pancreatic insufficiency confirms cystic fibrosis. The sweat test (stimulation of sweat glands, collection of samples, and laboratory analysis) shows that the volume of sweat is normal, but that its weight is increased because of increased chloride and sodium concentration. (Normal sodium concentration of sweat in mEq/L is less than 40; in cystic fibrosis, it rises to more than 60.) The sodium and chloride concentration of sweat normally rises with age, but any value greater than 50, even in adults, strongly suggests cystic fibrosis and calls for repeated testing.

Examination of duodenal contents for pancreatic enzymes and stools for trypsin can confirm pancreatic insufficiency; trypsin is absent in over 80% of children with cystic fibrosis. Chest X-rays, pulmonary function tests, and arterial blood gas determination assess the patient's pulmonary status. Sputum culture can detect concurrent infectious diseases. Family history may show siblings or other relatives with cystic fibrosis.

Treatment and additional considerations

Since cystic fibrosis has no cure, the aim of treatment is to help the child lead as normal a life as possible. The child's family needs instruction about the nature and course of this disease and its complications; referral for genetic counseling will also be helpful. The emphasis of individualized treatment depends on the organ system involved.

• To combat sweat electrolyte losses, treatment includes generous salting of foods and, during hot weather, administration of salt supplements.

• To offset pancreatic enzyme deficiencies, treatment includes oral pancreatic enzymes with meals and snacks. Such supplements improve absorption and digestion, and satisfy hunger on a reasonable calorie intake. Other dietary measures include limiting fat intake while allowing the child to eat the family's normal foods as much as possible, and supplements of water-miscible, fat-soluble vitamins (A, D, E, and K).

• Pulmonary dysfunction management includes physical therapy, postural drainage, and breathing exercises several times daily, to aid removal of secretions from lungs. Patients with cystic fibrosis shouldn't receive antihistamines, since they have a drying effect on mucous membranes, making expectoration of mucus difficult or impossible. Aerosol therapy includes intermittent nebulizer treatments before postural drainage, to loosen secretions.

Treatment of pulmonary infection requires:

• loosening and removing mucopurulent secretions, and using an intermittent nebulizer and postural drainage to relieve obstruction. Using a mist tent is controversial, since mist particles may become trapped in the esophagus and stomach and never even reach the lungs.

• aggressively using broad-spectrum antimicrobials (usually only during acute pulmonary infections, since prophylactic use encourages resistant bacterial strains)

• using oxygen therapy as needed. Hot, dry air increases vulnerability to respiratory infections, so cystic fibrosis patients benefit from air conditioners and humidifiers.

Throughout this illness:
- the patient and his family should be taught about the disease and all treatment.
- emotional support is crucial. Hospital care schedule and visiting hours should be flexible to allow continuation of schooling and friendships.

For further information and support, the patient and his family should be referred to the Cystic Fibrosis Foundation, 6000 Executive Blvd., Suite 309, Rockville, MD 20852.

Tay-Sachs Disease
(Familial amaurotic idiocy)

The most common of the lipid storage diseases, Tay-Sachs disease results from a congenital enzyme deficiency. It's characterized by progressive mental and motor deterioration and is always fatal, usually before age 5.

Causes and incidence

Tay-Sachs disease is an autosomal recessive disorder in which the enzyme hexosaminidase A is deficient. This enzyme is necessary for metabolism of gangliosides, water-soluble glycolipids found primarily in CNS tissues. Without hexosaminidase A, accumulating lipid pigments distend and progressively destroy and demyelinate CNS cells. Tay-Sachs disease is quite rare and appears in fewer than 100 infants born each year in the United States. However, it strikes persons of Ashkenazic Jewish ancestry about 100 times more often than the general population, occurring in about 1 in 3,600 live births in this ethnic group. About 1 in 30 such persons are heterozygous carriers of this defective gene. If two such carriers have children, each of their offspring has a 25% chance of having Tay-Sachs disease.

Signs and symptoms

A newborn with Tay-Sachs disease appears normal at birth, but at age 3 to 6 months, he becomes apathetic and no longer responds to stimuli. Increasing physical and mental deterioration follow. His neck, trunk, arm and leg muscles grow weaker, so that soon he can't sit up or lift his head. He has difficulty turning over, can't grasp objects, and has progressive vision loss.

By 18 months, such an infant is usually deaf, and has seizures and generalized paralysis and spasticity. Although he's blind, he may hold his eyes wide open and roll his eyeballs. His pupils are always dilated and don't react to light.

Decerebrate rigidity and a complete vegetative state follow. From 2 years on, such a child suffers recurrent bronchopneumonia, which is commonly fatal before age 5.

Diagnosis

 Typical clinical features point to Tay-Sachs disease, but serum analysis showing deficient hexosaminidase A is the key to diagnosis. An ophthalmic examination showing optic nerve atrophy and a distinctive cherry-red spot on the retina further supports diagnosis.

Diagnostic screening is essential for all couples of Ashkenazic Jewish ancestry and for others with a familial history of the disease. A simple blood test evaluating hexosaminidase A levels can identify carriers. If carriers wish to have children, amniocentesis at 15 to 16 weeks of gestation is recommended to detect hexosaminidase A deficiency and, consequently, Tay-Sachs disease in the fetus.

Treatment

Tay-Sachs disease has no known cure. Supportive treatment includes tube feedings using nutritional supplements, suctioning and postural drainage to remove pharyngeal secretions, skin care to prevent decubiti in such children once they're bedridden, and mild laxatives to relieve neurogenic constipation. Unfortunately, anticonvulsants usually fail to prevent seizures. Because these children need round-the-clock physical care, their parents often place them in long-term special care facilities.

Additional considerations
To help the family deal with inevitably progressive illness and death:
• The parents should be directed to an appropriate agency for genetic counseling, and the mother should have an amniocentesis in future pregnancies. Siblings should be screened to determine if they're

carriers. If they are carriers and are past adolescence, they should also get genetic counseling. They should know, however, that there's no danger of transmitting the disease to their offspring if they don't marry another carrier.
• Parents may need psychological counseling, as well, since they may feel excessive stress or guilt due to their child's illness.
• Parents should be taught how to do suctioning, postural drainage, and tube feeding, if their child will live at home. They'll also need to know how to give good skin care to prevent decubitis ulcers.

For more information, write to National Tay-Sachs and Allied Diseases Association, Inc.

Phenylketonuria
(Phenylalaninemia, phenylpyruvic oligophrenia)

Phenylketonuria (PKU) is an inborn error in phenylalanine metabolism, resulting in high serum levels of phenylalanine, cerebral damage, and mental retardation.

Causes and incidence
In the United States, this disorder occurs once in approximately 14,000 births. (Approximately one person in 60 is an asymptomatic carrier.) It has a very low incidence in Finland and among Ashkenazi Jews and American Blacks.

PKU is transmitted by an autosomal recessive gene. Patients with this disorder have insufficient phenylalanine hydroxylase, an enzyme that acts as a catalyst in the conversion of phenylalanine to tyrosine. As a result, phenylalanine and its metabolites accumulate in the blood, causing mental retardation. The exact biochemical mechanism that causes this retardation isn't clearly understood.

Signs and symptoms
An infant with PKU appears normal at birth but by 4 months of age begins to show signs of arrested brain development, including mental retardation and,

later, personality disturbances (schizoid and antisocial personality patterns, and uncontrollable temper). Such a child may have a lighter complexion than unaffected siblings and often has blue eyes. He may also have macrocephaly; eczematous skin lesions or dry, rough skin; and a musty (mousy) odor due to skin and urinary excretion of phenylacetic acid. Approximately 80% of these children have abnormal EEG patterns, and about one third have seizures, which usually begin when they are 6 to 12 months old.

Children with this disorder show a precipitous decrease in IQ in their first year, are usually hyperactive and irritable, and show purposeless, repetitive motions. They have increased muscle tone and an awkward gait.

Although blood phenylalanine levels are normal at birth, they begin to rise within a few days. By the time they reach detectable significant levels (approximately 30 mg/dl), cerebral damage has begun. Such damage probably is complete by age 2 to 3 years and is irreversible. However, early detection and treatment can prevent or minimize this cerebral damage.

Diagnosis

Most states require screening for PKU at birth; the Guthrie screening test on a capillary blood sample (bacterial inhibition assay) reliably detects PKU. However, since phenylalanine levels may be normal at birth, the infant should be reevaluated after he has received dietary protein for 24 to 48 hours. Adding a few drops of 10% ferric chloride solution to a wet diaper is another method of detecting PKU. If the area turns a deep, bluish-green color, phenylpyruvic acid is present in the urine. Detection of elevated blood levels of phenylalanine and the presence of phenylpyruvic acid in the infant's urine confirm the diagnosis. (Urine should also be tested 4 to 6 weeks after birth, since urinary levels of phenylpyruvic acid vary with the amount of protein ingested.)

Treatment

Treatment consists of restricting dietary intake of the amino acid phenylalanine to keep phenylalanine blood levels below 3 to 7 mg/dl. Since most natural proteins contain 5% phenylalanine, they must be eliminated from the child's diet. Enzymatic hydrosylate of casein, such as Lofenalac powder or Progestimil powder, is substituted for milk in the diets of affected infants and should be continued at least until age 5 or 6. This milk substitute contains a minimal amount of phenylalanine, normal amounts of other amino acids, and added amounts of carbohydrate and fat.

Such a diet calls for careful monitoring. Since the body doesn't make phenylalanine, overzealous dietary restriction can induce phenylalanine deficiency, producing lethargy, anorexia, anemia, skin rashes, and diarrhea.

Additional considerations

The phenylketonuric child and his parents will need to be educated about this disease, and given emotional support and counseling. Such a child often develops psychologic and emotional problems because of his difficult dietary restrictions.

The patient and his parents must learn that adhering to his diet is of critical importance. The child must avoid breads, cheese, eggs, flour, meat, poultry, fish, nuts, milk, and legumes. As the child grows older and is supervised less closely, parents have less control over what he eats. As a result, deviation from the diet becomes more likely, parental anxiety increases, and so does the risk of further brain damage.

Parents need to develop a trusting relationship with their child. They can strengthen this trust by allowing the child some choices in the kinds of low-protein foods he wants to eat; this will help make him feel more responsible too. Parents must know about normal phys-

PHENYLALANINE, PROTEIN, AND CALORIE RECOMMENDATIONS IN PHENYLKETONURIA			
AGE	PHENYLALANINE (MG PER POUND)	PROTEIN (G PER POUND)	CALORIES (PER POUND)
0 to 3 months	20-22	1.75-2.0	60-65
4 to 12 months	18-20	1.5	55-60
1 to 3 years	16-18	32 g total	50-55
4 to 7 years	10-16	40 g total	40-50

From Corinne H. Robinson, *Normal and Therapeutic Nutrition*. Copyright © 1972 by Macmillan Publishing Co., Inc. Used by permission.

ical and mental growth and development, so they can recognize any developmental delay that may point to excessive phenylalanine intake.

To minimize or prevent this disorder:
• Infants should be routinely screened for PKU, since detection and control of phenylalanine intake soon after birth can prevent severe mental retardation.
• Phenylketonuric females who reach reproductive age should receive genetic counseling, since recent research indicates that their offspring may have a higher than normal incidence of brain damage; microcephaly; and major congenital malformations, especially of the heart and central nervous system. Such damage seems to be preventable by following a low-phenylalanine diet throughout pregnancy.

Albinism

Albinism is a rare inherited defect in melanin metabolism of the skin and eyes (oculocutaneous albinism) or just the eyes (ocular albinism). This ocular defect impairs visual acuity. Oculocutaneous albinism also causes severe intolerance to sunlight and increases susceptibility to skin cancer in exposed skin areas.

Causes and incidence
Oculocutaneous albinism results from autosomal recessive inheritance; ocular albinism from an X-linked recessive trait that causes hypopigmentation only in the iris and the ocular fundus.

Normally, melanocytes synthesize melanin. Melanosomes, melanin-containing granules within melanocytes, diffuse and absorb the sun's ultraviolet light (UVL), thus protecting the skin and eyes from the dangerous effects of UVL. In tyrosinase-negative albinism, the most common form, melanosomes don't contain melanin since they lack tyrosinase, the enzyme that stimulates melanin production. In tyrosinase-positive albinism, melanosomes contain tyrosine, a tyrosinase substrate, but a defect in the tyrosine transport system impairs melanin production. In tyrosinase-variable albinism, which is rare, an unidentified enzyme defect probably impairs synthesis of a melanin precursor. Even rarer forms of albinism include Hermansky-Pudlak syndrome (tyrosinase-negative albinism coexisting with platelet dysfunction and resultant bleeding abnormalities) and Cross-McKusick-Breen syndrome (tyrosinase-positive albinism coexisting with neurologic involvement).

Tyrosinase-negative albinism affects 1 in every 34,000 persons in the United States, and is equally common in Caucasians and Blacks. Tyrosinase-positive albinism affects more Blacks than Caucasians (1 in every 15,000 Blacks; 1 in every 40,000 Caucasians). American Indians have a high incidence of both forms of albinism.

Signs and symptoms
Light-skinned Caucasians with tyrosinase-negative albinism have pale skin, and hair color ranging from white to cream to yellow; their pupils appear red because of translucent irises. Blacks with the same disorder have hair that may be white, faintly tinged with yellow, or yellow-brown. Both Caucasians and Blacks with tyrosinase-positive albinism show signs of darker coloration as they age. For instance, their hair may become straw-colored or light brown, and their skin cream-colored or pink. Blacks with tyrosinase-positive albinism may also have freckles and pigmented nevi.

In tyrosinase-variable albinism, at birth the child's hair is white, his skin is pink, and his eyes are gray. As he grows older, though, his hair becomes yellow, his irises may become darker, and his skin may even tan slightly.

The skin of a person with albinism is easily damaged by the sun. It may look weather-beaten and is highly susceptible to precancerous and cancerous growths. Deficiency of pigment in the ocular fundi causes photophobia; other abnormalities include myopia, strabismus, and congenital horizontal nystagmus.

Diagnosis
Diagnosis is based on clinical observation and the patient's family history. Microscopic examination of the skin and of hair follicles determines the amount of pigment present. Testing plucked hair roots for pigmentation when incubated in tyrosine distinguishes tyrosinase-negative albinism from tyrosinase-positive albinism. Tyrosinase-positive hair bulbs will develop color.

Treatment and additional considerations
The child and his parents need to know what measures give the best protection from solar radiation. They must also learn solar radiation's danger signals (excessive drying of skin, crusty lesions on exposed skin, changes in skin color). For protection, the patient should wear full-spectrum sunblocks, dark glasses, and protective clothing.

If the patient's appearance causes him social and emotional problems, he may need psychiatric counseling. Such counseling may also be in order for his family, if they too find it difficult to accept his disorder. Parents may be able to work through initial feelings of guilt and depression by devoting themselves to early infant/parent bonding. Also, parents should know about cosmetic measures (glasses with tinted lenses, makeup foundation) that can minimize disfigurement when their child gets older. Their child will have to get frequent refractions and eye examinations to correct visual defects.

Sickle Cell Anemia

A congenital hemolytic anemia that occurs primarily but not exclusively in Blacks, sickle cell anemia results from a defective hemoglobin molecule (hemoglobin S) which causes red blood cells (RBCs) to roughen and become sickle-shaped. Such cells impair circulation, resulting in chronic ill health (fatigue, dyspnea on exertion, swollen joints), periodic crises, long-term complications, and premature death.

At present, only symptomatic treatment is available. Half of such patients die by their early 20s; few live to middle age.

Causes and incidence
Sickle cell anemia results from homozygous inheritance of the hemoglobin S-producing gene, which causes substitution of the amino acid valine for glutamic acid in the B hemoglobin chain. Heterozygous inheritance of this gene results in sickle cell trait, generally an asymptomatic condition. Sickle cell anemia is most common in tropical Africans and in persons of African descent; about 1 in 10 Afro-Americans carries the abnormal gene. If two such carriers have offspring, there is a 1 in 4 chance that each child will have the disease. Overall, 1 in every 400 to 600 Black children has sickle cell anemia. This disease also occurs in Puerto Rico, Turkey, India, the Middle East, and the Mediterranean area. Possibly, the defective hemoglobin S-producing gene has persisted because in areas where malaria is endemic, the heterozygous sickle cell trait provides resistance to malaria and is actually beneficial.

The abnormal hemoglobin S found in such patients' RBCs becomes insoluble whenever hypoxia occurs. As a result, these RBCs become rigid, rough, and elongated, forming a crescent or sickle shape. Such sickling can produce hemolysis (cell destruction). In addition, these

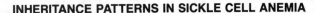

INHERITANCE PATTERNS IN SICKLE CELL ANEMIA

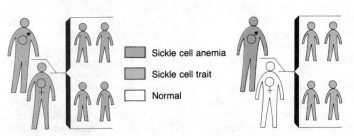

- ◼ Sickle cell anemia
- ◼ Sickle cell trait
- ☐ Normal

The most serious risk occurs when both parents have sickle cell anemia; childbearing—if possible at all—is dangerous for the mother, and all offspring will have sickle cell anemia.

When one parent has sickle cell anemia and one is normal; all offspring will be carriers of sickle cell anemia.

altered cells tend to pile up in capillaries and smaller blood vessels, making the blood more viscous. Normal circulation is impaired, causing pain, tissue infarctions, and swelling. Such blockage causes anoxic changes that lead to further sickling and obstruction.

Signs and symptoms

Characteristically, sickle cell anemia produces tachycardia, cardiomegaly, systolic and diastolic murmurs, pulmonary infarctions (which may result in cor pulmonale), chronic fatigue, unexplained dyspnea or dyspnea on exertion, hepatomegaly, jaundice, pallor, joint swelling, aching bones, chest pains, ischemic leg ulcers (especially around the ankles), and increased susceptibility to infection. Such symptoms usually don't develop until after 6 months of age, since large amounts of fetal hemoglobin protect infants for the first few months after birth. Low socioeconomic status and related problems, such as poor nutrition and low educational levels, may delay diagnosis and supportive treatment.

Infection, stress, dehydration, and conditions that provoke hypoxia—strenuous exercise, high altitude, unpressurized aircraft, cold, and vasoconstrictive drugs—may all provoke periodic crisis. A *painful crisis* (vaso-occlusive crisis, infarctive crisis), the most common crisis and the hallmark of this disease, usu-

ally doesn't appear until age 5 but recurs periodically thereafter. It results from blood vessel obstruction by rigid, tangled sickle cells, which causes tissue anoxia and possible necrosis. It's characterized by severe abdominal, thoracic, muscular, or bone pain and possibly increased jaundice, dark urine, or a low-grade fever. Autosplenectomy, in which splenic damage and scarring is so extensive that the spleen shrinks and becomes impalpable, occurs in patients with long-term disease. Such autosplenectomy can lead to increased susceptibility to *Diplococcus pneumoniae* sepsis, which can be fatal without prompt treatment. After the symptoms of crisis subside, infection may develop, so lethargy, sleepiness, fever, or apathy must be watched for.

An *aplastic crisis* (megaloblastic crisis) results from bone marrow depression and is associated with infection, usually viral. It's characterized by pallor, lethargy, sleepiness, dyspnea, possible coma, markedly decreased bone marrow activity, and RBC hemolysis.

In infants between 8 months and 2 years old, an *acute sequestration crisis* may cause sudden massive entrapment of red cells in the spleen and liver. This rare crisis causes lethargy and pallor, and if untreated, can progress to hypovolemic shock and death. In fact, it's the most common cause of death in sickle cell children under 1 year.

A *hemolytic crisis* is quite rare and usually occurs in patients who have glucose-6-phosphate dehydrogenase (G-6-PD) deficiency with sickle cell anemia. It probably results from complications of sickle cell anemia, such as infection, rather than from the disorder itself. Hemolytic crisis causes liver congestion and hepatomegaly as a result of degenerative changes. It worsens chronic jaundice, although increased jaundice doesn't always point to a hemolytic crisis.

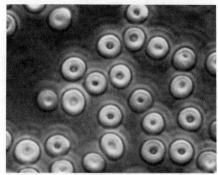
Normal red blood cells

Any of these crises should be suspected in a sickle cell anemia patient with pale lips, tongue, palms, or nail beds; lethargy; listlessness; sleepiness, with difficulty awakening; irritability; severe pain; temperature over 104° F. (40° C.) or a fever of 100° F. (38° C.) that persists for 2 days.

Sickle cell anemia also causes long-term complications. Typically, a sickle cell anemic child is small for his age, and puberty is delayed. (However, fertility isn't impaired.) If he reaches adulthood, his body build tends to be spiderlike—narrow shoulders and hips, long extremities, curved spine, barrel chest, and elongated skull. An adult usually has complications stemming from infarction of various organs, such as retinopathy and nephropathy. Premature death commonly results from infection, or repeated occlusion of small blood vessels and consequent infarction or necrosis of major organs. For example, cerebral blood vessel occlusion causes cerebrovascular accident.

Diagnosis

A positive family history and typical clinical features suggest sickle cell anemia; a stained blood smear showing sickle cells, and hemoglobin electrophoresis showing hemoglobin S confirm it. Ideally, electrophoresis should be done on umbilical cord blood samples at birth, especially if the parents are known to carry the sickle cell trait. Additional lab studies show low RBC, elevated WBC and platelet count, decreased erythrocyte sedimentation rate (ESR), increased

serum iron, decreased RBC survival, and reticulocytosis. Hemoglobin may be low or normal. During early childhood, palpation may reveal splenomegaly, but as the child grows older, the spleen shrinks and splenic function is impaired.

Treatment

Treatment is primarily symptomatic and can usually take place at home. If the patient's hemoglobin drops suddenly, as in an aplastic crisis, or if his condition deteriorates rapidly, hospitalization is needed for transfusion of packed red cells. In a sequestration crisis, treatment may include blood transfusion, oxygen administration, and large amounts of oral or I.V. fluids. So far, research to find an effective antisickling agent hasn't been successful.

Additional considerations

Supportive measures during periodic

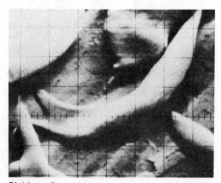
Sickle cells

SICKLE CELL TRAIT

This relatively benign condition results from heterozygous inheritance of the abnormal hemoglobin S–producing gene. Like sickle cell anemia, this condition is most common in Blacks. Sickle cell trait *never* progresses to sickle cell anemia.

In persons with sickle cell trait (also called carriers), 20% to 40% of their total hemoglobin is hemoglobin S; the rest is normal.

Such persons usually have no symptoms. They have normal hemoglobin and hematocrit values and can expect a normal life span. Nevertheless, they must avoid situations that provoke hypoxia, since these occasionally cause a sickling crisis similar to that in sickle cell anemia.

Genetic counseling is essential for sickle cell carriers. If two sickle cell carriers marry, each of their children has a 25% chance of inheriting sickle cell anemia.

exacerbations and precautions to avoid such crises can help these children live as normally and comfortably as possible. Here are some actions that can be taken to help the patient during a painful crisis:

• Applying warm compresses to painful areas, and covering the child with a blanket. (Cold compresses should never be used, since these cause vasoconstriction, further aggravating the condition.)

• Administering an analgesic-antipyretic, such as aspirin or acetaminophen.

• Encouraging bed rest, and placing the patient in a sitting position. If dehydration or severe pain occurs, hospitalization may be necessary.

• When cultures indicate, giving antibiotics as ordered.

During remission, the patient can prevent exacerbation of sickle cell anemia by:

• avoiding tight clothing that restricts circulation.

• avoiding strenuous exercise, vasoconstricting medications, cold temperatures (including drinking large amounts of ice water and swimming), unpressurized aircraft, high altitude, and other conditions that provoke hypoxia.

• getting the normal childhood immunizations, performing meticulous wound care and good oral hygiene, having regular dental checkups, and eating a balanced diet. Together, these act as safeguards against infection.

• getting prompt treatment of infection.

• increasing fluid intake to prevent dehydration that results from impaired ability to concentrate urine properly. Parents can encourage such a child to drink more fluids, especially in the summer, by offering milkshakes, Popsicles, and eggnog.

To encourage normal mental and social development, parents should avoid being overprotective. Although the child must avoid strenuous exercise, he can enjoy most everyday activities.

Parents of children with sickle cell anemia will need genetic counseling to answer their questions about the risk posed to future offspring. They should screen other family members to determine if they're heterozygote carriers as well. These parents may also need psychologic counseling to cope with their guilt feelings. They may find it helpful to join an appropriate community support group.

Sickle cell anemia calls for special precautions during pregnancy or surgery:

• Women with sickle cell anemia must know that they're poor obstetrical risks. However, their use of oral contraceptives is also risky; they should get birth control counseling by a gynecologist. If such women *do* become pregnant, they should maintain a balanced diet during pregnancy and may benefit from a folic acid supplement.

• During general anesthesia, a sickle cell anemia patient requires adequate ventilation, to prevent hypoxic crisis. Therefore, the surgeon and the anesthesiologist must be made aware that the patient has sickle cell anemia. Then, they can provide a preoperative transfusion of packed red cells, as needed.

X-LINKED INHERITANCE

Hemophilia

Hemophilia is a hereditary bleeding disorder resulting from deficiency of specific clotting factors. Hemophilia A (classic hemophilia), which affects over 80% of all hemophiliacs, results from deficiency of Factor VIII; hemophilia B (Christmas disease), which affects 15% of hemophiliacs, from deficiency of Factor IX.

Severity and prognosis of bleeding disorders vary with degree of deficiency and the site of bleeding. Overall prognosis is best in mild hemophilia, which doesn't cause spontaneous bleeding and joint deformities. Advances in treatment have greatly improved prognosis, but hemophilia can still be fatal, usually after surgery or trauma.

Causes and incidence

Hemophilia A and B are inherited as X-linked recessive traits. This means that female carriers have a 50% chance of transmitting the gene to each daughter, who would then be a carrier, and a 50% chance of transmitting the gene to each son, who would develop hemophilia. Hemophilia is the most common X-linked genetic disease and occurs in approximately 1.25 in 10,000 live male births. Hemophilia A is five times more common than hemophilia B; rarely, do both forms coexist. Hemophilia causes abnormal bleeding through absence or deficiency of a specific clotting factor. After a person with hemophilia forms a platelet plug at a bleeding site, clotting factor deficiency impairs capacity to form a stable fibrin clot.

Signs and symptoms

Hemophilia produces abnormal bleeding, which may be mild, moderate, or severe, depending on the degree of factor deficiency. Typically, mild hemophilia causes easy bruising, hematomas, a tendency toward nosebleeds, bleeding gums, and prolonged bleeding during and after even minor surgery, such as dental extractions. Usually, postoperative bleeding continues as a slow ooze, or may cease and start again, up to 8 days after surgery. Mild hemophilia may be overlooked until adolescence or adulthood.

Moderate hemophilia causes symptoms similar to mild hemophilia but produces more frequent bleeding episodes and occasional bleeding into joints.

Severe hemophilia causes spontaneous bleeding. Often, the first sign of severe hemophilia is excessive bleeding after circumcision. Later, spontaneous bleeding or severe bleeding after minor trauma may produce large subcutaneous and deep intramuscular hematomas. Bleeding into joints and muscles causes pain, swelling, extreme tenderness, and possibly, permanent deformity.

Bleeding near peripheral nerves causes peripheral neuropathies, pain, paresthesias, and muscle atrophy. If bleeding impairs blood flow through a major vessel, it can cause ischemia and gangrene. Anemia may follow all bleeding episodes. Genitourinary bleeding (hematuria), gastrointestinal bleeding (hematemesis or melena), and, more dangerously, pharyngeal, lingual, intracardial, intracerebral, and intracranial bleeding may all lead to shock and death.

Diagnosis

A clear diagnosis of hemophilia requires evidence of abnormal bleeding, a coagulation profile that points to clotting factor deficiency, and possibly, a positive family history. The following are characteristic findings in hemophilia A:

• Factor VIII assay 0 to 30% of normal

- prolonged partial thromboplastin time
- normal platelet count and function, bleeding time, and prothrombin time.

Characteristics of hemophilia B:
- deficient Factor IX assay
- baseline coagulation results similar to hemophilia A, with normal Factor VIII.

In hemophilia A or B, the degree of factor deficiency determines severity:
- mild hemophilia—factor levels 5% to 50% of normal

- moderate hemophilia—factor levels 1% to 5% of normal
- severe hemophilia—factor levels less than 1% of normal.

Treatment
Hemophilia is not curable, but treatment can prevent crippling deformities and prolong life expectancy. Correct treatment must quickly stop local bleeding, increase plasma levels of deficient factors

---

PARENT TEACHING AID

Helping the Parent Manage a Hemophilia Child

Your child has hemophilia, a serious lifelong condition that requires special care.
- Notify your doctor immediately after even minor injury, but especially after injury to the head, neck, or chest. Such injuries may require special blood factor replacement. Also, check with your doctor before you allow dental extractions or any other surgery. Get the names of other doctors you can contact in case your regular doctor isn't available.
- Teach your child the importance of regular, careful toothbrushing to prevent any need for dental surgery. Have him use a soft toothbrush to avoid gum injury.
- Always watch for signs of severe internal bleeding, such as severe pain or swelling in a joint or muscle, stiffness, joint movement, insomnia, severe abdominal pain, blood in urine, and black tarry stools.
- Because your child receives blood components, he risks hepatitis. Watch for early signs of this disease, which may appear 6 weeks to 6 months after treatment with blood components: headache, fever, decreased appetite, nausea, vomiting, abdominal tenderness, and pain over the liver.
- Make sure your child wears a medical identification bracelet at all times.
- *Never give him aspirin!* It can aggravate his tendency to bleed. Give

acetaminophen instead.
- Protect your child from injury, but avoid unnecessary restrictions that impair his normal development. For example, for a toddler, sew padded patches into the knees and elbows of clothing to protect these joints during frequent falls. You must forbid an older child to participate in contact sports such as football, but you can encourage him to swim or to play golf.
- After injury, apply cold compresses or ice bags and elevate the injured part, or apply light pressure to the bleeding site. To prevent recurrence of bleeding after treatment, restrict activity for 48 hours after bleeding is under control.
- If you've been trained to administer blood factor components at home to avoid frequent hospitalization, know proper venipuncture and infusion techniques, and don't delay treatment during bleeding episodes. Keep blood factor concentrate and infusion equipment with you at all times, even when you're on vacation. Don't let your child miss routine follow-up examinations at your local hemophilia center. To answer your questions about the vulnerability of future offspring, get genetic counseling. Your daughters should have genetic screening to determine if they're hemophilia carriers.

For more information, write to National Hemophilia Foundation.

This parent teaching aid is intended for distribution to patients by doctors and nurses. It should not be used without a doctor's approval.

during bleeding episodes, and prevent disabling deformities that result from bleeding into joints.

In hemophilia A, cryoprecipitated antihemophilic factor (AHF), lyophilized AHF, or both given in doses large enough to raise clotting factor levels above 25% of normal can permit normal hemostasis. After surgery, AHF must be given in doses that raise clotting factor levels about 50% of normal. If AHF is unavailable, treatment may include transfusions of fresh frozen plasma from normal humans or plasma fraction rich in AHF.

In hemophilia B, administration of fresh frozen plasma or Factor IX concentrate during bleeding episodes increases Factor IX levels. In both hemophilia A and B, if the patient has massive blood loss, whole blood transfusion is necessary to prevent hypovolemic shock. However, if the patient hasn't lost large amounts of blood, whole blood transfusion risks fluid over-load.

A person with hemophilia who undergoes surgery needs careful management by a hematologist. Then, the patient may require deficient factor replacement before and during surgery. Such replacement may be necessary even for minor surgery, such as a dental extraction. Indeed, if more than one tooth is to be extracted, adequate factor replacement must raise factor levels to 50% of normal and must continue after surgery. In addition, aminocaproic acid can inhibit fibrinolysis. Preventive treatment teaches the patient how to avoid trauma, manage minor bleeding, and recognize bleeding that requires immediate intervention. Genetic counseling helps parents and siblings who are carriers understand how this disease is transmitted.

Additional considerations

During bleeding episodes:
• Deficient clotting factor or plasma is given, as ordered. AHF remains effective from 48 to 72 hours, so transfusions are repeated, as ordered, until bleeding stops.
• Cold compresses or ice bags are applied, the injured part raised, the wound cleaned, and, if ordered, a thrombin-soaked fibrin

---

FACTOR REPLACEMENTS

In hemophilia, various blood components may augment deficient clotting factors.

Fresh frozen plasma
• Contains all coagulation factors except platelets
• Can be stored frozen up to 12 months but must be used within 2 hours after it thaws
• Given through a blood filter

Cryoprecipitated AHF
• Contains Factor I and Factor VIII
• Can be stored frozen up to 12 months but must be used within 4 to 6 hours after it thaws
• May cause hepatitis
• About 10% of patients develop circulating anticoagulants that inhibit AHF
• Given through a cryoprecipitate administration set

Lyophilized AHF
• Contains freeze-dried Factor VIII concentrate
• Can be stored up to 2 years at 36° to 46° F. (2° to 8° C.); up to 6 months at room temperature exceeding 88° F. (31° C.)
• May cause hepatitis and occasional allergic, febrile, or hemolytic reactions
• Given through a butterfly needle by syringe or infusion set

---

sponge applied to the wound.
• To prevent recurrence of bleeding, activity is restricted for 48 hours after bleeding is under control.
• Pain can be controlled with an analgesic, such as acetaminophen, propoxyphene, codeine, or meperidine, as ordered. I.M. injections should be avoided because of possible hematoma formation at the injection site. Aspirin is contraindicated, since it decreases platelet adherence and may increase the bleeding.

If the patient has bled into a joint:
• The joint is immediately elevated, and immobilized in slight flexion. Blood is aspirated from the joint or an elastic bandage is applied to reduce pain and spasms.

• Joint mobility can be restored through range-of-motion exercises. They can begin, if ordered, 48 hours after the bleeding is controlled. The patient should avoid weight bearing until bleeding stops and swelling subsides.

After bleeding episodes and surgery:
• The patient is watched closely for signs of further bleeding (increased pain and swelling, fever, or symptoms of shock). His prothrombin time is monitored.
• Parents should take special precautions to prevent bleeding episodes. But they should be reassured that with proper management, their child can lead a productive life.

CHROMOSOMAL ABNORMALITIES

Down's Syndrome
(Mongolism, trisomy 21)

The first disorder attributed to a chromosome aberration, Down's syndrome characteristically produces mental retardation, abnormal facial features, and other distinctive physical abnormalities. It's often associated with congenital heart defects and other congenital disorders.

Life expectancy for patients with Down's syndrome has increased significantly because of improved treatment for related complications (heart defects, tendency toward respiratory and other infections, acute leukemia). Nevertheless, up to one third die before they're 10 years old. Mortality is highest in patients with congenital heart disease.

Causes and incidence
Down's syndrome usually results from trisomy 21, an aberration in which chromosome 21 has three copies instead of the normal two because of faulty meiosis (nondisjunction) of the ovum, or sometimes the sperm. This results in a karyotype of 47 chromosomes instead of the normal 46. About 4% of the time, though, Down's syndrome results from an unbalanced translocation in which the long arm of chromosome 21 breaks and attaches to another chromosome.

One of the parents of a child with such an unbalanced translocation is a "balanced translocation carrier" with no physical or mental abnormalities. A mother who is a balanced translocation carrier has a 10% chance of having a Down's child; a carrier father has a less than 5% chance.

Overall, Down's syndrome occurs in 1 per 650 live births, but the incidence increases with maternal age, especially after age 35. For instance, at age 20, a mother has about one chance in 2,000 of having a child with Down's syndrome; by age 49, she has one chance in 12. Although women over age 35 account for fewer than 13.5% of all pregnancies, they bear 50% of all children with Down's syndrome. Paternal age doesn't seem to play a significant part. This suggests that sometimes the chromosome abnormality responsible for Down's syndrome results from deterioration of the oocyte because of age alone or because of the accumulated effects of environmental factors, such as radiation and viruses. Once a mother has had one child with Down's syndrome, the risk of recurrence is only 1% to 2%, unless trisomy results from translocation.

Signs and symptoms
The physical signs of Down's syndrome (especially hypotonia) are readily apparent at birth; mental retardation is obvious as such infants grow older. Typically, these persons have craniofacial

anomalies, such as slanting, almond-shaped eyes (epicanthic fold); protruding tongue; small open mouth; a single transverse palmar crease (simian crease), small white spots (Brushfield spots) on the iris; strabismus; small skull; flat bridge across the nose; slow dental development, with abnormal or absent teeth; flattened face; small external ears; short neck; and occasionally, cataracts.

Other physical abnormalities include dry skin with decreased elasticity, umbilical hernia, short stature, and short extremities, with broad, flat, and squarish hands and feet. These patients have clinodactyly (small little finger that curves inward), a wide space between the first and second toe, and abnormal fingerprints and footprints. Their hypotonic limb muscles impair reflex development, posture, coordination, and balance.

Such patients have an IQ between 30 and 50. So, as infants, they're slow to sit up, walk, and talk, but they're usually docile and easily managed. They often have congenital heart disease (septal defects, or pulmonary or aortic stenosis), duodenal atresia, megacolon, and pelvic bone abnormalities. Their genitalia are poorly developed, and puberty is delayed. In many males, the testicles fail to descend. These patients are especially susceptible to leukemia and to acute and chronic infections.

Diagnosis
Physical findings at birth, especially hypotonia, suggest this diagnosis.

 A karyotype showing the chromosome abnormality can confirm it. Amniocentesis allows prenatal diagnosis; 80% of all amniocenteses are done for this purpose and are recommended for pregnant women past age 35.

Treatment
Down's syndrome has no known cure. Surgery to correct heart defects and other related congenital abnormalities, and antibiotic therapy for recurrent infections have improved life expectancy considerably. Such patients may be cared for

at home and attend special education classes, or if profoundly retarded, may be institutionalized. As adults, some may work in a sheltered workshop.

Additional considerations
The parents of a child with Down's syndrome require special support. A health care professional can help them deal with their problems and meet their child's

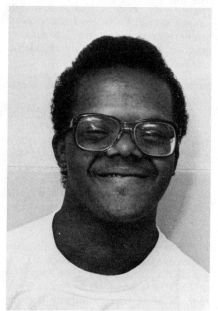

Down's syndrome is characterized by these facial abnormalities: epicanthal folds, slanting almond-shaped eyes, flat nose bridge, small ears.

physical and emotional needs by following these guidelines:
• Establishing a trusting relationship with parents, and encouraging communication during the difficult period soon after diagnosis, when parents face the difficult decision of whether or not to care for their child at home.
• Teaching parents the importance of a balanced diet and stressing the need for patience while feeding their child, since he may have difficulty sucking, and may be less demanding and seem less eager to eat than normal babies.

• Encouraging parents to hold and nurture their child, even though their first reaction may be to reject him because he isn't normal.

• Emphasizing the importance of adequate exercise and maximal environmental stimulation, and referring them for infant stimulation classes, which may begin at age 3 months.

• Assisting parents in setting realistic goals for their child. His mental development may seem normal at first, but parents should be warned not to view this early development as a sign of future progress. By the time he's 1 year old, the Down's child's development clearly lags behind that of normal children. Parents must learn to view their child's achievements positively, even though he's slow. The Denver Developmental Screening Test for noninstitutionalized Down's children can help chart progress.

• Referring parents and older siblings for genetic counseling and, if necessary, for psychologic counseling, to help them evaluate future risks and adopt a positive outlook.

• Warning parents not to overlook the emotional needs of other children in the family.

Klinefelter's Syndrome

This relatively common genetic abnormality results from one or more extra X chromosomes, and it affects only males. It usually becomes apparent at puberty, when the secondary sex characteristics develop; the penis and testicles fail to mature, and degenerative testicular changes begin that eventually result in irreversible infertility. Klinefelter's syndrome often causes gynecomastia and is also associated with a tendency toward mental deficiency.

Causes and incidence

Klinefelter's syndrome, probably the most common cause of hypogonadism, appears in approximately 1 in every 600 males. (For information on another common cause of hypogonadism, Turner's syndrome, see opposite.) Also, it accounts for roughly 10 in every 1,000 institutionalized mentally retarded males.

This disorder usually results from one extra X chromosome, giving such patients a 47,XXY complement instead of the normal 46,XY. Sometimes additional X chromosomes are present (XXXY, XXXXY). Usually, the larger the number of extra chromosomes, the more severe the disorder. In the rare, mosaic form of this syndrome, only some cells contain the extra X chromosomes, while others contain the normal XY complement.

The extra chromosome or chromosomes responsible for Klinefelter's syndrome probably result either from meiotic nondisjunction during parental gametogenesis or from meiotic nondisjunction in the zygote. The incidence of meiotic nondisjunction, like many other chromosome errors, increases with maternal age.

Signs and symptoms

Klinefelter's syndrome usually isn't apparent until puberty or later and many cases probably go undetected—espe-

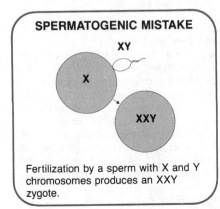

SPERMATOGENIC MISTAKE

Fertilization by a sperm with X and Y chromosomes produces an XXY zygote.

cially mild ones, with no abnormalities except infertility. Its characteristic features include a small penis and prostate; small, firm testicles; sparse facial and abdominal hair; feminine distribution of pubic hair; sexual dysfunction (impotence, lack of libido); and in less than 50% of patients, gynecomastia. Aspermatogenesis and infertility result from progressive sclerosis and hyalinization of the seminiferous tubules in the testicles and from testicular fibrosis during and after puberty. In the mosaic form, such changes and resulting infertility may be delayed.

In addition to these sex-related abnormalities, Klinefelter's syndrome is associated with mental retardation, osteoporosis, abnormal body build (long legs with short obese trunk), tall stature, and a tendency toward alcoholism, antisocial behavior, and other personality disorders. It's also linked with increased incidence of pulmonary disease, varicose veins, and breast cancer.

Diagnosis

Typical clinical features suggest Klinefelter's syndrome, but only a karyotype (chromosome analysis) determined by culturing lymphocytes from peripheral blood can clearly confirm it. In suspected Klinefelter's syndrome, a buccal smear can detect sex chromatin (Barr body); if present, a karyotype can definitively confirm the extra chromosomes.

Characteristically, Klinefelter's syndrome decreases urinary 17-ketosteroids, increases follicle-stimulating hormone (FSH) excretion, and decreases plasma testosterone levels after puberty.

Treatment and additional considerations

Depending on severity, treatment may include mastectomy in persistent gynecomastia, and supplemental testosterone in sexual dysfunction. However, not all such patients need hormonal treatment; not all patients respond to it. The degenerative testicular changes that eventually result in infertility can't be prevented. But research suggests that earlier

---

TURNER'S SYNDROME

In Turner's syndrome (ovarian dysgenesis) nondisjunction during an early phase of spermatogenesis results in a missing X chromosome. This produces a 45,XO karyotype instead of the normal 46,XX. Turner's syndrome occurs in approximately 1 in 10,000 live female births.

Characteristics of Turner's syndrome include short stature (patients seldom are taller than 5 feet), webbing of the neck, low hairline at the nape of the neck, wide chest with broadly spaced nipples and poor breast development, and underdeveloped genitalia. In fact, the ovaries of such a patient are no more than a streak of connective tissue; of course, she is sterile. Turner's syndrome also produces coarctation of the aorta and edema of the legs and feet. It's often unrecognized until primary amenorrhea and failure to develop secondary sex characteristics cause the patient to seek help.

Treatment consists of estrogen therapy to induce sexual maturation. Such therapy is usually deferred until age 13 to 15 to avoid early epiphyseal closure. Once menses occurs, cyclic estrogen-progestogen therapy creates a hormonal cycle but doesn't reverse sterility. Patients with Turner's syndrome also need genetic counseling and emotional support.

—SARA M. SUMNER, RN

---

treatment may be more effective.

Psychotherapy (including sexual counseling) is indicated when sexual dysfunction causes emotional maladjustment. If patients with the mosaic form of the syndrome are fertile, genetic counseling is essential, since they may transmit this chromosomal abnormality to their offspring.

To promote emotional well-being, patients should be encouraged to discuss feelings of confusion and rejection that may arise because of their disorder.

To improve compliance with hormonal therapy, these patients must understand testosterone's benefits and side effects.

Cri du Chat Syndrome
(Cat's cry syndrome, 5p— syndrome)

Cri du chat syndrome is a rare congenital disorder characterized by a catlike cry in infancy, and severe mental and physical retardation. Many cri du chat infants do not live past their first year, but of those who do survive, some may live to adulthood.

Causes and incidence
Cri du chat syndrome results from abnormal deletion of the short arm of chromosome 5 (5p–). About 10% of infants with this disorder have a parent who is a balanced carrier for a translocation of the short arm of chromosome 5. The risk of cri du chat does not increase with parental age. Incidence is probably about 1 in every 20,000 live births and is more common in females than in males.

Signs and symptoms
An infant with this disorder usually has a normal prenatal history and birth. At birth he is abnormally small and shows microencephaly, wide-set eyes, receding chin, high-arched palate, round face, and decreased muscle tone, which makes feeding difficult. The high-pitched catlike cry appears soon after birth and later disappears. Other symptoms include low-set ears, simian crease, epicanthal folds, severe mental retardation (IQ is less than 50), and associated defects, such as congenital heart disease, joint and bone deformities, and inguinal hernia.

Diagnosis
These typical clinical features (cat cry, facial disproportions, microencephaly, small birth size, poor physical and mental development) strongly suggest cri du chat syndrome. A karyotype showing deleted short arms of chromosome 5 confirms it.

Treatment
No specific treatment exists for cri du chat. Individualized treatment includes evaluation and treatment of congenital heart and eye defects. When these infants survive past their first year, management is primarily nonmedical and emphasizes education, training in self-care and socialization, recreational and social services, vocational training, and custodial arrangements. Ideally, such management requires the cooperation of a team of specialists to develop a personalized and realistic care plan. Whenever possible, such a plan should emphasize home care, early education (which may use behavior modification), and parent teaching to maximize stimulation.

Additional considerations
• Because an infant with cri du chat syndrome is usually a poor eater, fluid intake and output, caloric intake, and weight should be monitored closely. Frequent, small feedings will help him meet calorie requirements. Large meals are apt to tire him because of his decreased muscle tone.
• Amniocentesis can detect cri du chat syndrome prenatally. Parents of such a child should receive genetic counseling. If the male is the translocation carrier, artificial insemination may be a viable alternative.
• The family must understand the child's potential so they can make long-term plans (including whether or not to institutionalize the child). The parents may be interested in an infant stimulation program, which will help their child reach his potential. To avoid rejection or overprotection of such a child, the parents must learn to set realistic goals.
• If parents have trouble coping, they should seek psychological counseling.

MULTIFACTORIAL ABNORMALITIES

Cleft Lip and Palate

Cleft lip and cleft palate deformities occur in 1 in every 800 births. They originate in the second month of pregnancy, when the front and sides of the face and the palatine shelves fuse imperfectly. Cleft deformities fall into four categories: clefts of the lip (unilateral or bilateral); clefts of the palate (along the midline); unilateral clefts of the lip, alveolus (gum pad), and palate, which are twice as common on the left side as on the right; and bilateral clefts of the lip, alveolus, and palate. Cleft lip with or without cleft palate is more common in males, while cleft palate alone is more common in females.

Causes and incidence

Although cleft lips and palates occur in infants with chromosomal abnormalities, they are also found in infants who are otherwise normal. Incidence of cleft deformities is higher in children with a positive family history. If normal parents have a baby with a cleft, the risk that subsequent offspring will have the defect is 5%; if they have two children with this disorder, the risk in subsequent offspring climbs to 12%.

Signs and symptoms

Congenital clefts of the face occur most often in the upper lip. They range from a simple notch to a complete cleft, extending from the lip edge through the floor of the nostril, on either side of the midline. A cleft lip rarely runs along the midline itself, unless accompanied by other congenital anomalies.

A cleft palate may be partial or complete. A complete cleft includes the soft palate, the bones of the maxilla, and the alveolus on one or both sides of the premaxilla. A double cleft—the severest of all cleft deformities—runs from the soft palate forward to either side of the nose, separating the maxilla and premaxilla into free-moving segments. The tongue and other muscles can displace these bony segments, increasing the size of the cleft. In Pierre Robin syndrome, micrognathia and glossoptosis coexist with cleft palate.

Diagnosis

Typical clinical picture confirms diagnosis.

Treatment

Treatment consists of surgical correction, but the timing of surgery varies. Some plastic surgeons repair cleft lips within the first few days of life. This makes it easier to feed the baby and makes him more acceptable to his parents. However, many surgeons delay lip repairs for 8 to 10 weeks and sometimes as long as 6 to 8 months, to allow time for maternal bonding, and most important, to rule out associated congenital anomalies. Cleft palate repair is usually completed by the 12th to 18th month. Still other surgeons repair cleft palates in two steps, repairing the soft palate between 6 and 18 months and the hard palate as late as 5 years of age. In any case, surgery is performed only after the infant is gaining weight satisfactorily and is free of any respiratory, oral, or systemic infections.

When a wide horseshoe defect makes surgery impossible, a contoured speech bulb is attached to the posterior of a denture to occlude the nasopharynx and help the child develop intelligible speech. Surgery must be coupled with speech therapy. Because the palate is essential to speech formation, structural changes, even in a repaired cleft, can permanently affect speech patterns. To compound the problem, children with cleft palates often have hearing difficulties because of middle ear damage or infections.

Additional considerations

• A child with Pierre Robin syndrome (micrognathia, glossoptosis) must never be placed on his back, since his tongue can fall back and obstruct his airway. Therefore, such a baby must be trained to sleep on his side. All other cleft palate babies can sleep on their backs without difficulty.

• Adequate nutrition must be maintained for normal growth and development. A baby with a cleft palate has an excellent appetite but often has trouble feeding because of nasal regurgitation and air leaks around the cleft. He often feeds better from a nipple with a flange that occludes the cleft, a lamb's nipple (a big soft nipple with large holes), or just a regular nipple with enlarged holes.

To feed the infant, the mother should hold him in a near-sitting position, with the flow directed to the side or back of the baby's tongue. She should burp the baby frequently, since he tends to swallow a lot of air. If the underside of the nasal septum becomes ulcerated and the child refuses to suck because of the pain, the mother should direct the nipple to the side of his mouth, to give the mucosa time to heal. The palatal cleft can be cleaned with a cotton-tipped applicator dipped in half-strength hydrogen peroxide or water after each feeding.

• The mother of a baby with cleft lip can breast-feed if the cleft doesn't prevent effective sucking. Breast-feeding an infant with a cleft palate or one who has just had corrective surgery is impossible. (Postoperatively, the infant can't suck for up to 6 weeks.) However, if the mother desires, she can use a breast pump to express breast milk and then feed it to her baby from a bottle. Following surgery, the baby's intake and output should be recorded.

• To prevent atelectasis and pneumonia the doctor may gently suction the nasopharynx (this may be necessary before surgery too).

• The infant should be restrained so he doesn't hurt himself. Elbow restraints allow the baby to move his hands while keeping them away from his mouth. When necessary, an infant seat can keep the child in a comfortable sitting position. To entertain him, toys may be hung within reach of restrained hands.

• Surgeons sometimes place a curved metal Logan bow over a repaired cleft lip to minimize tension on the suture line. The gauze must be removed before feedings, and replaced often. It should be kept moistened with normal saline solution until the sutures are removed.

• The parents will need help dealing with their feelings about the child's deformity. They should be told about it immediately and shown their baby as soon as possible. Because society places undue importance on physical appearance, parents often feel shock, disappointment, and guilt when they see the child. The parents attention should be directed to their child's assets; being shown what is "right" about their baby and learning what his positive characteristics are.

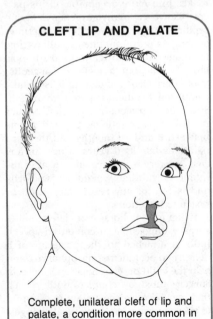

CLEFT LIP AND PALATE

Complete, unilateral cleft of lip and palate, a condition more common in males than in females

They should know that surgical repairs can be made.

The parents will need instruction in the care and feeding of the child right from the start to encourage normal bonding. In addition, they will need emotional support and reassurance to take proper care of the child at home. A social worker will be able to guide them to community resources for help.

Selected References

Bergsma, Daniel, ed. BIRTH DEFECTS COMPENDIUM, 2nd ed. New York: Alan R. Liss, Inc., 1979.

Bergsma, Daniel, and Harold Abramson. GENETIC COUNSELING. National Foundation of Birth Defects. Baltimore: Williams & Wilkins, 1970.

Division of Medical Sciences, National Research Council. GENETIC SCREENING: PROGRAMS, PRINCIPLES, AND RESEARCH. Washington: National Academy of Sciences, 1975.

Eppink, H. *Facts and Concepts for Genetic Counseling: Genetic Causes of Abnormal Fetal Development and Inherited Diseases,* JOURNAL OF OBSTETRICS, GYNECOLOGY, AND NEONATAL NURSING. 6:14-22, September/October 1977.

Goodman, Richard M., ed. GENETIC DISORDERS OF MAN. Boston: Little, Brown & Co., 1970.

Holum, John R. ORGANIC AND BIOLOGICAL CHEMISTRY. New York: John Wiley & Sons, Inc., 1978.

Huddart, A. *The Care and Management of the Newborn Cleft Palate Infant,* NURSING MIRROR. 140:61-65, January 16, 1975.

Kelly, Thaddeus. CLINICAL GENETICS AND GENETIC COUNSELING. Chicago: Year Book Medical Publishers, 1980.

Klaus, Marshall, and Avroy A. Fanaroff. CARE OF THE HIGH-RISK NEONATE, 2nd ed. Philadelphia: W.B. Saunders Co., 1979.

Longacre, J.J. CLEFT PALATE DEFORMATION: CAUSATION AND PREVENTION. Springfield, Ill.: Charles C. Thomas, Pubs., 1970.

McKusick, Victor. MENDELIAN INHERITANCE IN MAN: CATALOGS OF AUTOSOMAL DOMINANT, AUTOSOMAL RECESSIVE, AND X-LINKED PHENOTYPES, 4th ed. Baltimore: Johns Hopkins Press, 1975.

Nora, James J., and F. Clarke Fraser. MEDICAL GENETICS: PRINCIPLES AND PRACTICE. Philadelphia: Lea & Febiger, 1974.

Purtilo, D. A SURVEY OF HUMAN DISEASES. Menlo Park, Calif.: Addison-Wesley Pub. Co., 1978.

Ross, R. Bruce, and Malcolm C. Johnston. CLEFT LIP AND PALATE. Huntington, N.Y.: Robert E. Krieger Pub. Co., 1972.

Scipien, G., et al. COMPREHENSIVE PEDIATRIC NURSING, 2nd ed. New York: McGraw-Hill Book Co., 1979.

Singer, S. HUMAN GENETICS: AN INTRODUCTION TO THE PRINCIPLES OF HEREDITY. San Francisco: W.H. Freeman & Co., 1978.

Smith, David W. RECOGNIZABLE PATTERNS OF HUMAN MALFORMATION: GENETIC, EMBRYOLOGIC AND CLINICAL ASPECTS, Vol. 7, 2nd ed. Philadelphia: W.B. Saunders Co., 1976.

Sutton, Eldon H. AN INTRODUCTION TO HUMAN GENETICS. New York: Holt, Rinehart & Winston, 1975.

Thompson, James S., and Margaret W. Thompson. GENETICS IN MEDICINE, 2nd ed. Philadelphia: W.B. Saunders Co., 1973.

Vaughan, Victor C., and R. James McKay, eds. NELSON TEXTBOOK OF PEDIATRICS, 10th ed. Philadelphia: W.B. Saunders Co., 1975.

Whaley, L., and D. Wong. NURSING CARE OF INFANTS AND CHILDREN. St. Louis: C.V. Mosby Co., 1979.

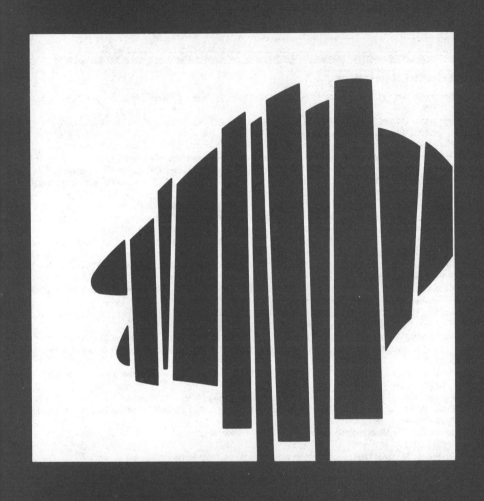

3 Mental and Emotional Disorders

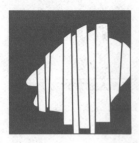

Mental and Emotional Disorders

Introduction

For the past 30 years, psychiatry has been changing in ways both dramatic and profound. In the 1950s, the discovery of chlorpromazine and, later, of other mood-altering drugs began a revolutionary new approach to the treatment of mental illness. In addition, behaviorist and humanist theorists supplemented the theories of Freudian psychoanalysis and developmental psychiatrists. In the 1960s, community mental health centers began to offer an alternative to inpatient psychiatric hospitals. These centers provided early community-based mental health services. The main goal for developing these centers was to minimize the negative effects of institutionalization; secondary goals included increasing public awareness of mental health, encouraging people to seek help early for milder forms of mental illness, and fostering a realistic and accepting community attitude toward mental patients. These community treatment centers made it possible to treat some severe forms of mental illness in various settings—not solely in the restricted milieu of the psychiatric hospital. More recently, research in genetics and biochemistry has contributed to the knowledge about causes and effects of mental illness. This new information has prompted many to question and revise traditional classifications of mental illness (especially of schizophrenia, manic-depressive psychosis, and involutional melancholia). As a result, psychiatrists may differ radically in their diagnostic evaluation of the same patient and, consequently, in the treatment they might recommend.

Changing roles

These developments and changes have profoundly affected the roles of other health care professionals, as well. The nurse's role, for example, has changed markedly from "caretaker" to care-planner and care-giver. With other members of the psychiatric team she sets treatment goals and implements plans for meeting them. Her enlarged responsibilities require a working knowledge of psychiatric terminology; well-developed skills in history-taking, assessment, and documentation (especially for recording changes in the patient's behavior in response to treatment); and a working knowledge of psychotropic drugs, including their administration, side effects, and related diet restrictions. Perhaps one of her most valuable assets is her ability to communicate. In all, she must develop a holistic approach to the patient, recognizing and caring for both his physical and emotional needs.

Assessing the patient's physical status is vital, because physical and mental health are interdependent. Just as physical illness can produce psychiatric behaviors such as anxiety, anger, depression, or denial, unresolved anxiety or conflict can be turned inward, to produce psychosomatic illnesses such as headaches, ulcers, or colitis.

How mental illness develops
Understanding mental illness and its nursing implications requires some understanding of the difference between mental health and mental illness, and how they develop. At birth, each person begins an endless process of developing a sense of self and self-esteem based on reactions and adaptations to environmental and internal biological stimuli. When these stimuli are stressful, psychologic (as well as physiologic) disequilibrium occurs, and the person must adapt to it to maintain his psychologic well-being. He can do this with coping (defense) mechanisms. Healthy use of coping mechanisms can minimize anxiety and other forms of mental illness; but their inappropriate or exclusive use can increase anxiety and maladaptation. Ultimately, continuing inability to cope with life and reality induces some degree of mental illness, and may bring the pa-

---

ASSESSMENT OF THE PSYCHIATRIC PATIENT

- Psychiatric interview
- Complete history, physical examination, and laboratory studies
- Mental status examination
- Special diagnostic tests
  A. *Psychologic tests:*
    —Intelligence tests
      (Wechsler Adult Intelligence Scale [WAIS], Wechsler Intelligence Scale for Children)
    —Minnesota Multiphasic Personality Inventory (MMPI)
    —California Test for Personality for Children
    —Bender gestalt
    —Aptitude tests (both vocation and interest)

    —Children's Aptitude Test (CAT)
    —Denver Developmental Test (DDST)
  B. *Projective tests:*
    —Rorschach
    —Thematic Apperception Test (TAT)
    —Draw-a-Person, complete-the-sentence tests
  C. *Neurologic tests:*
    —Electroencephalography
    —Echoencephalography
    —Computerized axial tomography (CAT) scan
    —Brain scan
    —Skull X-ray
    —Spinal tap

tient to a mental health care professional for help.

The nurse, along with other health care professionals, plays an integral role in providing this help by assessing the patient's physical and mental status, helping to formulate a treatment, implementing treatment, and evaluating the patient's response to treatment. She assesses physical and mental status through careful observation and detailed interview and history, recording only objective data. One essential tool for such assessment is the mental status exam. Other sources of information include the patient's family and friends, and the records of referral agencies.

Assessment of mental status

To assess mental status, a careful appraisal of appearance, speech patterns, emotional status, and sensorium and intelligence can be made by methodically evaluating the following areas:

• *Appearance and behavior:* Posture, personal hygiene, grooming and dress, facial expressions, body language and mannerisms, attitude, and general manner.

• *Speech:* Quality and quantity of speech, speed and manner of responses, changes during conversation, speech abnormalities (mutism, echolalia, neologisms, perseveration, flight of ideas).

• *Mood and affect:* Appropriateness to situation, intensity, range or emotional expression, signs of anxiety or depression.

• *Thought content:* presence of delusions or hallucinations, areas of preoccupation, use of defense mechanisms, whether processes are concrete, abstract, or autistic, presence of suicidal or homicidal thought. What the patient says directly should be recorded as well as what he implies, using direct quotes. Deliberate, leading questions help elicit thought content (For example, the patient can be asked, "Do you ever see or hear things that other people don't?").

• *Sensorium and intelligence:* orientation, short- and long-term memory, attention and concentration, general knowledge.

• *Insight and judgment:* patient's understanding of his own personality and illness. For example, does he understand why he's been hospitalized? A hypothetical situation, requiring sound judgment, should be posed and he should be asked what his response would be (For example, "What would you do if the building caught

---

COMMON DEFENSE MECHANISMS

• Denial—completely blocking out a painful reality

• Displacement—transferring feelings, emotions, or drives to a substitute object or person

• Projection—attributing one's own feelings to someone else

• Rationalization—using an acceptable, logical reason to explain unacceptable feelings or behavior

• Regression—returning (in the mind) to an earlier, safer mode of adapting (developmental stage) in response to severe anxiety

• Compensation—covering up inadequate aspects of character by overemphasizing other aspects to maintain self-respect and gain recognition

• Conversion—redirecting emotional reactions or anxiety to symbolic somatic complaints

• Identification—imitating a person who has the attributes the patient considers admirable

• Introjection—internalizing the feelings, values, and attitudes of another person, or using the hostility felt toward others against oneself

• Isolation—effectively separating emotions from a painful memory, thought, or experience

• Reaction formation—substituting an attitude with its opposite

• Sublimation—redirecting unacceptable impulses or energy into socially acceptable, constructive activities

• Fantasy—daydreaming as a temporary escape from a painful situation.

fire?").

After assessment, the psychiatric team member must develop a realistic, goal-directed treatment plan for the patient aimed at relieving anxiety or correcting unacceptable behavior. Allowing the psychiatric patient to help formulate this plan increases his motivation and feelings of self-worth and greatly increases its chance to succeed.

Throughout treatment, health care professionals must regularly reevaluate the treatment plan and the patient's progress (or lack of it—in treating the psychiatric patient, some goals will never be met) and be prepared to modify it, as needed. Above all, health care professionals who work with mental patients need to be flexible and nonjudgmental. They must be aware of and understand their own feelings and attitudes. By doing so, they can control their feelings, and respond to their patients in helpful constructive ways.

NEUROSES

Anxiety Reaction

Anxiety reaction (anxiety neurosis, chronic anxiety, acute anxiety attack) is an exaggerated feeling of apprehension, uncertainty, and fear. It may be mild, beginning slowly with general feelings of tension and nervousness; moderate; or severe, escalated to panic in a terrifying acute attack that can last from a few minutes to an hour. Chronic anxiety, mild or moderate, persists for long periods, often causing loss of interest in daily activities.

Anxiety reaction, one of the most prevalent neuroses in developed countries, affects twice as many women as men. If it's of recent onset, it's usually benign and transient, and the prognosis is good. But if it persists for several months after the precipitating stress, the outlook is uncertain.

Causes
Occasional anxiety is a normal part of life, and is a rational response to some real threat. However, anxiety reaction represents uncontrollable, unreasonable anxiety. It may result from a perceived physical threat (inability to meet needs for food, water, necessities of life) or a perceived psychologic threat (rejection, loss of approval from loved one; unmet emotional needs). In short, anxiety reaction stems from the patient's failure to cope rationally and effectively with a threatening situation. Some investigators suggest that physiologic symptoms of anxiety are related to high serum lactate levels.

Signs and symptoms
The patient with anxiety reaction experiences varying psychologic or physiologic symptoms. The mildly anxious patient shows mainly psychologic symptoms: restlessness, sleeplessness, appetite changes, irritability, repetitive questioning, and constant seeking of attention and reassurance. He may be unusually alert to his environment and to himself. The moderately anxious patient is selectively inattentive and is better able to concentrate on a single task. The severely anxious patient concentrates on small or scattered details of a task but can't concentrate on it as a whole. The acutely anxious, panicky patient can't concentrate at all, and most of his speech is unintelligible.

Again, varying according to severity, the morbidly anxious patient shows parasympathetic and sympathetic (mostly sympathetic) symptoms, including skeletal muscle tension (headache, muscle spasm in the back, neck, or chest); excessive perspiration; hyperventilation (sighing, dyspnea, dizziness); gastrointestinal disorders (abdominal pain, belching, heartburn, anorexia, nausea, diarrhea, constipation); cardiovascular symptoms (palpitations, precordial discomfort, tachycardia, transient hypertension); and occasionally, genitourinary dysfunction (frequent urination, dysuria, impotence, frigidity).

During an acute anxiety attack and panic, the same symptoms are possible but in intensely magnified form. The panic-stricken patient is likely to show facial flush, cold perspiration, and trembling extremities. He may say he's losing his mind, having a heart attack (because of palpitation and precordial chest pain), or dying. Almost invariably, he hyperventilates, sometimes to the point of respiratory alkalosis (dizziness, weakness, faintness, syncope). Also, when questioned after the attack, he may be unable to recall what precipitated his anxiety, perhaps because of repression.

Diagnosis

A careful history confirms anxiety reaction when it shows a pattern of failure to cope with past or current stress. However, careful evaluation must rule out organic causes of the patient's symptoms (hyperthyroidism, paroxysmal tachycardia, pheochromocytoma, coronary artery disease). Thus, if a patient complains of chest pain during anxiety reaction, he should have an EKG to rule out myocardial ischemia. An anxious patient also needs careful evaluation for depression, because its treatment differs from that for anxiety. Other tests should include complete blood count (CBC) and differential, and tests for serum lactate and calcium levels to rule out hypocalcemia.

Treatment

To ease the patient's distress while he learns better ways to cope with stress, the doctor may prescribe a minor tranquilizer, such as diazepam, chlordiazepoxide, or clorazepate. Treatment may also include psychotherapy or psychoanalysis.

Additional considerations

If the patient is taking tranquilizers, he must:
• understand that tranquilizers may cause drowsiness, fatigue, ataxia, blurred vision, slurred speech, tremors, and hypotension.
• avoid simultaneous use of alcohol or any CNS depressants and avoid driving and other hazardous tasks until he's developed a tolerance to the tranquilizer's sedative effects.
• take the tranquilizers as prescribed, and discontinue them only with his doctor's guidance, because abrupt withdrawal may cause severe symptoms.

A female patient should tell the doctor if she becomes pregnant.

When a patient has an acute attack, these measures may help calm him:
• offering reassurance, listening to him talk, and answering his questions
• protecting him from others who may increase his anxiety: for example, family members or health care professionals who can't control their feelings
• avoiding remarks like, "I don't understand why you're so upset," or, "Don't be so upset." Instead, the patient should be reassured that he's all right, that he's not having a heart attack, and that someone will stay with him until he's calmed down. He should not be pressured to change immediately.
• after the attack, encouraging him to do simple tasks or activities that will distract him from anxiety; for example, handicrafts, art therapy, or occupational therapy.

When a patient has a moderate anxiety attack he needs understanding to resolve the conflict that's causing his anxiety, so he can begin controlling his reaction to it. Then, he can look for alternative ways of dealing with the anxiety-provoking situation.

After the patient is discharged, his family should be as supportive as possible.

Depression

Depression (depressive reaction, reactive depression, depressive syndrome, neurotic depression, anaclitic depression, melancholia, postpartum depression, grief, psychotic depression) is an abnormal mental state marked by negative mood changes, such as sadness, loneliness, and apathy; persistent feelings of low self-esteem and self-blame; slow or agitated activity levels; and withdrawal and suicidal ideation. Some authorities classify depression by cause into endogenous (organic, biochemical, or psychotic) or exogenous (reactive, psychogenic, or neurotic); others classify it only according to degree of severity, regardless of cause. This discussion will cover mild to moderate depression, the kind likely to be psychogenic or reactive rather than organic. For a discussion of severe, psychotic depression, see MANIC-DEPRESSIVE ILLNESS *in this chapter.*

Depression is the most common psychiatric disorder and is a major health problem in the United States. It occurs in all age-groups and is common among children and elderly people. It occurs twice as often in women as in men at any age. Prognosis depends on the precipitating situation and on the patient's own stability and resilience. Patients who were reasonably stable before the onset of depression recover more quickly than those who were not.

Causes

Depression often follows certain stressful events in persons predisposed to depression. Such events usually impose loss or separation: bereavement, divorce, or a job loss. In postpartum depression, a woman may perceive her new baby as a source of loss of a former role and lifestyle. Other precipitating factors include physical illnesses, such as a viral infection, intra-abdominal neoplasm, or any chronic disfiguring illness, especially one that leaves the patient with a permanent handicap. Certain medications—especially antihypertensives, such as reserpine, and oral contraceptives—can induce depression.

Certain life factors predispose a person to develop depression. If a child loses a parent at an early age or grows up in a cold or hostile family environment, he may fail to develop self-esteem or to cope well with loss and disappointment. If he learns to expect rejection and continually feels hopeless and worthless, he is more likely to develop depression in reaction to loss and disappointment later in life. "Masked depression" describes depression in children who react to loss with aggressive, antisocial behavior.

Some authorities have suggested a hereditary factor in the development of depression, but studies have never confirmed it.

Signs and symptoms

Depression characteristically produces changes in physical appearance and affect, accompanied by somatic complaints. The depressed patient generally looks sad and old, and carries himself in a defeated, stooped posture.

Continually and obviously sad, he may be withdrawn and quiet, and have frequent crying spells. He has little energy and is apathetic and antisocial. He shows a hopeless, pessimistic attitude toward the future, is restless and irritable, and has difficulty talking, concentrating, and making decisions. Because of severe anorexia, he usually looks gaunt.

Associated somatic complaints include blurred vision, headaches, dry mouth, anorexia, constipation, abdominal pain, sexual difficulties (impotence and frigidity), and sleep disturbances (typically, insomnia and early morning wakening). The neurotically depressed patient's mood worsens progressively during the course of the day. He may express suicidal tendencies in obvious ways, or covertly in self-neglect, such as starvation, falling asleep in the bathtub, or not responding to a fire alarm.

Diagnosis

The diagnosis of depression requires evidence of sad affect, somatic complaints, and depressed activity levels. A history of severe personal loss supports this diagnosis. But the patient also needs evaluation for other psychiatric illnesses, for drug-induced depression (antihypertensives and oral contraceptives), and for physical illnesses that may produce depression. Especially in older patients, intra-abdominal neoplasms and viral infections may manifest themselves in depression before any physical signs and symptoms appear.

Early recognition of depression and prompt intervention can be lifesaving. According to a recent study, 50% of one group of patients who committed suicide sought medical treatment for their physical symptoms 1 week before they took their own lives.

Treatment

Treatment of depression aims to ease the patient's sad feelings and to relieve physical symptoms through drugs, psychotherapy, and in some cases, electroshock (electroconvulsive) treatment (ECT).

Drug therapy may include tricyclic antidepressants (TCAs), such as amitriptyline or imipramine, given under strict supervision because of suicide risk. Rarely, if tricyclic antidepressants are ineffective, the patient may benefit from a monoamine oxidase inhibitor (MAOI), such as phenelzine or tranylcypromine. For a discussion of these drugs, their side effects, and contraindications, see MANIC-DEPRESSIVE ILLNESS (page 90).

If the adult patient doesn't respond to drug therapy, treatment may also include ECT; however, this is generally used only for severe depression. ECT is administered two to three times a week for 3 to 4 weeks. After the patient is anesthetized, an electric current is passed through the temporal lobe. The patient then has a grand mal seizure. (Care must be taken to maintain an airway during this procedure.) Immediately after treatment, the patient is drowsy and lethargic, and has transient mental impairment but should become alert and communicative after 30 minutes (at the latest, 6 to 8 hours).

The patient's insight may be increased and his feelings of hopelessness and despair may be eased by individual psychotherapy, group therapy, or family therapy. The depressed child may benefit from individual treatment, play therapy, or group play therapy.

Additional considerations

A depressed patient must be assessed for suicide potential; intervention may be necessary to prevent a suicide attempt. Although the patient's depression should be accepted, he should also be reassured that it will eventually lift. Health care professionals and family members can help increase the patient's self-esteem by encouraging him to talk, by listening to him, and by allowing him time to formulate his thoughts. They should try to develop a trusting relationship with him and encourage him to accept noncompetitive, undemanding tasks with short-term goals. For example, if he's hospitalized, a nurse could ask him to give out drinks or deliver mail to other patients; to walk up and down the hall a certain number of times; or to get involved in crafts or hobbies.

Physical activity can help improve the patient's muscle tone and decrease his constipation. Solitary, noncompetitive sports, such as swimming or jogging, should be encouraged.

A depressed patient must be encouraged to eat. If he's constipated, bulk foods high in fiber should be added to his diet. Another person should stay with him while he eats. Small, frequent meals may help him regain weight.

If the patient has insomnia, measures such as drinking warm milk and getting a backrub may help him sleep.

Obsessive-compulsive States

Obsessive-compulsive states (obsessional states, obsessive-compulsive personality, obsessive-compulsive neuroses, phobic neuroses, obsessive-compulsive-ruminative states) are marked by recurrent thoughts, feelings, or impulses (obsessions) and by repetitive acts (compulsions) that the patient recognizes as unhealthy but cannot control. These abnormal mental states develop during adolescence or early adulthood. They affect both men and women, with a higher incidence among women. Overall, they account for fewer than 5% of all psychiatric patients.

The outlook for complete recovery from obsessive-compulsive states is only fair, because such patients have rigid and immature personalities, low stress tolerance, and poor insight. However, since they usually seek help earlier than many other psychiatric patients, about 50% of these patients do improve, especially if they can free their environment of any precipitating stress.

Causes

Obsessive-compulsive states seem to develop in certain personality types and under certain conditions. The person with an obsessional personality is usually rigid, conscientious, and has great aspirations; he takes responsibility seriously and finds decision-making difficult. He lacks creativity and the ability to find alternate solutions to his problems. One or both of his parents may have shown similar traits.

Obsessive-compulsive states develop slowly. For several years before overt illness begins, the patient can control his chronic obsessional preoccupation. Then some apparently trivial incident, often involving a clash between the patient's moral standards and his normal impulses, precipitates an acute onset of uncontrollable obsessive behavior.

Signs and symptoms

Obsessive-compulsive states characteristically produce obsessions, compulsions, and phobias leading to further anxiety. They cause a patient with such a disorder to complain that an unwanted, repetitive thought (obsession) keeps running through his mind. He often finds this thought (which may be an abstract idea or a negative impulse) unpleasant, frightening, or anxiety-provoking. He may analyze each thought or contemplated action in such detail

that he becomes incapacitated. Because of his underlying fears, he may also be preoccupied with unlikely dangers. For example, he may fear that a partially extinguished cigarette will start a house fire, and he will need to return to the house repeatedly to allay this fear. Or he may have a phobia (obsessive fear) of specific things, like closed places, venereal disease, insanity, or death. These fears lead the patient to compulsive actions to alleviate anxiety: ritualistic handwashing, placing objects in a certain order, or using a clean handkerchief to wipe off objects he touches. He may also show repetitive movements of the shoulders, arms, and hands, or facial spasms (tics).

Most obsessive-compulsive patients are tense, nervous, apprehensive. Usually, they recognize their rituals as irrational yet find them difficult to control, and may have acute anxiety attacks if others interfere with them. If untreated, ritualistic behavior eventually takes over their lives and makes normal function impossible.

Diagnosis

This diagnosis rests on evidence of compulsively repetitive patterns of thought or behavior. A careful history may identify previous obsessive-compulsive personality traits. Often, the patient's own description of his behavior offers the best clues to this diagnosis. However, he also needs evaluation for other psychiatric disorders, such as formal thought disorders (schizophrenia), confusion, disorientation, anxiety neurosis, and organic brain disease or other physical disorders. One difference between obsessive-compulsive states and schizophrenia, which may produce similar behavior patterns, is that schizophrenics have lower visible levels of anxiety.

Treatment
Treatment of obsessive-compulsive states aims to reduce anxiety, resolve inner conflicts, relieve depression, and teach more effective ways of dealing with stress. Such treatment (especially during an acute episode) may include a tranquilizer, such as meprobamate or chlordiazepoxide, and antidepressants or electroshock therapy, if the patient develops a secondary depressive reaction with suicidal tendency. But intensive long-term psychotherapy, brief supportive psychotherapy, or group therapy is the treatment of choice.

Additional considerations
Health care professionals can help by encouraging the patient to tell them his concerns and fears, and by offering him and his family support and reassurance. If the patient's compulsions interfere with his rest and with his meals, a strict daily schedule may satisfy his need for control and help provide adequate rest and nutrition.

The patient needs help to recognize his underlying fears, but he'll continue to need his ritualistic defenses until he feels strong enough to discard them. These rituals should be stopped only if they are dangerous to himself or others. Such intervention can precipitate an anxiety attack. To keep his compulsive behavior from interfering with the staff's daily routine, and to help redirect his actions and increase his self-esteem, he should be kept busy with special tasks requiring detailed efforts (for example, being the secretary or treasurer of a patient group).

If the patient needs a tranquilizer, he and his family should be warned that it may cause drowsiness, fatigue, ataxia, blurred vision, slurred speech, tremors, and hypotension. The patient must: avoid activities that require alertness until he can tolerate the tranquilizer's sedative effects; take the drug only as prescribed; and continue it as long as his doctor directs, since abrupt withdrawal may cause severe symptoms. Avoiding alcohol and any other CNS depressants is very important, since they potentiate the action of minor tranquilizers. Since tranquilizers may cause physical and psychologic dependence, the doctor must be notified if the patient elects to uses larger doses than the doctor prescribed.

Prevention
To prevent recurrence of the obsessive-compulsive state, the patient must understand the importance of developing better ways to cope with stress and anxiety. In addition, he may benefit from a maintenance dose of a minor tranquilizer and continued psychotherapy to reduce anxiety and make compulsive behavior unnecessary.

Hysteria

In hysterical states (hysterical neurosis, conversion hysteria, hysterical personality, dissociative reaction), the patient uses symptoms (conversion) to transfer emotional disturbances to body parts controlled by the voluntary nervous system. Thus hysteria can produce motor (paralysis) or sensory (blindness or deafness) disturbances; dissociative states, in which the patient experiences loss of consciousness or identity (fugue, amnesia, somnambulism, and multiple personality); and multiple and per-

sistent somatic symptoms, for which the patient seeks medical and surgical treatment. Hysteria tends to run in families, suggesting that it may be learned or inherited. It occurs mostly in women; less often in men. It usually begins in adolescence, in response to a definable emotional stress, and it ends when the precipitating stress subsides. Once hysteria is established, it tends to recur intermittently throughout a patient's lifetime, decreasing in frequency as the patient ages. Hysteria is most treatable if the patient is older at onset and previously well adjusted.

Causes

Although the exact cause of hysteria isn't known, two theories are widely accepted. The first is the classical, or Freudian, view: When a repressed experience or a sexual impulse (that the patient perceives as negative or anxiety-producing) conflicts with the patient's conscience, he converts the resulting anxiety into a physical symptom, which may be symbolic of the underlying mental conflict. For example, a man who wants to hit someone during an argument may develop hysterical paralysis of an arm, making the forbidden act impossible to carry out. Freud considered hysteria the result of psychic trauma in a patient who was genetically predisposed to developing it.

The second theory holds that hysteria is an escape from unsatisfactory interpersonal relationships and an attempt to satisfy unmet dependency needs. By being physically ill, the hysterical patient obtains secondary gains: sympathy, or relief from responsibility and work. When a man develops hysteria, he is often the victim of an industrial or an auto accident in which workers' compensation or other monetary or legal settlement is involved (compensation hysteria). Unlike the patient who malingers or consciously pretends to be ill to achieve a specific goal, the hysterical patient *unconsciously* relieves his anxiety through a physical illness.

Signs and symptoms

Typically, the hysterical patient is emotionally immature, unstable, and dependent. He shows a calm affect toward his illness (la belle indifference) and becomes extremely anxious when confronted with the fact that his illness has no physical basis. Such a patient may express hysteria

by conversion symptoms, dissociative states, or multiple vague somatic symptoms. Conversion symptoms include aphonia, blindness, tremors, paralysis, hemiplegia, and dramatic public seizures or convulsions. These seizures can be either generalized or localized; however, the patient experiences no aura, no hurtful fall, and no incontinence.

The patient with dissociative states has fugue (stupor-like states), amnesia (memory loss), or double or multiple personalities. In a fugue, which often follows a crisis, the patient wanders around for days, carrying out complex acts, such as taking a long trip, without remembering his past life. The patient with multiple personalities shows two or more different personalities with different values and behavior, with possible sudden shifts from one personality to another.

The patient with multiple vague somatic symptoms commonly complains of recurrent headaches and backaches or gastrointestinal disturbances, for which repeated physical examinations fail to establish an organic cause. Blurred vision, lump in the throat, dyspnea, palpitations, anxiety attacks, anorexia, nausea, vomiting, urinary retention, loss of libido, dyspareunia, menstrual irregularities, nervousness, and easy crying are all common complaints in such patients.

Some patients experience these somatic complaints in a definite, recognizable hysterical syndrome of pain, vomiting, or paralysis. These patients can have severe, hysterical pain, generalized or localized, in any part of the body. They overdramatize this pain, complain about it endlessly, but can't describe it clearly. Usually, they complain of lower abdominal pain and ten-

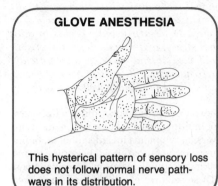

GLOVE ANESTHESIA

This hysterical pattern of sensory loss does not follow normal nerve pathways in its distribution.

derness, and vomiting after meals. Oddly enough, they don't usually lose weight, because they immediately become hungry and eat again. During pregnancy, such patients will vomit throughout the entire 9 months.

In hysterical paralysis, the extent of numbness reflects the patient's own knowledge of anatomy instead of known organic patterns of paralysis. This hysterical phenomenon is called paralysis with "stocking and glove" distribution. For instance, such a patient may experience numbness in both legs, from the knees down—a distribution of paralysis that's physiologically impossible.

Diagnosis

A reliable diagnosis of hysteria requires an accurate patient history, physical examination, and appropriate diagnostic tests to rule out other psychiatric and organic diseases with similar key symptoms (temporal lobe epilepsy, multiple sclerosis, brain tumor, parkinsonism, pernicious anemia, Ménière's disease, cortical blindness, myasthenia gravis, depression). For example, the neurologic workup on the blind hysterical patient will confirm blindness that is inconsistent with known anatomic principles and nerve patterns; that is, pupils continue to react to light, and the patient avoids harmful collisions with objects. Past medical history usually shows that he has been hospitalized and possibly has had surgery for similar somatic complaints, and that he has experienced recent stress. Often, his symptoms can be symbolically linked to the stress.

Special diagnostic tests may include an EEG, hypnosis, complete blood count and differential, urinalysis, and an EKG. A patient with conversion hysteria may be tested with I.V. amobarbital. Under its influence, psychogenic signs tend to disappear, while organic signs persist and may even be exaggerated.

Treatment

Correct treatment of hysteria provides immediate relief by removing symptoms through persuasion or hypnosis, and long-range control by helping the patient recognize the sources of his anxiety, so he can develop constructive ways of dealing with it. After symptoms subside, the doctor may order short-term therapy with small doses of benzodiazepines, such as chlordiazepoxide or diazepam, under strict supervision. Psychotherapy may also be helpful.

Additional considerations

If tranquilizers are prescribed for the patient, he must know that they may cause drowsiness, fatigue, ataxia, blurred vision, slurred speech, tremors, hypotension, and psychologic dependency. He should take the drug only as prescribed and not stop taking it without his doctor's guidance (abrupt withdrawal may cause severe symptoms). In addition, he must avoid hazardous tasks until he has developed a tolerance to the sedative effects, and avoid alcohol or other CNS depressants (they potentiate the action of minor tranquilizers).

Even though the hysterical patient has no organic illness, his function is really impaired. He should be treated as though he's been sick and is now getting well. Family members can reduce his anxiety by listening to him, by encouraging him, and by helping him to clarify his thoughts and feelings. Since he complains and makes excessive demands, he may make them feel hostile. Nevertheless, they should try to maintain a nonjudgmental attitude.

Hypochondriasis

Hypochondriasis is an exaggerated and obsessive concern about the body and health, with delusion of disease or bodily dysfunction. It's often associated with a multitude of symptoms and complaints that reflect real suffering—despite the absence of organic pathology. Hypochondriasis is fairly common and accounts for many of the patients who regularly visit general practitioners and outpatient clinics. It is usually chronic and unresponsive to treatment.

Causes

The source of hypochondriasis is a particularly high level of anxiety that the patient can't manage effectively. The patient with hypochondriasis displaces this anxiety onto body organs and gratifies his needs by magnifying the intensity of normal sensations, such as fatigue. Hypochondriasis can develop in the person who is narcissistic and egocentric and in the person with obsessive-compulsive traits, such as one who is unusually preoccupied with bodily health, fitness, dietary fads, and sometimes with elimination. It's often associated with mild depression and, when clearly related to endogenous depression, tends to subside when the depression lifts. Hypochondriasis is also associated with schizophrenia or, in the absence of other psychiatric symptoms, with recent recovery from severe illness, when the patient is temporarily preoccupied with his body. In women, hypochondriasis is most likely to appear transiently during the menopause, when regressive body functions and changing life conditions magnify stress.

Signs and symptoms

The most telling characteristics of hypochondriasis are persistent, multiple symptoms and detailed complaints that don't fit any specific pattern of disease, in an agitated person peculiarly preoccupied with his symptoms. These symptoms often include difficulty in swallowing or breathing, epigastric distress, bloating, belching, rectal pain, abdominal cramps and fullness, pressure in the genital organs, fatigue, backache, chest pains, and insomnia.

The patient with hypochondriasis attributes the symptoms he feels to a life-threatening disease and remains convinced he is ill, despite any number of negative examinations and laboratory tests. He finds his doctor's inability to find any disease depressing and frustrating—not reassuring—and persistently fears invalidism and death.

Diagnosis

The suspected hypochondriacal patient needs a thorough physical examination and appropriate laboratory studies to clearly rule out underlying organic disease. Usually, such examination shows no abnormality, or only insignificant signs of unrelated disease. But the most important diagnostic tool is a meticulously detailed health history. In some patients, such a history may reveal long-standing preoccupation with health problems and neurotically rigid personal habits related to food, elimination, or infection, but no other psychiatric symptoms. A careful health history is important in ruling out schizophrenia and underlying depression. Late-onset hypochondriasis is especially likely to obscure underlying depression unless the examiner asks carefully about the patient's mood, present capacity for work, and enjoyment of life.

Treatment

Treatment of hypochondriasis should include careful evaluation of symptoms, suitable measures to relieve distressing symptoms, and reassurance. For example, once he has ruled out organic disease, the doctor may prescribe a minor tranquilizer (such as chlordiazepoxide or clorazepate) to ease anxiety and may also refer the patient to a psychiatrist for treatment of underlying anxiety neuroses. But this kind of patient often resists such referral, and unless he has severe psychiatric symptoms, is usually managed by a general practitioner or an outpatient clinic.

Additional considerations
The patient with hypochondriasis feels real pain and distress, so the health care professional dealing with him shouldn't deny his symptoms or challenge his behavior. However, the professional should firmly state that the patient's medical tests were negative. Instead of reinforcing his symptoms, the professional should encourage him to discuss his other problems, and urge his family to do the same.

(If his family continues to reinforce the patient's hypochondriasis, family therapy may be necessary.)

If the patient is receiving a tranquilizer, both he and his family should know dosages, expected effects, and possible side effects; for example, drowsiness, fatigue, ataxia, blurred vision, slurred speech, tremors, and hypotension. While taking tranquilizers, the patient must avoid alcohol or other CNS depressants, since they may potentiate tranquilizer action.

The patient must be warned: to take the drug only as prescribed, since larger or more frequent doses may lead to dependence; to avoid hazardous tasks until he has a tolerance to the tranquilizer's sedative effects; and to continue the tranquilizer as his doctor directs, since abrupt withdrawal may be hazardous.

PERSONALITY DISORDERS

Paranoid Personality

The paranoid personality disorder is characterized by delusions of reference, influence, grandeur, morbid jealousy, or persecution. This disorder rarely develops before age 30; this age distinction separates paranoid personality from schizophrenia, which can occur much earlier. Paranoia occurs twice as often in women as in men, and has a higher incidence in immigrants and in urban populations than in natives and in rural populations. Prognosis is poor, because the paranoid patient seldom seeks treatment on his own; instead, relatives or friends urge him to seek help, because they find his actions and attitudes intolerable. Patients with this personality disorder represent 10% of psychiatric admissions in the United States.

Causes
Causes of paranoia include childhood predisposition, cultural factors, and physical trauma.

Many paranoid patients have a history of unrealistic parental expectations, unjust punishment, and punishment by withholding love. As children, they were constantly frustrated and grew up expecting hostility. As adults, they are wary, distrustful, and defensive; they find failure in competitive situations extremely painful. Because they regard failure as intolerable, they may eventually project the blame for it onto others. As their feelings of hostility and aggression grow, they become isolated and may develop a near-psychotic delusional system.

The high incidence of this disorder among immigrants, migrant workers, and other displaced people suggests a cultural factor. Possibly, the loneliness and isolation resulting from separation

---

PARANOID STATE VERSUS PARANOID SCHIZOPHRENIA
—Differential Diagnosis—

PARANOID STATE
- Delusional system reflects reality; well systematized
- Based on misinterpretations or elaborations of reality
- No hallucinations
- Affect and behavior normal

PARANOID SCHIZOPHRENIA
- Delusional system scattered, illogical, and poorly systematized
- No relationship to reality or real events
- Hallucinations possible
- Inconsistent and inappropriate affect
- Bizarre behavior

---

from the homeland encourage paranoid feelings in such groups. Studies have shown that if such displaced people return to their homelands, frequently their paranoia disappears.

Paranoia may also develop as a reaction to a physical deficit, such as a facial deformity, a crippling handicap, or deafness. In such cases, the patient begins to think that everyone is laughing at him or talking about him.

Signs and symptoms

The paranoid person is generally hostile and resentful. He is generally suspicious, insecure, and resents discipline. He is hypersensitive and tends to find hostility and evil intentions in others' innocuous or even kindly acts; he thinks that all society is "out to get him." He tends to be rigid, inflexible, and ambitious; he may be very efficient at his job because of his compulsive traits, but his efficiency is marred by jealousy and suspicion. He easily feels wronged, slighted, or ignored. He may think that the phone is tapped or that spies are watching him.

A person with paranoid personality disorder lacks a sense of humor and is often bitter or sarcastic. His criticism of others masks feelings of insecurity and inadequacy; he compensates for these feelings with an air of self-righteousness. These personality traits combine to make the paranoid person unlikable, and he is rejected by those around him, which tends to reinforce his delusions of persecution.

Diagnosis

The diagnosis of paranoid personality rests on evidence of delusions of persecution associated with hostility, suspiciousness, and resentfulness. A careful, in-depth history often provides the best clues to diagnosis, since these patients seldom seek treatment willingly.

They also need evaluation for hearing loss (since deafness may produce paranoid tendencies) and for paranoid schizophrenia.

Treatment

Treatment of paranoia can include psychotherapy and drug therapy, and aims to relieve the anxiety, hostility, suspicion, and fear that underlie the patient's delusions. Outpatient psychotherapy (group, family, or milieu) is generally more effective than hospitalization, since the paranoid patient tolerates restriction poorly. Drug therapy commonly includes tranquilizers, such as chlorpromazine, thioridazine, trifluoperazine, perphenazine, or promazine.

Additional considerations

If the patient needs a tranquilizer, he and his family should be warned that it may cause drowsiness, fatigue, ataxia, blurred vision, slurred speech, tremors, and hypotension. He will have to avoid activities that require alertness until he can tolerate the tranquilizer's sedative effects. In addition, he should take the drug only as prescribed and continue taking it as his doctor directs, since abrupt withdrawal may cause severe distress. Alcohol and other CNS depressants should be avoided, since they potentiate the action of tranquilizers. Tranquilizers may cause physical and psychologic dependence. If the patient begins to take larger doses than the doctor prescribed, the doctor should be notified.

By being open and nonjudgmental, health care professionals and the patient's family may be able to gain the patient's trust and confidence. To do so, they should speak to him in clear, simple language that he can't misinterpret. They should also minimize the patient's contact with people whom he imagines are plotting against him. Contact with such people may reinforce his delusions.

Attempts to reason with the patient or talk him out of his fears are useless (although his fears and delusions should be acknowledged). His attention should be redirected to activities such as ceramics, or crossword or jigsaw puzzles. When his delusions are active, care must be taken to prevent him from hurting himself or others.

If the patient imagines he's being poisoned, he may refuse to eat. Serving food in original containers, letting him prepare his own meals, or having another person eat with him may help.

A patient who's afraid to sleep for fear of being attacked may benefit from a tranquilizer with strong sedative effects.

Schizoid Personality

Schizoid (schizothymic) personality disorder is characterized by withdrawn, eccentric, or aloof behavior and failure to interact with others and form relationships because of insecurity and a fear of being hurt. This personality disorder may occur alone or with other neuroses or psychoses. For example, it appears in 40% of schizophrenics before the onset of their psychosis, but not all schizoid patients develop schizophrenia.

Prognosis is good, and patients can usually live in a community setting.

Causes
The cause of schizoid personality is unknown, but it commonly runs in families. However, it's not clear whether an inherited factor predisposes a person to the disease, or whether stilted childhood relationships with schizoid family members are to blame. In any event, at an early age the schizoid patient learns to deal with stress by withdrawing from other people.

Signs and symptoms
The schizoid patient is a loner: cold, aloof, and withdrawn. He's preoccupied with his own thoughts and feelings but is unwilling or unable to express himself or develop close relationships with others. He often prefers daydreaming to facing reality and may exhibit signs of depression. He may complain of feeling depressed or isolated (he has few friends), or of losing interest in his family or the world around him.

Diagnosis
Observation of schizoid behavior patterns supports this diagnosis. A careful family history (including interviews with family members) can provide further evidence. Schizophrenia, paranoid personality, and depression must be carefully ruled out.

Treatment and additional considerations
Psychotherapy is the standard treatment for the schizoid patient. It's successful only if the patient recognizes his disorder and cooperates. Through psychotherapy the schizoid patient may gain enough insight into his maladaptive be-

havior patterns to attempt to change them. But his progress is usually slow. Treatment is most successful when the patient develops a trusting, long-term relationship with one therapist; it's least successful in severe cases, when the patient is completely withdrawn. Young children with the disorder may become more social and less isolated during therapy, but this improvement may be temporary.

During treatment, such a patient needs help learning to trust others. Health care professionals should try to establish a balanced emotional relationship with him: not too close, not too distant. They also should follow up on their promises to him, and encourage him to express his feelings (even hostility or frustration). The patient should be assigned just one primary nurse. When she goes off duty at the end of her shift, she should introduce her replacement so the patient won't feel abandoned.

Passive-aggressive Personality

Passive aggression (passive dependence, aggression) is a personality trait disturbance characterized by avoidance of normal, healthy, open expression of feelings, especially confrontation, anger, or hostility. It's not always a serious disorder; however, it may interfere with the patient's life-style, since his behavior makes others resent him and want to avoid him.

Causes
The cause of passive-aggressive personality is probably purely psychosocial. It may be the result of not being allowed, as a child, to directly confront one's parents in an emotionally healthy way. The fathers of many passive-aggressive and aggressive patients were domineering, demanding, rigid, unapproachable, and hard to please; and aggressive patients were often openly hostile to their fathers.

Signs and symptoms
The patient with this disorder hasn't attained mature emotional development and attempts to manipulate others in one of three ways: by being passive-dependent, passive-aggressive, or aggressive. The passive-dependent patient is not self-confident or self-reliant; instead, he behaves childishly and leans on others for support and approval. Unconsciously hostile, he is mild, timid, and fearful on the surface, and withdraws from situations that will likely produce negative emotions such as anger or hostility. Through this behavior, he directs attention to himself, or controls others or the situation around him.

The passive-aggressive patient is stubborn, sullen, inefficient, and tends to procrastinate, while appearing to cooperate. He doesn't work well with others and tends to have a demoralizing effect on the group. Instead of confronting others openly, he accomplishes his goals by subversion.

The aggressive patient reacts to frustration with irritability, aggression, and even destructiveness. He tends to be hostile and antagonistic, demands special attention, and assumes authority he doesn't deserve, especially with authority figures. This type of patient uses his aggressiveness to hide marked dependency needs.

Diagnosis
Diagnosis of passive-aggressive personality rests on evidence of manipulative behavior, such as indecisiveness requiring assistance from others; unusual passivity or timidity (passive-dependent); sullenness, stubbornness, or chronic complaining (passive-aggressive); and inappropriate or chronic irritability, aggression, and temper tantrums (aggressive).

TYPICAL PASSIVE-AGGRESSIVE STATEMENTS

"I don't want you to be mad at me, but you aren't giving me the kind of attention I need."

"I know you've lost ten pounds, and you look pretty good. Still, you've got 50 more pounds to go."

"I don't mean to be critical, but you're late with my lunch."

"I'm a top-level executive at my company, and I don't have time to lie around here while these medical people try to figure out what's wrong with me."

Treatment
Intensive psychotherapy is of limited value, because the passive-aggressive patient seldom comes to treatment willingly, requires treatment for a long time, and gains insight slowly. Group therapy is beneficial for this patient, because the group gives support but doesn't tolerate excessive manipulation.

Additional considerations
In a hospital setting, a passive-aggressive patient tends to be disruptive and demand special attention and care. The staff should try to extablish a trusting relationship with the patient, and use behavior modification techniques and patience when dealing with him.

The patient needs to know limits for acceptable behavior. These may be formalized in a contract and should be consistently enforced by the staff. He should be confronted directly with the consequences of his actions, and alternative patterns of behavior should be discussed with him. Additionally, he should be encouraged to openly express anger and negative opinions.

Sociopathic/Psychopathic Personality
(Antisocial personality, constitutional psychopathic state)

The patient with sociopathic/psychopathic personality is grossly impulsive and demands immediate gratification through behavior that usually goes against the mores, laws, and customs of society. He resists rehabilitation and chronically repeats his socially unacceptable, and sometimes illegal, actions. Incidence is high among males, especially in minority, socially deprived, or low-income groups. Prognosis is poor, because the sociopath sees nothing wrong with his behavior. Under pressure he may promise to improve but soon reneges. Sociopathic behavior may level off at ages 40 to 50, perhaps as a result of maturation, but many sociopaths remain maladjusted throughout life.

Causes
Although the cause of sociopathic/psychopathic personality is unknown, many consider it a lifelong pattern that begins in childhood but is often not recognized until the patient is in his 20s (2% to 7% are identified in the court system). Studies show a high correlation of incidence of sociopathic behavior between twins and between fathers and sons.

Factors in upbringing have bearing on sociopathic behavior. For instance, the parents of many sociopathic patients were indifferent or hostile to them as children. Such deprived children became narcissistic, never learning empathy or sympathy. Lack of clearly defined authority figures, and of mutual trust and respect among family members, led to confusion. Another recurring factor in the history of the sociopath is inconsistent parental response; the same action received disapproval at one time, and indifference or even approval at another. From this the child learned that his actions had no bearing on the way he was treated, and that he need not be held responsible for his behavior. In some cases, the parents may even have derived vicarious pleasure from the child's antisocial behavior.

Signs and symptoms

The sociopath is a social misfit, lacking the ability to adjust normally to life. In his search for instant gratification, he engages in socially unacceptable activities, such as alcohol and drug abuse, and tends to be sexually promiscuous. Superficially charming and usually intelligent, he is completely self-centered, unable to tolerate frustration, and capable of violence or other criminal behavior. He is amoral and irresponsible, and he lacks the capacity for normal emotional responses, including guilt or remorse. Typically, such a person has a long history of sociopathic behavior, such as rebelliousness, temper tantrums, or cruelty to animals or children, even in childhood. As a teenager, he was destructive, sneaky, stubborn, or defiant; he repeatedly ran away from home and almost invariably had school problems.

Diagnosis

Evidence of lifelong antisocial behavior patterns confirms this diagnosis. Such evidence comes from a careful family history and observation that may reveal information about home environment, family interaction, and peer group influences. Of course, the patient suspected of sociopathic personality also needs evaluation for other physical illnesses, such as epilepsy and hyperkinesis; for other psychiatric illness or mental retardation; or for injury resulting from his impulsive and sometimes violent actions.

Treatment

Treatment of the sociopathic personality aims to eliminate the patient's destructive, harmful, or socially unacceptable behavior, and to encourage the formation of trust and emotional warmth. Psychotherapy is of limited value, because such a patient seldom seeks treatment on his own; instead, such treatment is imposed by relatives or legal authorities. Effective psychotherapy often requires long-term placement in an institution or a group residential environment. During such long-term care, the patient should receive emotional support and reassurance, with firmly applied pressure to conform to acceptable behavior patterns, using rewards and withdrawal of rewards for behavior modification. At the same time, treatment can include antidepressants (amitriptyline), phenothiazines (chlorpromazine) or minor tranquilizers (diazepam).

Especially if the patient is young, the family may be the source of abnormal behavior. If so, all the family members should receive treatment; if they refuse treatment, the child should be removed from them temporarily.

Additional considerations

If a sociopath is hospitalized, he'll use his charm to try to manipulate other patients and the hospital staff; or he'll try to set staff, family, or other patients against one another to get what he wants. Frequent meetings with the family and other staff members should be held; an exchange of information may eliminate this problem. Other patients need protection from him; he will readily supply them with drugs, alcohol, or dangerous objects. Staff members must be calm and impartial when dealing with the sociopath. They need to set limits on his behavior, perhaps by making a contract with him, and enforce these limits consistently. When explaining procedures, they should answer questions briefly and simply. Lengthy explanations may lead to temper tantrums on his part or undesirable concessions by the staff. The patient's manipulative or abusive behavior reflects mental illness. Remembering this may help staff and family to avoid feeling angry, offended, or hurt.

PSYCHOSES

Manic-depressive Illness
(Manic-depressive reaction or psychosis)

Manic-depressive illness is marked by pathologic mood swings from euphoria to sadness, by spontaneous recoveries, and by a tendency to recur. The cyclic (bipolar) form consists of separate episodes of mania (elation) and depression; however, either the manic or the depressive episodes can be predominant, producing few, if any, mood swings. When depression is the predominant mood, the patient has the unipolar form of the disease. The overall incidence is 1% to 2% in the general population. Manic-depressive illness occurs twice as often in women as in men and is more common in higher socioeconomic groups. It can begin any time after adolescence, but most first attacks occur in persons 20 to 35 years old. Peak onset is at age 30 for the bipolar form and at 50 for the unipolar. Manic-depressive illness recurs in 80% of patients; as they grow older, the attacks of illness recur more frequently and last longer. Twenty percent of these patients die as a result of suicide; many, just as the depression lifts.

Causes

The exact cause of manic-depressive illness isn't known, but hereditary, biologic, and psychologic factors may play a part. Although a hereditary factor has never been proven, 10% to 15% of parents, siblings, and children of patients with the bipolar form also develop the manic-depressive illness. The bipolar form is probably transmitted by a dominant sex-linked gene. A higher incidence in females also suggests a sex-linked genetic cause. Other familial influences, especially the early loss of a parent and other childhood problems, seem to predispose a person to this illness, especially the unipolar type.

Emotional or physical trauma may precede the onset of manic-depressive illness, but most often it appears with no easily identified precipitating factors. Lack of mature personality development and an inability to love (similar to that of obsessive-compulsive patients) may predispose the patient to this illness.

Although certain biochemical changes accompany mood swings, it's not clear whether these changes cause the mood swings or result from them. In both mania and depression, intracellular sodium concentration increases; these levels fall to normal after recovery. In depression, brain catecholamines decrease; in mania, they increase. These changes can accompany abnormal adrenal steroid levels and other metabolic anomalies.

Signs and symptoms

Both the manic and the depressive phases of manic-depressive illness produce characteristic mood swings and other behavioral and physical changes. The depressive phase (manic-depressive, psychotic, or endogenous depression; involutional melancholia) has a rapid onset and progression. In this phase, the patient experiences loss of self-esteem and overwhelming feelings of inertia, hopelessness, and despondency. He appears withdrawn and apathetic. He usually feels worse in the morning, often awakening early after restless sleep. He may also have anorexia, causing weight loss of 20 lb (9 kg) or more, and may become constipated. He may also show psychomotor retardation (slow movement and slow speech, with low vocal tones and one-word answers) and difficulty in concentrating, usually without disorientation or intellectual impairment.

The depressed patient may also express hypochondriacal concern over somatic complaints such as constipation, fatigue, pressure in the head or chest, and heaviness in the limbs. He may feel guilt and self-reproach over trivial past events and, in severe cases, may have delusions of being wicked or persecuted, a disgrace to his family. Suicide is an ever present risk in such patients, especially in the early phase of depression and during recovery. Before killing himself, the patient may kill his family to spare them agony and disgrace.

The manic phase of the illness (acute mania) is less common than the depressive. In half the cases, the patient is depressed for a few days just before he enters this manic phase, but then his mood changes, bringing a sense of well-being, more self-confidence, and more energy. As his mood escalates to mania, he becomes overactive and excessively talkative (although his speech may be incoherent and contain numerous disparate ideas), but he also has periods of rationality and insight. In acute mania, he loses inhibitions and may make tactless remarks and inappropriate sexual advances that damage his relationships with others. He may forget to eat and sleep, and becomes easily exhausted. Although he appears happy, he may become abruptly hostile if his grand schemes are hindered or his views questioned. As mania subsides, he may become depressed and is at slight risk for suicide.

Hypomania, a moderate mood elevation, is more common than acute mania. It too causes patients to be elated, overactive, easily distracted, talkative, irritable, impatient, impulsive, and full of energy but doesn't induce flight of ideas or delusions. Luckily, hyperacute (delirious) mania, the most severe form, is rare. The patient with hyperacute mania is totally incoherent and uncontrollable, has hallucinations and delusions, has no insight into his illness, and may be incontinent (both urine and feces).

The duration and course of manic-depressive illness vary, but the typical manic episode lasts from 3 to 6 months; the typical depressive episode from 6 to 9 months. These episodes alternate, and transition from one episode to another may bring an interim normal period. Recovery from each episode is usually complete, but fluctuating mania and chronic depression may occasionally persist, especially in elderly persons.

Diagnosis

Evidence of pathologic mood swings from elation to sadness confirms manic-depressive illness. Careful history may identify previous mood swings or a family history of manic-depressive illness. Nevertheless, the patient needs careful physical evaluation to rule out intra-abdominal neoplasm, hypothyroidism, cardiac failure, cerebral arteriosclerosis, parkinsonism, brain tumor, and uremia; and for drug-induced depression, since antihypertensives, such as reserpine and methyldopa, and oral contraceptives can induce clinical depression in an otherwise healthy person. Amphetamine addiction may cause mania; alcohol abuse may cause depression or result from it.

The diagnosis should distinguish between depression of manic-depressive illness and neurotic depression. Both produce anxiety, crying, and self-pity, but the manic-depressive patient shows psychomotor retardation and persistent delusions and guilt feelings. Another telling difference: before onset, the manic-depressive patient is characteristically warm, energetic, and outgoing; whereas the neurotically depressed patient is unstable and rigid. Furthermore, the depression of manic-depressive illness usually has no known cause; but neurotic depression often follows recent loss and bereavement. The depressed manic-depressive feels worse in the morning; the neurotically depressed person, worse in the afternoon. Also, the depressed manic-depressive patient may experience anxiety and agitation severe enough to suggest anxiety neurosis.

Manic-depressive illness may also be confused with schizophrenia. An aggressive, irritable manic-depressive patient experiencing mania with delusions of persecution but no readily apparent mood elevation, is often misdiagnosed as schizophrenic, but distinguishing signs do exist. For example, the manic patient shows greater activity, infectious happiness, and thought content consistent with mood elevation; the schizophrenic patient shows withdrawal from reality, emotional incongruity, incoherent thoughts, and bizarre behavior. While the manic-depressive patient relates to others fairly easily, the schizophrenic patient cannot. Although depressive symptoms may develop during the onset of schizophrenia, true schizophrenic symptoms soon dominate.

Treatment and additional considerations

Long-term treatment with lithium carbonate may control recurrent manic episodes; long-term use of tricyclic antidepressants (TCAs) may control recurrence of unipolar depression. Drugs, electroshock (electroconvulsive or ECT) therapy (especially in the depressive phase), psychotherapy, and short-term hospitalization may all be useful during acute episodes of illness.

During the depressive phase, treatment aims to relieve depression and accompanying physical and psychomotor symptoms; during the manic phase, to control hyperactive behavior and ensure adequate supervision, rest, hydration, and nutrition.

To help relieve severe depression, the doctor may order a tricyclic antidepressant, such as imipramine or amitriptyline. If these fail, phenelzine or tranylcypromine (MAOIs) may be effective. TCAs and MAOIs are seldom used together due to possible drug interactions. If insomnia persists despite the sedative effects of the tricyclic antidepressant, a sedative may be appropriate.

Psychotherapy can also help relieve depression, but deep, probing psychotherapy may aggravate the patient's depression and is contraindicated until the depression lifts. To prevent possible suicide, health care professionals or his family should remove harmful objects from the patient's environment (glass, belts, rope, bobby pins), observe him closely but unobtrusively, and strictly supervise his medications.

The depressed patient needs continual positive reinforcement to improve his self-esteem. He should be encouraged to talk, or to write down his feelings if he has trouble expressing them orally. He should be listened to attentively and respectfully, and allowed time to formulate his thoughts. A structured routine, including activities to increase his confidence and interaction with others (for instance, group therapy), should be provided, along with repeated assurances that his depression *will* lift. All observations and appropriate conversations with the patient should be recorded, since these are valuable for evaluating his condition.

Such a patient's physical needs must not be neglected. If he's too depressed to care for himself, he'll need help with personal hygiene. He may also need help and encouragement to eat. If he's constipated, high-fiber foods should be added to his diet. Small, frequent feedings and physical activity will also help.

If drug treatment fails, the doctor may order ECT, in which an electric current, passed through the temporal lobe, produces a grand mal seizure. Such therapy usually brings a dramatic improvement after only one or two treatments and paves the way for psychotherapy. A course of ECT usually includes two to three treatments per week for 3 to 4 weeks.

Before each ECT, the patient is given a sedative, and a nasal or oral airway is inserted. Afterward, the patient may be drowsy and have transient amnesia, but usually within 30 minutes, he should be alert, with a good memory.

During the manic phase of manic-depressive illness, a patient usually resists treatment, because he feels well and lacks insight into his condition. However, he may need hospitalization during this phase to prevent exhaustion. During the acute manic phase, the doctor may

DRUG PRECAUTIONS
DURING MANIC-DEPRESSIVE ILLNESS

Tricyclic antidepressants (TCAs)

• Because TCA may cause drowsiness and fatigue, the patient should take the drug only as prescribed by the doctor, and avoid hazardous tasks until he can tolerate its sedative effects. If the patient's drowsiness persists, the doctor may prescribe a single daily dose at bedtime.
• The patient must avoid using alcohol and should use other CNS depressants only as the doctor prescribes.
• If the patient's been taking large doses for a long time, the patient must not discontinue the drug without the doctor's guidance. Abrupt withdrawal may cause severe nausea and headache.
• The patient should expect a lag time of 10 days to a month before the antidepressant effects begin; however, the following side effects may occur within 24 hours: dry mouth, urinary retention, blurred vision, tachycardia, arrhythmias, sweating, dizziness, and hallucinations.
• TCAs are contraindicated in males with prostatic hypertrophy and are very seldom used with MAO inhibitors, due to possible drug interactions.

MAO inhibitors (MAOIs)

• A patient taking an MAOI must not eat foods containing tryptophan, tyramine, vasopressors, or caffeine. For example, he must avoid cheese, especially strong or aged; sour cream; beer, chianti, or sherry; pickled herring; liver; canned figs; raisins, bananas, or avocados; chocolate; soy sauce; fava beans; yeast extracts; meat tenderizers; coffee. These foods may cause severe hypertension.
• The patient's blood pressure must be monitored at the beginning and throughout MAOI therapy. Phentolamine must be available to treat hypertensive crisis.
• To avoid dizziness, the patient should sit up for at least a minute before attempting to get out of bed, and then rise slowly. He should lie down or squat if he feels dizzy or faint.
• The patient must not discontinue medication without a doctor's guidance, since abrupt withdrawal may cause severe symptoms; he must also avoid combining MAOIs with any other medications, especially over-the-counter cold, hay fever, or weight-reducing medications.
• The patient should expect a lag time of 1 to 3 weeks before antidepressant effects begin.
• MAOIs are rarely given with TCAs, due to possible drug interactions.
• Any patient taking antidepressants should be closely supervised. He may attempt suicide when his depression lifts.

Lithium carbonate

• Lithium carbonate is used cautiously with haloperidol, (the patient must be observed for early signs of encephalopathy, such as lethargy or fever), diuretics, sodium bicarbonate, and I.V. solutions containing sodium chloride.
• The patient's daily salt intake must remain constant. He should be observed for excessive perspiration, vomiting, or diarrhea.
• Fluid intake and output, and serum electrolyte levels must be monitored closely, since lithium interferes with ADH and is contraindicated in fluid or electrolyte imbalance.
• The patient must be watched for side effects (fine tremor, orthostatic hypotension, polyuria, nausea, and diarrhea) and early signs of toxicity (coarse tremor, slurred speech, nystagmus, drowsiness, and ataxia).
• The patient should avoid hazardous tasks until drug response is determined and should carry a Medic-Alert card.
• The patient shouldn't stop taking the drug abruptly without doctor's supervision.

order chlorpromazine or haloperidol. However, haloperidol should be used cautiously in a patient who takes lithium. Chlorpromazine and haloperidol are sometimes given with an antiparkinson agent, such as benztropine, to prevent dystonic and extrapyramidal reactions. After this acute manic phase subsides, these drugs are reduced to maintenance levels and combined with lithium carbonate.

The manic patient's physical needs require special attention. He may need encouragement to eat, especially if he jumps up and walks around the room after every mouthful. If he is reminded to eat, he may sit down again. Short naps during the day, and help with personal hygiene may be necessary. He needs emotional support, a calm environment, and realistic goals for his behavior. Activities suited to the patient's short attention span should be provided, and he must avoid overextending himself. When necessary, the patient should be reoriented to reality, and tactfully diverted when conversations become intimately involved with other patients or staff members. Treatment sometimes includes ECT, but this is less effective for mania than for depression; the results are better with frequent treatments.

Schizophrenia

Schizophrenia refers to a group of psychotic states (paranoid, hebephrenic, catatonic, and simple) marked mainly by withdrawal into self and failure to distinguish reality from fantasy. It begins insidiously or suddenly, usually between the ages of 12 and 40, and is most often chronic, although it can be acute.

The schizophrenic suffers from personality disorganization that severely handicaps his usually already difficult social relations, causing extreme withdrawal into a self-contained world where no guidelines prevail for reality testing. As a result, his communications with others are highly idiosyncratic and often bizarrely inappropriate, making sense only to himself.

Prognosis varies according to onset, observable precipitating factors, conscious anxiety, prepsychotic personality, general attitude, affect, presence or absence of hopelessness and depression, content of hallucinations and delusions, and nature of treatment. Adolescent schizophrenics rarely recover completely. Schizophrenics with close, personal relationships have social skills that improve their prognosis.

Causes
Schizophrenia probably results from a combination of biochemical, psychologic, and sociologic factors. It is the psychosis that most often causes institutionalization. Approximately 1% of the U.S. population is schizophrenic. Research into fundamental causes has been controversial because of significant differences in theoretical approaches, and has failed to isolate a single cause.

Signs and symptoms
In a schizophrenic patient, the first signs of illness may be neurotic symptoms of fatigue, insomnia, and headache. Later, he loses interest in his life, despite a preoccupation with physical well-being or some detail of his appearance, and may concentrate obsessively on a specific problem. He begins to have ideas of reference; events and objects have special meaning or relation for him. Eventually, he experiences bouts of confusion, excitement, or agitation, and he's increasingly incapable of abstract thought, becoming progressively more literal-minded, and displaying concrete thinking. His visual and auditory perceptions are distorted (illusions). He has hallucinations and delusions that are often negative, because he imagines others

think badly of him or want to persecute him and control his thoughts and actions. The schizophrenic substitutes puns, rhymes, and alliterations (clang) for ordinary conversation. He may abruptly make unusual and unexpected life-altering decisions. Interestingly, his overall behavior may seem normal, despite his abnormal ideas.

The most telling sign of schizophrenia is an apparently inexplicable personality change, causing dramatic mood swings and strange emotional responses. The schizophrenic's behavior may show regression and include deterioration in living habits; routine and stereotypical actions without purpose; impulsive gestures, strange mannerisms, or contorted facial expressions; loss of concentration and memory; disorientation; odd speech habits (neologism, mutism, blocking, evasion, clang, echolalia, word-salad, verbigeration, and perseveration). However, no single patient displays all these symptoms.

Paranoid schizophrenic

The paranoid schizophrenic shows less regression of mental faculties, emotional response, and behavior than is common in other forms of schizophrenia. He is fearful and suspicious, and projects his negative feelings about himself onto others. His delusions are systematized according to a scientific, philosophic, or theologic structure consistent with his perceptions of himself. These delusions reflect his cultural, familial, and socioeconomic background and may become disordered. Such delusions are often rooted in hostility and aggression, and may cause the schizophrenic to think himself persecuted; to believe great, near-cosmic things of himself; to be hypochondriacal; or to think himself transformed, controlled, or poisoned.

Paranoid schizophrenia is the most common form of schizophrenia. It's usually diagnosed later in life in highly intelligent people, whose prognosis is reasonably good. Paranoid schizophrenics with a single delusion are called monosymptomatic. In exceptional cases, they're dangerous, often perpetrating unmotivated crimes. But because of their single delusion, their prognosis is good.

Hebephrenic schizophrenic

The hebephrenic has the most severely disorganized personality and has no contact with reality; his world is all fantasy. His mannerisms are manic and bizarre, and he's absorbed by trivial preoccupations. He is more often a hypochondriac than the paranoid schizophrenic, and more likely to have grandiose delusions. Generally, his delusions are poorly systematized, kinesthetic, and concerned with body image. (He may think his brain is shrinking, for example.) His hallucinations are pleasurable and frequent, causing inappropriate giggling and laughing. At the same time, he's depressed, appearing apathetic and detached. His personal habits so deteriorate that he exhibits grotesque infantilism and needs excessive personal care.

The onset of hebephrenic schizophrenia is insidious and usually begins in adolescence. Once established, it brings rapid and progressive personality disintegration. Hebephrenic schizophrenia carries a *very* poor prognosis.

Catatonic schizophrenic

The catatonic schizophrenic's most outstanding characteristic is his overwhelming failure of will (negativity); he's literally incapable of motion for long periods and can maintain rigid and contorted postures (catatonic stupor). However, current drug therapy makes this stuporous phase rare. The catatonic is usually obedient, easily following someone else's will. But in an agitated phase, he does the opposite of what he's told and may become uncontrollable, pacing, shouting, and being generally destructive. He avoids new activities and shows no spontaneity, but he may perform repetitious actions that have special meaning for him. Generally, he can't communicate his delusions and hallucinations to the therapist until he begins to improve. These delusions tend to be cosmic: "The sky is falling." He may

CHILDHOOD SCHIZOPHRENIA

Schizophrenic reactions that occur before the age of puberty (12 years) are included in this group; some children have these reactions as early as ages 2 to 3.

Schizophrenic children may be confused and anxious but may be responsive to those who are taking care of them and to their environment. Usually, they've learned to talk but don't always feel the need to communicate. When they do speak, their language isn't always meaningful. These children aren't able to differentiate between what's real and what isn't. Those who become ill when they're very young aren't able to distinguish themselves from others around them (autistic tendency) and are usually hospitalized.

A health care professional involved with a schizophrenic child must work to establish a loving, secure, accepting relationship with him. The professional can help him distinguish his own body from those of others. Only after he begins to improve or to develop *some* concept of himself, is it advisable to involve him in a daily routine. One goal is to provide time intervals for when he rests and when he works or plays. Another important goal is to have such a child learn to eat, dress, and bathe himself. His family may need family counseling.

make monosyllabic responses and uses echolalia and neologisms. His handwriting is usually exceptionally disorganized and peculiar, even for a schizophrenic; its characters are exotic and often indecipherable.

Acute catatonic patients are the most likely to recover completely; chronic catatonics generally continue to regress.

Simple schizophrenic

The simple schizophrenic lacks the irrational thoughts common to other schizophrenics; indeed, he lacks abstract thought entirely. Consequently, he doesn't suffer delusions, hallucinations, ideas of reference, or other such obvious

symptoms. Simple schizophrenia begins in early childhood, and its onset is usually slow and insidious; rarely, acute. The patient who develops this form of schizophrenia suffers total physical and emotional withdrawal and may never be hospitalized or formally treated. He's much more likely to be quietly tolerated by his family, playing the role of the strange, withdrawn relative. Without a family, he may become a street person or a chronic drifter, never forming permanent attachments.

Diagnosis

Diagnosis must first rule out organic brain and metabolic disorders, and psychiatric disorders such as manic-depression, asocial personality, and psychoneurosis. Then, the most critical aspect of diagnosis is recognizing a *constellation* of symptoms (psychologic, intellectual, behavioral) that correspond to the patient's overall presentation. A diagnosis of schizophrenia requires the presence of one or more of the following mental aberrations: loose associations, changes in affect (inappropriate moods, actions, or responses), ambivalence (inability to make decisions because two opposite wishes exist at the same time), and autism (withdrawal, total fantasy, or narcissism). No psychologic tests clearly confirm schizophrenia, but some tests help the therapist get a better overall assessment of the patient, his family, and his background to evaluate borderline or doubtful cases. The most commonly used tests are the Rorschach test, Thematic Apperception Test (TAT), Wechsler Adult Intelligence Scale (WAIS), and the Minnesota Multiphasic Personality Inventory (MMPI). However, the contemporary drug and counter cultures have sometimes confused the division between schizophrenic and nonschizophrenic young people.

Treatment

The prescribed treatment for schizophrenia is directly linked to the therapist's theory about what causes it. Most psychiatrists tend to prescribe drug therapy initially for the schizophrenic rather than recommend long-term psychotherapy. However, treatment varies greatly and is very often controversial. Don't be surprised if two similar schizophrenic patients with different therapists receive totally opposite treatment. Drug therapy is usually restricted to phenothiazines, such as trifluoperazine and chlorpromazine. When phenothiazines fail, other antipsychotics, like haloperidol, are used instead. Other forms of therapy include behavioral therapy, based on operant conditioning (most effective in acute schizophrenia); electroshock (electroconvulsive) therapy (ECT) (most effective in stuporous catatonics); psychosurgery (lobotomy); and psychotherapy. Psychosurgery is rarely performed, and improved drug therapy makes ECT increasingly unpopular.

Additional considerations

When caring for a schizophrenic patient, members of the hospital staff must stay in touch with their own feelings, and react honestly to the patient's behavior. (Honest responses are best; otherwise, the patient's undesirable behavior may be reinforced.)

Staff members should not try to talk a patient out of his delusions or hallucinations; nor should they compel the patient to reason with them. Instead, they should deal with his feelings while reinforcing reality. For example, a staff member might say, "I don't see the bugs, but I understand that you're afraid."

Staff members must use discretion when talking within the hearing of a schizophrenic patient. Even a catatonic patient can hear.

Care for the schizophrenic patient also includes:
• providing chewing gum or hard candy to relieve dry mouth caused by drug therapy, and watching for drug side effects, particularly orthostatic hypotension. The patient *and his family* must know about the drugs' side effects and the perils of combining the prescribed drugs with other drugs or alcohol.
• establishing and maintaining communication with the patient.
• undertaking reality orientation, when appropriate.
• providing adequate safety precautions.
• supervising occupational and recreational activities.
• assisting at mealtimes, because the patient may be too distracted or disinterested to feed himself.
• helping the patient maintain personal hygiene.
• *observing, assessing,* and *documenting* whenever possible.

MISCELLANEOUS DISORDERS

Infantile Autism

Infantile autism is a syndrome beginning in infancy and marked by extreme withdrawal, unresponsiveness, and severely impaired speech. Some autistic children can't participate in any organized routine, while others have an obsessive need for a rigidly uniform environment. About one third of autistic children show moderate social adaptation by age 15. However, most of those who can function socially are persistently considered somewhat peculiar. Outlook for improvement is best if they can be taught to use meaningful speech before age 5; improvement after that is rare.

Causes and incidence

The causes of infantile autism remain unclear but are thought to include both mental and physical factors. The autistic child's parents are commonly intelligent, educated people of high socioeconomic

TREATMENT GOALS IN INFANTILE AUTISM

To help the autistic child, the health care professional (or other adult) should:
• encourage and document interaction with adults. Any response by the child, no matter how tentative, should be acknowledged quickly and warmly. If the child is especially responsive to one adult, contact between them should be maintained on a regular schedule.
• encourage interaction with other children. Spontaneous play should be allowed, but the children must be supervised and protected from excessive roughness. The adult should help resolve conflicts by presenting alternatives.
• discourge withdrawn, repetitive behavior. The adult can try distracting him by rolling a ball with him, or encouraging him to join group activity. At times, joining the child in repetitive behavior, such as rocking, may help.
• discourage self-destructive behavior. When the adult observes an attempt at self-injury, he should express concern and stop the activity. If he can't stop it, restraints may be necessary.
• encourage self-care skills, such as dressing and washing. The adult needs to give the child time to help with these activities, and praise the child for doing so. The child must learn that he's responsible for basic self-care.
• discourage the obsessive need for uniformity. The child has to learn to accept changes in his surroundings or daily routine. If changes provoke a temper tantrum, the child must be encouraged to try the new activity or investigate changes in his surroundings.
• ensure adequate nutrition. The child should be given a variety of foods at meals, and allowed to eat what he wants. Vitamins must be provided daily.
• encourage verbal and nonverbal communication. All words the child uses should be recorded, noting clarity and context. When the child talks, the adult should respond quickly and completely. Nonverbal clues need to be clarified verbally. For example, if the child points to the door, the adult should say, "You want to go outside, don't you?"

status. Parents' behavior toward their autistic child may appear distant and lack affection. However, because autistic children are clearly "different" from birth, and because they are unresponsive or respond negatively to touch and attention, parental remoteness may be a reaction to this disorder, not a cause. Autistic children often show abnormal but nonspecific EEG findings, suggesting that brain damage or other brain defect may play a part.

Infantile autism is almost three times more common in males than in females. In the United States and Great Britain, the incidence of infantile autism ranges from 2.1 to 7.25 per 10,000.

Signs and symptoms

The most characteristic sign of infantile autism is severe language impairment, both verbal and nonverbal. This includes total lack of speech, failure of language development beyond infantile level, and echolalia, in which the autistic child repeats the last phrase or word of a phrase he hears in a meaningless echo-like manner. An autistic child who does learn to speak normally rarely has a large vocabulary and may be remarkably proficient at rote learning.

The autistic child also shows characteristically bizarre behavior patterns, such as screaming fits, rituals, rhythmic rocking, arm-flapping, or crying without tears, and disturbed sleeping and eating patterns. His behavior may also be self-destructive, with hand-biting, eye-gouging, hair-pulling, or head-banging. Withdrawal from other people, avoidance of eye contact with others, and a compulsion for uniformity in the environment are also typical. As an infant, he may fail to respond to auditory stimuli, giving only a reflex smile response. He may appear to "look right through" his mother and other people as if they aren't present, and doesn't relate to the world around him. For instance, if left alone, an autistic child may remain quiet and passive. But if picked up, or if furniture or other objects in his environment are moved, he flies into a fit of rage.

Diagnosis

The diagnosis usually is clear when an infant fails to respond positively to touch and affection, exhibits repetitive behavior, and does not develop normal speech. Interviews with and observation of the family, along with screening tests to determine developmental delays are the major diagnostic tools. The autistic child's lack of responsiveness may at first be seen as a sign of mental retardation, but intelligence tests show that he usually possesses average to superior intelligence. EEG findings may be abnormal but nonspecific. Infantile autism is usually distinguishable from childhood schizophrenia. However, the latter may begin as infantile autism.

Treatment and additional considerations

Treatment aims to increase social adjustment, limit self-destructive and repetitive behavior, and most importantly, promote language development (since this is so clearly tied to eventual social adjustment). Behavioral techniques have proven most successful. For example, positive reinforcement using food or other rewards can promote language and social development; and maintaining a rigid daily routine seems to put least strain on the child.

Treatment may take place in a psychiatric institution, in a specialized school, or in a day-care program, but the current trend is to train parents to use behavioral techniques at home. Helping family members to develop strong one-to-one relationships with the autistic child often initiates responsive, imitative behavior. Because family members often feel inadequacy and guilt, they may need family counseling. Until the causes of infantile autism are known, prevention is not possible.

The doctor may order a tranquilizer such as chlorpromazine to control screaming fits and other hyperactive behavior.

For more information about this disorder, or for referrals to local organizations, parents should contact The National Society for Autistic Children, 1234 Massachusetts Ave., N.W., Suite 1017, Washington, D.C. 20005.

Chronic Brain Syndrome

Chronic (organic) brain syndrome results from irreversible, diffuse brain damage, and often has a slow and insidious onset characterized by progressive dementia and delirium. This disorder is most common in patients over age 70 and progresses until their death. Even when it results from a causative agent that can be eliminated, brain impairment usually persists.

Causes and incidence

Chronic brain syndrome may follow senile brain deterioration, neurologic disorders (such as Alzheimer's disease or Pick's disease), organic disorders (syphilis), metabolic disorders (hypothyroidism), vascular diseases leading to CVA, or chemical poisoning (lead, mercury, or organic solvents).

Signs and symptoms

The first signs of chronic brain syndrome are recurring errors in judgment; disregard for personal hygiene; impaired capacity for abstract thinking; disturbances of memory, imagination, and humor; apathy; disorientation; and reduced intellectual function. These signs may accompany depression (self-imposed isolation and social regression), anxiety, irritability, and progressively decreasing inhibitions. Many times the patient and his family are slow to recognize early symptoms, which are often more obvious to the casual observer. More dramatic symptoms include hallucinations (especially at night), incoherent speech, inappropriate response, restlessness (patient wanders away from home) and sleeplessness, exacerbated psychotic tendencies, occasional manic and hypermanic states, and in advanced stages, stupor and coma.

Diagnosis

Identifying chronic brain syndrome requires a careful patient history (taken from family interviews) and a thorough physical and neurologic exam, supplemented by relevant diagnostic tests to rule out other causes of impaired mental function. The history concentrates on the patient's general background (occupation, possible exposure to toxic elements, life-style, coping mechanisms) and changes in mental activity (time of occurrence, progression). The neurologic exam tests orientation, ability to use language, new memory, old memory, calculation, abstraction, judgment, mood, and thought content. Diagnostic measures usually include a lumbar puncture to examine cerebrospinal fluid; electrolyte determinations; and hepatic, renal, and thyroid function tests.

Treatment

Naturally, treatment varies according to the cause and extent of brain damage. It aims to relieve symptoms, to protect the patient from harming himself, to support self-esteem and dignity, and if possible, to reorient the patient to greater productivity. Rarely, the cause can be removed (for example, a tumor), but even then, return of normal function is unlikely. Preventive therapy tries to control the underlying cause, such as alcohol abuse, before it produces irreversible damage.

Additional considerations

A trusting relationship should be developed between the patient and hospital staff. His unacceptable behavior must be dealt with nonjudgmentally, and he should be treated with understanding and kindness.

Even though the patient's behavior is often childlike, he still should be treated as an adult. He needs to be as independent as possible (with appropriate safety measures). Restraints should be used as little as possible. The patient and his family will need goals for daily living.

COMMON TREATABLE CAUSES OF CHRONIC BRAIN SYNDROME

Endocrine disorders
- Thyroid, parathyroid, or adrenal dysfunction
- Hypoglycemia

Conditions that cause metabolic disorders
- Hepatic, renal, or pulmonary insufficiency
- Hyponatremia
- Inappropriate antidiuretic hormone secretion
- Porphyria
- Wilson's disease
- Vitamin B deficiencies (pellagra)
- Alcoholism

Toxins
- Drug toxicity (barbiturates, bromides)
- Heavy metal exposure

Vascular disorders
- Postsubarachnoid hemorrhage
- Cerebral anoxia
- Hypertensive encephalopathies
- Anoxic or ischemic vascular derangements
- Vascular stenosis

Inflammation
- General paresis
- Brain abscess
- Meningoencephalitis
- Various types of chronic inflammation
- Postinflammatory arachnoiditis, with hydrocephalus
- Fungal and parasitic infections

Miscellaneous
- Recurrent seizures
- Hematologic disorders
- Occult or communicating hydrocephalus
- Lupus erythematosus
- Trauma (subdural hematoma)
- Neoplasm (brain tumor)

Recreational, occupational, and physical therapies encourage social interaction.

The patient needs to be oriented to reality. A direct, simple explanation of any change in routine; a clock and calendar; and a regular schedule for hygiene, nutrition, and elimination, will help orient him. All members of the hospital staff should provide consistent and continuous care. Staff and family may need help coping with the continuing frustration of managing the patient's chronic condition.

Alcoholism

Alcoholism is a chronic illness characterized by a physical and mental dependence on alcoholic beverages. Such dependence has severely detrimental effects on physical, emotional, and economic well-being, which may combine to shorten the alcoholic's life span by 10 to 12 years. An estimated 10 million Americans over 18 years old are alcoholics (that's about 10% of all men and 3% of all women).

Causes

No one knows exactly what causes alcoholism, but family background seems to play a part. Actually, about half of all alcoholics have at least one alcoholic parent, but it's not yet clear whether alcoholism stems primarily from biochemical or genetic abnormalities, or from environmental tensions resulting from parental alcohol abuse. However, many alcoholics also come from families in which use of any alcohol is strictly forbidden.

Alcoholics have certain personality traits in common: they lack self-esteem and are easily frustrated, which may lead to dependency, guilt, and depressive or self-destructive tendencies.

Signs and symptoms

Chronic alcohol abuse brings with it a vast array of physical and mental complications: gastritis, acute pancreatitis, malnutrition and other nutritional deficiencies, fatty liver, cirrhosis, cardiomyopathy, and organic brain damage. Indeed, 10% of all alcoholics develop cirrhosis of the liver. Such hepatic damage may be visible in the telltale signs of jaundice, spider telangiectasia, ascites, and edema. Liver damage may lead to hypoglycemia and ultimately to hepatic coma (in persons who have abused alcohol for many years).

Alcoholics tend to abuse other drugs besides alcohol, adding a host of additional problems. Major complications of chronic alcoholism include organic brain damage, grand mal seizures (also called "alcoholic epilepsy" or "rum fits"), and *Wernicke-Korsakoff syndrome*, an organic brain disorder stemming from thiamine deficiency. The alcoholic with this disorder is mentally confused, apathetic, listless, and unable to concentrate. He has large memory gaps and can't put time into sequence; he then confabulates to fill the gaps. Wernicke-Korsakoff syndrome also may cause ocular nerve paralysis and ataxia. Prognosis is fair with vitamin replacement, but restoration of memory may take a year or longer.

After abstinence during sleep, alcoholics experience a mild form of alcohol withdrawal (morning hangover). Its well-known symptoms include jitters, irritability, profuse sweating, nausea, and vomiting. All these symptoms can be temporarily relieved by drinking alcohol, but they will recur the following morning.

The most acute complication of alcohol abuse is delirium tremens (DTs)—*alcohol withdrawal syndrome*—a condition of severe distress that follows abrupt withdrawal after prolonged or massive use. Delirium tremens usually begins 12 to 36 hours after the patient's last drink. Its earliest signs are coarse tremors, accompanied by depression, disorientation, and decreased attention span; later signs include anorexia, insomnia, tachycardia, fever, tachypnea, and profuse sweating. It also produces bizarre visual or tactile hallucinations. The alcoholic may see bugs crawling on the wall and feel them crawling on his body, or he may feel that the floor is moving. This potentially dangerous condition, if untreated, carries a 15% to 20% mortality rate and calls for close medical supervision. Normally, its acute phase begins to subside after 12 to 24 hours, but milder withdrawal symptoms may continue as long as 2 weeks. After all symptoms disappear, the patient usually falls into a deep sleep and wakes up feeling better.

Since alcohol can alter the effects of treatment and drugs, health care professionals need to watch for clues that can identify an alcoholic; for example, traumatic injuries the patient can't fully explain, or unexplained poor personal hygiene. Secretive behavior may be an attempt by the patient to hide his disease or his alcohol supply. Alcoholism should be suspected when a patient *always* smells of aftershave lotion or mouthwash. Deprived of his usual supply, an alcoholic will consume alcohol in any form he can find it.

When confronted about his drinking problem, an alcoholic characteristically becomes hostile and may even sign out of the hospital, against medical advice.

Diagnosis

To diagnose alcoholism requires that the patient have a history of chronic and excessive ingestion of alcohol. However, a complete evaluation—including physical examination, pertinent laboratory results, and observation for typical signs and symptoms of alcoholism or alcohol withdrawal— can support the diagnosis. If the patient is unwilling or unable to give a history, his family should be asked how much he drinks, how often, when he had his last drink, if he uses other drugs, if he has any emotional problems, if there have been suicide attempts, or if he's received any treatment for alcoholism.

A complete physical examination can identify complications of alcohol abuse and other physical problems related to alcoholism. The patient's gastrointestinal, hepatic, cardiac, and pulmonary systems need assessment, and his skin should be checked for changes characteristic of hepatic damage (spider telangiectasia).

Lab data can document recent alcohol ingestion (blood alcohol levels may be as high as 400 to 500 mg/ml if the patient has been drinking recently) but can't confirm alcoholism. However, the onset of withdrawal symptoms can be predicted by how long ago the patient stopped drinking.

A complete serum electrolyte count may be necessary to identify electrolyte abnormalities (in severe hepatic disease, BUN is increased and serum glucose is decreased). Further testing may show increased serum ammonia levels and increased serum amylase levels. Urine toxicology may help to determine if the alcoholic with DTs or another acute complication abuses other drugs as well. Hepatic function studies revealing increased serum cholesterol, LDH, SGOT, SGPT, and CPK may all point to hepatic damage, while elevated serum amylase and lipase point to acute pancreatitis. Hematologic workup can identify anemia, thrombocytopenia, increased prothrombin time and increased partial thromboplastin time.

Treatment

Initial treatment during acute withdrawal aims to protect the patient and those around him, to relieve withdrawal symptoms, and to treat associated illnesses. This therapy may take place in a general hospital or a special detoxification center. Later, the alcoholic may receive rehabilitation in a psychiatric hospital or a detoxification center. This may include outpatient care combined with membership in Alcoholics Anonymous (AA).

Treatment during acute withdrawal may include I.V. glucose, for hypoglycemia; I.V. fluids containing thiamine and other B complex vitamins, to correct nutritional deficiencies and help metabolize glucose. I.V. therapy must be monitored to prevent congestive heart failure. However, if symptoms develop, treatment may include furosemide I.V.

Care for a patient in acute alcohol withdrawal includes monitoring mental status, heart rate, lung sounds, blood pressure, and rectal temperature every 4 to 6 hours, depending on the severity of symptoms. Since the patient may experience hallucinations, he should be oriented to reality. If he's combative or disoriented, temporary restraints may be necessary.

Once the alcoholic is sober, treatment aims to help him stay sober. He should be warned that he'll be tempted to drink again and won't be able to control himself after the first drink. Therefore, he must abstain from alcohol totally for the rest of his life. Two forms of treatment may help him abstain: aversion therapy, if ordered, and supportive counseling. Unfortunately, these treatments aren't effective for every patient.

Aversion, or *deterrent,* therapy employs a daily oral dose of disulfiram. This drug interferes with alcohol metabolism and allows toxic levels of acetaldehyde to accumulate in the patient's blood, producing immediate and potentially fatal distress if the patient drinks alcohol within 12 hours of taking it. The reaction includes nausea, vomiting, facial flushing, headache, shortness of breath, red eyes, blurred vision, sweating, tachycardia, hypotension, and fainting, and may last from 30 minutes to 3 hours or longer. The patient needs close medical supervision during this time. He must understand that even a small amount of alcohol will induce this adverse reaction and that the longer he takes the drug, the greater will be his sensitivity to alcohol. Because of this, he must avoid even medicinal sources of alcohol, such as mouthwash, cough syrups, liquid vitamins, or cold remedies. Paraldehyde, a sedative, is chemically similar to alcohol and may also provoke a disulfiram reaction.

Aversion therapy is contraindicated during pregnancy and in patients with diabetes, heart disease, severe hepatic disease, or any disorder in which such a reaction could be especially dangerous. Patients taking this drug should be told that they may continue this treatment for months or years, and that they should remain under medical supervision.

Another form of deterrent therapy attempts to induce aversion by administering alcohol with an emetic. However, for long-term success with deterrent therapy, the sober alcoholic must learn to fill the place alcohol once occupied in his life with something constructive. Indeed, for patients with abnormal dependency needs or for those who also abuse other drugs, deterrent therapy with disulfiram may only substitute one drug dependency for another; so it should be used prudently.

Additional considerations

Supportive counseling or individual, group, or family psychotherapy may improve the alcoholic's ability to cope with stress, anxiety, and frustration, and may help him gain insight into the personal problems and internal conflicts that led him to alcohol abuse. Occasionally, a doctor may order a tranquilizer to relieve overwhelming anxiety during rehabilitation, but such drugs are dangerous because of their potential for transferring addiction, and for coma and death following their combined use with alcohol.

In AA, a self-help group with more than a million members worldwide, the alcoholic finds emotional support from others with similar problems. Approximately 40% of AA's members stay sober as long as 5 years, and 30% stay sober longer than 5 years. Spouses of alcoholics can find encouragement in Al-Anon, another self-help group; children in Al-Ateen. Family involvement in rehabilitation can reduce family tensions.

For alcoholics who've lost all contact

with family and friends and who have a long history of unemployment, trouble with the law, or other problems associated with alcohol abuse, rehabilitation may involve job training, sheltered workshops, halfway houses, or other supervised facilities.

Until the primary causes of alcoholism are discovered, prevention isn't possible.

Banning alcoholic beverages, as during Prohibition, has proved spectacularly unsuccessful in preventing alcohol abuse. Providing comprehensive treatment for alcoholics can help them maintain sobriety. This, in turn, may limit family disruptions that possibly contribute to the development of alcoholism in offspring.

Drug Abuse

Drug abuse is the chronic or occasional use of drugs for other than their prescribed medical purpose. This disorder is widespread, from high-school students who abuse heroin, methaqualone, and phencyclidine (PCP), to adults who misuse tranquilizers and barbiturates. Virtually any drug can be abused. Prognosis varies with the drug and the extent of abuse.

Causes and incidence

Although the causes of drug abuse aren't clear, certain elements affect the degree of dependence: the abuser's psychologic and physiologic makeup, the drug's pharmacologic composition, and external social and cultural factors.

Inability to cope with stress, frustration, or anxiety; desire for immediate gratification; immaturity; insecurity; and low self-esteem characterize the drug abuser. Usually, the person who abuses one drug abuses others (including alcohol) as well.

Narcotics, barbiturates, and certain other drugs pharmacologically induce physical dependence (distressing symptoms follow abstinence), so the abuser uses the drug to avoid discomfort. Physical dependence may lead to abuse, even in persons who originally received the drug for therapeutic reasons.

Society encourages drug use while discouraging abuse. However, certain societal factors contribute to improper use of drugs: casual prescribing practices, inadequate controls to prevent fraudulent prescriptions, and easy access to drugs by medical professionals. Peer pressure is an important contributory factor among adolescents.

Treatment

Emergency treatment varies according to the type of drug abuse. In treating narcotics abuse, the immediate goal is to prevent shock and maintain respirations by intubation with an endotracheal tube and mechanical ventilation. Other emergency treatment includes oxygen to correct hypoxemia, I.V. fluids and plasma expanders, and naloxone to reverse the narcotic effect. For treating the patient with methadone toxicity, repeated doses of naloxone are necessary. For many patients, detoxification in a hospital or outpatient program is required.

ASSESSING DRUG USE

With *all* types of drug abuse, assessment of the patient's drug use pattern is critical. For example:
- What drugs is the patient using.
- How much is used, and how often.
- How long has he been using them.

Such a patient may be unwilling or unable to give a history of his drug use. Further information may be gathered from his family or friends, from a physical examination, and from blood and urine tests. Accompanying disorders that also require treatment may be identified at the same time.

SIGNS AND SYMPTOMS OF DRUG ABUSE

DRUG	CLINICAL FEATURES	COMPLICATIONS
Narcotic analgesics: codeine, heroin, meperidine, morphine, opium. Butorphanol and pentazocine, though not narcotics, have similar effects and addictive potential	*Acute:* coma, hypotension, tachycardia, pinpoint pupils *Chronic (after injection):* needle marks, scars from skin abscesses, thrombophlebitis *Withdrawal:* sweating, nausea, vomiting, diarrhea, anxiety, insomnia, dilated pupils, runny nose, tearing eyes, yawning, goosebumps, persistent back and abdominal pain, anorexia, cold flashes; spontaneous orgasm (in women) or ejaculation (in men), fever, tachycardia, rising BP and respiration rate. Symptoms subside within 7 to 10 days after the last dose.	Viral hepatitis (resulting in hepatic dysfunction), osteomyelitis, pulmonary edema, bacterial endocarditis, coma (resulting in organic brain damage or seizures), secondary infection Physical and psychologic dependence
Amphetamines: amphetamine, dextroamphetamine, methamphetamine	*After high doses:* anxiety, hyperactivity, irritability, insomnia, muscle tension, repeated compulsive movement, tooth grinding, aggressive or violent behavior, paranoia, psychotic symptoms resembling schizophrenia, fever, hypertension, dilated pupils, tachycardia, convulsions, cardiovascular collapse, malnutrition, and threatening visual, auditory, and tactile hallucinations *After injection:* needle marks, scars from skin abscesses, thrombophlebitis *Withdrawal:* depression, overwhelming fatigue.	Little or no physical dependence, but tolerance and psychologic dependence possible
Cocaine	*Acute intoxication (after I.V. injection):* tremors, seizures, convulsions, delirium, potentially fatal cardiovascular or respiratory failure *Chronic intoxication:* hallucinations, formication, dilated pupils, tachycardia, muscle twitching, violent behavior, tachycardia, elevated respiratory rate, perforation of the nasal septum *Withdrawal:* depression, irritability, disorientation, tremors, muscle weakness	Psychologic dependence
Barbiturates: amobarbital, pentobarbital, secobarbital. Methaqualone is not a barbiturate, but symptoms and treatment are similar	*Acute intoxication:* progressive CNS and respiratory depression *Chronic intoxication:* slurred speech, impaired coordination, decreased mental alertness and attention span, memory disturbances, depressed pulse rate and tendon reflexes, mood swings, nystagmus or strabismus, diplopia, dizziness, hypotension, dehydration, and aggressive, combative, or suicidal behavior *Withdrawal:* jitteriness, anxiety, irritability, grand mal seizures, status epilepticus, orthostatic hypotension, tachycardia, auditory and visual disturbances. Symptoms subside within 1 week.	Apnea, shock, coma, death Physical and psychologic dependence
Phencyclidine	*Acute intoxication:* apnea, status epilepticus, coma, death *"Bad trip":* paralysis, numbness, frightening hallucinations (may mimic schizophrenia), anxiety, dissociative reaction, feeling of imminent death, paranoid or violent behavior *Chronic intoxication:* confusion, fatigue, irritability, depression, hallucinations	Psychologic dependence and tolerance
Marijuana: hashish, marijuana, tetrahydrocannabinol (THC)	*Acute transient reaction* (rare): panic and paranoid reactions (with first-time use); pseudopsychotic reaction (with THC)	Psychologic dependence possible
Hallucinogens: LSD, mescaline, psilocybin	*Acute intoxication ("bad trip"):* anxiety, frightening hallucinations, and depression (possible suicidal tendencies)	Tolerance and psychologic dependence possible

For amphetamine abuse, immediate therapy may consist of an alpha-adrenergic blocking agent to inhibit life-threatening autonomic effects; ammonium chloride to promote amphetamine excretion; and haloperidol, chlorpromazine, or another antipsychotic agent to control amphetamine-induced psychosis. The hospitalized patient may be detoxified by abrupt withdrawal. Symptoms of stimulant abuse do not usually require treatment because of these drugs' short duration of action. However, if necessary, excessive stimulation may be quickly controlled with intravenous barbiturates or intramuscular phenothiazines. Supportive therapy includes hydration with I.V. fluids and intubation to support respiration.

The goal of treatment in barbiturate abuse is to restore CNS and respiratory function and to prevent shock. Treatment usually includes endotracheal intubation, I.V. fluids to correct hypotension and dehydration, and I.V. sodium bicarbonate to promote diuresis and counteract intoxication. Extreme intoxication may require dialysis. Gastric lavage or administration of activated charcoal followed by a cathartic is usually recommended to eliminate the toxic drug. During detoxification, pentobarbital-challenge test determines the patient's tolerance level. An appropriate pentobarbital dose lessens withdrawal symptoms until dosage can gradually be reduced and finally totally withdrawn.

After phencyclidine abuse, support of vital systems is essential. Continuous gastric suctioning is necessary to remove phencyclidine and other drugs (PCP abusers seldom take PCP alone). Endotracheal intubation supports respiration. Acidification with ammonium chloride promotes PCP excretion. Meanwhile, diazepam, haloperidol, or other antipsychotic drugs alleviate psychotic symptoms. *Caution:* Repeated doses of diazepam can prolong drug effects. In severe reactions to marijuana, pentobarbital or diazepam reduces anxiety. After hallucinogen abuse, pentobarbital, diazepam, or chlordiazepoxide relieves anxiety. After abuse of volatile solvents, pulmonary crisis is abrupt and severe, and requires rigorous support of vital systems and I.V. fluids.

Additional considerations

During withdrawal from any drug, the patient needs a quiet, safe environment. Harmful objects should be removed from the room and restraints used judiciously. Side rails are necessary for comatose patients. The patient should be reassured that medication will control most symptoms of withdrawal. Other supportive care varies with the drug.

• Narcotic intoxication: Since narcotics may impair hypoxic drive, the patient must be observed continuously. Pulmonary edema is a possible complication if the patient's receiving I.V. fluids and plasma expanders. Restraints should be applied before the patient is given naloxone. He may be disoriented and agitated as he emerges from coma.

• Amphetamine intoxication: Neurologic status must be monitored closely, since haloperidol and chlorpromazine lower seizure threshold. Vital signs must be monitored, and the patient watched for suicidal behavior.

• Cocaine intoxication: Respirations are monitored closely, because treatment can aggravate cocaine-induced respiratory depression.

• Barbiturate intoxication: If the patient isn't comatose, his level of consciousness is closely monitored; if comatose or nearly so, his airway and respirations must be maintained. During pentobarbital-challenge test, signs of intoxication may be observed. During detoxification, the patient is watched for signs of intoxication and withdrawal.

• Phencyclidine: Adequate hydration is needed to promote PCP excretion. A quiet, safe, isolated environment will help. Overt attempts to reassure an aggressive patient may provoke aggressive behavior.

• Marijuana or hallucinogen intoxication: A quiet environment minimizes sensory input until the reaction subsides. Someone should stay with the patient to

provide support and orientation.
• Volatile solvents: Vital signs, level of consciousness, and I.V. infusions are monitored. While immediate lifesaving treatment and detoxification are essential, they leave underlying problems unsolved. Consequently, after detoxification, drug abusers need zealous follow-up care (including individual, group, or family therapy). When drug abuse has thoroughly disrupted ability to function in society, court-supervised programs, or federally sponsored rehabilitation programs may be necessary.

Anorexia Nervosa

Anorexia nervosa, probably a mental disturbance, is characterized by self-imposed starvation and consequent emaciation, nutritional deficiency disorders, and atrophic changes. Gorging, vomiting, and purging may occur during starvation or after normal weight is restored, as a means of weight control instead of starvation. This disorder primarily affects adolescent females and young adults but is not uncommon among older women; occasionally, it also affects males. Prognosis varies but is improved if the diagnosis is made early or if the patient voluntarily seeks help and wants to overcome the disorder. Nevertheless, mortality ranges from 5% to 15%.

Causes and incidence

No one knows exactly what causes anorexia nervosa. Researchers in neuroendocrinology are seeking a physiologic cause but have found nothing definite yet. Clearly, however, social attitudes that equate slimness with beauty play some role in provoking this disorder, as do internal and family conflicts.

Anorexia nervosa most often strikes girls from achievement-oriented, upwardly mobile families, but it can occur among those of lower socioeconomic status. It may have a higher incidence in families that stress the importance of certain foods or who have rituals involving them.

Signs and symptoms

Anorexia nervosa usually develops in a patient whose weight is usually normal or who may be only 5 pounds (2.3 kg) overweight. One of its cardinal symptoms is a 20% *or more* weight loss for no organic reason, coupled with a morbid dread of being fat and a compulsion to be thin. The anorectic shows multiple and severe sequelae of chronic undernourishment: skeletal muscle atrophy, loss of fatty tissue, hypotension, constipation, dental caries, susceptibility to infection, blotchy or sallow skin, intolerance to cold, lanugo on the face and body, dryness or loss of scalp hair, and amenorrhea. Oddly, the patient usually demonstrates restless activity and vigor (despite undernourishment), and often exercises avidly without apparent fatigue. Paradoxically, even though she may be obsessed with food or cooking, she refuses to eat and is convinced she's too fat, despite all evidence to the contrary. Gorging, followed by spontaneous or self-induced vomiting or self-administration of laxatives or diuretics, may lead to dehydration, or metabolic alkalosis or acidosis. Circulatory collapse (signaled by a drop in systolic pressure below 50 mmHg) may prove fatal. Cardiac arrhythmias due to electrolyte imbalance may cause cardiac arrest.

While anorexia nervosa is not necessarily an expression of a death wish, feelings of despair, hopelessness, and worthlessness produce a higher rate of attempted suicides in these patients.

Diagnosis

Diagnosis requires careful interpretation of clinical status to rule out endocrine, metabolic, and CNS abnormalities; malignancy; malabsorption syndrome; and other disorders that also cause physical wasting. The patient's obvious physical vigor (despite her emaciated appearance) simplifies this task, and a history of compulsive dieting and bulimic episodes help confirm the diagnosis.

Initial laboratory analysis should probably include a complete blood count (CBC); measurement of serum levels of creatinine, BUN, uric acid, cholesterol, total protein, albumin, sodium, potassium, chloride, CO_2 content, calcium, SGOT, and SGPT; determination of fasting blood glucose levels; a urinalysis; and an electrocardiogram (EKG). The necessity for periodic repetition of these studies depends on the severity of malnutrition, emesis, and laxative or diuretic abuse, as well as the degree of abnormality of the test results. Laboratory data are usually normal, unless weight loss exceeds 30%.

Treatment

Treatment aims to promote weight gain or control the patient's compulsive gorging and purging, and to correct the underlying dysfunction. Hospitalization in a medical or a psychiatric unit may be required to improve the patient's precarious physical state. The required length of stay may be as brief as 2 weeks or may stretch from a few months to 2 years or longer.

Specific approaches to treatment may include behavior modification (privileges are dependent on weight gain); curtailing activity for physical reasons (such as cardiac arrhythmias); vitamin and mineral supplements; a reasonable diet, with or without liquid supplements; hyperalimentation (subclavian, peripheral, or enteral [enteral and peripheral routes carry less risk of infection]); and group, family, or individual psychotherapy.

All forms of psychotherapy, from psychoanalysis to hypnotherapy, have been used in treating anorexia nervosa, with varying success. To be successful, such therapy should address the patient's underlying problems of low self-esteem, guilt, and anxiety; feelings of hopelessness and helplessness; and depression. Most therapists consider task-centered approaches and therapeutic flexibility important requirements for success in treating anorexia nervosa.

Additional considerations

• During hospitalization, the patient's vital signs and intake and output are monitored. The patient's weighed daily—before breakfast, if possible. However, since such a patient often fears being weighed, the routine for this may differ greatly.

• The patient should be frequently offered small portions of food or drinks. Many times nutritionally complete liquid feedings are more acceptable, since they eliminate choices between foods—something the anorectic often finds difficult.

• If tube feedings or other special feeding measures become necessary, they should be fully explained to the patient, and her fears or reluctance discussed; however, the discussion about food itself should be limited.

• The patient's need for food should be discussed with her matter-of-factly; she should know that improved nutrition can correct abnormal laboratory findings.

• If edema or bloating occurs after the patient has returned to normal eating behavior, she should be reassured that this phenomenon is temporary, since she'll probably find this condition frightening.

• The patient should recognize and assert her feelings freely. If she understands that she can be assertive, she may gradually learn that expressing her true feelings will not result in her losing control or love. The anorectic uses exercise, preoccupation with food, ritualism, manipulation, and prevarication as mechanisms that preserve the only control she feels she has in her life.

• The patient's family may need therapy to uncover and correct faulty interactions. Family members should avoid discussing food. The patient's weight should be monitored by someone who is acceptable to the patient, her family, and her therapist.

The doctor may refer the patient and her family to Anorexia Nervosa and Associated Disorders (ANAD), a national information and support organization. This organization will help them understand what anorexia is, and find a psychotherapist or medical doctor who is experienced in treating it.

Sexual Deviation

In sexual deviation, sexual satisfaction requires manipulation of material objects or abnormal sexual behavior. Usually, such behavior harms others or takes the place of normal sexual activity. Sexual deviation is more common in men than in women. Prognosis varies with the kind of deviation and with the person's motivation to change his behavior.

Causes
The causes of sexual deviation are thought to include a combination of sociocultural, physical, and psychologic factors —for example, an overly intimate relationship with parents, or rejection, hostile treatment, and social deprivation during childhood—all of which diminish self-esteem. They provoke feelings of inadequacy or hostility expressed through sexually deviant behavior.

Signs and symptoms
Most sexual deviants are outwardly quiet and reserved. Their poor self-image, low frustration level, and overwhelming feelings of fear and inadequacy prevent them from experiencing normal relationships and effective interactions with others.

Kinds of sexual deviation
Exhibitionism. The exhibitionist derives sexual satisfaction from exposing his genitals in public. While he is not dangerous and does not participate in more serious deviations, his need to reinforce his masculinity in this manner cannot be treated by reassurance alone; psychiatric treatment is necessary.

Voyeurism. The voyeur obtains sexual satisfaction by watching others engaged in sexual activity or by observing a woman nude or undressing. Since normal sexual activity may include an element of voyeurism, this is considered a deviation only when it disturbs others or replaces normal sexual activity. The voyeur only occasionally engages in dangerous sexual deviations.

Fetishism. The fetishist receives gratification by manipulating a material object, usually an article of women's clothing. Often this object becomes the sole focus of sexual desire.

Transvestism. For the transvestite, sexual stimulation is achieved by wearing clothes of the opposite sex, often in public. Some transvestites are homosexual, but others lead fairly contented married lives and engage in normal sexual activity. The transvestite is not dangerous to others and seldom seeks treatment.

Rape. The rapist uses violence to sexually assault a nonconsenting partner. Rape is a violent crime—an expression of hostility, power, and rage—not just sexual gratification. It may occur as an isolated incident but is more often part of a recurring behavior pattern. The rapist needs psychotherapy. For more information, see RAPE CRISIS SYNDROME.

Necrophilia. The necrophiliac engages in sexual intercourse with a corpse. This rare deviation usually involves a murderer and his recently killed victim, and requires psychotherapy.

Pedophilia. The pedophiliac has sexual relations with children, frequently those of friends or relatives. The pedophiliac may be homosexual or heterosexual, and needs psychotherapy.

Sadism. The sadist obtains sexual satisfaction by inflicting physical or mental pain on the sexual partner, is likely to commit murder or other violent crimes, and is dangerous. Psychiatric treatment is necessary.

Masochism. The masochist achieves sexual gratification through physical or mental abuse before, during, after, or instead of sexual intercourse. Masochism results from feelings of guilt and the desire to be punished, and calls for psychiatric treatment.

Incest. Incest (sexual relations with family members) most often involves a father and his daughter. The wife/mother may tacitly approve of the activity. Once begun, incest tends to persist and may extend to include several children. An incestuous father was often socially deprived during his childhood. He seldom commits other crimes. As a rule, all members of an incestuous family need psychiatric treatment.

Diagnosis

Diagnosis requires careful interpretation of clinical assessment, including the patient's history and physical examination. Often a referral from the criminal justice system leads to diagnosis.

Treatment and additional considerations

When dealing with a sexual deviant, the health care professional must remain nonjudgmental, avoid activity requiring close physical contact (if possible), firmly stop all sexual overtures, and avoid reinforcing deviant behavior. The professional should maintain a safe, nonthreatening environment, and set realistic treatment goals. If the patient has other associated psychiatric disorders, they must be treated appropriately.

Transsexualism

Transsexualism is a form of gender dysphoria; it's not the same as homosexuality or transvestism, nor is it a type of these two disorders. The transsexual patient believes his anatomical sexual determination is mistaken, because it doesn't correspond with his psychologic perception of his own sexuality. He sincerely believes himself trapped in the wrong body, physically coerced by it to accept inappropriate sexual identification. His feelings of sexual misidentification are so strong that he seeks surgical correction, sex-reassignment.

Most transsexuals who seek sex-reassignment are men, possibly because male-to-female reassignment is more widely publicized, and because the surgical procedure is simpler than it is for female-to-male reassignment.

Prognosis depends upon the transsexual's success with personal and social readjustment. Failure to readjust could cause long-term psychologic problems.

Causes

Despite continuing medical investigation, much disagreement still exists about the causes of transsexualism. Possible causes are hormonal imbalance, chromosome anomaly, gonadal lesions, and an early psychological defect in the mother-child bond.

Signs and symptoms

During childhood, the transsexual may be more comfortable playing games dominated exclusively by children of the opposite sex, or there may be nothing abnormal about his play activities. He may express a wish to be a child of the opposite sex, or he may keep his feelings to himself. He may be accepted by the other children as if he were no different from themselves, or he may be teased by them. In adolescence and puberty, the transsexual may become increasingly withdrawn and may experience severe psychologic problems, because he can't find social acceptance as the person he believes himself to be. This lack of social acceptance may precipitate a potentially dangerous identity crisis, if the transsexual despairs of finding a solution to his problem and thinks the situation hopeless.

Diagnosis

Standard guidelines for diagnosing transsexualism are still tentative. However, the Harry Benjamin International Gender Dysphoria Association recommends diagnosis based on the patient's persistent feelings of discomfort and sexual misidentification and a desire for surgical correction. The patient's feelings should be verified by a psychiatrist or psychologist in a psychotherapeutic relationship with the transsexual. To do this, the therapist must have independent knowledge of the patient's claims (interviews with family, friends, work associates); he can't rely upon the patient's word alone. He must determine that the patient's feelings of discomfort and misidentification have existed unabated *for at least 2 years*. Also, he must have known the patient for *at least 3 months* before recommending hormonal sex-reassignment, and for *at least 6 months* before recommending surgical reassignment. Final diagnosis is made by a medical team that includes a psychotherapist, a social worker, and doctors from the hospital where the patient is to be treated.

During the final diagnosis, the medical team must determine that no signs of physical intersex or genetic abnormality are present, and that the patient's feelings don't indicate another psychiatric disorder (the patient must take a battery of psychologic tests). Of course, a transsexual may have a coexisting psychiatric disorder. If so, he is treated *first* for the other disorder. If the medical team recommends surgery, its decision is subject to peer review.

Treatment

Most hospitals have no established policies and procedures for treating transsexuals. In those that do, treatment varies. The Harry Benjamin International Gender Dysphoria Association, hoping to standardize treatment, recommends therapy that can be divided into three categories: hormonal and nongenital, nongenital alone (superficial assumption of opposite sex identity that may include limited plastic surgery), and hormonal and genital combined.

All treatment begins with confirmation and screening, which overlap with team diagnosis. Hormonal therapy begins after the team has confirmed that the patient is, in fact, a transsexual; that the transsexual wants a more profound change than modified life-style; that hormonal therapy isn't ill-advised because of health reasons; and the patient has completed a successful trial run of living full-time, professionally and socially, in the role of the opposite sex. While role-playing as a member of the opposite sex before and during hormone therapy, the patient may carry an identity card to avoid being penalized by civil authorities for use of public facilities (restrooms, dressing rooms) where gender is a discriminating factor.

Before hormonal reassignment therapy can begin, the patient must be advised that it may lead to serious and

---

COMMON MISCONCEPTIONS CORRECTED

- Transsexuals may dress in clothing suitable for the opposite sex, but they don't derive sexual pleasure from this, as do transvestites.
- Their sexual preference for others of their own sex is determined by the belief that they're truly members of the opposite sex.
- Homosexuals and transvestites may qualify for sex-reassignment, but by definition, they're not transsexuals.
- The transsexual is sometimes misdiagnosed as a schizophrenic because of serious psychologic difficulties.
- No true transsexual ever changes his mind about sexual identity as a result of psychotherapy.

SURGICAL SEX-REASSIGNMENT (Male to Female)

- Removal of internal penile structures

- Use of remaining inverted penile skin tube for a vaginal lining

- Removal of testicles and spermatic cord

- Formation of the vagina between the prostate gland and rectum (prostate gland left intact, so orgasm is possible as a result of prostatic stimulation)

- Insertion of vaginal stent, consisting of a polyurethane foam insert covered with a silicone elastomer, to maintain vaginal opening

potentially fatal health complications, and that its effects are irreversible. Female-to-male hormonal reassignment causes infertility, hair growth, deepening of voice, and clitoral enlargement. The patient who experiences dissatisfaction with hormonal reassignment may be disqualified for further treatment.

Before surgery for hormonal and genital reassignment, the following tests must be performed: preliminary routine blood studies, urinalysis, chest X-ray, electrocardiogram (EKG), excretory urogram (to rule out anatomical abnormalities in the genitourinary tract), and electroencephalogram (to rule out an occult tumor of the temporal lobe, which can cause personality disorders; preoperative screening of transsexuals has sometimes disclosed these tumors). A 2-day bowel preparation is also necessary.

Immediately after surgery, the patient is given intravenous fluids and nothing by mouth; later, a clear liquid diet. If the patient has had a male-to-female reassignment, she will come back from the operating room with the vaginal stent in place. The stent must be checked periodically to make sure it hasn't dislodged. She has a Foley catheter inserted to enable the staff to check urinary output and help keep the operative site clean.

For the first 5 days postop, she receives a broad-spectrum antibiotic intravenously (usually one of the cephalosporins); then, she receives an oral antibiotic for 2 or 3 weeks. On the fifth postop day, the transsexual recovering from surgery has her dressing changed under anesthesia. If no complications are visible at the surgical site, the catheter is removed. (The vaginal stent is removed during the dressing change and when the patient voids, defecates, or bathes, but it's reinserted each time for at least 6 weeks. Then, the stent must be kept in place *almost all the time* for an additional 3 months.)

The most common postoperative complications are infection of the suture line, fistula, sloughing of the graft, and osteitis pubis. Barring such complications, the patient is usually discharged on the seventh day after surgery and returns for an outpatient office visit in 3 weeks.

Additional considerations

The nurse-patient relationship is extremely important both before and after surgery. The nurse is one of the first people the patient sees after sex-reassignment; her help and acceptance are crucial to the patient's physical and emotional well-being.

Before surgery, the transsexual often overcompensates for, denies, and distorts the reality of the planned surgery with a cavalier attitude. Such a patient expresses eagerness for surgery, with little attendant anxiety, and seems relieved to be finally having sexual identity corrected. After surgery, this attitude may change abruptly. For example, following male-to-female reassignment, the patient may have emotional outbursts and behave as a stereotypical female. Health care professionals should be prepared for such a change and bear with it, making sure beforehand that the patient knows exactly what to expect about the surgery and its consequences (pain, catheterization, I.V., antibiotics), and has no unanswered questions about it. The patient must be asked about allergies to antibiotics before receiving the first dose. It's also very important to begin addressing the patient immediately according to the new gender to show acceptance of the patient's new identity.

Medical care during postoperative recovery includes:

• keeping the patient NPO (nothing by mouth).

• checking the patient's vital signs until they're stable or until the patient's awake.

• checking the dressing for excessive bleeding, or infection, and reporting it to the doctor.

• medicating the patient for pain, as ordered.

• monitoring intravenous fluids; keeping track of intake and output.

• helping the patient maintain privacy.

• holding staff conferences, including social services personnel and psychotherapists, to help the staff deal with their unusual patient.

• continuing to communicate with the patient, using the new identity; watching for signs of depression.

• providing patient teaching about the necessary lifelong hormone therapy and its side effects (acne, fluid retention, changes in libido), the signs and symptoms of infection (fever, red and swollen suture line), and the importance of any pertinent follow-up tests (urinalysis, hepatic function studies, blood).

• emphasizing how important the stent is in preventing vaginal stenosis or retraction (if the patient has had a male-

---

SURGICAL SEX-REASSIGNMENT (Female to Male)

First operation
• Bilateral reduction mammoplasty

Second operation
• Total hysterectomy and bilateral salpingo-oophorectomy

Third operation
• First stage of phallus formation
• Penis formation
• Release of urethra from its normal position to place behind the new phallus

Three to six months later
• Attachment of urethra to phallus; patient no longer must sit to void

---

to-female reassignment). Using the stent will be painful, particularly just after surgery. To relieve pain and promote the healing process, the patient should take warm baths three times daily. When necessary, she should wash the stent in hot water and a *very mild* detergent. The patient may engage in sexual intercourse during the final 3 months that the stent is in place.

• providing further psychological therapy, if necessary, and suggesting that the patient learn relevant legal rights (the social services agency can help).

• advising the patient to obtain a new social security card.

Selected References

Freedman, Alfred M., and Harold I. Kaplan. COMPREHENSIVE TEXTBOOK OF PSYCHIATRY, 2nd ed. Baltimore: Williams & Wilkins Co., 1975.

Giannini, A., et al. PSYCHIATRIC, PSYCHOGENIC AND SOMATOPSYCHIC DISORDERS HANDBOOK. Garden City, N.Y.: Medical Examination Publishing Co., Inc., 1978.

Kneisl, Carol R., and H. Wilson. LEARNING ACTIVITIES IN PSYCHIATRIC NURSING. Menlo Park, Calif.: Addison-Wesley Publishing Co., 1979.

Minuchin, Salvatore, et al. PSYCHOSOMATIC FAMILIES, ANOREXIA NERVOSA IN CONTEXT. Cambridge, Mass.: Harvard University Press, 1978.

Payne, Doris B., ed. PSYCHIATRIC-MENTAL HEALTH NURSING. Garden City, N.Y.: Medical Examination Publishing Co., Inc., 1977.

Stuart, G., and S. Sundeen. PRINCIPLES AND PRACTICES OF PSYCHIATRIC NURSING. St. Louis: C.V. Mosby Co., 1979.

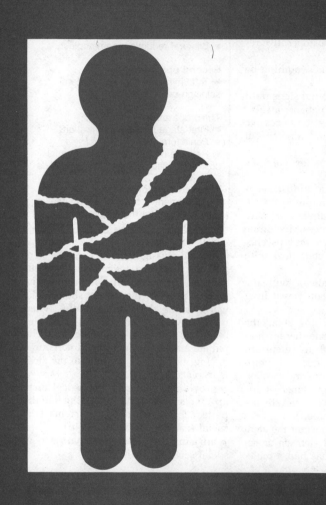

4 Trauma

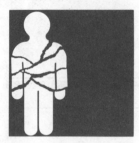

Trauma

Introduction

After cardiovascular disease and cancer, trauma is the leading cause of death in the United States; in persons under age 40, it is *the* leading cause of death. The proper way to deal with trauma victims varies, depending on each hospital's emergency department protocol, but the basics include triage; assessing and maintaining airway, breathing, and circulation (the ABCs); and, as necessary, preparing the patient for transport and possibly surgery.

Triage: First things first

Basically, triage is the setting of medical priorities for emergency care by making sound, rapid assessments. The need for triage often arises at the scene of injury and continues in the emergency department. Usually, each emergency department assigns triage responsibilities to one person, for example, a triage nurse. That person, following hospital protocol, will decide which patient to treat first, which injury to treat first, how to best utilize other members of the medical team, and how to control patient and staff traffic. Preferably, triage should be performed in a well-lighted central area where patient traffic can flow freely.

Generally, patients are assigned to the following categories:

1. Emergent—Life-threatening injury requiring treatment within a few minutes to prevent death or further injury. This includes patients with respiratory distress or cardiopulmonary arrest, and severe hemorrhage or shock.

2. Urgent—Serious but not immediately life-threatening injury that should receive treatment within 1 hour; for example, stable head, chest, or abdominal injuries and long bone fractures.

3. Delayed—Minor injuries, such as lacerations or abrasions, that can wait 4 to 6 hours for treatment.

4. Indefinite—Treatment can wait indefinitely; patient can be referred to a clinic. In disaster or military situations, this applies to patients with massive injuries who have marginal chance for recovery even with immediate care.

Trauma care generates a great deal of stress, and much of it falls on the shoulders of the triage nurse. She must deal with patients and families who are emotionally upset, angry, belligerent, intoxicated, or frightened; some patients speak only a foreign language. Therefore, she must work calmly and rationally and must avoid becoming easily upset or angered. She can help the patient a great deal by talking to him while giving him care—even if he's unconscious. She should tell the patient what she's going to do before she touches him. She must also handle difficult situations diplomatically and intelligently, recognizing personal limitations, and asking help when its needed.

Beginning with the ABCs

Suppose you were responsible for instructing the triage nurse in her duties. You'd list them as follows:

Always begin your care of an injured patient with a brief assessment of the ABCs: Airway, Breathing, and Circulation. To help establish your priorities, obtain a brief history from the patient, family, or friends. Also, find out how, when, and where the injury occurred.

To assess airway patency, routinely check for respiratory distress or signs of obstruction, such as stridor or choking. Be especially alert for respiratory distress in a patient who inhaled chemicals, was in a fire, or has upper body burns. If the airway's obstructed, remove vomitus, dentures, blood clots, or foreign bodies from the patient's mouth. To open the airway, use a head-tilt maneuver (unless you suspect a neck injury; then, use the jaw-thrust maneuver). Then, insert an oropharyngeal or nasopharyngeal airway. As necessary, assist with the insertion of an esophageal obturator airway or an endotracheal tube. The agitated patient may try to pull out his airway; watch for this and prevent it. Consider that he may just be trying to talk, or he may not be getting enough oxygen.

Next, make sure the patient's breathing is adequate. Look, listen, and feel for respirations. If the patient isn't breathing, call for help and begin mouth-to-mouth or mouth-to-nose respiration.

To assess circulation, check for carotid and peripheral pulses. If carotid pulse is absent, apply external cardiac massage. If external hemorrhage is evident, apply direct pressure to the bleeding site, and if the wound is on an extremity, elevate it above heart level, if possible. Apply a tourniquet only if hemorrhage is life-threatening. (Traumatic amputation usually requires a tourniquet.)

Assess vital signs

Monitor vital signs even if the patient appears stable. Because vital signs may change rapidly, taking them serially can point out subtle and overt changes. Document your own baseline readings, and obtain new readings every 5 to 15 minutes, until the patient is stable.

Your assessment should also include level of consciousness, and pupillary and motor response to assess neurologic status. Determine and report level of consciousness by using a stimulus-response method of reporting, rather than categorizing; don't use words like "semiconscious" or "stuporous." Report decorticate or decerebrate responses immediately. The patient need not have a head injury to show abnormal neurologic response. Any injury that impairs ventilation or perfusion can cause cerebral edema and can raise intracranial

MANAGING TETANUS PROPHYLAXIS

HISTORY	PROPHYLAXIS REQUIRED
Booster within last 12 months	Tetanus prophylaxis not necessary.
Booster more than 5 years ago but within 10 years	For a recent or clean small wound, 0.5 ml tetanus toxoid adsorbed is administered.
Booster within last 10 years	If wound is severe or more than 24 hours old, 0.5 ml tetanus toxoid adsorbed and 250 units tetanus immune globulin, human, are administered. Separate syringes and different injection sites should be used.
No immunization or booster within last 10 years	If wound is small and clean, 0.5 ml tetanus toxoid adsorbed is administered. The patient should be instructed to return for immunization series. (0.5 ml I.M. is repeated 1 month after initial dose and again 1 year later.)
	For a larger wound, 250 units tetanus immune globulin, human, and 0.5 ml tetanus toxoid adsorbed are administered. Separate syringes and sites should be used.
	For a severe wound, 500 units tetanus immune globulin, human, and 0.5 ml tetanus toxoid adsorbed are administered. Separate syringes and sites should be used.

pressure. If the patient has neurologic symptoms and is *hypotensive*, look for an extracranial cause, since intracranial bleeding rarely causes hypotension.

Quickly and carefully look for multiple injuries by systematically examining the patient. If no cervical injury exists, carefully roll the patient over to examine his back. Such an examination could reveal other wounds.

As necessary, give oxygen and draw samples for arterial blood gas measurement, to establish a baseline for oxygen therapy. Multiple injuries always create a need for supplementary oxygen because of blood loss and overwhelming physiologic stress. Actually, the conscious multiple-injury patient should show compensatory hyperventilation. If he doesn't, expect neurologic involvement or chest injury.

In multiple injuries, always suspect cervical spinal trauma until proven otherwise. Immobilize the cervical spine, using a cervical collar, a backboard, or sandbags, and obtain a lateral cervical spine film of all seven cervical vertebrae before moving the patient again.

In open or blunt wounds, administer tetanus prophylaxis, as needed, type and cross-match blood, give blood products, as ordered, and monitor hematocrit, hemoglobin, CBC, prothrombin time, partial thromboplastin time, and serum amylase.

In chest trauma, assess for open wounds, tension pneumothorax, hemothorax, cardiac tamponade, bruises and hematomas, flail chest, and fractured larynx. Cover open wounds, and as necessary, apply direct pressure to the wound, begin cardiac monitoring, and be ready to assist with insertion of chest tubes, needle thoracotomy, pericardiocentesis, cricothyreotomy, or tracheotomy.

As indicated, insert a Foley catheter and a nasogastric tube, give prophylactic antibiotics, obtain an order for appropriate diagnostic studies—such as peritoneal lavage or intravenous pyelography—and notify medical or surgical specialists.

Combat shock

Since severe injuries often lead to shock, check skin temperature, color, and moisture. To control shock, administer I.V. fluids (lactated Ringer's solution or normal saline) and consider using Medical Anti-shock Trousers (MAST).

In all massive external bleeding or suspected internal bleeding, watch for hypovolemia, and estimate blood loss. Remember, however, a 500 to 1,000 ml blood loss might not change systolic blood pressure, but it may decrease diastolic pressure and elevate the pulse rate. Stay alert for signs of occult bleeding, common in the chest, abdomen, pelvis, and thigh. Assess for such bleeding by taking serial girth measurements at these sites. Use a tape measure, and mark its placement on the body with a marking pen, so you measure in exactly the same place each time. This way you can accurately detect any enlargement. Increased diameter of the legs, abdomen, or pelvis often means leakage of blood into these tissues (as much as 4,000 ml into the abdomen, 3,000 ml into the chest, and 500 ml into a thigh). Such blood loss will induce textbook signs of hypovolemic shock (tachycardia, tachypnea, hypotension, restlessness, falling urinary output, and cold clammy skin).

If the patient has renal injuries or a fractured pelvis, look for the classic sign of retroperitoneal hematoma—numbness or pain in the leg on the affected side, which is the result of pressure on the lateral femoral cutaneous nerve in L1 to L3. Retroperitoneal bleeding may not cause abdominal tenderness. If the patient shows clinical signs of hypovolemia, immediately begin I.V. therapy with two or more large-bore catheters, and regulate fluids according to the severity of hypovolemia. Assist with insertion of a central venous pressure (CVP) or pulmonary artery catheter to monitor circulating blood volume.

Splinting for transport

Look for limb fractures and dislocations, and check circulation and neurovascular status distal to injury by palpating pulses distal to the injury and looking for the classic signs of arterial insufficiency: decreased or absent pulse, pallor, paresthesia, pain, and paralysis. Splint and apply traction, as needed.

Prepare the victim for transport. Use special care in suspected cervical spinal injury. If necessary, after splinting the injury site, also splint the areas above and below it, to prevent further soft-tissue and neurovascular damage and to minimize pain. Example: if the forearm is injured, splint wrist and elbow too.

Types of splints include:
- *soft splint*—a nonrigid splint (example: pillow or blanket)
- *hard splint*—rigid splint with a firm surface (example: long or short board, aluminum ladder splint, cardboard splint, padded board splint, plaster)
- *air splint*—inflatable splint
- *traction splint*—uses traction to decrease angulation and reduce pain (examples: Hare and Thomas splints).

Tips on applying a splint

- Splint most injuries "as they lie," except when the neurovascular status is compromised.
- Whenever possible, have two people apply the splint—one to support the injured part, the other to apply padding and the splint.
- Secure the splint to the injured extremity with straps or gauze. *Don't* use an elastic bandage.
- To apply an air splint, slide the splint over your arm backward, and with that same arm, grasp the distal portion of the injured limb. Then, slip the splint from your arm onto the injured extremity, and inflate the splint. Always use an air splint that's open at both ends, to permit neurovascular assessment.

HEAD INJURIES

Concussion

By far the most common head injury, concussion results from a blow to the head—a blow hard enough to jostle the brain and make it hit against the skull, causing temporary neural dysfunction, but not hard enough to cause a cerebral contusion. Most concussion victims recover completely within 24 to 48 hours. Repeated concussions, however, exact a cumulative toll on the brain.

Causes
The blow that causes a concussion is usually sudden and forceful—a fall to the ground, a punch to the head, an automobile accident. Also, such a blow sometimes results from child abuse. Whatever the cause, the resulting injury is mild compared to the damage done by cerebral contusions or lacerations.

Signs and symptoms
Concussion may produce a short-term loss of consciousness, vomiting, and both anterograde and retrograde amnesia; the patient not only can't recall what happened immediately after the injury, but also has difficulty recalling events that led up to the traumatic incident. The presence of anterograde amnesia and the duration of retrograde amnesia reliably correlate with the severity of the injury. The injury often causes adults to behave irritably, lethargically, or simply out of character, and usually brings complaints of dizziness, nausea, or severe headache. Some children have no apparent ill effects, but many grow lethargic and somnolent in a few hours. All these signs occur normally with a concussion, and don't necessarily indicate a serious injury. Postconcussion syndrome—headache, dizziness, vertigo, anxiety, fatigue—may persist for several weeks after the injury.

Diagnosis
Differentiating between concussion and more serious head injuries requires a

PATIENT TEACHING AID

What to Do After Concussion

You have suffered a concussion. Since it has not caused any serious brain injury, you are being discharged. For safety's sake, however, follow these instructions:
• Return to the hospital immediately if you experience a persistent or worsening headache, forceful or constant vomiting, blurred vision, any change in personality, abnormal eye movements, staggering gait, or twitching.
• Don't take any pain killer stronger than aspirin or acetaminophen.

• If vomiting occurs, eat lightly until it stops. (*Occasional* vomiting is normal after concussion.)
• Relax for 24 hours. Then, if you feel well, resume normal activities.
• Give this note to your parents, guardian, spouse, or roommate: *Wake me every 2 hours during the night, and ask me my name, where I am, and whether I can identify you. If you can't awaken me, or I can't answer these questions, bring me back to the hospital immediately.*

This patient teaching aid is intended for distribution to patients by doctors and nurses.
It must not be used without a doctor's approval.

thorough history of the trauma and a neurologic examination. Such an examination must evaluate the level of consciousness, mental status, cranial nerve and motor functions, deep tendon and abdominal reflexes, and orientation as to time, place, and person. If no abnormalities are found, the patient has probably suffered nothing worse than a concussion but should be observed for signs of more severe cerebral trauma. Observation provides a baseline for gauging any deterioration in the patient's condition. Skull X-rays may rule out fractures.

Treatment and additional considerations

• The patient should be asked for a thorough history of the trauma. If he's suffering from amnesia or can't speak, the history can be supplied by his family, eyewitnesses, or ambulance personnel.

To determine if the injury involved the head (this may not be apparent in the absence of a laceration or surface hematoma), the patient must be asked whether he lost consciousness and, if so, for how long.

• Vital signs must be monitored, and additional injuries ruled out. The skull should be palpated for tenderness or hematomas.

• If a neurologic examination reveals no abnormalities, the patient, while still in the emergency room, should be checked for vital signs, level of consciousness, and pupil size every 15 minutes. The patient who remains stable can be discharged with an instruction sheet. If his condition worsens or fluctuates, or if he develops an altered state of consciousness, or a neurologic examination reveals abnormalities, the injury may be more severe than a concussion; the patient should be admitted for neurosurgical consultation.

Cerebral Contusion

Cerebral contusion is a bruising of brain tissue as a result of a severe blow to the head. More serious than a concussion, contusion disrupts normal nerve functions in the bruised area, and may cause loss of consciousness, hemorrhage, edema, and even death.

Causes

Cerebral contusion results from acceleration-deceleration or coup-contrecoup injuries. Such injuries can occur directly beneath the site of impact when the brain rebounds against the skull from the force of a blow (a beating with a blunt instrument, for example), when the force of the blow drives the brain against the opposite side of the skull, or when the head is hurled forward and stopped abruptly (as in an automobile accident, when a driver's head strikes the windshield). The brain continues moving and slaps against the skull (acceleration), then rebounds (deceleration). These injuries can also cause the brain to strike against bony prominences inside the skull (especially the

sphenoidal ridges), causing intracranial hemorrhage or hematoma that may result in tentorial herniation.

Signs and symptoms

With cerebral contusion, the patient may sustain severe scalp wounds and display labored respirations. He may lose consciousness for a few minutes or for as long as an hour. If he remains conscious, he may be drowsy, confused, and/or disoriented, agitated, or even violent. He may also exhibit hemiparesis and decorticate or decerebrate posturing, and unequal pupillary response. Eventually, he should return to a relatively alert state, perhaps with temporary aphasia, slight hemiparesis, or unilateral numbness. A lucid period after head injury, followed by rapid dete-

rapid deterioration, suggests epidural hematoma.

Diagnosis

A history of the trauma and a neurologic examination are the principal diagnostic tools. Skull X-rays rule out fractures and may help to show a shift in brain tissue from the midline. Cerebral angiography outlines vasculature, and a CAT scan identifies ischemic or necrotic tissue. Intracranial hemorrhage contraindicates lumbar puncture.

Treatment and additional considerations

• First, a patent airway should be established; a tracheotomy may be necessary but is seldom undertaken on an emergency basis. Next, a neurologic examination should be performed, focusing on the level of consciousness, motor responses, and intracranial pressure.

• I.V. fluids should be started. Hypotonic fluids, such as 5% dextrose in water, are not indicated; they may aggravate cerebral edema. Mannitol I.V. may be given to reduce cerebral edema. Dexamethasone I.V. or I.M. will be given for several days to control cerebral edema.

• Blood will be typed and cross-matched for a patient suspected of having intracerebral hemorrhage. A blood transfusion may be needed and possibly a craniotomy, to control bleeding and to aspirate blood.

• A Foley catheter may be ordered to help monitor intake and output. With unconscious patients, a nasogastric tube is also inserted to prevent aspiration.

• Absolute bed rest must be enforced. The patient should be observed for CSF leaks. His bed sheets need to be checked for "halo" sign. If CSF leaks develop, the

HEMORRHAGE, HEMATOMA, AND TENTORIAL HERNIATION

Among the most serious consequences of a head injury are hemorrhage, hematoma, and tentorial herniation. An epidural hemorrhage or hematoma results from a rapid accumulation of blood between the skull and the dura mater; a subdural hemorrhage or hematoma, from a slow accumulation of blood between the dura mater and the subarachnoid membrane. Intracerebral hemorrhage or hematoma occurs within the cerebrum itself. Tentorial herniation occurs when injured brain tissue swells and squeezes itself through the tentorial notch, constricting the brain stem, impairing vital centers and cranial nerves, and reducing the brain's blood supply.

Epidural hemorrhage or hematoma causes immediate loss of consciousness, followed by a lucid interval lasting minutes to hours, which eventually gives way to a rapidly progressive decrease in the level of consciousness. Accompanying symptoms include hemiparesis, progressively severe headache, unilateral pupillary dilation (all on the same side as the lesion), as well as signs of increased intracranial pressure (ICP): decreasing pulse and respirations, and increasing systolic blood pressure. Because the blood accumulates slowly, symptoms of subdural hemorrhage or hematoma may not occur until days after the injury. Loss of consciousness again occurs, often with weakness or paralysis on one or both sides. Intracerebral hemorrhage or hematoma usually causes nuchal rigidity, photophobia, nausea, vomiting, dizziness, convulsions, decreased respiratory rate, and progressive obtundation.

Tentorial herniation causes drowsiness, confusion, dilation of one or both pupils, hyperventilation, nuchal rigidity, bradycardia, and decorticate or decerebrate posturing. Irreversible brain damage or death can occur rapidly.

Intracranial hemorrhage may require a craniotomy, to locate and control bleeding and to aspirate blood. Epidural and subdural hematomas are usually drained by aspiration through burr holes in the skull. Increased ICP may be controlled with mannitol I.V., steroids, or diuretics, but emergency surgery is usually required to save the patient's life.

head of the bed must be raised 30°. If CSF leaks from the nose (rhinorrhea), a gauze pad is placed under the nostrils. The patient should wipe his nose, *not* blow it. If CSF leaks from the ear, the patient needs to be positioned so the ear drains naturally. No packs should be placed in the ear or nose.

• Vital signs and respirations require regular monitoring (usually every 15 minutes). Abnormal respirations could indicate a breakdown in the respiratory center in the brain stem and a possible impending tentorial herniation—a critical neurologic emergency.

• Frequent neurologic checks should be performed. Restlessness, level of consciousness, and orientation as to time, place, and person must also be assessed.

• After the patient's condition has stabilized, superficial scalp wounds require cleaning and dressing. Administering tetanus prophylaxis, if the skin's broken, and suturing may be needed.

Skull Fractures

A skull fracture is considered a neurosurgical condition, since possible damage to the brain is the first concern, rather than the fracture itself. Skull fractures may be closed (simple) or open (compound) and may or may not displace bone fragments. Skull fractures are further described as linear, comminuted, or depressed. A linear fracture is a common hairline break, without displacement of structures; a comminuted fracture splinters or crushes the bone into several fragments; a depressed fracture pushes the bone toward the brain. Depressed fractures are of significance only if they compress underlying structures. In children, thinness and elasticity of the skull allow a depression without fracture (linear fracture across a suture line in an infant increases the possibility of epidural hematoma). Skull fractures are also classified according to location, such as a cranial vault fracture; a basilar fracture is at the base of the skull and involves the cribriform plate and the frontal sinuses. Because of the danger of grave cranial complications and meningitis, basilar fractures are usually far more serious than vault fractures.

Causes

Like concussions and cerebral contusions or lacerations, skull fractures invariably result from a traumatic blow to the head. Motor vehicle accidents, bad falls, and severe beatings (especially in children) top the list of causes.

Signs and symptoms

Skull fractures are often accompanied by scalp wounds—abrasions, contusions, lacerations, or avulsions. If the scalp has been lacerated or torn away, bleeding may be profuse, because the scalp contains many blood vessels. Bleeding is rarely heavy enough to induce hypovolemic shock, although the patient may be in shock from other injuries or from medullary failure in severe head injuries. Linear fractures associated only with concussion don't produce loss of consciousness (although the patient may appear dazed) and don't require treatment. A fracture that results in cerebral contusion or laceration, however, may cause the classic signs of brain injury: agitation and irritability, with loss of consciousness and changes in respiratory pattern (labored respirations).

If the patient with a skull fracture remains conscious, he is apt to complain of persistent, localized headache. Skull fracture also may result in cerebral edema, which may "jam" the reticular activating system, cutting off the normal flow of impulses to the brain and resulting in possible respiratory distress. The patient may have alterations in level of consciousness or may lose consciousness for hours, days, weeks, or indefinitely. When jagged bone fragments pierce the dura mater or the cerebral cortex, skull fractures may cause subdural, epidural, or intracerebral hemorrhage or hematoma. With the resulting space-occupying lesions, clinical findings may include hemiparesis, dizziness, convulsions, projectile vomiting, decreased pulse and respirations, and progressive unresponsiveness. Sphenoidal fractures may also damage the optic nerve, causing blindness, while temporal fractures can cause unilateral deafness or facial paralysis. Symptoms reflect the severity and the extent of the head injury. However, some elderly patients may have brain atrophy; therefore, they have more space for brain swelling under the cranium and, as a result, may not show signs of increased intracranial pressure (ICP).

A vault fracture often produces soft-tissue swelling in the area of the fracture, making it difficult to detect without X-rays.

A basilar fracture often produces hemorrhage from the nose, pharynx, or ears; blood under the periorbital skin ("raccoon's eyes") and under the conjunctiva; and Battle's sign (supramastoid ecchymosis), sometimes with bleeding behind the eardrum. This type of fracture may also cause CSF, or even brain tissue, to leak from the nose or ears.

Depending on the extent of brain damage, the patient could suffer residual effects, such as convulsive disorders (epilepsy), hydrocephalus, and organic brain syndrome. Children may develop headaches, giddiness, easy fatigability, neuroses, and behavior disorders.

Diagnosis

Brain injury shuld be suspected in all skull fractures until clinical evaluation proves otherwise. Therefore, every suspected skull injury calls for a thorough history of the trauma and skull X-rays to attempt to locate the fracture (vault fractures often aren't visible or palpable). A fracture also requires a neurologic examination, to check cerebral function (mental status and orientation to time, place, and person), level of consciousness, pupillary response, motor function, and deep tendon and abdominal reflexes. Using reagent strips, a dipstick test should be performed on the draining nasal or ear fluid for CSF. The tape turns blue if CSF is present; there is no change in the presence of blood alone. However, the tape will also turn blue if the patient is hyperglycemic. Also, the patient's bedsheets should be checked for the "halo sign"—a blood-tinged spot surrounded by a lighter ring—from leakage of CSF.

Brain damage can be assessed through:
• cerebral angiography, which reveals vascular disruptions from internal pressure or injury.
• CAT scan, echoencephalography, air encephalography, and radioactive scan, which disclose intracranial hemorrhage from ruptured blood vessels (carotid arteries, venous sinuses, middle meningeal artery) or cranial nerve injury, or will indicate or localize subdural or intracerebral hematomas.

Except for angiography, these tests are indicated only for patients not requiring neurosurgery. Expanding lesions contraindicate lumbar puncture.

Treatment

Although occasionally even a simple linear skull fracture can tear an underlying blood vessel or cause a CSF leak, linear fractures generally require only supportive treatment, including mild analgesics (aspirin or acetaminophen), and cleansing and debridement of any wounds after a local injection of procaine and shaving of the scalp around the wound. If the patient hasn't lost consciousness, he should be observed in the emergency room for at least 4 to 6 hours. Afterward, if vital signs are stable, he can be discharged and given an instruction sheet for 24 hours of observation at home.

More severe vault fractures, especially depressed fractures, usually require a craniotomy to elevate or remove fragments that have been driven into the brain, and to extract foreign bodies and necrotic tissue, thereby reducing the risk of infection and further brain damage.

Cranioplasty follows the use of tantalum mesh or acrylic plates to replace the removed skull section. Antibiotic therapy and, in profound hemorrhage, blood transfusions are often required.

Basilar fractures call for immediate prophylactic antibiotics to prevent the onset of meningitis from CSF leaks, and close observation for secondary hematomas and hemorrhages. Surgery may be necessary. In addition, both basilar and vault fractures require dexamethasone I.V. or I.M. to reduce cerebral edema and minimize brain tissue damage.

Additional considerations

• A patent airway must be established; a tracheotomy may be necessary. Aspiration must be done through the mouth, not the nose, to prevent introduction of bacteria in case a CSF leak is present.
• A complete history of the trauma must be obtained from the patient, his family, eyewitnesses, and ambulance personnel. The patient should be asked whether he lost consciousness and, if so, for how long. Diagnostic tests, including a neurologic examination, will be ordered. Abnormal reflexes, such as Babinski's reflex, must be checked.
• CSF draining may occur from the ears, nose, or mouth. Pillowcases and linens should be checked for CSF leaks and "halo" sign. If the patient's nose is draining CSF, he must wipe it—*not* blow it. If an ear is draining, it should be covered lightly with sterile gauze—*not* packed.
• A patient with a head injury should be positioned so secretions can drain properly. With CSF leaks, the head of the bed must be elevated 30°; without CSF leaks, the head of the bed can be left flat, but the patient should be positioned on his side or abdomen. Such a patient risks jugular compression leading to increased ICP, if he's not positioned on his back, so his head must be kept properly aligned. Scalp wounds need to be covered with a sterile dressing; and bleeding controlled, as necessary.
• Seizure precautions should be taken, but not to the point of restraining the patient. Hypoxia or increased ICP, which can also cause agitated behavior, must be watched for. Sudden moves around the patient must be avoided.
• Narcotics or sedatives can't be given, because they may depress respirations, increase CO_2, and lead to increased ICP, as well as mask changes in neurologic status. Instead, a mild analgesic for pain should be given as ordered.

When a fracture requires surgery:
• Consent is needed to shave the patient's head, to provide a clean area for surgery. Blood must be typed and cross-matched. Baseline laboratory studies, such as CBC, electrolytes, and urinalysis, may be ordered.
• After surgery, vital signs and neurologic status must be monitored often (usually every 5 minutes until stable, and then every 15 minutes for 1 hour). Any changes in level of consciousness require reporting. Since skull fractures and brain injuries heal slowly, dramatic postop improvement can't be expected.
• Intake and output needs to be monitored frequently. Foley catheter patency must be maintained. Hypotonic fluids (even 5% dextrose in water) can increase cerebral edema, so they should be given only as ordered.
• If the patient is unconscious, he should get parenteral nutrition. (The patient may regurgitate and aspirate food if a nasogastric tube is used.)

When the fracture doesn't require surgery:
• The scalp laceration should be examined. The wound can be probed with a gloved finger for foreign bodies and palpable fracture. Lacerations and surrounding area should be gently cleansed and covered with sterile gauze. Suturing may be necessary.
• The patient and his family will need emotional support. They should understand the need for procedures to reduce the risk of brain injury.
• Before discharge, the patient's family must be instructed on how to identify changes in mental status, level of consciousness, or respirations, and how to relieve the patient's headache with aspirin or acetaminophen. The patient's family

should bring the patient to the hospital immediately if his level of consciousness decreases, if his headaches persist (after several doses of mild analgesics), if he vomits more than once, or if weakness develops in his arms or legs. The family must know how to care for his scalp wound. Finally, they should be told when to return for suture removal and follow-up evaluation.

Fractured Nose

The most common facial fracture, a fractured nose usually results from blunt injury and is often associated with other facial fractures. The severity of the fracture depends on the direction, force and type of the blow. Severe, comminuted fracture may cause extreme swelling or bleeding that may jeopardize the airway and require tracheotomy during early treatment. Inadequate or delayed treatment may cause permanent nasal displacement, septal deviation, and obstruction.

Signs and symptoms
Immediately after injury, nosebleed may occur (ranging from minimal trickling to full nasal hemorrhage), and soft-tissue swelling may quickly obscure the break. After several hours, pain, periorbital ecchymoses, and nasal displacement and deformity are prominent. Possible complications include septal hematoma, which may lead to abscess formation, resulting in avascular and septic necrosis.

Diagnosis
Clinical findings, palpation, and X-rays confirm a nasal fracture. Diagnosis also requires a complete patient history, including the cause of the injury and the amount of nasal bleeding. Watch for clear fluid drainage, which may suggest a CSF leak.

Treatment
Treatment restores normal facial appearance and reestablishes bilateral nasal passage after swelling subsides. Reduction of the fracture corrects alignment; immobilization (intranasal packing and an external splint shaped to the nose and taped) maintains it. Such reduction is best accomplished in the operating room, with local anesthetic for adults and general anesthetic for children. Severe swelling may delay treatment for several days to a week. In addition, CSF leakage calls for close observation and antibiotic therapy; septal hematoma requires incision and drainage to prevent necrosis.

Additional considerations
• Treatment must start immediately. While waiting for X-rays, ice packs should be applied to the nose to minimize swelling (these packs must first be wrapped in a light towel to prevent direct contact with the skin.) To control anterior bleeding, gentle, local pressure should be applied. Posterior bleeding is rare and requires an internal tamponade applied in the emergency department.
• Since the patient will find breathing more difficult as the swelling increases, he should breathe slowly through his mouth. To warm the inhaled air during cold weather, he will need to cover his mouth with a handkerchief or scarf. To prevent subcutaneous emphysema or intracranial air penetration (and potential meningitis), he must not blow his nose.
• Following packing and splinting, ice in a plastic bag should be applied over the bandages.
• Before discharge, the patient should know that ecchymoses will fade after about a week.

Dislocated or Fractured Jaw

Dislocation of the jaw is a displacement of the temporomandibular joint. A fracture of the jaw is a break in one or both of the two maxillae (upper jawbones) or the mandible (lower jawbone). Treatment can usually restore jaw alignment and function.

Causes
Simple fractures or dislocations are usually caused by a manual blow along the jawline; more serious compound fractures often result from car accidents.

Signs and symptoms
Malocclusion is the most obvious sign of dislocation or fracture. Other signs include mandibular pain, swelling, ecchymosis, loss of function, and asymmetry. In addition, mandibular fractures that damage the alveolar nerve produce paresthesia or anesthesia of the chin and lower lip. Maxillary fractures produce infraorbital paresthesia and often accompany fractures of the nasal and orbital complex.

Diagnosis
Abnormal maxillary or mandibular mobility during physical examination and a history of trauma suggest fracture or dislocation; X-rays confirm it.

Treatment
As in all trauma, checking for a patent airway, adequate ventilation, and pulses takes priority; then, controlling hemorrhage, and checking for other injuries should follow. As necessary, the doctor will order an oropharyngeal airway, nasotracheal intubation, or a tracheotomy. Pain should be relieved with analgesics, as needed. After the patient stabilizes, surgical reduction and fixation by wiring restores mandibular and maxillary alignment. Maxillary fractures may also require reconstruction and repair of soft-tissue injuries. Teeth or bone are never removed during surgery unless unavoidable. If the patient has lost teeth due to trauma, the surgeon will decide whether they can be reimplanted. If they can, they'll only be viable within 6 hours after injury. Dislocations are usually manually reduced under anesthesia.

Additional considerations
After reconstructive surgery:
• The patient should be positioned on his side, with his head slightly elevated. A nasogastric tube is usually in place, with low suction to remove gastric contents and prevent nausea, vomiting, and aspiration of vomitus. As necessary, the nasopharynx should be suctioned through the nose, or by inserting a small suction catheter through any natural gap between teeth.
• If the patient isn't intubated, nourishment must be provided through a straw. If a natural gap occurs between teeth, the straw can be inserted there; if not, one or two teeth may have to be extracted. However, such extraction is avoided when possible. Feeding should start with clear liquids; after the patient can tolerate fluids, milk shakes, eggnog, broth, juices, blenderized foods, and commercial nutritional supplements are appropriate.
• If the patient is unable to tolerate oral fluids, I.V. therapy can maintain hydration postoperatively.
• Antiemetics may be ordered to minimize nausea and prevent aspiration of vomitus (a very real danger in a patient whose jaw is wired). A pair of wire cutters must be kept at the bedside to snip the wires should the patient vomit.
• A dental water-pulsator may be used for mouth care while the wires are intact.
• Since the patient will have difficulty talking while his jaw is wired, he should be given a Magic Slate or pencil and paper so he can communicate.

Perforated Eardrum

Perforation of the eardrum is a rupture of the tympanic membrane. Such injury may cause otitis media and hearing loss.

Causes
The usual cause of perforated eardrum is trauma: the deliberate or accidental insertion of sharp objects (cotton swabs, bobby pins) or sudden excessive changes in pressure (explosion, a blow to the head, flying, or diving). The injury may also result from untreated otitis media, and in children, from acute otitis media.

Signs and symptoms
Sudden onset of severe earache and bleeding from the ear are the first signs of a perforated eardrum. Other symptoms include hearing loss, tinnitus, and vertigo. Purulent otorrhea within 24 to 48 hours of injury signals infection.

Diagnosis
 Severe earache and bleeding from the ear with a history of trauma strongly suggest perforated eardrum; direct visualization of the perforated tympanic membrane with an otoscope confirms it. Additional diagnostic measures include audiometric testing and a check of voluntary facial movements to rule out facial nerve damage.

Treatment and additional considerations
If there is bleeding from the ear, a sterile, cotton-tipped applicator can be used to absorb the blood and any purulent drainage or CSF leakage. A culture of the specimen may be ordered. *Irrigation of the ear is absolutely contraindicated.* A sterile dressing should be applied over the outer ear. Then, the patient should see an ear specialist for follow-up care.

A large perforation accompanied by uncontrolled bleeding may require immediate surgery to approximate the ruptured edges. Treatment may include a mild analgesic to relieve pain, a sedative to decrease anxiety, and an oral antibiotic.

If the suspected cause of the injury is child abuse, the matter must be reported to the local police. Before discharge, the patient must know not to blow his nose or get water in his ear canal until the perforation heals.

External Ear Laceration

External ear laceration is a common injury. Its severity ranges from earlobe laceration (often caused by a sharp pull on a hoop-shaped earring) to almost complete external ear avulsion.

Signs and symptoms
Symptoms include pain, swelling, and bleeding; clinical examination confirms this diagnosis. If the injury is severe, clinical evaluation should include skull X-rays and a neurologic examination for possible facial nerve damage and head trauma.

Treatment
After careful and gentle cleansing, earlobe laceration requires suturing to join separated edges, and to correct alignment and cover exposed cartilage (such cartilage is highly susceptible to severe infection). Some lacerations may require shaving a small area of surrounding

scalp. After suturing, the application of antibiotic ointment and a small sterile dressing is appropriate to maintain ear alignment and prevent skin surfaces from touching. Because injured ears tend to swell significantly, a bulky dressing is preferred to prevent pressure necrosis. Tetanus prophylaxis may also be necessary.

Additional considerations
The patient should:
• apply ice packs intermittently for 1 to 2 days to reduce pain and swelling.
• change the dressing and reapply antibiotic ointment, as prescribed (usually two to four times daily).
• see the doctor for follow-up care, including suture removal.

NECK & SPINAL INJURIES

Acceleration-deceleration Cervical Injuries
(Whiplash)

Acceleration-deceleration cervical injuries result from sharp hyperextension and flexion of the neck that damages muscles, ligaments, disks, and nerve tissue in the cervical area. Prognosis is excellent; symptoms usually subside with symptomatic treatment.

Causes
Commonly, whiplash results from rear-end automobile accidents. However, the padded headrests and seat belts with shoulder harnesses required in new cars have reduced the risk.

Signs and symptoms
Although symptoms may develop immediately, if the injury is mild they're often delayed 12 to 24 hours. Whiplash produces moderate to severe anterior and posterior neck pain. Within several days, the anterior pain diminishes, but posterior pain persists or even intensifies, causing patients to seek medical attention if they didn't do so before. Whiplash may also cause dizziness, gait disturbances, vomiting, headache, nuchal rigidity, neck muscle asymmetry, and rigidity or numbness in the arms.

Diagnosis
An X-ray of the lateral cervical spine is required to rule out cervical fractures. If the X-ray is negative, examination emphasizes motor ability and sensation below the cervical spine, to detect possible signs of nerve root compression.

Treatment and additional considerations
In all suspected spinal injuries, the spine should be considered injured until proven otherwise. The patient with suspected whiplash or other injuries who can't walk requires careful transportation from the accident scene on a spine board, with sandbags on both sides of his head to prevent rotation. If he can walk, a soft cervical collar provides support and minimizes pain during transport. Until an X-ray rules out cervical fracture, the patient should be moved as little as possible and be encouraged to remain still. Jewelry must be removed before an x-ray's taken but the patient should not be undressed.

Symptomatic treatment includes:
• mild analgesic—such as aspirin with codeine—and possibly a muscle relaxant—such as diazepam, or chlorzoxazone with acetaminophen
• hot showers, or warm compresses to the neck to relieve pain
• immobilization with a soft, padded cervical collar for several days or weeks
• in severe muscle spasms, short-term cervical traction.

Most whiplash patients are discharged immediately. Before discharge, patients need to know how to identify their drug's side effects; must be told to avoid alcohol if they're receiving diazepam; and should rest for a few days and avoid lifting heavy objects. They should return immediately to the hospital for further neurologic evaluation if they experience persistent pain or if they develop numbness, tingling, or weakness on one side.

Spinal Injuries
(Without cord damage)

Spinal injuries include fractures, contusions, and compressions of the vertebral column, usually the result of trauma to the head or neck. The real danger lies in possible spinal cord damage. Spinal fractures most commonly occur in the fifth, sixth, and seventh cervical, twelfth thoracic, and first lumbar vertebrae, where there's a greater range of mobility than elsewhere in the vertebral column.

Causes
Most serious spinal injuries result from motor vehicle accidents, falls, diving into shallow water, and gunshot wounds; less serious injuries, from lifting heavy objects and minor falls. Spinal dysfunction may also result from hyperparathyroidism and neoplastic lesions.

Signs and symptoms
The most obvious symptom of spinal injury is muscle spasm, and back pain that worsens with movement. In cervical fractures, pain may produce point tenderness; in dorsal and lumbar fractures, it may radiate to other body areas, such as the legs. If the injury damages the spinal cord, clinical effects range from mild paresthesia to quadriplegia and shock. After milder injuries, such symptoms may be delayed for several days or weeks.

Diagnosis
Diagnosis rests on patient history, neurologic examination, X-rays, and possibly, lumbar puncture and myelography.
• *History* may reveal trauma, metastatic lesion, infection that could produce a spinal abscess, or endocrine disorder.
• *Physical examination* (including a neurologic evaluation) locates the level of injury and detects cord damage.
• *Spinal X-rays*, the most important diagnostic measure, locate the fracture.
• In spinal compression, a *lumbar puncture* may show increased CSF pressure from a lesion or trauma; *myelography* locates the spinal mass.

Treatment
The primary treatment after spinal injury is immediate immobilization to stabilize the spine and prevent cord damage; other treatment is supportive. Cervical injuries require immobilization, using sandbags on both sides of the patient's head, a plaster cast, hard cervical collar, or skeletal traction, using skull tongs (Crutchfield, Barton, Vinke) or a halo device.

Treatment of stable lumbar and dorsal fractures consists of bed rest on firm support (such as a bed board), analgesics, and muscle relaxants until the fracture stabilizes (usually 10 to 12 weeks). Later treatment includes exercises to strengthen the back muscles, and a back brace or corset to provide support while walking.

An unstable dorsal or lumbar fracture requires a plaster cast, turning frame, and in severe fracture, a laminectomy and spinal fusion. When the damage results in compression of the spinal column, neurosurgery may relieve the pressure. If the cause of compression is a metastatic lesion, chemotherapy and radiation may relieve it. Surface wounds accompanying the spinal injury require tetanus prophylaxis unless the patient has had recent immunization.

Additional considerations
In all spinal injuries, suspect cord damage until proven otherwise.
• During initial assessment and during X-rays, the patient must be immobilized on a firm surface, with sandbags on both sides of his head. He should not move or be moved, since hyperflexion can damage the cord. But if he *must* be moved, he should be logrolled, to avoid disturbing body alignment.
• Throughout assessment, the patient will need comfort and reassurance. His fear of possible paralysis may be overwhelming. A family member who isn't too distraught should be allowed to accompany him and talk to him quietly.
• If the injury necessitates surgery, prophylactic antibiotics and catheterization (to avoid urinary retention) may be ordered. Defecation patterns require monitoring to avoid impaction.
• Traction methods should be explained to the patient and his family. They should know that traction devices don't penetrate the brain. If the patient has a halo or skull-tong traction device, pin sites should be cleaned daily, hair trimmed short, and analgesics provided for persistent headaches. During traction, the patient must be turned often to prevent pneumonia, embolism, and skin breakdown; and must perform passive range-of-motion exercises to maintain muscle tone. Using a CircOlectric bed or Stryker frame facilitates turning and avoids further spinal cord injury.
• The patient should be turned on his side during feedings, to prevent aspiration. A relaxed atmosphere is best at mealtimes.
• Diversionary activities can help fill the long hours of immobility. Prism glasses will help the patient read comfortably.
• Neurologic status requires close scrutiny and changes must be reported immediately. Skin sensation and loss of muscle strength, for example, could point to pressure on the spinal cord, possibly as a result of edema or shifting bone fragments.
• The patient should walk as soon as the doctor allows; he'll probably have to wear a back brace.
• Before discharge, the patient must know the importance of taking his medication on schedule and getting regular follow-up examinations.
• To help prevent spinal injury from becoming spinal *cord* injury, firemen, policemen, paramedics, and the general public should know the proper way to handle such injuries.

THORACIC INJURIES

Blunt Chest Injuries

Chest injuries account for one fourth of all trauma deaths in the United States. Many are blunt chest injuries, which include myocardial contusion, and rib and sternal fractures that may be simple, multiple, displaced, or jagged. Such fractures may cause potentially fatal complications, such as hemothorax, pneumothorax, hemorrhagic shock, and diaphragmatic rupture.

Causes
Most blunt chest injuries result from automobile accidents in which the driver is thrown against the steering wheel.

Signs and symptoms
Rib fractures produce tenderness, slight edema over the fracture site, and pain that worsens with deep breathing and

FLAIL CHEST: PARADOXICAL BREATHING

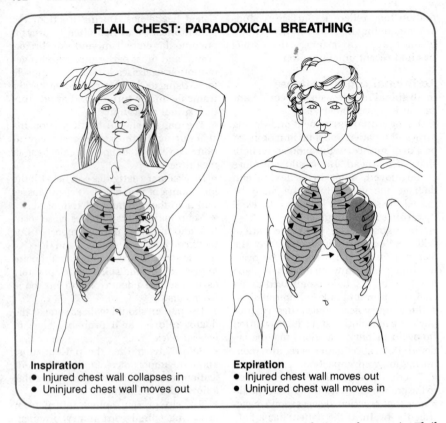

Inspiration
- Injured chest wall collapses in
- Uninjured chest wall moves out

Expiration
- Injured chest wall moves out
- Uninjured chest wall moves in

movement; this painful breathing causes the patient to display shallow, splinted respirations that may lead to hypoventilation. Sternal fractures, which are usually transverse and located in the middle or upper sternum, produce persistent chest pains, even at rest. If a fractured rib tears the pleura and punctures a lung, it causes pneumothorax, which usually produces severe dyspnea, cyanosis, agitation, extreme pain, and when air escapes into chest tissue, subcutaneous emphysema.

Multiple rib fractures may cause flail chest: a portion of the chest wall caves in, which causes a loss of chest wall integrity, and prevents adequate lung inflation. Bruised skin, extreme pain caused by rib fracture and disfigurement, paradoxical chest movements, and rapid, shallow respirations are all signs of flail chest, as are tachycardia, hypotension,

respiratory acidosis, and cyanosis. Flail chest can also cause tension pneumothorax, a condition in which air enters the chest but can't be ejected during exhalation; life-threatening thoracic pressure buildup causes lung collapse and subsequent mediastinal shift. The cardinal symptoms of tension pneumothorax include tracheal deviation (away from the affected side), cyanosis, severe dyspnea, absent breath sounds (on the affected side), agitation, distended jugular veins, and shock.

Hemothorax occurs when a rib lacerates lung tissue or an intercostal artery, causing blood to collect in the pleural cavity, thereby compressing the lung and limiting respiratory capacity. Massive hemothorax is the most common cause of shock following chest trauma. Although slight bleeding occurs even with mild pneumothorax, such bleeding resolves very quickly, usually without changing the patient's condition. Rib fractures may also cause pulmonary contusion (resulting in hemoptysis, anoxia, dyspnea, and possible obstruction), large myocardial tears (rapidly fatal), and small myocardial tears (causing pericardial effusion). Myocardial contusions produce tachycardia, arrhythmia, conduction delays, and ST-T segment changes. Laceration or rupture of the aorta is nearly always immediately fatal. Rarely, laceration of the aorta may develop 24 hours after blunt injury, so vigilant patient observation is critical. Diaphragmatic rupture (usually on the left side because the liver protects the right side) causes severe respiratory distress. Unless treated early, abdominal viscera may herniate through the rupture into the thorax, compromising both circulation and the lungs' vital capacity.

Diagnosis

History of trauma with dyspnea, chest pain, and other typical clinical features suggest a blunt chest injury. To determine the extent of the injury, however, a thorough physical examination and other diagnostic measures are necessary.
• Chest X-rays may confirm rib and sternal fractures, pneumothorax, flail chest, pulmonary contusions (nonsegmental infiltrate resembling pulmonary edema), lacerated or ruptured aorta (widened mediastinum), tension pneumothorax (mediastinal shift), diaphragmatic rupture, and lung compression, or atelectasis with hemothorax.
• In hemothorax, percussion reveals a dullness that shifts when the patient changes position. In tension pneumothorax, percussion reveals a hyperresonant or tympanic note; auscultation may reveal a change in position of the loudest heart sound, indicating possible mediastinal shift.
• With cardiac damage, EKG changes are usually nonspecific but may show a right bundle branch block.
• Serial SGOT, SGPT, LDH, creatine phosphokinase (CPK), and MB fraction are elevated.

• Retrograde aortography reveals aortic laceration or rupture.
• Contrast studies, and liver and spleen scans help detect diaphragmatic rupture.

Treatment and additional considerations

Blunt chest injuries call for immediate physical assessment, control of bleeding, maintenance of a patent airway, adequate ventilation, and fluid and electrolyte balance.
• The following should be evaluated: Pulses (including peripheral pulses); level of consciousness; color and temperature of skin; depth of respiration; use of accessory muscles; length of inspirations compared to expirations; tracheal position, jugular vein distension and paradoxical chest motion; heart and lung sounds; and structural rib integrity.
• A quick history of the injury should be obtained. (If it involved a weapon, the police must be notified.) Unless severe dyspnea is present, the patient should locate the pain, and say if he's having trouble breathing. The doctor will order appropriate lab studies, such as arterial blood gases, cardiac enzymes, CBC, and typing and crossmatching.
• For simple rib fractures, a mild analgesic, bed rest, and heat applied to the affected area is usually ordered. The chest should not be strapped or taped.
• For more severe fractures, the doctor may administer intercostal nerve blocks. (He'll order X-rays both before and after to rule out pneumothorax.) The patient will be intubated in the event of excessive bleeding or hemopneumothorax. Chest tubes may also be inserted. To prevent atelectasis, the patient must be turned frequently, and encouraged to cough and deep breathe.
• For pneumothorax, the doctor will place a large-bore needle into the second intercostal space—in the midclavicular line on the affected side, or in the midaxillary line at the fourth intercostal space—to aspirate as much air as possible from the pleural cavity and to reexpand the lungs. When time permits,

chest tubes will be inserted and attached to water-seal drainage and suction.

• For flail chest, the patient is placed in semi-Fowler's position. The affected area is wrapped with an elastic bandage, or padded with a thick dressing and, then, taped with wide adhesive, to stabilize the chest wall. As temporary first aid, sandbags should be placed on the affected side, or manual pressure exerted over the flail segment on exhalation. An endotracheal tube must be used to give oxygen at a high-flow rate under positive pressure. The patient should: be repositioned and suctioned frequently, receive postural drainage, have his acid-base balance maintained, and be put on controlled mechanical ventilation until paradoxical motion of the chest wall ceases. The patient must be watched for signs of tension pneumothorax. I.V. therapy may be ordered using lactated Ringer's or normal saline solution.

• For hemothorax, shock is treated with I.V. infusions of lactated Ringer's or normal saline solution. Oxygen is administered and chest tubes are inserted into the fifth or sixth intercostal space at the midaxillary line, to remove blood. Vital signs and blood loss are monitored. Falling blood pressure, rising pulse rate, and uncontrolled hemorrhage all mandate thoracotomy to stop bleeding.

• For pulmonary contusions, the doctor may order limited amounts of colloids (salt-poor albumin, whole blood, or plasma) to replace volume and maintain oncotic pressure; analgesics; diuretics; and if necessary, corticosteroids (the use of steroids is controversial). Blood gases must be monitored to ensure adequate ventilation. Oxygen therapy, mechanical ventilation, and chest tube care should be provided, as needed.

• For suspected cardiac damage, close intensive care or telemetry may detect dysrhythmias and prevent cardiogenic shock. The patient should be put on bed rest in semi-Fowler's position (unless the patient requires shock position); and, as needed, receive oxygen, analgesics, and supportive drugs, such as digitalis, to control heart failure or supraventricular arrhythmia. If cardiac tamponade occurs, the doctor will perform pericardiocentesis. Essentially, this patient should get the same care that's given a patient who's suffered a myocardial infarction.

• For myocardial rupture, septal perforations, and other cardiac lacerations, immediate surgical repair is mandatory; less severe ventricular wounds require a digital or balloon catheter; atrial wounds, a clamp or balloon catheter.

• For the patient with aortic rupture or laceration who reaches the hospital alive, immediate surgery is mandatory, using synthetic grafts or anastomosis to repair the damage. The patient will be given large volumes of I.V. fluids (lactated Ringer's or normal saline solution), and whole blood, along with oxygen at very high flow rates; placed in Medical Antishock Trousers (MAST suit); and transported to the operating room.

• For tension pneumothorax, the doctor will insert a spinal or 14- to 16-gauge needle into the second intercostal space at the midclavicular line, to release pressure in the chest. A chest tube will also be inserted to normalize pressure and reexpand the lung. The patient should receive oxygen under positive pressure, along with I.V. fluids.

• For a diaphragmatic rupture, a nasogastric tube should be inserted to temporarily decompress the stomach. The diaphragm will need surgical repair.

Penetrating Chest Wounds

Penetrating chest wounds, depending on their size, may cause varying degrees of damage to bones, soft tissue, blood vessels, and nerves. Mortality and morbidity from a chest wound depend on the size and severity of the wound. Gunshot wounds are usually more serious than stab wounds, both because they cause more severe lacerations and cause rapid blood loss and because ricochet often damages large areas and multiple organs. With prompt, aggressive treatment, up to 90% of patients with penetrating chest wounds recover.

Causes

Stab wounds from a knife or ice pick are the most common penetrating chest wounds; gunshot wounds are a close second. Wartime explosions or firearms fired at close range are the usual source of large, gaping wounds.

Signs and symptoms

Aside from the obvious chest injuries, penetrating chest wounds cause:
• a sucking sound, as the diaphragm contracts and air enters the chest cavity through the opening in the chest wall.
• varying levels of consciousness, depending on the extent of the injury. If the patient is awake and alert, he may be in severe pain, which will cause him to splint his respirations, thereby reducing his vital capacity.
• tachycardia, due to anxiety and blood loss.
• weak, thready pulse, from massive blood loss and hypovolemic shock.

Penetrating chest wounds may also cause lung lacerations (bleeding and substantial air leakage through the chest tube); arterial lacerations (loss of more than 100 ml blood/hour through the chest tube); exsanguination; pneumothorax (air in pleural space causes loss of negative intrathoracic pressure and lung collapse); tension pneumothorax (intrapleural air accumulation causes potentially fatal mediastinal shift); and hemothorax, arrhythmias, cardiac tamponade, mediastinitis, subcutaneous emphysema, esophageal perforation, and bronchopleural fistula.

Diagnosis

 An obvious chest wound and a sucking sound during breathing confirm the diagnosis. Any lower thoracic chest injury should be considered a thoracicoabdominal injury until proven otherwise. Baseline data include:

• arterial blood gases to assess respiratory status.
• chest X-rays before and after chest tube placement to evaluate injury and tube placement.
• CBC, including hemoglobin, hematocrit, and differential. Low hemoglobin and hematocrit reflect severe blood loss.
• palpation and auscultation of chest and abdomen to evaluate damage to adjacent organs and structures.

Treatment and additional considerations

Penetrating chest wounds require immediate support of respiration and circulation, prompt surgical repair of tissue injury, and appropriate measures to prevent complications. The following actions should also be taken:
• Immediately assessing airway, breathing, and circulation (ABCs); establishing a patent airway and support ventilation, as needed; monitoring pulses frequently for rate and quality.
• Placing an occlusive dressing (for example, petrolatum-impregnated gauze) over the sucking chest wound; monitoring for signs of tension pneumothorax, which are tracheal shift, respiratory distress, tachycardia, tachypnea, and diminished or absent breath sounds on the affected side (if tension pneumothorax develops, the occlusive dressing should be temporarily removed to create an open pneumothorax).
• Controlling blood loss; typing and cross-matching blood; replacing blood and fluids, as necessary.
• Taking a chest X-ray; placing chest tubes (using water-seal drainage) to reestablish intrathoracic pressure, and to drain blood in hemothorax. (A second X-ray will evaluate the position of tubes and their function.)
• Monitoring central venous pressure and blood pressure to detect hypovolemia; assessing vital signs. (Analgesics

should be provided, as appropriate. Tetanus and antibiotic prophylaxis may be necessary.)
• Comforting the patient, especially if he's been the victim of a violent crime. Such incidents must be reported to the police in accordance with local laws. The patient's family must be contacted and comforted, as well.

After the patient's condition has stabilized, surgery can repair the damage caused by the wound.

ABDOMINAL & PELVIC INJURIES

Blunt and Penetrating Abdominal Injuries

Blunt and penetrating abdominal injuries may damage major blood vessels and internal organs. Their most immediate life-threatening consequence is hemorrhage and hypovolemic shock; later threats include infection. Prognosis depends on the extent of injury and the organs damaged, but is generally improved by prompt diagnosis and surgical repair.

Causes
Blunt (nonpenetrating) abdominal injuries usually result from automobile accidents, falls from heights, or athletic injuries; penetrating abdominal injuries, from stab and gunshot wounds.

Signs and symptoms
Symptoms vary with the degree of injury and the organs damaged. Penetrating abdominal injuries cause obvious wounds (gunshots often produce both entrance and exit wounds), with variable blood loss, pain, and tenderness. These injuries often cause pallor, cyanosis, tachycardia, shortness of breath, and hypotension.

Blunt abdominal injuries cause severe pain (such pain may radiate beyond the abdomen, for instance, to the shoulders), bruises, abrasions, contusions, or distention. They may also result in tenderness, abdominal splinting or rigidity, nausea, vomiting, pallor, cyanosis, tachycardia, and shortness of breath. Rib fractures often accompany blunt injuries.

In both blunt and penetrating injuries, massive blood loss may cause hypovolemic shock, diaphragm injury, respiratory distress, rupture of the colon, or peritonitis. In general, damage to solid abdominal organs (liver, spleen, pancreas, and kidneys) causes hemorrhage; damage to hollow organs (stomach, intestine, gallbladder, and bladder) causes rupture and release of the organs' contents (including bacteria) into the abdomen, with resultant inflammation.

Diagnosis
A history of abdominal trauma, clinical features, and laboratory results confirm the diagnosis and determine organ damage. Any upper abdominal injury should be considered a thoracicoabdominal injury until proven otherwise. Laboratory studies vary with the patient's condition but usually include:
• chest X-rays (preferably done with the patient upright, to show free air)
• abdominal films
• examination of the stool and stomach aspirate for blood
• blood studies (decreased hematocrit and hemoglobin point to blood loss; coagulation studies evaluate hemostasis; an elevated WBC doesn't necessarily mean infection; typing and crossmatching are done prior to a transfusion)
• arterial blood gases to evaluate respiratory status
• serum amylase levels, which often may be elevated in pancreatic injury

- ultrasound examination
- intravenous pyelography to detect renal and urinary tract damage
- radioisotope scanning and ultrasound to detect liver, kidney, or spleen injury
- angiography to detect specific injuries, especially to the kidneys
- abdominal paracentesis (peritoneal lavage), with a midline insertion of a lavage catheter to check for blood, urine, pus, ascitic fluid, bile, and chyle (a milky fluid absorbed by the intestinal lymph vessels during digestion). In blunt trauma, with equivocal abdominal findings, this procedure helps establish the need for exploratory surgery.
- exploratory laparotomy to detect specific injuries when other clinical evidence is incomplete
- other lab studies to rule out associated injuries, such as head injuries.

Treatment

Emergency treatment of abdominal injuries controls hemorrhage and prevents hypovolemic shock by the infusion of I.V. fluids and possibly, blood components. After stabilization, most abdominal injuries require surgical repair. Analgesics and antibiotics increase patient comfort and prevent infection. Most patients with a history of abdominal trauma require hospitalization; if they're asymptomatic, they may require observation for only 6 to 24 hours.

Additional considerations

Emergency care in abdominal injuries has, as its aim, the support of vital functions by maintaining airway, breathing, and circulation. At admission, respiratory and circulatory status must be evaluated immediately and if possible, a history of the trauma obtained.

- To maintain airway and breathing, the patient should be intubated and put on mechanical ventilation, or given supplemental oxygen as necessary.
- One or more I.V. lines should be started using a large-bore needle. They'll be needed for monitoring and for rapid fluid infusion, using a normal saline solution. Then, a blood sample must be drawn for laboratory studies. Also, a nasogastric tube and, if necessary, a Foley catheter should be inserted; stomach aspirate and urine should be monitored for blood.

- Vital signs are needed for baseline data and require frequent monitoring.
- A sterile dressing should be applied to open wounds. A suspected pelvic injury can be splinted on arrival by tying the patient's legs together with a pillow between them. Such a patient should be moved as little as possible.
- Analgesics can be administered, as ordered. Usually, narcotics aren't recommended; but if the pain is severe, narcotics may be given in small titrated I.V. doses.
- Tetanus prophylaxis and prophylactic I.V. antibiotics may be ordered.
- To prepare the patient for surgery, a consent form is needed, signed by the patient or a responsible relative. Any dentures must be removed. Blood should be typed and crossmatched.
- If the injury was caused by a motor vehicle accident, or a shooting or stabbing, the police must be notified. In the case of a shooting or stabbing, all of the patient's clothes must be retained for the police. The number and sites of the wounds must also be documented.

PROJECTILE PATHWAY

Probable internal damage can be estimated by determining the organs lying on the pathway between the entry and exit sites.

INJURIES OF THE EXTREMITIES

Sprains and Strains

A sprain is a complete or incomplete tear in the supporting ligaments surrounding a joint that usually follows a sharp twist. A strain is an injury to a muscle or tendinous attachment. Both injuries usually heal without surgical repair.

Signs and symptoms

A sprain causes local pain (especially during joint movement), swelling, loss of mobility (which may not occur until several hours after the injury), and a black-and-blue discoloration, from blood extravasating into surrounding tissues. A sprained ankle is the most common joint injury.

A strain may be acute (an immediate result of vigorous muscle overuse or overstress) or chronic (a result of repeated overuse). An acute strain causes a sharp, transient pain (the patient may say he heard a snapping noise) and rapid swelling. When severe pain subsides, the muscle is tender; after several days, ecchymoses appear. A chronic strain causes stiffness, soreness, and generalized tenderness; these conditions appear several hours after the injury.

Diagnosis

History of recent injury or chronic overuse, clinical findings, and an X-ray to rule out fractures establish the diagnosis.

Treatment and additional considerations

Treatment of sprains consists of controlling pain and swelling, and immobilizing the injured joint to promote healing. Immediately after the injury, swelling can be controlled by elevating the joint above the level of the heart, and by intermittently applying ice packs, wrapped in towels to prevent cold injury to the patient's skin.

The joint can be immobilized using an elastic bandage, or if the sprain is severe, a soft cast. Depending on the severity of the injury, codeine or another analgesic may be necessary. If the patient has a sprained ankle, he may need crutches and crutch gait training. Because patients with sprains seldom require hospitalization, comprehensive patient teaching should be provided.

• The patient should elevate the joint for 48 to 72 hours after the injury (while sleeping, joint can be elevated with pillows), and should apply ice intermit-

MUSCLE-TENDON RUPTURES

Perhaps the most serious muscle-tendon injury is a rupture of the muscle-tendon junction. These ruptures may occur at any such junction, but they're most common at the Achilles tendon, which extends from the posterior calf muscle to the foot. An Achilles tendon rupture produces a sudden sharp pain, and until swelling begins, a palpable defect. Such ruptures typically occur in men between ages 35 and 40, especially during physical activities such as jogging or tennis.

To distinguish Achilles tendon rupture from other ankle injuries, the doctor performs this simple test: With the patient prone and his feet hanging off the foot of the table, the doctor squeezes the calf muscle. If this causes plantar flexion, the tendon is intact; if ankle dorsiflexion, it's partially intact; if there's no flexion of any kind, the tendon is ruptured.

Usually an Achilles tendon rupture requires surgical repair, followed first by a long leg cast for 4 weeks, and then by a short cast for an additional 4 weeks.

tently for 12 to 48 hours.

• If an elastic bandage has been applied, the patient must know how to reapply it by wrapping from below to above the injury, forming a figure eight. For a sprained ankle, the bandage is applied from the toes to midcalf. The patient must not sleep with the bandage on and should loosen it if it causes the leg to become pale, numb, or painful.

• If pain worsens or persists, the patient should call the doctor. An additional X-ray may detect a fracture originally missed.

An immobilized sprain usually heals in 2 to 3 weeks, and the patient can then gradually resume normal activities. Occasionally, however, torn ligaments don't heal properly and cause recurrent dislocation, necessitating surgical repair. Some athletes may request immediate surgical repair to hasten healing; to prevent sprains, they may tape their wrists and ankles before sports activities.

Acute strains require analgesics and immediate application of ice for up to 48 hours, followed by heat application. Complete muscle rupture may require surgical repair. Chronic strains usually don't require treatment, but local heat application, aspirin, or an analgesic-muscle relaxant relieves discomfort.

Arm and Leg Fractures

Arm and leg fractures usually result from trauma and often cause substantial muscle, nerve, and other soft-tissue damage. Prognosis varies with extent of disablement or deformity, amount of tissue and vascular damage, adequacy of reduction and immobilization, and the patient's age, health, and nutrition. Children's bones usually heal rapidly and without deformity. Bones of adults in poor health and with impaired circulation may never heal properly. Severe open fractures, especially of the femoral shaft, may cause substantial blood loss and life-threatening hypovolemic shock.

Causes

Most arm and leg fractures result from major trauma; for example, a fall on an outstretched arm, a skiing accident, or child abuse (shown by multiple or repeated episodes of fractures). However, in a person with a pathologic bone-weakening condition, such as osteoporosis, bone tumors, or metabolic disease, a mere cough or sneeze can also produce a fracture. Prolonged standing, walking, or running can cause stress fractures of the foot and ankle—usually in nurses, postal workers, soldiers, and joggers.

Signs and symptoms

Arm and leg fractures may produce any or all of the "5 Ps": pain and point tenderness, pallor, pulse loss, paresthesia, and paralysis. (The last three are distal to the fracture site.) Other signs include deformity, swelling, discoloration, crep-itus, and loss of limb function. Numbness and tingling, mottled cyanosis, cool skin at the end of the extremity, and loss of pulses distal to the injury indicate possible arterial compromise or nerve damage. Open fractures also produce an obvious skin wound.

Complications of arm and leg fractures include:

• permanent deformity and dysfunction if bones fail to heal (nonunion) or heal improperly (malunion)

• aseptic necrosis of bone segments from impaired circulation

• hypovolemic shock as a result of blood vessel damage (this is especially likely to develop in patients with fractured femur)

• muscle contractures

• renal calculi from decalcification (produced by prolonged immobility)

• fat embolism.

Diagnosis

History of trauma and physical examination, including gentle palpation and a cautious attempt by the patient to move parts distal to the injury, suggest an arm or leg fracture. (Physical examination should also check for other injuries.)

Anteroposterior and lateral X-rays of the suspected fracture, as well as X-rays of the joints above and below it, confirm the diagnosis.

Treatment

Emergency treatment consists of splinting the limb above and below the suspected fracture, applying a cold pack, and elevating the limb, to reduce edema and pain. In severe fractures that cause blood loss, direct pressure should be applied to control bleeding, and fluid replacement (including blood products) should be administered to prevent or treat hypovolemic shock.

After confirming diagnosis of a fracture, treatment begins with reduction (restoring displaced bone segments to their normal position), followed by immobilization by splint, cast, or traction. In closed reduction (manual manipulation), a local anesthetic—such as lidocaine—and an analgesic—such as

---

TYPES OF FRACTURES

Incomplete: Break extends only partially through the bone; for example, in a greenstick fracture (common in children), bone splinters fibers on one side of the bone, leaving the other side intact

Complete: Bone breaks into two or more pieces

Closed (simple): Overlying skin remains unbroken

Open (compound): Wound is present overlying the fracture, creating the risk of infection

Nondisplaced: Fractured bones remain in alignment

Displaced: Break knocks bone ends out of alignment, creating the risk of muscle contractures and deformities

Transverse: Break runs transversely across the bone shaft

Spiral: Break winds around bone like a coil

Linear: Break runs the length of the bone

Comminuted: Bone shatters or is compressed into fragments

Impacted: Bone ends are driven into each other

Compression: Bone collapses (vertebrae) under excessive pressure

Avulsion: Overexertion tears a muscle or ligament away from a bone, pulling a small bone fragment with it

Depression: Trauma drives bone fragments inward (usually refers to a skull fracture)

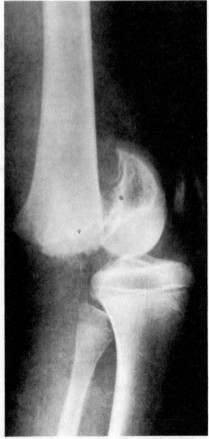

This X-ray shows a complete, displaced fracture at the epiphyseal line at the distal end of the femur.

meperidine I.M.—minimize pain, while a muscle relaxant—such as diazepam I.V.—facilitates muscle-stretching necessary to realign the bone. (An X-ray confirms reduction and proper bone alignment.) When closed reduction is impossible, open reduction during surgery reduces and immobilizes the fracture by means of rods, plates, or screws. Afterward, a plaster cast is usually applied.

When a splint or cast fails to maintain the reduction, immobilization requires skin or skeletal traction, using a series of weights and pulleys. In skin traction, elastic bandages and moleskin coverings are used to attach traction devices to the patient's skin. In skeletal traction, a pin or wire inserted through the bone distal to the fracture and attached to a weight allows more prolonged traction.

Open fractures also require careful wound cleansing, tetanus prophylaxis, prophylactic antibiotics, and possibly, surgery, to repair soft-tissue damage.

Additional considerations

• The patient with a severe open fracture of a large bone, such as the femur, may exhibit signs of shock: rapid pulse, decreased blood pressure, cool clammy skin, and pallor. His vital signs must be monitored and I.V. fluids administered, as ordered.

• With any fracture the patient is apt to be frightened and in pain. The pain can be eased with analgesics, as needed. The fear can be minimized with reassurance. The patient may require help to set realistic goals for recovery.

• If the fracture requires long-term immobilization with traction, the patient should be repositioned often to increase comfort and prevent decubitus ulcers. He must perform active range-of-motion exercises to prevent muscle atrophy, and deep breathing and coughing to avoid hypostatic pneumonia.

• The patient must maintain an adequate fluid intake to prevent urinary stasis and constipation. He should be watched for signs of renal calculi (flank

FAT EMBOLISM

Fat embolism, a potentially fatal complication of arm or leg fractures, may follow the release of fat droplets from bone marrow, or the release of catecholamine after trauma, which mobilizes fatty acids. Fat embolism can lodge in the lungs or even the brain, and often occurs within 24 hours after the fracture, although it may be delayed up to 72 hours. Its typical symptoms include apprehension, sweating, fever, tachycardia, pallor, dyspnea, pulmonary effusion, tissue hypoxia, cyanosis, convulsions, and coma. The most distinctive sign, however, is a petechial rash on the chest and shoulders.

In fat embolism, arterial blood gases show low PO_2, and chest X-ray may disclose a typical "snowstorm" pattern of infiltrates scattered over the lungs. Treatment consists of oxygen delivery by nasal catheter or mask, immobilization (if the fracture isn't already immobilized), and administration of heparin, corticosteroids, and a diuretic, such as furosemide, to reduce interstitial or pulmonary edema. Extensive pulmonary damage may require insertion of chest tubes, a tracheotomy, or use of a ventilator. Throughout treatment arterial blood gases and vital signs should be monitored.

pain, nausea, and vomiting).

• Good cast care is important. While the cast is wet, it should be supported with pillows. The skin near the edges of the cast must be watched for signs of irritation or discharge. The patient should know signs of impaired circulation (skin coldness, numbness, tingling, or discoloration) and report them immediately. Also, the patient must not get the cast wet or insert foreign objects under the cast.

• The patient must start moving around as soon as he is able. He should be taught proper crutch use—putting weight on hands, not axillary areas.

• After cast removal, he should see a physical therapist, to restore limb mobility.

Dislocations and Subluxations

Dislocations displace joint bones so their articulating surfaces totally lose contact; subluxations partially displace the articulating surfaces. Dislocations and subluxations occur at the joints of the shoulders, elbows, wrists, digits, hips, knees, ankles, and feet; the injury may accompany fractures of these joints or result in deposition of fracture fragments between joint surfaces. Prompt reduction can limit the resulting damage to soft tissue, nerves, and blood vessels.

Causes
A dislocation or subluxation may be congenital (as in congenital dislocation of the hip), or it may follow trauma or disease of surrounding joint tissues (for example, Paget's disease).

Signs and symptoms
Dislocations and subluxations produce deformity around the joint, change the length of the involved extremity, impair joint mobility, and cause point tenderness. When the injury results from trauma, it is extremely painful and often accompanies joint surface fractures. Even in the absence of concomitant fracture, the displaced bone may damage surrounding muscles, ligaments, nerves, and blood vessels, and may cause bone necrosis, especially if reduction is delayed.

Diagnosis
Patient history, X-rays, and clinical examination rule out or confirm fracture.

Treatment
Immediate reduction (before tissue edema and muscle spasm make reduction difficult) can prevent additional tissue damage and vascular impairment. Closed reduction consists of manual traction, under general anesthetic, or local anesthetic and sedatives. During such reduction, meperidine I.V. controls pain; diazepam I.V. controls muscle spasm and facilitates muscle-stretching during traction. Occasionally, such injuries require open reduction under regional block or general anesthetic. Such surgery may include wire fixation of the joint, skeletal traction, and ligament repair.

After reduction, a splint, cast, or traction immobilizes the joint. Generally, immobilizing the digits for 2 weeks, hips for 6 to 8 weeks, and other dislocated joints for 3 to 6 weeks allows surrounding ligaments to heal.

Additional considerations
• Until reduction immobilizes the dislocated joint, manipulation should not be attempted. Ice will help ease the patient's pain and edema. The extremity should be splinted "as it lies," even if the angle is awkward. If severe vascular compromise is present or is indicated by pallor, pain, loss of pulses, paralysis, and paresthesia, then an orthopedic examination is necessary.
• When a patient receives meperidine I.V. or diazepam I.V., he may develop respiratory depression or even respiratory arrest. So during reduction, an airway and hand-held resuscitator (AMBU bag) should be kept in the room, and respirations should be monitored closely.
• To avoid injury from a dressing that is too tight, the patient should report numbness, pain, cyanosis, or coldness of the extremity below the cast or splint.

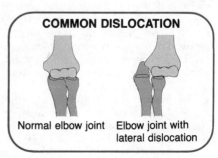

COMMON DISLOCATION

Normal elbow joint   Elbow joint with lateral dislocation

• To avoid skin damage, the patient should watch for pain, or soreness under and around the dressing.

• After removal of the cast or splint, the patient may gradually return to normal joint activity.

• If the patient has a dislocated hip, reduction should take place without delay. At discharge, he should understand the need for regular follow-up visits to detect aseptic femoral head necrosis from vascular damage.

Traumatic Amputation

Traumatic amputation is the accidental loss of a body part, usually a finger, toe, arm, or leg. In complete amputation, the member is totally severed; in partial amputation, some soft-tissue connection remains. Prognosis has improved as a result of early improved emergency and critical care management, new surgical techniques, early rehabilitation, prosthesis fitting, and new prosthesis design. New limb reimplantation techniques have been moderately successful, but incomplete nerve regeneration remains a major limiting factor.

Causes
Traumatic amputations usually result directly from factory, farm, or power tools, or a motor vehicle accident.

Assessment
Every traumatic amputee requires careful monitoring of vital signs. If amputation involves more than just a finger or toe, assessment of airway, breathing, and circulation is also required. Since profuse bleeding is likely, the patient may experience hypovolemic shock. A blood sample should be drawn for hemoglobin, hematocrit, and type and crossmatch analysis. In partial amputation, pulses distal to the amputation should be checked. After any traumatic amputation, other traumatic injuries must be given attention as well.

Treatment
Because the greatest immediate threat after traumatic amputation is blood loss and hypovolemic shock, emergency treatment consists of local measures to control bleeding, fluid replacement with normal saline solution, crystalloids and colloids, and blood replacement, as needed. Reimplantation remains controversial, but it's becoming more common and successful because of advances in microsurgery. If reconstruction or reim-

plantation is possible, surgical intervention attempts to preserve usable joints. When arm or leg amputations are done, the surgeon attempts to create a stump that can be fitted with a prosthesis. A rigid dressing allows for early prosthesis fitting and rehabilitation.

Additional considerations
During emergency treatment the following steps should be taken: monitoring vital signs (especially in hypovolemic shock); cleaning the wound; and giving tetanus prophylaxis, analgesics, and antibiotics, as ordered. After complete amputation, the extremity should be preserved in a sterile plastic bag filled with cooled sterile normal saline solution (the limb must *not* be frozen). After partial amputation, the limb should be positioned in normal alignment, and draped with towels or dressings soaked in sterile normal saline solution.

Preoperative care includes thorough wound irrigation and debridement (using a local block with lidocaine). Postoperative care includes dressing changes using sterile technique to prevent skin infection and to ensure skin graft viability. The amputee will need reassurance to cope with his altered body image.

During rehabilitation, the patient's stump should be protected from trauma.

WHOLE BODY INJURIES

Burns

A major burn is a horrifying injury, necessitating painful treatment and a long period of rehabilitation. It is often fatal or permanently disfiguring and incapacitating (both emotionally and physically). In the United States, about 2 million persons annually suffer burns. Of these, 300,000 are burned seriously and over 6,000 are fatalities, making burns this nation's third largest cause of accidental death.

Causes

Thermal burns, the most common type, are frequently the result of residential fires, automobile accidents, playing with matches, improperly stored gasoline, space heater or electrical malfunctions, or arson. Other causes include improper handling of firecrackers, scalding accidents, and kitchen accidents (for example, a child climbing on top of a stove or grabbing a hot iron). Burns in children are sometimes traced to parental abuse.

Chemical burns result from the contact, ingestion, inhalation, or injection of acids, alkalis, or vesicants. Electrical burns usually occur after contact with faulty electrical wiring or with high-voltage power lines, or when electric cords are chewed (by young children). Friction, or abrasion, burns happen when the skin is rubbed harshly against a coarse surface. Sunburn, of course, follows excessive exposure to sunlight.

Assessment

One goal of assessment is to determine the *depth* of skin and tissue damage. A partial-thickness burn damages only part of the dermis, while a full-thickness burn extends into subcutaneous tissue. However, a more traditional method gauges burn depth by degrees, although most burns are a combination of different degrees and thicknesses.

- *First degree*—Damage is limited to the epidermis, but it produces erythema and pain.
- *Second degree*—The epidermis and part of the dermis are damaged, producing blisters and mild to moderate edema and pain.
- *Third degree*—Both the epidermis and the dermis are damaged. No blisters appear, but white, leathery tissue and thrombosed vessels are visible.
- *Fourth degree*—Damage extends through subcutaneous tissue to muscle and bone. The tissue appears deeply charred.

Both the Lund and Browder chart (most accurate, since it also takes the victim's age into account) and the Rule of Nines chart (most common) allow an estimate of the *size* of the burn, usually measured as the percentage of body surface area (BSA) covered by the burn. A correlation of the burn's depth and size permits an estimate of its severity.

- *Major*—Third-degree burns on more than 10% of BSA; second-degree burns on more than 25% of adult BSA (more than 20% in children); burns of hands, feet, or genitalia; burns complicated by fractures or respiratory damage; electrical burns; all burns in poor-risk patients
- *Moderate*—third-degree burns on 2% to 10% of BSA; second-degree burns on 15% to 25% of adult BSA (over 10% in children)
- *Minor*—third-degree burns on less than 2% of BSA; second-degree burns on less than 15% of adult BSA (10% in children).

Here are other important factors in assessing burns:

BURN SEVERITY

Extent of injury in deep 2nd degree burn

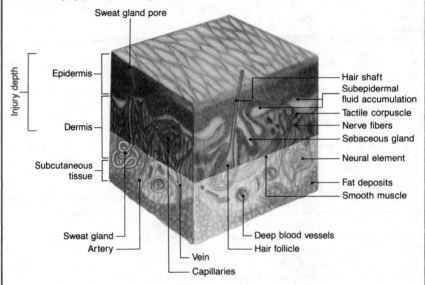

Injury depth

Epidermis

Dermis

Subcutaneous tissue

Sweat gland pore

Hair shaft
Subepidermal fluid accumulation
Tactile corpuscle
Nerve fibers
Sebaceous gland
Neural element
Fat deposits
Smooth muscle

Sweat gland
Artery
Vein
Capillaries
Deep blood vessels
Hair follicle

Extent of injury in 3rd degree burn

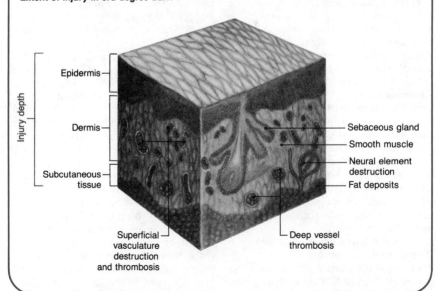

Injury depth

Epidermis

Dermis

Subcutaneous tissue

Sebaceous gland
Smooth muscle
Neural element destruction
Fat deposits

Superficial vasculature destruction and thrombosis

Deep vessel thrombosis

FLUID REPLACEMENT: THE FIRST 24 HOURS POSTBURN

One of these two formulas is used as a guideline for the amount of fluid replacement necessary, but they are varied according to the patient's clinical response, especially urinary output.

• *Baxter formula*: 4 ml lactated Ringer's solution/kg/% BSA/24 hours. One half of total is given over first 8 hours postburn and remainder over next 16 hours.

• *Brooke formula*: colloids (plasma, plasmanate, dextran) 0.5 ml/kg/% BSA + lactated Ringer's solution 1.5 ml/kg/% BSA + 2,000 ml dextrose in water for adults (less for children). One half of total is given over first 8 hours postburn and remainder over next 16 hours.

• Configuration—Circumferential burns can cause total occlusion of circulation in the area as a result of edema.

• History of complicating medical problems—Disorders that impair peripheral circulation, especially diabetes, coronary artery disease, and chronic alcohol abuse will hinder recovery.

• Other injuries sustained at the time of the burn.

• Patient age—Victims under age 4 or over age 60 have a higher incidence of complications and, consequently, a higher mortality.

Treatment and additional considerations

Immediate, aggressive burn treatment increases the patient's chance for survival. Later, supportive measures and strict aseptic technique can minimize infection. Because burns necessitate such comprehensive bedside care, the nurse, who has the most frequent contact with the patient, can make the difference between life and death.

When the burns are minor, the nurse should do the following:

• Immerse the burned area in cool tap water (55° F. [12.8° C.]) or apply cool compresses.

• Soak the wound in a mild soap solution to cleanse it, and give pain medication, as ordered.

• Debride the devitalized tissue, taking care not to break any blisters.

• Cover the wound with an antimicrobial agent (nonstick) and a bulky dressing; administer tetanus prophylaxis, as ordered.

• Provide aftercare instructions for the patient, especially keeping the dressing dry and clean, elevating the burned extremity for the first 24 hours, taking ordered analgesics, and returning for a wound check in 2 days.

When the burns are moderate or major, the nurse should do the following:

• Immediately assess for airway, breathing, and smoke inhalation injuries, remembering that neck and facial burns may cause extensive edema that impairs respirations.

• Look for singed nasal hair, soot in the mouth or nose, and darkened sputum; these signs point to smoke inhalation and possible lung damage.

• Ask the patient or witnesses what caused the burn, what was the length of exposure, where it occurred (smoke inhalation is more likely if the patient was burned in an enclosed area, and he may need 100% oxygen by mask), and the exact time of the burn (used to gauge treatment).

• Control bleeding, and remove smoldering clothing (soak it first in saline solution if it's stuck to the patient's skin), rings, and other constricting items.

• Cover burns with a clean, dry, preferably sterile bed sheet. (*Never* cover large burns in saline-soaked dressings, since they can drastically lower body temperature.)

• Begin I.V. therapy immediately to prevent hypovolemic shock and maintain cardiac output. If available at the scene of the burn (and if an emergency room is more than an hour away), use 3 to 4 ml/lb/hr of lactated Ringer's solution if the burn covers less than 30% of the patient's BSA or use a fluid replacement formula, such as the Baxter formula, if burn covers more than 30%.

• Closely monitor intake and output, and frequently check vital signs, including the patient's blood pressure even on a burned limb. Check pupillary response.

In the hospital, a central venous pressure (CVP) line and additional I.V. lines, (using venous cutdown, if necessary,) and a Foley catheter may be inserted. To combat fluid evaporation through the burn and the release of fluid into interstitial spaces (possibly resulting in hypovolemic shock), fluid therapy will be continued.

Whether at the scene or in the hospital, a burn assessment should be made. Tissue damage from electrical burns is difficult to assess, because internal destruction along the conduction pathway is usually greater than the surface burn would indicate. Electrical burns that ignite the patient's clothes may cause thermal burns as well. If the electric shock caused ventricular fibrillation, and cardiac and respiratory arrest, cardiopulmonary resuscitation (CPR) should be started at once. The estimated voltage, and whether or not the patient was grounded, should be determined.

If the burn resulted from an automobile accident or an explosion, a brief neurologic examination and additional injury check are necessary. For example, loss of consciousness and hemorrhage indicate other injuries.)

In a chemical burn, the wound should be irrigated with copious amounts of water or normal saline solution. Using a weak base ($NaHCO_3$) to neutralize hydrofluoric acid, hydrochloric acid, or sulfuric acid on skin or mucous membrane is controversial, particularly in the emergency phase, since seeking the neutralizing agent can waste precious time.

If the chemical entered the patient's eyes, they must be flushed with large amounts of water or saline solution for 30 minutes and covered with a dry, sterile dressing. The type of chemical causing the burn should also be noted.

Vital signs should be checked every 15 minutes (the doctor may insert an arterial line if blood pressure is unobtainable with a cuff). Blood typing and crossmatching must be done and all baseline laboratory studies should be performed. To decompress the stomach and avoid aspiration of stomach contents, a nasogastric tube may be used.

The burn wound itself shouldn't be treated in the emergency department if the patient is to be transferred to a specialized burn care unit within 4 hours after the burn. Instead, the patient should be wrapped in a sterile sheet and a blanket for warmth, have the burned extremity elevated to decrease edema, and be transported immediately.

Electric Shock

When an electric current passes through the body, the damage it does depends on the intensity of the current (amperes, milliamperes, or microamperes), which tissues the current passes through, the narrowness of the current pathway, the kind of current (AC, DC, or mixed), and the frequency and duration of current flow. Accordingly, electric shock may cause ventricular fibrillation, respiratory paralysis, burns, and death. Prognosis depends on the site and extent of damage, the patient's state of health, and the speed and adequacy of treatment. In the United States, each year about 1,000 people die of electric shock.

Causes

Electric shock usually follows accidental contact with exposed parts of electrical appliances or wiring, but may also result from lightning or the flash of electric arcs from high-voltage power lines or machines. The increased use of electrical medical devices in the hospital, many of which are connected directly to the patient, has raised serious concern for electrical safety and has led to the development of electrical safety standards. But even well-designed equipment with reliable safety features can cause electric shock if mishandled.

Signs and symptoms

Severe electric shock usually causes muscle contraction, followed by unconsciousness and loss of reflex control, sometimes with respiratory paralysis (by way of prolonged contraction of respiratory muscles, or a direct effect on the respiratory nerve center). After momentary shock, hyperventilation may follow initial muscle contraction. Passage of even the smallest electric current—if it passes through the heart—may induce ventricular fibrillation or other dysrhythmia that progresses to fibrillation.

Electric shock from a high-frequency current (which generates more heat in tissues than a low-frequency current) usually causes burns, and local tissue coagulation and necrosis. Low-frequency currents can also cause serious burns if the contact with the current is concentrated in a small area (for example, when a toddler bites into an electrical cord). Contusions, fractures, and other injuries can result from violent muscle contractions or falls during the shock; later, the patient may develop renal shutdown. Residual hearing impairment, cataracts, and vision loss may persist after severe electric shock.

Diagnosis

Usually, the cause of electrical injuries is either obvious or suspected. However, an accurate history can define the voltage and the length of contact. If the shock has caused ventricular fibrillation, frequent EKGs are in order to monitor cardiac function until it returns to normal.

Treatment and additional considerations

Immediate emergency treatment includes separating the victim from the current source, quick assessment of vital functions, and emergency measures, such as cardiopulmonary resuscitation (CPR) and defibrillation.

To separate the victim from the current source, the source should be turned off or unplugged immediately. If this isn't possible, the victim should be pulled free with a nonconductive device, such as a loop of dry cloth or rubber, a dry rope, or a leather belt.

• A quick assessment should be made of vital functions. If a pulse or breathing can't be detected, CPR should be started at once and continued until vital signs return or until emergency help arrives with a defibrillator and other life-support equipment.

• Since internal tissue destruction in burns may be much greater than skin damage might indicate, I.V. lactated Ringer's solution may be ordered to maintain a urine output of 50 to 100 ml/hour. Mannitol may also be ordered to prevent acute tubular necrosis and renal shutdown. The patient's intake and output should be measured hourly. His extremities should be observed for color changes since this may point to peripheral circulatory failure. Remember: If the electrical current passes through dry, calloused, or unbroken skin, there is less chance of internal tissue damage than if it passes through mucous membrane, an open wound, or thin, moist skin.

• After vital functions stabilize, the extent of the injury should be assessed and the patient's EKG monitored for dysrhythmia. Splinting may be needed to prevent contractures and treat accompanying injuries (burns, fractures).

Anyone can prevent electric shock by following these electrical precautions:
• Check for cuts, cracks, or frayed insulation on electric cords, and electric devices; keep them away from hot or wet surfaces and sharp corners. Don't set glasses of water, damp towels, or other wet items on electrical equipment. Wipe up accidental spills before they leak into electrical equipment. Avoid using extension cords, since they may circumvent grounding; if extension cords are abso-

lutely necessary, don't place them under carpeting or in areas where they'll be walked on.
• Make sure ground connections on electrical equipment are intact. Line cord plugs should have three prongs; the prongs should be straight and firmly fixed. Check to make sure prongs fit wall outlets properly. Don't use adapters on three-prong plugs. Also, avoid using outlets that are loose or broken.
• Get faulty equipment repaired promptly. If a machine sparks, smokes, seems unusually hot, or gives off a slight shock, unplug it immediately, if doing so isn't a hazard in itself. Check inspection labels, if present, and report equipment overdue for inspection.
• Be especially careful when using electrical equipment near a person with a pacemaker, since a pacemaker can create a direct, low-resistance path to the heart; even a small shock may cause ventricular fibrillation.
• Avoid electrical hazards at home and at work by putting safety guards on all electrical outlets. Warn children to keep away from electrical devices. Do not use electrical appliances while showering or while wet. Also, *never* touch electrical appliances while touching faucets or cold water pipes in the kitchen, since these pipes often provide the ground for all circuits in the house.
• If you're certified to operate a defibrillator, make sure defibrillator paddles are free of dry, caked gel before applying fresh gel, since poor electrical contact between the paddles and the patient's skin can cause burns or electrical arcing. Also, don't apply too much gel. If the gel runs over the edge of the paddle and touches your hand, you'll receive some of the defibrillator shock, while the patient loses some of the energy in the discharge.

Cold Injuries

Cold injuries result from overexposure to cold air or water, and occur in two major forms: localized injuries (such as frostbite) and systemic injuries (such as hypothermia). Untreated or improperly treated frostbite can lead to gangrene and may necessitate amputation; severe hypothermia can be fatal.

Causes
Localized cold injuries occur when ice crystals form in the tissues and expand extracellular spaces. With compression of the tissue cell, the cell membrane ruptures, interrupting enzymatic and metabolic activities. Increased capillary permeability accompanies the release of histamine, resulting in aggregation of red blood cells and microvascular occlusion. Hypothermia effects chemical changes that slow the functions of most major organ systems, such as decreased renal blood flow and decreased glomerular filtration. Frostbite results from prolonged exposure to dry temperatures far below freezing; hypothermia, from cold-water near-drowning and prolonged exposure to cold temperatures.

The risk of serious cold injuries, especially hypothermia, is increased by youth, lack of insulating body fat, wet or inadequate clothing, old age, drug abuse, cardiac disease, smoking, fatigue, hunger and depletion of caloric reserves, and excessive alcohol intake (which draws blood into capillaries and away from body organs).

Signs and symptoms
Frostbite may be deep or superficial. Superficial frostbite affects skin and subcutaneous tissue, especially of the face, ears, and other exposed body areas. Although it may go unnoticed at first, upon returning to a warm place, it produces burning, tingling, numbness, skin mottling, and a grayish skin color. Deep

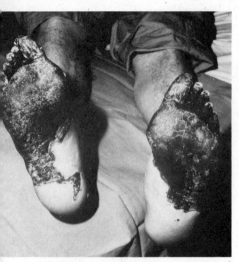

Frostbite of the feet. Blackened areas in photo show tissue necrosis and gangrene—the result of deep frostbite that extends beyond subcutaneous tissue.

frostbite extends beyond subcutaneous tissue and usually affects the hands or feet. The skin becomes white until it's thawed; then it turns purplish-blue. Deep frostbite also produces pain, skin blisters, tissue necrosis, and gangrene.

Indications of hypothermia vary with severity:

• *Mild hypothermia*: Drop in body temperature to 95° to 98° F. (35° to 36.6° C.), shivering, and loss of firm muscle coordination
• *Moderate hypothermia*: Drop to 89.6° to 95° F. (32° to 35° C.), severe shivering, slurred speech, and amnesia
• *Marked hypothermia*: Drop to 82.4° to 89.6° F. (28° to 32° C.), muscle rigidity, peripheral cyanosis, and with improper rewarming, signs of shock
• *Severe hypothermia*: Drop to 77° to 82.4° F. (25° to 28° C.), loss of deep tendon reflexes and ventricular fibrillation. The patient may appear dead, with no palpable pulse, audible heart sounds, or deep tendon reflexes. His pupils may dilate, and he appears to be in a state of rigor mortis. Body temperature drop below 77° F. (25° C.) causes cardiopulmonary arrest and death.

Diagnosis
A history of severe and prolonged exposure to cold may make this diagnosis obvious. But often, hypothermia may be easily overlooked, especially if the patient is comatose.

Treatment and additional considerations
In a localized cold injury, treatment consists of rewarming the injured part, providing supportive measures, and sometimes performing a fasciotomy to increase circulation by decreasing edemic tissue pressure. However, if gangrene occurs, amputation may be necessary. In hypothermia, therapy consists of immediate resuscitative measures, careful monitoring, and gradual rewarming of the entire body. Cold injuries in children suggest neglect or abuse and mandate a thorough history.

To treat localized cold injuries:
• Constrictive clothing is removed, and the affected part is gradually rewarmed in tepid water (100° to 105° F. [37.7° to 40.5° C.]). The patient is given warm fluids to drink. The injured area is *never* rubbed, since this aggravates tissue damage.
• When the affected part begins to rewarm (the patient will feel a tingling sensation), pulse is checked, and the area is wrapped in a bulky sterile dressing. If the injury is on the foot, cotton or gauze sponges are placed between the toes to prevent maceration. The patient must not put pressure on injured feet in any way.
• Analgesics may be given for pain. If the injury has caused an open skin wound, antibiotics and tetanus prophylaxis may also be given.
• If pulse fails to return, the patient may require a fasciotomy, to allow adequate circulation; if gangrene develops, he may be prepared for amputation.
• The patient should know that there may be long-term residual effects: increased sensitivity to cold, burning and tingling, and increased sweating. He should not smoke, since this causes vasoconstriction and slows healing.

To treat systemic hypothermia:
- If there's no pulse or respiration, cardiopulmonary resuscitation (CPR) is started immediately, and if necessary, continued for 2 to 3 hours. (Remember: hypothermia protects the brain from anoxia, which normally accompanies prolonged cardiopulmonary arrest. Therefore, even after the patient has been unresponsive for a long time, resuscitation may be possible, especially after cold-water near-drownings.)
- The patient should then be moved to a warm area, undressed and kept dry. If he's conscious, he should drink warm fluids with high sugar content, such as tea with sugar.
- The patient's body core and surface should be rewarmed at 1° to 2° C. per hour concurrently. (If the surface is rewarmed first, rewarming shock can cause potentially fatal ventricular fibrillation.) To warm the body core, I.V. solutions are infused, after having passed through a warming coil at 98.6° F. (37° C.), and nasogastric lavage is performed with normal saline solution that has been warmed to the same temperature. Additional procedures may include: peritoneal lavage, using a normal saline solution (full or half strength) warmed to 98.6° F. (37° C.); and, in severe hypothermia, heart/lung bypass, at controlled temperatures, and thoracotomy with direct cardiac warm-saline bath.
- Body surface can be warmed by bathing the patient in water that is 104° F. (40° C.), covering him with a heating blanket set at 97.9° to 99.9° F. (36.6° to 37.7° C.), and cautiously applying hot water bottles at 104° F. (40° C.) to groin and axillae, guarding against burns.
- Throughout treatment, the following should be monitored: arterial blood gases, intake and output, central venous pressure, temperature, neurologic status, and lab results such as CBC, BUN, electrolytes, prothrombin time, and partial thromboplastin time.

To prevent cold injuries:
- In cold weather, wear mittens (not gloves); windproof, water-resistant, many-layered clothing; two pairs of socks (cotton next to skin, then wool); and a scarf and a hat that cover the ears (to avoid heat loss through the head).
- Before anticipated prolonged exposure to cold, don't drink alcohol or smoke, and get adequate food and rest.
- If caught in a severe snowstorm, find shelter early or increase physical activity to maintain body warmth.

Patients who have developed cold injuries because of inadequate clothing or housing may appreciate assistance from a community social service agency.

Heat Syndrome

Heat syndrome may result from environmental or internal conditions that impair dissipation of heat. Heat syndromes fall into three categories: heat cramps, heat exhaustion, and heatstroke.

Causes
Normally, humans accommodate excessive temperatures by several mechanisms, which are probably regulated by the hypothalamus. These mechanisms include the ability to secrete sweat of low sodium chloride content and concentration; dilation of peripheral blood vessels; decrease in total circulating blood volume; and increased secretion of antidiuretics hormone (ADH). When one or more of these mechanisms fail and high environmental temperature persists, the body retains heat and develops heat syndrome.

Precautions
Heat illnesses are easily preventable, and it's important that the public know what causes these illnesses. The following in-

HOW TO MANAGE HEAT SYNDROME

TYPE AND SIGNS AND SYMPTOMS	CONFIRMING DIAGNOSIS	MANAGEMENT
Heat cramps • Muscle twitching and spasms, weakness, severe muscle cramps • Nausea • Falling blood pressure • Rapid, pounding pulse • Cool, pallid skin; diaphoresis • Normal or slight fever	• History of recent prolonged or extreme exposure to heat • Typical clinical picture • CBC: hemoconcentration • Decreased sodium	• Hospitalization usually unnecessary. • To replace fluid and electrolytes, take salt tablets and electrolyte drink, such as Gatorade. • Loosen clothing, and lie down in a cool place. Have muscles massaged. If muscle cramps are severe, a health care professional will start an I.V. infusion of normal saline solution.
Heat exhaustion • Muscle cramps • Nausea and vomiting • Decreased blood pressure • Thready, rapid pulse • Cool, pallid skin • Headache, mental confusion, syncope, giddiness • Dilated pupils • Oliguria, thirst • No fever • May progress to heatstroke	• History of recent prolonged or extreme exposure to heat • Typical clinical picture • CBC: hemoconcentration • Decreased sodium	• Hospitalization usually unnecessary. • To replace fluids and electrolytes, and prevent progression, *immediately* take salt tablets and balanced electrolyte drink. • Loosen clothing, and lie in shock position in a cool place. Have muscles massaged. If cramps are severe, a health care professional will start an I.V. infusion with normal saline solution or lactated Ringer's. • Oxygen may be given.
Heatstroke • Severe headache and muscle cramps early; later disappear • Vomiting • Hypertension, followed by hypotension • Atrial or ventricular tachycardia • Hot, dry, red skin, which later turns gray; no diaphoresis • Confusion, progressing to loss of consciousness • Temperature higher than 102.2° F. (39° C.) • Dilated pupils • Slow, deep respiration; then Cheyne-Stokes • Body odor of burned flesh	• History of recent prolonged or extreme exposure to heat • Typical clinical picture • Increased serum glucose • Arterial blood gases: metabolic acidosis, decreased P_{CO_2} • Increased potassium • Meningitis, malaria, encephalitis, typhoid, typhus, hypothalamic hemorrhage must be ruled out.	• Hospitalization necessary. • To replace fluids and electrolytes, a health care professional will start an I.V. infusion with appropriate solution. • ABCs of life support will be initiated, along with high-flow O_2. • Body temperature will be cooled rapidly with ice packs on arterial pressure points. • Diazepam or chlorpromazine I.V. may be given to reduce shivering; mannitol or corticosteroids may be given to treat edema. • A nasogastric tube should be inserted to prevent aspiration.

formation is especially vital for athletes involved in rigorous sports or for soldiers on maneuvers.

• To avoid heat syndrome in hot weather, wear loose-fitting, lightweight clothing, rest frequently, avoid hot places, and drink fluids.

• The patient who is obese, elderly, or taking drugs that impair heat regulation must not overexert himself in hot weather, since this will cause overheating. Heat illness is often related to phenothiazines.

• The patient who has been treated for heat syndrome must not go out in the sun again for awhile.

• The patient with heatstroke must recognize the fact that residual hypersensitivity to high temperatures may persist for several months.

Asphyxia

A condition of insufficient oxygen and accumulating carbon dioxide in the blood and tissues due to interference with respiration, asphyxia results in cardiopulmonary arrest. Without prompt treatment it is fatal.

Causes
Asphyxia results from any internal or external condition or substance that inhibits respiration. Some examples:

• hypoventilation as a result of narcotic abuse, medullary disease or hemorrhage, respiratory muscle paralysis, or cardiopulmonary arrest

• intrapulmonary obstruction, as in airway obstruction, pulmonary edema, pneumonia, and near-drowning

• extrapulmonary obstruction, as in tracheal compression from a tumor, strangulation, or suffocation

• inhalation of toxic agents, as in carbon monoxide poisoning, smoke inhalation, profound anesthesia, and excessive oxygen inhalation.

Signs and symptoms
Depending on the duration and degree of asphyxia, common symptoms include anxiety, dyspnea, agitation and confusion leading to coma, altered respiratory rate (apnea, bradypnea, occasional tachypnea), decreased breath sounds, central and peripheral cyanosis (cherry-red mucous membranes in late-stage carbon monoxide poisoning), convulsions, and fast, slow, or absent pulse.

Diagnosis
Diagnosis rests on patient history (including possible strangulation or other trauma) and laboratory results. Arterial blood gas measurement, the most important test, shows decreased PO_2 (less than 60 mmHg) and increased PCO_2 (more than 50 mmHg). Other test results vary. Chest X-rays may show a foreign body, pulmonary edema, or atelectasis. Toxicology tests may show drugs, chemicals, or abnormal hemoglobin.

Treatment
Asphyxia requires immediate support of respiration—with cardiopulmonary resuscitation, endotracheal intubation, and supplemental oxygen, as needed—and removal of the underlying cause: bronchoscopy for the extraction of a foreign body, a narcotic antagonist like naloxone for narcotic overdose, gastric lavage for poisoning, and discontinuation of supplemental oxygen for CO_2 narcosis that results from excessive oxygen therapy.

Additional considerations
Respiratory distress is frightening so the patient will need reassurance throughout treatment. Careful suctioning should be done, as needed. Vital signs and lab results must be monitored closely. To prevent drug-induced asphyxia, patients should never mix alcohol with other drugs.

Near-drowning

Near-drowning refers to surviving—temporarily, at least—the physiologic effects of hypoxemia and acidosis that result from submersion in fluid. Hypoxemia and acidosis are the primary problems in victims of near-drowning.

Near-drowning occurs in three forms: (1) "dry"—the victim doesn't aspirate fluid but suffers respiratory obstruction or asphyxia (10% to 15% of patients); (2) "wet"— the victim aspirates fluid and suffers from asphyxia or secondary changes due to fluid aspiration (about 85% of patients); (3) secondary—the victim suffers recurrence of respiratory distress (usually aspiration pneumonia or pulmonary edema) within minutes or 1 to 2 days after a near-drowning incident.

Causes and incidence

In the United States, drowning claims nearly 8,000 lives annually. No statistics are available for near-drowning incidents. Near-drowning results from an inability to swim or, in swimmers, from panic, a boating accident, a heart attack or a blow to the head while in the water, or drinking heavily before swimming. It may also be the outcome of a suicide attempt.

Regardless of the tonicity of the fluid aspirated, hypoxemia is the most serious consequence of near-drowning, followed by metabolic acidosis. But other consequences depend on the kind of water aspirated. After fresh water aspiration, changes in the character of lung surfactant result in exudation of protein-rich plasma into the alveoli. This, plus increased capillary permeability, eventually leads to secondary pulmonary edema and hypoxemia. After saltwater aspiration, the hypertonicity of sea water exerts an osmotic force, which pulls fluid from pulmonary capillaries into the alveoli. The resulting intrapulmonary shunt damages the lung parenchyma and induces hypoxemia and secondary pulmonary edema. In both kinds of near-drowning, pulmonary edema and hypoxemia are secondary to aspiration.

Signs and symptoms

Near-drowning victims can display a host of clinical problems: apnea, shallow or gasping respirations, substernal chest pain, asystole, tachycardia, bradycardia, restlessness, irritability, lethargy, fever, confusion, unconsciousness, vomiting, abdominal distention, and a cough that produces a pink frothy fluid.

Diagnosis

Diagnosis requires a history of near-drowning, along with characteristic clinical features and auscultation showing rales and rhonchi. Supportive diagnostic tests include:

• blood tests: arterial blood gases show decreased oxygen content, low HCO_3- and pH (reflecting metabolic acidosis). Leukocytosis is present.

• EKG: supraventricular tachycardia, occasional premature contractions, non-specific ST segment, and T wave abnormalities.

Treatment and additional considerations

Emergency treatment begins as soon as the victim is pulled from the water. Treatment includes cardiopulmonary resuscitation (CPR) and administration of oxygen (100%).

• When the patient arrives at the hospital, he's assessed for a patent airway. One will be established, if necessary. Then, as CPR continues, the patient may be intubated and given respiratory assistance. Arterial blood gases are assessed. Then, if the patient's abdomen is distended, a nasogastric tube is inserted. (Intubation is done first if the patient's unconscious.) I.V. lines are started and a Foley catheter inserted.

• The doctor may order drugs. Much controversy exists about the benefits of treating near-drowning victims with drugs. However, such treatment may include sodium bicarbonate for acidosis, corticosteroids for cerebral edema, antibiotics to prevent infections, and bronchodilators to ease bronchospasms.

• Pulmonary complications, signs of infection, and signs of delayed drowning (confusion, substernal pain, adventitious breath sounds) require watching; as do vital signs, intake and output, and peripheral pulses. Pulmonary artery catheters may be useful in assessing cardiopulmonary status. To facilitate the patient's breathing, the head of the bed can be raised slightly.

• All near-drowning victims should be admitted for an observation period of 24 to 48 hours because of the possibility of delayed drowning.

• To prevent near-drowning, swimmers should avoid drinking alcohol before swimming, observe water safety measures, and take a water safety course sponsored by the Red Cross or the YM/YWCA.

Decompression Sickness
"The bends," caisson disease

Decompression sickness is a painful condition that results from too rapid change from high- to low-pressure environments (decompression). Usually, victims are scuba divers who ascend too quickly from water deeper than 33 feet, and pilots and passengers of unpressurized aircraft who ascend too quickly to high altitudes.

Causes
Decompression sickness results from an abrupt change in air or water pressure that causes nitrogen to spill out of tissues faster than it can be diffused through respiration. It causes gas bubbles to form in blood and body tissues, which produce excruciating joint and muscle pain, neurologic and respiratory distress, and skin changes.

Signs and symptoms
Usually, symptoms appear during or within 30 minutes of rapid decompression, although they may be delayed up to 24 hours. Typically, decompression sickness results in:

• "the bends," which is deep and usually constant joint and muscle pain so severe that it may be incapacitating.

• transitory neurologic disturbances, such as difficult urination (from bladder paralysis), hemiplegia, deafness, visual disturbances, dizziness, aphasia, paresthesia and hyperesthesia of the legs, unsteady gait, and possibly, coma.

• respiratory distress, known as the "chokes," which includes chest pain, retrosternal burning, and a cough that may become paroxysmal and uncontrollable.

Such symptoms may persist for days and result in dyspnea, cyanosis, fainting, and occasionally, shock. Other symptoms include decreased temperature, pallor, itching, burning, mottled skin, and fatigue. In some patients, tachypnea may occur.

Diagnosis
History of rapid decompression and a physical examination showing characteristic clinical features confirm the diagnosis.

Treatment and additional considerations
Treatment consists of recompression and oxygen administration, followed by gradual decompression, and supportive measures.

Recompression takes place in a hyperbaric chamber (not available in all hospitals), in which air pressure is increased to 2.8 absolute atmospheric pressure over 1 to 2 minutes. This rapid rise in pressure reduces the size of the circulating nitrogen bubbles, and relieves pain and other clinical effects. During recompression, intermittent oxygen administration, with periodic maximal exhalations, promotes gas bubble diffusion. Once symptoms subside and diffusion is complete, a slow air pressure decrease in the chamber allows for gradual, safe decompression.

Supportive measures include fluid replacement in hypovolemic shock and sometimes corticosteroids to reduce the risk of spinal edema. Narcotics are contraindicated, since they further depress impaired respiration.

• To prevent toxicity, the patient who's receiving oxygen by mask must periodically exhale maximally for 5 minutes or more (the patient on a ventilator requires periodic "sighing").

• The following must be avoided in the patient's room during oxygen administration: improperly grounded electrical equipment; smoking; use of electric razors and other electrical appliances; use of wool or other static-electricity–producing blankets.

• If the patient with bladder paralysis needs catheterization, intake and output must be monitored accurately.

• To prevent decompression sickness, divers and fliers should follow the ascent guidelines developed and tested by the U.S. Navy.

Radiation Exposure

Expanded use of ionized radiation in medicine and in the nuclear power industry has vastly increased the incidence of radiation exposure. Cancer patients receiving radiation therapy and nuclear power plant workers are the most likely victims of this distinctly modern anomaly. The amount of radiation absorbed by a human body is measured in rads (short for "radiation absorbed dose"), not to be confused with roentgens, which are used to measure radiation emissions. A person can absorb up to 200 rads without fatal consequences. A dose of 450 rads is fatal in half the cases; more than 600 rads is nearly always fatal. However, when radiation is focused on a small area, the body can absorb and survive many thousands of rads, providing they are administered in carefully controlled doses over a long time. This is the key to safe and successful radiation therapy.

Causes
Exposure to radiation can occur by inhalation, ingestion, or direct contact. Whether or not such exposure damages tissue, and the severity of the damage, depend on the amount of body area exposed (the smaller, the better), length of exposure, dosage absorbed, distance from the source, and presence of protective shielding. Ionized radiation (X-rays, protons, neutrons, and alpha, beta, and gamma rays) may cause immediate cell necrosis or disturbed DNA synthesis, which impairs cell function and division. Rapidly dividing cells—bone marrow, hair follicles, gonads, lymph tissue—are most susceptible to radiation damage; highly differentiated cells—nerve, bone, muscle—resist radiation more successfully.

Signs and symptoms
The effects of ionized radiation can be immediate and acute, or delayed and chronic. Acute effects may be hematopoietic (after 200 to 500 rads), gastrointestinal (after 400 rads or more), or cerebral (after 1,000 rads or more). These effects depend strictly on the *amount* of radiation absorbed, not the site of absorption; they can follow absorption of radiation by any part of the body.

Acute hematopoietic radiation exposure induces nausea, vomiting, diarrhea, and anorexia, which subside after 24 to 48 hours. During the latent period that follows, pancytopenia develops. Within 2 to 3 weeks, thrombocytopenia, leukopenia, lymphopenia, and anemia produce nosebleeds, hemorrhage, petechiae, pallor, weakness, oropharyngeal abscesses, and increased susceptibility to infection because of impaired immunologic response. Thrombocytopenia becomes pronounced after 3 to 4 weeks.

Gastrointestinal radiation exposure causes ulceration, infection, intractable nausea, vomiting, and diarrhea, resulting in severe fluid and electrolyte imbalance. Breakdown of intestinal villi eventually produces plasma loss, which can lead to circulatory collapse and death.

Cerebral radiation poisoning after brief exposure to large amounts of radiation causes nausea, vomiting, and diarrhea within hours. Lethargy, tremors, convulsions, confusion, coma, and death may follow within hours or days.

Delayed or chronic effects from repeated, prolonged exposure to small doses of radiation over a long time can seriously damage skin, causing dryness, erythema, atrophy, and malignant lesions. (Such damage can also follow acute exposure.) Other delayed effects include alopecia, brittle nails, hypothyroidism, amenorrhea, cataracts, decreased fertility (in both sexes), anemia, leukopenia, thrombocytopenia, malignant neoplasms (leukemia, for example), and a shortened life span. In addition, long-term exposure to radiation may retard fetal growth or may cause serious genetic defects, but this remains a matter of intense controversy.

Diagnosis

An accurate history offers the best clues to radiation exposure. Supportive lab findings show decreased hematocrit, hemoglobin, WBC, platelet, and lymphocyte counts, and decreased serum electrolytes (K and Cl) from vomiting and diarrhea. Bone marrow studies show bone dyscrasia; X-rays may reveal bone necrosis. When radiation exposure produces open wounds, a Geiger counter may help determine the amount of exposure.

Treatment

Treatment is essentially symptomatic, and includes antiemetics to counter nausea and vomiting, fluid and electrolyte replacement (especially in cases of gastrointestinal radiation exposure), antibiotics, and possibly, sedatives if convulsions occur (most likely in cerebral radiation poisoning). Transfusions of plasma, platelets, and RBCs may be necessary if blood studies so indicate. Bone marrow transplant remains a highly controversial treatment but may be the only recourse in certain extreme cases. When radiation exposure results from inhalation or ingestion of large amounts of radioiodine, potassium iodide or a strong iodine solution may be given to block thyroid uptake.

Additional considerations

• To minimize radiation exposure, contaminated clothing must be disposed of following hospital guidelines. If the pa-

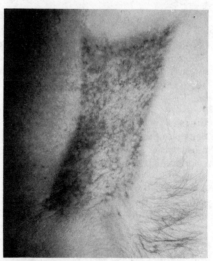

Radiation dermatitis of the axilla. Repeated prolonged exposure to radiation—even small doses—often induces erythematous dermatitis and atrophy of skin at site of radiation treatment.

tient's skin is contaminated, his entire body should be washed thoroughly with a chelating solution (calcium trisodium penetate or calcium disodium edetate) and plenty of water. Open wounds should be debrided and irrigated. If the patient recently ingested radioactive material, vomiting must be induced and lavage begun.

• Intake and output must be monitored, and fluid and electrolyte balance maintained. I.V. fluids and electrolytes may be administered. If the patient can tolerate oral feedings, he should be put on a high-protein, high-calorie diet. The patient will need to use a soft toothbrush to minimize bleeding from gums, and may find lidocaine helpful in easing the pain of mouth ulcers.

• To prevent skin breakdown, the patient must avoid extreme temperatures, tight clothing, and drying soaps. In the hospital, rigid aseptic technique and double preps for venipunctures and injections must be used.

• The patient and his family will need emotional support. After cerebral radiation poisoning, they must face the prospect of imminent death. After less severe exposure, they must learn to cope with distressing side effects.

Hospital personnel can avoid exposure to radiation by wearing proper shielding devices when supervising X-ray and radiation treatments. Those who work in these vulnerable areas should wear radiation detection badges and should be required to turn them in periodically for readings. Persons who have been exposed to significant amounts of radiation should be encouraged to receive genetic counseling and screening.

MISCELLANEOUS INJURIES

Poisoning

Inhalation, ingestion, injection, or skin contamination with any harmful substance is a common problem. In fact, in the United States, approximately 10 million persons are poisoned annually, 4,000 of them fatally. Prognosis depends on the amount of poison absorbed, its toxicity, and the time interval between poisoning and treatment.

Causes
Because of their curiosity and ignorance, most poison victims are children. In fact, accidental poisoning—usually from the ingestion of salicylates (aspirin), cleaning agents, insecticides, paints, and cosmetics—is the fourth leading cause of death in children.

In adults, poisoning is most common among chemical company employees, particularly those in companies that use chlorine, carbon dioxide, hydrogen sulfide, nitrogen dioxide, and ammonia; and in companies that ignore safety standards. Other causes of poisoning in adults include improper cooking, canning, and storage of food; ingestion of, or skin contamination from, plants; and accidental or intentional drug overdose (usually barbiturates).

Signs and symptoms
Symptoms vary according to the poison.

Diagnosis
A history of ingestion, inhalation, injection, or skin contact with a poisonous substance, and typical clinical features suggest the diagnosis. Poisoning should be suspected in any unconscious patient with no history of diabetes, seizure disorders, or trauma.

Toxicologic studies (including drug screens) of poison levels in the mouth,

COMMON POISONOUS PLANTS

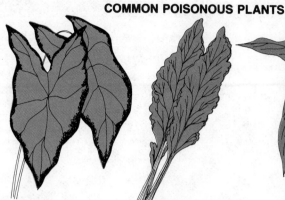

ELEPHANT EAR PHILO-DENDRON
Sx: burning throat and GI distress
Rx: gastric lavage or emesis; antihistamines and lime juice; symptomatic treatment

RHUBARB
Sx: GI and respiratory distress, internal bleeding, coma
Rx: gastric lavage or emesis with lime water; calcium gluconate and force fluids

DIEFFENBACHIA
Sx: burning throat, edema, GI distress
Rx: gastric lavage or emesis; antihistamines and lime juice; symptomatic treatment

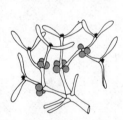

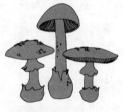

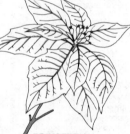

MISTLETOE
Sx: GI distress and slow pulse
Rx: gastric lavage or emesis; cardiac drugs, potassium, and sodium

MUSHROOMS
Sx: GI, respiratory, CNS, parasympathomimetic effects
Rx: lavage with potassium permanganate; saline catharsis; atropine

POINSETTIA
(milky juice)
Sx: inflammation and blisters
Rx: none; condition will disappear after several days

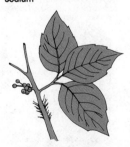

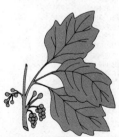

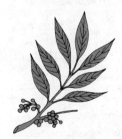

POISON IVY, POISON SUMAC, POISON OAK (sap)
Sx: allergic skin reactions; if ingested, GI distress, liver and kidney damage
Rx: if ingested: demulcents, morphine, fluids; high-protein low-fat diet. For skin reactions: antihistamine, topical antipyretics.

Poisonous parts of the plant appear in color. If the poisonous part can't be shown, it appears in parentheses after the plant's name.

MANAGEMENT OF COMMON POISONING

1. No treatment necessary after ingestion of small amounts. Fluids may be given.

2. Induce vomiting. Give syrup of ipecac in the following dosages:
   Under 1 year of age:
   2 teaspoons followed by at least 2 to 3 glasses of fluid.
   1 year and older:
   Give 1 tablespoon followed by at least 2 to 3 glasses of fluid.
   Do not induce vomiting if the patient is semicomatose, comatose, or convulsing.
   Call Poison Center for additional information.

3. Dilute or neutralize with water or milk. *Do not induce vomiting.* Gastric lavage is indicated. Call Poison Center for specific instructions.

4. Treat symptomatically unless botulism is suspected. Call Poison Center for specific information regarding botulism.

5. Dilute or neutralize with water or milk. *Do not induce vomiting.* Gastric lavage should be avoided. This substance may cause burns of the mucous membranes. Consult ENT specialist following emergency treatment. Call Poison Center for specific information.

Suggested general treatment for poisoning

6. Immediately wash skin thoroughly with running water. Call Poison Center for further treatment.

7. Immediately wash eyes with a gentle stream of running water. Continue for 15 minutes. Call Poison Center for further treatment.

8. Specific antagonist may be indicated. Call Poison Center.

9. Remove to fresh air. Support respirations. Call Poison Center for further treatment.

10. Call Poison Center for specific instructions.

11. Symptomatic and supportive treatment. *Do not induce vomiting* for *ingestion.* I.V. naloxone hydrochloride to be given as indicated for respiratory depression.
    Dosage:
    Adult—0.4 mg I.V.
        May be repeated at 2- to 3-minute intervals.
    Child—0.01 mg/kg I.V.
        May be repeated at 5- to 10-minute intervals.

Permission to reproduce this chart granted by the National Poison Center Network, Children's Hospital of Pittsburgh.

vomitus, urine, feces, blood, or on the victim's hands or clothing confirm the diagnosis. If possible, the family or patient should bring the container holding the poison to the emergency room for comparable study. In inhalation poisoning, chest X-rays may show pulmonary infiltrates or edema; in petroleum distillate inhalation, X-rays may show aspiration pneumonia.

Treatment
Treatment includes emergency resuscitation and support, prevention of further absorption of poison, continuing supportive or symptomatic care, and when possible, a specific antidote.

Additional considerations
A health care professional treating a poison victim should:
• assess cardiopulmonary and respiratory function, and if necessary, begin cardiopulmonary resuscitation (CPR); monitor vital signs and level of consciousness.
• depending on the poison, prevent further absorption of ingested poison by inducing emesis one of these ways: using syrup of ipecac; stimulating the gag reflex with a finger or tongue blade, or administering gastric lavage and cathartics (magnesium sulfate [Epsom salt], phosphate soda). The effectiveness of such treatment depends on the speed of absorption and the time that's elapsed between ingestion and removal.

When syrup of ipecac is used to induce vomiting, the patient should drink warm water (usually less than 1 quart [less than 1 liter]) until vomiting occurs, or be given another dose of ipecac, as ordered. If activated charcoal is ordered to neutralize the poison, it must not be administered until *after* emesis, since the charcoal absorbs ipecac.

When gastric lavage is used, 30 ml fluid is instilled by nasogastric tube; and then aspirated. This is repeated until aspirate is clear. Vomitus and aspirate should be saved for analysis. (To prevent aspiration in the unconscious patient, an endotracheal tube should be in place before lavage.)
• never induce emesis if corrosive acid poisoning is suspected, if the patient is unconscious or has convulsions, or if the gag reflex is impaired even in a conscious patient. Instead, the poison should be neutralized by instilling the appropriate antidote by nasogastric tube. Common antidotes include milk, magnesium salts (milk of magnesia), activated charcoal, or other chelating agents (deferoxamine, edetate disodium [EDTA]). When possible, the antidote is added to water or juice. (Note: The removal of hydrocarbon poisoning is controversial. In the conscious patient, since there is a lower risk of aspiration with ipecac-induced emesis than with lavage, emesis is becoming the preferred treatment, but some doctors still use lavage. Moreover, some believe that because of poor absorption, kerosene [a hydrocarbon] does not require removal from the gastrointestinal tract; others believe removal depends on the amount ingested.)
• use large quantities of I.V. fluids to diurese the patient, if several hours have passed since the patient ingested the poison. The kind of fluid used depends on the patient's acid-base balance, the I.V. set flow rate, and on his cardiovascular status.
• be prepared to perform peritoneal dialysis or hemodialysis in cases of severe ingested poisoning.
• to prevent further absorption of inhaled poison, remove the patient to fresh or uncontaminated air; alert the anesthesia department; and provide supplemental oxygen. Some patients may require intubation.
• to prevent further absorption from skin contamination, remove the clothing covering the contaminated skin, and immediately flush the area with large amounts of water.
• for the patient in severe pain, give analgesics, as ordered; and monitor fluid intake and output, vital signs, and level of consciousness.
• refer the patient for psychiatric counseling, if the poison was ingested intentionally.

• instruct patients to prevent accidental poisoning by reading the label before they take medicine; by storing all medications and household chemicals properly; by keeping them out of reach of children; by discarding old medications; by not taking medicines prescribed for someone else; by not transferring medicines from their original bottles to other containers without labeling them properly; by never transferring poisons to food containers.

Parents of young children should not take medications in front of their children or call medications "candy" to get children to take them. Also, toxic sprays must only be used in well-ventilated areas, following instructions carefully. Pesticides, as well, must be used carefully. Finally, the phone number of the local poison control center should be kept handy.

Poisonous Snakebites

Each year, poisonous snakes bite about 7,000 persons in the United States. Such bites are most common during summer afternoons, in grassy or rocky habitats. Poisonous snakebites are medical emergencies. With prompt, correct treatment, they need not be fatal.

Causes
The only poisonous snakes in the United States are pit vipers (Crotalidae) and coral snakes (Elapidae). Pit vipers include rattlesnakes, water moccasins (cottonmouths), and copperheads. They have a pitted depression between their eyes and nostrils, and two fangs ¾" to 1¼" (2 to 3 cm) long. Since the fangs are delicate and may break off, some snakes have only one fang; but since new fangs often grow behind old ones, some have three or four. Pit vipers can strike at a speed from 6 to 45 mph, and they do not have to rattle or be coiled to strike.

Since coral snakes are nocturnal and placid, their bites are less common than pit viper bites; pit vipers are also nocturnal but are more active. The fangs of coral snakes are short but have teeth behind them. Coral snakes tend to bite with a chewing motion and may leave multiple fang marks, small lacerations, and much tissue destruction.

Signs and symptoms
Most snakebites happen on the arms and legs, below the elbow or knee. Bites to the head or trunk are most dangerous, but any bite into a blood vessel is dangerous, regardless of location.

Most pit viper bites that result in envenomation cause immediate and progressively severe pain and edema (the entire extremity may swell within a few hours), local elevation in skin temperature, fever, skin discoloration, petechiae, ecchymoses, blebs, blisters, bloody discharge from the wound, and local necrosis.

Because pit viper venom is neurotoxic, pit viper bites may cause local and facial numbness and tingling, fasciculation and twitching of skeletal muscles, convulsions (especially in children), extreme anxiety, difficulty in speaking, fainting, weakness, dizziness, excessive sweating, occasional paralysis, mild to severe respiratory distress, headache, blurred vision, marked thirst, and in severe envenomation, coma and death. Pit viper venom may also impair coagulation and cause hematemesis, hematuria, melena, bleeding gums, and internal bleeding. Other symptoms of pit viper bites include nausea, vomiting, diarrhea, tachycardia, lymphadenopathy, hypotension, and shock.

The reaction to coral snake bite is usually delayed—perhaps up to several hours. Unlike pit viper bites, these snakebites cause little or no local tissue reaction (local pain, swelling, or necrosis). However, because their venom is neurotoxic, after a reaction develops, it progresses swiftly, producing such neurotoxic effects as local paresthesia, weakness, euphoria, drowsiness, nausea, vomiting, difficulty swallowing, marked salivation, dysphonia, ptosis, blurred vision, miosis, respiratory distress and possible respiratory failure, loss of muscle coordination, abnormal reflexes, peripheral paralysis, and possibly, shock with cardiovascular collapse and death. Coral snake bites can also cause coagulotoxicity.

Diagnosis

Patient history, observation of fang marks, snake identification (when possible), and progressive symptoms of envenomation all point to snakebite. Lab values help identify the extent of envenomation and provide guidelines for supportive treatment. Abnormal lab results may include prolonged bleeding time and partial thromboplastin time, decreased hemoglobin and hematocrit, sharply decreased platelet count (less than 200,000/mm³), urinalysis showing hematuria, and in infection (snake mouths contain gram-negative bacteria), increased WBC. In addition, chest X-ray may show pulmonary edema or emboli, an EKG may show tachycardia and ectopic beats, and severe envenomation may produce an abnormal EEG. (Usually, an EKG is necessary only in severe envenomation, especially when the patient is over age 40.)

Treatment

Prompt, appropriate first aid can reduce venom absorption and prevent severe symptoms. A health care professional on the scene should:
• identify the snake, if possible, but not waste time trying to find it.
• immobilize the limb below heart level immediately; instruct the victim to remain as quiet as possible.
• apply a slightly constrictive tourniquet (one that obstructs only lymphatic and superficial venous blood flow) about 4″ (10 cm) above the fang marks, or just above the first joint proximal to the bite. Caution: This constrictive tourniquet must only be applied if less than 30 minutes has elapsed since the bite. Also, total constrictive tourniquet time should not exceed 2 hours; nor should it delay antivenin administration. During that time, the tourniquet must be released for 60 to 90 seconds every 30 minutes, especially if swelling progresses rapidly. A tight tourniquet should be applied only for extremely severe envenomation by a coral snake. In this case, the tight tourniquet must be released every 10 minutes for 90 seconds until antivenin is administered. Remember, use of a tourniquet makes loss of limb likely.
• wash the skin over the fang marks; make an incision through the marks approximately ½″ (1 cm) long and ⅛″ (3 mm) deep (being especially careful if the bite is on the hand, where blood vessels and tendons are close to the skin surface); and apply suction using a bulb syringe—or if no other means is available, mouth suction—for 20 to 30 minutes, or for up to 2 hours in the absence of antivenin administration. Remember: This method is effective only in pit viper bites, and only within 30 minutes of the bite; also the rescuer must not mouth suction if he has oral ulcers.
• never give the victim alcoholic drinks

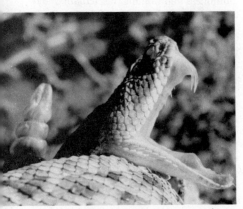

A pitted depression between eyes and nostrils, and two long fangs are characteristic of pit vipers, the most common poisonous snakes.

or stimulants, since these speed venom absorption; also, never apply ice to a snakebite.

• transport the victim as quickly as possible, keeping him warm and at rest. The signs and symptoms of progressive envenomation and when they develop must be recorded. Most snakebite victims are hospitalized for only 24 to 48 hours, but some remain longer after severe envenomation. Usually, treatment consists of antivenin administration, though minor snakebites may not require antivenin. Other treatment includes tetanus toxoid or tetanus immune globulin, human; broad-spectrum antibiotics; and depending on respiratory status, severity of pain, and type of snakebite (narcotics are contraindicated in coral snake bites), aspirin, codeine, morphine, or meperidine. Usually, necrotic snakebites need surgical debridement after 3 or 4 days. Intense, rapidly progressive edema requires fasciotomy within 2 or 3 hours of the bite; extreme envenomation may require limb amputation and subsequent reconstructive surgery, rehabilitation, and physical therapy.

When the patient arrives at the hospital, a hospital staffer there should:
• immobilize the extremity if this hasn't been done already. If a tight tourniquet has been applied within the past hour, he should apply a loose tourniquet proximally, and remove the tight tourniquet. The loose tourniquet must be gradually released during antivenin administration. A sudden release of venom into the bloodstream may cause cardiorespiratory compromise or collapse. That's why emergency equipment is kept available.
• start a flow sheet documenting vital signs, level of consciousness, skin color, respiratory status, description of the bite, the area surrounding it, and symptoms; monitor vital signs every 15 minutes; start an I.V. with a large-bore needle for antivenin administration. Severe bites that cause coagulotoxic symptoms may require two I.V. lines: one for antivenin, another for blood products.
• obtain a patient history of allergies (especially to horse serum) and other medical problems *before* antivenin administration; do hypersensitivity tests and desensitization, if needed. During antivenin administration, epinephrine, oxygen, and vasopressors may be used to combat anaphylaxis from horse serum.
• give packed cells, whole blood, I.V. fluids, and possibly, fresh frozen plasma or platelets, to counteract coagulotoxicity and maintain blood pressure. If respiratory distress requires endotracheal intubation or tracheotomy, good tracheostomy care will also be required.
• give analgesics, as needed. Remember: Narcotics must not be given to victims of coral snake bites. Instead, the snakebite should be cleansed using sterile technique. If blebs and blisters form, they should be opened, debrided, and drained since they may contain venom. Dressings must be changed daily.

Additional considerations

• If the patient requires hospitalization for longer than 24 to 48 hours, he'll need to be positioned carefully to avoid contractures. Passive exercises should be done until the fourth day after the bite, followed by active exercises and whirlpool treatments, as ordered.
• Hikers and campers should carry a snakebite kit if they'll be more than a half hour from the nearest hospital.

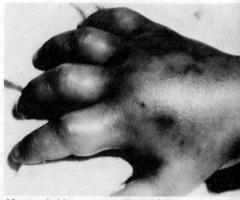

After snakebite, severe edema of the affected extremity occurs within hours.

Insect Bites and Stings

Among the most common traumatic complaints are insect bites and stings, the more serious of which include those of a tick, brown recluse spider, black widow spider, scorpion, bee, wasp, or yellow jacket.

GENERAL INFORMATION

CLINICAL FEATURES

Tick

- Common in woods and fields throughout the United States
- Attaches to host in any of its life stages (larva, nymph, adult). Fastens to host with its teeth, then secretes a cementlike material to reinforce attachment.
- Flat, brown, speckled body about 0.25" (6.25 mm) long; has eight legs
- Also transmits diseases such as Rocky Mountain spotted fever.

- Itching may be sole symptom; or after several days, host may develop tick paralysis (acute flaccid paralysis, starting as paresthesia and pain in legs and resulting in respiratory failure from bulbar paralysis).

Brown recluse (violin) spider

- Common to south-central United States; usually found in dark areas (outdoor privy, barn, woodshed)
- Dark brown violin on its back, three pairs of eyes; female more dangerous than male
- Most bites occur between April and October.

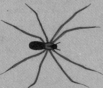

Venom is coagulotoxic. Reaction begins within 2 to 8 hours after bite.
- Localized vasoconstriction causes ischemic necrosis at bite site. Small, reddened puncture wound forms a bleb and becomes ischemic. In 3 to 4 days, center becomes dark and hard. Within 2 to 3 weeks, an ulcer forms.
- Minimal initial pain increases over time.
- Other symptoms: fever, chills, malaise, weakness, nausea, vomiting, edema, convulsions, joint pains, petechiae, cyanosis, phlebitis
- Rarely, thrombocytopenia and hemolytic anemia develop and lead to death within first 24 to 48 hours (usually in a child or patient with previous history of cardiac disease). Prompt and appropriate treatment results in recovery.

Black widow spider

- Common throughout the United States, particularly in warmer climates; usually found in dark areas (outdoor privy, barn, woodshed)
- Female is coal black with a red or orange hourglass on her ventral side; she is larger than male (male does not bite).
- Mortality less than 1% (increased risk among the elderly, infants, and those with allergies).

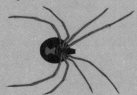

Venom is neurotoxic. Age, size, and sensitivity of patient determines severity and progression of symptoms
- Pinprick sensation, followed by dull, numbing pain (may go unnoticed)
- Edema and tiny, red bite marks
- Rigidity of stomach muscles and severe abdominal pain (10 to 40 minutes after bite)
- Muscle spasms in extremities
- Ascending paralysis, causing difficulty in swallowing and labored, grunting respirations
- Other symptoms: extreme restlessness, vertigo, sweating, chills, pallor, convulsions (especially in children), hyperactive reflexes, hypertension, tachycardia, thready pulse, circulatory collapse, nausea, vomiting, headache, ptosis, eyelid edema, urticaria, pruritus, and fever

After brown recluse (violin) spider bite, localized vasoconstriction causes ischemic necrosis at bite site. Small, reddened puncture wound forms a bleb and becomes ischemic.

TREATMENT	TECHNIQUES AND CONSIDERATIONS
• Removal of tick • Local antipruritics for itching papule • Mechanical ventilation for respiratory failure	• To remove tick, cover it with mineral, salad, or machine oil, or alcohol on a tissue or gauze pad. This blocks the tick's breathing pores and causes it to withdraw from the skin. If the tick doesn't disengage after the pad has been in place for ½ hour, carefully remove it with tweezers, taking care to remove all parts. • To reduce risk of being bitten, patients should keep away from wooded areas, wear protective clothes, and carefully examine body for ticks after being outdoors.
• No known specific treatment • Combination therapy with corticosteroids, antibiotics, antihistamines, tranquilizers, I.V. fluids, and tetanus prophylaxis • Lesion excision in first 10 to 12 hours relieves pain. A split-thickness skin graft closes the wound. Without grafting, healing may take 6 to 8 weeks. • A large chronic ulcer may require skin grafting.	• A health care professional should: cleanse the lesion with a 1:20 Burow's aluminum acetate solution, and as ordered, apply antibiotic ointment; take complete patient history, including allergies and other preexisting medical problems; monitor vital signs, patient's general appearance, and any changes at bite site. • The patient with disfiguring ulcer should know that skin grafting can improve appearance. • To prevent brown recluse bites, patients should spray areas of infestation with creosote at least every 2 months, wear gloves and heavy clothes when working around woodpiles or sheds, inspect outdoor working clothes for spiders before use, and discourage children from playing near infested areas.
• Neutralization of venom using antivenin I.V., preceded by desensitization when skin or eye tests show sensitivity to horse serum • Calcium gluconate I.V. to control muscle spasms. • Muscle relaxants like methocarbamol for severe muscle spasms • Adrenalin or antihistamines • Oxygen by nasal cannula or mask • Tetanus immunization • Antibiotics to prevent infection	• A health care professional should: take complete patient history, including allergies and other preexisting medical problems; have epinephrine and emergency resuscitation equipment on hand in case of anaphylactic reaction to antivenin; keep patient quiet and warm, and the affected part immobile; cleanse bite site with antiseptic, and apply ice to relieve pain and swelling and to slow circulation; check vital signs frequently during first 12 hours after bite; report any changes (symptoms usually subside in 3 to 4 hours); when giving analgesics, monitor respiratory status. • To prevent black widow spider bites, the patient should spray areas of infestation with creosote at least every 2 months; wear gloves and heavy clothing when working around woodpiles or sheds; inspect outdoor working clothes for spiders before putting them on; discourage children from playing near infested areas.

GENERAL INFORMATION	CLINICAL FEATURES

Scorpion
- Common throughout the United States (30 different species); two deadly species in southwestern states
- Curled tail with stinger on end; eight legs; 3″ (7.5 cm) long
- Most stings occur during warmer months.
- Mortality less than 1% (increased risk among the elderly and children).

Nonlethal reaction: anaphylaxis (rare)
- Local swelling and tenderness, sharp burning sensation, skin discoloration, paresthesia, lymphangitis with regional gland swelling
Lethal reaction (neurotoxic): immediate sharp pain; hyperesthesia; drowsiness; itching of nose, throat, and mouth; impaired speech (due to sluggish tongue); generalized muscle spasms (including jaw muscle spasms, laryngospasms, incontinence, convulsions, nausea, vomiting, drooling)
- Symptoms last from 24 to 78 hours. Bite site recovers last.
- Death may follow cardiovascular or respiratory failure.
- Prognosis is poor if symptoms progress rapidly in first few hours.

Bee, wasp, and yellow jacket
- When a honeybee (rounded abdomen) or a bumblebee (over 1″ [2.5 cm] long; furry, rounded abdomen) stings, its stinger remains in the victim; the bee flies away and dies.
- A wasp or yellow jacket (slender body with elongated abdomen) retains its stinger and can sting repeatedly.

Localized reaction: painful wound (protruding stinger from bees), edema, urticaria, pruritus
Systemic reaction (anaphylaxis): symptoms of hypersensitivity usually appear within 20 minutes and may include weakness, chest tightness, dizziness, nausea, vomiting, abdominal cramps, and throat constriction. The shorter the interval between the sting and systemic symptoms, the worse the prognosis. Without prompt treatment, symptoms may progress to cyanosis, coma, and death.

Open Trauma Wounds
(Abrasions, avulsions, crush wounds, lacerations, missile injuries, punctures)

Open trauma wounds are common injuries that often result from home, work, or motor vehicle accidents, and acts of violence. For information on specific types of wounds, see chart.

Assessment

In all open wounds, the following should be assessed: the extent of injury, vital signs, level of consciousness, obvious skeletal damage, local neurologic deficits, and general patient condition. An accurate history of the injury from the patient or witnesses will be needed, including: when and where it occurred, if it involved a weapon (if so, notify the police), and if the patient has already received any treatment.

The following should also be assessed: peripheral nerve damage (common complication in lacerations and other open trauma wounds) fractures, and dislocations. Signs of peripheral nerve damage vary with location as follows:
- *Radial nerve:* weak forearm flexion, inability to extend thumb in a hitchhiker's sign
- *Median nerve:* numbness in tip of in-

TREATMENT	TECHNIQUES AND CONSIDERATIONS
• Antivenin (made from cat serum), if available. (Contact Poisonous Animals Research Lab, Arizona State University, Tempe, Arizona.) • Calcium gluconate I.V. for muscle spasms • Phenobarbital I.M. for convulsions • Emetine subcutaneously to relieve pain (opiates such as morphine and codeine are contraindicated)	• A health care professional should: take complete patient history, including allergies and other preexisting medical conditions; immobilize patient, and apply tourniquet proximal to sting; pack area extending beyond tourniquet in ice. After 5 minutes of ice pack, remove tourniquet; monitor vital signs. (Watch closely for signs of respiratory distress and keep emergency resuscitation equipment available.)
• Antihistamines and corticosteroids (in urticaria) • Tetanus prophylaxis *In anaphylaxis:* • Oxygen by nasal cannula or mask • Epinephrine 1:1,000 subcutaneously or I.M. • In bronchospasm, aminophylline and hydrocortisone • In hypotension, metaraminol and isoproterenol	• If stinger is in place, it should be scraped off, not pulled; this releases more toxin. Then, the site should be cleansed and ice applied. The victim should be watched carefully for signs of anaphylaxis, and emergency resuscitation equipment kept available. • The patient who is allergic to bee stings must wear a medical identification bracelet or carry a card, and carry an anaphylaxis kit. • To prevent bee stings, the patient should: not wear fragrant cosmetics when outdoors during insect season; avoid wearing bright colors and going barefoot; avoid contact with flowers and fruit that attract bees; use insect repellent.

dex finger; inability to place forearm in prone position; weak forearm, thumb, and index finger flexion
• *Ulnar nerve:* numbness in tip of little finger, clawing of hand
• *Peroneal nerve:* inability to extend the foot or big toe, footdrop
• *Sciatic and tibial nerves:* paralysis of ankles and toes, footdrop, weakness in leg, numbness in sole.

Most open wounds require emergency treatment. In those with suspected nerve involvement, however, electromyography, nerve conduction, and electrical stimulation tests can provide more detailed information about possible peripheral nerve damage.

Treatment and additional considerations

• If hemorrhage occurs, bleeding must be stopped by applying direct pressure on the wound and, if necessary, on arterial pressure points. If the wound is on an extremity, the extremity should be elevated, if possible. A tourniquet must not be applied except in life-threatening hemorrhage. In such a case, the patient may lose his limb.
• Patients with major wounds require frequent vital signs assessment, with special attention paid to: a 20% drop in blood pressure and a 20% increase in pulse (taken when the patient's sitting *and* when he's lying down); increased respirations; decreasing level of consciousness; thirst; and cool, clammy skin—all indications of blood loss and hypovolemic shock.
• Oxygen should be administered.
• Blood samples must be typed and cross-matched and analyzed for CBC (including hematocrit, hemoglobin) and prothrombin and partial thromboplas-

HOW TO MANAGE OPEN TRAUMA

TYPE	CLINICAL ACTION

Abrasion
Open surface wounds (scrapes) of epidermis and possibly the dermis, resulting from friction. Nerve endings exposed.

Diagnosis based on scratches, reddish welts, bruises, pain, and history of friction injury.

- Obtaining a history to distinguish injury from second-degree burn.
- Cleansing gently with topical germicide, and irrigating. Too vigorous scrubbing of abrasions will increase tissue damage.
- Removing all imbedded foreign objects, and applying a local anesthetic if cleansing is very painful.
- Applying light, water-soluble antibiotic cream to prevent infection.
- If wound is severe, applying loose protective dressing that allows air to circulate.
- Administering tetanus prophylaxis, if necessary.

Avulsion
Complete tissue loss that prevents approximation of wound edges, resulting from cutting, gouging, or complete tearing of skin. Frequently affects nose tip, earlobe, fingertip, and penis.

Diagnosis based on full-thickness skin loss, hemorrhage, pain, history of trauma. X-ray required to rule out bone damage; CBC and differential before surgery.

- Checking history for bleeding tendencies and anticoagulant use.
- Recording time of injury to help determine if tissue is salvageable. Preserving tissue (if available) in cool saline solution for possible split-thickness graft or flap.
- Controlling hemorrhage with pressure, absorbable gelatin sponge, or topical thrombin.
- Cleansing gently, irrigating with saline solution, and debriding, if necessary. Covering with a bulky dressing.
- Telling patient to leave dressing in place until return visit, to keep area dry, and to watch for signs of infection (pain, fever, redness, swelling).
- Administering analgesic and tetanus prophylaxis, if necessary.

Crush wound
Heavy falling object splits skin and causes necrosis along split margins and damages tissue underneath. May look like laceration.

Diagnosis based on history of trauma, edema, hemorrhage, massive hematomas, damage to surrounding tissues (fractures, nerve injuries, loss of tendon function), shock, pain, history of trauma. X-rays required to determine extent of injury to surrounding structures. CBC and differential, and electrolyte count also required.

- Checking history for bleeding tendencies and use of anticoagulants.
- Cleansing open areas gently with soap and water.
- Controlling hemorrhage with pressure and cold packs.
- Applying dry, sterile bulky dressing; wrapping entire extremity in compression dressing.
- Immobilizing injured extremity; encouraging patient to rest; monitoring vital signs; and checking peripheral pulses and circulation often.
- Administering tetanus prophylaxis, if necessary.
- If wound is severe, giving I.V. infusion of lactated Ringer's or saline solution with large-bore catheter, and surgically exploring, debriding, and repairing.

Puncture wound
Small-entry wounds that probably damage underlying structures, resulting from sharp, pointed objects.

Diagnosis based on hemorrhage (rare), deep hematomas (in chest or abdominal wounds), ragged wound edges (in bites), small-entry wound (in very sharp object), pain, and history of trauma. X-rays can detect retention of injuring object.

- Checking history for bleeding tendencies and anticoagulant use.
- Obtaining description of injury, including force of entry.
- Assessing extent of injury.
- Leaving impaling objects in place until injury is completely evaluated. (If the eye is injured, an ophthalmologist should be called immediately.)
- Thoroughly cleansing injured area with soap and water; irrigating all minor wounds with saline solution after removing foreign object.
- Leaving human bite wounds open; applying dry, sterile dressing to other minor puncture wounds.
- Telling patient to apply warm soaks daily.
- Administering tetanus prophylaxis and, if necessary, rabies vaccine.
- For deep wounds that damage underlying tissues, performing exploratory surgery; in the case of retention of injuring object, performing surgical removal.

Laceration

Open wound, possibly extending into deep epithelium, resulting from penetration with knife or other sharp object or from a severe blow with a blunt object.

Diagnosis based on hemorrhage, torn or destroyed tissues, pain, and history of trauma.

In laceration less than 8 hours old, and in all lacerations of face and areas of possible functional disability (such as the elbow):
- Applying pressure and elevating injured extremity to control hemorrhage.
- Cleansing wound gently with soap and water; irrigating with normal saline solution.
- As necessary, debriding necrotic margins, and closing wound, using strips of tape or sutures.
- If laceration is severe and is accompanied by underlying structural damage, performing surgery.

In grossly contaminated laceration or laceration more than 8 hours old (except laceration of face and areas of possible functional disability):
- Administering broad-spectrum antibiotic, such as tetracycline, for at least a 5-day course, as ordered.
- Leaving wound open for several days.
- Instructing patient to elevate injured extremity for 24 hours after injury to reduce swelling.
- Telling patient to keep dressing clean and dry and to watch for signs of infection.
- After 5 to 7 days, closing wound with sutures or butterfly dressing if it appears uninfected and contains healthy granulated tissue.
- Applying sterile dressing and splint, as necessary.

In all lacerations:
- Checking history for bleeding tendencies and anticoagulant use.
- Determining approximate time of injury, and estimating blood loss.
- Assessing for neuromuscular, tendon, and circulatory damage.
- Administering tetanus prophylaxis, as necessary.
- Stressing the need for follow-up and suture removal.
- If sutures become infected, culturing the wound and scrubbing with surgical soap preparation; removing some or all sutures; giving broad-spectrum antibiotic, as ordered; instructing patient to soak wound in warm, soapy water for 15 minutes, three times daily, and to return for follow-up every 2 to 3 days, until the wound heals.
- If injury is the result of foul play, reporting it to police department.

Missile injury

High velocity issue penetration, such as a gunshot wound.

Diagnosis based on entry and possibly exit wounds, signs of hemorrhage, shock, pain, and history of trauma. X-ray, CBC, and differential and electrolyte levels required to assess extent of injury and estimate blood loss.

- Checking history for bleeding tendencies and use of anticoagulants.
- Controlling hemorrhage with pressure, if possible; if injury is near vital organs, using large-bore catheters to start two I.V.s, using lactated Ringer's or normal saline solution for volume replacement, and preparing for possible exploratory surgery.
- Maintaining airway, and monitoring for signs of hypovolemia, shock, and cardiac arrhythmias; checking vital signs and neurovascular response often.
- Covering sucking chest wound during exhalation with petrolatum gauze and an occlusive dressing.
- Cleansing wound gently with soap and water; debriding as necessary.
- If damage is minor, applying dry sterile dressing.
- Administering tetanus prophylaxis, if necessary.
- Obtaining X-rays to detect retained fragments.
- If possible, determining caliber of weapon.
- Reporting injury to police department.

tin times.
• In accompanying peripheral nerve damage, the extremity should be immobilized to prevent further damage.
• To prepare the patient for surgery, I.V. lines are started, using two large-bore catheters, for the infusion of lactated Ringer's, normal saline solution, or whole blood. A central venous pressure (CVP) line is inserted, and the patient is placed in a modified V position (head flat, legs elevated). If modified V position doesn't help and Medical Anti-shock Trousers (MAST) aren't available, the Trendelenburg position is an alternative.
• In suspected internal bleeding, a nasogastric tube is inserted; if systolic blood pressure is less than 90 mmHg, a MAST suit may be used to *temporarily* restore blood volume to vital organs.

Rape Crisis Syndrome

The term rape refers to illicit sexual intercourse without consent. It's a violent assault, in which sex is used as a weapon. Rape inflicts varying degrees of physical and psychologic trauma. Rape crisis syndrome occurs during the period following the rape or attempted rape; it refers to the victim's short-term and long-term reactions and to the methods she uses to cope with this trauma.

In the United States, rape is the fastest-growing violent crime, with one reported every 7 minutes, or occurring at the rate of 200 per day, 62,500 per year. Incidence is highest in large cities and is rising. This rise may reflect the fact that more women now report rape. However, possibly over 90% of assaults are never reported.

Known victims of rape range in age from 2 months to 97 years. The age-group most affected are the 10- to 19-year-olds; the average victim's age is 13½. Over 50% of rapes occur in the home; about one third of these involve a male intruder, who forces his way into a home. Approximately half the time, the victim has some casual acquaintance with the attacker. Most rapists are 15 to 24 years old. Usually, the attack is planned.

In most cases, the rapist is a man and the victim is a woman. However, rapes do occur between persons of the same sex, especially in prisons, schools, hospitals, and other institutions. Also, children are often the victims of rape; most of the time these cases involve manual, oral, or genital contact with the child's genitals. Usually, the rapist is a member of the child's family. In rare instances, the rapist-victim roles are reversed: a man or child is sexually abused by a woman.

Prognosis is good if the rape victim receives physical and emotional support and counseling to help her deal with her feelings. Victims who articulate their feelings are able to cope with fears, interact with others, and return to normal routines faster than those who do not.

Causes
Some of the cultural, sociologic, and psychologic factors that contribute to rape are increasing exposure to sex, permissiveness, cynicism about relationships, feelings of anger, and powerlessness amid social pressures. The rapist often has feelings of violence or hatred toward women, or sexual problems, such as impotence or premature ejaculation. Frequently, he's socially isolated and unable to form warm, loving relationships. Some rapists seem to be psychopaths who seek pleasure, regardless of how it affects their victims; others rape to satisfy a need for power. Some have been abused as children.

Assessment
When a rape victim arrives in the emergency department, the health care professional working there should do the

following:

Assess her physical injuries. If she's not *seriously* injured, allow her to remain clothed, and take her to a private room, where she can talk with a counselor before the necessary physical examination. Remember, immediate reactions to rape differ and include crying, laughing, hostility, confusion, withdrawal, or outward calm; often anger and rage don't surface until later. During the assault, the victim may have felt demeaned, helpless, and afraid for her life; afterward, she may feel ashamed, guilty, shocked, and vulnerable, and have a sense of disbelief and lowered self-esteem. Offer support and reassurance. Help her explore her feelings; listen, convey trust and respect, and remain non-judgmental. Don't leave her alone unless she requests it.

Being careful to upset the victim as little as possible, obtain an accurate history of the rape, pertinent to physical assessment. (Remember: these notes may be used as evidence if the rapist is tried.) Record the victim's statements in the first person, using quotation marks. Also document objective information provided by others.

Never speculate as to what may have happened or record subjective thoughts. Include in your notes the time the victim arrived at the hospital, the date and time of the alleged rape, and the time the victim was examined. Ask the victim about allergies to penicillin and other drugs, if she's had recent illnesses (especially venereal disease), if she was pregnant before the attack, and the date of her last menstrual period.

Thoroughly explain the examination she'll have, and tell her why it's necessary (to rule out internal injuries and obtain a specimen for venereal disease testing). Obtain her informed consent for treatment and for the police report. Allow her some control, if possible; for instance, ask her if she's ready to be examined or if she'd rather wait a few minutes.

Before the examination, ask the victim whether she douched, bathed, or washed before coming to the hospital. Note this on her chart. Have her change into a hospital gown, and place her clothing in *paper bags*. (*Never* use plastic bags, because secretions and seminal stains will mold, destroying valuable evidence.) Label each bag and its contents carefully.

IF THE RAPE VICTIM IS A CHILD

The child must be interviewed with special care to assess how well he or she will be able to deal with the situation after going home. A young child will place only as much importance on an experience as others do, unless there is physical pain. A good question to ask is, "Did someone touch you when you didn't want to be touched? Does anyone ever do this?" As with other rape victims, information should be recorded in the child's own words.

The interview should not involve the parents; this is done for the child's comfort, not to keep secrets from them. The parents should be asked to supply the names that the child uses to refer to parts of the anatomy. A complete pelvic examination is necessary only if penetration has occurred; such an examination requires an analgesic or local anesthetic.

Both the child and the parents need counseling to minimize possible emotional disturbances. The child should be encouraged to talk about the experience, and be corrected when confused. A young victim may regress; an older child may become fearful about being left alone. If a parent needs additional counseling, a counselor of the same sex may be more beneficial.

Parents need to understand that it's normal for them to feel angry and guilty, but they must not project these feelings onto the child. They should assure the child that they're not angry with her or him; that the child is good, and did not cause the incident; that they're sorry it happened but glad the child's all right; and that the family will work out the problems together.

Tell the victim she may urinate, but warn her not to wipe or otherwise cleanse the pubic area. Stay with her, or ask the counselor to stay with her, throughout the examination.

Even if the victim wasn't beaten, physical examination (including a pelvic examination by a gynecologist) will probably show signs of physical trauma, especially if the assault was prolonged. Depending on specific body areas attacked, a patient may have a sore throat, mouth irritation, difficulty swallowing, or rectal pain and bleeding.

If additional physical violence accompanied the rape, the victim may have hematomas, lacerations, bleeding, severe internal injuries and hemorrhage, and if the rape occurred outdoors, she may suffer from exposure. X-rays may reveal fractures. If severe injuries require hospitalization, introduce the victim to her primary nurse, if possible.

If the health care professional is female, she should do the following:

Before the victim's pelvic area is examined, take vital signs, and if the patient is wearing a tampon, remove it, wrap it, and label it as evidence. This exam is often very distressing to the rape victim. Reassure her, and allow her as much control as possible. During the exam, assist in specimen collection, including those for semen and gonorrhea. Carefully label all specimens with the patient's name, the doctor's name, and the location from which the specimen was obtained. List all specimens in your notes. If the case comes to trial, specimens will be used for evidence, so accuracy is vital.

Carefully collect and label fingernail scrapings, and foreign material obtained by combing the victim's pubic hair; these also provide valuable evidence. Note to whom these specimens are given.

Assist in photographing the patient's injuries (this may be delayed until a day later, when bruises and ecchymoses become more apparent).

Most states require the hospital to report all incidents of rape. The patient may elect not to press charges, and not to assist the police investigation. If the patient does *not* go to the hospital, she may not report the rape.

During the police interview, be supportive, and encourage the patient to recall events of the rape. Your kindness and empathy are invaluable at this time.

The patient may also want you to call her family. Help her to verbalize anticipation of her family's response.

Treatment and additional considerations

Treatment consists of supportive measures and protection against venereal disease, and if the patient wishes, against pregnancy. The latter should be discussed to allay fears. Probenicid P.O., with penicillin G procaine I.M., may be ordered, to prevent venereal disease.

Since cultures can't detect gonorrhea for 5 to 6 days after the rape, or syphilis for 6 weeks, the patient must return for follow-up venereal disease testing. If the patient wishes to prevent possible pregnancy as a result of the rape, she may be given small doses of oral diethylstilbestrol (DES) for 5 days. Immediately inserting an intrauterine device (IUD) may prevent pregnancy; however, this carries infection risks. Adverse effects of DES and IUD insertion should be explained. The victim may wait 3 to 4 weeks and have a D&C or a vacuum aspiration to abort a pregnancy.

If the patient has vulvar lacerations and hair cuts, the doctor will clean the area and repair the lacerations after all the evidence is obtained. He may order topical application of ice packs to reduce vulvar swelling.

Recovery from rape, which may be prolonged, consists of the acute phase (immediate reaction) and the reorganization phase. During the acute phase, physical aspects include pain, loss of appetite, and wound healing; emotional reactions typically include shaking, crying, and mood swings. Feelings of grief, anger, fear, or revenge may color the victim's social interactions. Counseling helps the victim identify the coping mechanisms she's using. The victim may relate more easily to a counselor of the same sex.

During the reorganization phase, which usually begins a week after the rape and may last months or years, the victim is concerned with restructuring her life. Initially, she often has nightmares in which she's powerless; later dreams show her gradually gaining more control. She may also suffer from "daymares"—frightening thoughts about the

rape that occur when she's alone.

Legal proceedings during this time force the victim to relive the trauma, leaving her feeling lonely and isolated, perhaps even temporarily halting her emotional recovery. To help her cope, she should write her thoughts, feelings, and reactions in a daily diary, and know how to contact organizations such as Women Against Rape or a local crisis center for empathy and advice.

Selected References

Alspach, J. *The Patient with Chest Trauma*, CRITICAL CARE UPDATE, 6:18-26, 1979.

Budassi, Susan A. *Chest Trauma*, NURSING CLINICS OF NORTH AMERICA. 13:533-541, 1978.

Budassi, Susan A., and Janet Barber. EMERGENCY NURSING: PRINCIPLES AND PRACTICE. St. Louis: C.V. Mosby Co., 1980.

GIVING EMERGENCY CARE COMPETENTLY. Nursing Skillbook™ Series. Springhouse, Pa.: Intermed Communications, Inc., 1978.

Hoff, B.H. *Multisystem Failure: A Review with Special Reference to Drowning*, CRITICAL CARE MEDICINE. July 1979.

Ipema, D. *Rape: The Process of Recovery*, NURSING RESEARCH. 28:272, September-October 1979.

Kohn, M.S. *Management of Chest Injuries*, TOPICS IN EMERGENCY MEDICINE. 1:79-94, 1979.

Larson, Carroll B., and Marjorie Gould. ORTHOPEDIC NURSING, 8th ed. St. Louis: C.V. Mosby Co., 1974.

McCrady, V. L., Issue Ed. *Burn Management*, CRITICAL CARE QUARTERLY. Vol. 1, No. 3, 1978.

Miller, Robert H., and James R. Cantrell. TEXTBOOK OF BASIC EMERGENCY MEDICINE. St. Louis: C.V. Mosby Co., 1975.

Mills, Patrick, ed. RAPE INTERVENTION RESOURCE MANUAL. Springfield, Ill.: Charles C. Thomas, 1977.

Strauss, Richard H., *Diving Medicine*, AMERICAN REVIEW OF RESPIRATORY DISEASE (Decompression Sickness). 119:1001-1023, 1979.

Van Microp, L. *Poisonous Snakebite: A Review*, JOURNAL OF FLORIDA MEDICAL ASSOCIATION. 63:199-208, March 1976.

Warner, Carmen Germaine. EMERGENCY CARE, 2nd ed. St. Louis: C.V. Mosby Co., 1978.

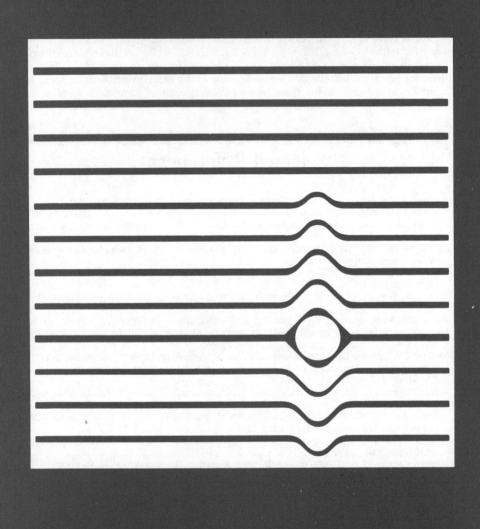

5 Neoplasms

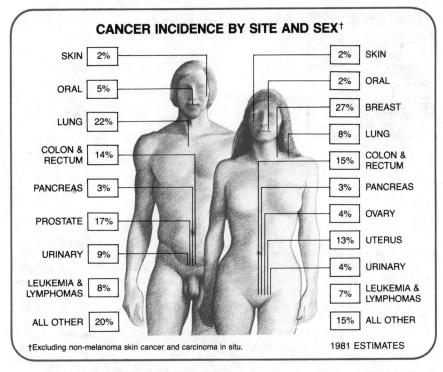

CANCER INCIDENCE BY SITE AND SEX†

SKIN	2%		2%	SKIN
ORAL	5%		2%	ORAL
			27%	BREAST
LUNG	22%		8%	LUNG
COLON & RECTUM	14%		15%	COLON & RECTUM
PANCREAS	3%		3%	PANCREAS
			4%	OVARY
PROSTATE	17%		13%	UTERUS
URINARY	9%		4%	URINARY
LEUKEMIA & LYMPHOMAS	8%		7%	LEUKEMIA & LYMPHOMAS
ALL OTHER	20%		15%	ALL OTHER

†Excluding non-melanoma skin cancer and carcinoma in situ.

1981 ESTIMATES

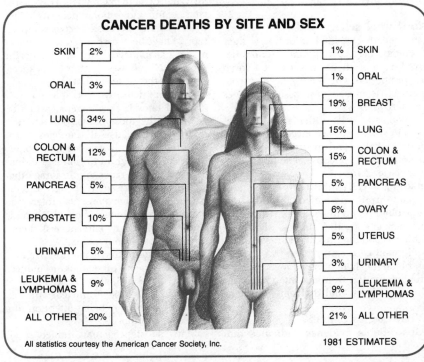

CANCER DEATHS BY SITE AND SEX

SKIN	2%		1%	SKIN
ORAL	3%		1%	ORAL
			19%	BREAST
LUNG	34%		15%	LUNG
COLON & RECTUM	12%		15%	COLON & RECTUM
PANCREAS	5%		5%	PANCREAS
			6%	OVARY
PROSTATE	10%		5%	UTERUS
URINARY	5%		3%	URINARY
LEUKEMIA & LYMPHOMAS	9%		9%	LEUKEMIA & LYMPHOMAS
ALL OTHER	20%		21%	ALL OTHER

All statistics courtesy the American Cancer Society, Inc.

1981 ESTIMATES

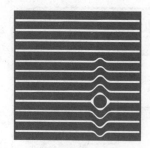

Neoplasms

Introduction

Cancer is second only to cardiovascular disease as the leading cause of death in the United States (over 350,000 deaths annually). Predominately a disease of older adults (incidence increases geometrically with age), it's generally more common among men but is also relatively common in children (only accidental death exceeds it as the leading cause of death in this age-group).

Abnormal cell growth

Conveniently classified according to their histologic origin, malignant tumors derived from epithelial tissues are known as carcinomas, while those arising from connective, muscle, and osseous tissues are sarcomas.

Neoplastic cells differ from normal cells in size—they are larger and divide more quickly—and in function, as they serve no useful purpose. The most characteristic difference, however, is the malignant cells'.ability to grow and spread throughout the body rapidly, uncontrollably, and independently from the primary site to other tissues, and to establish secondary foci called metastases. Malignant cells can metastasize by way of blood or lymphatics, by accidental transplantation from one site to another during surgery, and by local extension.

What causes cancer?

All available evidence indicates that malignant transformation of cells (carcinogenesis) may result from complex interactions of viruses, physical and chemical carcinogens, genetic predisposition, immunologic factors, and diet. Through studies on animals that monitor the ability of viruses to transform cells, some human viruses have been shown to have carcinogenic potential; particularly the Epstein-Barr virus (EBV), the cause of infectious mononucleosis. Other DNA viruses (such as herpes simplex, type 2) have been associated with cancer of the nasopharynx and of the uterine cervix; RNA viruses, with breast cancer. However, the evidence that viruses cause cancer isn't definitive.

Of all known carcinogens, radiation is by far the most dangerous and unpredictable because it damages DNA, inducing genetically transferable abnormalities. Although radiation can induce many different types of tumors, other factors, such as tissue type, age, and the patient's hormonal state, also interact to promote its carcinogenic effect. Even the sun's ultraviolet rays can cause skin cancer on exposed body areas.

While trauma and irritation are also linked to cancer (pipe smoking induces cancer of the lip), their mechanism of carcinogenic action is unclear. In fact, trauma may merely bring attention to a preexisting tumor.

Many substances may induce carcinogenesis by damaging the DNA. Although many produce tumors in experimental animals, only a few have been proven carcinogenic in humans:

- asbestos—mesothelioma of the lung
- vinyl chloride—angiosarcoma of liver
- aromatic hydrocarbons and benzopyrene (from polluted air)—lung cancer
- nitrogen mustard—leukemia
- cigarettes—cancer of the lung, the oral cavity and upper airways, the esophagus, the pancreas, the kidneys, and the bladder.

Diet has also been implicated, especially in the development of colon cancer as a result of a high protein and fat diet; and liver tumors from additives composed of nitrates and aflatoxin B_1, a fungus that grows on stored grains and other foodstuffs.

The role of hormones in carcinogenesis is still controversial, but it seems that excessive use of some hormones, especially estrogen, produces cancer in animals. Also, the synthetic estrogen diethylstilbestrol (DES) causes vaginal cancer in some daughters of women who were treated with it. It's unclear, however, whether changes in human hormonal balance retard or stimulate cancer development.

Some forms of cancer and precancerous lesions result from genetic predisposition either directly (as in Wilms' tumor and retinoblastoma) or indirectly (in association with inherited conditions such as Down's syndrome or immunodeficiency diseases). Expressed as autosomal recessive, X-linked, or autosomal dominant disorders, their common characteristics include:

- early onset of malignant disease
- increased incidence of bilateral cancer in paired organs (breasts, adrenal glands, kidneys, and eighth cranial nerves [acoustic neuroma])
- increased incidence of multiple primary malignancies in nonpaired organs
- abnormal chromosome complement in tumor cells.

Immune tumor response

Other factors that interact to increase susceptibility to carcinogenesis are immunologic competence, age, nutritional status, hormonal balance, and response to stress. Theoretically, the body develops cancer cells continuously, but the immune system recognizes them as foreign cells and destroys them. This defense mechanism, known as immunologic surveillance, has two major components: humoral immune response and cellular immune response; their interaction promotes antibody production, cellular immunity, and immunologic memory. Presumably, the intact human immune system is responsible for spontaneous regression of tumors.

Theoretically, the *cellular immune re-*

sponse begins when T lymphocytes become sensitized by contact with a specific antigenic substance—in this case, cancer cells. After repeated contacts, sensitized T cells release chemical factors called *lymphokines,* which begin to destroy the antigen. This reaction triggers the transformation of an additional population of uncommitted T lymphocytes into "killers" of antigen-specific cells—in this case, cancer cells.

Similarly, *humoral immune response* reacts to an antigen by causing the release of antibodies from plasma cells and activating the serum-complement system, which destroys the antigen-bearing cell. An opposing immune factor, a "blocking antibody," enhances tumor growth by protecting malignant cells from immune destruction.

Theoretically, cancer arises when certain factors inhibit the immune system.
• *Aging cells,* when copying their genetic material, may begin to err, giving rise to mutations; the aging immune system may not recognize these mutations as foreign, and thus may allow them to proliferate and form a malignant tumor.
• *Cytotoxic drugs or steroids* decrease antibody production and destroy circulating lymphocytes.
• *Stress* stimulates adrenal cortex to produce cortisol, causing destruction of lymphocytes.
• *Overwhelming systemic infection* depresses the immune system.
• *Increased susceptibility to infection* often results from radiation, cytotoxic drug therapy, and lymphoproliferative and myeloproliferative diseases, such as lymphatic and myelocytic leukemia. These cause bone marrow depression, which can impair leukocyte function.
• *Cancer* itself is immunosuppressive; advanced cancer exhausts the immune response. (The absence of immune reactivity is known as *anergy.*)

Diagnostic methods
A thorough medical history and physical examination should precede sophisticated diagnostic procedures. Tests that are useful in the early detection and staging of tumors include X-rays, isotope scan, and CAT scan, but the single most important diagnostic tool is a biopsy for direct histologic study of tumor tissue. Biopsy tissue samples can be taken by curettage, fluid aspiration (pleural effusion), needle aspiration biopsy (breast), dermal punch (skin or mouth), endoscopy (rectal polyps), and surgical excision (visceral tumors and nodes).

An important tumor marker, carcinoembryonic antigen (CEA), although not diagnostic by itself, can signal malignancies of the large bowel, the stomach, the pancreas, lungs, breasts, and sometimes, sarcomas, leukemias, and lymphomas. CEA titers range from normal (less than 2.5 ng), to suspicious (5 to 10 ng), to very suspect (over 10 ng). CEA provides a valuable baseline during chemotherapy to evaluate the extent of spread, regulate drug dosage, prognosticate after surgery or radiation, and detect tumor recurrence.

Although no more specific than CEA, alpha-fetoprotein (AFP), a fetal antigen uncommon in adults, can suggest testicular, ovarian, gastric, pancreatic, and primary lung cancers. Like CEA titers, AFP titer levels may correlate with tumor size.

Staging and grading
Choosing effective therapeutic options depends on correct *staging* of malignant disease, often with the internationally known TNM-staging system (tumor size, nodal involvement, metastatic progress). This classification allows an accurate tumor description that's adjustable as the disease progresses. TNM staging allows reliable comparison of treatment and survival among large groups; it also identifies nodal involvement and metastasis to other areas. TNM staging is applicable to most cancers (but not Hodgkin's disease and other lymphomas).

Grading is another objective way to define a tumor. Grading takes into account resemblance of tumor tissue to normal cells (differentiation) and its estimated growth rate (for example, a well-differentiated tumor with a slow

ESSENTIAL DIFFERENCES
BETWEEN BENIGN AND MALIGNANT TUMORS

	BENIGN	MALIGNANT
Growth	Slow expansion; push aside surrounding tissue but do not infiltrate	Usually infiltrate surrounding tissues rapidly, expanding in all directions
Limitation	Frequently encapsulated	Seldom encapsulated; often poorly delineated
Recurrence	Rare after surgical removal	When removed surgically, frequently recur due to infiltration into surrounding tissues
Morphology	Cells closely resemble cells of tissue of origin	Cells may differ considerably from those of tissue of origin
Differentiation	Well differentiated	Poor or no differentiation
Mitotic activity	Slight	Extensive
Tissue destruction	Usually slight	Extensive due to infiltration and metastatic lesion
Spread	No metastasis	Spread via blood and/or lymph systems; establish secondary tumors
Effect on body	Cachexia rare; usually not fatal but may obstruct vital organs, exert pressure, produce excess hormones; can become malignant	Cachexia typical—anemia, loss of weight, weakness, etc.; fatal if untreated

growth rate would be termed "low grade"). Grading also names the lesion according to corresponding normal cells, such as lymphoid or mucinous.

Three major therapies

The major therapies used to treat cancer are surgery, radiation, and chemotherapy, employed independently or in combination; immunotherapy to bolster the patient's immune response to cancer is still considered an adjuvant form of therapy. In every case, treatment depends on the type, stage, localization, and responsiveness of the tumor.

1.–*Surgery,* once the mainstay of cancer treatment, is now more often combined with radiation and chemotherapy. For example, surgery removes the bulky tumor, while chemotherapy and radiation discourage proliferation of residual cells. Surgery can also be used to relieve pain, correct obstruction, and alleviate pressure. Today's less radical surgery (for example, a lumpectomy instead of a radical mastectomy) is more acceptable to patients.

2.–*Radiation* therapy aims to alter the membranes of the rapidly dividing cancer cells and to destroy them, while damaging normal cells as little as possible. Radiation consists of two types: ionizing radiation (gamma-ray) and particle radiation (beta-ray). Both have the cellular DNA as their target; however, particle radiation produces less skin damage.

Radioactive isotope therapy (strontium, cobalt, cesium) includes external beam radiation and intracavitary and interstitial implants. Such therapy necessitates surface contact or a mold applicator.

Normal and malignant cells respond to radiation differently, depending on

RADIATION SIDE EFFECTS

AREA RADIATED	EFFECT	MANAGEMENT
Abdomen/pelvis	Cramps, diarrhea	Opium tincture, camphorated; diphenoxylate with atropine; low-residue diet; fluid and electrolyte balance maintenance
Head	Alopecia	Wig or head covering.
	Mucositis	Viscous lidocaine mouthwash; cool carbonated drinks; ice pops; soft, nonirritating diet
	Monilia	Nystatin mouthwash—avoidance of commercial mouthwash
	Dental caries	Prophylactic application of flouride to teeth; gingival care
Chest	Lung tissue devitalization	No smoking; avoidance of people with upper respiratory infections; provide humidifier, if necessary
	Pericarditis	Control arrhythmias with appropriate agents (procainamide, disopyramide phosphate); monitor for heart failure.
Kidneys	Nephritis, lassitude, headache, edema, dyspnea on exertion, hypertensive nephropathy, azotemia, secondary anemia	Maintain fluid and electrolyte balance; watch for signs of renal failure.

blood supply, oxygen saturation, previous irradiation, and immune status. Generally, normal cells recover from radiation faster than malignant cells. The success of the treatment and damage to normal tissue also vary with the intensity of the radiation. Although the cellular effects of a large single dose of radiation are greater than fractions of the same amount delivered sequentially, a protracted schedule allows normal tissue to recover in the intervals between individual sublethal doses.

Radiation is often used palliatively—to relieve pain, obstructions, malignant effusions, cough, dyspnea, ulcerative lesions, and hemorrhage; it can also promote the repair of pathologic fractures and delay tumor spread. Radiation can give a cancer patient an important psychologic lift just by shrinking a visible tumor.

Combining radiation and surgery can minimize radical surgery, prolong survival, and preserve anatomical function.

For example, small preoperative doses of radiation shrink a tumor, making it operable, while preventing further spread of the disease during surgery. After the wound has healed, larger postoperative doses prevent residual neoplastic cells from multiplying or metastasizing. Postoperative radiation can also minimize radical surgery, for instance, by saving a limb in osteogenic sarcoma.

Systemic side effects after radiation include weakness and fatigue, and possibly, anorexia, nausea, vomiting, anemia, and diarrhea, which usually begin after 1 week of therapy. (For other radiation side effects, see above.) These symptoms are called "radiation sickness" and subside with dose reduction. They also respond to treatment with antiemetics, sedatives, steroids, frequent small meals, fluid maintenance, medications to control diarrhea (diphenoxylate with atropine or camphorated opium tincture), and bed rest. Radiation sickness is seldom severe enough to cause discontinuation of treatment, but often necessitates careful adjustment of radiation dosage. Radiation therapy also requires frequent blood counts (with particular attention to WBC and platelets).

3.–*Chemotherapy* includes a wide array of drugs and may induce regression of a tumor and its metastasis. It is particularly useful in controlling residual disease or as an adjunct to surgery or radiotherapy, and can induce long remissions and probably also effect some cures, especially in patients with childhood leukemia, Hodgkin's disease, choriocarcinoma, and testicular cancer. As palliative treatment, chemotherapy aims to improve the patient's quality of life by temporarily relieving pain or other symptoms. The major cancer chemotherapeutic agents are as follows:

• *Alkylating agents* inhibit cell growth and division by reacting with DNA (antineoplastic agents of the nitrosurea group act in the same way).

• *Antimetabolites* prevent cell growth by competing with metabolites in the production of nucleic acid.

• *Anticancer antibiotics* block cell growth by binding with DNA, except for bleomycin sulfate and procarbazine, which directly affect DNA.

• *Plant alkaloids* prevent cellular reproduction by altering protein synthesis and nucleic acids through some still-unknown mechanism.

• *Steroid hormones* inhibit the growth of hormone-susceptible tumors by changing their chemical environment.

Chemotherapy side effects

Although antineoplastic agents exert selective toxicity against cancer cells, they can also cause transient changes in normal tissues, especially among rapidly proliferating body cells. For example, they often depress bone marrow, causing anemia, leukopenia, and thrombocytopenia; irritate gastrointestinal epithelial cells, causing ulceration, bleeding, and vomiting; and destroy the cells of the hair follicles and skin, causing alopecia and dermatitis. Many I.V. drugs cause pain on administration and vein sclerosis, and if extravasated can lead to deep cutaneous necrosis requiring debridement and skin grafting.

Therefore, the health care professional caring for the patient undergoing chemotherapy must:

• watch for any signs of infection, and report them immediately (especially if the patient is receiving simultaneous radiation treatment); be especially alert for fever when the granulocyte count falls below 500/mm³; take the patient's temperature frequently, and call the doctor if fever develops.

• force fluids to 2 to 3 liters daily.

• warn of the possibility of hair loss (if patient is receiving drugs that cause this condition), and give reassurance that hair should grow back in 8 weeks after therapy ends, although it may then be a different color and texture. (Before treatment begins, the patient should obtain a hairpiece, scarf, or other head covering).

• check skin for petechiae, ecchymoses, and chemical cellulitis, and for secondary infection during treatment with sclerosing drugs.

• minimize the possibility of vein sclerosis by frequently checking for blood return during I.V. push administration and by maintaining a properly running I.V.; notify the doctor immediately, in case of extravasation (he should order local infiltration with a rapid-acting steroid for vesicant agents); apply an ice pack to the site, and repeat at regular intervals for the next 24 hours; then, apply a warm, moist soak.

Chemotherapy can be administered orally, subcutaneously, I.M., I.V., intracavitarily, intrathecally, and by arterial infusion, depending on the drug and its pharmacologic action; usually, administration is intermittent to allow for bone marrow recovery between doses. Dosage is calculated according to the patient's body surface area with adjustments for general condition and degree of myelosuppression. When calculating dosage, information must be current, since chemotherapy dosages may change due to constant research.

Because patients approach chemotherapy with fear and apprehension, its beneficial results need to be emphasized along with its possible side effects. To minimize nausea and vomiting during treatment, the power of suggestion may downplay these side effects, but an effective antiemetic should be on hand in case they occur. The patient will need support and encouragement throughout the cycle of drug treatment, and may wish to be referred to the chaplain or social service worker for further support.

Experimental immunotherapy

Such treatment may be active, passive, or adoptive. *Active immunotherapy* stimulates the patient's own immune mechanisms to control or reject his malignant cells by producing antibodies plus lymphocytes. It can be specific, responding to a particular tumor-associated antigen; or nonspecific, responding to multiple antigens. Active nonspecific immunotherapy has the widest clinical application today, because it augments the patient's own immunosurveillance, and combats the immunosuppressive effects of cancer and its treatment. Several biologic products are available to stimulate the reticuloendothelial system, including BCG vaccine (bacille Calmette-Guérin), methanol extraction residue of BCG (MER), *Corynebacterium parvulum*, levamisole, and dinitrochlorobenzene (DNCB). BCG has been reported particularly effective in acute childhood leukemia, regionally recurrent melanoma, squamous cell carcinoma of the head and neck, and bronchogenic carcinoma. BCG is best introduced as close to the tumor as possible, and may be administered by scarification, intralesionally (for recurrent melanotic nodules), intracavitarily (for pleural or peritoneal tumors), intravesically (for bladder tumors), intrapulmonarily (by aerosol), orally (for upper GI tumors), and intradermally. Exactly how BCG and MER work is still unclear, but their use during or after primary treatment may well prolong remissions. However, BCG produces its own complications, such as transient malaise, fever, chills, ulcers at the sites of injection, systemic BCG infections, granulomatous hepatitis, and occasionally, anaphylaxis and seizures. Complications are most common when BCG enters the circulatory system rapidly. MER, however, isn't a live vaccine and doesn't induce systemic BCG infection.

Care for the patient receiving nonspecific immunostimulation varies with the site and dose. After scarification or intradermal administration, the patient may have no side effects or may experience flulike symptoms, with lymph node swelling in the drainage area of the treated site in the first 48 hours after treatment. Intralesional administration can precipitate profound reactions, and requires careful monitoring for hyperthermia and anaphylaxis.

Passive immunity is transient, and is achieved with an antiserum or the transfer of immunologically active cells from donors with established immunity. In *adoptive immunity*, transferred passive immunity subsequently stimulates active immunity.

Maintaining nutrition and fluid balance

Tumors grow at the expense of normal tissue by competing for nutrients and vitamins; consequently, the cancer patient often suffers protein deficiency and may also be hypermetabolic from the large number of dividing cells. Moreover, cancer treatments themselves produce fluid and electrolyte disturbances, such as vomiting, diarrhea, draining fistulae, and anorexia. Understandably, maintaining adequate nutrition, fluid intake, and electrolyte balance should be a major health care focus.

• A comprehensive dietary history of the patient is needed to pinpoint nutritional problems and their past causes, such as diabetes; a diet should be planned accordingly.

• The dietitian should provide a liquid, high-protein, high-carbohydrate, high-

HOW TO PREPARE THE PATIENT
FOR EXTERNAL RADIATION THERAPY

A hospital staff member preparing a patient for external radiation therapy should:

• show the patient where radiation therapy takes place, and introduce him to the radiation therapist.

• tell him to remove all metal objects (pens, buttons, jewelry) that may interfere with therapy; explain that the areas to be treated will be marked with water-soluble ink, and that *he must not scrub these areas,* because the same areas must be radiated each time.

• reinforce the doctor's explanation of the procedure; answer all questions the patient has as honestly as possible or refer the patient to someone who can answer them.

• teach the patient to watch for and report possible side effects; warn him to avoid persons with colds or other infections during therapy, since radiation therapy may increase susceptibility to infection; emphasize the benefits (such as outpatient treatment) instead of the side effects.

• reassure the patient that treatment is painless and won't make him radioactive; stress that he'll be under constant surveillance during radiation administration and need only call out if he needs anything.

---

calorie diet if the patient can't tolerate solid foods. If the patient has stomatitis, he'll need soft, bland, nonirritating foods. The patient's family should be encouraged to bring his favorite foods from home.

• Mealtime should be as relaxed and pleasant as possible. Visitors may eat with the patient (in most hospitals, the dietary department will gladly send an extra tray if it's requested) or, if possible, the patient may want to dine with other patients. He should be able to choose from a varied menu.

• With the doctor's approval, a glass of wine or a cocktail before dinner may help the patient relax and may stimulate his appetite.

• The patient should drink juice or other caloric beverages instead of water.

If the patient can't eat

An alternate method of providing nourishment for the patient who has had recent head, neck, or gastrointestinal surgery, or who has dysphagia or pain when swallowing is through a nasogastric tube. If the patient still needs to use the tube after he's discharged, he must know how to insert it, how to test its position in the stomach by aspirating stomach contents, and how to use it to feed himself.

If a nasogastric tube isn't appropriate, other alternatives are gastrostomy, jejunostomy, and occasionally, esophagotomy. These make it possible for the patient to be fed prescribed protein formulas and semiliquids, such as cream soups and eggnog, and also make it easier for him to feed himself. The patient must remember to wash off any spilled gastric or intestinal juices that come in contact with the skin, since they will cause abdominal excoriation. Some patients may prefer to chew their food before it's placed with the liquid in the tube. While this may be a distasteful procedure, it should be the patient's option. The tube *must* be well flushed with water after each feeding. Also, to provide adequate hydration, 4 to 6 ounces (118 to 177 ml) water or other clear liquid should be instilled between meals. After jejunostomy, feedings should begin very small, slowly and carefully increase in amount and variety over 10 days until they're normal. Additional fluids and calories can be provided during these days of limited food intake by supplementing jejunostomy feedings with I.V. fat emulsions or alcohol.

Hyperalimentation is becoming increasingly important in cancer care, since patients who receive it during aggressive chemotherapy or radiotherapy experience less nausea, vomiting, diarrhea, and weight loss than patients who don't; and because of better nutritional status, they may respond better to the therapeutic effects of these drugs. Hyperalimentation can also bring a severely debilitated patient into positive protein balance so he can tolerate surgery better. It can cause a slight weight gain in the patient receiving radiation therapy, provide optimum nutrition for wound healing, and help the patient combat infection after radical surgery.

Pain control critical

Cancer patients have a great fear of overwhelming pain. Therefore, controlling pain is a major consideration at every stage of cancer—from localized cancer to advanced metastasis. Cancer pain may result from inflammation of or pressure on pain-sensitive structures, tumor infiltration of nerves or blood vessels, or metastatic extension to bone. Its chronic, unrelenting character can wear down the patient's tolerance and interfere with eating and sleeping; it can color the patient's life with anger, despair, and anxiety, and totally prevent enjoyment of life.

Narcotic analgesics are the mainstay of pain relief in advanced cancer. They are effective alone or with phenothiazines, such as chlorpromazine, prochlorperazine, and promazine. In terminal illness, narcotic dosages may be quite high, since drug addiction is no longer a consideration. Such analgesia should be generously provided. The patient will need pain relief, and it must be provided on a schedule that relieves the pain before it becomes severe. The patient should know that he can have pain medication whenever he needs it.

Surgery or treatment with antibiotics can relieve the pressure and pain caused by inflamed necrotic tissue; radiation can shrink metastatic tissue and control bone pain. When a tumor invades nervous tissue, pain control requires anesthetics, destructive nerve blocks, electronic stimulation with a dorsal column or transcutaneous nerve stimulator,

rhizotomy, or chordotomy.

A new, controversial treatment for intractable pain of terminally ill patients is Brompton's cocktail, a mixture containing varying amounts of cocaine (or amphetamine), methadone (or morphine), alcohol, a phenothiazine, chloroform water, and a flavoring syrup (or honey). Since cocaine is absorbed through the oral mucosa instead of the GI tract, the patient should swish this mixture in his mouth for a few minutes before swallowing it.

The hospice approach

A holistic approach to patient care modeled after St. Christopher's Hospice in London, hospice care provides comprehensive physical, psychologic, social, and spiritual care for terminally ill patients. Many hospices are associated with hospitals, but some are independent or use home care programs. The goal of the hospice is to maintain the patient's quality of life by providing treatment in as homelike an atmosphere as possible. Pain control is considered the first priority, with the use of methadone or Brompton's cocktail. Hospice care also emphasizes a coordinated team effort to overcome the anxiety, fear, and depression that often overcome the terminally ill patient. Hospice staffs encourage family members to assume an active role in the patient's care, provide warmth and security, and help them begin to work out their grief before the patient dies.

Every health care professional involved in this new method of care must be committed to high quality care, unafraid of emotional involvement, and comfortable with their own feelings about death and dying. Good hospice care also requires open communication among team members, not just for the evaluation of care, but also to help the staff cope with their own feelings. As a variation of the hospice approach, several large cities in the United States have facilities that offer children with leukemia and their families a homelike environment during outpatient treatment at a nearby hospital.

Psychologic aspects

No illness evokes as profound an emotional response as the diagnosis of cancer. Patients express this response in several ways. A few face this difficult reality immediately, from the outset of treatment. Many use denial as a coping mechanism and simply refuse to accept the truth, but this stance is increasingly difficult for them to maintain. As evidence of the tumor becomes inescapable, the patient may plunge into deep depression. Family members may express denial in attempts to cope by encouraging unproven methods of cancer treatment, which often delay effective care. Some patients cope by intellectualizing about their disease, enabling them to obscure the reality of the cancer and regard it as unrelated to themselves. Intellectualization is a more productive coping behavior than denial, because throughout, the patient is receiving treatment. Awareness of these possible behavioral responses will make dealing with them easier. For many malignancies, the patient can entertain realistic hope for long-term survival or remission; even in advanced disease, he can entertain short-term achievable goals.

To help a patient cope with cancer, a health care professional must get his own feelings about it under control. Then, he can listen sensitively to the patient and give appropriate understanding and support.

HEAD, NECK, AND SPINE

Malignant Brain Tumors

Malignant brain tumors (gliomas, meningiomas, and schwannomas) are common (slightly more so in men than in women), with an incidence of 4.5 per 100,000.

Tumors may occur at any age. In adults, incidence is generally highest between ages 40 and 60. The most common tumor types in adults are gliomas and meningiomas; these tumors are usually supratentorial (above the covering of the cerebellum). In children, incidence is generally highest before age 1 and then again between ages 2 and 12. The most common tumors in children are astrocytomas, medulloblastomas, ependymomas, and brain stem gliomas. In children, brain tumors are one of the most common causes of death from cancer.

Causes

The cause of brain tumors is unknown.

Signs and symptoms

Brain tumors cause changes in the CNS by invading and destroying tissues, and by secondary effect—mainly compression of the brain, cranial nerves, and cerebral vessels; cerebral edema; and increased intracranial pressure (ICP). Generally, clinical features result from increased ICP. Specifically, they vary with the type of tumor, its location, and the degree of invasion. Onset of symptoms is usually insidious and commonly misdiagnosed.

 Definitive diagnosis is made from biopsy of the lesion to identify the histologic type. Patient history, neurologic assessment, and the following tests can locate the tumor: skull X-rays, encephalography and echoencephalography, brain scan, CAT scan, and cerebral angiography. Lumbar puncture shows increased pressure and protein, decreased glucose, and occasionally, tumor cells in CSF.

Treatment

Treatment includes removing a resectable tumor, reducing the size of a non-

Glioblastoma multiforme
(spongioblastoma multiforme)
- Peak incidence at 50 to 60 years. Twice as common in males. Most common glioma
- Unencapsulated, highly malignant, grows rapidly and infiltrates the brain extensively. May become enormous before diagnosed
- Occurs most often in cerebral hemispheres, especially frontal and temporal lobes (rarely in brain stem and cerebellum)
- Occupies more than one lobe of affected hemisphere; may spread to opposite hemisphere by corpus callosum; may metastasize into CSF, producing tumors in distant parts of the nervous system
- *Prognosis:* median survival, 6 months; maximum 1 to 2 years

Early:
- Increased ICP (nausea, vomiting, headache)
- Subtle behavioral changes

Localizing:
- Midline: headache (bifrontal or bioccipital); worse in A.M.; intensified by coughing, straining, or sudden head movements
- Temporal lobe: psychomotor seizures
- Central region (motor-sensory strip of opposite hemisphere): focal and Jacksonian seizures
- Optic and oculomotor nerves: visual defects
- Frontal lobe: abnormal reflexes and motor responses (paralyses or paresthesias, ataxia, uncoordinated movements)
- Obstruction of CSF pathways: secondary hydrocephalus

Late:
- Altered vital signs (increased systolic pressure; widened pulse pressure)

Astrocytoma
- Second most common malignant glioma (approximately 30% of all gliomas)
- Occurs at any age; incidence higher in males
- Occurs most often in white matter of cerebral hemispheres; may originate in any part of the CNS
- Cerebellar astrocytomas usually confined to one hemisphere
- *Prognosis:* median survival, 6 to 7½ years

Early:
- Headache; mental activity changes for years before diagnosis
- Seizures (first symptom if tumor is in cerebral hemispheres)

Localizing:
- Third ventricle: early—changes in mental activity and level of consciousness, nausea, pupillary dilation and sluggish light reflex; later—paresis or ataxia, seizures, increased systolic blood pressure, widened pulse pressure, respiratory changes
- Brain stem and pons: early—ipsilateral trigeminal, abducens, and facial nerve palsies; later—cerebellar ataxia, tremors, other cranial nerve deficits
- Third or fourth ventricle or aqueduct of Sylvius: secondary hydrocephalus
- Thalamus or hypothalamus: variety of endocrine, metabolic, autonomic, and behavioral changes

Oligodendroglioma
- Third most common glioma
- Occurs in middle adult years; more common in women
- Slow growing
- *Prognosis:* median survival, 5 years

Localizing:
- Temporal lobe: hallucinations of memory, vision, smell, and taste; contralateral homonymous hemianopia; repetitive grand mal seizures; jerking; psychomotor seizures
- Central region (motor-sensory strip of opposite hemisphere): convulsive seizures (confined to one muscle group or unilateral)
- Midbrain or third ventricle: early—behavior and personality changes: later—increased ICP; pyramidal tract symptoms (dizziness, ataxia, paresthesias of the face)
- Brain stem and cerebrum: papilledema, nystagmus, hearing loss, flashing lights, dizziness, ataxia, paresthesias of face, cranial nerve palsies (V, VI, VII, IX, X, primarily sensory), hemiparesis, suboccipital tenderness; compression of supratentorial area produces other general and focal symptoms

TUMOR	CLINICAL FEATURES

Ependymoma
- Rare glioma
- Most common in children and young adults
- Locates most often in fourth and lateral ventricles
- *Prognosis:* median survival, 5 years

General:
- Similar to oligodendroglioma
- Increased ICP and obstructive hydrocephalus, depending on tumor size

Medulloblastoma
- Rare glioma
- Incidence highest in children aged 4 to 6 years
- Affects males more than females
- Frequently metastasizes via CSF
- *Prognosis:* median survival, 5 years

General:
- Increased ICP
Localizing:
- Brain stem and cerebrum: papilledema, nystagmus, hearing loss, flashing lights, dizziness, ataxia, paresthesias of face, cranial nerve palsies (V, VI, VII, IX, X, primarily sensory), hemiparesis, suboccipital tenderness; compression of supratentorial area produces other general and focal symptoms

Meningioma
- Most common nongliomatous brain tumor (15% of primary brain tumors)
- Peak incidence among 50-year-olds; rare in children; more common in females (ratio 3:2)
- Arises from the meninges
- Common locations include parasagittal area, sphenoidal ridge, anterior part of the base of the skull, cerebellopontile angle, spinal canal
- Benign, well-circumscribed highly vascular tumors compress underlying brain tissue by invading overlying skull
- *Prognosis:* median survival, 1 to 2 years or less; if treated, neurologic deficits likely to be completely reversible.

General:
- Headache
- Seizures (in ⅔ of patients)
- Vomiting
- Changes in mental activity
- Similar to schwannomas
Localizing:
- Skull changes (bony bulge) over tumor
- Sphenoidal ridge, indenting optic nerve: unilateral visual changes and papilledema
- Prefrontal parasaggital: personality and behavior changes
- Motor cortex: contralateral motor changes
- Anterior fossa compressing both optic nerves and frontal lobes: headaches and bilateral vision loss
Late:
- Pressure on other cranial nerves produces varying symptoms

Schwannoma
(acoustic neurinoma, neuriloma, cerebellopontile angle tumor)
- Accounts for approximately 10% of all intracranial tumors
- Higher incidence in women
- Onset of symptoms at ages 30 to 60 years
- Affects the craniospinal nerve sheath, usually the eighth (VIII) cranial nerve; also, the V and VII, and to a lesser extent, the VI and X on the same side as the tumor
- Benign, but often classified as malignant because of its growth patterns. Slow-growing, may be present for years before symptoms occur
- Prognosis: adequately treated, excellent chance of permanent cure

Early: unilateral hearing loss with or without tinnitus
General:
- Stiff neck and suboccipital discomfort
- Secondary hydrocephalus
Localizing:
- V: early—hypoesthesia or paresthesia of face on same side as hearing loss; unilateral loss of corneal reflex
- VI: diplopia or double vision
- VII: paresis progressing to paralysis (Bell's palsy)
- X: weakness of palate, tongue, and nerve muscles on same side as tumor
Late (due to pressure on brain stem and cerebellum):
- Ataxia
- Uncoordinated movements of one or both arms

Adapted with permission from CANCER NURSING—A HOLISTIC MULTIDISCIPLINARY APPROACH, 2nd ed., by Ardelina A. Baldonado and Dulcelina A. Stahl. (Garden City, N.Y.: Medical Examination Publishing Co., Inc., 1980)

resectable tumor, relieving cerebral edema or ICP, relieving symptoms, and preventing further neurologic damage (and consequent impaired motor or sensory function).

Mode of therapy depends on the tumor's histologic type, its radiosensitivity, and its anatomic location, and may include surgery, radiation, chemotherapy, or decompression of increased ICP with diuretics, corticosteroids, or possibly ventriculoatrial or ventriculoperitoneal shunting of CSF.

A glioma usually requires resection by craniotomy, followed by radiation therapy. Recently, a combination of carmustine (BCNU), lomustine (CCNU), methyl-CCNU, or procarbazine combined with postoperative radiation has proven to be more effective than radiation alone.

For low-grade cystic cerebellar astrocytomas, surgical resection brings long-term survival. For other astrocytomas, treatment consists of repeated surgery, radiation therapy, and shunting of fluid from obstructed CSF pathways. Some astrocytomas are highly radiosensitive; others are radioresistant.

Treatment for oligodendrogliomas and ependymomas includes surgical resection and radiation therapy; medulloblastomas, surgical resection, and possibly, intrathecal infusion of methotrexate or another antineoplastic drug. Meningiomas require surgical resection, including dura mater and bone (operative mortality may reach 10% because of large tumor size).

For schwannomas, microsurgical technique allows complete dissection of tumor and preservation of facial nerves. Although schwannomas are moderately radioresistant, postoperative radiation therapy is necessary.

Chemotherapy for malignant brain tumors includes methotrexate, nitrogen mustard, cyclophosphamide, vincristine, hydroxyurea, thiotepa, and doxorubicin. Intrathecal administration of such drugs is still under investigation.

Palliative measures for gliomas, astrocytomas, oligodendrogliomas, and ependymomas include dexamethasone for ICP and antacids for stress ulcers. These tumors and schwannomas may also require anticonvulsants, such as phenytoin and phenobarbital.

Additional considerations

A patient with a brain tumor requires comprehensive neurologic assessment, teaching, and supportive care. During the health professional's first contact with the patient, he should perform a comprehensive assessment (including a complete neurologic evaluation) to provide baseline data and to help develop a care plan. He'll need a thorough health history concerning the onset of symptoms. Additionally, he should assist the patient and his family in coping with the diagnosis, treatment, potential disabilities, and changes in life-style resulting from his tumor.

Throughout hospitalization, proper care includes:

• carefully documenting seizure activity, such as occurrence, nature, and duration.

• maintaining airway.

• monitoring patient safety.

• administering anticonvulsive drugs, as ordered.

• checking continuously for changes in neurologic status, and watching for increase in ICP.

 • watching for and immediately reporting sudden unilateral pupillary dilation with loss of light reflex; this ominous change indicates imminent transtentorial herniation.

• monitoring respiratory changes carefully (anoxia, and abnormal respiratory rate and depth may point to rising ICP or herniation of the cerebellar tonsils from expanding infratentorial mass).

• monitoring temperature carefully. Fever commonly follows hypothalamic anoxia but might also indicate meningitis. Hypothermia blankets should be used pre- and postoperatively to keep the patient's temperature down and minimize cerebral metabolic demands.

• administering steroids and antacids,

as ordered; observing and reporting signs of stress ulcer: abdominal distention, pain, vomiting, and tarry stools.

• restricting fluids to 1,500 ml/24 hours; administering osmotic diuretics, such as mannitol or urea, as ordered; carefully monitoring fluid and electrolyte balance, because rapid diuresis can precipitate heart failure.

• observing the wound carefully for infection and sinus formation during radiation therapy, because it can induce wound breakdown; monitoring closely for signs of rising ICP, because radiation may cause brain inflammation.

• before chemotherapy, giving prochlorperazine or another antiemetic, as ordered, to minimize nausea and vomiting. (Remember, however, that phenothiazines, such as prochlorperazine, are contraindicated with procarbazine.)

• during chemotherapy, watching for and reporting any signs of infection or bleeding, since the nitrosoureas—carmustine (BCNU), lomustine (CCNU), methyl-CCNU, and procarbazine—used as adjuncts to radiotherapy and surgery cause delayed bone marrow depression.

• teaching patient and family early signs of recurrence; urging compliance with therapy.

• beginning rehabilitation early, since brain tumors may cause residual neurologic deficits that handicap the patient physically or mentally; encouraging independence in daily activities; as necessary, providing aids for self-care and mobilization, such as bathroom rails for wheelchair patients; arranging for consultation with a speech pathologist for the aphasic patient.

Surgery necessitates additional health care, including:

• after craniotomy, continuing to monitor general neurologic status, and watching for signs of increased ICP, such as an elevated bone flap and typical neurologic changes; reducing the risk of increased ICP by restricting fluids to 1,500 ml/24 hours.

• after supratentorial craniotomy, promoting venous drainage and reducing cerebral edema by elevating the head of the bed about 30° and positioning the patient on his side; withholding oral fluids, since they may provoke vomiting, which could, in turn, raise ICP.

• after infratentorial craniotomy, keeping the patient flat for 48 hours, but logrolling him every 2 hours to minimize complications of immobilization; preventing other complications by careful attention to ventilatory status, and cardiovascular, gastrointestinal, and musculoskeletal functions.

Pituitary Tumors

Pituitary tumors, which comprise 10% of intracranial neoplasms, originate most often in the anterior pituitary (adenohypophysis). They occur in adults of both sexes, usually during the third and fourth decades of life. The three tissue types of pituitary tumors include chromophobe adenoma (90%), basophilic adenoma, and eosinophilic adenoma.

Prognosis is fair to good, depending on the extent to which the tumor spreads beyond the sella turcica.

Causes

Although the exact cause is unknown, some experts believe patients with pituitary tumors have inherited a predisposition to them through an autosomal dominant trait. Pituitary tumors aren't malignant in the strict sense, but because their growth is invasive, they're considered a neoplastic disease.

Chromophobe adenoma may be associated with production of adrenocorticotrophic hormone (ACTH),

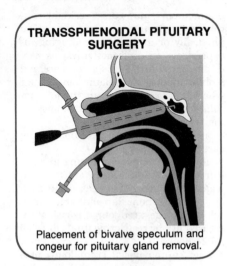

TRANSSPHENOIDAL PITUITARY SURGERY

Placement of bivalve speculum and rongeur for pituitary gland removal.

melanocyte-stimulating hormone (MSH), growth hormone, and prolactin; basophilic adenoma, with evidence of excess ACTH production and, consequently, with signs of Cushing's syndrome; eosinophilic adenoma, with excessive growth hormone.

Signs and symptoms

As pituitary adenomas grow, they replace normal glandular tissue and enlarge the sella turcica, which houses the gland. The resulting pressure on adjacent intracranial structures produces these typical clinical manifestations:

Neurologic
• frontal headache
• visual symptoms, beginning with blurring and progressing to field cuts (hemianopias) and then unilateral blindness
• cranial nerve involvement (III, IV, VI) from lateral extension of the tumor, resulting in strabismus; double vision, with compensating head tilting and dizziness; conjugate deviation of gaze; nystagmus; lid ptosis; and limited eye movements
• increased intracranial pressure (secondary hydrocephalus)
• personality changes or dementia, if the tumor breaks through to the frontal lobes
• seizures

• rhinorrhea, if the tumor erodes the base of the skull
• pituitary apoplexy secondary to hemorrhagic infarction of the adenoma. Such hemorrhage may lead to both cardiovascular and adrenocortical collapse.

Endocrine
• hypopituitarism, to some degree, in all patients with adenoma, becoming more obvious as the tumor replaces normal gland tissue. Symptoms include amenorrhea, decreased libido and impotence in men, skin changes (waxy appearance, decreased wrinkles, and pigmentation), decreased axillary and pubic hair, lethargy, weakness, increased fatigability, intolerance to cold, and constipation (because of decreased ACTH and thyroid-stimulating hormone [TSH] production).
• addisonian crisis, precipitated by stress and resulting in nausea, vomiting, hypoglycemia, hypotension, and circulatory collapse
• diabetes insipidus, resulting from extension to the hypothalamus
• prolactin-secreting adenomas (in 70% to 75%), with amenorrhea and galactorrhea; growth-hormone–secreting adenomas, with acromegaly; and ACTH-secreting adenomas, with Cushing's syndrome.

Diagnosis

• *Skull X-rays* with tomography show enlargement of the sella turcica or erosion of its floor; if growth hormone secretion predominates, they show enlarged paranasal sinuses and mandible, thickened cranial bones, and separated teeth.
• *Pneumoencephalography* shows the degree of extension of the tumor out of the sella turcica, as well as involvement of the third ventricle.
• *Carotid angiogram* shows displacement of the anterior cerebral and internal carotid arteries if the tumor mass is enlarging; also rules out intracerebral aneurysm.
• *CAT scan* confirms the existence of the adenoma and accurately depicts its size.
• *Spinal fluid* may show increased protein.

• *Endocrine function tests* may contribute helpful information, but results are often ambiguous and inconclusive.

Treatment
Surgical options include transfrontal surgical removal of large tumors impinging on the optic apparatus, and transsphenoidal resection for smaller tumors confined to the pituitary fossa. Radiation is the primary treatment for small, nonsecretory tumors that don't extend beyond the sella turcica, or for patients who may be poor postoperative risks; otherwise, it's an adjunct to surgery.

Postoperative treatment includes hormone replacement with cortisone, thyroid, and sex hormones; correction of electrolyte imbalance; and as necessary, insulin therapy.

Drug therapy may include a still-investigational drug—bromocriptine—an ergot derivative that shrinks prolactin-secreting and growth-hormone–secreting tumors. Cyproheptadine, an antiserotonin drug, can reduce increased corticosteroid levels to normal in the patient with Cushing's syndrome.

Adjuvant radiotherapy is used when only partial removal of the tumor is possible. Cryohypophysectomy (freezing the area with a probe inserted by transsphenoidal route) is a promising alternative to surgical dissection of the tumor.

Additional considerations
• A comprehensive health history and physical assessment should first establish the onset of neurologic and endocrine dysfunction, and provide baseline data for later comparison.
• A trusting relationship must be established with the patient and family to assist them in coping with the diagnosis, treatment, and potential long-term changes. They must understand that the patient will need lifelong evaluations and, possibly, hormone replacement.
• The patient should know that some of the distressing physical and behavioral signs and symptoms caused by pituitary dysfunction will disappear with treat-

---

POSTCRANIOTOMY CARE
• Monitoring vital signs (especially level of consciousness), and performing a baseline neurologic assessment from which to plan further care and assess progress.
• Maintaining the patient's airway; suctioning as necessary.
• Monitoring intake and output carefully.
• Giving the patient nothing by mouth for 24 to 48 hours, to prevent aspiration and vomiting, which increases intracranial pressure.
• Observing for cerebral edema, bleeding, and CSF leakage.
• Providing a restful, quiet environment.

---

ment (for example, altered sexual drive, impotence, infertility, loss of hair, and emotional lability).
• A safe, clutter-free environment should be maintained for the visually impaired or acromegalic patient. He will be relieved to know that he'll probably recover his sight.
• The patient who has undergone supratentorial or transsphenoidal hypophysectomy should have the head of his bed elevated about 30°, to promote venous drainage and reduce cerebral edema. Placing the patient on his side allows secretions to drain and prevents aspiration.
• Oral fluids must be withheld because of the possibility of vomiting, which increases intracranial pressure. A patient who's had transsphenoidal surgery must *not* blow his nose. Spinal fluid may drain from the nose. Signs of infection from the contaminated upper respiratory tract must be monitored. If infection occurs, the patient will lose his sense of smell.
• The patient's postoperative neurologic status should be compared regularly with his baseline assessment.
• Before discharge, the patient needs to purchase and wear a Medic-Alert bracelet or necklace to identify his hormone deficiencies and their treatment.
• Intake and output require monitoring to detect fluid and electrolyte imbalances.

Cancers of the Upper Aerodigestive Tract

Cancers of the upper aerodigestive tract account for approximately 3% of all cancer in the United States. They are most common in men over age 50, and usually occur as squamous cell carcinomas of the mouth, pharynx, larynx, or sinuses. Such cancers often begin with lesions that appear benign in early stages but progress to fungating masses or ulcerations, which spread by direct extension, lymphatic invasion, dissemination, and ultimately, distant metastasis. Common sites of upper aerodigestive tract cancers—each with its own clinical characteristics, diagnostic criteria, and treatment—include paranasal sinuses, mouth and oropharynx, salivary glands, nasopharynx, and rarely, the tonsils.

Causes

Although their causes are unknown, predisposing factors include heavy tobacco use (major factor) and alcohol abuse, especially when used together.

Treatment

Treatment consists of radiation therapy, including radioactive implants (molds or needles); surgery, including radical neck dissection (removal of all nonvital neck structures, including cervical lymph nodes on side of cancer, some muscles [sternomastoid], and connecting vessels); or chemotherapy, as an adjunct to surgery or to treat recurrence after radiation.

Additional considerations

A strong care plan should provide for relief of symptoms, general support, monitoring of special treatments, and thorough patient teaching; for example:
• Before radiation therapy, the patient should know its expected benefits and side effects (dental caries, mucositis, and mouth dryness). Before treatment with radioactive implants, the patient must know that talking with needles or molds in place will be difficult or impossible. He must avoid sudden movements that could dislodge the implant, and should seek help before moving.
• During treatment, he can counteract mouth dryness by chewing gum or lozenges, avoiding alcohol and tobacco, and using a humidifier. To maintain good oral hygiene, the patient should use a

soft toothbrush, eat a dental-soft, non-spicy diet without temperature extremes, and use an antimicrobial mouthwash. Mouth irrigation with diluted hydrogen peroxide or normal saline may be beneficial.
• After mouth or facial surgery, the patient must cope with excessive drooling. This can be done by swallowing frequently, having easy access to tissues, and taping a bag for tissue disposal to the bed. If severe drooling continues, the doctor should be notified. He may order plastic reconstruction of oral structures.
• Before radical neck dissection, the patient must know about the possibility of a tracheotomy, its purpose, how to care for it, how it will affect his speech, and about other postoperative procedures (catheter drainage system, suture removal). He should know that after surgery he will experience shoulder weakness (which can cause shoulder drop) unless he does prescribed exercises.
• After radical neck dissection, the patient must be watched for any complications: airway obstruction (wheezing, stridor, retraction, respiratory difficulty), infection (fever), carotid rupture or chylous fistula (milky drainage seen especially after meals).
• To avoid airway obstruction, the patient must cough frequently. If he can't, he should be suctioned at least hourly.
• To avoid infection, sterile technique must be used in tracheostomy care and suctioning. Also to prevent infection, bacitracin may be applied (using aseptic

REHABILITATION EXERCISES
AFTER HEAD AND NECK SURGERY

After head and neck surgery, exercises, as allowed by the doctor, help restore maximum shoulder and neck motion. The patient should do the exercises shown below, initially doing them once and gradually increasing the number of times each exercise is done.

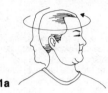

1a

Gently turn head to each side and look as far as possible.

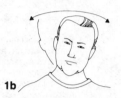

1b

Gently tip right ear toward right shoulder as far as possible. Repeat on left side.

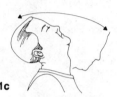

1c

Move chin to chest, and then lift head up and back.

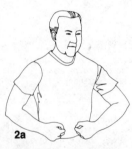

2a

Place hands in front, with elbows at right angles away from body.

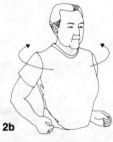

2b

Rotate shoulders back, bringing elbows to side.

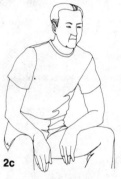

2c

Relax whole body.

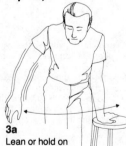

3a

Lean or hold on to low table or chair with hand on the unoperated side. Bend body slightly at waist, and swing shoulder and arm from left to right.

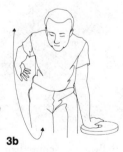

3b

Swing shoulder and arm from front to back.

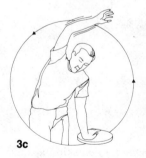

3c

Swing shoulder and arm in a wide circle, gradually bringing arm above head.

Adapted from EXERCISES FOR RADICAL NECK SURGERY, with the permission of Memorial Sloan-Kettering Cancer Center, New York, N.Y.

UPPER AERODIGESTIVE TRACT CANCERS

LOCATION	CLINICAL CHARACTERISTICS
Paranasal sinuses • Maxillary sinuses (most common) • Ethmoidal sinuses • Sphenoidal sinuses • Frontal sinuses (Tumor often spreads to orbit, infratemporal space, mouth, external cheek structure)	• Chronic sinusitis (splitting headache; tender, swollen forehead; fever; chills) • In advanced stages, cheek mass, eye displacement, facial paresthesia, nasal airway obstruction
Mouth and oropharynx • Lips • Tongue • Mouth floor • Buccal	• Painful, local leukoplakia (whitish plaques); erythroplasia (velvety red hyperplasias); or persistent ulcer (2 weeks) that expands to adjacent structures • Other symptoms: impaired tongue function, swallowing difficulty, aspiration of saliva; with vessel involvement, hemorrhage • Advanced stage: lymph node enlargement, with eventual breakdown of overlying skin
Salivary glands • Parotid • Submaxillary (most common) • Sublingual (rare)	• Firm, local mass spreads to adjacent structures • With parotid cancer, facial nerve paralysis; with submaxillary cancer, mandible attachment
Nasopharynx	• Metastatic nodes beneath the ear • With nodes compressing eustachian tube, secretory otitis media; with nasal airway obstruction, bloody discharge, postnasal discharge, and nasal speech; with skull and cranial nerve involvement (frequent, especially sixth cranial nerve), diplopia and rectus muscle paralysis of eye
Tonsils	• Carcinomas poorly differentiated; cause metastatic upper neck nodes, local ulceration, and ear pain; metastasize early • Lymphoepitheliomas occur early, grow large; seldom ulcerate tonsils, and tonsils often remain small • Histiocytic lymphoma produces greatly enlarged tonsils, metastasizes early to neck and other parts of the lymph system, but usually doesn't ulcerate or cause pain.

technique) on skin flaps twice daily.
• To avoid carotid rupture and chylous fistula, the suture line should be kept intact and free from infection, and an effective drainage system maintained (normal drainage equals 240 to 300 ml during the first 24 hours, followed by scant drainage thereafter). If carotid rupture occurs, pressure must be applied to the site immediately; the patient will die without immediate surgery. To decrease venous pressure on the skin flap, ease breathing, and promote drainage, the patient should be placed in Fow-

DIAGNOSIS	TREATMENT
• Chronic sinusitis • X-rays of sinuses reveal bone destruction or masses • Biopsy for histologic confirmation	• Preoperative radiation • Maxillectomy with or without orbital exenteration • Chemotherapy adjunctive to surgery
• Leukoplakia, erythroplasia, or persistent ulcers • Tissue biopsy confirms diagnosis	• Lip cancer: surgery (to remove lesion) or radiation • Tongue (small primary lesion): surgery to remove lesion, or en bloc resection of tumor, mouth floor, mandible, and neck contents • Buccal mucosa or gums: en bloc resection of tumor, mouth floor, mandible, and side of neck; or with mandible involvement, en bloc dissection of neck and resection of mouth floor, in combination with partial mandibulectomy • Chemotherapy adjunctive to surgery
• Salivary gland mass • X-rays show malignancy or simple duct obstruction	• Radical salivary gland resection • Supplementary radiation therapy • Chemotherapy adjunctive to surgery
• Metastatic nodes beneath the ear • Anterior and posterior rhinoscopy to identify tumor • Biopsy for histologic confirmation • Skull X-rays determine extent of disease	• Radiation • Radical neck dissection for residual or recurrent metastasis (if primary cancer is controlled) • Chemotherapy adjunctive to surgery
• Biopsy for histologic confirmation	• Radiation therapy (however, local or distant metastases recur)

ler's position.
• The patient's acceptance of his altered body image will be eased if the health care professional caring for him shows his own acceptance of the patient by talking with him or simply keeping him company. His adjustment will be easier if he has a means of communication, such as a Magic Slate, until he can speak again.
• To improve his self-image, he should learn to do his own tracheostomy care.
• Because of the possibility of recurrence, the patient must report any new lesions immediately.

Laryngeal Cancer

The most common form of laryngeal cancer is squamous cell carcinoma (95%); rare forms include adenocarcinoma, sarcoma, and others. Such cancer may be intrinsic or extrinsic. An intrinsic tumor is on the true vocal cord and does not have a tendency to spread, because underlying connective tissues lack lymph nodes. An extrinsic tumor is on some other part of the larynx and tends to spread early. Laryngeal cancer is nine times more common in males than in females; most victims are between ages 50 and 65.

Causes and incidence

In laryngeal cancer, major predisposing factors include smoking (it's especially common in heavy smokers and rare in nonsmokers) and alcoholism; minor factors, chronic inhalation of noxious fumes, familial tendency, and less commonly, a history of frequent laryngitis and vocal straining.

Laryngeal cancer is classified according to its location:
• supraglottis (posterior surface of the epiglottis, aryepiglottic folds, false vocal cords)
• glottis (true vocal cords)
• subglottis (downward extension from vocal cords [rare]).

Signs and symptoms

In intrinsic laryngeal cancer, the dominant and earliest symptom is hoarseness that persists longer than 3 weeks; in extrinsic cancer, it's a lump in the throat, or pain or burning in the throat when drinking citrus juice or hot liquid. Later clinical effects of metastases include dysphagia, dyspnea, cough, enlarged cervical lymph nodes, and pain radiating to the ear.

Diagnosis

Any hoarseness that lasts longer than 2 weeks requires visualization of the larynx, by indirect laryngoscopy (mirror visualization) or direct laryngoscopy. Depending on the hospital, firm diagnosis also requires xeroradiography, laryngoscopy, biopsy, laryngeal tomography, or laryngography to define the borders of the lesion, and chest X-ray to detect metastases.

Treatment

In laryngeal cancer, the goal of treatment is to eliminate the cancer through surgery, radiation, or both, and to preserve speech. If speech preservation isn't possible, speech rehabilitation may include esophageal speech or prosthetic devices; surgical techniques to construct a new voice box are still experimental. Surgical procedures vary with tumor size, and can include cordectomy, partial or total laryngectomy, supraglottic laryngectomy, or total laryngectomy with laryngoplasty.

Additional considerations

Psychologic support and good pre- and postoperative care can minimize complications and speed recovery.

Before partial or total laryngectomy:
• The patient should maintain good oral hygiene; a bearded male may have to shave to facilitate postoperative care.
• The patient should verbalize his concerns before surgery temporarily cuts off effective verbal communication. Before surgery, he should choose an alternate method of communication that he finds comfortable (such as pencil and paper, sign language, or alphabet board).
• If the patient is going to have a total laryngectomy, he may find that visiting with a laryngectomee will reassure him. He should be told about postoperative procedures (suctioning, nasogastric feeding, care of laryngectomy tube) and their results (breathing through neck,

speech alteration).

After partial laryngectomy:
• The patient should get I.V. fluids and, usually, tube feedings for the first 2 days postoperatively; then oral fluids. The tracheostomy tube (inserted during surgery) should remain in place until tissue edema subsides.
• The patient must *not* use his voice until the doctor gives permission (usually 2 to 3 days postop). Then the patient should whisper until healing is complete.

After total laryngectomy:
• The patient should be immediately positioned on his side, with his head elevated 30° to 45°. When he's moved, the back of his neck must receive constant support, to prevent tension on sutures and possible wound dehiscence.
• The patient will probably have a laryngectomy tube in place until his stoma heals (about 7 to 10 days). This tube is shorter and thicker than a tracheostomy tube but requires the same care. Crusting and secretions around the stoma must be prevented since they can cause skin breakdown. This can be done by providing adequate room humidification. The crust can be removed by using a thin coating of petrolatum, antimicrobial ointment, and moist gauze.
• Complications to watch for and report include: fistula formation (redness, swelling, secretions on suture line), ca-

---

PATIENT TEACHING AID

Neck Stoma Care

After you're discharged, you'll have to do your own neck stoma care.
• To prevent infection, wash your hands before touching your stoma.
• Then, wet a washcloth with warm water (don't use wet cotton or soap); wring it out, and place it over the stoma.
• To keep the stoma moist, apply petrolatum thinly around its edges. Wipe off any excess.
• Use a stoma bib (crocheted cover or cotton cloth) over the stoma to filter and warm air before it enters the stoma. Fasten the bib with a tie around your neck. You can wear an ascot, a turtleneck sweater, or a regular shirt (sew the second button from the top over the buttonhole as though it were fastened, to leave access for a handkerchief when coughing); you can also wear jewelry or scarves.
• If you're a man, be careful when shaving, as some of your sensory nerve endings may have been cut in surgery. These endings will regenerate in about 6 months.

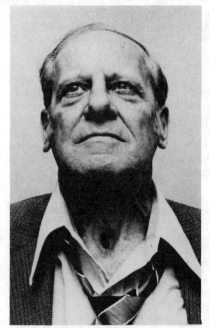

Patient shows well-healed neck stoma.

This patient teaching aid is intended for distribution to patients by doctors and nurses.
It should not be used without a doctor's approval.

rotid artery rupture (bleeding), and tracheostomy stenosis (constant shortness of breath). A fistula may form between reconstructed hypopharynx and the skin. This eventually heals spontaneously but may take weeks or months.

Carotid artery rupture usually occurs in patients who have had preoperative radiation, particularly those with a fistula that bathes the carotid artery with oral secretions. If carotid rupture occurs, pressure must be applied to the site; the patient will be taken to the operating room for carotid ligation.

Tracheostomy stenosis occurs weeks to months after laryngectomy. Treatment for tracheostomy stenosis includes fitting the patient with successively larger tracheostomy tubes until he can tolerate insertion of a large one. If the patient has a fistula, he should be fed through a nasogastric tube; otherwise, food will leak through the fistula and delay healing. Vital signs must be monitored, with special attention paid to temperature, since fever, indicates infection. Fluid intake and output require recording to avoid dehydration.

• The patient will need frequent mouth care. The patient's tongue and the sides of his mouth should be scrubbed with a soft toothbrush and his mouth rinsed with a deodorizing mouthwash.

• The patient may require gentle suctioning; deep suctioning must not be done because it could penetrate the suture line. Both tube and nose may be used, since the patient can no longer blow air through his nose; his mouth must be suctioned gently.

• After insertion of drainage catheter (usually connected to a blood drainage system or a gastrointestinal drainage system), suctioning should continue until a stop order is given. After catheter removal, dressings should be checked for drainage.

• Analgesics should be given as ordered. Keep in mind, narcotics depress respiration and inhibit coughing.

• To feed the patient through a nasogastric tube, the health care professional should check tube placement, elevate the patient's head to prevent aspiration, and be ready to suction after tube removal or oral fluid intake, since the patient may have difficulty swallowing.

• The patient will be able to speak again through speech rehabilitation (laryngeal speech, esophageal speech [air bolus techniques], artificial larynx, various mechanical aids). More information on speech rehabilitation can be supplied by the American Speech and Hearing Association, the International Association of Laryngectomees, the American Cancer Society, or the local chapter of the "Lost Chord Club" or the "New Voice Club."

• The patient will probably go through some grieving. Remember, he has not only lost his voice, he also can't smell, blow his nose, whistle, gargle, sip soup, or suck on a straw. If the depression seems severe, psychiatric referral may be in order.

Thyroid Cancer

Thyroid carcinoma occurs in all age-groups, especially in persons who have had radiation treatment to the neck area. Papillary and follicular carcinomas are most common and are usually associated with prolonged survival.

Papillary carcinoma accounts for half of all thyroid cancers in adults; it can occur at any age but is most common in adult females during childbearing years. It is usually multifocal and bilateral, and metastasizes slowly into regional nodes of the neck, mediastinum, lungs, and other distant organs. It is the least virulent form of thyroid cancer. Follicular carcinoma is less common (30% of all cases), but is more likely to recur and metastasize to the regional nodes, and through blood vessels into the bones, liver, and lungs. Medullary (solid) carcinoma originates in *the parafollicular cells derived from the last branchial pouch and contains amyloid and calcium deposits. It can produce calcitonin, histaminase, ACTH (producing Cushing's syndrome), and prostaglandin E_2 and F_3 (producing diarrhea). This form of thyroid cancer is familial, possibly inherited as an autosomal dominant trait, and is often associated with pheochromocytoma. This rare (5%) form of thyroid cancer usually occurs in women over age 40. It is completely curable when detected before it causes symptoms. Untreated, it grows rapidly, frequently metastasizing to bones, liver, and kidneys.*

Giant and spindle cell cancer (anaplastic tumor) resists radiation and is almost never curable by resection. It metastasizes rapidly and causes death by tracheal invasion and compression of adjacent structures.

Causes and incidence

Predisposing factors include radiation, prolonged TSH stimulation (through radiation or heredity), familial predisposition, or chronic goiter.

Radiation therapy in childhood, a high-risk factor, was common in the 1950s to shrink enlarged thymus gland, tonsils, or adenoids, and to treat acne and other skin disorders. Twenty-five percent of those so treated later developed thyroid nodules; 25% of those nodules became malignant. Risk of malignancy after radiation correlates with dose (a threshold dose has not been defined) and age (malignancy is rare in patients who begin radiation treatment after age 21).

Signs and symptoms

The dominant signs of thyroid cancer are a painless nodule, a hard nodule in an enlarged thyroid gland, or palpable lymph nodes with thyroid enlargement. Eventually, the pressure of such a nodule or enlargement causes hoarseness, dysphagia, dyspnea, and pain on palpation. If the tumor is large enough to destroy the gland, hypothyroidism follows, with its typical signs of low metabolism (mental apathy, cold sensitivity). However, if the tumor stimulates excess thyroid hormone production, it induces signs of hyperthyroidism (heat sensitivity, restlessness, overactivity). Other clinical features include diarrhea, weight loss, anorexia, irritability, vocal cord paralysis, and symptoms of distant metastases.

Diagnosis

The first clue to thyroid cancer is usually an enlarged, palpable node in the thyroid gland, neck, lymph nodes of the neck, or vocal cords. Patient history of radiation therapy or a family history of thyroid cancer supports diagnosis. However, tests must rule out nonmalignant thyroid enlargements, which are much more common. Thyroid scan differentiates between functional nodes (rarely malignant) and hypofunctional nodes (commonly malignant) by measuring

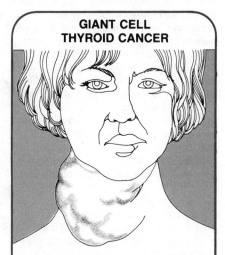

GIANT CELL THYROID CANCER

The most disfiguring, destructive, and deadly form of thyroid carcinoma, giant (or spindle) cell cancer has the poorest prognosis. Although this tumor rarely metastasizes to distant organs, its size produces severe anatomical distortion of nearby structures. Treatment usually consists of a total thyroidectomy but is rarely successful.

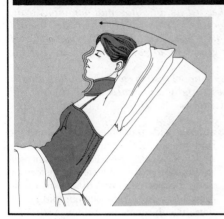

how readily nodules trap isotopes compared with the rest of the thyroid gland. In thyroid cancer, the scintiscan shows a "cold," nonfunctioning nodule. Other tests include ultrasonic scan and serum calcitonin assay (other serum tests are useless) to diagnose medullary cancer. Calcitonin assay is a reliable clue to silent medullary carcinoma. Calcitonin level is measured during a resting state and during an infusion of calcium (15 mg/kg) over a 4-hour period. An elevated fasting calcitonin and an abnormal response to calcium stimulation (high release of calcitonin from the node in comparison with the rest of the gland) are indicative of medullary cancer.

Treatment

Treatment varies and may include any or a combination of the following:
• Total or subtotal thyroidectomy, with modified node dissection (bilateral or homolateral) on the side of the primary cancer (papillary or follicular cancer)
• Total thyroidectomy and radical neck excision (for medullary, or giant and spindle cell cancer)
• Radiation (^{131}I), with external radiation (for large inoperable cancer and sometimes postoperatively in lieu of radical neck excision) or by itself (for local or distant metastases)

• Adjunctive thyroid suppression, with exogenous thyroid hormones suppressing TSH production, and simultaneous administration of an adrenergic blocking agent, such as propranolol, increasing tolerance to surgery and radiation
• Chemotherapy, which is experimental; doxorubicin is sometimes beneficial with metastasizing thyroid cancer.

Additional considerations

Before surgery, the patient should:
• expect temporary voice loss or hoarseness lasting several days after surgery.
• understand the operation and postoperative procedures.
• know proper postop positioning.
• have a normal functioning thyroid gland, as demonstrated by a normal EKG, thyroid function tests, and pulse rate.

After surgery, the patient should:
• be placed in semi-Fowler's position, with his head neither hyperextended nor flexed, to avoid pressure on the suture line, and his head and neck supported with sandbags and pillows. When he's moved, hands should be used to continue this support. If the patient is out of bed within 24 hours after surgery, support may be discontinued.
• have his dressing, neck, and back checked, following vital signs monitor-

ing, for bleeding. If he complains that the dressing feels tight (whether bleeding's present or not), the dressing should be loosened and the doctor called immediately. Serum calcium levels must be checked daily. Other complications to watch for and report include: hemorrhage and shock (elevated pulse and hypotension); tetany (carpopedal spasm, twitching, convulsions); thyroid storm (high fever, severe tachycardia, delirium, dehydration, and extreme irritability), and respiratory obstruction (dyspnea, crowing respirations, retraction of neck tissues). In case of respiratory obstruction, a tracheotomy set and oxygen equipment should be kept handy. Continuous steam inhalation can be used until his chest clears.

• receive I.V. fluids or be put on a soft diet, as needed, though he may be able to tolerate a regular diet within 24 hours after surgery.

Care of the patient after extensive tumor and node excision is identical to other radical neck postoperative care.

Intraorbital Malignant Melanoma

Intraorbital tumors develop in the globe of the eye. The two most common types are malignant melanoma and retinoblastoma. About 6% to 8% of intraorbital malignant melanomas affect the iris; 9%, the ciliary body; and 85%, the choroid.

Malignant melanoma is the most common intraorbital tumor in Caucasian adults aged 50 to 60; it's rare in Blacks and Asians. Prognosis depends on the location and tumor type; for example, tumors of the iris allow longer survival than those in the choroid.

Causes
Possible predisposing factors include inflammation or trauma. Malignant melanomas often stem from melanocytes of the uvea, retina, or iris.

Signs and symptoms
Since malignant melanoma of the iris is usually asymptomatic, discovery of the lesion is often accidental. Its most common symptom is hemorrhage into the anterior chamber. Others include:
• history of change in size and color of a pigmented lesion
• appearance of discrete, pigmented, fleshy mass in the iris, or diffuse discoloration or thickening
• loss of peripheral vision
• floaters
• glaucoma later in the disease.

Malignant melanoma of the ciliary body appears as a black, subconjunctive mass. It may produce blurred vision, loss of visual field, and pain from associated glaucoma or inflammation.

Malignant melanoma of the choroid produces a brown or gray, somewhat elevated lesion, which frequently becomes mushroom-shaped as it grows. The most common symptom is a change in visual acuity due to retinal detachment. Less common clinical features include metamorphopsia (distortion of shapes) and photopsia (sensation of flashes or sparks).

Diagnosis
Transillumination and retroillumination confirm the diagnosis. Other tests include ophthalmoscopy, florescein angiography to evaluate tumor size, ultrasonography to define tumor location, and skull X-ray to determine bone involvement.

Treatment
Treatment depends on the location of the lesion:
• iridectomy for iris tumors
• iridocyclectomy (removal of a portion of the iris and all the ciliary body) for small lesions of the ciliary body

- enucleation for most malignant melanomas of the choroid.

New treatment methods for small tumors include photocoagulation, laser therapy, cryosurgery, radon seed implants, and cobalt applicators.

Additional considerations

A health care professional caring for a patient with intraorbital malignant melanoma should:

- help prevent eye disease by encouraging patients to have regular eye examinations, and by teaching them to watch for early clinical effects of eye disease (blurred vision, change in acuity, and pain).
- prepare the patient carefully for special eye tests by explaining exactly what to expect and why the tests are needed.
- teach the patient to be realistic about eye tumors. Many eye tumors are noninvasive and not necessarily life-threatening. A normal life is possible with impaired vision or with only one eye. Understandably, the thought of vision loss is frightening, so the patient will need emotional support.
- recommend a rehabilitation center for a visually handicapped patient, when appropriate. These centers help patients return to normal levels of activity, for example, by reteaching important skills and providing vocational training.

- include the patient's family and friends in any teaching; their primary goal should be to foster independence.
- if the patient needs radiation, drug, or laser therapy, teach him how to recognize side effects, how to perform skin care (gentle cleansing with warm water around irradiated area), how to cope with photophobia (wearing dark glasses helps), and how to prevent eye strain.
- warn the patient to report any vision changes to the doctor immediately, since these may signal treatment-induced damage or tumor recurrence.

Before eye surgery, the patient must be prepared for his eye's postoperative appearance. Iridectomy doesn't leave an obvious external scar. After enucleation, the patient may wear a prosthesis. The patient must know safety measures to compensate for loss of visual field and depth perception.

After eye surgery, the patient may experience complications of enucleation (hemorrhage, thrombosis, infection). A pressure dressing must be kept on for approximately 5 days to prevent hemorrhage. The patient should know about available prostheses, most of which are plastic and must be replaced every 2 years. An oculist can supply more information. Finally, the patient must be able to care for the eye socket and the prosthesis.

Intraorbital Eye Tumors

Except for malignant melanoma and retinoblastoma, intraorbital eye tumors are relatively rare. They include hemangiomas (most common), gliomas of the optic nerve (occur most often in children and young adults), and rhabdomyosarcomas (most common primary orbital malignant tumor in children aged 6 months to 13 years).

Causes

The causes of these tumors remain unknown.

Signs and symptoms

The hallmark of these tumors is exophthalmos. Other signs depend on tumor size and growth rate (rapid growth produces edema of lid, for example). Tumors near the orbital apex produce early vision loss and retinal striae; tumors outside the muscle core, restricted ocular movements without vision loss.

In children, hemangiomas are nonen-

PATIENT TEACHING AID

How to Insert and Remove an Artificial Eye

To insert the artificial eye:
• Carefully pull down the lower lid. Slip the narrower end of the artificial eye into the inner corner of the orifice.
• Pinch the upper eyelashes between your fingers and carefully lift the upper lid.

• Gently push the artificial eye into the orifice with your other hand.
To remove the artificial eye:
• Carefully pull down the lower lid. Push up under the artificial eye with the fingers of your other hand. Keep this hand cupped to catch it.

This patient teaching aid is intended for distribution to patients by doctors and nurses. It should not be used without a doctor's approval.

capsulated and grow rapidly during the first 6 to 12 months of life, then regress over the next 6 to 7 years. In adults, hemangiomas are encapsulated and cavernous. Hemangiomas are commonly accompanied by lesions elsewhere.

Gliomas of the optic nerve are slow-growing tumors that produce early vision loss. Rhabdomyosarcomas grow rapidly and commonly appear as a mass in the inner portion of the upper lid.

Diagnosis

Although patient history and physical examination usually suggest these tumors, confirmation requires orbital and skull X-rays, ultrasound, or tomography.

Treatment

For children with hemangiomas, treatment consists of radiation and systemic steroids; for adults, surgical excision, since these tumors are radioresistant. Gliomas require excision and radiation; rhabdomyosarcomas, radiation or exenteration.

Additional considerations

The health care professional caring for the patient with an intraorbital eye tumor should:
• help in the early detection of eye disease by encouraging patients to have regular eye examinations, and by teaching them to watch for early clinical effects of eye disease (blurred vision, change in acuity, and pain).

• prepare patients carefully for eye examination by explaining exactly what to expect and why the tests are needed.
• teach the patient to be realistic about eye tumors. Many eye tumors are non-invasive and not necessarily life-threatening. A normal life is possible with impaired vision or with only one eye. Understandably, the thought of vision loss is frightening, so the patient will need emotional support.
• recommend a rehabilitation center for a visually handicapped patient, when appropriate. These centers help patients return to normal levels of activity by re-teaching important skills and providing vocational training.
• include the patient's family in any teaching; their primary goal should be to foster independence.
• if the patient undergoes radiation or drug therapy, teach him about side effects, good skin care (gentle cleaning with warm water around irradiated area), photophobia (wearing dark glasses helps), and prevention of eye strain.
• warn the patient to report any vision changes to the doctor immediately, since these may signal treatment-induced damage or tumor recurrence.

Before surgery, the patient must be prepared for his eye's postoperative appearance. Removal of part or all of the lid is deforming; however, reconstructive surgery may lessen deformity for some patients. Exenteration means removal of the eyelid, the eyeball, and the orbital contents. Such a patient can't wear a prosthesis and must wear an eyepatch. He'll have to learn safety measures to compensate for some loss of visual field and depth perception. The patient will have to cope with the depression that normally follows exenteration. He'll need the health care professional's help. To protect the remaining eye, the patient should wear safety glasses.

Extraorbital Basal Cell Carcinoma of the Eye

The most common extraorbital cancer of the eye, basal cell carcinoma affects the lid, conjunctivae, and cornea. Basal cell carcinoma occurs most often in men, and incidence rises with age. With surgery, its cure rate is excellent.

Causes
Although the exact cause remains unclear, predisposing factors include exposure to direct sunlight, radiation, chemicals, and other carcinogens.

Extraorbital basal cell carcinoma spreads by direct invasion and readily invades the bony orbit. It rarely metastasizes outside the eye.

Signs and symptoms
Basal cell carcinoma of the eye characteristically begins as a small, elevated nodule on the inner canthus of the lower lid, which later becomes dimpled with a pearly border. The invasive form typically produces ulceration and visual defects, such as blurring.

Diagnosis
External examination suggests extraorbital basal cell carcinoma; biopsy, to determine cell type, confirms it. X-rays are necessary to detect invasion of bony orbit.

Treatment
Generally, treatment consists of surgical excision of the tumor. Radiation therapy is usually necessary with orbital invasion, although possible complications include cataracts, corneal ulcers, and skin necrosis.

Additional considerations
To prevent eye disease, patients should have regular eye examinations, and should seek prompt medical evaluation if they experience any early clinical effects of eye dysfunction, such as blurred vision, or notice any changes in the external appearance of the eye.

Spinal Neoplasms

Spinal neoplasms may be any one of many tumor types similar to intracranial tumors; they involve the cord or its roots and, if untreated, can eventually cause paralysis. As primary tumors, they originate in the meningeal coverings, the parenchyma of the cord or its roots, the intraspinal vasculature, or the vertebrae. They can also occur as metastatic foci from primary tumors.

Causes and incidence
Primary tumors of the spinal cord may be extramedullary (occurring outside the spinal cord) or intramedullary (within the cord itself). Extramedullary tumors may be intradural (meningiomas and schwannomas), which account for 60% of all primary spinal cord neoplasms; or extradural (metastatic tumors from breasts, lungs, prostate, leukemia, or

lymphomas), which account for 25%. These metastases deposit in the extradural space and produce neurologic deficits by compressing the cord. They may also invade the vertebrae, which subsequently collapse and directly compress the cord.

Intramedullary tumors, or gliomas (astrocytomas or ependymomas), are comparatively rare, accounting for only about 10%; in children, they're low-grade astrocytomas.

Cord tumors are rare compared with intracranial tumors (ratio of 1:4). They occur with equal frequency in both men and women, with the exception of meningiomas, which occur most often in women. Spinal cord tumors can occur anywhere along the length of the cord.

Signs and symptoms

Extramedullary tumors produce symptoms by pressing on nerve roots, spinal cord, and spinal vessels; intramedullary tumors, by destroying the parenchyma and compressing adjacent areas. Because intramedullary tumors may extend over several spinal cord segments, their symptoms are more variable than those of extramedullary tumors.

The following clinical effects are likely with all spinal cord neoplasms:
• *Pain*—Most severe directly over the tumor, radiates around the trunk or down the limb on the affected side, and is unrelieved by bed rest
• *Motor symptoms*—Asymmetric spastic weakness, decreased muscle tone, exaggerated reflexes, and a positive Babinski's sign. If the tumor is at the level of the cauda equina, flaccidity, muscle wasting, weakness, and progressive diminution in tendon reflexes are characteristic.
• *Sensory deficit*—Contralateral loss of pain, temperature, and touch sensation (Brown-Séquard syndrome). These losses are less obvious to the patient than functional motor changes. Caudal lesions invariably produce paresthesias in the distribution of the involved roots.
• *Bladder symptoms*—Urinary retention is an inevitable late sign with cord compression. Early signs include incomplete emptying or difficulty with the urinary stream, which is usually unnoticed or ignored. Cauda equina tumors cause bladder and bowel incontinence due to flaccid paralysis.

Diagnosis

• A *spinal tap* shows clear yellow cerebrospinal fluid (CSF) as a result of increased protein levels if the flow is completely blocked. If the flow is partially blocked, protein levels rise, but the fluid is only slightly yellow in proportion to the CSF protein level. A Pap smear of the CSF may show malignant cells of metastatic carcinoma.
• *X-rays* show distortions of the intervertebral foramina; changes in the vertebrae or collapsed areas in the vertebral body; and localized enlargement of the spinal canal, indicating an adjacent block.
• *Myelography* identifies the level of the lesion by outlining it if the tumor is causing partial obstruction; it shows anatomic relationship to the cord and the dura. If obstruction is complete, the injected dye can't flow past the tumor. (This study is dangerous if cord compression is nearly complete, since withdrawal or escape of CSF will actually allow the tumor to exert greater pressure against the cord.)
• A *bone scan* demonstrates metastatic invasion of the vertebrae by showing a characteristic increase in osteoblastic activity.
• *CAT scan* shows cord compression and location of the tumor.
• *Frozen section biopsy* at surgery identifies the tissue type.

Treatment

Treatment of spinal cord tumors generally includes laminectomy or radiation. Laminectomy is indicated for primary tumors that produce spinal cord or cauda equina compression; it's *not* usually indicated for metastatic tumors. If the tumor is slowly progressive, or if it's treated before the cord degenerates from compression, symptoms are likely to disappear, and complete restoration of function

INTRADURAL EXTRAMEDUL-LARY SPINAL NEOPLASM

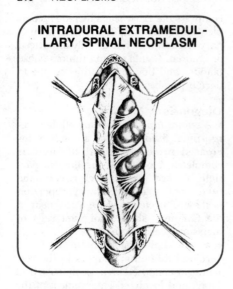

is possible. In a patient with metastatic carcinoma or lymphoma who suddenly experiences complete transverse myelitis with spinal shock, functional improvement is unlikely, even with treatment, and his outlook is ominous. If the patient has incomplete paraplegia of rapid onset, emergency surgical decompression may save cord function. Steroid therapy minimizes cord edema until surgery can be performed. Partial removal of intramedullary gliomas, followed by radiation, may alleviate symptoms for a short time. Metastatic extradural tumors can be controlled with radiation, analgesics, and (in the case of hormone-mediated tumors [breast and prostate]) appropriate hormone therapy. Transcutaneous nerve stimulation (TENS) may control radicular pain from spinal cord tumors and is a useful alternative to narcotic analgesics. In TENS, an electrical charge is applied to the skin to stimulate large-diameter nerve fibers and thereby inhibit transmission of pain impulses through small-diameter nerve fibers.

Additional considerations

Care plans for patients with spinal cord tumors should emphasize early recognition of the disease or its recurrence, skilled support and intervention during the acute and chronic phases, prevention and treatment of complications, and maintenance of the patient's quality of life.

On first contact with the patient, a complete neurologic evaluation is needed to obtain the data base for planning future care and evaluating clinical status.

Care for the patient with a spinal cord tumor is basically the same as that for the patient with spinal cord injury, requiring psychologic support, rehabilitation (including bowel and bladder retraining), and prevention of infection and skin breakdown. After laminectomy, care includes checking neurologic status frequently, changing position by logrolling, administering analgesics, monitoring frequently for infection, and aiding in early walking.

• The patient and his family must learn to understand and cope with the diagnosis, treatment, potential disabilities, and necessary changes in life-style.

• Safety precautions should be taken for the patient with impaired sensation and motor deficits, such as using side rails if the patient is bedridden, or encouraging him to wear flat shoes if he's not, and removing scatter rugs and clutter to prevent falls.

• The patient must try being independent in performing daily activities. Aggravating pain can be avoided by moving the patient slowly and by making sure his body is well aligned when giving personal care. He should use TENS to block radicular pain.

• Steroids and antacids may be administered for cord edema after radiation therapy. Sensory or motor dysfunction may occur, which indicates the need for more steroids.

• The patient with vertebral body involvement must be on strict bed rest until the doctor says he can safely walk, because body weight alone can cause cord collapse and cord laceration from bone fragments.

• The patient should be logrolled and positioned on his side every 2 hours to prevent decubitus ulcers.

• If the patient is to wear a back brace, he must wear it whenever he gets out of bed.

THORAX

Lung Cancer

Lung cancer usually develops within the wall or epithelium of the bronchial tree. Its most common types are epidermoid (squamous cell) carcinoma, small-cell (oat cell) carcinoma, adenocarcinoma, and large-cell (anaplastic) carcinoma. Although, generally, prognosis is poor, it varies with the extent of spread at the time of diagnosis and cell type growth rate. Only 8% of men and 12% of women with lung cancer survive 5 years. Lung cancer is the most common cause of cancer death in men and is fast becoming the most common cause in women, even though it's largely preventable.

Causes and incidence

Most experts agree that lung cancer is attributable to inhalation of carcinogenic pollutants by a susceptible host. Who is most susceptible? Any smoker over age 40, especially if he began to smoke before age 15, has smoked a whole pack or more per day for 20 years, or works with or near asbestos.

As a result of smoking, pollutants in tobacco cause progressive cellular degeneration in lung tissue. Lung cancer is 10 times more common in smokers than in nonsmokers; indeed, 80% of lung cancer patients are smokers. Cancer risk is determined by the number of cigarettes smoked daily, the depth of inhalation, how early in life smoking began, and the nicotine content of cigarettes. Two other factors also increase susceptibility: exposure to carcinogenic industrial and air pollutants (asbestos, uranium, arsenic, nickel, iron oxides, chromium, radioactive dust, and coal dust), and familial susceptibility.

Signs and symptoms

Because early-stage lung cancer usually produces no symptoms, this disease is often in an advanced state at diagnosis. The following late-stage symptoms often lead to diagnosis:
• With epidermoid and small-cell carcinomas—smoker's cough, wheezing, dyspnea, hemoptysis, and chest pain
• With adenocarcinoma and large-cell carcinoma—fever, weakness, weight loss, and anorexia.

In addition to their obvious interference with respiratory function, lung tumors may also alter the production of hormones that regulate body function or homeostasis. Clinical conditions that result from such changes are known as hormonal paraneoplastic syndromes:
• *Gynecomastia* may result from large-cell carcinoma.
• *Hypertrophic pulmonary osteoarthropathy* (bone and joint pain from cartilage erosion due to abnormal production of growth hormone) may result from large-cell carcinoma and adenocarcinoma.
• *Cushing's and carcinoid syndromes*, from small-cell carcinoma.
• *Hypercalcemia*, from epidermoid tumors.

Metastatic symptoms vary greatly, depending on the effect of tumors on intrathoracic and distant structures:
• *bronchial obstruction*: hemoptysis, atelectasis, pneumonitis, dyspnea
• *recurrent nerve invasion*: hoarseness, vocal cord paralysis
• *chest wall invasion*: piercing chest pain; increasing dyspnea; severe shoulder pain, radiating down arm
• *local lymphatic spread*: cough, hemoptysis, stridor, pleural effusion
• *phrenic nerve involvement*: dyspnea; shoulder pain; unilateral paralyzed diaphragm, with paradoxical motion

- *esophageal compression*: dysphagia
- *vena caval obstruction*: venous distention and edema of face, neck, chest, and back
- *pericardial involvement*: pericardial effusion, tamponade, arrhythmias
- *cervical thoracic sympathetic nerve involvement*: miosis, ptosis, exophthalmos, reduced sweating.

Distant metastases may involve any part of the body, including the CNS, abdomen, bone, and connective and vascular tissues.

Diagnosis

Typical clinical findings may strongly suggest lung cancer, but firm diagnosis requires further evidence.

- *Chest X-ray* usually shows an advanced lesion, but it can detect a lesion up to 2 years before symptoms appear. It also indicates tumor size and location.
- *Sputum cytology*, which is 75% reliable, requires specimen coughed up from lungs and tracheobronchial tree, *not* postnasal secretions or saliva.
- *Bronchoscopy* can locate the tumor site. Bronchoscopic washings provide material for cytologic and histologic examination. The flexible fiberoptic bronchoscope increases scope of vision and test effectiveness.
- *Needle biopsy* of the lungs can detect peripherally located tumors. It is performed under local anesthetic and employs biplane fluoroscopic visual control. This allows firm diagnosis in 80% of patients.
- *Tissue biopsy* of accessible metastatic sites includes pleural biopsy, and biopsy of supraclavicular and mediastinal nodes.
- *Thoracentesis* allows chemical and cytologic examination of pleural fluid.

Additional studies include chest tomography, bronchography, esophagography, angiocardiography (contrast studies of bronchial tree, esophagus, and cardiovascular tissues). Tests to detect metastasis include bone scan (positive scan may lead to bone marrow biopsy; bone marrow biopsy is also recommended in small-cell carcinoma); CAT scan of the brain; liver function studies; and gallium scan (noninvasive nuclear scan) of liver, spleen, and bone.

After histologic confirmation, staging determines the extent of the disease and helps in planning treatment and understanding prognosis.

Treatment

Recent treatment—which consists of combinations of surgery, radiation, and chemotherapy—may improve prognosis and prolong survival. Nevertheless, because treatment usually begins at an advanced stage, it is largely palliative.

Surgery is the primary treatment for Stage I, Stage II, or selected Stage III squamous cell carcinoma; adenocarcinoma; and large-cell carcinoma, unless the tumor is nonresectable or other conditions (such as cardiac disease) rule out surgery. Surgery may include partial removal of a lung (wedge resection, segmental resection, lobectomy, radical lobectomy) or total removal (pneumonectomy, radical pneumonectomy).

Preoperative radiation therapy may reduce tumor bulk to allow for surgical resection, but this is of questionable value. Radiation therapy is ordinarily recommended for Stage I and Stage II lesions if surgery is contraindicated, and for Stage III when the disease is confined to the involved hemithorax and the ipsilateral supraclavicular lymph nodes. Generally, radiation therapy is delayed until 1 month after surgery, to allow the wound to heal, and is then directed to the part of the chest most likely to develop metastasis.

Chemotherapy, with other treatment measures, induces remission in over 65% of patients with small-cell carcinoma. It's less effective in adenocarcinoma and large-cell carcinoma; its effectiveness in epidermoid carcinoma is still unknown. Normally, chemotherapy employs combinations of methotrexate, cyclophosphamide, lomustine, doxorubicin, bleomycin, carmustine, procarbazine, and vincristine.

Immunotherapy is still experimental. Nonspecific immunotherapy using BCG (bacille Calmette-Guérin) vaccine or,

STAGING LUNG CANCER

TO: No evidence of primary tumor

TX: Tumor proven by the presence of malignant cells in bronchopulmonary secretions but not visualized roentgenographically or bronchoscopically, or any tumor that cannot be assessed

TIS: Carcinoma in situ

T1: A tumor that is 3 cm or less in greatest diameter, surrounded by lung or visceral pleura, and without evidence of invasion proximal to a lobar bronchus at bronchoscopy.

T2: A tumor more than 3 cm in greatest diameter, or a tumor of any size that invades the visceral pleura or has associated atelectasis or obstructive pneumonitis extending to the hilar region. At bronchoscopy, the proximal extent of demonstrable tumor must be within a lobar bronchus or at least 2 cm distal to the carina. Any associated atelectasis or obstructive pneumonitis must involve less than an entire lung, and there must be no pleural effusion.

T3: A tumor of any size with direct extension into an adjacent structure such as the parietal pleura, the chest wall, the diaphragm, or the mediastinum and its contents; or a tumor demonstrable bronchoscopically to involve a main bronchus less than 2 cm distal to the carina; or any tumor associated with atelectasis, obstructive pneumonitis of an entire lung, or pleural effusion.

N0: No demonstrable metastasis to regional lymph nodes

N1: Metastasis to lymph nodes in the peribronchial or the ipsilateral hilar region, or both, including direct extension

N2: Metastasis to lymph nodes in the mediastinum

M0: No distant metastasis

M1: Distant metastasis such as in scalene, cervical, or contralateral hilar lymph nodes, brain, bones, liver, or contralateral lung.

Occult Carcinoma	Stage I	Stage II	Stage III
TX N0 M0	TIS N0 M0	T2 N1 M0	T3 any N or M
	T1 N0 M0		N2 any T or M
	T1 N1 M0		M1 any T or N
	T2 N0 M0		

From David T. Carr and C. Rosenow, "Bronchogenic Carcinoma," *Basics of Respiratory Disease*, Vol. 5, No. 5, 1977, p. 5. Used by permission of the authors and the American Lung Association.

possibly, C Parvum (*Corynebacterium parvulum*) appears most promising.

Additional considerations

Comprehensive supportive care, patient teaching, and psychologic support can minimize complications and speed recovery from surgery, radiation, and chemotherapy.

Before surgery, a hospital staff member should:

• supplement and reinforce what the doctor has already told the patient.

• explain expected postop procedures, such as insertion of a Foley catheter, endotracheal tube, dressing changes, and I.V. therapy; instruct the patient in coughing, deep diaphragmatic breathing, and range-of-motion exercises; reassure him that analgesics and proper positioning will control postop pain.

• give the patient nothing by mouth

DISTRIBUTION OF THE SIX MOST COMMON CANCER SITES

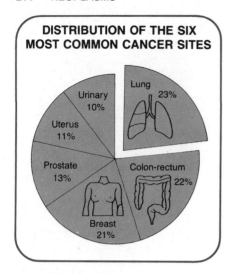

Lung 23%
Urinary 10%
Uterus 11%
Prostate 13%
Colon-rectum 22%
Breast 21%

(NPO) after midnight the night before surgery; give the patient a povidone-iodine shower the night or morning before surgery; give the patient preop medications, such as a sedative, and an anticholinergic to dry secretions.

After thoracic surgery, a staff member should:

• maintain a patent airway; monitor chest tubes to reestablish normal intrathoracic pressure; prevent postoperative and pulmonary complications.

• check vital signs every 15 minutes during the first hour after surgery, every 30 minutes during the next 4 hours, and then every 2 hours; watch for and report abnormal respiration and other changes.

• suction patient often, and encourage him to begin deep breathing and coughing as soon as possible; check secretions often. Initially, sputum will be thick and dark with blood, but it should become thinner and grayish-yellow within a day.

• monitor and record closed chest drainage; keep chest tubes patent and draining effectively (fluctuation in the water seal chamber on inspiration and expiration indicates that the chest tube is patent); watch for air leaks, and report them immediately; position the patient on the surgical side to promote drainage and lung reexpansion.

• watch for and report foul-smelling discharge and excessive drainage on dressing. Usually, the dressing is removed after 24 hours, unless the wound appears infected.

• monitor intake and output; maintain adequate hydration.

• watch for and treat infection, shock, hemorrhage, atelectasis, dyspnea, mediastinal shift, and pulmonary embolus; prevent pulmonary embolus by applying antiembolism stockings and encourage range-of-motion exercises.

If the patient is receiving chemotherapy and radiation, a staff member should:

• explain possible side effects of radiation and chemotherapy; watch for, treat, and, when possible, try to prevent them.

• ask the dietary department to provide soft, nonirritating foods that are high in protein, and encourage the patient to eat high-calorie between-meal snacks.

• give antiemetics and antidiarrheals, as needed.

• schedule patient care to help the patient conserve his energy.

• impose reverse isolation if patient develops bone marrow suppression.

• give good skin care to minimize skin breakdown, during radiation therapy. If the patient receives radiation therapy as an outpatient, he must avoid wearing tight clothing, getting sunburned, and putting harsh ointments on his chest. He should be taught exercises to prevent shoulder stiffness.

Health care professionals should educate high-risk patients about how to reduce their chances of developing lung cancer:

• Smokers who want to quit should be referred to local branches of the American Cancer Society, Smoke Enders, I Quit Smoking Clinics, or I'm Not Smoking Clubs; or to group therapy, individual counseling, or hypnosis.

• All heavy smokers over age 40 should have a chest X-ray annually and sputum cytology every 6 months.

• Patients with recurring or chronic respiratory infections and those with chronic lung disease who detect any change in the character of a cough should see their doctor promptly for evaluation.

Breast Cancer

Breast cancer is the most common malignancy affecting women and is their number one killer. It occurs in men, but rarely. The 5-year survival rate has improved from 53% in the 1940s to 65% in the 1970s. This is probably because of earlier diagnosis and the variety of treatment modes now available. The death rate, however, has not changed in the past 50 years.

Although breast cancer may develop any time after puberty, it's uncommon before age 35.

Causes and incidence

The cause of breast cancer isn't known, but its high incidence in women implicates estrogen. Certain predisposing factors are clear; women at *high risk* include those who:

- have a family history of breast cancer.
- have long menstrual cycles; began menses early or menopause late.
- were first pregnant after age 35.
- have had unilateral breast cancer.
- have endometrial or ovarian cancer.
- are Caucasians of middle or upper socioeconomic class.
- are under constant stress or undergo unusual disturbances in their home or work lives.

Many other predisposing factors have been researched, such as radiation, hair dyes, estrogen therapy, antihypertensives, diet, and fibrocystic disease of the breasts. However, none of these has been demonstrated conclusively.

Women at *lower risk* include those who:

- were pregnant before age 20.
- had multiple pregnancies.
- are Indian or Asian.
- are of lower socioeconomic class.

Pathophysiology

Breast cancer occurs more often in the left breast than the right, and more often in the upper outer quadrant. Growth rates vary. Theoretically, slow-growing breast cancer may take up to 8 years to become palpable at ⅜″ (1 cm) in size. It spreads by way of the lymphatic system and the bloodstream, through the right heart to the lungs, and to the liver, bone, adrenals, kidneys, and brain.

Many refer to the estimated growth rate of breast cancer as "doubling time," or the time it takes the malignant cells to double in number.

Often, these patients die with evidence of distant metastases, so many view breast cancer as a chronic disease.

Classified by histologic appearance and location of the lesion, breast cancer may be:

- *adenocarcinoma*—arising from the epithelium
- *intraductal*—developing within the ducts
- *infiltrating*—occurring in parenchymal tissue of the breast
- *inflammatory (rare)*—rapid tumor growth, in which the overlying skin becomes edematous, inflamed, and indurated
- *medullary or circumscribed*—large tumor with rapid growth rate
- *Paget's disease*—cancer of the nipple, in which erosion and bleeding of the nipple occur.

These classifications should be coupled with a staging or nodal status classification system for a clearer understanding of the extent of the cancer. The most common system for staging, both before and after surgery, is the tumor-nodes-metastasis (TNM) system.

Signs and symptoms

Warning signals of possible breast cancer include:

- a lump or mass in the breast (a hard, stony mass is usually malignant).
- change in breast symmetry or size.

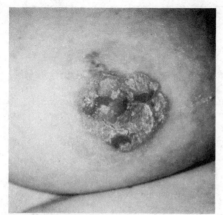

Paget's disease (cancer of the nipple), in which erosion and bleeding of the nipple occur

- change in breast skin, such as thickening, dimpling, edema (peau d'orange), or ulceration.
- change in skin temperature (a warm, hot, or pink area; suspect cancer in such a nonlactating woman past childbearing age until proven otherwise).
- unusual drainage or discharge (a spontaneous discharge of any kind in a nonnursing, nonlactating woman warrants investigation; so does any discharge produced by breast manipulation [greenish-black, white, creamy, serous, or bloody]). If a nursing infant rejects one breast, this may suggest possible breast cancer.
- change in the nipple, such as itching, burning, erosion, or retraction.
- pain (not usually a symptom of breast cancer unless the tumor is advanced, but it should be investigated).
- bone metastasis, pathologic bone fractures, and hypercalcemia.

Diagnosis

The most reliable method of detecting breast cancer is the regular breast exam (self breast exam [SBE]), followed by immediate evaluation of any abnormality. Other dependable diagnostic measures include mammography, xeromammography, ultrasonography, thermography, and surgical biopsy.

Mammography is indicated for any woman whose physical exam might suggest breast cancer. It should be done as a baseline on women between ages 35 and 40 (some say all women over 50), and annually on women who've had unilateral breast cancer, to check for new disease. However, the value of mammography is questionable for women under 35 (because of the density of the breasts), except those who are strongly suspected of having breast cancer.

Bone scan, carcinoembryonic antigen (CEA) tests, measurement of alkaline phosphatase levels, liver function studies, and liver biopsy can detect distant metastases. A hormonal reception assay done on the tumor can determine if the tumor is estrogen- or progesterone-dependent. (This test is important in making therapy decisions. Such therapy then aims to block the action of the estrogen hormone that supports tumor growth.) Infrequently, injection galactography may be done on a patient with abnormal nipple drainage to investigate the possibility of intraductal papilloma.

Treatment

Controversy exists over treatment of breast cancer at every stage of the disease; however, therapy should take into consideration the stage of the disease, the woman's age and menopausal status, and the disfiguring effects of the surgery. Treatment may include any or a combination of the following:

Surgery:
Lumpectomy (excision of the tumor) is the initial surgery, which also aids in determining tumor cell type. This procedure is often done on an outpatient basis and is all the surgery some patients require, especially those with a small tumor, with no evidence of axillary node involvement.

A two-stage procedure, in which the surgeon removes the lump, confirms that it's malignant, and discusses treatment options with the patient, is desirable, because it allows the patient to participate in her treatment plans. Sometimes, if the tumor is diagnosed as clinically malignant, such planning can be done before surgery. In lumpectomy and dissection of the axillary lymph nodes, the tumor and the axillary lymph nodes are removed, leaving the breast intact. A simple mastectomy removes the breast but not the lymph nodes or pectoral muscles. Modified radical mastectomy removes the breast and the axillary lymph nodes. Radical mastectomy removes the breast, pectoralis major and minor, and the axillary lymph nodes (the use of radical mastectomy has declined).

Postmastectomy, reconstructive surgery can create a breast mound if the patient desires it and doesn't demonstrate evidence of advanced disease. Additional surgery to modify hormone production may include oophorectomy, adrenalectomy, and hypophysectomy (with the latter two procedures, the patient is required to take daily cortisone supplements permanently).

Chemotherapy:
Various drug combinations are being used, either as adjuvant therapy (when no evidence of metastasis exists) or as primary therapy (when metastasis has occurred), based on a number of factors, including the patient's pre- or postmenopausal status. The most commonly used drugs are cyclophosphamide, 5-fluorouracil, methotrexate, doxorubicin, vincristine, and prednisone. A common combination of such drugs, for example, is cyclophosphamide, methotrexate, and 5-fluorouracil (or CMF); it's used in both pre- and postmenopausal women.

Radiation therapy:
Primary radiation therapy *after* tumor removal has been effective only for small tumors in early stages, with no evidence of metastasis; it's also used to prevent or treat local recurrence.

Other methods:
Breast cancer patients may also receive estrogen, progesterone, or androgen therapy; or anti-estrogen therapy, specifically tamoxifen—a new drug with few side effects, which inhibits DNA syn-

---

PATIENT TEACHING AID

Preventing Infection After Axillary Node Dissection

Dear Patient:
Because edema makes tissue especially vulnerable to injury, take special care of the arm and hand on the surgical side.

Some don'ts
• Don't hold a cigarette in the affected hand.
• Don't use it to carry your purse or anything heavy.
• Don't wear a wristwatch or other jewelry on it.
• Don't cut or pick at cuticles or hangnails.
• Don't work near thorny plants or dig in the garden, without heavy gloves.
• Don't reach into a hot oven with it.
• Don't permit injection into it.
• Don't permit blood to be drawn from it.

• Don't allow your blood pressure to be taken on it.

Some do's
• Do wear a loose rubber glove on this hand when washing dishes.
• Do wear a thimble when sewing.
• Do apply lanolin hand cream daily if your skin is dry.
• Do wear your Life Guard Medical Aid tag engraved with CAUTION OR PREVENT—LYMPHEDEMA ARM—NO TESTS—NO HYPOS.
• Do contact your doctor immediately if your arm gets red, feels warm, or is unusually hard or swollen.
• Do elevate your arm if it feels heavy.
• Do show this hand care sheet to your surgeon.

This patient teaching aid is intended for distribution to patients by doctors and nurses.
It should not be used without a doctor's approval.
Information courtesy of the Cleveland Clinic, Department of Physical Medicine and Rehabilitation.

POSTOPERATIVE ARM AND HAND CARE

Hand exercises for the patient who is prone to lymphedema can begin on the day of surgery. The doctor should help plan arm exercises, because he can anticipate potential problems with the suture line.
- The patient should open her hand and close it tightly six to eight times every 3 hours while she's awake.
- Her arm on the affected side should be elevated on a pillow above her heart.
- The patient should be encouraged to wash her face and comb her hair—an effective exercise.
- The circumference of the patient's arm must be measured and recorded 2¼" (6 cm) from her elbow. The exact place measured should be indicated. By remeasuring at that exact place at regular intervals it can be determined whether lymphedema is present.
The patient may complain that her arm is heavy—an early sign of lymphedema.
- When the patient is home, she can elevate her arm and hand by supporting it on the back of a chair or a couch.

thesis. Tamoxifen is used in postmenopausal women and is most effective against estrogen-receptor positive tumors. Marijuana may relieve nausea and vomiting caused by some drugs, but this treatment is controversial due to legal questions.

Additional considerations

To provide good care for a breast cancer patient, a health care professional should begin with a history, assess the patient's feelings about her illness, and determine what she knows about it and what she expects.

A woman should not go to surgery expecting removal of a lump and wake up to find that one of her breasts has been removed. Preoperatively, the patient must be told what kind of surgery she is going to have. If the surgery is to be a mastectomy, in addition to the usual preoperative preparation (skin prepa-

rations, not allowing the patient anything by mouth), the patient should be told:
- to deep breathe and cough, to prevent pulmonary problems. She must not suppress full inhalation to avoid pain in the incision. She'll be given adequate pain medication to control it. Remember: pain relief is essential for the patient's well-being.
- to further ease her pain by lying on the affected side, or by placing a hand or pillow on the incision. (Preoperatively, she should be shown where the incision will be.) A small pillow placed anteriorly under the arm may provide increased comfort for the patient.
- to rotate her ankles to help prevent thromboembolism.
- she may move about and get out of bed as soon as possible (even as soon as the anesthesia wears off or the first evening after surgery).
- after mastectomy, an incisional drain or some type of suction (Hemovac) is used to remove accumulated serous, sanguineous fluid from the site and to keep the tension off the suture line.

To provide good postoperative care, a health care professional should:
- inspect the dressing anteriorly and posteriorly, and report excessive bleeding promptly.
- measure and record the amount and color of drainage. The drainage is bloody during the first 4 hours and then becomes serous.
- monitor circulatory status (blood pressure, pulse, respirations, and bleeding).
- monitor intake and output for at least 48 hours after general anesthesia.
- prevent lymphedema of the arm. This may be a complication of any treatment of breast cancer involving lymph node dissection. The patient can prevent this by exercising her hand and arm, and by avoiding activities that might cause infection in this hand or arm (infection increases the chance of developing lymphedema). Such prevention is very important, because lymphedema can't be treated effectively.

- inspect the incision and encourage the patient and her husband to look at her incision as soon as feasible, perhaps when the first dressing is removed.
- advise the patient about reconstructive surgery. She should ask her doctor, or call the local or state medical society for the names of plastic reconstructive surgeons who regularly perform surgery to create breast mounds. Such reconstruction may be done at the same time as the mastectomy.
- instruct the patient about the prosthesis she will wear. The American Cancer Society's Reach to Recovery group can provide instruction, emotional support, and a list of area stores that sell prostheses.
- give psychologic support. Many patients react to the fear of cancer and to disfigurement, and worry about loss of sexual function. Breast surgery doesn't interfere with sexual function; the patient may resume sexual activity as soon as she wants to after surgery.

The patient may experience "phantom breast syndrome" (a temporary phenomenon in which a tingling or a pins-and-needles sensation is felt in the area of the amputated breast tissue) or depression following mastectomy. The health care professional should listen, offer support, and refer the patient to an appropriate organization, such as the American Cancer Society, and Reach to Recovery—which run caring and sharing groups to help breast cancer patients in the hospital and at home.

ABDOMEN AND PELVIS

Gastric Carcinoma

Gastric carcinoma is common throughout the world and affects all races; however, unexplained geographic and cultural differences in incidence occur; for example, mortality rates are high in Japan, Iceland, Chile, and Austria. In the United States, during the past 25 years, incidence has decreased 50%, with the resulting death rate from gastric carcinoma one third that of 30 years ago. Incidence is higher in males over 30. Prognosis depends on the stage of the disease at the time of diagnosis; however, overall, the 5-year survival rate is approximately 10%.

Causes

The cause of gastric carcinoma is unknown, but predisposing factors include gastritis with gastric atrophy, achlorhydria, hypochlorhydria, and pernicious anemia. Polyps and chronic ulcers are occasionally associated with carcinoma of the stomach, but the data linking them is insubstantial. (Apparently, no correlation exists between duodenal ulcers and carcinoma of the stomach.) Genetic factors have also been implicated, since this disease occurs more frequently among people with type A blood than among those with type O; similarly, it occurs more frequently in people with a family history of such carcinoma. Dietary factors also seem related, including types of food preparation, physical properties of some foods, and certain methods of food preservation (especially smoking, pickling, or salting).

The parts of the stomach affected by gastric carcinoma, listed in order of decreasing frequency, are the pylorus and antrum, the lesser curvature, the cardia, the body of the stomach, and the greater curvature.

Gastric carcinoma infiltrates rapidly to regional lymph nodes, omentum, liver, and lungs by the following routes: walls of the stomach, duodenum, and esophagus; lymphatic system; adjacent organs; bloodstream; and peritoneal cavity.

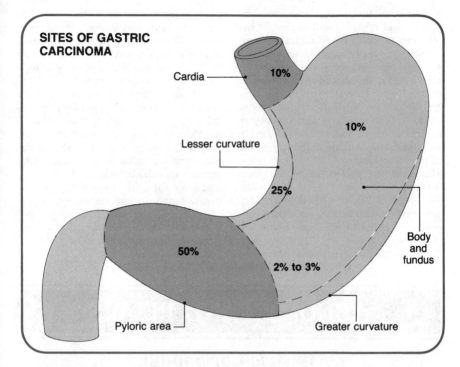

SITES OF GASTRIC CARCINOMA

Cardia — 10%

10%

Lesser curvature

25%

50%

2% to 3%

Body and fundus

Pyloric area —

Greater curvature

The decrease in the frequency of gastric carcinoma during the past 25 years in the United States has been attributed, without proof, to the improved and well-balanced diets most Americans enjoy from infancy through adulthood.

Signs and symptoms

Early clues to gastric cancer are chronic dyspepsia and epigastric discomfort, followed in later stages by weight loss, anorexia, feeling of fullness after eating, anemia, and fatigue. If the carcinoma is in the cardia, the first symptom may be dysphagia, and later vomiting (often coffee grounds vomitus). Affected patients may also have blood in their stools.

The course of gastric cancer may be insidious or fulminating. Unfortunately, the patient typically treats himself with antacids until the symptoms of advanced stages appear.

Diagnosis

Diagnosis depends primarily on reinvestigations of any persistent or recurring gastrointestinal changes and complaints. To rule out other conditions producing similar symptoms, diagnostic evaluation must include the testing of blood, stool, and stomach fluid samples.

Diagnosis of carcinoma of the stomach often requires these studies:
• *Barium X-rays of the GI tract, with fluoroscopy* show changes (tumor or filling defect in the outline of the stomach; loss of flexibility and distensibility; and abnormal gastric mucosa with or without ulceration).
• *Gastroscopy with fiberoptic endoscopy* helps rule out other diffuse gastric mucosal abnormalities by allowing direct visualization and gastroscopic biopsy to evaluate gastric mucosal lesions.
• *Photography with fiberoptic endoscope* provides a permanent record of gastric lesions that can later be used to determine disease progression and effect of treatment.

Certain other studies may rule out specific organ metastases: chest X-rays, liver and bone scans, and liver biopsy.

Treatment

Surgery is often the treatment of choice. Excision of the lesion with appropriate margins is possible in over one third of patients. Even in patients whose disease isn't considered surgically curable, resection offers palliation and improves potential benefits from chemotherapy and radiation.

The nature and extent of the lesion determine what kind of surgery is most appropriate. Common surgical procedures include subtotal gastric resection (subtotal gastrectomy) and total gastric resection (total gastrectomy). When carcinoma involves the pylorus and antrum, gastric resection removes the lower stomach and duodenum (gastrojejunostomy or Billroth II). If metastasis has occurred, the omentum and spleen may also have to be removed.

If gastric cancer has spread to the liver, peritoneum, or lymph glands, palliative surgery may include gastrostomy, jejunostomy, or a gastric or partial gastric resection. Such surgery may temporarily relieve vomiting, nausea, pain, and dysphagia, while allowing enteral nutrition to continue.

Chemotherapy for gastrointestinal malignancies may help to control symptoms and prolong survival. Adenocarcinoma of the stomach has responded to several agents including 5-fluorouracil, BCNU, and doxorubicin. Antiemetics can control nausea, which increases as the malignancy grows. In later stages, sedatives and tranquilizers may be necessary to control overwhelming anxiety. Narcotics are often necessary to relieve pain. However, morphine itself may produce nausea, so a synthetic derivative has been used more often recently.

Radiation has not been highly effective against carcinoma of the stomach but is still used occasionally. It should be given on an empty stomach, and shouldn't be used preoperatively, since it may damage viscera and impede healing.

Patients for whom extensive spread of malignancy rules out surgery may benefit from a medical regimen. Antispasmodics and antacids may relieve distress.

Additional considerations

Before surgery, the patient should be prepared for its effects and for postsurgical procedures, such as having a nasogastric tube in place for drainage, and getting intravenous feedings.

While the patient who is having a partial gastric resection may eventually be able to eat normally, the patient who is having a total gastrectomy must prepare for a slow recovery and only partial return to a normal diet.

The patient must understand the importance of changing position every 2 hours and of deep breathing.

After surgery, meticulous supportive care is needed to promote recovery and prevent complications. The family should be included in all phases of the patient's care.

Following any type of gastrectomy, pulmonary complications may result. The patient may need oxygen postoperatively. He should cough, deep breathe, and be turned hourly. These actions, along with judicious use of analgesic narcotics (which depress respiration), may prevent pulmonary problems. If the patient isn't able to breathe effectively on his own, intermittent positive pressure breathing (IPPB) or incentive spirometry breathing may help. Proper patient positioning is important; the semi-Fowler's position facilitates breathing and drainage.

After gastrectomy, little (if any) drainage comes from the nasogastric tube,

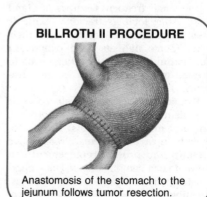

BILLROTH II PROCEDURE

Anastomosis of the stomach to the jejunum follows tumor resection.

DUMPING SYNDROME

After gastric resection, rapid emptying of gastric contents into the small intestine produces the following:

• *Early dumping syndrome,* which may be mild or severe, occurs a few minutes after eating and lasts up to 45 minutes. Onset is sudden, with nausea, weakness, sweating, palpitations, dizziness, flushing, borborygmi, explosive diarrhea, and increased blood pressure and pulse rate.

• *Late dumping syndrome,* which is less serious, occurs 2 to 3 hours after eating. Similar symptoms include profuse sweating, anxiety, fine tremor of the hands and legs accompanied by vertigo, exhaustion, lassitude, palpitations, throbbing headache, faintness, sensation of hunger, glycosuria, and marked decrease in blood pressure and blood sugar.

These symptoms may persist for 1 year after surgery or for the rest of the patient's life.

---

because no secretions form after the stomach is removed. Since the stomach's storage function has been eliminated, the patient often suffers from a dumping syndrome. In addition, intrinsic factor, manufactured in the stomach lining, is absent. This causes malabsorption of vitamin B_{12}. To prevent vitamin B_{12} deficiency, the patient needs to replace this vitamin, as well as an iron supplement, the rest of his life.

During radiation treatment, the patient needs to eat high-calorie, well-balanced meals. Fluids, such as orange juice, grapefruit juice, or ginger ale, will minimize nausea and vomiting. Radiation side effects include: nausea, vomiting, hair loss, malaise, and diarrhea.

Patients who experience poor digestion and absorption after gastrectomy need a special diet: frequent feedings of small amounts of clear liquids, increasing to small frequent feedings of bland food. After total gastrectomy, patients must eat small meals for the rest of their lives. (Some patients need pancreatin and sodium bicarbonate after meals to prevent or control steatorrhea and dyspepsia.)

Wound dehiscence and delayed healing, stemming from decreased protein, anemia, and avitaminosis, occur frequently in cancer patients. Preoperative vitamin and protein replacement can prevent such complications. The wound must be checked regularly for redness, swelling, failure to heal, or warmth. Parenteral administration of vitamin C may improve wound healing.

Vitamin deficiency results from obstruction, diarrhea, or an inadequate diet. Ascorbic acid, thiamine, riboflavin, nicotinic acid, and vitamin K supplements may be beneficial. Good nutrition promotes weight gain, strength, independence, and positive emotional outlook, and promotes tolerance for surgery, radiotherapy, or chemotherapy. Aside from meeting caloric needs, good nutrition must provide adequate protein, fluid, and potassium intake to facilitate glycogen and protein synthesis. Anabolic agents, such as methandrostenolone, may induce nitrogen retention. Steroids, antidepressants, wine, or brandy may stimulate the appetite.

When all treatment has failed, care should concentrate on keeping the patient comfortable and free of unnecessary pain, and on providing as much psychologic support as possible. He should be encouraged to verbalize his feelings and fears. When he asks questions about his illness, they should be answered honestly. Evasive answers will make him retreat and feel isolated. Family members should be treated with the same honesty and understanding. They should let the patient talk about his future but, at the same time, encourage a realistic outlook.

If the patient is going home, he may need the services of a visiting nurse or homemaker, as well as furnishings for his sickroom (for example, a bedside commode or a walker).

Esophageal Cancer

Esophageal cancer usually develops in men over 60 years of age and is nearly always fatal. This disease occurs worldwide, but incidence varies geographically. It's most common in Japan, Russia, China, the Middle East, and in the Transkei region of South Africa, where esophageal cancer has reached almost epidemic proportions. More than 8,000 cases of esophageal cancer are reported annually in the United States alone.

Causes

The cause of esophageal cancer is unknown, but predisposing factors have been identified: chronic irritation, as in heavy smoking and excessive use of alcohol; stasis-induced inflammation, as in achalasia or stricture; previous head and neck tumors; and nutritional deficiency, as in untreated sprue and Plummer-Vinson syndrome. Esophageal tumors are usually fungating and infiltrating. Most arise in squamous cell epithelium; a few are adenocarcinomas; fewer still, melanomas and sarcomas.

About half the squamous cell cancers occur in the lower portion of the esophagus, about 40% in the midportion, and the remaining 10% in the upper or cervical esophagus. Regardless of cell type, prognosis for esophageal cancer is grim. Five-year survival rates don't exceed 10%.

In most cases, the tumor partially constricts the lumen of the esophagus. Regional metastasis occurs early, by way of submucosal lymphatics, and often fatally invades adjacent vital intrathoracic organs. Direct invasion of adjoining structures may lead to dramatic complications: mediastinitis, tracheo- or bronchioesophageal fistulas (causing an overwhelming cough induced by swallowing liquids); or aortic perforation with sudden exsanguination. If the patient survives primary extension, the liver and lungs are the usual sites of distant metastasis. Rarer sites of metastasis include bone, kidneys, and adrenals.

Signs and symptoms

Dysphagia and weight loss are the most common presenting symptoms. At first,
dysphagia is usually mild and intermittent, occurring only after ingestion of solid food (especially meat). Before long, however, dysphagia becomes constant, with pain on swallowing, hoarseness, coughing, and glossopharyngeal neuralgia. In later stages, signs of esophageal obstruction appear—sialorrhea, nocturnal aspiration, regurgitation, and inability to swallow even liquids. Cachexia usually develops.

Diagnosis

X-rays of the esophagus, with barium swallow and motility studies, reveal structural and filling defects and reduced peristalsis.

 Endoscopic examination of the esophagus, punch and brush biopsies, and exfoliative cytologic tests confirm esophageal tumors.

Treatment

Whenever possible, treatment includes resection to maintain a passageway for food. This often involves radical surgery, such as esophagogastrectomy with jejunal or colonic bypass grafts. Palliative surgery may include a feeding gastrostomy. Treatment also consists of radiation; chemotherapy with, for example, bleomycin; or installation of prosthetic tubes (such as the Mousseau Barbin or Celestin tubes), to bridge the tumor and alleviate dysphagia. Unfortunately, none of these methods is completely successful. Surgery can cause its own complications (anastomotic leak, fistula formation, pneumonia, empyema, malnutrition); radiation can cause esophageal perforation, pneumonitis and fibrosis of the lungs, or myelitis of the spinal cord; and prosthetic tubes can become blocked or dislodged, causing a perforation of the mediastinum, or can precipitate tumor erosion.

Additional considerations

Before surgery, a health care professional should answer the patient's questions and let him know what to expect during surgery and afterwards.

After surgery, a health care professional should monitor vital signs, report any unexpected changes, and, if surgery has included an anastomosis, position the patient flat on his back to prevent tension on the suture line.

The primary goal in caring for the esophageal cancer patient is to promote adequate nutrition. Good nutritional care includes:
• assessing the patient's nutritional and hydrational status for possible supplementary parenteral feedings.
• preventing aspiration of food by plac-

ing the patient in Fowler's position for meals and allowing plenty of time to eat.
• providing high-calorie, high-protein, blenderized food, as needed.
• since the patient will probably regurgitate some food, cleaning his mouth carefully after each meal and keeping mouthwash handy.
• if the patient has a gastrostomy tube, giving food slowly—by gravity—in prescribed amounts (usually 200 to 500 ml); offering something to chew before each feeding (this promotes gastric secretions and provides some semblance of normal eating); encouraging the patient's family to participate in the feedings; instructing the family in the care of the gastrostomy tube (checking to see that the tube is patent before each feeding, providing skin care around the tube, having the patient remain upright during and after feedings).
• providing emotional support for the patient and family; referring them to appropriate organizations such as the American Cancer Society.

Pancreatic Cancer

Second only to cancer of the colon as the deadliest gastrointestinal cancer, pancreatic cancer now ranks fourth among all fatal carcinomas. Prognosis is poor, and most patients die within a year after diagnosis.

Tumors of the pancreas are almost always adenocarcinomas, and arise most frequently (2 out of 3) in the head of the pancreas. Rarer tumors are those of the body and tail of the pancreas and islet cell tumor. The two main tissue types of pancreatic cancer, both of which form fibrotic nodes, are cylinder cell (which arises in ducts and degenerates into cysts) and large, fatty, granular cell (which arises in parenchyma).

Causes and incidence

Pancreatic adenocarcinoma occurs most often among Blacks, particularly in men between ages 35 and 70. Geographically, incidence of pancreatic cancer is highest in Israel, the United States, Sweden, and Canada; lowest in Switzerland, Belgium, and Italy.

Evidence suggests that pancreatic cancer is linked to inhalation or absorption of carcinogens which are then excreted

by the pancreas:
• cigarette smoking—pancreatic cancer is three to four times more common among smokers
• diets high in fat and protein—induce chronic hyperplasia of the pancreas with increased turnover of cells
• food additives
• exposure to industrial chemicals, such as beta-naphthalene, benzidine, and urea.

TYPES OF PANCREATIC CANCER

PATHOLOGY	CLINICAL FEATURES
Head of pancreas • Often obstructs ampulla of Vater and common bile duct • Directly metastasizes to duodenum • Adhesions anchor tumor to spine, stomach, and intestines.	• Jaundice (predominant symptom)—slowly progressive, unremitting; may cause skin (especially of the face and genitals) to turn olive green or black • Pruritus—often severe • Weight loss—rapid and severe (as great as 30 lbs [13.6 kg]); may lead to emaciation, weakness, and muscle atrophy • Slowed digestion, gastric distention, nausea, diarrhea, and steatorrhea with clay-colored stools • Liver and gallbladder enlargement from lymph node metastasis to biliary tract and duct wall results in compression and obstruction; gallbladder may be palpable (Courvoisier's sign). • Dull, nondescript, continuous abdominal pain radiating to upper right quadrant; relieved by bending forward • GI hemorrhage and biliary infection common
Body and tail of pancreas • Large nodular masses become fixed to retropancreatic tissues and spine. • Direct invasion of spleen, left kidney, suprarenal gland, diaphragm • Involvement of celiac plexus results in thrombosis of splenic vein and spleen infarction.	**Body** • Pain (predominant symptom)—usually epigastric, develops slowly and radiates to back; relieved by bending forward or sitting up; intensified by lying supine; most intense 3 to 4 hours after eating; when celiac plexus is involved, pain is more intense and lasts longer • Venous thrombosis and thrombophlebitis—frequent; may precede other symptoms by months • Splenomegaly (from infarction), hepatomegaly (occasionally), and jaundice (rarely) **Tail** Symptoms result from metastasis: • Abdominal tumor (most common finding) produces a palpable abdominal mass; abdominal pain radiates to left hypochondrium and left chest. • Anorexia leads to weight loss, emaciation, and weakness. • Splenomegaly and upper GI bleeding

Other possible predisposing factors are chronic pancreatitis, diabetes mellitus, and chronic alcohol abuse.

Signs and symptoms

The most common features of pancreatic carcinoma are weight loss and abdominal or low back pain. Other generalized symptoms include fever, skin lesions (usually on the legs), and emotional disturbances, such as depression, anxiety, and premonition of fatal illness.

Diagnosis

Definitive diagnosis requires a laparotomy with a biopsy. However, a biopsy may miss relatively small or deep-seated cancerous tissue or create a pancreatic fistula. Other tests that suggest cancer include:

• *X-rays*—retroperitoneal insufflation, cholangiography, scintillagraphy, and particularly, barium swallow (to locate neoplasm and detect changes in the duodenum or stomach relating to carcinoma of the head of the pancreas)

• *ultrasound*—can identify a mass but not its histology

• *CAT scan*—similar to ultrasound but shows greater detail

• *angiography*—shows vascular supply of tumor

• *endoscopic retrograde cannulization of the pancreas* (ERCP) *or endoscopic pancreatography*—allows visualization, instillation of contrast medium, and possible specimen

• *secretin test*—shows absence of pancreatic enzymes; suggests pancreatic duct obstruction and tumors of body and tail.

ISLET CELL TUMORS

Relatively uncommon, islet cell tumors (insulinomas) may be benign or malignant and produce symptoms in three stages:
1. *Slight hypoglycemia*—fatigue, restlessness, malaise, and excessive weight gain
2. *Compensatory secretion of epinephrine*—pallor, clamminess, perspiration, palpitations, finger tremors, hunger, decreased temperature, increased pulse and blood pressure

3. *Severe hypoglycemia*—ataxia, clouded sensorium, diplopia, episodes of violence and hysteria.
   Usually, insulinomas metastasize to the liver alone but may metastasize to bone, brain, and lungs. Death results from a combination of hypoglycemic reactions and wide dissemination of the neoplasm. Treatment consists of enucleation of tumor (if benign) and resection to include pancreatic tissue (if malignant).

Laboratory values supporting this diagnosis include increased carcinoembryonic antigen (CEA) and serum bilirubin, serum amylase-lipase (occasionally elevated); prolonged prothrombin time; SGOT and SGPT (elevation of enzymes indicates necrosis of liver cells); alkaline phosphatase (marked elevation with biliary obstruction); plasma insulin immunoassay (shows measurable serum insulin in presence of islet cell tumors); hemoglobin/hematocrit (may show mild anemia); fasting blood sugar (hypoglycemia, hyperglycemia); and stools (occult blood with ulceration in GI tract or ampulla of Vater).

Treatment
Treatment of pancreatic cancer is rarely successful, because this disease is often widely metastasized at diagnosis. Therapy consists of surgery, and possibly, radiation and chemotherapy.

Small advances have been made in the survival rate with surgery:
• Total pancreatectomy has perhaps increased survival time by resecting a localized tumor or by controlling postop gastric ulceration.
• Cholecystojejunostomy, choledochoduodenostomy, and choledochojejunostomy have partially replaced radical resection to bypass obstructing common bile duct extensions, and thereby ease jaundice and pruritus. They aim to improve the quality of survival.
• Whipple's procedure, or pancreatico-

duodenectomy, has a high mortality rate, but can obtain wide lymphatic clearance except with tumors located near the portal vein, superior mesenteric vein and artery, and celiac axis. This rarely used procedure removes the head of the pancreas, duodenum, and portions of the body and tail of pancreas, stomach, jejunum, pancreatic duct, and distal portion of the bile duct.
• Gastrojejunostomy is performed if radical resection isn't indicated and duodenal obstruction is expected to develop later.

Although pancreatic carcinoma generally responds poorly to chemotherapy, recent studies using combinations of carmustine (BCNU), 5-fluorouracil, and doxorubicin show a trend toward longer survival time. Other medications used in pancreatic cancer include:
• antibiotics (oral, I.V., or I.M.)—prevent infection and relieve symptoms
• anticholinergics—particularly propantheline, decrease GI tract spasm and motility, and reduce pain and secretions
• antacids (oral or by nasogastric tube)—decrease secretions of pancreatic enzymes by neutralizing acid from gastric contents; they also suppress peptic activity and thereby reduce stress-induced damage to gastric mucosa
• diuretics—mobilize extracellular fluid from ascites
• insulin—provides adequate exogenous insulin supply after pancreatic resection

• narcotics—relieve pain; but since morphine, meperidine, and codeine can lead to biliary tract spasm and increase common bile duct pressure, they're used only after other analgesics fail

• pancreatic enzymes—(average dose 0.5 to 1 mg with meals) assist digestion of proteins, carbohydrates, and fats when pancreatic juices are insufficient due to surgery or obstruction.

Radiation therapy is usually ineffective except when used as an adjunct to 5-fluorouracil chemotherapy; then it may prolong survival time from 4 to 9 months. It can also ease the pain associated with nonresectable tumors.

Additional considerations

Supportive health care can prevent surgical complications, increase patient comfort, and help the patient and his family cope with inevitable death.

Before surgery, a hospital staff member should:

• ensure that the patient is medically stable, particularly regarding nutrition (this may take 4 to 5 days). If the patient can't tolerate oral feedings, total parenteral nutrition and I.V. fat emulsions can be used to correct deficiencies and maintain positive nitrogen balance.

• give blood transfusions (to combat anemia), vitamin K (to overcome prothrombin deficiency), antibiotics (to prevent postoperative complications), and gastric lavage (to maintain gastric decompression), as ordered.

• tell the patient about expected postop procedures and expected side effects of radiation and chemotherapy.

After surgery, a staff member should:

• watch for and report complications, such as fistula, pancreatitis, fluid and electrolyte imbalance, infection, hemorrhage, skin breakdown, nutritional deficiency, hepatic failure, renal insufficiency, and diabetes.

• watch for and treat chemotherapy's toxic effects, if applicable.

Throughout the illness, to provide meticulous supportive care, the staff member should:

• monitor fluid balance, abdominal girth, metabolic state, and weight daily; replace nutrients I.V., P.O., or with a nasogastric tube if weight loss occurs; impose dietary restrictions, such as a low-sodium or fluid retention diet, if weight gain (due to ascites) occurs, maintaining a 2,500-calorie/day diet.

• serve small, frequent meals; consult the dietitian in planning meals to ensure proper nutrition, make mealtimes as pleasant as possible; administer an oral pancreatic enzyme at mealtimes, if needed; give an antacid to prevent stress ulcers, if needed.

• prevent constipation by administering laxatives, stool softeners, and cathartics, as ordered; modify diet; and increase fluid intake.

• increase GI motility by positioning the patient properly during and after meals, and assisting him with walking when he's able.

• ensure adequate rest and sleep (with a sedative, if warranted); assist with range-of-motion exercises and isometrics; make sure the patient rests after exertion.

• administer analgesics for pain, and antibiotics and antipyretics for fever, as ordered; note time, site (if injected), and response.

• observe closely for signs of hypoglycemia or hyperglycemia; administer glucose or a hypoglycemic agent, such as tolbutamide, as ordered; monitor blood glucose concentration, urine sugar, acetone, and response to treatment; document progression of jaundice.

• provide scrupulous skin care to avoid pruritus and necrosis; keep skin clean and dry; prevent excoriation in severe proritus by clipping his nails and persuading him to wear light, cotton gloves.

• watch for signs of upper GI bleeding; hematest stools and emesis; maintain flow sheet of frequent hemoglobin/hematocrit determinations; control active bleeding by promoting gastric vasoconstriction with medication and iced saline lavage through a nasogastric or duodenal tube; replace any fluid loss; ease discomfort from pyloric obstruction with a nasogastric tube.

- prevent thrombosis by applying anti-embolism stockings and assisting in range-of-motion exercises; treat thrombosis by elevating legs, applying moist heat to thrombus site and giving an anticoagulant or aspirin, as ordered, to prevent further clot formation and pulmonary embolus.
- provide psychologic support; encourage the patient to verbalize his fears; promote family involvement; offer the assistance of a chaplain or psychologist; stay in touch with the patient and his feelings to help him and his family deal with the impending reality of death; examine and work out personal feelings about death to provide maximum support to the dying patient.

Colorectal Cancer

Colorectal cancer is the third most common visceral neoplasm in the United States and in Europe. Incidence is equally distributed between men and women.

Colorectal malignant tumors are almost always adenocarcinomas. About half of these are sessile lesions of the rectosigmoid area; the rest are polypoid lesions.

Colorectal cancer tends to progress slowly and remains localized for a long time. Consequently, it's potentially curable in 80% to 90% of patients if early diagnosis allows resection before nodal involvement. With improved diagnosis, the overall 5-year survival rate is nearing 50%.

Causes

The exact cause of colorectal cancer is unknown, but studies showing concentration in areas of higher economic development suggest a relationship to diet (excess animal fat, particularly beef, and low fiber). Other factors that magnify the risk of developing colorectal cancer include:

- other diseases of the digestive tract.
- age (over 40).
- history of ulcerative colitis (average interval before onset of cancer is 11 to 17 years).
- familial polyposis (cancer almost always develops by age 50).

Signs and symptoms

Symptoms of colorectal cancer result from local obstruction and, in later stages, from direct extension to adjacent organs (bladder, prostate, ureters, vagina, sacrum) and distant metastasis (usually liver and lungs). In the early stages, symptoms are typically vague, and depend on the anatomical location and function of the bowel segment containing the tumor. Later, they generally include pallor, cachexia, ascites, hepatomegaly, or lymphadenopathy.

On the right side of the colon (which absorbs water and electrolytes), early tumor growth causes no signs of obstruction, since it tends to grow along the bowel rather than surround the lumen and the fecal content in this area is normally liquid. It may, however, cause black, tarry stools; anemia; and abdominal aching, pressure, or dull cramps. As the disease progresses, the patient develops weakness, fatigue, exertional dyspnea, vertigo, and eventually, diarrhea, obstipation, anorexia, weight loss, vomiting, and other signs of intestinal obstruction. In addition, a tumor on the right side may be palpable.

On the left side, a tumor causes signs of an obstruction even in early stages, since in this area stools are of a formed consistency. It commonly causes rectal bleeding (often ascribed to hemorrhoids), intermittent abdominal fullness or cramping, and rectal pressure. As the disease progresses, the patient develops obstipation, diarrhea, or "ribbon" or pencil-shaped stools. Typically, he notices that passage of a stool or flatus relieves the pain. At this stage, bleeding from the colon becomes obvious, with dark or bright red blood in the feces and mucus in or on the stools.

With a rectal tumor, the first symptom is a change in bowel habits, often beginning with an urgent need to defecate on arising ("morning diarrhea") or obstipation alternating with diarrhea. Other signs are blood or mucus in stool and a sense of incomplete evacuation. Late in the disease, pain begins as a feeling of rectal fullness that later becomes a dull, and sometimes constant, ache confined to the rectum or sacral region.

Diagnosis

Only tumor biopsy can verify colorectal cancer, but other tests help detect it:

• *Digital examination* can detect almost 50% of tumors in the anus, rectum, or lower sigmoid.

• *Hemoccult test* (guaiac) can detect blood in stools.

• *Proctoscopy or sigmoidoscopy* can detect more than 50% of colorectal cancers.

• *Colonoscopy* permits visual inspection (and photographs) of the colon up to the ileocecal valve, and gives access for polypectomies and biopsies of suspected lesions.

• *Intravenous pyelography* verifies bilateral renal function and checks for any displacement of the kidneys, ureters, or bladder.

• *Barium X-ray,* utilizing a dual contrast with air, can locate lesions undetectable manually or visually. Barium examination should *follow* endoscopy or intravenous pyelography, because the barium interferes with these tests.

• *Carcinoembryonic antigen (CEA),* though not specific or sensitive enough for early diagnosis, is helpful in monitoring patients before and after treatment to detect metastasis or recurrence.

Treatment

The most effective treatment for colorectal cancer is surgery to remove the malignant tumor and adjacent tissues, and any lymph nodes that may contain cancer cells. The type of surgery depends on the location of the tumor:

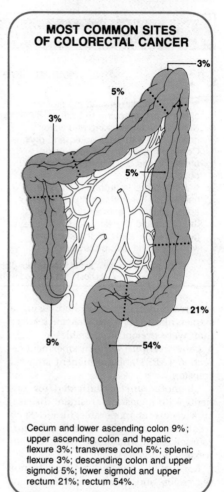

MOST COMMON SITES OF COLORECTAL CANCER

3%
5%
3%
5%
21%
9%
54%

Cecum and lower ascending colon 9%; upper ascending colon and hepatic flexure 3%; transverse colon 5%; splenic flexure 3%; descending colon and upper sigmoid 5%; lower sigmoid and upper rectum 21%; rectum 54%.

• *Cecum and ascending colon*—right hemicolectomy (for advanced disease) may include resection of the terminal segment of the ileum, cecum, ascending colon, and right half of the transverse colon with corresponding mesentery

• *Proximal and middle transverse colon*—right colectomy to include transverse colon and mesentery corresponding to midcolic vessels, or segmental resection of transverse colon and associated midcolic vessels

• *Sigmoid colon*—surgery is usually limited to sigmoid colon and mesentery

• *Upper rectum*—anterior or low ante-

PATIENT TEACHING AID

How to Care for a Stoma

• Keep the skin around the stoma clean after removing the pouch by washing with mild soap and water, rinsing well with clear water, and drying. Coat the skin with a silicone skin protector and cover with a collection pouch.
• Keep the skin around the stoma unirritated. For irritation and breakdown, apply a layer of antacid precipitate to the clean and dry skin, dust with karaya gum powder, allow to dry, and coat with a silicone skin protector.

• Measure the stoma, and prepare the face plate of the pouch to clear the stoma, with a ⅛" (3.2 mm) margin.
• Protect the skin from the effluent and abrasiveness of the adhesive.
• Cut the opening in the barrier the same size as the stoma to prevent skin irritation.
• Check the pouch frequently to make sure the skin seal is still intact.
• Control odor within the pouch with any of the commercial products available.

This patient teaching aid is intended for distribution to patients by doctors and nurses.
It should not be used without a doctor's approval.

---

rior resection (newer method, using a stapler, allows for resections much lower than were previously possible)
• *Lower rectum*—abdominoperineal resection (APR) and permanent sigmoid colostomy.

Chemotherapy is indicated for patients with metastasis, residual disease, or a recurrent inoperable tumor. Such treatment commonly includes 5-fluorouracil, lomustine, mitomycin, methotrexate, and vincristine.

Radiation therapy induces tumor regression and may be used before or after surgery. Immunotherapy using BCG (bacille Calmette-Guérin) vaccine is still experimental.

Additional considerations

Before colorectal surgery, the patient will need diet modifications, laxatives, enemas, and antibiotics—all used to cleanse the bowel and to decrease abdominal and perineal cavity contamination during surgery. If the patient is to have a colostomy, he and his family should be taught what they need to know about the procedure, such as:
• how the stoma will appear: red, moist, and swollen; how postoperative swelling will eventually subside.

• how the intestine looks before and after surgery; how much of the bowel remains intact. (Helpful instruction booklets are available for a fee from the United Ostomy Association and free from various ostomy supply companies.)
• how other ostomates function; a postsurgical visit from a recovered ostomate may help.
• what the patient will return from the operating room with: I.V.s, nasogastric tube, and Foley catheter.
• how important it is for him to cooperate during coughing and deep breathing exercises.

After surgery, the patient's family must be aware of how their positive reactions will affect the patient's adjustment. An enterostomal therapist, if available, can help set up a regimen for the patient.

The patient should look at the stoma and participate in its care as soon as possible. He must learn good hygiene and skin care. He may shower or bathe as soon as the incision heals. The patient with a sigmoid colostomy should learn how to do his own irrigation 5 to 7 days after surgery. He should schedule colostomy irrigation for the time of day when he normally evacuated before the colostomy surgery. Many find that irrigating every other day or every third day is sufficient for regulation. If flatus, diarrhea, or constipation occurs, suspected causative foods can be eliminated from the patient's diet.

After several months, many ostomates establish control with irrigation and no longer need to wear a pouch. A stoma cap or gauze sponge placed over the stoma protects it and absorbs mucoid secretions.

Before achieving such control, the patient can resume physical activities, including sports, providing there is no threat of injury to the stoma or surrounding abdominal muscles. He can place a pouch or stoma cap (if regulated) over the stoma when swimming. However, he should permanently avoid heavy lifting, as herniation may occur through weakened muscles in the abdominal wall.

A visiting nurse should call on the patient at home to check on his physical care. Sexual counseling may be appropriate for male patients; most are impotent after an APR, and suffer fear of rejection.

Anyone who has had colorectal cancer runs an increased risk of developing another primary cancer, and should have yearly screening and follow-up testing, as well as a diet high in fiber (bulk).

Wilms' Tumor
(Congenital nephroblastoma, embryoma, adenomyosarcoma)

Wilms' tumor is a malignant mixed tumor of the kidneys, which occurs primarily in children. In fact, it's the most common intra-abdominal malignant tumor of childhood. With treatment, prognosis is good. Wilms' tumor has the highest survival rate of all childhood cancers: when the tumor is localized, the 5-year survival rate is 90%; after metastasis, it's 50%.

Causes and incidence
The cause of Wilms' tumor isn't known, but it's generally considered a developmental anomaly that forms in the embryo and then lies dormant for years. It's common in children with other congenital anomalies.

Wilms' tumor affects both sexes equally, and usually appears before age 7, with peak incidence occurring at 3 to 4 years. Commonly, it affects only one kidney, but 10% of the time affects both. This tumor tends to grow rapidly, and often becomes large enough to distend and rupture the kidney capsule and invade perirenal tissues, such as the large intestine, the liver, vena cava, or vertebrae.

Signs and symptoms
The most distinctive signs of Wilms' tumor are a firm, smooth, palpable abdominal mass in an enlarged abdomen, and commonly, hypertension and vomiting. Clinical effects include nonspecific abdominal pain (in 10% of patients), fever (in 20%), gross hematuria (in a few), and microscopic hematuria (in about 25%). Late-stage symptoms include pallor, weight loss, anorexia, and lethargy, indicating metastases, usually to the liver, lungs, bone, or brain.

Diagnosis
A large, palpable abdominal mass appearing during childhood suggests Wilms' tumor, but intravenous pyelography must rule out an extrarenal mass, especially neuroblastoma, which also often affects children. For the same reason, the doctor routinely orders a 24-hour urine specimen (increased catecholamines point to neuroblastoma, not Wilms' tumor) and a chest X-ray to check for pulmonary nodules. Some doctors routinely use venacavography, followed by intravenous pyelography to determine tumor size and possible extension into the vena cava or renal vein. Further diagnostic evaluation

STAGING WILMS' TUMOR

Stage I: Well-encapsulated tumor that can be removed surgically

Stage II: Extension of tumor beyond renal capsule into abdominal cavity; total removal by surgery still possible

Stage III: Extension of tumor beyond renal capsule into abdominal cavity to such an extent that it can't be totally removed by surgery

Stage IV: Distant metastasis to lungs, liver, bone, or brain

Stage V: Bilateral kidney metastasis

during resection, including histologic examination, rules out other intrarenal masses and allows accurate staging.

Treatment

Treatment depends on staging, and consists of tumor resection, radical nephrectomy, and excision of accessible metastatic sites, such as the adrenal glands; radiation therapy beginning within days of this surgery; and chemotherapy using vincristine, actinomycin D, doxorubicin, and possibly, cyclophosphamide.

Additional considerations

Good preparation, postoperative care, and supportive measures during radiation and chemotherapy can prevent complications and minimize side effects.

Before surgery, a health care professional should:
• *never* palpate the abdomen of a child or infant suspected of having Wilms' tumor, since Wilms' tumor tends to be fragile and can rupture and disseminate easily; use extreme caution when turning, burping, or otherwise handling the infant; warn his parents to use similar caution, and place a large sign over his bed to warn other staff members to do the same.
• prepare the child and his family psychologically by describing the surgery and other procedures. Such a child should have a primary nurse to assure continuity of care. If the child is old enough to understand, dolls and puppets or body outlines may help to explain the placement of tubes after surgery. He should be prepared for the size of the incision and dressing.
• encourage the parents and child to talk about their feelings; help the child play out some of his fears, using dolls or puppets; tell parents what side effects they should expect (such as alopecia), and realistically describe the benefits of radiation and chemotherapy.
• use a self-adhesive pediatric urine bag to facilitate collection of a 24-hour urine specimen if the child isn't toilet-trained.

After surgery, a health care professional should:
• accurately measure intake and output; watch for signs of circulatory overload, interstitial fluid accumulation, and diminished urinary output; monitor blood pressure; watch for infection.
• watch for signs of bone marrow depression (anemia, bleeding, and infection) and other side effects, throughout radiation and chemotherapy.
• give a mild analgesic (if necessary) and a stool softener, and monitor bowel sounds, since vincristine causes peripheral neuropathy (jaw and joint pain), constipation, and paralytic ileus; keep a record of bowel movements; watch for vomiting, bowel distention, and abdominal pain.
• check the radiation site daily for signs of burns or increased pigmentation, since actinomycin D may cause permanent skin damage; keep the site clean and dry.
• suggest that parents provide a wig or scarf for the child, since doxorubicin causes alopecia; monitor for signs of congestive heart failure, since doxorubicin is cardiotoxic in large doses.
• make sure his parents understand the importance of continuing chemotherapy and other outpatient treatment, before the child is discharged; tell them to notify the doctor of any changes in the child's condition and to try scheduling outpatient treatment so it doesn't interfere with school.

Kidney Cancer

(Nephrocarcinoma, renal cell carcinoma, hypernephroma, Grawitz's tumor)

Kidney cancer usually occurs in older adults and accounts for about 85% of all primary kidney cancers. Other kidney cancers include metastases from other primary-site carcinomas. Renal pelvic tumors and Wilms' tumor occur primarily in children.

Usually, kidney tumors, which may affect either kidney, are large, firm, nodular, encapsulated, unilateral, and solitary. Occasionally, they're bilateral or multifocal. Kidney cancer can be separated histologically into clear cell, granular, and spindle cell types. In the clear cell type, prognosis is sometimes considered better than it is for the other two types; in general, however, prognosis seems more dependent on the stage of the disease than on the type.

Prognosis has improved considerably, with the 5-year survival rate now at about 50% of patients, and the 10-year survival at 18% to 23% of patients.

Causes and incidence

The causes of kidney cancer aren't known. However, the incidence of this malignancy is rising, possibly as a result of exposure to environmental carcinogens as well as increased longevity. Even so, such cancer accounts for only about 2% of all adult cancers. Kidney cancer is twice as common in men as in women, and usually strikes after age 40, with peak incidence between ages 50 and 60.

Signs and symptoms

Kidney cancer produces a classic clinical triad: hematuria, pain, and a palpable mass. Any one of these may occur as the first sign of cancer. Microscopic or gross hematuria (which may be intermittent) often indicates that the cancer has spread to the renal pelvis. Constant abdominal or flank pain may be dull, or if the cancer causes bleeding or clot formation, acute and colicky. The palpable mass is generally smooth, firm, and nontender. All three major signs coexist in only about 10% of patients.

Other symptoms include fever (perhaps a result of hemorrhage or tumor necrosis); hypertension (a result of compression of the renal artery with renal parenchymal ischemia); rapidly progressing, and occasionally fatal, hypercalcemia (possibly due to ectopic parathyroid hormone production by the tumor); and urinary retention, from an obstructing blood clot. Weight loss, edema in the legs, nausea, and vomiting point to advanced disease.

Diagnosis

Studies to identify kidney cancer usually include intravenous pyelography, retrograde pyelography, ultrasound studies, cystoscopy (to rule out associated bladder cancer), and nephrotomography or renal angiography to distinguish a kidney cyst from a tumor. (In angiography, pooling of the contrast medium points to a tumor.)

STAGING KIDNEY CANCER

Stage I: Tumor confined to kidney

Stage II: Perirenal spread confined to Gerota's space (fascia around the kidney)

Stage III: Spread to renal vein or inferior vena cava, with or without lymphatic involvement

Stage IV: Advanced disease, with spread to adjacent organs (except for adrenal glands) or metastases, usually to distant lymph nodes, lungs, liver, and bone

NEPHROCARCINOMA

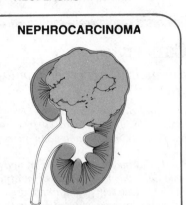

Tumors such as these in the upper kidney pole usually occur unilaterally.

Other relevant tests include liver function studies, showing increased alkaline phosphatase, bilirubin, transaminase, and prolonged prothrombin time. Such results may point to liver metastasis, but if the tumor hasn't metastasized, these abnormalities reverse after tumor resection.

Routine lab studies that show hematuria, anemia (unrelated to blood loss), polycythemia, hypercalcemia, and increased erythrocyte sedimentation rate (ESR) call for further testing to rule out kidney cancer.

Treatment

Radical nephrectomy, including regional lymph node dissection, offers the only chance of being cured for a patient with kidney cancer. Since this disease is radiation resistant, radiation is used only when the cancer has spread into the perinephric region or the lymph nodes, or when the primary tumor or metastatic sites can't be completely excised. Then, high radiation doses are necessary.

Drug therapy has been only erratically effective against kidney cancer. Chlorambucil, 5-fluorouracil, cyclophosphamide, vinblastine, lomustine, vincristine, cis-platinum, tamoxifen, and hormones, such as medroxyprogesterone and testosterone, have been used with varying success.

Additional considerations

Meticulous postoperative care, supportive treatment (including relief from associated symptoms and side effects) during radiation and chemotherapy, and psychologic reassurance can hasten recovery and minimize complications.

Before surgery:
• The patient should express his anxieties and fears. He may need assurance that his body will adequately adapt to the loss of a kidney.
• He must be aware of the possible side effects of radiation and chemotherapy.
• The patient should know about the expected postop procedures, as well as diaphragmatic breathing, how to cough properly, and how to splint his incision while coughing.

After surgery:
• The patient must do diaphragmatic breathing and coughing.
• The patient must perform leg exercises to reduce the risk of emboli, and be turned every 2 hours.
• The patient should be positioned on the operative side to allow the pressure of adjacent organs to fill the dead space at the operative site and thus improve dependent drainage. If possible, the patient should try walking within 24 hours after surgery.
• Dressings require frequent checking for excessive bleeding. Signs of internal bleeding include: restlessness, sweating, and increased pulse rate.
• Adequate fluid intake is essential, so intake and output must be monitored. Lab results must also be monitored for anemia, polycythemia, or abnormal chemistries. They may point to bone or hepatic involvement, or may result from radiation or chemotherapy.
• All drug side effects should be treated symptomatically.

When a patient's being prepared for discharge, he must be made to understand the importance of complying with any prescribed outpatient treatment. This includes an annual follow-up chest X-ray to rule out lung metastasis and intravenous pyelography every 6 to 12 months to check for contralateral tumors.

Liver Cancer
(Primary hepatic carcinoma)

Liver cancer is a rare form of cancer with a high mortality rate. It's responsible for roughly 2% of all malignancies in the United States, and for 10% to 50% in Africa and parts of Asia. Liver cancer is most prevalent in men (particularly over age 60); incidence increases with age. It is rapidly fatal, usually within 6 months from gastrointestinal hemorrhage, progressive cachexia, hepatic failure, or metastatic spread.

Most primary liver tumors (90%) originate in the parenchymal cells and are hepatomas (hepatocellular carcinoma, primary lower-cell carcinoma). Some primary tumors originate in the intrahepatic bile ducts and are known as cholangiomas (cholangiocarcinoma, cholangiocellular carcinoma). Rarer tumors include a mixed-cell type, Kupffer cell sarcoma, and hepatoblastomas (which occur almost exclusively in children and are usually resectable and curable). The liver is one of the most common sites of metastasis from other primary cancers, particularly colon, rectum, stomach, pancreas, esophagus, lung, breast, or melanoma. In the United States, metastatic carcinoma occurs over 20 times more often than primary carcinoma, and after cirrhosis, is the leading cause of fatal hepatic disease. At times, liver metastasis may appear as a solitary lesion, the first sign of recurrence after a remission.

Causes

The immediate cause of liver cancer is unknown, but many consider it a congenital disease in children. Adult liver cancer may result from environmental exposure to carcinogens, such as the chemical compound aflatoxin (a mold that grows on rice and peanuts), thorium dioxide (a contrast dye medium used in liver radiography in the past), Senecio alkaloids, and possibly, androgens and oral estrogens.

Roughly 30% to 70% of patients with hepatomas also have cirrhosis, and it is estimated that a person with cirrhosis is 40 times more likely to develop hepatomas than someone with a normal liver. Whether cirrhosis is a premalignant state, or alcohol and malnutrition predispose the liver to develop hepatomas, is still unclear. Another high-risk factor is Australia antigen-positive blood.

Signs and symptoms

Clinical effects of liver cancer include:
- a mass in the right upper quadrant
- tender, nodular liver on palpation
- severe pain in epigastrium or right upper quadrant
- bruit, hum, or rubbing sound if tumor involves a large part of the liver
- weight loss, weakness, anorexia, fever
- occasional jaundice or ascites
- occasional evidence of metastatic spread through venous system to lungs, from lymphatics to regional lymph nodes, or by direct invasion of portal veins
- dependent edema.

Diagnosis

The definitive or confirming test for liver cancer is a liver biopsy by needle or open biopsy. Liver cancer is difficult to diagnose in the presence of cirrhosis, but several tests can help identify it:
- SGOT, alkaline phosphatase, lactic dehydrogenase (LDH), and bilirubin all show abnormal liver function.
- Alpha-fetoprotein (AFP) rises to a level above 500 mcg/ml.
- Chest X-ray may rule out metastasis.
- Liver scan may show filling defects.
- Arteriography may define large tumors. Electrolyte studies may indicate an

increased retention of sodium (resulting in functional renal failure), and hypoglycemia, leukocytosis, hypercalcemia, or hypocholesterolemia.

Treatment

Because liver cancer is often in an advanced stage at diagnosis, few hepatic tumors are resectable. A resectable tumor must be a single tumor in one lobe, without cirrhosis, jaundice, or ascites. Resection is done by lobectomy or partial hepatectomy.

Radiation therapy for unresectable tumors is usually palliative. But because of the liver's low tolerance for radiation, this therapy has not increased survival.

Another method of treatment is chemotherapy with intravenous 5-fluorouracil, methotrexate, doxorubicin, or with regional infusion of 5-fluorouracil or methotrexate (catheters are placed directly into the hepatic artery or left brachial artery for continuous infusion for 7 to 21 days).

Appropriate treatment for liver metastasis may include resection by hepatic lobectomy or chemotherapy for palliation (with results similar to those in hepatoma). Liver transplants have been attempted without success.

Additional considerations

A good health care plan should emphasize meeting supportive and emotional needs, as well as:

• controlling edema and ascites, and monitoring the patient's diet. Most patients need a special diet restricting sodium, fluids (no alcohol allowed), and protein. The patient should be weighed daily, with intake and output noted. Signs of ascites include peripheral edema, orthopnea, or dyspnea on exertion. If ascites is present, abdominal girth must be measured and recorded daily. To increase venous return and prevent edema, the patient's legs should be elevated whenever possible.

• monitoring respiratory function. Increase in respiratory rate or shortness of breath should be noted. Bilateral pleural effusion (noted on chest X-ray) is common, as is metastasis to the lungs. Signs of hypoxemia may result from intrapulmonary arteriovenous shunting.

• relieving fever. Low-grade fever is common. Sponge baths and aspirin suppositories will treat it, if there are no signs of gastrointestinal bleeding. Acetaminophen must not be given since the diseased liver is unable to metabolize it. High fever indicates infection and requires antibiotics.

• giving meticulous skin care. This includes: turning the patient frequently; keeping skin clean to avoid decubitus ulcers; applying lotion to prevent chafing; and giving an antipruritic (diphenhydramine) for severe itching.

 • watching for encephalopathy. Many patients develop end-stage symptoms of ammonia intoxication, including confusion, restlessness, irritability, agitation, delirium, asterixis, lethargy, and finally, coma. Serum ammonia level, vital signs, and neurologic status require monitoring. If ammonia accumulation occurs, it should be controlled with sorbitol (to produce osmotic diarrhea), neomycin (to reduce bacterial flora in the GI tract), lactulose (to control bacterial elaboration of ammonia), and sodium polystyrene sulfonate (to lower potassium level).

• frequently irrigating a transhepatic catheter, used to relieve obstructive jaundice with prescribed solution (normal saline or, sometimes, 5,000 U heparin in 500 ml 5% dextrose in water). Vital signs must be monitored for any indication of bleeding or infection.

After surgery, the patient should get standard postop care. Special hazards include intraperitoneal bleeding and sepsis (factors which precipitate coma). Renal failure can be prevented by checking urine output, BUN, and creatinine levels hourly. Throughout the course of this intractable illness, the patient's comfort should be the primary concern.

Bladder Cancer

Bladder tumors can develop on the surface of the bladder wall (papillomas, benign or malignant), or grow within the bladder wall (generally more virulent) and quickly invade underlying muscles. Almost all bladder tumors (90%) are transitional cell carcinomas, arising from the transitional epithelium of mucous membranes. They may result from malignant transformation of benign papillomas. Less common bladder tumors include adenocarcinomas, epidermoid carcinomas, squamous cell carcinomas, sarcomas, tumors in bladder diverticula, and carcinoma in situ.

Bladder tumors are most prevalent in people over age 50, and are more common in men than in women. The incidence of bladder tumors rises in densely populated industrial areas. Bladder cancer accounts for about 2% to 4% of all cancers.

Causes

Certain environmental carcinogens, such as 2-naphthylamine, benzidine, tobacco, nitrates, and coffee, are known to predispose to bladder tumors. Thus, certain industrial groups are at high risk for developing such tumors: rubber workers, cable workers, weavers, aniline dye workers, hairdressers, petroleum workers, spray painters, and leather finishers. The latent period between exposure to the carcinogen and development of symptoms is approximately 18 years.

Squamous cell carcinoma of the bladder also occurs with great frequency in geographic areas where schistosomiasis is endemic (such as Egypt). It's also associated with chronic bladder irritation and infection in people with kidney stones, Foley catheters, and chemical cystitis caused by cyclophosphamide.

Signs and symptoms

In early stages, approximately one fourth of patients with bladder tumors have no symptoms. Commonly, the first sign is gross, painless, intermittent hematuria (often with clots in the urine). Patients with invasive lesions often have suprapubic pain after voiding. Other clinical effects include bladder irritability, urinary frequency, nocturia, and dribbling.

Diagnosis

Only cystoscopy and biopsy confirm bladder cancer. Cystoscopy should be performed when hematuria first appears. When it is performed under anesthesia, a bimanual examination is usually done to determine if the bladder is fixed to the pelvic wall. A careful history and thorough physical examination may help determine whether the tumor has invaded the prostate or the lymph nodes.

The following tests can provide essential information about the size and location of the tumor:

• *Intravenous pyelography* can identify a large, early-stage tumor, or an infiltrating tumor; can delineate functional problems in the upper urinary tract; and can assess the degree of hydronephrosis.

• *Urinalysis* can detect blood in the urine and malignant cytology.

• *Excretory urography* can detect ureteral obstruction or rigid deformity of the bladder wall.

• *Pelvic arteriography* can reveal tumor invasion into the bladder wall.

• *CAT scan* demonstrates the thickness of the involved bladder wall and detects enlarged retroperitoneal lymph nodes.

Treatment

Superficial bladder tumors are removed through transurethral (cystoscope) resection and fulguration (electrical destruction). This procedure is adequate when the tumor has not invaded the muscle. However, additional tumors may develop, and the fulguration may have to be repeated every 3 months for years. Once the tumors penetrate the muscle layer or recur frequently, cystoscopy with

TWO TYPES OF URINARY DIVERSION

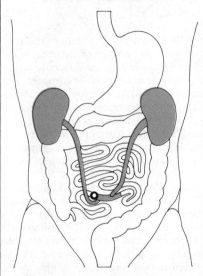

Ileal conduit (preferred method)—diversion of urine through a loop in the ileum to a stoma on the abdomen.

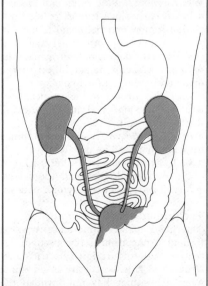

Ureterosigmoidoscopy (alternative method)—anastomosis of the ureters to the sigmoid, to direct urine flow through the colon.

fulguration is no longer appropriate.

Tumors too large to be treated through a cystoscope require segmental bladder resection to remove a full-thickness section of the bladder. This procedure is feasible only if the tumor isn't near the bladder neck or ureteral orifices. Bladder instillations of thiotepa after transurethral resections may also help control such tumors.

For infiltrating bladder tumor, radical cystectomy is the treatment of choice. The week before cystectomy, treatment may include 2,000 rads of external beam therapy to the bladder. Then, resection removes the bladder with perivesical fat, lymph nodes, urethra, and in males, the prostate and seminal vesicles; in females, the uterus and adnexa. The surgeon forms a urinary diversion, usually an ileal conduit (permanent ostomy). The patient must then wear an external pouch continuously. Other diversions include ureterostomy, nephrostomy, vesicostomy, ileal bladder, ileal loop, and sigmoid conduit.

Males are impotent following radical cystectomy and urethrectomy, because such resection damages the sympathetic and the parasympathetic nerves that control erection and ejaculation. At a later date, the patient may desire a penile implant, to make sexual intercourse (without ejaculation) possible.

Treatment for patients with advanced bladder cancer includes cystectomy to remove the tumor, radiation therapy, and systemic chemotherapy, such as cyclophosphamide, 5-fluorouracil, doxorubicin, and cis-platinum. This combined treatment has sometimes been successful in arresting this disease.

Additional considerations

A health care professional caring for a patient with bladder cancer should:
• provide psychologic support; encourage the patient to have a positive outlook about the stoma.
• assist in selection of the stoma site preoperatively by assessing the patient's abdomen in varying positions (the usual site is in the rectus muscle to minimize

subsequent herniation); make sure the selected site is visible to the patient.

• encourage the patient postoperatively to look at the stoma. If he has difficulty doing this, he should be left alone for a few minutes with the stoma exposed. A mirror will make viewing easier.

• catheterize the patient, using sterile technique, to obtain a specimen for culture and sensitivity. This can be done by inserting the lubricated tip of the catheter into the stoma about 2″ (5 cm). (In many hospitals, a double telescope-type catheter is available for ileal conduit catheterization.)

• elicit psychologic support and understanding from the spouse of the patient with surgically induced impotence. They'll have to learn alternate methods of sexual expression.

• assure the patient with a urinary stoma that he may participate in various athletics and physical activities, except for heavy lifting and contact sports.

• arrange for follow-up home care from a visiting nurse, when a patient with a urinary diversion is discharged.

• make a referral to the enterostomal therapist, if available, who will teach the patient stoma management, including skin care and pouch changes. Instruction usually begins 5 to 6 days after surgery. The patient's spouse, friend, or relative should attend the teaching session, and should know beforehand that a negative reaction to the stoma can impede the patient's adjustment.

Teaching the patient about a urinary stoma involves these steps:

The patient first learns to prepare the pouch and then to apply it. The pouch may be either reusable or disposable. If the patient chooses the reusable type, at least two are needed.

Selecting the right sized pouch is important; the stoma will be measured and a pouch ordered with an opening that clears the stoma with a ⅛″ (3.2 mm) margin. The patient should remeasure the stoma after he goes home, in case the size changes. The pouch will have a push-button or twist-type valve at the bottom that will allow for drainage. The patient should empty the pouch when it is one third full, or every 2 to 3 hours.

Assuring a good skin seal is important. Since urine tends to destroy skin barriers that contain a lot of karaya, a skin barrier that contains synthetics and little or no karaya is best. The pouch must be checked frequently to ascertain that the skin seal is still intact. A good skin seal with a skin barrier may last for 5 to 7 days, so the pouch only needs to be changed that often. The patient can wear an elastic belt to help secure the pouch.

The ileal conduit stoma reaches its permanent size about 2 to 4 months after surgery. Since the intestine is normally mucus-producing, mucus will appear in the draining urine. The patient should know that this is normal.

The skin around the stoma must be kept clean and free of irritation. After removing the pouch, the patient should wash the skin with water and mild soap; rinse with clear water to remove soap residue, and then gently pat, *not* rub, the skin dry. A gauze sponge soaked with vinegar-water (1 part: 3 parts) and placed over the stoma for a few minutes is recommended to prevent uric acid crystal buildup. While preparing the skin, the patient should place a rolled-up dry sponge over the stoma to collect draining urine. The skin is then coated with a silicone skin protector, and covered with the collection pouch. If skin irritation or breakdown occur, applying a layer of antacid precipitate to the clean, dry skin, and then coating it with silicone skin protector will help.

The patient can level uneven surfaces on his abdomen, such as gullies, scars, or wedges, with a variety of specially prepared products or skin barriers.

All high-risk people—for example, aniline dye or chemical workers, those in areas where schistosomiasis is endemic, and those with histories of benign bladder tumors or persistent unexplained cystitis—should have periodic cytologic examinations, and should know about the danger of significant exposure to irritants, toxins, and carcinogens. Many industries have taken measures to protect workers from possible exposure to aromatic amines, such as 2-naphthylamine and benzidine, and have reduced incidence of bladder cancer among their workers.

For added information, ostomates may write to the American Cancer Society or to the United Ostomy Association.

Gallbladder and Bile Duct Carcinoma

Gallbladder carcinoma is rare, comprising less than 1% of all malignancies. It's normally found coincidentally in patients with cholecystitis; 1 in 400 cholecystectomies reveals malignancy. This disease is most prevalent in females over age 60. It's rapidly progressive and usually fatal; patients seldom live a year after diagnosis. Poor prognosis is due to late diagnosis; gallbladder cancer is usually not diagnosed until after cholecystectomy, when it is often in an advanced, metastatic stage.

Extrahepatic bile duct carcinoma is the cause of approximately 3% of all cancer deaths in the United States. It occurs in both males and females (incidence is slightly higher in males) between ages 60 and 70. The usual site is at the bifurcation in the common duct. Carcinoma at the distal end of the common duct is often confused with carcinoma of the pancreas. Characteristically, metastatic spread occurs to local lymph nodes, the liver, lungs, and the peritoneum.

Causes

Many consider gallbladder carcinoma a complication of gallstones. However, this inference rests on circumstantial evidence from postmortem examinations: from 60% to 90% of gallbladder carcinoma patients also have gallstones; but postmortem data from patients with gallstones show gallbladder carcinoma in only 0.5%.

The predominant tissue type in gallbladder cancer is adenocarcinoma, 85% to 95%; squamous cell, 5% to 15%. Mixed-tissue types are rare.

Lymph node metastasis is present in 25% to 70% of patients at diagnosis. Direct extension to the liver is common (in 46% to 89%); direct extension to both the cystic and the common bile ducts, stomach, colon, duodenum, and jejunum also occurs, and produces obstructions. Metastasis also spreads by portal or hepatic veins to the peritoneum, ovaries, and lower lung lobes.

The cause of extrahepatic bile duct carcinoma isn't known; however, statistics report an unexplained increased incidence of this carcinoma in patients with ulcerative colitis. This association may be due to a common cause—perhaps an immune mechanism, or chronic use of certain drugs by the colitis patient.

Signs and symptoms

Clinically, gallbladder cancer is almost indistinguishable from cholecystitis: pain in the epigastrium or right upper quadrant, weight loss, anorexia, nausea, vomiting, and jaundice. However, chronic, progressively severe pain in an afebrile patient suggests malignancy. In patients with simple gallstones, pain is sporadic. Another telling clue to malignancy is palpable gallbladder (right upper quadrant), with obstructive jaundice. Some patients may also have hepatosplenomegaly.

Progressive profound jaundice is commonly the first sign of obstruction due to extrahepatic bile duct cancer. The jaundice is usually accompanied by chronic pain in the epigastrium or the right upper quadrant, radiating to the back. Other common symptoms, if associated with active cholecystitis, include pruritus, skin excoriations, anorexia, weight loss, chills, and fever.

Diagnosis

No test or procedure is, in itself, diagnostic of gallbladder carcinoma. However, the following laboratory tests support this diagnosis when they suggest hepatic dysfunction and extrahepatic biliary obstruction:

• *baseline studies* (CBC, routine urinalysis, electrolyte studies, enzymes)
• *liver function tests* (bilirubin, urine bile and bilirubin, and urobilinogen are elevated in more than 50% of patients; serum alkaline phosphatase levels are consistently elevated)
• *liver scan*
• *upper GI series* (shows abnormality of pylorus or duodenum)
• *occult blood in stools* (linked to the associated anemia)
• *cholecystography* (may show stones or calcification—a "porcelain" gallbladder)
• *cholangiography* (may locate the site of common duct obstruction)
• *chest X-ray* (may show elevation [displacement by the tumor] of right side of diaphragm).

The following tests help confirm extrahepatic bile duct carcinoma:

• *liver function studies* indicate biliary obstruction; elevated bilirubin (5 to 30 mg/ 100 ml), alkaline phosphatase, and blood cholesterol; prolonged prothrombin time; response to vitamin K.
• *barium studies* and *cholangiography* (may help locate the obstruction but are not diagnostic).

Treatment

Surgical treatment of gallbladder cancer is essentially palliative, and includes cholecystectomy, common bile duct exploration, T-tube drainage, and wedge excision of hepatic tissue. If the cancer has invaded gallbladder musculature, the survival rate is generally less than 5%, even with massive resection.

Although some long-term survivals (4 to 5 years) have been reported, few patients survive longer than 6 months after surgery. Generally, radiation therapy and chemotherapy (usually 5-fluorouracil) have been relatively ineffective, but 5-fluorouracil probably provides the best results of any drug.

Surgery is normally indicated to relieve obstruction and jaundice that result from extrahepatic bile duct carcinoma. The procedure depends on the site of the carcinoma, and may include cholecystoduodenostomy, or T-tube drainage of the common duct.

Other palliative measures for both kinds of carcinomas include radiation (mostly used for local and incisional recurrences) and chemotherapy (especially 5-fluorouracil), both of which have limited effects.

Additional considerations

After biliary resection, the health care professional should:
• monitor vital signs.
• use strict aseptic technique when caring for incision and surrounding area.
• place the patient in low Fowler's position.
• prevent respiratory problems by encouraging deep breathing and coughing. The high incision makes the patient want to take shallow breaths; analgesics and an abdominal binder may aid in greater respiratory efforts.
• monitor bowel sounds and bowel movements; observe patient's tolerance to diet.
• provide pain control.
• check intake and output carefully; watch for electrolyte imbalance; monitor I.V. solutions to avoid overloading the cardiovascular system.
• monitor the nasogastric tube, which will be in place for 24 to 72 hours postop to relieve distention, and the T tube; record amount and color of drainage each shift; secure the T tube to minimize tension on it and prevent it from being pulled out.
• help the patient and his family cope with their initial fears and reactions to the diagnosis by offering information and support.
• advise the patient of the side effects of both chemotherapy and radiation therapy. The patient on radiation therapy must be monitored closely for side effects. The patient on drug therapy must be watched closely for toxic side effects.

MALE GENITALIA

Prostatic Cancer

After skin cancer, prostatic cancer is the most common neoplasm found in men over age 50. Adenocarcinoma is the form it appears in most frequently, and only rarely does it occur as a sarcoma. About 85% of prostatic carcinomas originate in the posterior part of the prostatic gland; the rest, near the urethra. Malignant prostatic tumors are seldom a result of the benign hyperplastic enlargement that commonly develops around the prostatic urethra in elderly men.

Prostatic carcinoma seldom produces symptoms until it's well advanced. When treated in its localized form, the 5-year survival rate is 70%; after metastasis, it's under 35%. When prostatic cancer is fatal, it's usually the result of widespread bone metastases.

Causes and incidence

While androgens regulate prostatic growth and function and may also speed tumor growth, a definite link between androgens and prostatic cancer hasn't been found. Typically, when primary prostatic lesions spread beyond the prostate gland, they invade the prostatic capsule, and then spread along the ejaculatory ducts in the space between the seminal vesicles, or perivesicular fascia.

Prostatic cancer accounts for 17% of all cancers. Incidence is highest among Blacks, and in men with blood type A; it is lowest in Orientals. Its occurrence is unaffected by socioeconomic status or fertility.

Signs and symptoms

Symptoms appear only in the advanced stages of the disease. Clinical effects include difficulty in starting urinary stream, dribbling, urine retention, unexplained cystitis, and rarely, hematuria.

Diagnosis

A rectal examination that reveals a small, hard nodule may help diagnose prostatic cancer before symptoms develop (except in Stage I of the disease, when the cancer is still occult). A routine physical examination of men over age 40 should *always* include a rectal examination to check for prostatic cancer.

 Biopsy confirms this diagnosis. Serum acid phosphatase is usually elevated in prostatic cancer, and provides a baseline to monitor the effectiveness of therapy. Successful therapy returns the serum acid phosphatase level to normal; a subsequent rise points to recurrent disease.

Elevated alkaline phosphatase levels and a positive bone scan point to bone metastasis; routine bone X-rays don't always show evidence of such metastasis.

Treatment

Correct management of prostatic cancer depends on clinical assessment, tolerance to therapy, expected life span, and the stage of the disease. Treatment must be chosen carefully, since prostatic cancer usually affects older men, who frequently have serious coexisting disorders, such as hypertension, diabetes, or cardiac disease.

Therapy varies with each stage of the disease, and generally includes radiation, prostatectomy, orchiectomy (removal of the testes) to reduce androgen production, and synthetic estrogen (diethylstilbestrol [DES]). Prostatic carcinoma often responds favorably to supervoltage radiation; such radiation can cure locally invasive and even more extensive cancer. Radiation also relieves bone pain from metastatic skeletal involvement, and is sometimes used for locally extensive tumors that don't respond to hormonal therapy. Chemotherapy is now achieving some success in treating advanced stages of the disease.

Treatment for Stage I prostatic cancer consists of radiation; however, occasionally, no treatment is required. In Stage II, therapy includes radical prostatectomy if the patient is otherwise healthy, or radiation in small-field areas if sexual potency is to be preserved. Treatment in Stage III includes orchiectomy, radiation, and hormonal therapy; in Stage IV, hormonal therapy, and combination chemotherapy with cyclophosphamide, doxorubicin, and tamoxifen.

Additional considerations

A supplemental care plan should emphasize psychologic support of patients facing prostatectomy, good postoperative care, and symptomatic treatment of radiation side effects.

Before prostatectomy, a hospital staff member should:
• explain the expected effects of surgery (such as impotence and incontinence), as well as the side effects of radiation.
• encourage the patient to express his fears.
• instruct the patient about postoperative procedures, such as placement of tubes and dressing changes.
• teach perineal exercises (done either sitting or standing) to minimize incontinence. To develop perineal muscles, patient should squeeze his buttocks together and hold this position for a few seconds; then relax. He should do this exercise 1 to 10 times an hour.

After prostatectomy, a staff member should:
• regularly check dressing, incision, and drainage systems for excessive bleeding and watch for signs of bleeding (cold clammy skin, pallor, restlessness, falling blood pressure, and rising pulse rate).
• watch for signs of infection (fever, chills, inflamed incisional area) and maintain adequate fluid intake (at least 2,000 ml daily).
• give antispasmodics, as ordered, to control postoperative bladder spasms, and give analgesics, as needed.
• keep the patient's skin clean and dry, since urinary incontinence is a frequent problem after prostatectomy.

After a suprapubic prostatectomy:
• keep the skin around the suprapubic drain dry, and free from drainage and urine leakage. (The patient can begin perineal exercises within 24 to 48 hours after surgery.)
• allow the patient's family to assist in his care, and encourage their psycho-

---

STAGING PROSTATIC CANCER

Staging procedures for prostatic cancer include X-rays, laboratory and radioisotopic studies for clinical diagnosis; laparotomy, bone marrow aspiration, open or needle biopsy; surgical resection and histologic examination of the prostate gland and, possibly, the regional lymph nodes as well.

Stage I: Occult cancer without symptoms.

Stage II: Cancer nodule confined within prostatic capsule; usually no symptoms.

Stage III: Cancer extends beyond the prostatic capsule into surrounding tissues and, possibly, pelvic lymph nodes, or is confined within the capsule with elevated serum acid phosphatase levels, pointing to high levels of tumor activity. The patient often has some urinary symptoms: difficulty in starting urinary stream, unexplained cystitis, dribbling, urine retention, and rarely, hematuria.

Stage IV: Bone or other extrapelvic involvement (nodes, lungs). The patient has signs of advanced disease, such as bladder outlet obstruction, urine retention, uremia, anemia, anorexia, and if bone metastasis has occurred, skeletal pain (which may be extremely severe).

logic support.
• give meticulous catheter care. After prostatectomy, a patient often has a three-way catheter with a continuous irrigation system. The tubing must be checked for kinks, mucus plugs, and clots, especially if the patient complains of pain. The patient must not pull on the tubes or the catheter.

After transurethral resection, a staff member should:
• watch for signs of urethral stricture (dysuria, small urinary stream, and straining to urinate) and for abdominal distention (a result of urethral stricture or catheter blockage by a blood clot).
• irrigate catheter, as ordered.

After a perineal prostatectomy, a staff member should:

• avoid taking rectal temperature, or inserting rectal tubes of any sort.
• provide pads to absorb urinary drainage and a rubber ring for sitting.
• give frequent sitz baths to relieve pain and inflammation.

After perineal and retropubic prostatectomy, a staff member should:
• give reassurance that urine leakage after catheter removal is normal and will disappear in time.
• watch for and treat nausea, vomiting, dry skin, and alopecia, when a patient receives radiation or hormonal therapy; watch for side effects of DES, (gynecomastia, fluid retention, nausea, and vomiting) and keep alert for thrombophlebitis (pain, tenderness, swelling, warmth, and redness in calf).

Testicular Cancer

Malignant testicular tumors primarily affect young to middle-aged adults, and are the leading cause of death from solid tumors in men between the ages of 15 and 34. In testicular tumors occurring in children, although rare, 50% are detectable before age 5. With few exceptions, testicular tumors are of gonadal cell origin. Such tumors may be seminomas (about 40%), in which uniform, undifferentiated cells resemble primitive gonadal cells; or nonseminomas, in which tumor cells show various degrees of differentiation.

Prognosis varies with the cancer cell type and staging. When treated with surgery and radiation, 100% of patients with Stage I or II seminomas and 90% of those with Stage I nonseminomas survive beyond 5 years. Even with proper treatment, the 5-year survival rate is 55%. Prognosis is poor if this disease is advanced beyond stage II at diagnosis.

Causes and incidence
The cause of testicular cancer isn't known, but incidence is higher in men with cryptorchidism (even when this condition has been surgically corrected). Testicular cancer rarely occurs in non-Caucasian males, and accounts for less than 1% of all male cancer deaths. Peak incidence of the disease is at age 32. Typically, when testicular cancer extends beyond the testes, it spreads through the lymphatic system to the iliac, para-aortic, mediastinal, and left cervical nodes, with metastases to the lungs, the liver, viscera, and bone.

Signs and symptoms
Characteristically, testicular cancer becomes apparent with the development of a firm, painless, and smooth testicular mass, which may be as small as a pea or as large as a grapefruit. Often there is also a feeling of testicular heaviness. When such a tumor produces chorionic gonadotropin or estrogens, it may also cause gynecomastia and nipple tenderness. In late stages, lymph node involvement and distant metastases lead to ureteral obstruction, abdominal mass, cough, hemoptysis, shortness of breath, weight loss, fatigue, pallor, and lethargy.

Diagnosis

The most effective means for detection of testicular cancer early are regular self-examination, and palpation of the testes as part of a routine physical examination. When such examination reveals a testicular mass, transillumination can distinguish between a tumor (which will *not* transilluminate) and a hydrocele or spermatocele (which will). Further diagnostic measures should include a breast examination for gynecomastia and abdominal palpation to detect abdominal masses.

Confirming lab tests include intravenous pyelography to search for ureteral deviation resulting from para-aortic node involvement, determination of urinary or serum luteinizing hormone (LH) levels, lymphangiography followed by ultrasound examination, and a hematologic workup, including a CBC. Serum alpha-fetoprotein and beta-human chorionic gonadotropin are important indicators of testicular tumor activity, and can provide a baseline to measure response to therapy and to help determine prognosis.

 When a tumor is present, surgical removal of the entire testis for biopsy permits histologic verification of tumor cell type—essential for effective treatment. Inguinal exploration determines nodal involvement.

Treatment

Treatment includes surgery, radiation, and chemotherapy; the intensity of such therapy varies with tumor cell type and staging. Surgery includes orchiectomy and retroperitoneal node dissection to prevent extension of the disease and to aid in staging. Most surgeons remove just the testis, not the scrotum, which allows for a prosthetic testicular implant at a later date. Hormone replacement may be necessary to supplement depleted hormonal levels, especially after bilateral orchiectomy.

Treatment of seminomas involves postoperative radiation to the retroperitoneal and homolateral iliac nodes, and in patients with retroperitoneal extension, prophylactic radiation to the mediastinal and supraclavicular nodes. In nonseminomas, treatment includes radiation to all positive nodes.

Chemotherapy is essential in patients with large abdominal or mediastinal nodes and frank distant metastases, or in others at high risk of developing metastases. Cyclophosphamide produces excellent results in seminomas; and combinations of vinblastine, bleomycin, cisplatinum, methotrexate, actinomycin D, and chlorambucil in nonseminomas.

Additional considerations

The patient's care plan should emphasize dealing with psychologic response to the disease, preventing postoperative complications, and minimizing and controlling the side effects of radiation and chemotherapy. The young patient with testicular cancer faces particularly difficult treatment, and probably fears sexual impairment and disfigurement.

Before orchiectomy, the health care professional should:
* encourage the patient to talk about his fears; try to establish a trusting relationship.
* give reassurance that sterility and impotence do not follow unilateral orchiectomy; explain that synthetic hormones can supplement depleted hormonal lev-

---

STAGING TESTICULAR CANCER

Staging work-up in testicular cancer combines surgical evaluation with pathologic staging. Usually, it includes testicular and tumor resection with lymph node dissection (especially inguinal exploration) to determine nodal involvement.

Stage I: Tumor confined to one testis, with no clinical or radiographic evidence of extratesticular spread

Stage II: Cancer metastasized to regional lymph nodes but not beyond

Stage III: Metastasis beyond regional nodes, usually to abdominal, mediastinal, supraclavicular, or pulmonary nodes

els; inform the patient that most surgeons don't remove the scrotum, and that implant of a testicular prosthesis can correct disfigurement; assure him that testicular cancer isn't contagious.

After orchiectomy, the health care professional should:
• apply an ice pack to the scrotum for the first day after surgery; provide analgesics, as ordered.
• check for excessive bleeding, swelling, and signs of infection. (Drainage should be minimal.)
• provide a scrotal athletic supporter to minimize pain during ambulation.
• know what side effects to expect during chemotherapy, and how to prevent or ease them; give antiemetics, as needed, to prevent severe nausea and vomiting; give small, frequent feedings to maintain oral intake despite anorexia; develop a good mouth care regimen, and check for stomatitis; watch for signs of myelosuppression; if the patient receives vinblastine, assess for neurotoxicity (peripheral paresthesias, jaw pain, muscle cramps); if the patient receives cisplatinum, check for ototoxicity; prevent renal damage by increasing fluid intake, giving I.V. hydration, as ordered, with a potassium supplement, and providing diuresis, with furosemide or mannitol.

Penile Cancer

Penile carcinoma rarely affects circumcised men in modern cultures; when it does occur, it's usually in men who are over age 50. The most common form, epidermoid squamous cell carcinoma, is usually found in the glans, but may also occur on the corona sulcus, and, rarely, in the preputial cavity. This malignancy produces ulcerative or papillary (wartlike, nodular) lesions, which may become quite large before spreading beyond the penis; such lesions may destroy the glans prepuce and invade the corpora.

Prognosis varies. Regional lymph node involvement, which is common, decreases the 5-year survival rate to under 40%; distant metastases almost invariably cut survival time to an average of 3 years. Unfortunately, many men delay treatment of penile cancer, because they fear disfigurement and loss of sexual function.

Causes
The exact cause of penile cancer is unknown; however, it's generally associated with poor personal hygiene, and phimosis in uncircumcised men. This may account for the low incidence among Jews, Muslims, and people of other cultures that practice circumcision at birth or shortly thereafter. (Incidence isn't decreased in cultures that practice circumcision at a later date.) Early circumcision seems to prevent penile cancer by allowing for better personal hygiene and minimizing inflammatory (and often premalignant) lesions of the glans and prepuce. Such lesions include:
• *leukoplakia*—inflammation, with thickened patches that may fissure
• *balanitis*—inflammation of the penis associated with phimosis
• *erythroplasia of Queyrat*—squamous cell carcinoma in situ; velvety, erythematous lesion that becomes scaly and ulcerative
• *penile horn*—scaly horn-shaped growth.

Signs and symptoms
In a circumcised man, early signs of penile cancer include a small circumscribed lesion, a pimple, or a sore on the penis. In an uncircumcised man, however, such early symptoms may go unnoticed, so penile cancer first becomes apparent when it causes late-stage symptoms, such as pain, hemorrhage, dysuria, purulent discharge, and obstruction of the urinary meatus. Rarely are metastases the first signs of penile cancer.

Diagnosis

Diagnosis of penile cancer requires tissue biopsy. Preoperative baseline studies include CBC, urinalysis, EKG, and a chest X-ray. Enlargement of inguinal lymph nodes because of infection from the primary lesion makes lymphangiographic preoperative evaluation of lymph node metastasis difficult.

Treatment

Depending on the stage of progression, treatment includes surgical resection of the primary tumor, and possibly, chemotherapy and radiation. Local tumors of the prepuce only require circumcision. Invasive tumors, however, require partial penectomy (unless contraindicated because of the patient's young age); tumors of the base of the penile shaft require total penectomy and inguinal node dissection (done less often in the United States than in other countries where incidence is higher). Radiation therapy may improve treatment effectiveness after resection of localized lesions without metastasis; it may also reduce the size of lymph nodes before nodal resection. It's not adequate primary treatment for groin metastasis, however. Bleomycin and methotrexate are generally used in chemotherapy but are not very effective.

Additional considerations

Penile cancer calls for good patient teaching, psychologic support, and comprehensive postoperative care. The patient with penile cancer fears disfigurement, pain, and loss of sexual function.

Before penile surgery, the health care professional should:
• spend time with the patient, and encourage him to talk about his fears.
• supplement and reinforce what the doctor has told the patient about the surgery and other treatment measures; explain expected postoperative procedures, such as dressing changes and catheterization; show the patient diagrams of the surgical procedure and pictures of the results of similar surgery to help him adapt to an altered body image.
• call in an enterostomal therapist if the patient needs urinary diversion. The therapist will help prepare the patient for his change in body image and teach him stoma and pouch care.

After penectomy, the health care professional should:
• monitor vital signs, and intake and output.
• give good skin care to prevent skin breakdown from urinary diversion or suprapubic catheterization; keep the skin dry and free from urine; make sure if the patient has a suprapubic catheter, that the catheter remains patent at all times.
• give analgesics, as ordered; elevate the penile stump with a small towel or pillow to minimize edema.
• check the surgical wound often for signs of infection, such as foul odor or excessive drainage on dressing.
• watch the patient who has had inguinal node dissection for signs of lymphedema, such as decreased circulation or disproportionate swelling of a leg.
• reassure the patient who's had a partial penectomy that the penile stump should be sufficient for urination and sexual function. He may need sexual counseling.

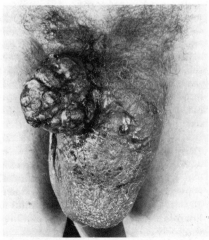

Penile carcinoma

FEMALE GENITALIA

Cervical Cancer

The third most common cancer of the female reproductive system, cervical cancer is classified as either preinvasive or invasive.

Preinvasive carcinoma ranges from minimal cervical dysplasia, in which the lower third of the epithelium contains abnormal cells, to carcinoma in situ, in which the full thickness of epithelium contains abnormally proliferating cells (also known as cervical intraepithelial neoplasia [CIN]). Preinvasive cancer is curable 75% to 90% of the time with early detection and proper treatment. If untreated (and depending on the form in which it appears), it may progress to invasive cervical cancer.

In invasive carcinoma, cancer cells penetrate the basement membrane, and can spread directly to contiguous pelvic structures or disseminate to distant sites by lymphatic routes. Invasive carcinoma of the uterine cervix is responsible for 8,000 deaths annually in the United States alone. In almost all cases (95%), the histologic type is squamous cell carcinoma, which varies from well-differentiated cells to highly anaplastic spindle cells. Only 5% are adenocarcinomas. Usually invasive carcinoma occurs between ages 30 and 50; rarely under age 20.

Causes

While the cause is unknown, several predisposing factors have been related to the development of cervical cancer: intercourse at a young age, multiple sexual partners, multiple pregnancies, and herpesvirus II and other bacterial or viral venereal infections.

Signs and symptoms

Preinvasive cervical cancer produces no symptoms or other clinically apparent changes. Early invasive cervical cancer causes abnormal vaginal bleeding, persistent vaginal discharge, and postcoital pain and bleeding. In advanced stages, it causes pelvic pain, vaginal leakage of urine and feces from a fistula, anorexia, weight loss, and anemia.

Diagnosis

A cytologic examination (Pap smear) can detect cervical cancer before clinical evidence appears. (Systems of Pap smear classification may vary from hospital to hospital.) Abnormal cervical cytology routinely calls for colposcopy, which can detect the presence and extent of pre- clinical lesions requiring biopsy and histologic examination. Staining with Lugol's solution (strong iodine) or Schiller's solution (iodine, potassium iodide, and purified water) may identify areas for biopsy when the smear shows abnormal cells but there's no obvious lesion. While the tests are nonspecific, they do distinguish between normal and abnormal tissues: normal tissues absorb the iodine and turn brown; abnormal tissues are devoid of glycogen and won't change color. Additional studies, such as lymphangiography, cystography, and scans, can detect metastasis.

Treatment

Appropriate treatment depends on accurate clinical staging. Preinvasive lesions may be treated with total excisional biopsy, cryosurgery, conization (and frequent Pap smear follow-up), or, rarely, hysterectomy. Therapy for invasive squamous cell carcinoma may include radical hysterectomy, radiation therapy (internal, external, or both), and invasive laser therapy.

Additional considerations

Management of cervical cancer requires skilled pre- and postop care, comprehensive patient teaching, and psychologic support.

When assisting with a biopsy, the health care professional should:

• drape and prepare the patient as for a routine Pap smear and pelvic examination; have a container of formaldehyde ready to preserve the specimen during transfer to the pathology lab.

• tell the patient she may feel pressure, minor cramps, or a pinch from the punch forceps; reassure her that pain will be minimal, because the cervix has few nerve endings; explain that the procedure may cause some spotting, and advise her to refrain from sexual intercourse for at least the rest of the day to reduce irritation to the excised area.

When assisting with cryosurgery, the health care professional should:

• drape and prepare the patient as if for a routine Pap smear and pelvic examination; explain that the procedure takes approximately 15 minutes, during which time the doctor will use coolant to freeze the cervix.

• warn the patient that she may experience abdominal cramps, headache, and sweating, but reassure her that she'll feel little, if any, pain; tell her to expect a heavy, watery, yellowish discharge for about 2 weeks after the procedure, and advise her not to douche, use tampons, or engage in sexual intercourse during this time.

When assisting with both excisional biopsy and cryosurgery, the health care

---

INTERNAL RADIATION SAFETY PRECAUTIONS

There are three cardinal safety rules in internal radiation therapy:

• *Time.* A radiosensitive badge must be worn. Remember, exposure increases with time, and the effects are cumulative. Therefore, hospital staff members must plan the time they spend with the patient to prevent overexposure. (However, they should not rush procedures, ignore the patient's psychologic needs, or give the impression that they can't get out of the room fast enough.)

• *Distance.* Radiation loses its intensity with distance. The staff members must avoid standing at the foot of the patient's bed, where they're in line with the radiation.

• *Shield.* Lead shields reduce radiation exposure. They should be used whenever possible.

In internal radiation therapy, the patient should be considered radioactive while the source is in place. Pregnant women should not be assigned to care for these patients.

The position of the source applicator must be checked every 4 hours. If it appears dislodged, the doctor should be notified immediately. If it's completely dislodged, the staff member must remove the patient from the bed, pick up the applicator with long forceps, and place it on a lead-shielded transport cart. (The source must *never* be picked up with bare hands.) The doctor and radiation safety officer must be notified when there's been an accident.

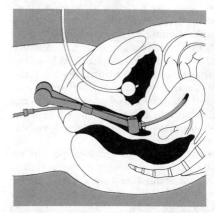

Positioning of internal radiation applicator for uterine cancer

STAGING CERVICAL CANCER

Stage 0: Carcinoma in situ, intraepithelial carcinoma

Stage I: Carcinoma is strictly confined to the cervix (extension to the corpus should be disregarded)

Stage Ia: Microinvasive carcinoma (early stromal invasion)

Stage Ib: All other cases of Stage I. Occult cancer should be marked "occ."

Stage II: Carcinoma extends beyond the cervix but has not extended to the pelvic wall. The carcinoma involves the vagina, but not as far as the lower third.

Stage IIa: No obvious parametrial involvement

Stage IIb: Obvious parametrial involvement

Stage III: Carcinoma has extended to the pelvic wall. On rectal examination, there is no cancerfree space between the tumor and the pelvic wall.

The tumor involves the lower third of the vagina. All cases with a hydronephrosis or nonfunctioning kidney are included, unless they are known to be due to other cause.

Stage IIIa: No extension to the pelvic wall

Stage IIIb: Extension to the pelvic wall and/or hydronephrosis or nonfunctioning kidney

Stage IV: Carcinoma has extended beyond the true pelvis or has clinically involved the mucosa of the bladder or rectum. A bullous edema as such does not permit a case to be allotted to Stage IV.

Stage IVa: Spread of the growth to adjacent organs

Stage IVb: Spread to distant organs

Reprinted from *Manual for Staging of Cancer* (Chicago: American Joint Committee for Cancer Staging and End Results Reporting, 1978). Used with permission.

professional should:
• tell the patient to watch for and report signs of infection; stress the need for a follow-up Pap smear and a pelvic examination within 3 to 4 months after these procedures and periodically thereafter.
• inform the patient what to expect postoperatively if a hysterectomy is necessary; monitor postop vital signs every 4 hours; watch for and immediately report signs of complications, such as bleeding, abdominal distention, severe pain, wheezing, or other breathing difficulties; administer analgesics, prophylactic antibiotics, and subcutaneous heparin, as ordered; encourage deep breathing and coughing.
• explain that external outpatient radiation therapy, when necessary, continues for about 4 to 6 weeks. The patient may be hospitalized for a 2- to 3-day course of internal radiation treatment (an intracavitary implant of radium, cesium, or some other radioactive material). The patient may have internal or external therapy, or both. Usually, internal radiation therapy is the first procedure; if this is so, the patient will require a private room.
• check to see if the radioactive source will be inserted while the patient is in the operating room (preloaded) or at bedside (afterloaded).
• explain the internal radiation application procedure, and answer the patient's questions. Internal radiation requires a 2- to 3-day hospital stay, a bowel prep, a povidone-iodine vaginal douche, a clear liquid diet, nothing by mouth the night before the implantation, and a Foley catheter. The procedure is performed in the operating room under general anesthesia, during which time she is placed in the lithotomy position, and a radium applicator is inserted. For *preloading*, the source is implanted in the applicator at this time by the doctor. For *afterloading*, a member of the radiation team will implant the source in the applicator after the patient is returned to her room from surgery.
• *remember* the safety precautions—time, distance, and shielding—begin as

soon as the radioactive source is in place (if the source is preloaded, the patient returns to her room *hot*, and safety precautions must begin immediately); inform visitors of safety precautions, and hang a sign listing these precautions on the patient's door.
• encourage the patient to lie flat and limit movement while the source is in place; elevate the head of the bed slightly if she prefers.
• check vital signs every 4 hours; watch for skin reaction, vaginal bleeding, abdominal discomfort, or evidence of dehydration; make sure the patient can reach everything she needs without stretching or straining; assist her in range-of-motion *arm* exercises (leg exercises and other body movements could dislodge the source); administer a tranquilizer, if ordered, to help the patient relax and remain still; organize the time you spend with the patient to minimize your exposure to radiation.
• teach the patient to watch for and report uncomfortable side effects; warn the patient during therapy to avoid persons with obvious infections, since radiation therapy may increase susceptibility to infection by lowering WBCs.
• reassure the patient that this disease and its treatment shouldn't radically alter her life-style or prohibit sexual intimacy.

Uterine Cancer

Uterine cancer (cancer of the endometrium) is the most common gynecologic cancer. Usually, it affects postmenopausal women between ages 50 and 60; it's uncommon between ages 30 and 40, and extremely rare before age 30. Most premenopausal women who develop uterine cancer have a history of anovulatory menstrual cycles or other hormonal imbalance. An average of 37,000 new cases of uterine cancer are reported annually; of these, 3,300 are eventually fatal.

Causes
Uterine cancer seems linked to several predisposing factors:
• low fertility index and anovulation
• abnormal uterine bleeding
• obesity, hypertension, or diabetes
• familial tendency
• history of uterine polyps or endometrial hyperplasia
• estrogen therapy (still controversial).
Generally, uterine cancer is an adenocarcinoma that metastasizes late, usually from the endometrium to the cervix, ovaries, fallopian tubes, and other peritoneal structures. It may spread to distant organs, such as the lungs and the brain, through the blood or the lymphatic system. Lymph node involvement can also occur. Less common uterine tumors include adenoacanthoma, endometrial stromal sarcoma, lymphosarcoma, mixed mesodermal tumors (including carcinosarcoma), and leiomyosarcoma.

Signs and symptoms
Uterine enlargement, and persistent and unusual premenopausal bleeding, or any postmenopausal bleeding, are the most common indications of uterine cancer. The discharge may at first be watery and blood-streaked but gradually becomes more bloody. Other symptoms, such as pain and weight loss, don't appear until the cancer is well advanced.

Diagnosis
Unfortunately, a Pap smear, so useful for detecting cervical cancer, doesn't dependably predict early-stage uterine cancer. Diagnosis of uterine cancer requires endometrial, cervical, and endocervical biopsies. Negative biopsies call for a fractional dilatation and curettage (D & C) to determine diagnosis. Positive diagnosis requires the following tests to provide baseline data and permit staging:

- multiple cervical biopsies and endocervical curettage to pinpoint cervical involvement
- Schiller's test, staining the cervix and vagina with an iodine solution that turns healthy tissues brown; cancerous tissues resist the stain, because they don't contain glycogen
- complete physical examination
- chest X-ray
- intravenous pyelography and, possibly, cystoscopy
- complete blood studies
- EKG
- proctoscopy or barium enema studies (rarely used).

Treatment

Treatment varies, depending on the extent of the disease:

- *Surgery* generally involves total abdominal hysterectomy, bilateral salpingo-oophorectomy, or possibly omentectomy with or without pelvic or para-aortic lymphadenectomy. Total exenteration removes all pelvic organs, including the vagina, and is done only when the disease is sufficiently contained to allow surgical removal of diseased parts. Partial exenteration may retain an unaffected colorectum or bladder.
- *Radiation therapy.* When the tumor isn't well differentiated, intracavitary or external radiation or both, given 6 weeks before surgery, may inhibit recurrence and lengthen survival time.
- *Hormonal therapy* using progesterone or chemotherapy with doxorubicin. Other combinations are useful for recurrence, especially vincristine, cyclophosphamide, and actinomycin D.

Additional considerations

A care plan for patients with uterine cancer should emphasize: comprehensive patient teaching to help them cope with surgery, radiation, and chemotherapy; good postoperative care; and psychologic support.

Before surgery:

- The patient should be told all about the surgery, the routine tests (e.g., repeated blood tests the morning after surgery), and postoperative care, including foley catheter care. If the patient is to have a lymphadenectomy *and* a total hysterectomy, she'll probably have a blood drainage system for about 5 days after

---

STAGING UTERINE CANCER

Stage-0: Carcinoma in situ. Histologic findings are suspicious of malignancy; cases of Stage 0 should not be included in any therapeutic statistics.

Stage I: Carcinoma confined to the corpus

Stage Ia: Length of the uterine cavity 8 cm or less

Stage Ib: Length of the uterine cavity more than 8 cm

    Stage I cases should be subgrouped by histologic type of the adenocarcinoma as follows:

- G1: Highly differentiated adenomatous carcinoma
- G2: Moderately differentiated adenomatous carcinoma with partly solid areas
- G3: Predominantly solid or entirely undifferentiated carcinoma

Stage II: Carcinoma has involved the corpus and the cervix but has not extended outside the uterus.

Stage III: Carcinoma has extended outside the uterus but not outside the true pelvis.

Stage IV: Carcinoma has extended outside the true pelvis or has obviously involved the mucosa of the bladder or rectum. A bullous edema as such does not permit a case to be allotted to Stage IV.

Stage IVa: Spread of the growth to adjacent organs

Stage IVb: Spread of the growth to distant organs

MANAGING PELVIC EXENTERATION

Before pelvic exenteration, a hospital staff member should:
• teach the patient about ileal conduit and colostomy, and make sure she understands that her vagina will be removed.
• minimize the risk of infection by supervising a rigorous bowel and skin preparation procedure, by decreasing the residue in the patient's diet for 48 to 72 hours, then maintaining a diet ranging from clear liquids to nothing by mouth, by administering oral or I.V. antibiotics, as ordered, and by prepping skin daily with antibacterial soap.
• instruct the patient about postop procedures, such as I.V. therapy, and an unsutured perineal wound with gauze packing.

After pelvic exenteration, a staff member should:
• check the stoma, incision, and perineal wound for drainage; be especially careful to check the perineal wound for bleeding after the packing is removed; expect red or serosanguineous drainage, but notify the doctor immediately if drainage is excessive, continuously bright red, foul-smelling, or purulent, or if there's bleeding from the conduit.
• provide excellent skin care; use warm water and saline solution to clean the skin, because soap may be too drying and may increase skin breakdown.

surgery. The patient should be fitted with antiembolism stockings for use during and after surgery. The patient's blood must be typed and cross-matched. If the patient is premenopausal, she must be told that removal of her ovaries will induce menopause.

After surgery:
• Fluid contents of the blood drainage system must be measured every shift. The doctor should be called immediately if drainage exceeds 400 ml.
• If the patient has received subcutaneous heparin, administration should continue until the patient is fully ambulatory again. Prophylactic antibiotics may also be ordered.
• Vital signs require checking every 4 hours. Signs of complications include: bleeding, abdominal distention, severe pain, wheezing, or other breathing difficulties. Analgesics may be ordered.
• The patient must breathe deeply and cough regularly to help prevent complications. The use of an incentive spirometer once every waking hour will help keep lungs expanded.
• The patient may be scheduled for internal or external radiation or both. Usually, internal radiation therapy is done first. The radioactive source will be in-

serted while the patient is in the operating room (preloaded) or at bedside (afterloaded). If the source is preloaded, the patient returns to her room "hot," and safety precautions begin immediately.
• The patient must understand the internal radiation procedure, and be given a chance to ask questions. Internal radiation requires a 2- to 3-day hospital stay, bowel prep, povidone-iodine vaginal douche, clear liquid diet, and nothing taken by mouth the night before the implantation; it also requires a Foley catheter.

If the patient is to have *preload* radiation therapy, the procedure is performed in the operating room under general anesthetic. The patient will be placed in a dorsal position, with knees and hips flexed, heels resting in footrests. The source is implanted in the vagina by the doctor.

If the patient is to have *afterloaded* radiation therapy, a member of the radiation team will implant the source while the patient is in her room.
• *Remember* that safety precautions— time, distance, and shielding—must be imposed as soon as the patient's radioactive source is in place. The patient will

require a private room.
- The patient must limit movement while the source is in place. If she prefers, the head of the bed may be slightly elevated. The patient should be able to reach everything she needs (call bell, telephone, water) without stretching or straining. She should engage in range-of-motion *arm* exercises. (Leg exercises and other body movements could dislodge the source.) If ordered, a tranquilizer will help the patient relax and remain still. Time that others spend with the patient must be restricted to minimize exposure to radiation.
- The patient's vital signs must be checked every 4 hours. Possible complications include skin reaction, vaginal bleeding, abdominal discomfort, or evidence of dehydration.
- Visitors must know safety precautions. A sign listing these precautions should be posted on the patient's door.

If the patient receives external radiation:
- The patient and her family must be taught about the therapy before it begins. The treatment is usually given 5 days a week for 6 weeks. She must not scrub body areas marked with indelible ink for treatment, because treatment must be directed to exactly the same area each time.

- The patient must maintain a high-protein, high-carbohydrate, low-residue diet to reduce bulk and yet maintain calories. Diphenoxylate with atropine may be ordered, to minimize diarrhea, a possible side effect of pelvic radiation.
- To minimize skin breakdown and reduce the risk of skin infection, the patient must keep the treatment area dry, avoid wearing clothes that rub against the area, and avoid using heating pads, alcohol rubs, or irritating skin creams. Since radiation therapy increases susceptibility to infection (possibly by lowering white blood cell (WBC) count), the patient should avoid people with colds or other infections.

Remember, a uterine cancer patient needs special counseling and psychologic support to help her cope with this disease and the necessary treatment measures. Fearful about her survival, she may also be concerned that treatment will alter her life-style and prevent sexual intimacy. She should know that, except in total pelvic exenteration, the vagina remains intact and, once she recovers, sexual intercourse is possible. A health care professional's presence and interest alone will help the patient, even if the professional can't answer every question she may ask.

Vaginal Cancer

Vaginal cancer accounts for approximately 2% of all gynecologic malignancies. It usually appears as squamous cell carcinoma, but occasionally as melanoma, or sarcoma, or adenocarcinoma (clear cell adenocarcinoma has an increaced incidence in young women whose mothers took diethylstilbestrol). Vaginal cancer generally occurs in women in their early to mid-50s, but some of the rarer types do occur in younger women, and rhabdomyosarcoma appears in children.

Pathophysiology
Vaginal cancer varies in severity according to its location and effect on lymphatic drainage. (The vagina is a thin-walled structure with a rich lymphatic drainage.) Vaginal cancer is similar to cervical cancer in that it may progress from an intraepithelial tumor to an invasive cancer. However, it spreads more slowly than cervical cancer.

A lesion in the upper third of the vagina (the most common site) usually metastasizes to the groin nodes; a lesion in the lower third (the second most common site) usually metastasizes to the hypogastric and iliac nodes; but a lesion in the middle third metastasizes erratically. A posterior lesion displaces and distends the vaginal posterior wall before spreading to deep layers. By contrast, an anterior lesion spreads more rapidly into other structures and deep layers, because unlike the posterior wall, the anterior vaginal wall is not flexible.

Signs and symptoms

Commonly, the patient with vaginal cancer has experienced abnormal bleeding and discharge. Also, she may have a small or large, often firm, ulcerated lesion in any part of the vagina. As the cancer progresses, it commonly spreads to the bladder (producing frequent voiding and bladder pain), the rectum (bleeding), vulva (lesion), pubic bone (pain), or other surrounding tissues.

Diagnosis

The diagnosis of vaginal cancer is based on the presence of abnormal cells on a vaginal Pap smear. Careful examination and biopsy rule out the cervix and vulva as the primary sites of the lesion. In many cases, however, the cervix contains the primary lesion that has metastasized to the vagina. Then, any visible lesion is biopsied and evaluated histologically. It is sometimes difficult to visualize the entire vagina because the speculum blades may hide a lesion, or the patient may be uncooperative because of discomfort. When lesions are not visible, colposcopy is used to search out abnormalities. Painting the suspected vaginal area with Lugol's solution (strong iodine solution) also helps identify malignant areas by staining glycogen-containing normal tissue, while leaving abnormal tissue unstained.

Treatment

Early-stage treatment aims to treat the malignant area, while preserving the normal parts of the vagina. Radiation or surgery varies with the size, depth, and location of the lesion, and the patient's desire to maintain a functional vagina.

STAGING VAGINAL CANCER

Stage 0: Carcinoma in situ; intraepithelial carcinoma

Stage I: Carcinoma limited to vaginal wall

Stage II: Carcinoma involves subvaginal tissue but not the pelvic wall.

Stage III: Carcinoma has extended to the pelvic wall.

Stage IV: Carcinoma has extended beyond the true pelvis or has involved the mucosa of the bladder or rectum. Bullous edema as such does not permit assignment to Stage IV.

Stage IVa: Spread to adjacent organs

Stage IVb: Spread to distant organs.

Reprinted from *Manual for Staging of Cancer* (Chicago: American Joint Committee for Cancer Staging and End Results Reporting, 1978). Used with permission.

Preservation of a functional vagina is generally possible only in the early stages. Survival rates are the same for patients treated with radiation as for those with surgery.

Surgery is usually recommended only when the tumor is so extensive that exenteration is needed, because close proximity to the bladder and rectum permits only minimal tissue margins around resected vaginal tissue.

Radiation therapy is the preferred treatment for advanced vaginal cancer. Most patients need preliminary external

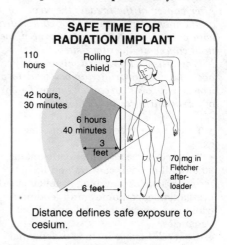

SAFE TIME FOR RADIATION IMPLANT

110 hours

Rolling shield

42 hours, 30 minutes

6 hours 40 minutes

3 feet

6 feet

70 mg in Fletcher afterloader

Distance defines safe exposure to cesium.

radiation treatment to shrink the tumor before internal radiation can begin. Then, if the tumor is localized to the vault and the cervix is present, radiation (radium or cesium) can be given with an intra-uterine tandem or ovoids; if the cervix is absent, then a specially designed vaginal applicator is used instead. To minimize complications, radioactive sources and filters are carefully placed away from radiosensitive tissues, such as the bladder and the rectum. Such treatment lasts 48 to 72 hours, depending on dosage.

Additional considerations
• Before treatment begins, hospital staff members caring for the patient should find out if the radiation source will be preloaded in the operating room or afterloaded while the patient is in her bed. Learning this will help the staff plan the patient's care to minimize their exposure to radiation.
• Before radiation treatment, the patient must understand the necessity of immobilization, and what it entails (such as no linen changes and the use of a Foley catheter).

• Since the effects of radiation are cumulative, each staff member must wear a radiosensitive badge and a lead shield (if available), when entering the patient's room. The radiation therapist will know the maximum recommended time that a staff member can safely spend with the patient when giving direct care.
• While the radiation source is in place, the patient must lie flat on her back. A Foley catheter should be inserted (usually done in the operating room). The patient's linens don't need to be changed routinely; only when they get soiled. The patient should have a call bell, phone, water, or anything else she needs within easy reach. The doctor will order a clear liquid or low-residue diet and an antidiarrheal drug to prevent bowel movements.
• To compensate for immobility, the patient must do active range-of-motion exercises with both arms.
• The patient should use a stent or prescribed candle exercises to prevent vaginal stenosis. Coitus is also helpful in preventing such stenosis.
• Finally, the patient should be encouraged to express her anxieties and fears.

Ovarian Cancer

After cancer of the breast, the colon, or the lung, primary ovarian cancer ranks as the most common cause of cancer deaths among American women. In women with previously treated breast cancer, metastatic ovarian cancer is more common than cancer at any other site.

Prognosis varies with the histologic type and staging of the disease, but is generally poor, because ovarian tumors tend to progress rapidly. Although about 25% of women with ovarian cancer survive for 5 years, prognosis may be improving because of recent advances in chemotherapy.

Three main types of ovarian cancer exist:
• *Primary epithelial tumors* account for 90% of all ovarian cancers and include serous cystoadenocarcinoma, mucinous cystoadenocarcinoma, and endometrioid and mesonephric (clear-cell) malignancies.
• *Germ cell tumors* include endodermal sinus malignancies, embryonal carcinoma (a rare ovarian cancer that appears in children), immature teratomas, and dysgerminoma.
• *Sex cord (stromal) tumors* include granulosa cell tumors (which produce estrogen and may have feminizing effects), thecomas, and the rare arrhenoblastomas (which produce androgen

STAGING OVARIAN CANCER

Stage I: Growth limited to the ovaries
Stage Ia: Growth limited to one ovary; no ascites*
Stage Iai: No tumor on the external surface; capsule intact
Stage Iaii: Tumor on the external surface, or capsule(s) ruptured, or both
Stage Ib: Growth limited to both ovaries; no ascites
Stage Ibi: No tumor on the external surface; capsule intact
Stage Ibii: Tumor on the external surface, or capsule(s) ruptured, or both
Stage Ic: Tumor either Stage 1a or 1b, but with ascites present or with positive peritoneal washings
Stage II: Growth involving one or both ovaries with pelvic extension
Stage IIa: Extension and/or metastases to the uterus and/or tubes

Stage IIb: Extension to other pelvic tissues
Stage IIc: Tumor either stage IIa or Stage IIb, but with ascites present or with positive peritoneal washings
Stage III: Growth involving one or both ovaries with intraperitoneal metastases outside the pelvis, or positive retroperitoneal nodes, or both. Tumor limited to the true pelvis with histologically proven malignant extension to small bowel or omentum.
Stage IV: Growth involving one or both ovaries with distant metastasis. If pleural effusion is present, there must be positive cytology to allot a case to Stage IV. Parenchymal liver metastasis signifies Stage IV.
Special Category: Unexplored cases thought to be ovarian carcinoma

---

*Ascites is peritoneal effusion that, in the opinion of the surgeon, is pathologic, clearly exceeds normal amounts, or both.

Reprinted from *Manual for Staging of Cancer* (Chicago: American Joint Committee for Cancer Staging and End Results Reporting, 1978). Used with permission.

and have virilizing effects).

Causes and incidence

Exactly what causes ovarian cancer isn't known, but its incidence is noticeably higher in women of upper socioeconomic level between ages 40 and 65, and in single women (although the disease may occur anytime, including childhood or during pregnancy). In a study involving a limited number of patients, a history of endometrial carcinoma seemed linked with ovarian cancer.

Primary epithelial tumors arise in the müllerian epithelium; germ cell tumors, in the ovum itself; and sex cord tumors, in the ovarian stroma (the ovary's supporting framework). Ovarian tumors spread rapidly intraperitoneally by local extension or surface seeding, and occasionally, through the lymphatics and the bloodstream. Generally, extraperitoneal spread is through the diaphragm into the chest cavity, which may cause pleural effusions. Other metastasis is rare.

Signs and symptoms

Typically, symptoms vary with the size of the tumor. Occasionally, in the early stages, ovarian cancer causes vague abdominal discomfort, dyspepsia, and other mild gastrointestinal disturbances. As it progresses, it causes urinary frequency, constipation, pelvic discomfort, distention, and weight loss. Tumor rupture, torsion, or infection may cause pain, which, in young patients, may mimic appendicitis. Granulosa cell tumors have feminizing effects (such as bleeding between periods in premenopausal women); conversely, arrhenoblastomas have virilizing effects. Advanced ovarian cancer causes ascites, rarely postmenopausal bleeding and pain, and symptoms relating to metastatic sites (most often pleural effusions).

Diagnosis

Diagnosis of ovarian cancer requires clinical evaluation, complete patient history, surgical exploration, and histologic studies.

Preoperative evaluation includes:
- a complete physical examination, including pelvic examination with Pap smear (an inconclusive test, as it is positive in only a small number of women with ovarian cancer)
- ultrasound studies or an X-ray of the abdomen (may help delineate tumor size)
- CBC, blood chemistries, and EKG
- intravenous pyelography for information on renal function and possible urinary tract anomalies and ureteral obstruction
- chest X-ray for distant metastasis and pleural effusions
- barium enema (especially in patients with gastrointestinal symptoms) to reveal obstruction and size of tumor
- lymphangiography to show lymph node involvement
- mammography to rule out primary breast cancer
- liver function studies or a liver scan in patients with ascites
- ascites fluid aspiration for identification of typical cells by cytology.

Despite extensive testing, accurate diagnosis and staging are impossible without exploratory laparotomy, including lymph node evaluation and tumor resection.

Treatment
According to the staging of the disease and the patient's age, treatment of ovarian cancer requires varying combinations of surgery, chemotherapy, and in some cases, radiation.

Occasionally, in girls or young women with a unilateral encapsulated tumor who wish to maintain fertility, a conservative approach may be appropriate:
- resection of the involved ovary
- biopsies of the omentum and the uninvolved ovary
- peritoneal washings for cytologic examination of pelvic fluid
- careful follow-up, including periodic chest X-rays to rule out lung metastasis.

Ovarian cancer usually requires more aggressive treatment, including total abdominal hysterectomy and bilateral salpingo-oophorectomy with tumor resection, omentectomy, appendectomy, lymph node palpation with probable lymphadenectomy, tissue biopsies, and peritoneal washings. Complete tumor resection is impossible if the tumor has matted around other organs or if it involves organs that can't be resected. Bilateral salpingo-oophorectomy in a girl who hasn't reached puberty necessitates hormone replacement therapy, beginning at the age of puberty, to induce the development of secondary sex characteristics.

Chemotherapy extends the length of survival time in most ovarian cancer patients but is largely palliative in advanced disease. However, prolonged remissions are being achieved in some patients. Chemotherapeutic drugs useful in ovarian cancer include melphalan, chlorambucil, thiotepa, methotrexate, cyclophosphamide, doxorubicin, vincristine, vinblastine, actinomycin D, bleomycin, and cis-platinum. These drugs are usually given in combination.

In early-stage ovarian cancer, instillation of a radioisotope, such as ^{32}P, is occasionally useful when peritoneal washings are positive. Radiation treatment is likely to be more than merely palliative only if residual tumor size is $3/4''$ (2 cm) or less; if there's no evidence of ascites or no metastatic deposits on the peritoneum, the liver, or kidneys; and if there are no distant metastases, and no prior history of abdominal radiation. Immunotherapy is controversial, and consists of I.V. or, in chronic ascites, intraperitoneal injection of *Corynebacterium parvulum* or BCG vaccine (bacille Calmette-Guérin).

Additional considerations
Because treatment for ovarian cancer varies widely, so must the care that the patient receives.

Before surgery:
- The patient must be told about all preoperative tests, the expected course of treatment, and surgical and postoperative procedures.
- All surgical procedures the patient will undergo are listed in the surgical

consent form. The patient must understand that this form lists multiple procedures because the extent of the surgery can only be determined after surgery has begun.

• Premenopausal women should know that bilateral oophorectomy artificially induces early menopause, so they may experience hot flashes, headaches, palpitations, insomnia, depression, and excessive perspiration.

After surgery:

• Vital signs require frequent monitoring. I.V. fluids must be checked often and intake and output monitored regularly. Good catheter care and regular dressing checks will minimize excessive drainage or bleeding, and infection.

• Abdominal distention must be avoided. To this end, coughing and deep breathing should be encouraged. The patient must be repositioned often, given abdominal support, and encouraged to walk shortly after surgery.

• Side effects of radiation and chemotherapy need to be monitored and treated.

• If the patient is receiving immunotherapy, she must be watched for flulike symptoms that may last 12 to 24 hours after drug administration. Aspirin or acetaminophen will combat fever. The patient should remain well covered with blankets, and be given warm liquids to relieve chills. An antiemetic may also be needed.

• The patient and her family will need psychologic support. Open communication is important but overcompensation or "smothering" of the patient by her family should be discouraged. If the patient is a young woman who grieves for her lost ability to bear children, she must be helped to overcome feelings that "there's nothing else to live for." If the patient is a child, she should be told she has cancer, and be given an opportunity to ask questions. Also, the social worker, chaplain, and other members of the health-care team can help provide for additional supportive care.

Cancer of the Vulva

Cancer of the vulva accounts for approximately 5% of all gynecologic malignancies. It can occur at any age, even in infants, but its peak incidence is in the mid-60s. The most common vulval cancer is squamous cell carcinoma. Early diagnosis increases the chance of effective treatment and survival. Lymph node dissection allows 5-year survival in 85% of patients if it reveals no positive nodes; otherwise, the survival rate falls to less than 75%.

Causes

Although the cause of cancer of the vulva is unknown, several factors seem to predispose women to this disease:

• leukoplakia (white epithelial hyperplasia)— in about 25% of patients

• chronic vulval granulomatous disease, including venereal disease

• chronic pruritus of the vulva (for months or years), with friction, swelling, and dryness

• pigmented moles that are constantly irritated by clothing or perineal pads

• irradiation of the skin, such as nonspecific treatment for pelvic cancer

• obesity

• hypertension

• diabetes

• nulliparity.

Signs and symptoms

Cancer of the vulva usually begins with vulval pruritus, bleeding, or a small vulval mass (which may start as a small ulcer on the surface; eventually, it becomes infected and painful), so such symptoms call for immediate diagnostic evaluation. Less common indications include a mass in the groin, abnormal urination or defecation, or cachexia.

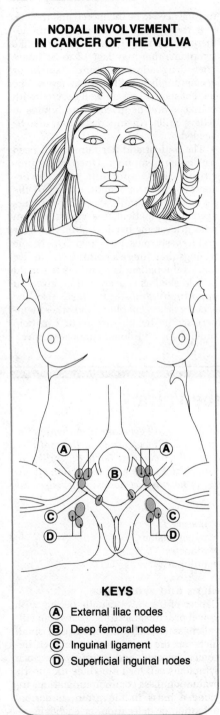

NODAL INVOLVEMENT IN CANCER OF THE VULVA

KEYS
Ⓐ External iliac nodes
Ⓑ Deep femoral nodes
Ⓒ Inguinal ligament
Ⓓ Superficial inguinal nodes

Diagnosis
A Pap smear that reveals abnormal cells or the typical clinical picture (pruritus, bleeding, or small vulval mass) strongly suggests vulval cancer.

Firm diagnosis requires histologic examination. Abnormal tissues for biopsy are first identified by: colposcopic examination to pinpoint vulvar lesions or abnormal skin changes; and by staining with toluidine blue dye, which is then retained by diseased tissues. (The stain is applied with a cotton swab, then rinsed with acetic acid solution.)

Other diagnostic measures include CBC, chest X-ray, EKG, and thorough physical (including pelvic) examination. Occasionally, lymphangiography may pinpoint lymph node involvement.

Treatment
Depending on the stage of the disease, cancer of the vulva usually calls for radical or simple vulvectomy. Radical vulvectomy requires bilateral dissection of superficial and deep inguinal lymph nodes. Depending on the extent of metastasis, resection may include the urethra, vagina, and bowel, leaving an open perineal wound until healing—about 2 to 3 months. After such surgery, the patient remains hospitalized from 10 days to several weeks, depending on how well her incision is healing. Plastic surgery, including mucocutaneous graft to reconstruct pelvic structures, may be done at a later date.

Small, confined lesions with no lymph node involvement may require a simple vulvectomy or hemivulvectomy (without pelvic node dissection). Personal considerations (young age of patient, active sexual life) may also necessitate such conservative management. However, a simple vulvectomy mandates careful postoperative surveillance, since it leaves the patient at higher risk of developing a new lesion.

If extensive metastasis, advanced age, or fragile health rules out surgery, irradiation of the primary lesion offers palliative treatment.

Additional considerations

Patient teaching, pre- and postoperative care, and psychologic support can help prevent complications, speed recovery, and return the patient to as nearly normal a life as possible.

Before surgery:

• The patient should be told about the surgery and the postop procedures, such as the use of a Foley catheter, a blood drainage system, preventive respiratory care, and exercises to prevent venous stasis.

• The patient should have the opportunity to ask questions, and get honest answers. She is sure to be frightened about this sexually mutilating surgery.

After surgery:

• Scrupulous routine gynecologic care is essential, particularly special care aimed at reducing pressure at the operative site, reducing tension on suture lines, and promoting healing through better air circulation.

• The patient should be placed on an air mattress or egg crate mattress, with a cradle supporting the top covers.

• The patient must be repositioned periodically, using pillows. Her bed should be equipped with a half-frame trapeze bar to help her move and she should know how to use it.

• For several days after surgery, the patient will be maintained on I.V. fluids or a clear liquid diet. She may also be given an antidiarrheal drug three times daily to reduce the discomforts and possible infection caused by defecation, a constant problem after such surgery. Later, she may need stool softeners and a low-residue diet to combat constipation.

• The operative site will need a thorough cleansing. The patient should be taught the procedure.

• The operative site must be checked regularly for bleeding, foul-smelling discharge, or other signs of infection. As a result of extensive skin retraction, the wound area will look lumpy, bruised, and battered, making it difficult to detect occult bleeding. This situation calls for a primary nurse, who can more easily

---

STAGING VULVAR CANCER

Stage 0: Carcinoma in situ
Stage I: Tumor confined to vulva—2 cm or less in diameter. Nodes are not palpable or are palpable in either groin, not enlarged, mobile (not clinically suspicious of neoplasm).
Stage II: Tumor confined to the vulva— more than 2 cm in diameter. Nodes are not palpable or are palpable in either groin, not enlarged, mobile (not clinically suspicious of neoplasm).
Stage III: Tumor of any size with (1) adjacent spread to the urethra and any or all of the vagina, the perineum, and the anus, and/or (2) nodes palpable in either or both groins (enlarged, firm, and mobile, not fixed but clinically suspicious of neoplasm).
Stage IV: Tumor of any size (1) infiltrating the bladder mucosa or the rectal mucosa or both, including the upper part of the urethral mucosa, and/or (2) fixed to the bone or other distant metastases. Fixed or ulcerated nodes in either or both groins.

Reprinted from *Manual for Staging of Cancer* (Chicago: American Joint Committee for Cancer Staging and End Results Reporting, 1978). Used with permission.

---

detect subtle changes in appearance.

• Within 5 to 10 days after surgery, the patient should try to walk. She should also engage in coughing and range-of-motion exercises.

• To prevent urine contamination, the patient will have a Foley catheter in place for 2 weeks. Fluid intake and output must be recorded.

The patient and her spouse will need counseling. They must realize that, postoperatively, the vulva will be numb and have a different appearance. Sensation will eventually return after the nerve endings heal, and the couple will probably be able to have sexual intercourse 6 to 8 weeks following surgery. They may need to experiment with different sexual techniques, because surgery generally removes the clitoris.

Choriocarcinoma

Choriocarcinoma is a rapidly metastasizing malignant tumor of placental tissue Like other gestational trophoblastic diseases, it's characterized by the secretion of large amounts of human chorionic gonadotropin (HCG). With modern treatment, prognosis is good; untreated choriocarcinoma can be fatal within 3 to 12 months. Choriocarcinoma was the first disseminated malignancy cured by chemotherapy.

Causes

Choriocarcinoma usually follows hydatidiform mole or abortion, but it may also occur during extrauterine or normal intrauterine pregnancy. Choriocarcinoma and other trophoblastic diseases are most common in Mexico and the Far East, and may be linked to fetal-maternal histoincompatibility, inherited factors, or infections such as viruses and toxoplasmosis.

Signs and symptoms

Choriocarcinoma causes profuse, and potentially fatal, vaginal and intra-abdominal bleeding; occasionally, tumor necrosis results in pancytopenia and sepsis. Metastasis occurs early and progresses rapidly, causing weight loss, cachexia, and anemia. Such metastasis usually appears first in the vagina and vulva, where it produces dark hemorrhagic nodules; other common metastatic sites include the lungs (resulting in cough and hemoptysis), the liver, bone, and skin.

Diagnosis

This disease is suspected if HCG levels rise or remain elevated after evacuation of hydatidiform mole or abortion, or if these levels are abnormally high in a pregnant woman with clinical features of this disease. Pretreatment workup includes:

- complete physical examination
- CBC
- urinalysis
- liver and kidney function studies and liver scan and thyroid tests
- 24-hour urine and serum collection to assay HCG levels

- EEG and CAT scan of the brain
- ultrasound of the pelvis
- intravenous pyelography
- EKG
- chest X-ray.

Treatment

When possible, treatment often takes place in a hospital designated as a regional trophoblastic disease center. In low-risk patients (those with no evidence of hepatic, renal, or CNS involvement), treatment consists of chemotherapy; in high-risk patients (those with metastases) it may also include radiation to metastatic sites (the primary site isn't irradiated since choriocarcinoma is radioresistant) and hysterectomy. Severe bleeding requires transfusion of packed red cells and platelets, as needed; infection requires antibiotics, and in the occasional patient with disseminated intravascular coagulation (DIC), high-dose corticosteroids, and heparin.

Chemotherapy employs methotrexate, actinomycin D, and in high-risk patients, chlorambucil, and continues until three consecutive weekly titers show normal HCG levels.

If HCG levels don't respond to these drugs, a combination of vinblastine, bleomycin, and cis-platinum may help. If all chemotherapy fails or if severe hemorrhage intervenes, a hysterectomy or resection of radiation-resistant metastatic tumors may be appropriate. Following treatment, periodic HCG titers are necessary.

Additional considerations

Supplemental care for the choriocarcinoma patient is largely supportive and highly variable, depending on the stage of the disease and the patient's condition. The patient may be hospitalized for as long as several months. Care following surgery includes:

• giving meticulous postop care and watching for signs of adverse reactions after transfusion to minimize complications.

• monitoring intake and output.

• watching for and treating side effects of radiation and chemotherapy; minimizing complications by encouraging adequate nutrition or providing total parenteral nutrition.

• emphasizing the need for periodic HCG titers, chest X-rays, physical examinations, pelvic examinations, and other follow-up studies to the patient being discharged.

CHORIOADENOMA DESTRUENS

Chorioadenoma destruens (invasive mole) is a hydatidiform mole in which the chorionic villi penetrate the uterine wall and, occasionally, adjacent tissues. Unlike choriocarcinoma, chorioadenoma destruens rarely metastasizes.

Rising HCG levels suggest trophoblastic disease, but a clear diagnosis of chorioadenoma destruens must rule out choriocarcinoma by microscopic tissue examination. Treatment consists of chemotherapy.

• reassuring the patient that she *can* resume sexual activity. However, she must use contraception for a full year after treatment ends, since pregnancy interferes with HCG follow-up titers.

Fallopian Tube Cancer

Primary fallopian tube cancer is extremely rare, and accounts for fewer than 0.5% of all gynecologic malignancies. It usually occurs in postmenopausal women in their 50s and 60s, but occasionally is found in younger women. Because this disease is generally well advanced before diagnosis (up to 30% of such cancers are bilateral with extratubal spread), prognosis is poor.

Causes

The causes of fallopian tube cancer aren't clear, but this disease appears to be linked with nulliparity. In fact, over half the women with this disease have never had children.

Signs and symptoms

Generally, early-stage fallopian tube cancer produces no symptoms. Late-stage disease is characterized by an enlarged abdomen with a palpable mass, amber-colored vaginal discharge, excessive bleeding during menstruation or at other times, abdominal cramps, frequent urination, bladder pressure, persistent constipation, weight loss, and unilateral colicky pain produced by hydrops tubae profluens. (This last symptom occurs when the abdominal end of the fallopian tube closes, causing the tube to become greatly distended until its accumulated secretions suddenly overflow into the uterus.) Metastases develop by local extension or by lymphatic spread to the abdominal organs or to the pelvic, aortic, and inguinal lymph nodes. Extra-abdominal metastases are rare.

Diagnosis

 Unexplained postmenopausal bleeding and an abnormal Pap smear (suspicious or positive in up to 50% of all cases) suggest this diagnosis, but laparotomy is usually necessary to confirm fallopian tube cancer. When such cancer involves both the ovary and fallopian tube, the primary site is very difficult to identify.

Preoperative workup includes:

• an ultrasound or plain film of the ab-

domen to help delineate tumor mass
• intravenous pyelography to assess renal function, and show urinary tract anomalies and ureteral obstruction
• chest X-ray to rule out metastases
• barium enema to rule out intestinal obstruction
• routine blood studies
• EKG.

Treatment

Treatment of fallopian tube cancer consists of total abdominal hysterectomy, bilateral salpingo-oophorectomy, and omentectomy; chemotherapy with progestogens, 5-fluorouracil, melphalan, and cyclophosphamide; and external radiation for 5 to 6 weeks. All patients should receive some form of adjunctive therapy (radiation or chemotherapy), even when surgery has removed all evidence of the disease.

Additional considerations

Good preoperative patient preparation and postoperative care, patient instruction, psychologic support, and symptomatic measures to relieve radiation and chemotherapy side effects can promote a successful recovery and minimize complications.

Before surgery, the health care professional caring for the fallopian tube cancer patient should:
• reinforce the doctor's explanation of the diagnostic and treatment procedures.
• explain the need for preoperative studies, and tell the patient what to expect: fasting the night before surgery; an enema to clear the bowel, using a Foley catheter attached to a drainage bag; an abdominal and possibly a pelvic prep; an I.V. line; and, possibly, a sedative.
• describe the tubes and dressings the patient can expect to have in place when she returns from surgery.
• teach the patient deep breathing and coughing techniques to prepare for postoperative exercises.

After surgery the health care professional should:
• check vital signs every 4 hours and report fever, tachycardia, and hypotension to the doctor.
• monitor I.V. fluids.
• change dressings regularly, and check for excessive drainage, bleeding, and infection.
• provide antiembolism stockings, as ordered.
• encourage deep breathing and coughing, and if necessary, institute intermittent positive pressure breathing (IPPB).
• turn and reposition the patient often, using pillows for support.
• auscultate for bowel sounds. (When the patient's bowel function returns, the dietitian will provide a clear liquid diet, and, when it can be tolerated, a regular diet.)
• encourage the patient to walk within 24 hours after surgery, reassuring her that she won't harm herself or cause wound dehiscence by doing so.
• provide psychologic support and encourage the patient to express anxieties and fears. (If she seems worried about the effect of surgery on her sexual life, she should be reassured that this surgery will not inhibit sexual function.)
• before radiation therapy begins, explain that the area to be irradiated is marked with water-soluble ink to precisely locate the treatment field.
• explain that radiation may cause a skin reaction, bladder irritation, myelosuppression and other systemic reactions, or a drop in blood pressure. (During and after treatment, side effects of radiation and chemotherapy must be watched for and treated).
• before discharge, advise the patient to maintain a high-carbohydrate, high-protein, low-fat, low-bulk diet to maintain caloric intake but reduce bulk. She should eat several small meals a day instead of three large ones.
• include the patient's husband or other close relatives in patient care and teaching as much as possible.

To help detect fallopian tube and other gynecologic cancers early, the patient must get regular pelvic examinations and should contact a doctor promptly about any gynecologic symptom.

BONE

Primary Malignant Bone Tumors
(Sarcomas of the bone, bone cancer)

Primary malignant bone tumors are rare, comprising less than 1% of all malignant tumors. Most bone tumors are secondary, caused by seeding from a primary site. Primary malignant bone tumors are more common in males, especially in children and adolescents, although some types do occur in persons between ages 35 and 60. They may originate in osseous or nonosseous tissue. Osseous bone tumors arise from the bony structure itself, and include osteogenic sarcoma (the most common), parosteal osteogenic sarcoma, chondrosarcoma, and malignant giant cell tumor. Together they make up 60% of all malignant bone tumors. Nonosseous tumors arise from hematopoietic, vascular, and neural tissues, and include Ewing's sarcoma, fibrosarcoma, and chordoma. Osteogenic and Ewing's sarcomas are the most common bone tumors in childhood.

Causes

Causes of primary malignant bone tumors remain unknown. Some suggest that primary malignant bone tumors arise in areas of rapid growth, since children and young adults with such tumors seem to be much taller than average. Additional theories point to heredity, trauma, and excessive radiotherapy.

Signs and symptoms

Bone pain is the most common indication of primary malignant bone tumors. It's often more intense at night and is not usually associated with mobility. The pain is dull and is usually localized, although it may be referred from the hip or spine and result in weakness or a limp. Another common sign is the presence of a mass or tumor. The tumor site may be tender and may swell; the tumor itself is often palpable. Pathologic fractures are common. In late stages, the patient may be cachectic, with fever and impaired mobility.

Diagnosis

A biopsy (by incision or by aspiration) is essential for confirming primary malignant bone tumors. Bone X-rays, and radioisotope bone and CAT scanning show the size of the tumor. Serum alkaline phosphatase is usually elevated in patients with sarcoma.

Treatment

Surgery (usually amputation) and radiation are the treatments of choice, sometimes combined with chemotherapy and immunotherapy. Sometimes radical surgery is necessary (such as hemipelvectomy, interscapulothoracic amputation). However, surgical resection of the tumor (often with preop radiation) *and* postop chemotherapy has proven successful and has saved limbs that would otherwise be amputated. Chemotherapeutic drugs include doxorubicin, actinomycin D, vincristine, cyclophosphamide, and melphalan. Immunotherapy using BCG vaccine (bacille Calmette-Guérin) is still being investigated, as is a new bone transplant technique using freeze-dried bone graft.

Additional considerations

• Health care professionals must be sensitive to the enormous strain caused by the threat of amputation, encourage communication, and help the patient set realistic goals. If amputation seems inevitable, he'll have to learn how to readjust his body weight so he'll be able to get in and out of a bed and a wheelchair. There are exercises he can perform even before surgery that will help him accomplish this.

• Before surgery, I.V. infusions should be used to maintain fluid and electrolyte balance, and to keep a vein open if blood or plasma is needed during surgery.

• After surgery, vital signs must be checked every hour for the first 4 hours; then every 2 hours for the next 4 hours; and then every 4 hours if the patient is stable. A tourniquet should be kept handy in case of hemorrhage. Dressing must be checked periodically for oozing. The foot of the bed should be elevated or the stump placed on a pillow for the first 24 hours; but the stump must not be left elevated for more than 48 hours, as this may lead to contractures.

• To ease the patient's anxiety, analgesics should be given for pain before morning care. The patient may need to be braced with pillows to keep the affected part at rest.

• The patient must eat foods high in protein, vitamins, and folic acid, and to get plenty of rest and sleep to promote recovery. Some physical exercise is also beneficial. Laxatives may be necessary to maintain proper elimination.

• Since the patient may have thrombocytopenia, he must use a soft toothbrush and an electric razor to avoid bleeding. He should not get I.M. injections or have his temperature taken rectally. He must also avoid bumping his arms or legs; his low platelet count causes bruising.

• Adequate fluid intake will prevent dehydration. This makes intake and output records important. After a hemipelvectomy, the insertion of a nasogastric tube will prevent abdominal distention. Low gastric suction should be continued for 2 days after surgery or until the patient can tolerate a soft diet. Administering antibiotics will prevent infection of the rectum. Transfusions may be needed. Drugs should be given to control pain. Drains will be inserted to aid wound drainage and prevent infection. A Foley catheter will be left in place until the patient can void voluntarily.

• Adverse reactions to radiation treatment include nausea, vomiting, and dryness of skin with excoriation.

To encourage early rehabilitation:

• Physical therapy should begin 24 hours postop. Pain is usually not severe after amputation. If it is, a wound complication, such as hematoma, excessive stump edema, or infection may be the problem.

• The "phantom limb" syndrome is when the patient "feels" an itch or tingling in an amputated extremity. This may occur for only a few hours or persist for years. The patient should know this sensation is normal and usually subsides.

• To avoid contractures and assure the best conditions for wound healing, the patient must not hang the stump over the edge of the bed; sit in a wheelchair with the stump flexed; place a pillow under his hip, knee, or back, or between his thighs; lie with knees flexed; rest an above the knee (AK) stump on the crutch handle; or abduct an AK stump.

• The stump should be washed, gently massaged, and kept dry until it heals. The bandage must be firm and worn day and night. The bandage should be applied so that it shapes the stump for a prosthesis.

• The patient, in selecting a prosthesis, should understand the needs to be considered and know the types of prostheses available. The rehabilitation staff will make the final decision, but since most patients are totally uninformed about choosing a prosthesis, some guidelines are needed. The patient's age and possible vision problems should be kept in mind. Generally, children need relatively simple devices, while elderly patients may require prostheses that provide more stability. Personal and family finances are also factors. Children outgrow prostheses, so parents should select inexpensive ones.

• Hospital staff members should encourage a positive attitude toward recovery. The patient should be urged to resume an independent life-style. Elderly patients may need the help of a community health services.

PRIMARY MALIGNANT BONE TUMORS

TYPE	CLINICAL FEATURES	TREATMENT
OSSEOUS ORIGIN		
Osteogenic sarcoma	• Osteoid tumor present in specimen • Tumor arises from bone-forming osteoblast and bone-digesting osteoclast • Occurs most often in femur, but also tibia and humerus; occasionally, in fibula, ilium, vertebra, or mandible • Usually in males, aged 10 to 30 years	• Surgery (tumor resection, high thigh amputation, hemipelvectomy, interscapulothoracic surgery) • Radiation • Chemotherapy • Combination of above
Parosteal osteogenic sarcoma	• Develops on surface of bone instead of interior • Progresses slowly • Occurs most often in distal femur, but also in tibia, humerus, and ulna • Usually in females, aged 30 to 40 years	• Surgery (tumor resection, possible amputation, interscapulothoracic surgery, hemipelvectomy) • Radiation • Chemotherapy • Combination of above
Chondrosarcoma	• Develops from cartilage • Grows slowly but is locally recurrent and invasive • Occurs most often in pelvis, proximal femur, and ribs • Usually in males, aged 30 to 50 years	• Hemipelvectomy, surgical resection (ribs) • Radiation (palliative) • Chemotherapy
Malignant giant cell tumor	• Arises from benign giant cell tumor • Found most often in long bones, especially in knee area • Usually in males, aged 40 to 60 years	• Amputation • Radiation (palliative) • Chemotherapy
NONOSSEOUS ORIGIN		
Ewing's sarcoma	• Originates in bone marrow and invades shafts of long and flat bones, instead of ends • Usually affects lower extremities, most often femur, innominate bones, ribs, tibia, humerus, vertebra, and fibula • Pain increasingly severe and persistent • Usually in males, aged 10 to 20 years • Prognosis poor	• High-voltage radiation (tumor is very radiosensitive) • Chemotherapy to slow growth • Amputation only if there's no evidence of metastases
Fibrosarcoma	• Relatively rare • Originates in fibrous tissue of bone • Invades long or flat bones (femur, tibia, mandible), but also involves periosteum and overlying muscle • Usually in males, aged 30 to 40 years	• Amputation • Radiation • Chemotherapy • Bone grafts (with low-grade fibrosarcoma)
Chordoma	• Derived from embryonic remnants of notochord • Progresses slowly • Usually found at end of spinal column and in spheno-occipital, sacrococcygeal, and vertebral areas • Characterized by constipation and visual disturbances • Usually in males, aged 50 to 60 years	• Surgical resection (often resulting in neural defects) • Radiation (palliative, or when surgery not applicable, as in occipital area)

Multiple Myeloma
(Malignant plasmacytoma, plasma cell myeloma, myelomatosis)

Multiple myeloma is a disseminated neoplasm of immature plasma cells that infiltrates bone to produce osteolytic lesions throughout the skeleton (flat bones,. vertebrae, skull, pelvis, ribs); in late stages, it infiltrates the body organs (liver, spleen, lymph nodes, lungs, adrenal glands, kidneys, skin, and gastrointestinal tract). Multiple myeloma strikes about 7,000 people yearly—mostly men in their 50s to 70s. Prognosis is usually poor, because diagnosis is often made after the disease has already infiltrated the vertebrae, pelvis, skull, ribs, clavicles, and sternum. By then, skeletal destruction is widespread and, without treatment, leads to vertebral collapse; 52% of patients die within 3 months of diagnosis, 90% within 2 years. Early diagnosis and treatment prolong the lives of many patients by 3 to 5 years. Finally, death usually follows complications, such as infection, renal failure, hematologic imbalance, fractures, hypercalcemia, hyperuricemia, or dehydration.

Signs and symptoms

The earliest indication of multiple myeloma is severe, constant back pain that increases with exercise. Arthritic symptoms may also occur: achiness, joint swelling, and tenderness, possibly resulting from vertebral compression. Other clinical effects include fever, malaise, slight evidence of peripheral neuropathy (such as peripheral paresthesias), and pathologic fractures. As multiple myeloma progresses, symptoms of vertebral compression may become acute, and are accompanied by anemia, weight loss, thoracic deformities (ballooning), and loss of body height—5" (12.7 cm) or more due to vertebral collapse. Renal complications, such as pyelonephritis (caused by tubular damage from large amounts of Bence Jones protein, hypercalcemia, and hyperuricemia), may occur. Severe, recurrent infection such as pneumonia may follow damage to nerves associated with respiratory function.

Diagnosis

After the patient has had a physical examination and a careful medical history has been obtained, the following diagnostic tests and nonspecific laboratory abnormalities are appropriate criteria for confirming the presence of multiple myeloma.

• *CBC* shows moderate or severe anemia. The differential may show 40% to 50% lymphocytes but seldom more than 3% plasma cells. Rouleaux formation (often the first clue) seen on differential smear results from elevation of the red cell sedimentation rate.

• *Urine studies* may show Bence Jones protein and hypercalciuria. Absence of Bence Jones protein doesn't rule out multiple myeloma, because this protein doesn't appear in the urine of all such patients; however, its presence almost invariably confirms the disease.

• *Bone marrow aspiration* confirms the diagnosis of the disease by detecting myeloma cells (abnormal number of immature plasma cells).

• *Serum electrophoresis* shows elevated globulin spike that is electrophoretically and immunologically abnormal.

• *X-rays* during early stages may show only diffuse osteoporosis. Eventually, they show multiple, sharply circumscribed osteolytic (punched out) lesions, particularly on the skull, pelvis, and spine—the characteristic lesions of multiple myeloma.

• *Intravenous pyelography* can assess renal involvement. To avoid precipitation of Bence Jones protein, iothalamate or diatrizoate is used instead of the usual contrast medium. And although oral fluid restriction is usually the standard procedure before an intravenous pyelogram (IVP), patients with multiple myeloma receive large quantities of fluid, generally orally but sometimes intravenously, before this test.

Treatment

Long-term treatment of multiple myeloma consists mainly of chemotherapy, which is used to suppress plasma cell growth and control pain. Combinations of melphalan and prednisone, or cyclophosphamide and prednisone may be used. Also, local radiation, used as an adjunct, reduces acute lesions, such as collapsed vertebrae, and relieves localized pain. Other treatment usually includes a melphalan-prednisone combination in high intermittent doses for 4 days every 4 to 6 weeks or in low continuous daily doses, and analgesics for pain. If the patient develops spinal cord compression, he may require a laminectomy; if he has renal complications, he may need dialysis.

Because the patient may have bone demineralization and may lose large amounts of calcium into blood and urine, he is a prime candidate for renal stones, nephrocalcinosis, and eventually, renal failure due to the hypercalcemia. Hypercalcemia is managed with hydration, corticosteroids, oral phosphate, and mithramycin I.V. to decrease serum calcium levels.

Additional considerations

• The patient should drink 3,000 to 4,000 ml fluids daily, particularly before his IVP. Fluid intake and output must be monitored; daily output should not be less than 1,500 ml.

• The patient must be encouraged to walk. (Immobilization increases bone demineralization and vulnerability to pneumonia.) He must not walk unaccompanied and he should use a walker or other supportive aid to prevent falls. To lessen the pain, he'll need analgesics. Since the patient is particularly vulnerable to pathologic fractures, he may understandably be fearful. He should be allowed to move at his own pace and not be hurried.

• Complications can be prevented by watching for fever or malaise, which may signal the onset of infection, and for signs of other problems, such as severe anemia and fractures.

• If the patient is bedridden, he should engage in passive range-of-motion and deep breathing exercises. When the patient can tolerate them, he should begin active exercises. In addition, his position must be changed every 2 hours.

• If the patient is taking melphalan (a phenylalanine derivative of nitrogen mustard that depresses bone marrow), his blood count (platelet and WBC) must be taken before each treatment. If he is taking prednisone, he must be watched closely for infection, since this drug often masks it.

• Whenever possible, the patient should get out of bed within 24 hours after a laminectomy. He must be checked for hemorrhage, motor or sensory deficits, and loss of bowel or bladder function. When he's being turned, he must be log-rolled to maintain his body alignment.

• The patient and his family will need

ALL ABOUT BENCE JONES PROTEIN

The hallmark of multiple myeloma, this protein (a light chain of gamma globulin) was named for Henry Bence Jones, an English doctor who in 1848 noticed that patients with a curious bone disease excreted a unique protein— unique in that it coagulated at 113° to 131° F. (45° to 55° C.), then redissolved when heated to boiling. It remained for Otto Kahler, an Austrian, to demonstrate in 1889 that Bence Jones protein was related to myeloma. Bence Jones protein is not found in the urine of *all* multiple myeloma patients, but it is almost never found in patients without this disease.

emotional support, as they are likely to be very anxious. Their anxiety can be relieved somewhat by getting truthful information about diagnostic tests (including painful procedures, such as bone marrow aspiration and biopsy), treat-ment, and prognosis. They may need help to work through their feelings of anger and grief, and perhaps, should be referred to an appropriate community resource for additional comfort and support.

Soft-tissue Sarcoma

Almost all soft-tissue malignancies are sarcomas. These tumors of muscle, fat, connective tissue, blood vessels, and synovium are made up of tightly packed cells similar to embryonic connective tissue. Soft-tissue sarcomas occur in both males and females, but they are rare. In fact, they account for only 1% of all malignancies and for 6% of all malignancies in persons under age 25. Prognosis varies with staging, and is best when the disease is diagnosed early.

Causes
The causes of soft-tissue sarcoma aren't known, but evidence suggests several still-unproven predisposing factors: trauma (sarcomas often arise in scars from burns, surgery, radiation, or penetrating wounds) and precursor tumors, such as benign angiomas.

Generally, sarcomas metastasize through the bloodstream; sometimes, through the lymphatic system. Usually, the more than 50 kinds of sarcomas are classified according to the site of origin. These are the most common types:
• *Liposarcoma* originates in fatty tissue, usually in the thigh, inguinal, and gluteal regions. It's the most common soft-tissue tumor and tends to become quite large. Although it's rare in children, when it does occur, it tends to develop during infancy or adolescence.
• *Fibrosarcoma* originates in subcutaneous fibrous tissue, scars, deep connective tissue, and around tendons, nerve sheaths, and muscle fascia. It's the second most common sarcoma but rarely occurs in children.
• *Rhabdomyosarcoma* originates in skeletal muscle and can be subdivided into four distinct, fast-growing types: the *pleomorphic* usually arises in the extremities in males; the *alveolar* generally affects adolescents and may occur anywhere; the *embryonal* most commonly

occurs on the head, neck, or within the eye orbit of children under 10 years old; and the *botryoidal* is frequently found in the muscles of the genital and urinary tracts at about age 7.
• *Leiomyosarcoma* originates in smooth muscle, usually in the uterus or retroperitoneal area. In children, it usually develops before age 5.
• *Synovial sarcoma* originates in the synovial tissue of tendon sheaths, joints (especially in the hands and feet), and bursa. It usually affects young adults and tends to recur.
• *Angiosarcoma* (angioendothelioma, hemangiosarcoma) originates in vascular tissue and is rare.
• *Mixed mesenchymal sarcoma* originates in primitive mesenchyme. It's usually subdivided into two types: *myxomas*, half of which occur in the extremities; and *mesenchymomas*, which occur in soft tissues anywhere in the body.

Signs and symptoms
Soft-tissue sarcomas are often painless in the early stages of the diseases (although some may be tender), so they're often overlooked until they're large enough to press against a nerve. Usually, they grow slowly, but some types grow so rapidly that they become quite large in a matter of weeks.

Soft-tissue sarcomas may be palpable

as a hard or soft mass; superficial tumors may cause local redness and heat. Palpation of regional nodes and the liver may reveal metastasis.

Diagnosis

An incisional or needle biopsy is absolutely essential for histologic determination of tumor type. Other tests include a chest X-ray (sarcomas often metastasize to the lungs), bone X-rays, and possibly, a CAT scan and arteriography.

Treatment

Treatment consists of surgical resection, and depending on the staging of the disease, radiation and chemotherapy. Treatment of rare tumors should take place in a medical center where the staff is experienced in complex multimodality therapy.
• Surgical resection varies with tumor location, and includes muscle resection, limb amputation, and radical local excision.
• Usually, in chemotherapy, combinations of actinomycin D, dacarbazine, doxorubicin, methotrexate, vincristine, and cyclophosphamide are used.
• Radiation to the tumor and, if necessary, to surrounding tissues may be ordered both pre- and postoperatively. However, these tumors are often radio-resistant.
• Immunotherapy is still being investigated to determine its effectiveness.
• After treatment, *all* patients require periodic follow-up examinations (including chest X-rays, local X-rays, and physical examination) to detect metastases and local recurrence.

Additional considerations

Patient teaching, meticulous postop care, and supportive measures can help the patient return to as nearly normal a life as possible. After diagnosis, information the doctor has given the patient and family about the disease and treatment should be supplemented and reinforced.

The patient must understand the expected surgery and postop procedures, and the possible side effects of radiation and chemotherapy.

After surgical resection, the health care professional should:
• check dressings frequently for bleeding and signs of infection, such as excessive swelling and foul odor.
• monitor vital signs regularly; watch for fever that may point to infection; encourage adequate fluid intake, and monitor intake and output carefully.
• provide good amputee care if amputation is necessary. (For more information, see PRIMARY MALIGNANT BONE TUMORS.)
• check the extremity for warmth, sensation, color, and movement; give good cast care, if applicable, to prevent skin breakdown; help the patient with casts, braces, or splints to position himself comfortably with pillows; assist with range-of-motion exercises; refer the patient for rehabilitation and physical therapy, as needed.

During radiation and chemotherapy, the dietary department must provide a diet high in protein. The patient will need supportive care to control toxic side effects, and an antiemetic, if ordered.

The patient and family should get psychologic support, answers to all questions, and help in setting realistic goals for recovery.

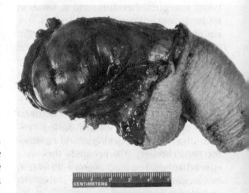

This is a specimen of liposarcoma (of the penis), the most common soft-tissue tumor.

SKIN

Basal Cell Epithelioma
(Basal cell carcinoma)

Basal cell epithelioma (BCE) is a slow-growing destructive skin tumor. This carcinoma usually occurs in people over age 40; it's more prevalent in blond, fair-skinned males and is the most common malignant tumor affecting Caucasians.

Causes
Prolonged sun exposure is the most common cause of basal cell epithelioma, but arsenic ingestion, radiation, burns, and rarely, vaccinations are other possible causes. Most of these tumors (94%) occur on parts of the body with abundant pilosebaceous follicles, especially on the face.

Although the pathogenesis of basal cell epithelioma is uncertain, some experts now hypothesize that it originates when, under certain conditions, undifferentiated basal cells become carcinomatous instead of differentiating into sweat glands, sebum, and hair.

Signs and symptoms
The lesions of basal cell epithelioma are of three types:

• *Nodulo-ulcerative* lesions occur most often on the face, particularly the forehead, margins of eyelids, and nasolabial folds. In early stages, these lesions are small, smooth, pinkish, and translucent papules. Telangiectatic vessels cross the surface, and the lesions are occasionally pigmented. As they enlarge, the centers of the lesions become depressed, while the borders become firm and elevated. Ulceration and local invasion occur next; these ulcerated tumors are called "rodent ulcers." These lesions rarely metastasize; however, if untreated, they can spread to vital areas, become infected, or cause massive hemorrhage if they invade large blood vessels.

• *Superficial BCEs* are often multiple and commonly occur on the chest and back. They're oval or irregularly shaped, lightly pigmented plaques, with sharply defined, threadlike borders that are slightly elevated. Due to superficial erosion, these lesions appear scaly and have small, atrophic areas in the center, resembling psoriasis or eczema. They're usually chronic and don't tend to invade other areas. This type of lesion is related to ingestion of or exposure to arsenic-containing compounds.

• *Sclerosing BCEs (morphealike epitheliomas)* occur on the head and neck. They appear yellow to white in color, and are waxy, sclerotic plaques without distinct borders. They may look like small patches of scleroderma.

Diagnosis
All basal cell epitheliomas are diagnosed by clinical appearance, incisional or excisional biopsy, and histologic study.

Treatment
Depending on the size, location, and depth of the lesion, treatment may include curettage and electrodesiccation, chemotherapy, surgical excision, irradiation, or chemosurgery.

• Curettage and electrodesiccation offer good cosmetic results for small lesions.

• Topical 5-fluorouracil is often used if the lesions are superficial. It produces marked local irritation or inflammation in the involved tissue but no systemic effects.

• Surgery may require skin grafting if the lesion is large.

• Irradiation is used for elderly or debilitated patients who might not withstand surgery.

• Chemosurgery is often necessary for persistent or recurrent lesions. It consists of periodic applications of a fixative paste (such as zinc chloride) and subsequent removal of fixed pathologic tissue. Treatment continues until complete tumor removal.

Additional considerations

• The patient should eat frequent small meals high in protein. If the lesion has invaded the oral cavity and produced eating problems, the patient can drink egg nog, blenderized foods, or liquid protein supplements to fulfill his protein requirements.
• The patient must avoid excessive sun exposure and use a sunscreen or sunshade to protect his skin from damage by ultraviolet rays. This helps to prevent disease recurrence.
• The patient can relieve local inflammation, following topical 5-fluorouracil application, by applying cool compresses or corticosteroid ointment to the skin.
• The patient with nodulo-ulcerative

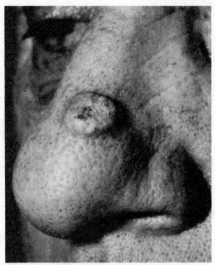

The photograph above shows an enlarged nasal nodule in basal cell carcinoma.

BCE that has ulcerated and become encrusted should be careful when washing; the crust is friable, and scrubbing too vigorously may cause bleeding.

Squamous Cell Carcinoma

Squamous cell carcinoma of the skin is an invasive tumor with metastatic potential that arises from the keratinizing epidermal cells. It occurs most often in fair-skinned Caucasian males over age 60. Outdoor employment and living in a sunny, warm climate (southwestern United States, Australia, for example) greatly increase the risk of developing squamous cell carcinoma.

Causes

Predisposing factors associated with squamous cell carcinoma include solar radiation, the presence of premalignant lesions (actinic keratosis, Bowen's disease), X-ray therapy, ingestion of herbicides containing arsenic, chronic skin irritation and inflammation, exposure to local carcinogens (tar and oil), and hereditary diseases (xeroderma pigmentosa and albinism). Rarely, squamous cell carcinoma may develop on the site of smallpox vaccination, psoriasis, or chronic discoid lupus erythematosus.

Signs and symptoms

Squamous cell carcinoma commonly arises in the skin of the face, the ears, the dorsa of the hands and forearms, and other sun-damaged areas. Lesions on sun-damaged skin tend not to be as invasive, with less tendency to metastasize than lesions on unexposed skin. Notable exceptions to this rule are squamous cell lesions on the lower lip and the ears. These are almost invariably markedly invasive metastatic lesions, with a generally poor prognosis.

Transformation from a premalignant

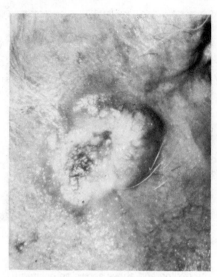

Ulcerated nodule with indurated base in squamous cell carcinoma

---

TREATING ACTINIC KERATOSES WITH TOPICAL 5-FLUOROURACIL

5-fluorouracil is available in different strengths (1%, 2%, and 5%) as a cream or solution. Local application causes immediate stinging and burning, followed later by erythema, vesiculation, erosion, superficial ulceration, necrosis, and re-epithelialization. The 5% solution induces the most severe inflammatory response, but provides complete involution of the lesions with little recurrence. 5-fluorouracil must be kept away from eyes, scrotum, or mucous membranes. In addition, the patient must avoid excessive exposure to the sun during the course of treatment because it intensifies the inflammatory reaction.

Application of 5-fluorouracil should continue until the lesions reach the ulcerative and necrotic stages (usually 2 to 4 weeks); then a corticosteroid preparation may be applied as an anti-inflammatory agent. Possible side effects of treatment include postinflammatory hyperpigmentation. Complete healing occurs within 1 to 2 months, with excellent results.

---

lesion to squamous cell carcinoma may begin with induration and inflammation of the preexisting lesion. When squamous cell carcinoma arises from normal skin, the nodule grows slowly on a firm, indurated base. If untreated, this nodule eventually ulcerates and invades underlying tissues. Metastasis can occur to the regional lymph nodes, producing characteristic systemic symptoms of pain, malaise, fatigue, weakness, and anorexia.

Diagnosis

 An excisional biopsy provides definitive diagnosis of squamous cell carcinoma. Other appropriate laboratory tests depend on systemic symptoms.

Treatment

The size, shape, location, and invasiveness of a squamous cell tumor, and the condition of the underlying tissue determine the treatment; a deeply invasive tumor may require a combination of techniques. All the major treatment methods have excellent rates of cure; generally, prognosis is better with a well-differentiated lesion than with a poorly differentiated one in an unusual location. Treatment may consist of:
• wide surgical excision
• electrodesiccation and curettage (offer good cosmetic results for smaller lesions)
• radiation therapy (generally for older or debilitated patients)
• chemosurgery (reserved for resistant or recurrent lesions).

Additional considerations

A care plan for patients with squamous cell carcinoma should emphasize meticulous wound care and thorough patient instruction. The health care professional should:
• coordinate a consistent care plan for changing the dressings; establish a standard routine to help the patient and family learn to care for the wound; explain any necessary changes in technique.
• keep the wound dry and clean.

PREMALIGNANT SKIN LESIONS

DISEASE	CAUSE	PATIENT	LESION	TREATMENT
Actinic keratosis	Solar radiation	Caucasian men with fair skin (middle-aged to elderly)	Reddish-brown lesions 1 mm to 1 cm in size (may enlarge if untreated) on face, ears, lower lip, bald scalp, dorsa of hands and forearms	Topical 5-fluorouracil, cryosurgery using liquid nitrogen, or curettage by electrodesiccation
Bowen's disease	Unknown	Caucasian men with fair skin (middle-aged to elderly)	Brown to reddish-brown lesions, with scaly surface on exposed and unexposed areas	Surgical excision, topical 5-fluorouracil
Erythroplasia of Queyrat	Bowen's disease of the mucous membranes	Men (middle-aged to elderly)	Red lesions, with a glistening or granular appearance on mucous membranes, particularly the glans penis in uncircumcised males	Surgical excision
Leukoplakia	Smoking, alcohol, chronic cheek-biting, ill-fitting dentures, misaligned teeth	Men (middle-aged to elderly)	Lesions on oral, anal, and genital mucous membranes vary in appearance from smooth and white to rough and gray	Elimination of irritating factors, surgical excision, or curettage by electrodesiccation (if lesion is still premalignant)

• pack deep, open lesions with dressings moistened in saline solution or povidine-iodine; allow the dressings to dry on the wound; debride the area by removing these dressings.

• try controlling odor with balsam of Peru, yogurt flakes, oil of cloves, or other odor-masking substances, even though they are often ineffective for long-term use. (Topical or systemic antibiotics also temporarily control odor and eventually will merely change the bacterial flora in the lesion.)

• be prepared for other problems that accompany a metastatic disease (pain, fatigue, weakness, anorexia).

• help the patient and family set realistic goals and expectations.

Disfiguring lesions are distressing to both the patient and hospital staff members who care for him. They must try to accept the patient as he is, and to increase his self-esteem and strengthen a caring relationship.

To prevent squamous cell carcinoma, a patient must:

• avoid excessive sun exposure.

• wear protective clothing (hats, long sleeves).

• have precancerous lesions removed promptly.

• use sunscreening agents containing para-aminobenzoic acid (PABA) in a 50% to 70% alcohol base, benzophenone (less effective), and zinc oxide (best known; cosmetically unsatisfactory).

• use lipscreens to protect the lips from sun damage.

Malignant Melanoma

A neoplasm which arises from pigment-producing melanocytes, malignant melanoma is relatively rare and accounts for only 1% to 2% of all malignancies. The three types of malignant melanomas are superficial spreading melanoma, nodular malignant melanoma, and lentigo maligna melanoma. Malignant melanoma is slightly more common in women than in men, and is rare in children. Peak incidence occurs between ages 50 and 70, although many expect the incidence in younger age-groups to increase in the future.

Melanoma spreads through the lymphatic and vascular systems, and metastasizes to the regional lymph nodes, the liver, lungs, and CNS. Its course is unpredictable, however, and recurrence and metastases may not appear for more than 5 years after resection of the primary lesion. Prognosis varies with tumor thickness. Generally, superficial lesions are curable, while deeper lesions tend to metastasize. Two methods are currently used to measure tumor depth: the Clark level and the Breslow level. The Breslow level measures lesion depth from the granular level of the epidermis to the deepest melanoma cell. Melanoma lesions less than 0.76 mm deep have an excellent prognosis, while deeper lesions (more than 0.76 mm) are at risk for metastasis. Prognosis is better for a tumor on an extremity (which is drained by one lymphatic network) than for one on the head, neck, or trunk (drained by several networks).

Causes

Several factors seem to influence the development of melanoma:

• *Excessive exposure to sunlight.* Melanoma is most common in sunny, warm areas, and often develops on parts of the body that are exposed to the sun.

• *Skin type.* Most persons who get melanoma have blond or red hair, fair skin, and blue eyes; sunburn easily; and are of Celtic or Scandinavian ancestry. Melanoma is rare among Blacks; when it does develop, it usually arises in lightly pigmented areas (the palms, plantar surface of the feet, or mucous membranes).

• *Hormonal factors.* Pregnancy may increase incidence and exacerbate growth.

• *Family history.* Melanoma may occur slightly more often within families, but this may merely reflect ethnic background, climate, and other factors.

• *Past history of melanoma.* A person who has had one melanoma is at greater risk of developing a second.

Signs and symptoms

Common sites for melanoma are on the head and neck in men, on the legs in women, and the backs of persons exposed to excessive sunlight. Up to 70% arise from a preexisting nevus. It rarely appears in the conjunctiva, choroid, pharynx, mouth, vagina, or anus.

Suspect melanoma when any skin lesion or nevus enlarges, changes color, becomes inflamed or sore, itches, ulcerates, bleeds, undergoes textural changes, or shows signs of surrounding pigment regression (halo nevus or vitiligo).

Each type of melanoma has special characteristics:

• *Superficial spreading melanoma* (SSM), the most common, usually develops between ages 40 and 50. Often, such a lesion arises on an area of chronic irritation, such as the belt line. In women, it's most common between the knees and ankles; in Blacks and Orientals, on the toe webs and soles (lightly pigmented areas subject to trauma). Characteristically, this melanoma has a red, white, or blue color over a brown or black background, and an irregular, notched margin. Its surface is irregular, with small elevated tumor nodules that may ulcerate and bleed. Horizontal growth may continue for many years; when vertical growth begins, prognosis worsens.

• *Nodular malignant melanoma* (NMM) usually develops between ages 40 and 50, grows vertically, invades the dermis, and metastasizes early. Such a lesion is usually a polypoidal nodule, with uniformly dark discoloration (it may be grayish), and looks like a blackberry. Occasionally, this melanoma is flesh-colored, with flecks of pigment around its base (which may be inflamed).

• *Lentigo maligna melanoma* (LMM) is relatively rare. It arises from a lentigo maligna on an exposed skin surface and usually occurs between ages 60 and 70. Such a lesion looks like a large (3 to 6 cm) flat freckle of tan, brown, black, whitish, or slate color, and has irregularly scattered black nodules on the surface. It develops slowly, usually over many years, and eventually may ulcerate. This melanoma commonly develops under the fingernails, on the face, and on the back of the hands.

Diagnosis

A skin biopsy with histologic examination can distinguish malignant melanoma from a benign nevus, seborrheic keratosis, and pigmented basal cell epithelioma, and can also determine tumor thickness. Physical examination, paying particular attention to lymph nodes, can point to metastatic involvement.

Baseline lab studies include CBC with differential, erythrocyte sedimentation rate (ESR), platelet count, liver function studies, and urinalysis. Depending on the depth of tumor invasion and metastatic spread, baseline diagnostic studies may also include chest X-ray and lung tomography, a liver-spleen scan, a CAT scan of the body, and a gallium scan. Signs of bone metastasis may call for a bone scan; CNS metastasis, a CAT scan of the brain.

Treatment

Malignant melanoma always requires surgical resection to remove the tumor. A deep tumor requires wide resection, with margins extending at least 2″ (5

CLARK LEVELS FOR MELANOMA

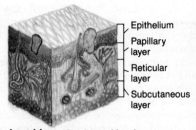

Epithelium
Papillary layer
Reticular layer
Subcutaneous layer

Level I—confined to epidermis
Level II—penetration of papillary layer

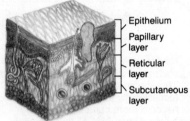

Epithelium
Papillary layer
Reticular layer
Subcutaneous layer

Level III—accumulation between papillary and reticular dermis

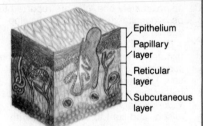

Epithelium
Papillary layer
Reticular layer
Subcutaneous layer

Level IV—extension into reticular dermis

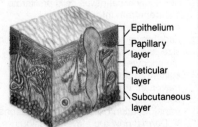

Epithelium
Papillary layer
Reticular layer
Subcutaneous layer

Level V—invasion of subcutaneous layer

cm) beyond the primary lesion's borders and into the deep fascia. Closure of such a resection may necessitate a skin graft. Treatment may also include regional lymphadenectomy.

Lesions deeper than 0.76 mm (Clark level III, IV, or V) may merit adjuvant chemotherapy with a cytotoxic agent to eliminate tumor cells.

Immunotherapy is being investigated and includes BCG vaccine (bacille Calmette-Guérin) or methanol extraction of residue of BCG (MER) given transcutaneously or intralymphatically to stimulate the patient's immune response. Another investigational form of immunotherapy consists of a topical application of a depigmenting agent, monobenzone ether of hydroquinone, which can destroy pigment cells and, hypothetically, triggers a systemic immunologic response to these cells. The benefit from these therapies has yet to be proven.

Radiation therapy is usually reserved for metastatic disease. It doesn't prolong survival but may reduce tumor size and relieve pain. Regardless of treatment, melanomas require close long-term follow-up to detect metastases and recurrences. Statistics show that 13% of recurrences develop more than 5 years after primary surgery.

RECOGNIZING POTENTIALLY MALIGNANT NEVI

Nevi (moles) are skin lesions that are often pigmented and may be hereditary. They begin to grow in childhood (occasionally they're congenital) and become numerous in young adults. Up to 70% of patients with melanoma have a history of a preexisting nevus at the tumor site. Of these, approximately one third are reported to be congenital; the remainder develop later in life.

Changes in nevi (color, size, shape, texture, ulceration, bleeding, or itching) suggest possible malignant transformation. The presence or absence of hair within a nevus has no significance.

• *Junctional nevi* are flat or slightly raised, and light to dark brown, with melanocytes confined to the epidermis. Usually, they appear before age 40. These nevi may change into compound nevi if junctional nevus cells proliferate and penetrate into the dermis.

• *Compound nevi* are usually tan to dark brown and slightly raised, although size and color vary. They contain melanocytes in both the dermis and epidermis, and they rarely undergo malignant transformation. Excision is necessary only to rule out malignant transformation or for cosmetic reasons.

• *Dermal nevi* are elevated lesions from 2 to 10 mm in diameter, and vary in color from flesh to brown. They usually develop in older adults and generally arise on the upper part of the body. Excision is necessary only to rule out malignant transformation.

• *Blue nevi* are slightly elevated lesions less than 0.5 cm in diameter. They appear on the head, neck, arms, and dorsa of the hands, and are twice as common in women as in men. Their blue color results from pigment and collagen in the dermis, which reflect blue light but absorb other wavelengths. Excision is necessary to rule out pigmented basal cell epithelioma or melanoma, or for cosmetic reasons.

• *Lentigo maligna* (melanotic freckles, Hutchinson's freckles) is a precursor to malignant melanoma. (In fact, about one third of them eventually give rise to malignant melanoma.) Usually, they occur in persons over age 40, especially on exposed skin areas, such as the face. At first, these lesions are flat, tan spots, but they gradually enlarge and darken, and develop black speckled areas against their tan or brown background. Each lesion may simultaneously enlarge in one area and regress in another. Histologic examination shows typical and atypical melanocytes along the epidermal basement membrane. Removal by simple excision (not electrodesiccation and curettage) is recommended.

Additional considerations

Management of the melanoma patient requires careful physical, psychologic, and social assessment. Preoperative teaching, meticulous postoperative care, and psychologic support can speed the patient's recovery and prevent complications.

• After diagnosis, the hospital staff member caring for the patient should: review the doctor's explanation of treatment alternatives; tell the patient what to expect before and after surgery, and what the wound will look like; warn him that the donor site for a skin graft may be as painful, if not more painful, than the tumor excision site itself; answer questions honestly regarding surgery, chemotherapy, and radiation.

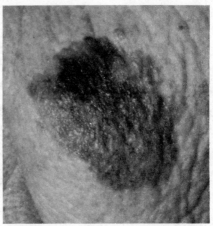
Lentigo maligna melanoma (LMM) of the cheek

• After surgery, the staff member should: be careful to prevent infection; check dressings on both donor and resection site often for excessive drainage, foul odor, redness, or swelling; minimize lymphedema (in case of lymphadenectomy) by applying a compression stocking, and instructing the patient to keep the extremity elevated.

• During chemotherapy, the staff member should know what side effects to expect and do what can be done to minimize them. For instance, giving an antiemetic will reduce nausea and vomiting. If treatment includes BCG, acetaminophen will relieve slight fever and malaise.

• To prepare the patient for discharge, the staff member should: emphasize the need for close follow-up to detect recurrences early; explain that recurrences and metastases, if they occur, are often delayed, so follow-up must continue for years; tell him how to recognize signs of recurrence; provide psychologic support to help the patient cope with anxiety; encourage him to verbalize his fears; answer his questions honestly without destroying hope.

• In advanced metastatic disease, the staff member should: control and prevent pain with consistent, regularly scheduled administration of analgesics, instead of relieving pain after it occurs; make referrals for home care, social ser-

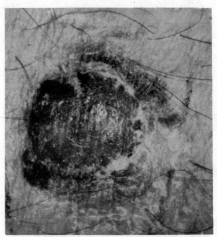
Superficial spreading melanoma (SSM) of the ankle

vices, and spiritual and financial assistance, as needed; identify the needs of patient, family, and friends, and provide appropriate support and care.

To help prevent malignant melanoma, patients must avoid overexposure to solar radiation, especially if they're fair-skinned and blue-eyed. They should use a sunblock or sunscreen. In all physical examinations, especially in fair-skinned persons, unusual nevi or other skin lesions may point to malignant melanoma.

BLOOD AND LYMPH

Hodgkin's Disease

Hodgkin's disease is a neoplastic disease characterized by painless, progressive enlargement of lymph nodes, spleen, and other lymphoid tissue resulting from proliferation of lymphocytes, histiocytes, eosinophils, and Reed-Sternberg's giant cells. The latter cells are its special histologic feature. Untreated, Hodgkin's disease follows a variable but relentlessly progressive and ultimately fatal course. However, recent advances in therapy make Hodgkin's disease potentially curable, even in advanced stages, and appropriate treatment yields a 5-year survival rate of approximately 54% of patients.

Causes and incidence
The cause of Hodgkin's disease is unknown. It is most common in young adults, with a higher incidence in males than in females. It occurs in all races but is slightly more common in Caucasians. Its incidence peaks in two age-groups: 15 to 38 and after age 50—except in Japan, where it occurs exclusively among people over 50.

Signs and symptoms
The first sign of Hodgkin's disease is usually a painless swelling of one of the cervical lymph nodes (but sometimes the axillary, mediastinal, or inguinal lymph nodes), occasionally in a patient who gives a history of recent upper respiratory infection. In older patients, the first symptoms may be nonspecific—persistent fever, night sweats, fatigue, weight loss, and malaise. Rarely, if the mediastinum is initially involved, Hodgkin's may produce respiratory symptoms.

Another early and characteristic indication of Hodgkin's disease is pruritus, which, while mild at first, becomes acute as the disease progresses. A rare symptom is the presence of the Pel-Ebstein fever pattern (intermittent fever of several days duration alternating with afebrile periods). Other symptoms depend on the degree and location of systemic involvement.

Lymph nodes may enlarge rapidly, producing pain and obstruction, or enlarge slowly and painlessly for months or years. It's not unusual to see the lymph nodes "wax and wane," but they usually don't return to normal. Sooner or later, most patients develop systemic manifestations, including enlargement of retroperitoneal nodes and nodular infiltrations of the spleen, the liver, and bones. At this late stage, other symptoms include edema of the face and neck, progressive anemia, possible jaundice, nerve pain, and increased susceptibility to infection.

Diagnosis
Diagnostic measures for confirming Hodgkin's disease include a thorough medical history, a thorough physical examination, followed by a lymph node biopsy checking for Reed-Sternberg's abnormal histiocyte proliferation, and nodular fibrosis and necrosis. Other appropriate diagnostic tests include bone marrow, liver, and spleen biopsies; and routine chest X-ray, intravenous pyelography, lung scan, bone scan, and lymphangiography, to detect lymph node or organ involvement.

Hematologic tests show mild to severe normocytic anemia; normochromic anemia (in 50%); elevated, normal, or reduced WBC and differential showing any combination of neutrophilia, lymphocytopenia, monocytosis, and eosinophilia. Blood chemistries show elevated serum alkaline phosphatase, indicating liver or bone involvement.

THE STAGES OF HODGKIN'S DISEASE

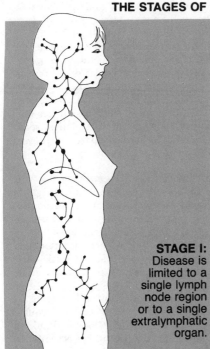

STAGE I:
Disease is limited to a single lymph node region or to a single extralymphatic organ.

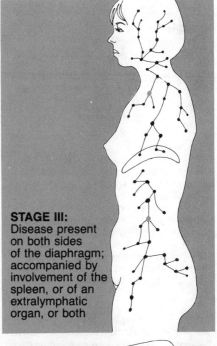

STAGE III:
Disease present on both sides of the diaphragm; accompanied by involvement of the spleen, or of an extralymphatic organ, or both

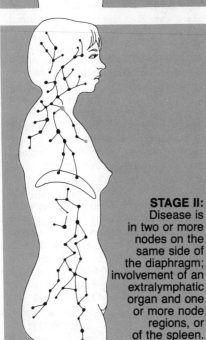

STAGE II:
Disease is in two or more nodes on the same side of the diaphragm; involvement of an extralymphatic organ and one or more node regions, or of the spleen.

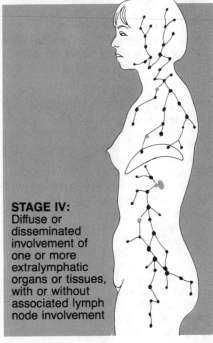

STAGE IV:
Diffuse or disseminated involvement of one or more extralymphatic organs or tissues, with or without associated lymph node involvement

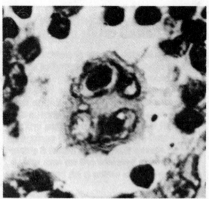

These enlarged, abnormal histocytes (Reed-Sternberg cells) from an excised lymph node suggest Hodgkin's disease. Note the large, distinct nucleoli. Reed-Sternberg cells indicate Hodgkin's disease when they coexist with one of these four histologic patterns: lymphocyte predominance, mixed cellularity, lymphocyte depletion, and nodular sclerosis.

The same diagnostic tests are also used for staging. A staging laparotomy is necessary for patients who are under age 55 or who don't have obvious Stage III or Stage IV disease, lymphocyte predominance subtype histology, or medical contraindications. Diagnosis must rule out other disorders that also enlarge the lymph nodes.

Treatment

Appropriate therapy (chemotherapy and/ or radiation varying with the stage of the disease) depends on careful physical examination with accurate histologic interpretation and proper clinical staging. Correct treatment allows longer survival and even induces an apparent cure in many patients. Radiation therapy is used alone for Stage I and Stage II, and in combination with chemotherapy for Stage III. Chemotherapy is used for Stage III and Stage IV, sometimes inducing complete remissions. Chemotherapy includes various combinations of mechlorethamine (nitrogen mustard), vincristine, procarbazine, prednisone, cyclophosphamide, vinblastine, carmustine, bleomycin, doxorubicin, and dacarbazine. The well-known MOPP protocol (mechlorethamine, vincristine [Oncovin], procarbazine, and prednisone) was the first to provide significant cures to patients with generalized Hodgkin's; another useful protocol is ABVD (adriamycin, bleomycin, vinblastine, and DTIC). Treatment with these drugs may require concomitant antiemetics, sedatives, or antidiarrheals to treat or prevent gastrointestinal side effects.

Additional considerations

Because many patients with Hodgkin's disease receive radiation or chemotherapy as outpatients, the patient must observe the following precautions:

• Watch for and report radiation and chemotherapy side effects (particularly anorexia, nausea, vomiting, and diarrhea).

• Minimize radiation side effects by good nutrition: eating small, frequent meals of his favorite foods; drinking plenty of fluids; pacing his activities to counteract therapy-induced fatigue; and making sure that the skin in irradiated areas stays dry.

• Control pain and bleeding of stomatitis by using a soft toothbrush, cotton swab, or anesthetic mouthwash such as viscous lidocaine (as prescribed); by applying petroleum jelly to his lips; and by avoiding astringent mouthwashes.

• If a woman patient is of childbearing age, she must delay pregnancy until prolonged remission, because radiation and chemotherapy can cause genetic mutations and spontaneous abortions.

Because the patient with Hodgkin's disease has usually been healthy up until this point, he is likely to be especially distressed. He'll need emotional support and appropriate counseling and reassurance. He should be encouraged by staff members and friends to be optimistic about his prognosis.

Both the patient and his family should know that the local chapter of the American Cancer Society is available for information, financial assistance, and supportive counseling.

Malignant Lymphomas

(Non-Hodgkin's lymphomas, lymphosarcomas)

Malignant lymphomas are a heterogeneous group of malignant diseases originating in lymph glands and other lymphoid tissue. Lymphomas are categorized by Rappaport histologic classification according to the degree of cellular differentiation and the presence or absence of nodularity. Nodular lymphomas yield a better prognosis than the diffuse form of the disease, but in both, prognosis is less hopeful than in Hodgkin's disease.

Causes and incidence

The cause of malignant lymphomas is unknown, although some researchers have suggested a viral source. Up to 8,000 new cases of malignant lymphoma appear annually in the United States alone. It's two to three times more common in males than in females, and occurs in all age-groups. Although it is rare in children, it occurs about one to three times more often and causes twice as many deaths as Hodgkin's lymphoma in children under 15. Incidence rises with increasing age (median age is 50). These lymphomas seem linked to racial or ethnic status, with increased incidence in Caucasians and people of Jewish ancestry.

Signs and symptoms

Usually, the first indication of malignant lymphoma is swelling of the lymph glands, enlarged tonsils and adenoids, and painless, rubbery nodes in the cervical supraclavicular areas. In children, these nodes are usually in the cervical region, and the disease causes dyspnea and coughing. As the lymphoma progresses, the patient develops symptoms specific to the area involved and systemic complaints of fatigue, malaise, weight loss, fever, and night sweats.

Diagnosis

 Diagnosis requires histologic evaluation of biopsied lymph nodes, or tonsils, bone marrow, liver, bowel, or skin; or, as needed, of tissue removed during exploratory laparotomy. (Biopsy differentiates malignant lymphoma from Hodgkin's disease.) Other relevant tests include bone and chest X-rays, lymphangiography, liver and spleen scan, CAT scan of the abdomen, and intravenous pyelography. Lab tests include CBC (may show anemia), uric acid (elevated or normal), serum calcium (elevated if bone

---

STAGING MALIGNANT LYMPHOMA

Stage I: Involvement of a single lymph node region or of a single extralymphatic organ or site

Stage II: Involvement of two or more lymph node regions on the same side of the diaphragm, or localized involvement of an extralymphatic organ or site of one or more lymph node regions on the same side of the diaphragm

Stage III: Involvement of lymph node regions on both sides of the diaphragm, which may also be accompanied by localized involvement of extralymphatic organ or site or by involvement of the spleen or both

Stage IV: Diffuse or disseminated involvement of one or more extralymphatic organs or tissues with or without associated lymph node enlargement.

Reprinted from *Manual for Staging of Cancer* (Chicago: American Joint Committee for Cancer Staging and End Results Reporting, 1978). Used with permission.

lesions present), serum protein (normal), and liver function studies.

Treatment
Treatment for malignant lymphomas may include radiotherapy or chemotherapy. Radiotherapy is used mainly in the early localized stage of the disease. Total nodal irradiation (usually for Stage III) is still experimental.

Chemotherapy is most effective with multiple combinations of antineoplastic agents. For example, cyclophosphamide, vincristine, and prednisone can induce a complete remission in 50% to 75% of patients with nodular histology, and in 20% to 55% of patients with diffuse histology. Encouragingly, other combinations—such as bleomycin, adriamycin, cytoxan, vincristine (Oncovin), and prednisone (BACOP)—induce prolonged remission and possible cure in patients with diffuse histology.

Additional considerations
• The patient receiving radiation or chemotherapy must be observed for side effects (anorexia, nausea, vomiting, diarrhea).
• The dietitian should plan small, frequent meals scheduled around the patient's treatment. If the patient can't tolerate oral feedings, I.V. fluids will be administered.
• If necessary, antiemetics and sedatives may be ordered. The patient must keep irradiated skin dry.
• Hospital staff members can provide emotional support by informing the patient and family about prognosis and diagnosis, and by listening to their concerns. If needed, they should be referred to the local chapter of the American Cancer Society for information, financial assistance, and counseling. They must understand the need for continued treatment and follow-up care.

Burkitt's Tumor
(Burkitt's lymphoma)

Burkitt's tumor is a highly undifferentiated malignant lymphoma that usually begins as a large osteolytic lesion in the jaw (African Burkitt's), or as an abdominal mass (American Burkitt's). Burkitt's tumor usually occurs in children (ages 2 to 11), with incidence peaking at age 7; occasionally it is found in adults. It strikes more males than females. In its advanced stage, the disease is rapidly fatal.

Causes and incidence
Burkitt's geographic distribution (yellow fever endemic areas) suggests a vectored, viral origin. It is most prevalent in the tropical, moist areas of Africa, Papua, and New Guinea, and occurs sporadically worldwide, except in mountainous or arid regions. It is rare in the United States.

The origin of Burkitt's tumor is unknown. Its probable cause, the Epstein-Barr virus (EBV)—a herpes-like virus —has been identified by electron microscopy of cultured Burkitt's lymphomas in most of the African and some of the American cases. (This represents the most direct link known for a viral etiology of human cancer.) EBV has a worldwide distribution, and appears to be associated with abacterial pharyngitis in children and infectious mononucleosis in adults.

Signs and symptoms
The African form of Burkitt's lymphoma generally begins with a jaw tumor as the major symptom; all other forms of the disease usually begin with an abdominal tumor. At first, the patient has no symptoms, but within 1 to 3 months, he develops nausea, vomiting, abdominal pain, and ascites (in 50%), often followed by neurologic deficits (paraplegia and loss of sphincter control).

Diagnosis

Diagnosis is based on patient history and physical assessment (presentation of jaw or of abdominal tumor), with characteristic histologic findings in the biopsy of the tumor; cytologic examination of peritoneal and pleural effusions, CSF, and bone marrow aspirates; and liver function studies to detect hepatic involvement. X-ray studies include intravenous pyelography to detect renal metastasis, abdominal lymphangiography to detect abdominal metastasis, and skeletal series to detect bone metastasis.

Treatment

Treatment includes chemotherapy (preferred treatment) and radiotherapy (effectiveness limited by multifocal nature of Burkitt's tumor). In a patient with extensive local disease, surgical resection of the tumor may be possible. Chemotherapy includes large intermittent I.V. doses of cyclophosphamide, an alkylating agent, and preceded by an antiemetic to prevent severe nausea.

Cyclophosphamide is given in single doses to patients with localized disease, (until remission occurs); in cyclic doses, to patients with Stage III and Stage IV disease; followed by methotrexate and cytosine arabinoside to patients who relapse while on the original drug regimen. Patients with CNS involvement are given intrathecal methotrexate, cytosine arabinoside, and vincristine.

Additional considerations

The Burkitt's lymphoma patient requires a great deal of special physical care and constant assessment. For example:
• Jaw tumors cause difficulty in swallowing and loosening of teeth which can result in malnutrition. So, the dietitian and the patient's family should plan giving the patient frequent, small meals of a soft diet.
• Both cyclophosphamide therapy and kidney metastases can cause renal failure with uremia, requiring dialysis. Kidney damage as a result of cyclophosphamide therapy can be minimized with adequate fluid intake. That makes accurate recording of fluid intake and output essential.
• Abdominal tumors can cause ascites, with hypoglycemia and lactic acidosis. Respiratory tumors can cause severe difficulty in breathing that may require tracheotomy and additional chemotherapy to shrink the respiratory tumor. Gastrointestinal mesentery tumors can cause bowel perforation requiring surgery, so the following complications must be watched for and reported promptly: hypoglycemia, lactic acidosis, respiratory distress, and abdominal perforation.
• Burkitt's lymphoma severely stresses the patient and his family. They should take hope in the positive aspects of treatment (expected good results from chemotherapy) without forming unrealistic expectations. Since recurrence is common, they must understand the importance of follow-up visits for early detection and treatment.

STAGING AFRICAN BURKITT'S LYMPHOMA

Stage I: Rapidly developing (2 to 4 weeks), painless jaw tumor (60%), frequently with mandible and maxilla involvement that distorts face and gingiva and loosens teeth (may be first symptom)
Stage II: Multiple facial tumors
Stage III: Concurrent (or without showing associated jaw tumor) intrathoracic, intra-abdominal, or osseous tumor, usually in the kidneys, ovaries, gonads, mesentery, or retroperitoneal tissue, excluding facial bones. Within 1 to 3 months, the patient with an abdominal tumor shows symptoms of nausea, vomiting, abdominal pain, and ascites (50%).
Stage IV: CNS involvement, with cranial nerve palsies and paraplegia (15%), begins with abrupt onset of leg weakness, progressing to sensory deficit and loss of sphincter control; and less commonly, bone marrow involvement with peripheral blood manifestations or enlarged peripheral lymph nodes (5%).

Mycosis Fungoides

(Malignant cutaneous reticulosis, granuloma fungoides)

Mycosis fungoides (MF) is a rare, chronic malignant lymphoma of unknown cause that originates in the reticuloendothelial system of the skin, eventually affecting lymph nodes and internal organs. In the United States, it strikes over 1,000 patients of all races annually; most are between ages 40 and 60. Unlike other lymphomas, MF allows an average life expectancy of 7 to 10 years after diagnosis. If correctly treated, particularly before it has spread past the skin, MF may go into remission for many years. However, after MF has reached the tumor stage, progression to severe disability or death is rapid.

Signs and symptoms

The first sign of MF may be generalized erythroderma, possibly associated with itching. Eventually, MF evolves into varied combinations of infiltrated, thickened, or scaly patches, tumors, or ulcerations.

Diagnosis

A clear diagnosis of mycosis fungoides depends on a history of multiple, varied, and progressively severe skin lesions associated with characteristic histologic evidence of lymphoma cell infiltration of the skin, with or without involvement of lymph nodes, or visceral organs. Consequently, this diagnosis is often missed during the early stages until lymphoma cells are sufficiently numerous in the skin to show up in biopsy.

Other diagnostic tests help confirm mycosis fungoides: CBC and differential; a finger stick smear for Sézary cells (abnormal circulating lymphocytes), which may be present in the erythrodermic variants of MF (Sézary syndrome); blood chemistries to screen for visceral dysfunction; chest X-ray; liver-spleen isotopic scanning; lymphangiography; and lymph node biopsy to assess histologic involvement. These tests also help to stage the disease—a necessary prerequisite to treatment.

Treatment

Depending on the stage of the disease and its rate of progression, past treatment and results, the patient's age and overall health, treatment facilities available, and other factors, treatment of MF can include topical, intralesional, or systemic corticosteroid therapy; phototherapy; methoxsalen photochemotherapy; radiation; topical, intralesional, or systemic nitrogen mustard (mechlorethamine), and other systemic chemotherapy.

Topical nitrogen mustard is the preferred treatment for inducing remission in pretumorous stages. However, this treatment calls for special patient preparation to reduce the risk of cutaneous allergy. For 5 weeks before topical administration, the patient receives small weekly doses (200 mcg) of nitrogen mustard I.V. If these are well tolerated, therapy can proceed. If the patient develops an allergic reaction, an alternative therapy is used.

The patient who can tolerate nitrogen

STAGING MYCOSIS FUNGOIDES

Mycosis fungoides develops in three often overlapping stages.

Stage I: Erythematous or premycotic lesions with itching; no internal involvement.

Stage II: Erythematous scaly patches, irregularly shaped plaques and nodes; no internal involvement.

Stage III: Painful, mucotic (fungoid) brownish-red tumors, with ulceration of infected area; lymph node and visceral involvement.

mustard applies this treatment himself to his entire skin surface (because the disease may be present in skin that appears normal). Generally, such treatment is applied once a day, but frequency can vary with the stage of the disease and the patient's response.

Additional considerations

• If the patient applying nitrogen mustard has difficulty reaching all skin surfaces, he'll need assistance. But hospital staff members or family member assisting must wear gloves to prevent contact sensitization.

• If nitrogen mustard induces skin irritation, the patient should apply it less often, less vigorously, and with corticosteroids, as ordered.

• If the patient is receiving drug treatment, he must be watched for side effects, particularly infection. The patient may need antibiotic therapy.

• If the patient is receiving radiation, he'll probably develop alopecia and erythema. He may want to wear a wig to boost his self-image until hair growth begins, and take medicated oil baths to ease erythema.

• When applying topical antipruritic preparations on denuded areas, aseptic technique must be used.

• Since pruritus is often worse at night, the patient may need larger bedtime doses of antipruritics or sedatives, as ordered, to ensure a good night's sleep. When the patient has had a difficult night's sleep, early morning care should be postponed to allow him to sleep as long as he can.

• The patient with pruritus has an overwhelming need to scratch—often to the point of removing epidermis and replacing pruritus with pain, which some patients find easier to endure. Such a patient can't be kept from scratching. The best that can be done is minimizing the damage. The patient should keep fingernails short and clean, and wear a pair of white gloves when he must scratch.

PATIENT TEACHING AID

How to Apply Nitrogen Mustard to the Skin

1. Each small vial of nitrogen mustard contains 10 mg of powder. Transfer the contents to a 2-oz. (57 ml) bottle. Add enough tap water to dissolve the powder, but do not fill the bottle.
2. Add 1 to 3 teaspoons (5 to 15 ml) of an emulsified oil. This will help prevent your skin from becoming too dry.
3. Fill the mixing bottle with water, shake well, and the nitrogen mustard solution is ready to use.
4. Using your hands, apply the nitrogen mustard solution to your *entire body surface* whether it shows any sign of disease or not. Be sure to include the skin on your scalp, eyelids, groin, and between the toes. If you have any nitrogen mustard solution left after coating your entire body, repeat the application until you have used up all of the prepared mixture.
5. You may apply nitrogen mustard solution at any time; however, after bathing is probably the most convenient time. Afterward, you may apply a soothing cream, if you wish.
6. To reduce irritation, remember to:
• Keep your eyes closed when applying the solution to your face.
• Apply the nitrogen mustard solution *lightly and just one time* to the sensitive intertriginous areas (under the arms, beneath the breasts, and in the groin), as the skin in these areas is thinner and may become irritated if you apply too much of the solution too vigorously.
• Wash your hands thoroughly after application to remove excess.
7. *Should you have any questions or problems, call your doctor.*

This patient teaching aid is intended for distribution to patients by doctors and nurses. It should not be used without a doctor's approval.

• The malignant skin lesions are likely to make the patient depressed, fearful, and self-conscious. The hospital staff should show a positive but realistic attitude, fully explaining the disease and its stages, to help the patient and family understand and accept the disease. They can reinforce their verbal support by touching the patient without any hint of anxiety or distaste.

Acute Leukemia

Acute leukemia is a malignant proliferation of white blood cell precursors (blasts) in bone marrow or lymph tissue and their accumulation in peripheral blood, bone marrow, and body tissues. Its most common forms are acute lymphoblastic (lymphocytic) leukemia (ALL), abnormal growth of lymphocyte precursors (lymphoblasts); acute myeloblastic (myelogenous) leukemia (AML), rapid accumulation of myeloid precursors (myeloblasts); and acute monoblastic (monocytic) leukemia, or Schilling's type, marked increase in monocyte precursors (monoblasts). Other variants include acute myelomonocytic leukemia and acute erythroleukemia.

Untreated, acute leukemia is invariably fatal, usually because of complications that result from leukemic cell infiltration of bone marrow or vital organs. With treatment, prognosis varies. In ALL, treatment induces remissions in 90% of children (average survival time: 5 years) and in 40% to 65% of adults (average survival time: 1 to 2 years). Children between ages 2 and 8 have the best survival rate. In fact, intensive therapy cures about 50% of these children. In AML, the average survival rate is only 1 year after diagnosis, even with aggressive treatment. In acute monoblastic leukemia, treatment induces remissions in 50% of children; these remissions last from 2 to 10 months. Even with treatment, adults with acute monoblastic leukemia survive only about 1 year after diagnosis.

Causes and incidence
Research indicates that viruses, radiation, and other factors may predispose patients to this disorder.

Pathogenesis isn't clearly understood, but immature, nonfunctioning white blood cells appear to accumulate first in the tissue where they originate (lymphocytes in lymph tissue, granulocytes in bone marrow). These immature WBCs then spill into the bloodstream, and from there infiltrate other tissues, eventually causing organ malfunction because of encroachment or hemorrhage.

Acute leukemia is more common in males than in females, in Caucasians (especially people of Jewish descent), in children (between ages 2 and 5; 80% of all leukemias in this age-group are ALL), and in persons who live in urban and industrialized areas. Acute leukemia ranks 20th in causes of cancer-related deaths among people of all age groups. Among children, however, it's the most common form of cancer. In the United States, an estimated 11,000 persons develop acute leukemia annually.

Signs and symptoms
Signs of acute leukemia are sudden onset of high fever accompanied by thrombocytopenia and abnormal bleeding, such as nosebleeds, gingival bleeding, purpura, ecchymoses, petechiae, easy bruising after minor trauma, and prolonged menses. Nonspecific symptoms, such as low-grade fever, weakness, and lassitude, may persist for days or months before visible symptoms appear. Other insidious signs include pallor, chills, and recurrent infections. In addition, ALL, AML, and acute monoblastic leukemia may cause dyspnea, anemia, fatigue, malaise, tachycardia, palpitations,

systolic ejection murmur, and abdominal or bone pain. When leukemic cells cross the blood-brain barrier and escape the effects of systemic chemotherapy, the patient may develop meningeal leukemia (confusion, lethargy, headache).

Diagnosis

 Typical clinical findings and bone marrow aspirate showing a proliferation of immature WBCs confirm acute leukemia. An aspirate that's dry or free of leukemic cells in a patient with typical clinical findings requires bone marrow biopsy, usually of the posterior superior iliac spine. Blood counts show thrombocytopenia and neutropenia. Differential leukocyte count determines cell type. Lumbar puncture detects meningeal involvement.

Treatment

Systemic chemotherapy aims to eradicate leukemic cells and induce remission (restore normal bone marrow function). Chemotherapy varies:
• Meningeal leukemia—intrathecal instillation of methotrexate or cytarabine in a sterile, preservative-free solution, or cranial radiation
• ALL—vincristine, prednisone, or both with intrathecal methotrexate or cytarabine; or I.V. asparaginase, daunorubicin, and doxorubicin; maintenance with mercaptopurine and methotrexate
• AML—a combination of I.V. daunorubicin or doxorubicin, cytarabine, and oral thioguanine; I.V. 5-azacytidine alone (investigational); or if these fail to induce remission, a combination of cyclophosphamide, vincristine, prednisone, or methotrexate; maintenance treatment is with additional chemotherapy or, possibly, immunotherapy using BCG vaccine (bacille Calmette-Guérin).
• Acute monoblastic leukemia—cytarabine and thioguanine with daunorubicin or doxorubicin.

Bone marrow transplant is under investigation. Treatment also must control complications of chemotherapy, such as hyperuricemia, cardiotoxicity, and bone marrow suppression.

Additional considerations

A health care plan for the leukemic patient should emphasize patient comfort, minimize the side effects of chemotherapy, promote preservation of veins, manage complications, and provide psychologic support and patient education. Because so many of these patients are children, a special part of the care is being sensitive to the patients' emotional needs and those of their families.

Before treatment begins:
• The patient should be told about the disease course, treatment and its side effects, and significance of blood values.

PREDISPOSING FACTORS IN ACUTE LEUKEMIA

Although the exact causes of most leukemias remain unknown, increasing evidence suggests a combination of contributing factors:

Acute lymphoblastic leukemia
• familial tendency
• monozygotic twins
• congenital disorders, such as Down's syndrome, Bloom's syndrome, Fanconi's anemia, ataxia-telangiectasia, and congenital agammaglobulinemia
• viruses

Acute myeloblastic leukemia
• familial tendency
• monozygotic twins
• congenital disorders, such as Down's syndrome, Bloom's syndrome, Fanconi's anemia, ataxia-telangiectasia, and congenital agammaglobulinemia
• ionizing radiation
• exposure to the chemical benzene and cytotoxins, such as alkylating agents
• viruses

Acute monoblastic leukemia
• unknown (irradiation, exposure to chemicals, heredity, and infections show little correlation to this disease)

He should understand terms, such as relapse and remission, that will be used to describe the effects of therapy.

• The patient and his family must know how to recognize infection (fever, chills, cough, sore throat) and abnormal bleeding (bruising, petechiae), and how to stop such bleeding (pressure, ice to area).

• The patient needs good nutrition. He should know that chemotherapy may cause weight loss and anorexia, so he needs to eat and drink high-calorie, high-protein foods and beverages. However, chemotherapy and adjunctive prednisone may cause weight gain, so dietary counseling is helpful.

During treatment a health care professional should:

• watch for signs of meningeal leukemia (confusion, lethargy, headache), after intrathecal chemotherapy, and, if these occur, know how to manage them. The patient must be placed in the Trendelenburg position for 30 minutes. He must drink much fluid, and stay supine for 4 to 6 hours. The lumbar puncture site should be checked often for bleeding. If the patient receives cranial radiation, he must know about potential side effects, and what can be done to minimize them.

• prevent hyperuricemia, a possible result of rapid chemotherapy-induced leukemic cell lysis, by forcing fluids to about 2 liters daily, and giving acetazolamide, $NaHCO_3$ tablets, and allopurinol. Urine pH must be checked often and should remain above 7.5. Rash or other hypersensitivity reactions to allopurinol must be watched for, as well.

• watch for early signs of cardiotoxicity, such as arrhythmias, and signs of heart failure if the patient receives daunorubicin or doxorubicin.

• control infection by placing the patient

TYPES OF LEUKEMIA

GENERAL CLASS	SUBCLASS AND CELL TYPE	HISTOCHEMISTRY OR OTHER FEATURES	PROGNOSIS
Acute leukemias	• Subclass: acute lymphatic (ALL) • Cell: lymphoblasts	• Sudan black and PAS +	• Children (2 to 8 years): 50% cured, 90% show response to therapy • Adults: average survival 5 years
	• Subclass: acute myeloblastic (AML) • Cell: myeloblasts	• Peroxidase +	• Adults (15 to 75 years): response to therapy 50% • Average survival 1 year
	• Subclass: acute monoblastic (monocytic) (AMOL) • Cell: monoblasts	• Muramidase +	• Children: response to therapy 50% • Adults: average survival 1 year
Chronic leukemias	• Subclass: chronic granulocytic (CGL) • Cell: granulocytic precursors	• Ph¹ chromosome • Low LAP	• After chronic phase: 3 to 4 years • After acute phase: 3 to 6 months
	• Subclass: lymphocytic • Cell: B type	• Immunoglobulin or surface markers	• Average survival 5 years

in a private room and imposing reverse isolation, if necessary. (The benefits of reverse isolation are controversial.) Patient care must be coordinated so the leukemic patient doesn't come in contact with staff who also care for patients with infected surgical wounds or infectious diseases. Using Foley catheters and giving I.M. injections should be avoided, since they provide an easy avenue for infection. Staff and visitors must be screened for contagious diseases, and signs of infection watched for.

• provide thorough skin care by keeping the patient's skin and perianal area clean, applying mild lotions or creams to keep skin from drying and cracking, and thoroughly cleaning skin before all invasive skin procedures. I.V. tubing should be changed according to hospital policy. Strict aseptic technique and a metal scalp vein needle (metal butterfly needle) must be used when starting I.V.s. If the patient receives total parenteral nutrition, scrupulous subclavian catheter care is necessary.

• plan the patient's care to ensure adequate rest and minimize weakness from anemia.

• watch for bleeding and treat it immediately by applying ice compresses and pressure and elevating the extremity. Giving I.M. injections and aspirin or aspirin-containing compounds should be avoided; so, too, should taking rectal temperatures, giving rectal suppositories, and doing digital examinations.

• prevent constipation with adequate hydration, a high-residue diet, stool softeners, and mild laxatives. The patient should be encouraged to walk.

• control mouth ulceration by checking often for obvious ulcers and gum swelling, and by providing frequent mouth care and saline rinses. The patient must use a soft toothbrush and avoid hot, spicy foods and overuse of commercial mouthwashes. His rectal area should be checked daily for induration, swelling, erythema, skin discoloration, or drainage.

• provide psychologic support by establishing a trusting relationship to promote communication; allow the patient and his family to verbalize their anger and depression; let the family participate in his care as much as possible.

• minimize stress by providing a calm, quiet atmosphere. For children particularly, patient care and visiting hours should be flexible to promote maximum interaction with family and friends, and allow time for schoolwork.

For those patients who are refractory to chemotherapy and in the terminal phase of the disease, supportive health care is directed to pain, fever, and bleeding, management, and patient and family support. The patient may need religious counseling. He should know about the option of home or hospice care.

Chronic Granulocytic Leukemia
(Chronic myelogenous [or myelocytic] leukemia [CML])

Chronic granulocytic leukemia (CGL) is characterized by the abnormal overgrowth of granulocytic precursors (myeloblasts, promyelocytes, metamyelocytes, and myelocytes) in bone marrow, peripheral blood, and body tissues. CGL is most common in young and middle-aged adults, and is slightly more common in men than in women; it is rare in children. In the United States, approximately 3,000 to 4,000 cases of CGL develop annually, accounting for roughly 20% of all leukemias.

CGL's clinical course proceeds in two distinct phases: the insidious chronic phase, *with anemia and bleeding abnormalities, and eventually, the* acute phase (blastic crisis), *in which myeloblasts, the most primitive granulocytic precursors, proliferate rapidly. This disease is invariably fatal. Average survival time is 3 to 4 years after onset of the chronic phase, and 3 to 6 months after onset of the acute phase.*

Causes

Almost 90% of patients with CGL have the Philadelphia (Ph[1]) chromosome, an abnormality discovered in 1960 in which the long arm of chromosome 22 is translocated, usually to chromosome 9. Radiation and carcinogenic chemicals may induce this chromosome abnormality. Myeloproliferative diseases also seem to increase the incidence of CGL, and some clinicians suspect that an unidentified virus causes this disease.

Signs and symptoms

Typically, CGL induces the following clinical effects:
- anemia (fatigue, weakness, decreased exercise tolerance, pallor, dyspnea, tachycardia, and headache)
- thrombocytopenia, with resulting bleeding and clotting disorders (retinal hemorrhage, ecchymoses, hematuria, melena, bleeding gums, nosebleeds, and easy bruising)
- hepatosplenomegaly, with abdominal discomfort and fullness and pain in splenic infarction from leukemic cell infiltration.

Other symptoms include sternal and rib tenderness from leukemic infiltrations of the periosteum; low-grade fever; weight loss; anorexia; renal calculi or gouty arthritis from increased uric acid excretion; occasionally, prolonged infection and ankle edema; and rarely, priapism and vascular insufficiency.

Diagnosis

In patients with typical clinical changes, chromosomal analysis of peripheral blood or bone marrow showing the Philadelphia chromosome and low leukocyte alkaline phosphatase levels confirm CGL. Other relevant lab results show:
- WBC abnormalities: leukocytosis (leukocytes more than 50,000/mm³, ranging as high as 250,000/mm³), occasional leukopenia (leukocytes less than 5,000/mm³), neutropenia (neutrophils less than 1,500/mm³) despite high leukocyte count, and increased circulating myeloblasts

- hemoglobin often below 10 g
- hematocrit low (less than 30%)
- platelets: thrombocytopenia common (< 50,000/mm³), but platelet levels may be normal or elevated
- serum uric acid: possibly > 8 mg
- bone marrow aspirate or biopsy: hypercellular, shows bone marrow infiltration by increased number of myeloid elements (biopsy is done only if aspirate is dry); in the acute phase, myeloblasts predominate.

Treatment

Control of abnormal myeloid proliferation requires rigorous treatment with chemotherapy. During the chronic phase, outpatient chemotherapy induces excellent remissions and is often continued at lower doses during remissions. Such chemotherapy usually includes busulfan and, occasionally, melphalan, other nitrogen mustards, thioguanine, and hydroxyurea.

Ancillary treatments may include:
- local splenic radiation to reduce peripheral blood counts and splenic size, or splenectomy (controversial)
- leukopheresis (selective leukocyte removal) to reduce leukocyte count
- allopurinol to prevent hyperuricemia or colchicine to relieve gouty attacks caused by elevated serum uric acid
- prompt treatment of infections that may result from chemotherapy-induced bone marrow suppression.

During the acute phase, treatment is the same as for acute myeloblastic leukemia (although it is less likely to induce remission) and emphasizes supportive measures and chemotherapy with doxorubicin or daunorubicin, thioguanine, cyclophosphamide, vincristine, methotrexate, cytarabine, or daunorubicin with prednisone. Despite vigorous treatment, CGL is rapidly fatal after onset of the acute phase.

Additional considerations

In patients with CGL, meticulous supportive care, psychologic support, and careful patient teaching help make the most of remissions and minimize complications. When the disease is diagnosed, the doctor's explanation of the disease and its treatment should be repeated and reinforced to the patient and his family.

Throughout the chronic phase of CGL when the patient is hospitalized:

• If the patient has persistent anemia, he must avoid exhaustion. Lab tests and physical care should be scheduled with frequent rest periods in between. The patient may need assistance with walking. The patient's skin and mucous membranes should be checked regularly for pallor petechiae and bruising.

• To minimize bleeding, the patient must use a soft-bristle toothbrush and an electric razor, and follow other safety precautions.

• To minimize the abdominal discomfort of splenomegaly, the patient should eat small frequent meals. For the same reason, he may need a stool softener or laxative to prevent constipation. The dietary department will provide a high-bulk diet, and encourage adequate fluid intake.

• To prevent atelectasis, the patient must do coughing and deep breathing exercises regularly.

Because the patient with CGL often receives outpatient chemotherapy throughout the chronic phase, sound patient teaching is essential:

• The patient must be told the expected side effects of chemotherapy, with attention paid to dangerous side effects, such as bone marrow suppression.

• The patient must watch for and immediately report signs and symptoms of infection: any fever over 100° F. (38.8° C.), chills, redness or swelling, sore throat, and cough.

• The patient must watch for signs of thrombocytopenia, immediately apply ice and pressure to any external bleeding site, and avoid aspirin and aspirin-containing compounds because of the risk of increased bleeding.

• The patient must get adequate rest and avoid strenuous activity to minimize the fatigue of anemia. The patient needs to understand the importance of a high-calorie, high-protein diet in minimizing the toxic effects of chemotherapy.

For more information on treatment during the acute phase, see ACUTE LEUKEMIA.

Chronic Lymphocytic Leukemia

A generalized, progressive disease that is common in the elderly, chronic lymphocytic leukemia is marked by an uncontrollable spread of abnormal, small lymphocytes in lymphoid tissue, blood, and bone marrow. Nearly all patients with chronic lymphocytic leukemia are men over age 50. According to the American Cancer Society, chronic lymphocytic leukemia accounts for almost a third of new leukemia cases annually.

Causes

Although the cause is unknown, researchers suspect heredity (higher incidence has been recorded within families), still undefined chromosome abnormalities, and immunologic defects (such as ataxia-telangiectasia or acquired agammaglobulinemia) as the possible causes of chronic lymphocytic leukemia. The disease does not seem to follow exposure to radiation.

Signs and symptoms

Chronic lymphocytic leukemia is the most benign and the most slowly progressive form of leukemia. Clinical signs derive from the infiltration of leukemic cells in bone marrow, lymphoid tissue, and organ systems.

In early stages, patients usually complain of fatigue, malaise, fever, and nodal enlargement. They're particularly susceptible to infection.

In advanced stages, patients may experience severe fatigue and weight loss, with liver or spleen enlargement, bone tenderness, and edema from lymph node obstruction. Pulmonary infiltrates may appear when lung parenchyma is involved. Skin infiltrations, manifested by macular to nodular eruptions, occur in about half the cases of chronic lymphocytic leukemia.

As the disease progresses, bone marrow involvement may lead to anemia, pallor, weakness, dyspnea, tachycardia, palpitations, bleeding, and infection. Opportunistic fungal, viral, and bacterial infections commonly occur in late stages.

Diagnosis
Typically, chronic lymphocytic leukemia is an incidental finding during a routine blood test that reveals numerous abnormal lymphocytes. In early stages, WBC count is mildly but persistently elevated. Granulocytopenia is the rule, but the WBC climbs as the disease progresses. Blood studies also show hemoglobin count under 11 g, hypogammaglobulinemia, and depressed serum globulins. Other common developments include neutropenia (under 1,500/mm³), lymphocytosis (over 10,000/mm³), and thrombocytopenia (under 150,000/mm³). Bone marrow aspiration and biopsy show lymphocytic invasion.

Treatment
Systemic chemotherapy includes alkylating agents, usually chlorambucil or cyclophosphamide, and sometimes steroids (prednisone) when autoimmunie hemolytic anemio or thrombocytopenia occurs.

When chronic lymphocytic leukemia causes obstruction, or organ impairment or enlargement, local radiation treatment can be used to reduce organ size. Allopurinol can be given to prevent hyperuricemia, a relatively uncommon finding.

Prognosis is poor if anemia, thrombocytopenia, neutropenia, bulky lymph-adenopathy, and severe lymphocytosis are present. Gross bone marrow replacement by abnormal lymphocytes is the most common cause of death, usually occurring within 4 to 5 years after diagnosis.

Additional considerations
The hospital staff member caring for the patient with lymphocytic leukemia should:
• plan patient care around relieving symptoms and preventing infection; clean patient's skin daily with mild soap and water; watch for signs of infection: temperature over 100° F. (37.8° C.), chills, redness, or swelling of any body part.
• watch for signs of thrombocytopenia (black tarry stools, easy bruising, nosebleeds, bleeding gums) and anemia (pale skin, weakness, fatigue, dizziness, palpitations).
• advise the patient to avoid aspirin and products containing aspirin; explain that innumerable medications contain aspirin, even though their names don't make this clear; teach him how to recognize aspirin variants on medication labels.
• explain chemotherapy and what its side effects are; tell him, upon discharge, to avoid coming in contact with obviously ill persons, especially children with childhood diseases; urge him to eat high-protein food and drink high-calorie beverages; stress the importance of follow-up care, frequent blood tests, and taking all medications exactly as prescribed; make sure the patient knows the signs of recurrence (swollen lymph nodes in the neck, axilla, and groin; increased abdominal size or discomfort) and tell him that, if he detects any of them, he should notify his doctor immediately.
• provide emotional support and be a good listener; try to keep the patient's spirits up by concentrating on little things like improving his personal appearance, providing pleasant environment, asking questions about his family; if possible, provide opportunities for his favorite activities.

Selected References

Baldonado, A., and D. Stahl. CANCER NURSING (Nursing Outline Series). Garden City, N.Y.: Medical Examination Publ. Co., 1977.

Bouchard, Rosemary, and Norma F. Owens. NURSING CARE OF THE CANCER PATIENT, 3rd ed. St. Louis: C.V. Mosby Co., 1976.

CANCER FACTS AND FIGURES. Boston: American Cancer Society, Inc., 1978.

CANCER: A MANUAL FOR PRACTITIONERS, 5th ed. Boston: American Cancer Society, Inc., 1978.

A CANCER SOURCE BOOK FOR NURSES. Boston: American Cancer Society, Inc., 1975.

Clark, Randolph Lee, et al. YEARBOOK OF CANCER, 1980 (Practical Medicine Year Books). Chicago: Year Book Medical Publishers, 1980.

Cooper, J. CONCEPTS IN CANCER CARE. Philadelphia: Lea & Febiger, 1980.

Cooper, Richard G., et al. *Adjuvant Chemotherapy of Breast Cancer*, JOURNAL OF CANCER. 44:793-798, September 1979.

Del Regato, Juan A., and Harlan J. Spjut. ACKERMAN AND DEL REGATO'S CANCER: DIAGNOSIS, TREATMENT, AND PROGNOSIS, 5th ed. St. Louis: C.V. Mosby Co., 1977.

Donovan, M., and S. Pierce. CANCER CARE NURSING. New York: Appleton-Century-Crofts, 1976.

HELPING CANCER PATIENTS EFFECTIVELY. Nursing Skillbook™ Series. Springhouse, Pa.: Intermed Communications, Inc., 1977.

Henderson, I. Craig, and George P. Canellos. *Cancer of the Breast*, NEW ENGLAND JOURNAL OF MEDICINE. 302:17-30, January 3, 1980.

Holland, J., and E. Frei. CANCER MEDICINE. Philadelphia: Lea & Febiger, 1973.

Lynch, H., et al. *Hereditary Cancer: Ascertainment and Management*, CA—A CANCER JOURNAL FOR CLINICIANS. 29:216-232, July/August 1979.

Markel, W., and V. Sinon. *The Hospice Concept*, CA—A CANCER JOURNAL FOR CLINICIANS. 28:225-237, July/August 1978.

Martini, N. *Lung Cancer: An Overview*, CANCER NURSING. 1:31-33, February 1978.

Rubin, P., and R. Bakemeiw. CLINICAL ONCOLOGY FOR MEDICAL STUDENTS AND PHYSICIANS. Boston: American Cancer Society, Inc., 1978.

Tully, J., and B. Wagner. *Breast Cancer: Helping the Mastectomy Patient to Live Life Fully*, NURSING78. 8:18-25, January 1978.

Valentine, A., et al. *Pain Relief for Cancer Patients*, AMERICAN JOURNAL OF NURSING. 78:2054-2056, December 1978.

Van Scott, E., and J. Kalmanson. *Complete Remissions of Mycosis Fungoides Lymphoma Induced by Topical Nitrogen Mustard (HN2)*, CANCER. 32:18-30, July 1973.

Wajsman, Z., et al. *Surgical Treatment of Penile Cancer: A Follow-up Report*, CANCER. 40:1697-1701, October 1977.

Williams, W., et al. HEMATOLOGY, 2nd ed. New York: McGraw-Hill, 1977, pp. 992-1085.

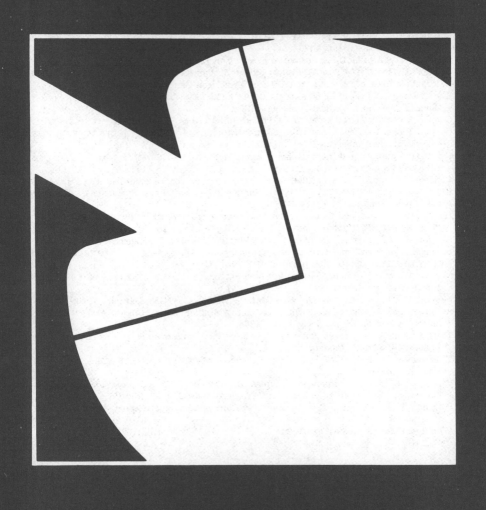

6 Infection

Infection

Introduction

Despite improved methods of treating and preventing infection—potent antibiotics, complex immunizations, and modern sanitation—infection still accounts for much serious illness, even in highly industrialized countries. In developing countries, infection competes with malnutrition as the most critical health problem.

What is infection?

Infection is the invasion and multiplication of microorganisms in or on body tissue. Such reproduction injures the host by causing cellular damage from microorganism-produced toxins or intracellular multiplication, or by competing with host metabolism. The host's own immune response may compound the tissue damage; such damage may be localized (as in infected decubitus ulcers) or systemic. The severity of the infection varies with the pathogenicity and number of the invading microorganisms, and the strength of host defenses.

Why are the microorganisms that cause infectious diseases so hard to overcome? There are many complex reasons:
- Some bacteria—especially, gram-negative bacilli—develop resistance to antibiotics.
- Some microorganisms—such as the influenza virus—include so many different strains that a single vaccine can't provide protection against them all.

- Most viruses resist available antiviral drugs.
- Also, some microorganisms localize in areas that make treatment difficult, such as the central nervous system and bone.

Moreover, the very factors that contribute to improved health—such as the affluence that allows good nutrition and living conditions, and advances in medical science—in some ways increase the risk of infection. For example, advanced age increases susceptibility to infection. Travel opportunities expose persons to diseases for which they have little or no natural immunity. Similarly, the expanded use of immunosuppressives, surgery, and other invasive procedures increases the risk of infection.

Kinds of infections

A laboratory-verified infection that fails to produce illness is called a *subclinical*, *silent*, *inapparent*, or *asymptomatic* infection (persons with such infections are called *carriers*, since they are not sick themselves but can transmit infection to others). A *latent* infection occurs after a microorganism has been dormant in the host, sometimes for years. An *exogenous* infection results from environmental pathogens; an *endogenous* infection, from the host's normal flora (e.g., *E. coli* displaced from the colon, causing a urinary tract infection).

The varied forms of microorganisms responsible for infectious diseases include bacteria, viruses, rickettsiae, chlamydiae, spirochetes, fungi (yeasts and molds), and protozoa; larger organisms, such as helminths (worms), may also cause disease.

Bacteria are single-cell microorganisms with well-defined cell walls, that can grow independently on artificial media without the need for other cells. In developing countries, where poor sanitation potentiates infection, bacterial diseases are prevalent sources of death and disability. In industrialized countries, bacterial infections are the most common fatal infectious diseases.

Bacteria can be classified according to shape. Spherical bacterial cells are called *cocci*; rod-shaped bacteria, *bacilli*; and spiral-shaped bacteria, *spirilla*. They can also be classified according to their response to staining (gram-positive, gram-negative, or acid-fast), their motility (motile or nonmotile), formation of a capsule (encapsulated or nonencapsulated), and their capacity to form spores (sporulating or nonsporulating).

Viruses are subcellular organisms made up only of an RNA or a DNA nu-

---

EPIDEMIOLOGY DEFINED

Epidemiology is the dynamic study of various factors as they relate to the occurrence, frequency, and distribution of disease in a given population. This includes the origin of the disease, how it's transmitted, and host and environmental factors that influence the development of the disease. Several terms describe the occurrence or frequency of a disease. In an *epidemic*, a disease occurs at a level that is higher than normal. An *outbreak*, however, is a sudden appearance of the disease, often in a small portion of the population. An *endemic* disease is persistently present in a given locale; a *hyperendemic* disease is persistent and has a high incidence. *Reservoir* refers to the natural habitat of the organism responsible for the disease; *source*, to the site (or milieu) from which the host (victim) directly acquires the disease. Infectious organisms can multiply within the source. A source includes a *vector*, which is usually an arthropod (for example, a mosquito) that transmits the disease indirectly from person to person, but it may be a person who has the disease, was recently exposed to it, or is a carrier. Transmission may also occur through a *vehicle*, like contaminated food or water. Infectious organisms can multiply within a vehicle.

HOW TO COLLECT CULTURE SPECIMENS

CULTURE SITE	SPECIMEN SOURCE	ADDITIONAL CONSIDERATIONS
Infected wound	• Aspiration of exudate with syringe (preferred technique)	• Use only sterile syringe. Pungent odor suggests the presence of anaerobes. Use oxygenfree collection tubes, if available.
	• Applicator swab	• Firmly but gently saturate swab with exudate from infected site. If surface is dry, moisten swab with sterile saline solution before taking culture.
Skin lesions	• Excision or puncture	• Thoroughly cleanse skin before excision or puncture.
Upper respiratory tract	• Nasopharyngeal swab (generally used to detect carriers of *Staphylococcus aureus*)	• Gently pass swab through nose into nasopharynx. Immediately send specimen to lab for culture.
	• Throat swab	• Under adequate light, swab the area of inflammation or exudation.
Lower respiratory tract	• Expectorated sputum	• Instruct patient to cough deeply and to expectorate into cup. Culture requires expectorated sputum, not just saliva from mouth.
	• Induced sputum (used when patient can't expectorate sputum)	• Use aerosol mist spray of saline solution or water to induce sputum production. Apply cupping and postural drainage, if needed.
	• Nasotracheal suction	• Measure approximate distance from patient's nose to his ear. Note the distance; then, insert a sterile suction catheter this length, with a collection vial attached, into his nose. Maintain suction during catheter withdrawal.
	• Pleural tap	• Advise patient that he may feel discomfort even though skin is anesthetized before this procedure. After tap, check site often for local swelling, and report dyspnea and other adverse reactions.
Lower intestinal tract	• Rectal swab	• Lesion on colon or on rectal wall may require colonoscopy or sigmoidoscopy to obtain specimen. If so, explain the procedure. Help patient to assume a left lateral decubitus or a knee-chest position.
	• Stool specimen	• Specimen should contain any pus or blood present in feces and a sampling of the first, middle, and last portion of stool. Urine with stool can invalidate results. Immediately send specimen to lab in a clean, tightly covered container, especially stools being examined for ova and parasites, which must be warm so that organisms remain viable.

cleus covered with proteins. They are the smallest known organisms (so tiny they're visible only through an electron microscope). Independent of host cells, viruses can't replicate. Rather, they invade a host cell and stimulate it to participate in the formation of additional virus particles. The estimated 400 viruses that infect

Proper identification of the causative organism requires proper culture collection. Label culture specimen with date, time, patient's name, suspected diagnosis, and source of culture.

CULTURE SITE	SPECIMEN SOURCE	ADDITIONAL CONSIDERATIONS
Eye	• Cotton swab	• Carefully retract lower lid, and gently swab sclera.
	• Corneal scrapings	• Doctor uses swab loop to scrape specimen from site of corneal infection. Reassure patient that procedure is short and discomfort minimal.
Genital tract	• Swab specimen	• In males, specimen should contain urethral discharge or prostatic fluid; in females, urethral or cervical specimens. Always collect specimens on two swabs simultaneously.
Urinary tract	• Midstream clean catch urine (avoids specimen contamination with microorganisms commonly found in the lower urethra and perineum)	• In an uninfected person, midstream clean catch should contain less than 10,000 bacteria/ml. • Instruct patient how to collect specimen or supervise collection. In males, retract foreskin and cleanse glans penis; in females, cleanse and separate labia so urinary meatus is clearly visible; then, cleanse meatus. Tell patient to void 25 to 30 ml and, without stopping urine stream, to collect specimen. • In infants, apply the collection bag carefully and check it frequently to avoid mechanical urethral obstruction. • Immediately send urine to lab, or refrigerate it to retard growth.
	• Foley catheter specimen	• Cleanse specimen port of catheter with alcohol, and aspirate urine with a sterile needle, or from a latex catheter, at a point distal to the "Y" branch.
Body fluids	• Needle aspiration	• Immediately send peritoneal and synovial fluid, and CSF to lab. *Don't* retard growth of CSF organisms by refrigerating specimen. After pericardial and pleural fluid aspiration, observe patient carefully, and check vital signs often. Watch for signs of pneumothorax or cardiac tamponade.
Blood	• Venous or arterial aspiration	• Cleanse aspiration site with alcohol, and prep skin according to your hospital's policy. • Using a sterile syringe, collect 12 to 15 ml blood, changing needles before injecting blood into the aerobic and anaerobic collection bottles. Continue the procedure according to your hospital's policy. • If patient is receiving penicillin, note this on lab slip, since lab may add penicillinase to culture to inactivate drug.

humans are classified according to their size, shape (spherical, rod-shaped, or cubic), or means of transmission (respirational, fecal, oral, or sexual).

Rickettsiae are relatively uncommon in the United States. They're small, gram-negative, bacterialike organisms that frequently induce life-threatening infections. Like viruses, they require a host cell for replication. Rickettsiae occur in three forms: *Rickettsia*, *Coxiella*, and *Rochalimaea*.

Chlamydiae are smaller than rickettsiae and bacteria but larger than viruses. They too depend on host cells for replication, but unlike viruses, they are susceptible to antibiotics.

Spirochetes are cellular organisms shaped like flexible, slender, undulating spiral rods. Most are anaerobic. The three forms pathogenic in humans are *Treponema*, *Leptospira*, and *Borrelia*.

IMMUNIZATION SCHEDULE

Usually, childhood immunizations are given on a fixed schedule, as follows:

AGE	IMMUNIZATION
2 months	First dose: diphtheria/tetanus/pertussis vaccine; polio vaccine
4 months	Second dose: diphtheria/tetanus/pertussis vaccine; polio
6 months	Third dose: diphtheria/tetanus/pertussis vaccine
15 months	Rubella vaccine; measles; mumps
18 months	Diphtheria/tetanus/pertussis; polio (third)
4-5 years	Diphtheria/tetanus/pertussis; polio

Before Immunization:
• The parents must be asked the child's immunization history; if the child is receiving corticosteroids or other immunosuppresive drugs; if he's had a recent febrile illness; or has a history of allergic reactions to antibiotics, eggs, or feathers.

After Immunization:
• Any reaction must be recorded. The child's parents must be taught how to recognize the signs of a severe reaction and should get a record of the immunization.

Fungi are single-cell organisms, with nuclei enveloped by nuclear membranes. They have rigid cell walls like plant cells but lack chlorophyll, the green matter necessary for photosynthesis; they also show relatively little cellular specialization. Fungi occur as yeasts (single-cell oval-shaped organisms) or molds (organisms with hyphae, or branching filaments). Depending on the environment, some fungi may occur in both forms. Fungal diseases in humans are called mycoses.

Protozoa are the simplest single-cell organisms of the animal kingdom but show a high level of cellular specialization. Like other animal cells, they have cell membranes rather than cell walls, and their nuclei are surrounded by nuclear membranes.

In addition to these microorganisms, infectious diseases may also result from larger parasites, such as round- or flatworms.

Modes of transmission

Most infectious diseases are transmitted in one of four ways.

1. In *contact transmission*, the susceptible host comes into direct contact (as in venereal disease) or indirect contact (contaminated inanimate objects or the close-range spread of respiratory droplets) with the source.

2. *Airborne transmission* results from inhalation of contaminated evaporated saliva droplets (as in pulmonary tuberculosis), which are sometimes suspended in airborne dust particles.

3. In *enteric* (fecal-oral) *transmission*, the organisms are found in feces and are ingested by susceptible victims, often through fecally contaminated food (as in salmonella infections).

4. *Vectorborne transmission* occurs when an intermediate carrier (vector), such as a flea or a mosquito, transfers an organism.

Much can be done to prevent transmission of infectious diseases:
• comprehensive immunization (including immunization required of travelers to or emigrants from endemic areas)

ISOLATION PRECAUTIONS

COMMON DISEASES THAT REQUIRE ISOLATION

	Private Room	Gown	Gloves	Mask	Linen Precautions	Dish Precautions
Strict isolation Smallpox, vaccinia, pneumonic plague, inhalation anthrax, varicella (chickenpox), disseminated herpes zoster, diphtheria, rabies, burns infected with *S. aureus*, and group A streptococci	X	X	X	X	X	X
Modified strict isolation Staphylococcal and streptococcal pneumonia; all patients with copious sputum production containing large numbers of coagulase positive staphylococci or group A beta-hemolytic streptococci	X	⊗	⊗	X	X	X
Respiratory isolation Pulmonary tuberculosis (if suspected, use respiratory isolation until three negative AFB smears are obtained), rubeola (measles), mumps, rubella (German measles), pertussis, chickenpox, meningococcal meningitis, meningococcemia; viral hepatitis A accompanied by copious respiratory secretions which require suctioning	X	—	—	X	—	—
Protective (reverse) isolation Agranulocytosis, lymphoma, leukemia, immunosupressant therapy, extensive noninfected burns; severe noninfected eczematous dermatitis	X	⊗ Use clean (not sterile)	⊗	X	—	—
Enteric precautions Infectious viral hepatitis (hepatitis A), salmonellosis, shigellosis, nonbacterial gastroenteritis, staphylococcal enterocolitis, cholera. (In patients with diarrhea of unknown origin, use enteric precautions until 3 days after diarrhea subsides or enteric infection is ruled out.)	D	⊗	⊗	—	X	X
Wound and skin precautions All wound and skin infections in which dressings can adequately contain drainage (*S. aureus*, and group A streptococcus infections, draining cellulitis, weeping lesions of herpes zoster)	X	⊗	⊗ During dressing changes	⊗ On contact with infected area	X	—
Blood precautions Type B hepatitis, type non-A, non-B hepatitis, arthropod-borne viral fever (dengue)	D	—	⊗ Contact with blood	—	⊗ contaminated with blood	⊗ contaminated with blood
Secretion precautions Infected ischemic ulcers, decubitus ulcers, stitch abscesses, infected wounds in which drainage is minimal, gas gangrene, impetigo	Double-bag soiled dressings and equipment. Use meticulous handwashing technique.					

Key

X = always necessary
⊗ = necessary only in direct contact with patient, his secretions or articles he's contaminated
D = desirable but optional
— = unnecessary

Adapted with permission from *Isolation Techniques for Use in Hospitals*, U.S. Public Health Service Publication stock #017-023-00094-2. (Washington, D.C.: Government Printing Office, Superintendent of Documents.)

REPORTABLE INFECTIOUS DISEASES

Most states require that certain diseases be reported to local public health authorities by mail, telephone, or telegraph. Such reports should include the patient's name, address, age, race, and sex, along with the disease or suspected disease and the means of exposure, if known.

The list of reportable diseases varies from state to state but usually includes acute respiratory viral diseases, anthrax, botulism, chancroid, cholera, neonatal inclusion conjunctivitis, keratoconjunctivitis, epidemic neonatal diarrhea, diphtheria, infectious encephalitis, gonorrhea, hepatitis A and B, histoplasmosis, influenza, leprosy, leptospirosis, listeriosis, malaria, rubeola (measles), meningococcal meningitis, meningococcemia, mumps, paratyphoid fever, pertussis (whooping cough), plague, poliomyelitis, psittacosis, Q fever, rabies, rat-bite fever, relapsing fever, rubella (German measles), shigellosis, smallpox, syphilis, tetanus, pulmonary and extrapulmonary tuberculosis, typhoid fever, typhus, and yersiniosis.

Some states also require the reporting of additional diseases, such as actinomycosis, amebiasis, lymphocytic choriomeningitis, coccidioidomycosis, acute bacterial conjunctivitis and epidemic hemorrhagic conjunctivitis, granuloma inguinale, hemorrhagic jaundice, impetigo contagiosa, lymphogranuloma venereum, pediculosis, bacterial and mycoplasmal pneumonia, ringworm, Rocky Mountain spotted fever, scabies, staphylococcal infections, streptococcal infections, trachoma, and tularemia.

Adapted from information provided by the American Public Health Association, 1015 18th St., N.W., Washington, D.C. 20036

- drug prophylaxis
- improved nutrition, living conditions, and sanitation
- correction of environmental factors.

Immunization can now control many diseases, including diphtheria, tetanus, pertussis, measles, rubella, some forms of meningitis, polio, and tetanus. One disease, smallpox (variola)—which has killed and disfigured millions—is believed to be successfully eradicated by a comprehensive World Health Organization program of surveillance and immunization.

Vaccines—which contain live but attenuated (weakened) or killed microorganisms—and toxoids—which contain bacterial exotoxins—induce active immunity against bacterial and viral diseases by stimulating antibody formation. Immune serums contain previously formed antibodies from hyperimmunized donors or pooled plasma, and provide temporary passive immunity. Antitoxins provide passive immunity to various toxins. Generally, passive immunization is used only when active immunization is perilous or impossible, or when complete protection requires both active and passive immunity.

While prophylactic antibiotic therapy may prevent certain diseases, the risks of superinfection and emergence of drug-resistant strains may outweigh the benefits. Prophylactic antibiotics, therefore, are usually reserved for patients at high risk of infection by or exposure to dangerous or fatal agents.

Nosocomial infections

A *nosocomial* infection is one that develops after a patient is admitted to a hospital or other health care institution. Most infections of this type are caused by group A *Streptococcus pyogenes*, *Staphylococcus aureus*, *Escherichia coli*, *Klebsiella*, *Proteus*, *Pseudomonas*, *Hemophilus influenzae*, hepatitis viruses, and *Candida albicans*. Transmission of nosocomial infection usually occurs by direct contact and, less often, by inhalation of or wound invasion by airborne organisms, or by contaminated equipment and solutions.

Despite hospital programs of infection control that include surveillance, prevention, and education, about 5% of patients who enter hospitals contract a nosocomial infection. Since the 1960s, staphylococcal infection has been declining, but gram-negative bacilli and fungal infections have been steadily increasing.

Nosocomial infections continue as a difficult problem, because most hospital patients are older and more debilitated than in the past. The very advances in treatment that increase longevity in many diseases which alter immune defenses also create a high-risk population. Moreover, the increased use of invasive and surgical procedures, immunosuppressives, and antibiotics predisposes patients to infection and superinfection. At the same time, the growing number of personnel that can come in contact with each patient makes the risk of exposure greater.

Nosocomial infections may be prevented by:

• following strict infection control procedures.

• documenting hospital infections as they occur.

• identifying outbreaks early, and implementing steps to prevent their spread.

• eliminating unnecessary procedures that contribute to infection.

• strictly following necessary isolation techniques.

• observing *all* patients for signs of infection, especially those at high risk.

• following good handwashing techniques, and encouraging other staff members to do the same.

• keeping staff and visitors with obvious infection, as well as known carriers, away from susceptible patients.

• taking special precautions with particularly vulnerable patients, for example those with Foley catheters, mechanical ventilators, or I.V.s, and those recuperating from surgery.

Accurate assessment is vital

Accurate health care assessment helps identify infectious diseases and prevents avoidable complications. Complete assessment consists of patient history, physical examination, and laboratory data. History should include the patient's sex, age, address, occupation, and place of work; known exposure to illness; and date of disease onset. It should also detail information about recent hospitalization, blood transfusions, blood donation refusal by Red Cross or other agencies, vaccination, travel or camping trips, and exposure to pets or other animals at home or work; also, if applicable, possible exposure to sexually transmitted diseases or drug abuse. Also, the patient's resistance to infectious disease should be determined, and usual dietary patterns, unusual fatigue, and any conditions, such as neoplastic disease or alcoholism, that may be a predisposition to infection, should be noted. Patient listlessness or unease, lack of concentration, or any obvious abnormality of mood or affect should also be included.

In suspected infection, a physical examination must include special attention to the skin, mucous membranes, liver, spleen, and lymph nodes. During the examination, the hospital staff member should check for and note the location and type of drainage from skin lesions (these are clues to infection); record skin color, temperature, and turgor; ask if the patient has pruritus; take temperature, using the same route consistently, and watch for a fever (the best indicator of many infections); note and record the pattern of temperature change and the effect of antipyretics; be aware that certain analgesics may contain antipyretics; watch for convulsions in high fever, especially in children.

During hospitalization of the patient with infection, the staff member should check the pulse rate. Infection often increases pulse rate, but some infections, notably typhoid fever and psittacosis, may decrease it. In severe infection or when complications are possible, he should watch for hypotension, hematuria, oliguria, hepatomegaly, jaundice, bleeding from gums or into joints, and altered level of consciousness.

GRAM-POSITIVE COCCI

Staphylococcal Infections

PREDISPOSING FACTORS	SIGNS AND SYMPTOMS	DIAGNOSIS
Bacteremia • Infected surgical wounds • Intra-abdominal or other abscesses • Infected I.V. or intra-arterial catheter sites or catheter tips • Infected vascular grafts or prostheses • Infected decubitus ulcers • Osteomyelitis • Parenteral drug abuse • Source unknown (primary bacteremia) • Subacute bacterial endocarditis (SBE), usually caused by coagulase-negative staphylococci, most often with infection of previously damaged or artificial heart valves, or infected intravascular shunts. Patients with continuous low-grade bacteremia often have vegetations on heart valves that seed into the bloodstream.	• Fever (high fever with no obvious source in children under age 1), shaking chills, tachycardia • Cyanosis or pallor • Confusion, agitation, stupor • Microabscesses in skin from emboli-containing bacteria • Complications: shock (likely in gram-negative bacteremia); acute bacterial endocarditis (in prolonged infection; indicated by new or changing systolic murmur); retinal hemorrhages (Roth's spots); splinter hemorrhages under nails, and small, tender red nodes on pads of fingers and toes (Osler's nodes); metastatic abscess formation in skin, bones, lungs, brain, and kidneys; pulmonary emboli if tricuspid valve is infected • Prognosis poor in patients over age 60 or with advanced malignancy	• Blood cultures (two to four samples from different sites taken at different times): Growing staphylococci and leukocytosis (usually 12,000 WBCs/mm³), with shift to the left of polymorphonuclear leukocytes (70% to 90% neutrophils) • Urinalysis shows microscopic hematuria. • ESR elevated, especially in chronic or subacute bacterial endocarditis • Severe anemia or thrombocytopenia (possible) • Prolonged PTT and PT, low fibrinogen and platelet counts, and low factor assays; possible DIC • Urine, sputum, and draining skin lesions should be cultured to identify primary infection site. Chest X-rays and scans of lungs, liver, abdomen, and brain may locate infection site.
Pneumonia • Immune deficiencies, especially in elderly and children under age 2 • Chronic lung diseases and cystic fibrosis • Malignancies • Antibiotics that kill normal respiratory flora but spare *S. aureus* • Viral respiratory infections, especially influenza • Hematogenous (bloodborne) bacteria spread to the lungs from primary sites of infections (such as heart valves, abscesses, and pulmonary emboli).	• High temperature: adults, 103° to 105° F. (39.5° to 40.5° C.); children, 101° F. (38.3° C.) • Cough, with purulent, yellow or bloody sputum • Dyspnea, rales, and decreased breath sounds • Pleural pain • In infants: mild respiratory infection that suddenly worsens: irritability, anxiety, dyspnea, anorexia, vomiting, diarrhea, spasms of dry coughing, marked tachypnea, expiratory grunting, sternal retractions, and cyanosis • Complications: necrosis, lung abscess, pyopneumothorax; empyema; pneumatocele; shock, hypotension, oliguria or anuria, cyanosis, loss of consciousness	• WBC elevated (15,000 to 40,000/mm³; 15,000 to 20,000/mm³ in children), with predominance of polymorphonuclear leukocytes • Sputum Gram's stain: mostly gram-positive cocci in clusters, with many polymorphonuclear leukocytes • Sputum culture: mostly coagulase-positive staphylococci • Chest X-rays: usually patchy infiltrates • Arterial blood gas (in shock): hypoxia and respiratory acidosis

Staphylococci are coagulase-negative (S. epidermidis) *or coagulase-positive* (S. aureus) *gram-positive bacteria. Coagulase-negative staphylococci, which grow abundantly as normal flora on skin and in the upper respiratory tract, are usually nonpathogenic, but can cause serious infections. Pathogenic strains of staphylococci are found in many adults—"carriers"—usually on the nasal mucosa, axilla, or groin. Sometimes, carriers shed staphylococci, infecting themselves or other susceptible people. Coagulase-positive staphylococci tend to form pus; they cause many types of infections.*

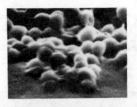

TREATMENT

CLINICAL INTERVENTION

● Semisynthetic penicillins (methicillin, nafcillin) or cephalosporins (cephalothin) given I.V.
● Probenecid may be given to partially prevent urinary excretion of penicillin and prolong blood levels.
● I.V. fluids to reverse shock

● *S. aureus* bacteremia can be fatal within 12 hours. It must be watched for in debilitated patients with Foley catheters, or those with history of drug abuse.
● Antibiotics must be administered on time to maintain adequate blood levels, but they also must be given slowly, using prescribed amount of diluent, to prevent thrombophlebitis.
● The patient must be watched for signs of penicillin allergy, especially pruritic rash (possible anaphylaxis). Epinephrine 1:1,000 and resuscitation equipment must be kept handy. Vital signs, urine output, and mental state require monitoring for signs of shock.
● Cultures must be carefully obtained, and observed for clues to primary site of infection. Blood cultures must not be refrigerated; it delays identification of organisms by slowing their growth.
● Isolation should be imposed if primary site of infection is draining. Special blood precautions are not necessary, since the number of organisms present, even in fulminant bacteremia, is minimal.
● Peak and trough levels are needed to determine the adequacy of treatment.

● Semisynthetic penicillins (methicillin, nafcillin), or cephalosporins, given I.V.
● Isolation until sputum shows minimal numbers of *S. aureus* (about 24 to 72 hours after starting antibiotics).

● Masks must be worn with isolated patients, because staphylococci from lungs spread by air as well as direct contact. Gown and gloves are needed when handling contaminated respiratory secretions.
● The door to the patient's room must be kept closed. The room shouldn't be used to store supplies. Suction bottles must be emptied carefully. Articles containing sputum (tissues, clothing, etc.) should be placed in a sealed plastic bag, marked "contaminated," and disposed of promptly by incineration.
● When obtaining sputum specimens, the sputum should be thick. If it's not, then it's probably saliva. Presence of epithelial cells (found in mouth, not lungs) indicates poor specimen.
● Antibiotics must be administered strictly on time, but slowly. The patient should be watched for signs of penicillin allergy and signs of infection at I.V. sites. I.V. site must be changed at least every third day.
● Frequent chest physical therapy should be performed. Chest percussion and postural drainage can follow IPPB treatments. Consolidated areas (revealed by X-rays or auscultation) need the most attention.

PREDISPOSING FACTORS	SIGNS AND SYMPTOMS	DIAGNOSIS
Enterocolitis • Broad-spectrum antibiotics (tetracycline, chloramphenicol, or neomycin) as prophylaxis for bowel surgery or treatment of hepatic coma • Usually occurs in elderly, but also in newborn infants (associated with staphylococcal skin lesions)	• Sudden onset of profuse, watery diarrhea usually 2 days to several weeks after start of antibiotic therapy, I.V. or P.O. • Nausea, vomiting, abdominal pain and distention • Hypovolemia and dehydration (decreased skin turgor, hypotension, fever)	• Stool Gram's stain: many gram-positive cocci and polymorphonuclear leukocytes, with few gram-negative rods • Stool culture: *S. aureus* • Sigmoidoscopy: mucosal ulcerations • Blood studies: leukocytosis, moderately increased BUN, and decreased serum albumin
Osteomyelitis • Hematogenous organisms • Skin trauma • Infection spreading from adjacent joint or other infected tissues • Usually occurs in growing bones, especially femur and tibia, of children under age 12 • More common in males	• Abrupt onset of fever—usually 101° F. (38.3° C.) or lower; shaking chills; pain and swelling over infected area; restlessness; headache • About 20% of children develop a chronic infection if not properly treated.	• Possible history of prior trauma to involved area • Positive bone and pus cultures (and blood cultures in about 50% of patients) • X-ray changes apparent after second or third week.
Food poisoning • Enterotoxin produced by toxogenic strains of *S. aureus* in contaminated food (second most common cause of food poisoning in U.S.)	• Anorexia, nausea, vomiting, diarrhea, and abdominal cramps 1 to 6 hours after ingestion of contaminated food • Symptoms usually subside within 18 hours, with complete recovery in 1 to 3 days.	• Clinical findings sufficient • Stool cultures usually negative for *S. aureus*
Skin infections • Decreased resistance • Burns or decubitus ulcers • Decreased blood flow • Possibly skin contamination from nasal discharge • Foreign bodies • Common in persons with poor hygiene living in crowded quarters	• Cellulitis—diffuse, acute inflammation of soft tissue (no drainage) • Pus-producing lesions of infectious or noninfectious origin (pyoderma) • Small pimples or boil-like lesions on skin or extending into subcutaneous tissues (furunculosis) • Small macule or skin bleb that may develop into vesicle containing pus (bullous impetigo); common in school-age children	• Clinical findings and analysis of pus cultures if sites are draining • Cultures of nondraining cellulitis taken from the margin of the reddened area by infiltration with 1 ml sterile saline solution and immediate fluid aspiration.

TREATMENT	CLINICAL INTERVENTION
• Broad-spectrum antibiotics should be discontinued. • Antistaphylococcal agents, such as vancomycin P.O., may be given.	• To prevent shock, vital signs require frequent monitoring. Fluids, in quantity, will correct dehydration. • Serum electrolyte levels must be determined. Bowel movements should be measured and recorded when possible. Serum chloride level monitoring may reveal alkalosis (hypochloremia). • Serial stool specimens will be collected for Gram's stain and culture for diagnosis and for evaluating effectiveness of treatment.
• Surgical debridement • Prolonged antibiotic therapy (4 to 8 weeks).	• Infected area must be identified and recorded. • The penetration wound from which organism originated may supply evidence of present infection. • Severe pain may render patient immobile. If so, passive range-of-motion exercises should be performed. Heat application or elevation may be needed. • Before procedures such as surgical debridement, the patient should be warned to expect some pain. He must understand that drainage is essential for healing, and that he will continue to receive analgesics and antibiotics after the surgery.
• No treatment necessary unless dehydration becomes a problem (usually in infants and elderly); then, I.V. therapy may be necessary to replace fluids.	• A complete history of symptoms, recent meals, and other known cases of food poisoning is required. • Vital signs, fluid balance, and serum electrolytes need to be monitored. • The patient may be dehydrated if vomiting is severe or prolonged. • The number and color of stools should be observed and reported.
• Topical ointments; bacitracin-neomycin-polymyxin or gentamicin • P.O. or I.V. antistaphylococcal drugs: erythromycin, cephalosporins, or vancomycin • Application of heat to reduce pain and speed healing • Surgical drainage • Identification and treatment of sources of reinfection (nostrils, perineum).	• The site and extent of infection must be identified. • Lesions should be kept clean with saline solution and peroxide irrigations. Infections near wounds or genitourinary tract should be covered with Telfa pads or gauze. Keeping pressure off the site will facilitate healing. • Extension of skin infections must be monitored. • Severe infection or abscess may require surgical drainage. The patient should understand the procedure. Cultures and specimens may be taken. • Impetigo is contagious. The patient must be isolated immediately. Secretion precautions should be used for all draining lesions.

Streptococcal Infections

CAUSES AND INCIDENCE

SIGNS AND SYMPTOMS

Pneumococcal pneumonia

• Infecting organism: *Streptococcus pneumoniae*. Mode of transmission: aspiration; possibly, inhalation
• Accounts for 70% of all bacterial pneumonia
• More common in men, in elderly and very young, and in cold, wet seasons (when 15% to 40% of persons may be carriers)
• Predisposing factors: trauma, viral infection, underlying pulmonary disease, overcrowded living quarters, chronic diseases, immunodeficiency

• Sudden onset with severe shaking chills, temperature of 102° to 105° F. (38.9° to 40.6° C.), bacteremia, cough (with thick, scanty, blood-tinged sputum) accompanied by pleuritic pain.
• Malaise, weakness, and prostration are common.
• Tachypnea, anorexia, nausea, and vomiting are less common.
• Severity of pneumonia is usually due to the host's cellular defenses, not bacterial virulence.

Streptococcal pharyngitis (strep throat)

• Infecting organism: *Streptococcus pyogenes* (group A beta-hemolytic streptococcus). Mode of transmission: inhalation, direct contact
• Accounts for 95% of all bacterial pharyngitis
• Most common in children aged 5 to 15, and during October to April
• Children with untreated strep throat will probably transmit the infection to more than half the members of their household
• Predisposing factors: overcrowded living quarters

• After 1- to 5-day incubation period: temperature of 101° to 104° F. (38.3° to 40° C.), sore throat with severe pain on swallowing, beefy red pharynx, tonsillar exudate, edematous tonsils and uvula, swollen glands along the jaw line, generalized malaise and weakness, nasal discharge, anorexia, occasional abdominal discomfort
• Up to 40% of small children have symptoms too mild for diagnosis.

Scarlet fever (scarlatina)

• Infecting organism: *Streptococcus pyogenes* (group A beta-hemolytic streptococcus). Mode of transmission: inhalation, direct contact
• Most common in children aged 2 to 10
• Predisposing factors: surgery, trauma, burns, childbirth; often follows pharyngitis, impetigo, superficial wound infection

• Streptococcal sore throat, nausea, vomiting, fever, strawberry tongue, fine erythematous rash that blanches on pressure and resembles sunburn with goosebumps
• Rash usually appears first on upper chest, then spreads to neck, abdomen, legs, and arms, sparing soles and palms; flushed cheeks, pallor around mouth
• Skin sheds during convalescence

Sydenham's chorea (St. Vitus' dance)

• Infecting organism: *Streptococcus pyogenes* (group A beta-hemolytic streptococcus). Mode of transmission: inhalation, direct contact
• Most common in children and in summer and early fall, after peak of rheumatic season
• Complication of 10% of rheumatic attacks several months after initial infection

• Choreiform movements (rapid, purposeless, involuntary movements), including facial grimacing during day that disappears during sleep (lasts about 6 to 8 months). These movements may affect writing and speech.

Streptococci are small, gram-positive spherical bacteria linked together in pairs (diplococci) or chains. Some species and serotypes of streptococci exist as normal flora in the respiratory and genitourinary tracts. When streptococci cause infection, drainage tends to be thin and serous.

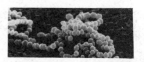

DIAGNOSIS	TREATMENT AND CONSIDERATIONS
• Gram's stain of sputum shows gram-positive lancet-shaped diplococci; culture shows *S. pneumoniae* • Chest X-ray shows lobular consolidation in adults; bronchopneumonia in children and elderly • Elevated WBC • Blood cultures often positive for group A beta-hemolytic streptococci	• Penicillin or erythromycin • Respiratory monitoring for depth and rate • Recording of sputum color and amount. Respiratory support with chest physiotherapy and intermittent positive pressure breathing (IPPB). • Dehydration prevention, especially during fever • To prevent spread: careful disposal of all purulent drainage. (High-risk patients [infants, elderly] must receive vaccine and avoid contact with infected persons.)
• Clinically indistinguishable from viral pharyngitis • Throat culture shows group A beta-hemolytic streptococci (carriers have positive throat culture) • Elevated WBC • Serology shows a fourfold rise in streptozyme titers during convalescence	• Penicillin or erythromycin • Bed rest and isolation from other children for the first 24 hours after antibiotic therapy begins. (The patient must finish prescription, which takes at least 10 days, since abscess, acute glomerulonephritis, and rheumatic fever can develop even if strep symptoms subside.) • Proper disposal of soiled tissues • Follow-up examination
• Characterisric rash and strawberry tongue • Culture and Gram's stain show *S. pyogenes* from nasopharynx • Granulocytosis	• Penicillin or erythromycin • Isolation for first 24 hours • Careful disposal of purulent discharge • Prompt and complete antibiotic treatment of any streptococcal infection
• Neurologic exam shows choreiform movements • Negative CSF	• Sedation to control choreiform movements (self-limiting complication); minimal environmental stimuli; protection against physical injury during episodes of forceful, involuntary movement • Penicillin I.M. or I.V. • Prevention: prompt treatment of all streptococcal infections

CAUSES AND INCIDENCE	SIGNS AND SYMPTOMS
Impetigo (streptococcal pyoderma) • Infecting organisms: *Streptococcus pyogenes* and *Staphylococcus aureus.* Mode of transmission: direct contact • More common in poor children, during hot humid weather, and in people who are frequently outdoors. High incidence of familial spread. • Predisposing factors: overcrowded living quarters, poor skin hygiene, minor skin trauma (usually draining wound)	• Small macules rapidly develop into vesicles, then become pustular and encrusted, causing pain, surrounding erythema, regional adenitis, cellulitis, and itching (scratching spreads infection).
Erysipelas (St. Anthony's fire) • Infecting organism: *Streptococcus pyogenes.* Mode of transmission: inhalation (only moderately communicable) • A rare disease; more common in infants and adults (ages 40 to 60), and during late spring and summer	• Sudden onset, with reddened, swollen, raised lesions (skin looks like an orange peel), usually on face and scalp, bordered by areas that often contain easily ruptured blebs filled with yellow-tinged fluid. Lesions sting and itch. • Other symptoms: vomiting, fever, headache, cervical lymphadenopathy, sore throat
Necrotizing fasciitis (cellulitis with necrosis of the fascia) • Infecting organism: *Streptococcus pyogenes* and other bacteria (often a mixed infection). Mode of transmission: direct contact • More common in elderly with arteriosclerotic vascular disease or diabetes • Predisposing factors: surgery, wounds, skin ulcers	• Mimics gas gangrene; within 72 hours of onset, patient shows red-streaked skin lesion, dusky red surrounding tissue (due to thrombosis of the blood vessels) • Other symptoms: fever, tachycardia, lethargy, prostration, disorientation, hypotension, jaundice, hypovolemia, severe pain followed by anesthesia (due to cutaneous nerve destruction) • Rapid progression of symptoms, usually leading to death
Rheumatic fever • Infecting organism: *Streptococcus pyogenes.* Mode of transmission: direct contact • Usually occurs a few days to 5 weeks after inadequately treated strep throat	• Major symptoms: carditis (prolonged apical systolic, apical middiastolic, basal diastolic murmurs), cardiomegaly, pericarditis, congestive failure, polyarthritis, chorea, erythema marginatum, subcutaneous nodules • Minor symptoms: fever, 101° to 104° F. (38.3° to 40° C.); arthralgia
Streptococcal neonatal meningitis and septicemia • Infecting organism: *Streptococcus agalactiae* (group B streptococcus). Mode of transmission: vaginal delivery, hands of nursery staff • One of the most common causes of neonatal meningitis and septicemia • Predisposing factors: 25% to 35% of pregnant women show cervical colonization during third trimester; 25% of their infants have nasopharyngeal or umbilical stump colonization; 1% develop symptoms	• Early syndrome (pulmonary): rapid onset of bacteremia and respiratory distress; mortality about 60% • Late syndrome (meningitis): fever, depressed CNS response develop 5 days to several weeks after birth; mortality 15% to 50%

DIAGNOSIS	TREATMENT AND CONSIDERATIONS
• Culture and Gram's stain of swabbed lesions show *S. pyogenes* and *S. aureus* • Characteristic lesions	• Penicillin I.V. or P.O., or erythromycin • Frequent washing of lesions with soap and water followed by thorough drying • Isolation of patient with draining wounds • Prevention: good hygiene and proper wound care
• Typical reddened lesions • Culture taken from edge of lesions shows group A beta-hemolytic streptococci	• Penicillin I.V. or P.O. • Cold packs, analgesics (aspirin and codeine for local discomfort) • Prevention: prompt treatment of streptococcal infections and secretion precautions
• Characteristic lesion • Culture and Gram's stain show *S. pyogenes*	• Immediate, wide, deep surgical excision of all necrotic tissues • High-dose penicillin I.V. • Good preoperative skin preparation; aseptic surgical and suturing technique
• Two major symptoms or diagnostic factors, or one major and two minor symptoms or diagnostic factors and a history of strep infection indicate high probability of rheumatic fever. • Major diagnostic factors: history of scarlet fever, positive culture for group A streptococci, increased antistreptolysin O or other streptococcal antibody • Minor diagnostic factors: history of previous rheumatic heart disease or rheumatic fever, increased erythrocyte sedimentation rate (ESR), positive C-reactive protein and leukocytosis	• Penicillin I.V. or I.M., with prophylactic penicillin continued indefinitely after onset of rheumatic fever • Aspirin to control inflammation, steroids to reduce fever and improve heart function • Bed rest in the acute phase, followed by slowly progressive rehabilitation and ambulation • Prevention: prompt treatment of strep throat with at least 10 days of oral penicillin therapy
• Chest X-ray showing massive infiltrate similar to respiratory distress syndrome or pneumonia; positive blood culture in bacteremia and culture of umbilicus, GI and respiratory tracts; and skin showing group B streptococci colonization	• Ampicillin or penicillin, or other semisynthetic penicillins I.V. • Patient isolation unnecessary, but careful handwashing essential • Vaccine in developmental stages

GRAM-NEGATIVE COCCI

Meningococcal Infections

Two major meningococcal infections (meningitis and meningococcemia) are caused by the gram-negative bacteria Neisseria meningitidis, *which also causes primary pneumonia, purulent conjunctivitis, endocarditis, sinusitis, and genital infection. Meningococcemia occurs as simple bacteremia, fulminant meningococcemia, and rarely, chronic meningococcemia. It often accompanies meningitis. (For more information on meningitis, see* MENINGITIS, NEUROLOGIC DISORDERS). *Meningococcal infections may occur sporadically or in epidemics; virulent infections may be fatal within a matter of hours.*

Causes and incidence
Meningococcal infections occur most often in children (ages 6 months to 1 year) and men, usually military recruits, due to overcrowding.

N. meningitidis has seven serogroups (A, B, C, D, X, Y, Z); group A causes most epidemics. These bacteria are often present in upper respiratory flora. Transmission takes place through inhalation of an infected droplet from a carrier (an estimated 2% to 38% of the population). The bacteria then localize in the nasopharynx. Following an incubation period of approximately 3 or 4 days, they spread through the bloodstream to joints, skin, adrenal glands, lungs, and the central nervous system. Resulting tissue damage (possibly due to bacterial endotoxin) produces the symptoms, and in fulminant meningococcemia and meningococcal bacteremia, progresses to hemorrhage, thrombosis, and necrosis.

Signs and symptoms
Clinical features of meningococcal infection vary. Symptoms of *meningococcal bacteremia* include sudden spiking fever, headache, sore throat, cough, chills, myalgia (in back and legs), arthralgia, tachycardia, tachypnea, mild hypotension, and a petechial, nodular, or maculopapular rash.

In about 10% to 20% of patients, this progresses to *fulminant meningococcemia*, with extreme prostration, enlargement of skin lesions, disseminated intravascular coagulation (DIC), and shock. Unless it is treated promptly, fulminant meningococcemia results in death from respiratory or heart failure in 6 to 24 hours.

Characteristics of the rare *chronic meningococcemia* include intermittent fever, maculopapular rash, joint pain, and enlarged spleen.

Diagnosis
Isolation of *N. meningitidis* through a positive blood culture, CSF culture, or lesion scraping confirms the diagnosis except in nasopharyngeal infections, since *N. meningitidis* exists as part of the normal nasopharyngeal flora.

Tests that support the diagnosis include counterimmunoelectrophoresis of CSF or blood, low WBC, and with skin or adrenal hemorrhages, decreased platelet and clotting levels. Diagnostic evaluation must rule out Rocky Mountain spotted fever and vascular purpuras.

Treatment
As soon as meningococcal infection is suspected, treatment begins with large doses of aqueous penicillin G or ampicillin; or for the patient who is allergic to penicillin, I.V. chloramphenicol. Therapy may also include mannitol for cerebral edema; I.V. heparin for DIC; dopamine for shock; and digoxin and a diuretic for congestive heart failure. Sup-

portive measures include fluid and electrolyte maintenance, proper ventilation (patent airway and oxygen, if necessary), insertion of an arterial or central venous pressure (CVP) line to monitor cardiovascular status, and bed rest.

Chemoprophylaxis with rifampin or minocycline is useful for hospital workers in close contact with the patient; minocycline can also temporarily eradicate the infection in carriers.

Additional considerations
When treating a patient with a meningococcal infection, the hospital staff member should:
• give I.V. antibiotics, as ordered, to maintain sufficient blood and CSF drug levels.
• enforce bed rest in early stages; provide a dark, quiet, restful environment.
• maintain adequate ventilation with oxygen or a ventilator, if necessary; suc-

tion and turn the patient frequently.
• keep accurate intake and output records to maintain proper fluid and electrolyte levels; monitor blood pressure, pulse, arterial blood gases, and CVP.
• watch for complications, such as DIC, arthritis, endocarditis, and pneumonia.
• check the patient's drug history for possible allergies before administering antibiotics.
• monitor CBC if the patient is receiving chloramphenicol.

To prevent the spread of meningococcal infection, the staff member should:
• isolate the patient until he has received antibiotic therapy for 24 hours.
• label all meningococcal specimens; deliver them to the laboratory quickly because meningococci are very sensitive to changes in humidity and temperature.
• report all cases of meningococcol infection to local public health department authorities.

GRAM-POSITIVE BACILLI

Diphtheria

Diphtheria is an acute, highly contagious toxin-mediated infection caused by Corynebacterium diphtheriae, a gram-positive rod that usually infects the respiratory tract, primarily involving the tonsils, nasopharynx, and larynx. Currently, both cutaneous and wound diphtherias are seen more frequently in the United States and are often caused by nontoxigenic strains. The gastrointestinal and the urinary tracts, conjunctivae, and ears are rarely involved.

Causes
Transmission usually occurs through intimate contact or by airborne respiratory droplets from apparently healthy carriers or convalescing patients, since many more people carry this disease than contract active infection. Diphtheria is more prevalent during the colder months due to closer person-to-person contact indoors. However, it may be contracted at any time during the year.

Thanks to effective immunization, diphtheria is rare in many parts of the world, including the United States. Since

1972, there has been an increase in cutaneous diphtheria, especially in the Pacific Northwest and the Southwest, particularly in areas where crowding and poor hygienic conditions prevail. Most victims are children under age 15. Diphtheria carries a mortality rate of up to 10%.

Signs and symptoms
Most infections are inapparent and go unrecognized, especially in partially immunized individuals. After an incubation period of less than a week, clinical

cases of diphtheria characteristically show a thick, patchy, grayish-green membrane over the mucous membranes of the pharynx, larynx, tonsils, soft palate, and nose; a rasping cough, hoarseness, and other symptoms similar to croup. Attempts to remove the membrane usually cause bleeding, which is highly characteristic of diphtheria. If this membrane causes airway obstruction (particularly likely in laryngeal diphtheria), symptoms include tachypnea, stridor, possibly cyanosis, suprasternal retractions, and suffocation, if untreated. In cutaneous diphtheria, skin lesions resemble impetigo.

Complications include myocarditis, neurologic involvement (primarily affects motor fibers but can also affect sensory neurons), renal involvement, and pulmonary involvement (bronchopneumonia) due to *C. diphtheriae* or other superinfecting organisms.

Diagnosis

 Examination showing the characteristic membrane and throat culture, or culture of other suspect lesions growing *C. diphtheriae* confirm this diagnosis.

Treatment

Standard treatment includes diphtheria antitoxin administered I.M. or I.V.; antibiotics, such as penicillin or erythromycin, to eliminate the organisms from the upper respiratory tract and other sites, to terminate the carrier state; and measures to prevent complications.

Additional considerations

Diphtheria requires comprehensive supportive care, including psychologic support.
• To prevent spread of this disease, the patient must be placed in strict isolation and taught how to properly dispose of nasopharyngeal secretions. Infection precautions must continue until after two consecutive negative nasopharyngeal cultures—at least 1 week after drug therapy stops. Treatment of exposed in-

dividuals with antitoxin remains controversial. Family members should receive diphtheria toxoid (usually given as combined diphtheria and tetanus toxoids [DT] and a combination including pertussis vaccine [DPT] for children under age 6) if they haven't already been immunized.

Although it is time-consuming and hazardous, desensitization should be attempted if tests are positive, since diphtheria antitoxin is the only *specific* treatment available. Since mortality increases directly with delay in antitoxin administration, the antitoxin may be given before laboratory confirmation of diagnosis if sensitivity tests are negative. Before giving diphtheria antitoxin, which is made from horse serum, eye and skin tests must be taken to determine sensitivity. Following antitoxin and/or penicillin administration, anaphylaxis may occur, so epinephrine 1:1,000 and resuscitative equipment should be kept available. In patients who receive erythromycin, thrombophlebitis is a possible complication.
• Respirations require careful monitoring, especially in laryngeal diphtheria (usually, such patients are in a high-humidity or croup tent). If signs of airway obstruction occur, immediate life support, including intubation and tracheotomy, will be necessary.
• Signs of shock can develop suddenly and must be watched for.
• If neuritis develops, it's usually transient. Peripheral neuritis may not develop until 2 to 3 months after onset of illness.

 • Signs of myocarditis, such as development of heart murmurs or EKG changes, must also be watched for. Ventricular fibrillation is a common cause of sudden death in diphtheria patients.
• A primary nurse, assigned to the patient, should make it her task to increase the effectiveness of isolation.
• Parents must understand the need for childhood immunization. Public health authorities must be notified of all cases.

Listeriosis

Listeriosis is an infection caused by the weakly hemolytic, gram-positive bacillus Listeria monocytogenes. It occurs most often in fetuses, in neonates (during the first 3 weeks of life), and in older or immunosuppressed adults. The infected fetus is usually stillborn or is born prematurely, almost always with fatal listeriosis. This infection produces milder illness in pregnant women, and varying degrees of illness in older and immunosuppressed patients; their prognoses depend on the severity of underlying illness.

Causes

The primary method of human-to-human transmission is neonatal infection *in utero* (through the placenta) or during passage through an infected birth canal. Other strongly suspected modes of transmission include inhaling contaminated dust; coming in contact with infected wild and domestic animals, contaminated sewage or mud, or soil contaminated with feces containing *L. monocytogenes*; and possibly, person-to-person transmission.

Signs and symptoms

In about 75% of patients, listeriosis produces meningoencephalitis of sudden onset, with or without bacteremia. Infected patients show signs of meningeal irritation (in infants tense fontanelles; in others, irritability, lethargy, convulsions, fever, headache, nausea, and vomiting); diarrhea; delirium and coma; circulatory collapse and shock; and dark red maculopapular skin lesions over the legs and trunk.

Listeriosis sometimes produces bacteremia and a febrile, generalized illness. In a pregnant woman, this infection produces an apparently mild illness, with general malaise and lethargy, but spells disaster for the fetus. Listeriosis may cause severe uterine fetal infection, abortion, premature delivery, stillbirth, or early neonatal death.

Diagnosis

L. monocytogenes is identified by its diagnostic tumbling motility on a wet mount of a culture. Other supportive diagnostic results include positive culture of blood, spinal fluid, drainage from cervical or vaginal lesions, or lochia from a mother with an infected infant, but isolation of the organism from these specimens is often difficult. Listeriosis also causes monocytosis.

Treatment

Treatment consists of combinations of ampicillin, penicillin G procaine, and erythromycin given I.V. or I.M. and continued for a minimum of 7 days after fever subsides.

Ampicillin and penicillin G are best for treating meningitis due to *L. monocytogenes*, since they more easily cross the blood-brain barrier. Pregnant women require prompt, vigorous treatment to combat fetal infection.

Additional considerations

When caring for a listeriosis patient, the hospital staff member should:
• use secretion precautions until a series of cultures of bodily discharges are negative; be especially careful when handling lochia from an infected mother, and secretions from her infant's eyes, nose, mouth, and rectum, including meconium.
• evaluate neurologic status at least every 2 hours; check an infant's fontanelles for bulging; maintain adequate I.V. fluid intake; measure intake and output accurately.
• provide respiratory assistance, check the rate and quality of respirations, and obtain frequent blood gas measurements if the patient has CNS depression and

becomes apneic.
• provide adequate nutrition by total parenteral nutrition, nasogastric tube feedings, or a soft diet, as appropriate for the patient's condition.
• allow parents to see and, if possible, hold their infant in the ICU; be flexible about visiting privileges; keep parents informed of the infant's status and prognosis at all times.
• reassure parents of an infected newborn who may feel guilty about the infant's illness.
• educate pregnant women to avoid infective materials on farms where listeriosis is endemic among livestock.

Tetanus
(Lockjaw)

Tetanus is an acute exotoxin-mediated infection caused by the anaerobic, spore-forming, gram-positive bacillus Clostridium tetani. *Usually, such infection is systemic; less often, localized. Tetanus is fatal in up to 60% of unimmunized persons, usually within 10 days of onset. When symptoms develop within 3 days after exposure, the prognosis is poor.*

Causes and incidence
Normally, transmission is through a puncture wound that is contaminated by soil, dust, or animal excreta containing *C. tetani*, or by way of burns and minor wounds. After *C. tetani* enters the body, it causes local infection and tissue necrosis. It also produces toxins which then enter the bloodstream and lymphatics, and eventually spread to CNS tissue.

Tetanus occurs worldwide, but it's more prevalent in agricultural regions and developing countries that lack mass immunization programs. It's one of the most common causes of neonatal deaths in developing countries, where infants of unimmunized mothers are delivered under unsterile conditions. In such infants, the unhealed umbilical cord is the portal of entry.

In the United States, approximately 75% of all cases occur between April and September.

Signs and symptoms
The incubation period varies from more than 10 days in mild tetanus to under 2 days in severe tetanus. When symptoms occur within 2 to 3 days after injury, the case fatality ratio is higher. If tetanus remains localized, signs of onset are spasm and increased muscle tone near the wound.

If tetanus is generalized (systemic), indications include marked muscle hypertonicity; hyperactive deep tendon reflexes; tachycardia; profuse sweating; low-grade fever; and painful, involuntary muscle contractions:
• neck and facial muscles, especially cheek muscles—locked jaw (trismus) and a grotesque, grinning expression called *risus sardonicus*
• somatic muscles—arched-back rigidity (opisthotonos), in which head and heels bend backward; boardlike abdominal rigidity
• intermittent tonic convulsions lasting several minutes, which may result in cyanosis and sudden death by asphyxiation.

Despite such pronounced neuromuscular symptoms, cerebral and sensory functions remain normal. Complications include atelectasis, pneumonia, pulmonary emboli, acute gastric ulcers, flexion contractures, and cardiac arrhythmias.

Neonatal tetanus is always generalized. The first clinical sign is difficulty in sucking, which usually appears 3 to 10 days after birth. It progresses to total inability to suck, accompanied by excessive crying, irritability, and nuchal rigidity.

Diagnosis

Frequently, diagnosis must rest on clinical features, and a history of trauma and no previous tetanus immunization. Blood cultures and tetanus antibody tests are often negative; only a third of patients have a positive wound culture. CSF pressure may rise above normal. Diagnosis also must rule out meningitis, rabies, phenothiazine or strychnine toxicity, and other conditions that mimic tetanus.

Treatment

Within 72 hours after a puncture wound, a patient with no previous history of tetanus immunization first requires tetanus immune globulin (TIG) or tetanus antitoxin, to confer temporary protection. Next, he needs active immunization with tetanus toxoid. A patient who has received tetanus immunization within 3 to 5 years needs a booster injection of tetanus toxoid. If tetanus develops despite immediate postinjury treatment, the patient will require airway maintenance and a muscle relaxant, such as diazepam, to decrease muscle rigidity and spasm. If muscle contractions are not relieved by muscle relaxants, a neuromuscular blocker may be needed. The patient with tetanus needs high-dose antibiotics (penicillin administered I.V. or I.M., if he is not allergic to it).

Additional considerations

When caring for the potential tetanus victim, the hospital staff member should:
• thoroughly debride and cleanse the injury site with 3% hydrogen peroxide, and check the patient's immunization history; record the cause of injury; report the case to local public health authorities if it's a dog bite.

• obtain an accurate history of allergies before giving TIG, antitoxin or toxoid, or penicillin; keep epinephrine 1:1,000 and resuscitative equipment available if the patient has a positive history.
• stress the importance of maintaining active immunization with a booster dose of tetanus toxoid every 10 years.

After tetanus develops, the staff member should:
• maintain an adequate airway and ventilation to prevent pneumonia and atelectasis; use suction often and watch for signs of respiratory distress; keep emergency airway equipment on hand, since the patient may require artificial ventilation or oxygen administration.
• maintain an I.V. line for medications and emergency care, if necessary.
• monitor EKG frequently for arrhythmias; accurately record intake and output, and check vital signs often.
• turn the patient frequently to prevent bedsores and pulmonary stasis.
• keep the patient's room dark and quiet, since even minimal external stimulation provokes muscle spasms; warn visitors not to upset or overly stimulate the patient, but don't make them too anxious about harming him.
• insert a Foley catheter if urinary retention develops.
• give muscle relaxants and sedatives, as ordered; schedule patient care to coincide with heaviest sedation.
• insert an artificial airway, if necessary, to prevent tongue injury and maintain airway during spasms.
• provide adequate nutrition to meet the patient's increased metabolic needs; be aware that the patient may need nasogastric tube feedings or hyperalimentation.

Botulism

Botulism, a severe form of food poisoning, results from ingestion of food contaminated by an exotoxin produced by the gram-positive, anaerobic bacillus Clostridium botulinum. The mortality rate from botulism is about 25%, with death most often caused by respiratory failure during the first week of illness.

Causes and incidence

Botulism is usually the result of ingesting inadequately cooked contaminated foods, especially those with low acid content, such as home-canned fruits and vegetables, sausages, and smoked or preserved fish or meat. Rarely, it is a result of wound infection with *C. botulinum.*

Botulism occurs worldwide and affects adults more often than children. Recently, findings have shown that an infant's GI tract can become colonized with *C. botulinum* from some unknown source, and then the exotoxin is produced within the infant's intestine. Incidence had been declining, but the current trend toward home canning has resulted in an upswing (approximately 250 cases per year in the United States) in recent years.

Signs and symptoms

Symptoms usually appear within 12 to 36 hours (range is 6 hours to 8 days) after the ingestion of contaminated food. Severity varies with the amount of toxin ingested. Generally, early onset (within 24 hours) signals critical and potentially fatal illness. Initial symptoms include dry mouth, sore throat, weakness, vomiting, and diarrhea. The cardinal sign of botulism, though, is acute symmetrical cranial nerve impairment (ptosis, diplopia, dysarthria), followed by descending weakness or paralysis of muscles in the extremities or trunk, and dyspnea from respiratory muscle paralysis. Such impairment doesn't affect mental or sensory processes and isn't associated with fever.

Infant botulism can produce the syndrome of the hypotonic (floppy) infant. The infant usually becomes ill between 3 to 20 weeks of age. Symptoms are constipation, feeble cry, depressed gag reflex, and inability to suck. Cranial nerve deficits also occur in infants and are manifested by a flaccid facial expression, ptosis, and ophthalmoplegia. Infants also develop generalized muscle weakness, hypotonia, and areflexia. Loss of head control may be striking. Respiratory arrest is likely.

Diagnosis

 Identification of the offending toxin in the patient's serum, stool, gastric content, or the suspected food confirms the diagnosis. An electromyogram (EMG) showing diminished muscle action potential after a single supramaximal nerve stimulus is also diagnostic.

Diagnosis also must rule out other diseases often confused with botulism, such as Guillain-Barré syndrome, myasthenia gravis, cerebrovascular accident (CVA), staphylococcal food poisoning, tick paralysis, chemical intoxications, carbon monoxide poisoning, fish poisoning, trichinosis, and diphtheria.

Treatment and additional considerations

Treatment consists of I.V. or I.M. administration of botulinum antitoxin (available through the Center for Disease Control).

If ingestion of contaminated food is suspected, the hospital staff member should:
• obtain a careful history of the patient's food intake for the past several days; check to see if other family members exhibit similar symptoms and share a common food history.
• observe the patient for abnormal neurologic signs; tell his family to watch for signs of weakness, blurred vision, and slurred speech after he returns home, and to bring him back to the hospital immediately if any of these signs appear.
• induce vomiting, begin gastric lavage, and give a high enema to purge any unabsorbed toxin from the bowel if ingestion has occurred within several hours.

If clinical signs of botulism appear, the staff member should:
• admit the patient to the ICU, and monitor cardiac and respiratory functions carefully.
• administer botulinum antitoxin, as ordered, to neutralize any circulating toxin; obtain an accurate patient history of allergies, and perform a skin test before giving antitoxin; watch for anaphy-

laxis or other hypersensitivity, and serum sickness after injection; keep epinephrine 1:1,000 (for subcutaneous administration) and emergency airway equipment available.
• closely assess and accurately record neurologic function, including bilateral motor status (reflexes, ability to move arms and legs).
• give I.V. fluids, as ordered; turn the patient often, and encourage deep breathing exercises.
• keep the patient and family informed regarding the course of the disease since it's sometimes fatal; warn the family of the patient's status.
• immediately report all cases of botulism to local public health authorities.

To help prevent botulism, the staff member should encourage patients to observe proper techniques in processing and preserving foods; and warn them to avoid even *tasting* food from a bulging can or one with a peculiar odor, and to sterilize by boiling any utensil that comes in contact with suspected food; eating even a small amount of food contaminated with botulism toxin can be fatal.

Gas Gangrene

Gas gangrene results from local infection with the anaerobic, spore-forming, gram-positive rod Clostridium perfringens *(or another clostridial species). It occurs in devitalized tissues and results from compromised arterial circulation following trauma or surgery. This rare infection carries a high mortality unless therapy begins immediately. However, with prompt treatment, 80% of patients with gas gangrene of the extremities survive; prognosis is poorer for gas gangrene in other sites, such as the abdominal wall or the bowel. The usual incubation period is 1 to 4 days but can vary from 3 hours to 6 weeks or longer.*

Causes

C. perfringens is a normal inhabitant of the gastrointestinal and the female genital tracts; it's also prevalent in soil. Transmission occurs by entry of organisms during trauma or surgery. Since *C. perfringens* is anaerobic, gas gangrene is most often found in deep wounds, especially those in which tissue necrosis further reduces oxygen supply. When *C. perfringens* invades soft tissues, it produces thrombosis of regional blood vessels, tissue necrosis, and localized edema. Such necrosis releases both carbon dioxide and hydrogen subcutaneously, producing interstitial gas bubbles. Gas gangrene most commonly occurs in the extremities and in abdominal wounds, and less frequently in the uterus.

Signs and symptoms

True gas gangrene produces myositis and another form of this disease, involving only soft tissue, called anaerobic cellulitis. Most signs of infection develop within 72 hours of trauma or surgery. The hallmark of gas gangrene is crepitation, a result of carbon dioxide and hydrogen accumulation as a metabolic by-product in necrotic tissues. Other typical indications are severe localized pain, swelling, and discoloration (often dusky brown or reddish), with formation of bullae and necrosis within 36 hours from onset of symptoms. Soon the skin over the wound may rupture, revealing dark red or black necrotic muscle, a foul-smelling watery or frothy discharge, intravascular hemolysis, thrombosis of blood vessels, and evidence of infection spread. In addition to these local symptoms, gas gangrene produces early signs of toxemia and hypovolemia (tachycardia, tachypnea, and hypotension), with moderate fever usually not above 101° F. (38.3° C.). Although pale, prostrate, and motionless, most patients remain alert and ori-

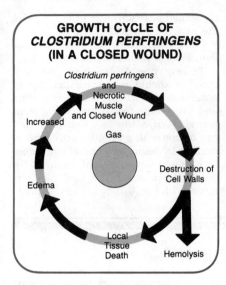

**GROWTH CYCLE OF
CLOSTRIDIUM PERFRINGENS
(IN A CLOSED WOUND)**

Clostridium perfringens
and
Necrotic
Muscle
and Closed Wound

Increased

Gas

Destruction of
Cell Walls

Edema

Local
Tissue
Death

Hemolysis

ented, and are extremely apprehensive. Usually death occurs suddenly, often during surgery for removal of necrotic tissue. Less often, death is preceded by delirium and coma, and is sometimes accompanied by vomiting, profuse diarrhea, and circulatory collapse.

Diagnosis

A history of recent surgery or a deep puncture wound and the rapid onset of pain and crepitation around the wound suggest this diagnosis. It is confirmed by anaerobic cultures of wound drainage showing *C. perfringens*; Gram's stain of wound drainage showing large, gram-positive, rod-shaped bacteria; X-rays showing gas in tissues; and blood studies showing leukocytosis and, later, hemolysis. Diagnosis must rule out synergistic gangrene and necrotizing fasciitis; however, unlike gas gangrene, both these disorders anesthetize the skin around the wound.

Treatment

Treatment includes careful observation for signs of myositis and cellulitis, and *immediate intervention*, if these signs appear; *immediate* wide surgical excision of all affected tissues and necrotic

muscle in myositis (delayed or inadequate surgical excision is a fatal mistake!); intravenous administration of high-dose penicillin; and, after adequate debridement, hyperbaric oxygenation, if available. For 1 to 3 hours every 6 to 8 hours, the patient is placed in a hyperbaric chamber and is exposed to pressures designed to increase oxygen tension and prevent multiplication of the anaerobic clostridia. Surgery may be done within the hyperbaric chamber if the chamber is large enough.

Additional considerations

Careful observation may result in *early* recognition. Signs of ischemia (cool skin temperature, pallor or cyanosis, sudden severe pain or edema, loss of pulses in involved limb) may be diagnostic.

Meticulous supportive care is necessary after diagnosis and throughout the illness.

• Fluid levels must be maintained.

• Pulmonary and cardiac functions should be watched closely, with maintenance of airway and ventilation.

• Good skin care can prevent skin breakdown and further infection. After surgery, meticulous wound care can prevent recurrence.

• A patient history of allergies is required before penicillin administration; afterward, the patient must be watched closely for signs of hypersensitivity.

• Psychologic support is critical, since these patients can remain alert until death, knowing that death is imminent and unavoidable.

• Room deodorization may be needed to control foul wound odor. The patient must be emotionally prepared for a large wound after surgical excision, and accept the possible need for physical rehabilitation.

• Wound precautions must be followed: proper disposal of drainage material (double-bag dressings in plastic bags for incineration); use of sterile gloves when changing dressings; and room cleaning with a germicidal solution after the patient's discharged.

Gas gangrene can be prevented by:

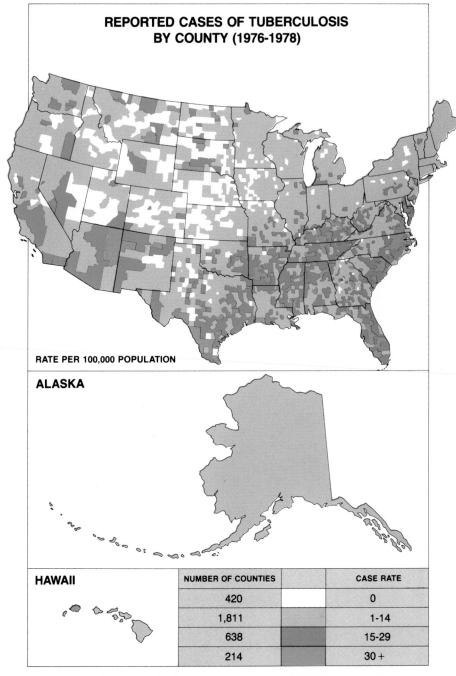

REPORTED CASES OF TUBERCULOSIS
BY COUNTY (1976-1978)

RATE PER 100,000 POPULATION

ALASKA

HAWAII

NUMBER OF COUNTIES		CASE RATE
420		0
1,811		1-14
638		15-29
214		30 +

Adapted with permission from MORBIDITY AND MORTALITY ANNUAL SUMMARY 1979
(Atlanta: Center for Disease Control, 1979).

EQUIPMENT FOR COLLECTING CULTURE SPECIMENS

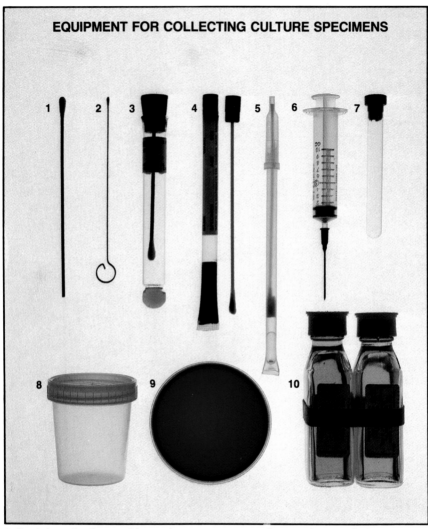

1. Swab for collecting aerobic specimens

2. Nasopharyngeal and urethral swab

3. Swab and tube containing carbon dioxide for collecting anaerobic specimens

4. Tube containing special medium and carbon dioxide for culturing *N. gonorrhoeae;* swab for collecting specimen

5. Culturette swab with transport medium for collecting aerobic specimens

6. Sterile syringe for collecting blood culture specimens; when needle is removed, syringe may also be used for aspirating wound drainage

7. Sterile, stoppered test tube for collecting cerebrospinal fluid

8. Sterile plastic container for urine or sputum specimens

9. Thayer-Martin plate with enriched media for isolating and culturing *N. gonorrhoeae*

10. Bottles containing appropriate media for blood culture

SPECIMEN COLLECTION AT A GLANCE

SPECIMEN	AMOUNT NEEDED	NORMAL FLORA	POSSIBLE PATHOGENS
Wound (fresh pus)	As much as possible (after cleansing wound to remove skin flora)	None (may have contamination from skin flora: *S. epidermidis*, diphtheroids, *P. acnes*)	Any organism (*S. aureus*, Group A streptococci, gram-negatives, yeast)
Blood	10 ml per culture (from two separate sites)	None	Any organism
Cerebrospinal fluid	1 ml (as much as possible)	None	Any organism (*S. pneumoniae, N. meningitidis*)
Eye	As much as possible	None (may have diphtheroids, *P. acnes, S. epidermidis*)	Herpes simplex, *S. aureus, S. pneumoniae, N. gonorrhoeae, C. trachomatis*
Ear	As much as possible	Mixed skin flora, diphtheroids, *S. epidermidis, P. acnes* (can have gram-negative rods)	*S. aureus, H. influenzae, P. aeruginosa*
Throat-nasopharynx	As much as possible (from tonsillar area, not tongue)	Streptococci, staphylococci, *Haemophilus, Neisseria*, diphtheroids	Group A beta-hemolytic streptococci, *C. diphtheriae, B. pertussis, H. influenzae, N. meningitidis*
Sputum	2 to 3 ml (of sputum, not saliva)	*S. epidermidis, Neisseria*, streptococci (nonhemolytic), diphtheroids	Any organism in pure or predominant culture (*S. pneumoniae, S. aureus*, gram-negatives, *M. tuberculosis*)
Urine	1 ml (5 ml for urine analysis)	*S. epidermidis, Neisseria, E. coli, T. vaginalis* (less than 100,000/ml)	Any organism greater than 100,000/ml, excluding the normal genital flora of lactobacilli, diphtheroids
Cervical-vaginal	As much as possible	Normal vaginal flora; lactobacilli, diphtheroids, *Candida, S. epidermidis*	*N. gonorrhoeae, T. vaginalis*, yeast (proliferative in pure culture)
Stool	A small amount; for *Shigella*, rectal swab may be used; for *Salmonella*, feces—not swab—must be obtained.	*E. coli* predominates (stool content is 98% bacteria; organisms are too numerous to list)	*Salmonella, Shigella, S. aureus* (greater than 50%), *C. albicans* (greater than 50%), *Campylobacter, Y. enterocolitica, V. cholerae, C. botulinum*, ova, and parasites
Skin (lesion or carbuncle)	As much as possible	Diphtheroids, *P. acnes, S. epidermidis*	Group A streptococci, *S. aureus*

GRAM'S STAINS OF BACTERIAL ORGANISMS

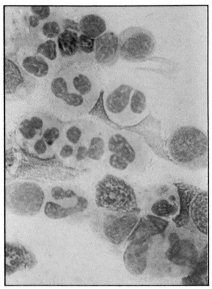

In *streptococcal pharyngitis,* the Gram's stain shows characteristic prevalence of pus cells.

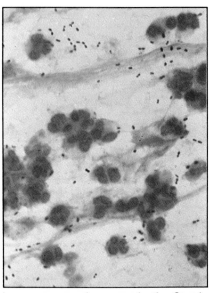

In *pneumococcal pneumonia,* the Gram's stain shows pus cells lined up in short chains, and gram-positive lancet- or helmet-shaped diplococci.

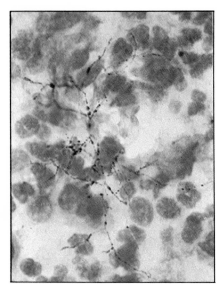

In *pulmonary nocardiosis,* the sputum Gram's stain shows many pus cells and the causative organism, *Nocardia* (fine filamentous, beaded and branching structure).

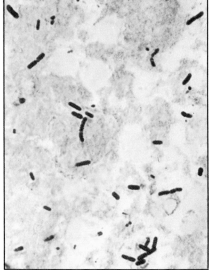

In *clostridial gas gangrene,* the Gram's stain shows cellular debris, degenerating cells, and characteristic, large, darkly staining gram-positive rods.

making all wound sites unsuitable for growth of clostridia by attempting to keep granulation tissue viable; reporting devitalized tissues; adequate debridement to minimize anaerobic growth conditions; patient positioning to facilitate drainage; and elimination of dead spaces in closed wounds.

Actinomycosis

Actinomycosis is an infection with the gram-positive anaerobic bacillus Actinomyces israelii *that produces granulomatous, suppurative lesions with abscesses. Most common sites of this infection are the head, neck, thorax, and abdomen, but it can spread to contiguous tissues, causing multiple draining sinuses.*

Occurring sporadically and infrequently throughout the world, actinomycosis most frequently affects males, ages 15 to 35; the ratio of males to females is 2 to 1. It is likely to infect people with dental disease.

Causes

A. israelii occurs as part of the normal flora of the throat, tonsillar crypts, and mouth (particularly around carious teeth); infection results from its traumatic introduction into body tissues.

Signs and symptoms

Symptoms appear from days to months after injury and may vary, depending on the site of infection.

In *cervicofacial actinomycosis* (lumpy jaw), painful, indurated swellings appear in the mouth or neck up to several weeks following dental extraction or trauma. They gradually enlarge and form fistulas that open onto the skin. Sulfur granules (yellowish-gray masses that are actually colonies of the *A. israelii*) appear in the exudate.

In *pulmonary actinomycosis*, aspiration of bacteria from the mouth into areas of the lungs already anaerobic from infection or atelectasis produces a fever, and a cough that becomes productive and occasionally causes hemoptysis. Eventually, empyema follows due to invasion of the pleura, and a sinus formation develops through the chest wall. Septicemia may also occur.

In *gastrointestinal actinomycosis*, ileocecal lesions are caused by swallowed bacteria, which produce abdominal discomfort, fever, sometimes a palpable mass, and an external sinus.

Rare sites of actinomycotic infection are the bones, brain, liver, kidneys, and female reproductive organs. Symptoms reflect the organ involved.

Diagnosis

Isolation of *A. israelii* in exudate or tissue confirms actinomycosis. Other procedures that can help identify actinomycosis include:

• *microscopic examination* of sulfur granules.
• *Gram's staining* of excised tissue or exudate, to reveal branching gram-positive rods.
• *chest X-ray* to show lesions in unusual locations, such as the shaft of a rib.

Treatment

High-dose I.V. penicillin or tetracycline therapy precedes surgical excision and drainage of abscesses in all forms of the disease, and continues for 3 to 6 weeks. Following parenteral therapy, treatment with oral penicillin or tetracycline may continue for 1 to 6 months.

Additional considerations

• All used dressings should be placed in a sealed plastic bag.
• Proper aseptic wound management must be maintained after surgery.
• Antibiotics will probably be ordered. An accurate patient history of allergies is necessary to prevent hypersensitivity

reactions such as rash, fever, itching, and signs of anaphylaxis. If the patient has a history of any allergies, epinephrine 1:1,000 and resuscitative equipment must be immediately available.
• Good oral hygiene and proper dental care are necessary in these patients to remove possible sources of reinfection.

Nocardiosis

Nocardiosis is an acute, subacute, or chronic bacterial infection caused by a weakly gram-positive species of the genus Nocardia—*usually* Nocardia asteroides. *It is most common in men, especially those with compromised immune defense mechanisms. Its mortality rate in brain infection exceeds 80%; in other forms, mortality rate is 50%, even with appropriate therapy.*

Causes
Nocardia are aerobic gram-positive bacteria, with branching filaments similar in appearance to fungi. Normally found in soil, these organisms cause occasional sporadic disease in humans and animals throughout the world. Their incubation period is unknown but is probably several weeks. Usual mode of transmission is presumably inhalation of organisms suspended in dust; less often, direct inoculation through puncture wounds or abrasions.

Signs and symptoms
Nocardiosis originates as a pulmonary infection, and causes a cough that produces thick, tenacious, purulent, mucopurulent, and possibly, blood-tinged sputum. It may also cause a fever as high as 105° F. (40.5° C.), chills, night sweats, anorexia, malaise, and weight loss. This infection may lead to pleurisy, intrapleural effusions, and empyema.

If the infection spreads through the blood to the brain, abscesses form, causing confusion, disorientation, dizziness, headache, nausea, and seizures. Rupture of a brain abscess can cause purulent meningitis. Extrapulmonary, hematogenous spread may cause endocarditis and lesions of kidneys, liver, subcutaneous tissue, and bone.

Diagnosis
Identification of *Nocardia* by culture of sputum or discharge is difficult. Special staining techniques often must be relied upon to make the diagnosis, in conjunction with a typical clinical picture (usually progressive pneumonia, despite antibiotic therapy). Occasionally, diagnosis requires biopsy of lung or other tissue. Chest X-ray (and sometimes sputum samples) shows pockets of infection that look like fungus balls. Unfortunately, up to 40% of nocardial infections elude diagnosis until postmortem examination.

In brain infection with meningitis, lumbar puncture shows nonspecific changes, such as increased opening pressure; CSF shows increased WBC and protein levels, and decreased glucose levels as compared to glucose levels in serum.

Treatment
Nocardiosis requires long-term (12 to 18 months) treatment, preferably with high doses of sulfonamides. In patients who do not respond to sulfonamide treatment, other drugs, such as ampicillin or erythromycin, may be added. Treatment also includes surgical drainage of abscesses and excision of necrotic tissue. The acute phase requires complete bed rest; as the patient's condition improves, activity can increase gradually.

Additional considerations
Nocardiosis doesn't require isolation, since it's not transmitted from person to person. Patient care is comprehensive.

- Adequate nourishment, through total parenteral nutrition, nasogastric tube feedings, or a balanced diet, is necessary.
- Tepid sponge baths and antipyretics will reduce fever.
- Antibiotics may cause allergic reactions.
- High-dose sulfonamide therapy (especially sulfadiazine) predisposes to crystalluria and oliguria; prevention requires frequent assessment and forced fluids. Alkalinization of the urine (sodium bicarbonate) may also be ordered as a preventive measure and will require urine pH determinations.
- Patients with pulmonary infection may need intermittent positive pressure breathing (IPPB) with chest physiotherapy. Daily auscultation is necessary, with checks for increased rales or consolidation. The amount, color, and thickness of sputum should be noted.
- Brain infection requires regular assessment of neurologic function. Signs of increased intracranial pressure include decreased level of consciousness and respiratory abnormalities.
- During long-term hospitalization, the patient should be turned often and assisted with range-of-motion exercises.

After hospitalization, the patient needs a regular medication schedule to maintain therapeutic blood levels; drug therapy must continue even after symptoms subside. Frequent follow-up examinations are important, as are support and encouragement to help the patient and his family cope with this long-term illness.

Erysipeloid

Erysipeloid is a rare, acute, self-limiting skin infection caused by the gram-positive rod Erysipelothrix insidiosa, *previously known as* E. rhusiopathiae. *Incidence is highest in summer and early fall. Erysipeloid usually subsides without complications within 3 weeks of onset.*

Causes
Transmission of this localized infection occurs through skin trauma, which allows penetration of *E. insidiosa* from infected meat, fish, poultry, animal hides or bones, or from manure of infected animals. Therefore, erysipeloid is most common in butchers, fishermen, and other persons (usually men) who handle infected tissues. Systemic infection (bacteremia) occasionally follows ingestion of undercooked contaminated pork, and can lead to septic arthritis and endocarditis.

Signs and symptoms
About 2 to 7 days after injury (often after the minor wound has healed), erysipeloid produces a purplish-red, clearly defined nonvesicular lesion (usually on the hand), with an irregular raised border. The lesion may burn and itch, and deep tissue inflammation may be intense enough to limit joint mobility. Relapse or complications, including those associated with systemic infection, rarely occur with erysipeloid.

Diagnosis
A characteristic skin lesion on a person with a history of occupational exposure and skin injury suggests erysipeloid. Isolation of *E. insidiosa* from a full-thickness skin biopsy from the edge of the lesion confirms it.

Treatment and additional considerations
Although erysipeloid is usually self-limiting, penicillin G or, in penicillin allergy, erythromycin, can prevent possible but rare complications. Hospitalization isn't necessary unless antibiotics

fail and complications occur. The outpatient should continue taking the prescribed antibiotic and finish the prescription even after symptoms subside to prevent the possibility of recurrence.

Anthrax
(Woolsorter's disease)

Anthrax is an acute infection caused by the nonmotile, encapsulated, gram-positive bacteria Bacillus anthracis. It occurs in oxen, sheep, goats, deer, and antelopes; it is transmitted to humans by contact with contaminated animals or their hides, bones, fur, hair, or wool. Anthrax spores that contaminate articles or soil can remain infective for years. Anthrax occurs in three different forms: cutaneous anthrax *(malignant pustule), the most common (95%);* inhalation anthrax, *rare (5%); and* gastrointestinal anthrax *(never reported in the United States). An estimated 100,000 cases of anthrax occur worldwide annually, most of them in countries that lack strict public health regulations. Anthrax is rare in the United States.*

With correct antibiotic treatment, cutaneous anthrax is rarely fatal. Without such therapy, it may spread to regional lymph nodes and even cause septicemia (it is fatal in 20% of untreated persons). Inhalation anthrax is usually fatal within 24 hours of onset.

Causes
Under aerobic conditions, *B. anthracis* produces oval spores that resist destruction by disinfectants, heat, or drying. Transmission to humans usually occurs by means of direct inoculation through skin wounds. About 80% of such infections result from industrial or agricultural workers' contact with the hair, wool, fur, hides, skin, and bones of animals, especially goats. Anthrax in veterinarians results from contact with infected animals or, occasionally, accidental self-inoculation with vaccine. Anthrax can also result from the inhalation of spores—an occasional event in dusty laboratories or textile mills—or, in rare cases, from the ingestion of contaminated, undercooked meat.

Signs and symptoms
In cutaneous anthrax, after a 1- to 7-day incubation period, a small papule appears at the site of inoculation and develops into a vesicle filled with clear fluid. Subsequently, a small, surrounding ring of similar vesicles develops and fuses. This fusion forms a single large lesion, causing erythema, pruritus, non-pitting edema, and rarely, pain. Eventually, this lesion ulcerates, and forms a deep crater with a crusted, blue-black central eschar. Untreated lesions persist for 2 weeks; then the eschar loosens and falls off, and granulation tissue forms a scar. Accompanying systemic symptoms include low-grade fever, malaise, and occasionally, lymphadenopathy.

After a 1- to 5-day incubation period, inhaled anthrax spores produce nonspecific symptoms (mild fever, myalgia, nonproductive cough, headache, malaise) that lead to high fever, prostration, and severe respiratory distress with cyanosis, stridor, and pleural effusion within 3 to 5 days. Untreated, it is often fatal within 24 hours of the acute phase.

Diagnosis
A history of exposure to wool, hides, or other animal products in a person with a large, pruritic, painless skin lesion clearly suggests anthrax. Gram's stains showing large gram-positive rods, drainage cultures growing *B. anthracis,* and a fourfold rise in titer (indirect hemagglutination) confirm it.

Treatment

Antibiotic therapy with high-dose penicillin I.V. is the primary treatment. Anthrax requires isolation to prevent possible spread by airborne or direct contact, even though person-to-person transmission is unlikely.

Additional considerations

• Patients suspected of exposure to anthrax will have to be under careful observation for at least 7 days.
• In the patient with inhalation anthrax, vital signs must be closely monitored, and respiratory support, including oxygen therapy and intubation, provided as needed.
• In the patient with cutaneous anthrax, lesions must be kept clean and covered with sterile dressings.
• Once the source of contamination is confirmed, the patient can be educated about the transmission and course of anthrax; also, to properly dispose of secretions and lesion exudate.
• Isolation precautions *must* be maintained: wash hands before and after giving care, place all contaminated objects in a closed plastic bag for incineration, and wear mask and gown when caring for a patient with inhalation anthrax.
• People at risk of contact with anthrax should clean and cover cuts, and when at work, wash their hands frequently and wear protective clothing. Persons employed in dusty textile mills should wear protective face masks. Vaccination is very important for high-risk persons.
• All cases of anthrax must be reported to local public health authorities.

GRAM-NEGATIVE BACILLI

Salmonellosis

One of the most common infections in the United States (over 2 million new cases appear annually), salmonellosis is caused by gram-negative bacilli of the genus Salmonella, *a member of the Enterobacteriaceae family. It occurs as enterocolitis, bacteremia, localized infection, typhoid, or paratyphoid fever. Nontyphoidal forms of salmonellosis usually produce mild to moderate illness, with low mortality.*

Typhoid, the most severe form of salmonellosis, usually lasts from 1 to 4 weeks. Mortality is about 3% of persons who are treated and 10% of those untreated, usually as a result of intestinal perforation or hemorrhage, cerebral thrombosis, toxemia, pneumonia, or acute circulatory failure. An attack of typhoid confers lifelong immunity, although the patient may become a carrier.

Causes and incidence

The most common species of *Salmonella* include *Salmonella typhi*, *Salmonella enteritidis*, and *Salmonella choleraesuis*. Of an estimated 1,700 serotypes of *Salmonella*, 10 cause the diseases most common in the United States; all 10 can survive for weeks in water, ice, sewage, or food. Nontyphoidal salmonellosis generally follows the ingestion of contaminated or inadequately processed foods, especially eggs, chicken, turkey, and duck. Proper cooking reduces the risk of contracting salmonellosis but doesn't eliminate it. Other causes include contact with infected persons or animals, or ingestion of contaminated dry milk, chocolate bars, or pharmaceuticals of animal origin. Salmonellosis may occur in children under age 5 from fecal - oral spread. Enterocolitis and bacteremia are especially common (and more virulent) among infants, the elderly, and people already weakened by other infections; paratyphoid fever is rare in the United States.

CLINICAL VARIANTS OF SALMONELLOSIS

VARIANT	CAUSE	CLINICAL FEATURES
Enterocolitis	Any species of nontyphoidal *Salmonella*, but usually *S. enteritidis*. Incubation period, 6 to 48 hours.	Mild to severe abdominal pain, diarrhea, sudden fever to 102° F. (38.8° C.), nausea, vomiting; usually self-limiting, but may progress to enteric fever (resembling typhoid), local abscesses (usually abdominal), dehydration, septicemia
Paratyphoid	*S. paratyphi* and *S. schottmüller* (formerly *S. paratyphi B*) Incubation period, 3 weeks or more.	Fever and transient diarrhea; generally resembles typhoid but less severe
Bacteremia	Any *Salmonella* species, but most commonly *S. choleraesuis*. Incubation period varies.	Fever, chills, anorexia, weight loss (without gastrointestinal symptoms), joint pains
Localized infections	Usually follows bacteremia caused by *S. choleraesuis*	Site of localization determines symptoms; localized abscesses may cause osteomyelitis, endocarditis, bronchopneumonia, pyelonephritis, and arthritis.
Typhoid fever	*S. typhi* enters GI tract and invades the bloodstream via the lymphatics, setting up intracellular sites. During this phase, infection of biliary tract leads to intestinal seeding with millions of bacilli. Involved lymphoid tissues (especially Peyer's patches in ileum) enlarge, ulcerate, and necrose, resulting in hemorrhage. Incubation period usually 1 to 2 weeks.	Symptoms of enterocolitis may develop within hours of ingestion of *S. typhi;* usually subside before onset of typhoid fever symptoms. **First week:** Gradually increasing fever, anorexia, myalgia, malaise, headache. **Second week:** Remittent fever up to 104° F. (40° C.) usually in the evening, chills, diaphoresis, weakness, delirium, increasing abdominal pain and distention, diarrhea or constipation, cough, moist rales, tender abdomen with enlarged spleen, maculopapular rash (especially on abdomen) **Third week:** Persistent fever, increasing fatigue and weakness; usually subsides end of third week, although relapses may occur **Complications:** Intestinal perforation or hemorrhage, abscesses, thrombophlebitis, cerebral thrombosis, pneumonia, osteomyelitis, myocarditis, acute circulatory failure, chronic carrier state

Typhoid results most frequently from drinking water contaminated by excretions of a carrier. Most typhoid patients are under age 30; most carriers are women over age 50. Incidence of typhoid in the United States is increasing due to the travelers returning from endemic areas.

Signs and symptoms
Clinical manifestations of salmonellosis vary but usually include fever, abdominal pain, and severe diarrhea with enterocolitis. Headache, increasing fever, and constipation are more common with typhoidal infection.

Diagnosis
Generally, diagnosis depends on isolation of the organism in a culture, particularly blood (in typhoid, paratyphoid, and bacteremia) or feces (in enterocolitis, paratyphoid, and typhoid). Other appropriate culture specimens include

urine, bone marrow, pus, and vomitus. In endemic areas, clinical symptoms of enterocolitis allow a working diagnosis before the cultures are positive. Presence of S. typhi in stool 1 or more years after treatment indicates that the patient is a carrier, which is true of 1% to 3% of patients.

Widal's test, an agglutination reaction against somatic and flagellar antigens, may suggest typhoid with a fourfold rise in titer. However, drug use or hepatic disease can also increase these titers and invalidate test results. Other supportive laboratory values may include transient leukocytosis during the first week of typhoidal salmonellosis, leukopenia during the third week, and leukocytosis in local infection.

Treatment
Antimicrobial therapy for typhoid, paratyphoid, and bacteremia depends on organism sensitivity. It may include ampicillin, amoxicillin, chloramphenicol, and in the severely toxemic patient, trimethoprim-sulfamethoxazole. Localized abscesses may also need surgical drainage. Enterocolitis requires a short course of antibiotics only if it causes septicemia or prolonged fever. Symptomatic treatment includes bed rest and, most important, replacement of fluids and electrolytes. Camphorated opium tincture or kaolin combined with pectin to relieve diarrhea may be necessary for patients who must remain active during the illness.

Additional considerations
The hospital staff member caring for the patient with salmonellosis should:
• follow enteric precautions; always wash hands thoroughly after any contact with the patient; teach the patient to use proper handwashing technique, especially after defecating and before eating or handling food; wear gloves and a gown when disposing of feces or fecally contaminated objects; continue enteric precautions until three consecutive stool cultures are negative—the first one, 24 hours after antibiotic treatment ends, followed by two more negative cultures at 24-hour intervals.
• observe the patient closely for signs of bowel perforation: sudden pain in the lower right abdomen, possibly after one

HUMAN SALMONELLA ISOLATES REPORTED IN THE UNITED STATES IN 1979

SEROTYPE	PERCENT	MEDIAN AGE
S. typhimurium*	32.6	9
Others	27.9	
S. enteritidis	8.5	19
S. heidelberg	8.0	4
S. newport	6.2	14
S. infantis	4.5	7
S. agona	3.5	3
S. saint-paul	2.8	19
S. typhi	2.1	26
S. montevido	2.0	12
S. oranienburg	1.9	17

*Includes S. typhimurium var. copenhagen

Adapted with permission from Morbidity and Mortality Weekly Report 29:189-191, 1980 C.D.C.

or more rectal bleeding episodes; sudden fall in temperature or blood pressure; rising pulse rate.

• plan care, during acute infection, to allow the patient as much rest as possible; raise the side rails and use other safety measures, because the patient may become delirious; assign the patient a room close to the nurses' station so he can be checked often; use a room deodorizer (preferably electric) to minimize odor from diarrhea and to provide a comfortable atmosphere for rest.

• accurately record intake and output; maintain adequate I.V. hydration; give high-calorie fluids, such as milkshakes, and watch for constipation once the patient can tolerate oral feedings.

• provide good skin and mouth care; turn the patient frequently; perform mild passive exercises, as indicated; apply mild heat to the abdomen to relieve cramps.

• *never* administer antipyretics. These mask fever and lead to possible hypothermia. Instead, heat loss can be promoted through the skin, without causing shivering (which keeps fever high by vasoconstriction), by applying tepid, wet towels (not alcohol or ice) to the patient's groin and axillae. To promote heat loss by vasodilation of peripheral blood vessels, additional wet towels can be used on the arms and legs. When done properly, this technique is very effective and promotes patient comfort.

• provide heat, elevation, and passive range-of-motion exercises, after draining the abscesses of a joint, to decrease swelling and maintain mobility.

On discharge, if the patient has positive stool cultures, he should use a different bathroom than other family members, if possible (while he's on antibiotics), and avoid preparing uncooked foods, such as salads, for healthy family members.

To prevent salmonellosis, all meat and cooked foods must be promptly refrigerated (or at least kept at room temperature for as short a time as possible). Proper handwashing is also important. Those at high risk (lab workers, travelers) should be vaccinated.

Shigellosis
(Bacillary dysentery)

Shigellosis is an acute intestinal infection caused by the bacteria Shigella, *a short, nonmotile, gram-negative rod.* Shigella *can be classified into four groups, all of which may cause shigellosis: group A* (Shigella dysenteriae), *which is most common in Central America and causes particularly severe infection and septicemia; group B* (Shigella flexneri); *group C* (Shigella boydii); *and group D* (Shigella sonnei). *Typically, shigellosis causes a high fever (especially in children), acute self-limiting diarrhea with tenesmus (ineffectual straining at stool), and possibly, electrolyte imbalance and dehydration. It's most common in children aged 1 to 4; however, adults often acquire the illness from children.*

Prognosis is good. Usually, mild infections subside within 10 days; severe infections may persist for 2 to 6 weeks. With prompt treatment, shigellosis is fatal in only 1% of cases, although in severe Shigella dysenteriae *epidemics, mortality may reach 8%.*

Causes and incidence

Shigellosis is endemic in North America, Europe, and the Tropics. In the United States, about 23,000 cases appear annually, usually in children or in elderly, debilitated, or malnourished persons. Shigellosis commonly occurs among confined populations, such as those in mental institutions; it's also common in hospitals. In Great Britain, incidence of shigellosis is rising, despite improved sanitation and infection control.

Transmission is through the fecal-oral route, by direct contact with contaminated objects, or through ingestion of contaminated food or water. Occasionally, the housefly is a vector.

Signs and symptoms

After an incubation period of from 1 to 4 days, *Shigella* organisms invade the intestinal mucosa and cause inflammation. In children, shigellosis usually produces high fever, diarrhea with tenesmus, nausea, vomiting, irritability, drowsiness, and abdominal pain and distention. Within a few days, the child's stool may contain pus, mucus, and—from the superficial intestinal ulceration typical of this infection—blood. Without treatment, dehydration and weight loss are rapid and overwhelming.

In adults, shigellosis produces sporadic, intense abdominal pain, which may be relieved at first by passing formed stools. Eventually, however, it causes rectal irritability, tenesmus, and in severe infection, headache and prostration. Stools may contain pus, mucus, and blood. In adults, shigellosis doesn't usually cause fever.

Complications of shigellosis are not common but may be fatal in children and debilitated patients, and include electrolyte imbalance (especially hypokalemia), metabolic acidosis, and shock. Less common complications include conjunctivitis, iritis, arthritis, rectal prolapse, secondary bacterial infection, acute blood loss from mucosal ulcers, and toxic neuritis.

Diagnosis

Fever (in children) and diarrhea with stools containing blood, pus, and mucus point to this diagnosis; microscopic bacteriologic studies help confirm it. Microscopic examination of a fresh stool may reveal mucus, RBCs, and polymorphonuclear leukocytes; direct immunofluorescence with specific antisera, *Shigella*. Severe infection increases hemagglutinating antibodies. In addition, sigmoidoscopy/proctoscopy may reveal typical superficial ulcerations.

Diagnosis must rule out other causes of diarrhea, such as enteropathogenic *Escherichia coli* infection, malabsorption diseases, and amebic or viral diseases.

Treatment

Treatment of shigellosis includes enteric precautions, low-residue diet, and most importantly, replacement of fluids and electrolytes with I.V. infusions of normal saline solution (with electrolytes) in sufficient quantities to maintain a urine output of 40 to 50 ml/hour. Antibiotics are of questionable value, but may be used in an attempt to eliminate the pathogen and thereby prevent further spread. Ampicillin, tetracycline, or sulfamethoxazole with trimethoprim may be useful in severe cases, especially in children with overwhelming fluid and electrolyte loss. Antidiarrheals that slow intestinal motility are contraindicated in shigellosis, since they delay fecal excretion of *Shigella* and prolong fever and diarrhea. An investigational vaccine containing attenuated strains of *Shigella* appears promising in preventing shigellosis.

Additional considerations

Supportive care can minimize complications and increase patient comfort.

• To prevent dehydration, I.V. fluids will be administered and intake and output (including stools) measured carefully.

• Correct identification of *Shigella* requires examination and culture of fresh stool specimens. Therefore specimens must be hand-carried directly to the laboratory. Since shigellosis is suspected, this information should be included on the lab slip.

• Using a hot-water bottle will help relieve abdominal discomfort. Careful scheduling can conserve patient strength.

• To help prevent spread of this disease, enteric precautions must be maintained until the stool specimen is negative. Before entering the patient's room, the hospital staff member must put on a gown and gloves, and wash hands on entering and leaving the room. The patient's nails should be kept short to avoid harboring organisms. Soiled linen require immediate changing and should be stored for laundering in an isolation container.

• During shigellosis epidemics, all potentially infected staff should provide stool specimens. Those infected should stay away from work until a stool specimen is negative.

Escherichia coli and Other Enterobacteriaceae Infections

Enterobacteriaceae—a group of mostly aerobic, gram-negative bacilli—cause local and systemic infections, including an invasive diarrhea resembling shigella and more often a noninvasive toxin-mediated diarrhea resembling cholera. With other Enterobacteriaceae, Escherichia coli *causes most nosocomial infections. Noninvasive, enterotoxin-producing* E. coli *infections may be a major cause of diarrheal illness in children in the United States.*

Prognosis in cases of mild to moderate infection is good, but severe infection requires immediate fluid and electrolyte replacement to avoid fatal dehydration, especially among children, in whom mortality may be quite high.

Causes and incidence

Although some strains of *E. coli* exist as part of the normal gastrointestinal flora, infection results from certain nonindigenous strains. For example, noninvasive diarrhea results from two toxins produced by strains called enterotoxic or enteropathogenic *E. coli* (EEC). These toxins interact with intestinal juices and promote excessive loss of chloride and water. In the invasive form, *E. coli* directly invades the intestinal mucosa, causing local irritation, inflammation, and diarrhea.

Transmission can occur either directly, from an infected person, or indirectly, by ingestion of contaminated food or water or contact with contaminated utensils. Incubation is from 24 to 48 hours.

Incidence of *E. coli* infection is highest among travelers returning from other countries, particularly Mexico (noninvasive), Southeast Asia, and South America (invasive). *E. coli* infection also induces other diseases, especially in persons whose resistance is low.

Signs and symptoms

Clinical effects of noninvasive diarrhea depend on the toxin causing the infection but generally include the abrupt onset of watery diarrhea with cramping abdominal pain, and in severe illness, symptoms of acidosis (hypotension, mental lethargy).

Invasive infection produces chills, abdominal cramps, and diarrheal stools that may contain blood and pus.

Infantile diarrhea from an *E. coli* infection is usually noninvasive; it begins with loose watery stools that change from yellow to green, and contain little mucus or blood. Vomiting, listlessness, irritability, and anorexia often precede diarrhea. This condition can progress to fever, severe dehydration, acidosis, and shock.

Diagnosis

Because certain strains of *E. coli* normally reside in the gastrointestinal tract, culturing is of little value; a working diagnosis depends on clinical observation alone. Firm diagnosis requires sophisticated identification procedures, such as bioassays, that are expensive, time-consuming, and consequently, not widely available. Diagnosis must rule out salmonellosis and shigellosis, other common infections which produce similar symptoms.

Treatment

Treatment consists of isolation, correction of fluid and electrolyte imbalance, and in an infant, I.V. antibiotics, such as tetracycline, chloramphenicol, and trimethoprim-sulfamethoxazole.

Additional considerations

Caring for a patient with *E. coli* includes:
• keeping accurate intake and output records; measuring stool volume and noting presence of blood and pus; replacing fluids and electrolytes, as needed; monitoring for decreased serum sodium and chloride levels and signs of gram-negative shock; watching for loss of skin turgor and other signs of dehydration.
• for infants, providing isolation, giving nothing by mouth, administering antibiotics, and maintaining body warmth.

Steps to prevent spread of this infection include:
• screening all hospital personnel and visitors for diarrhea, and preventing them from making direct patient contact during epidemics; reporting cases to local public health authorities.
• using proper handwashing technique; teaching personnel, patients, and their families to do the same.
• using enteric precautions (providing a private room, wearing gown and gloves while handling feces, and handwashing before entering and after leaving the patient's room).
• advising travelers to foreign countries to avoid unbottled water and uncooked vegetables.
• discarding all suction bottles, irrigating fluid, and open bottles of saline

---

ENTEROBACTERIAL INFECTIONS

The Enterobacteriaceae include *Escherichia coli, Arizona, Citrobacter, Enterobacter, Erwinia, Hafnia, Klebsiella, Morganella, Proteus, Providencia, Salmonella, Serratia, Shigella,* and *Yersinia.*

Enterobacterial infections are exogenous (from other people or the environment), endogenous (from one part of the body to another), or a combination of both. Enterobacteriaceae infections may cause any of a long list of bacterial diseases: bacterial (gram-negative) pneumonia, empyema, endocarditis, osteomyelitis, septic arthritis, urethritis, cystitis, bacterial prostatitis, urinary tract infection, pyelonephritis, perinephric abscess, abdominal abscesses, cellulitis, skin ulcers, appendicitis, gastroenterocolitis, diverticulitis, eyelid and periorbital cellulitis, corneal conjunctivitis, meningitis, bacteremia, and intracranial abscesses.

Appropriate antibiotic therapy depends on the results of culture and sensitivity test. Generally, the aminoglycosides, cephalosporins, and some penicillins—such as carbenicillin, ampicillin, and amoxicillin—are most effective.

---

solution once every 24 hours; changing I.V. tubing according to hospital policy; emptying ventilator water reservoirs completely before refilling them with sterile water; and using suction catheters one time only.

Pseudomonas Infections

Pseudomonas is a small gram-negative bacillus that produces nosocomial infections, superinfections of various parts of the body, and a rare disease called melioidosis. This bacillus is also associated with bacteremia, endocarditis, and osteomyelitis in drug addicts. In local pseudomonas infections, treatment is usually successful and complications rare. However, in patients with poor immunologic resistance—premature infants, the elderly, or those with debilitating disease, burns, or wounds—septicemic pseudomonas infections are serious—sometimes fatal.

Causes

The most common species of pseudomonas is *Pseudomonas aeruginosa*. Other species that cause disease in humans include *Pseudomonas maltophilia*, *Pseudomonas cepacia*, *Pseudomonas fluorescens*, *Pseudomonas testosteroni*, *Pseudomonas acidovorans*, *Pseudomonas alcaligenes*, *Pseudomonas stuzeri*, *Pseudomonas putrefaciens,* and *Pseudomonas putida*. These organisms are frequently found in hospital liquids that have been allowed to stand for a long time, such as benzalkonium chloride, hexachlorophene soap, saline solution, penicillin, water in flower vases, and fluids in incubators, humidifiers, and inhalation therapy equipment. In elderly patients, this infection usually enters through the genitourinary tract; in infants, through the umbilical cord, skin, and gastrointestinal tract.

Signs and symptoms

The most common infections associated with pseudomonas include skin infections (decubitus ulcers and some infections in burn patients), urinary tract infections, infant epidemic diarrhea and other diarrheal illnesses, bronchitis, pneumonia, bronchiectasis, meningitis, corneal ulcers, mastoiditis, otitis externa, otitis media, endocarditis, and bacteremia.

Drainage in pseudomonas infections has a distinct, sickly sweet odor, and a greenish-blue pus that forms a crust on wounds. Other symptoms depend on the site of infection. For example, when it invades the lungs, pseudomonas causes pneumonia with fever, chills, and a productive cough.

Diagnosis

Diagnosis requires isolation of the *Pseudomonas* organism in blood, spinal fluid, urine, exudate, or sputum culture.

Treatment

In the debilitated or otherwise vulnerable patient with clinical evidence of pseudomonas infection, treatment should begin immediately, without waiting for results of laboratory tests. Antibiotic treatment includes aminoglycosides, such as gentamicin or tobramycin, combined with a *Pseudomonas*-active penicillin, such as carbenicillin disodium or ticarcillin. An alternative combination is amikacin and colistimethate sodium. Such combination therapy is necessary because *Pseudomonas* quickly becomes resistant to carbenicillin alone. However, in urinary tract infections, carbenicillin indanyl sodium can be used alone if the organism is susceptible and the infection doesn't have systemic effects;

MELIOIDOSIS

Melioidosis results from wound penetration, inhalation, or ingestion of the gram-negative bacteria *Pseudomonas pseudomallei*. Once confined to Southeast Asia, Central America, South America, Madagascar, and Guam, incidence in the United States is rising due to the recent influx of Southeast Asians.

Melioidosis occurs in two forms: chronic melioidosis, causing osteomyelitis and lung abscesses; and acute melioidosis, which is rare, causing pneumonia, bacteremia, and prostration. Acute melioidosis is often fatal. However, most infections are chronic and asymptomatic, producing clinical symptoms only with accompanying malnutrition, major surgery, or severe burns.

Diagnostic measures consist of isolation of *P. pseudomallei* in a culture of exudate, blood, or sputum; serology tests (complement fixation, passive hemagglutination); and chest X-ray (findings resemble tuberculosis). Treatment includes oral tetracycline— and a sulfonamide, abscess drainage, and in severe cases, chloramphenicol— until X-ray shows resolution of primary abscesses.

Prognosis is good, since most patients have mild infections and acquire permanent immunity; aggressive use of antibiotics and sulfonamides has improved the prognosis in acute melioidosis.

it is excreted in the urine and builds up high urine levels that prevent resistance.

Local pseudomonas infections or septicemia secondary to wound infection requires 1% acetic acid irrigations, topical applications of colistimethate sodium and polymyxin B, and debridement or drainage of the infected wound.

Additional considerations
• The character of wound exudate and sputum may give indication of pseudomonas infection.
• Patient history of allergies, especially to penicillin, must be determined before administration of antibiotics. If combinations of carbenicillin or ticarcillin, and gentamicin or tobramycin, are ordered, doses should be scheduled 1 hour apart (carbenicillin and ticarcillin may decrease the antibiotic effect of gentamicin and tobramycin). The same administration set must not be used to give both antibiotics.
• Renal function changes will indicate aminoglycoside nephrotoxicity.
• Immunologically compromised patients are especially suspectible to this opportunistic infection. Careful attention to handwashing and aseptic techniques may prevent further spread.
• Pseudomonas infection may be prevented by: maintaining proper endotracheal/tracheostomy suctioning technique (strict sterile technique when caring for I.V.s, catheters, and other tubes); disposing of suction bottle contents properly; and labeling and dating solution bottles, and changing them frequently, according to hospital policy.

Cholera
(Asiatic cholera, epidemic cholera)

Cholera is an acute enterotoxin-mediated gastrointestinal infection caused by the gram-negative rod Vibrio cholerae. *It produces diarrhea, vomiting, massive fluid and electrolyte loss, and possibly, hypovolemic shock, metabolic acidosis, and death. A similar bacteria,* Vibrio parahaemolyticus, *causes food poisoning.*

Even with prompt diagnosis and treatment, cholera is fatal in up to 2% of children due to difficulty with fluid replacement; in adults, it is fatal in fewer than 1%. However, untreated cholera may be fatal in as many as 50% of victims. Cholera infection confers only transient immunity.

Causes
Humans are the only documented hosts and victims of *V. cholerae*, a motile, aerobic rod. It's transmitted directly through food and water contaminated with fecal material from carriers or persons with active infections. Cholera is most common in Africa, southern and Southeast Asia, and the Middle East, although isolated outbreaks have occurred in Japan, Australia, and Europe. It usually occurs during the warmer months, and is most prevalent among lower socioeconomic groups. In India, cholera is especially common among children aged 1 to 5, but in other endemic areas, it's equally distributed among all age-groups. Deficiency or absence of hydrochloric acid in gastric juices may increase susceptibility to cholera.

Signs and symptoms
After an incubation period ranging from several hours to 5 days, cholera produces acute, painless, profuse, watery diarrhea and effortless vomiting (without preceding nausea). As the number of stools increases, the stools contain white flecks of mucus ("rice water stools"). Because of massive fluid and electrolyte loss from diarrhea and vomiting (fluid loss in adults may reach 1 liter per hour), cholera causes intense thirst, weakness, loss of skin turgor, wrinkled skin, sunken

---

VIBRIO PARAHAEMOLYTICUS FOOD POISONING

V. parahaemolyticus is a common cause of gastroenteritis in Japan; outbreaks also occur on American cruise ships and in the eastern and southeastern coastal areas of the United States, especially during the summer.

V. parahaemolyticus, which thrives in a salty environment, is transmitted by ingesting uncooked or undercooked contaminated shellfish, particularly crabs and shrimp. After an incubation period of 2 to 48 hours, *V. parahaemolyticus* causes watery diarrhea, moderately severe cramps, nausea, vomiting, headache, weakness, chills, and fever. Food poisoning is usually self-limiting and subsides spontaneously within 2 days. Occasionally, however, it's more severe, and may even be fatal in debilitated or elderly persons.

Diagnosis requires bacteriologic examination of vomitus, blood, stool smears, or fecal specimens collected by rectal swab. Diagnosis must rule out not only other causes of food poisoning but also other acute gastrointestinal disorders.

Treatment is supportive, consisting primarily of bed rest and oral fluid replacement. I.V. replacement therapy is seldom necessary, but oral tetracycline may be prescribed. Thorough cooking of seafood prevents infection.

---

after 2 weeks.

Diagnosis

In endemic areas or during epidemics, typical clinical features strongly suggest cholera. A culture of *V. cholerae* from feces or vomitus indicates cholera, but definitive diagnosis requires agglutination and other clear reactions to group- and type-specific antisera. A dark-field microscopic examination of fresh feces showing rapidly moving bacilli (like shooting stars) allows for quick, tentative diagnosis. Immunofluorescence also allows rapid diagnosis. Diagnosis must rule out *Escherichia coli* infection, salmonellosis, and shigellosis.

Treatment

Improved sanitation and the administration of cholera vaccine to travelers in endemic areas can control this disease. Unfortunately, the vaccine now available confers only 60% to 80% immunity, and is effective for only 3 to 6 months. Consequently, vaccination is impractical for residents of endemic areas.

Treatment requires rehydration by rapid I.V. infusion of large amounts (50 to 100 ml/minute) of isotonic saline solution, alternating with isotonic sodium bicarbonate or sodium lactate. Potassium replacement may be added to the I.V. solution.

When I.V. infusions have corrected hypovolemia, fluid infusion decreases to quantities sufficient to maintain normal pulse and skin turgor or to replace fluid loss through diarrhea. An oral glucose-electrolyte solution can substitute for I.V. infusions. In mild cholera, oral fluid replacement is adequate. If symptoms persist despite fluid and electrolyte replacement, treatment includes tetracycline.

Additional considerations

A cholera patient requires isolation, enteric precautions, supportive care, and close observation throughout the disease's acute phase.

The hospital staff member caring for the cholera patient must:

eyes, pinched facial expression, muscle cramps (especially in the extremities), cyanosis, oliguria, tachycardia, tachypnea, thready or absent peripheral pulses, falling blood pressure, fever, and inaudible, hypoactive bowel sounds.

Patients usually remain oriented but apathetic, although small children may become stuporous or develop convulsions. If complications don't occur, the symptoms subside and the patient recovers in 1 to 3 days. But if treatment is delayed or inadequate, cholera may lead to metabolic acidosis, uremia, and possibly, coma and death. About 3% of patients who recover continue to carry *V. cholerae* in the gallbladder; however, most patients are free of the infection

• wear a gown and gloves when giving physical care, and wash hands before entering and after leaving the patient's room.

• monitor output (including stool volume) and I.V. infusion accurately, carefully observing neck veins and auscultating the lungs, to detect overhydration (fluid loss in cholera is massive—inadequate and delayed replacement may cause fatal renal insufficiency).

• protect the patient's family by administering oral tetracycline, if ordered.

• advise anyone traveling to an endemic area to boil all drinking water and avoid uncooked vegetables. If the doctor orders a cholera vaccine, the patient will need a booster 3 to 6 months later as well.

Septic Shock

Second only to cardiogenic shock as the leading cause of shock-death, septic shock (usually a result of bacterial infection) causes inadequate blood perfusion and circulatory collapse. It occurs most often among hospitalized patients, especially men over age 40 and women ages 25 to 45. About 25% of patients who develop gram-negative bacteremia go into shock. Unless vigorous treatment begins promptly, preferably before symptoms fully develop, septic shock rapidly progresses to death (often within a few hours) in up to 80% of these patients.

Causes

In two thirds of patients, septic shock results from infection with gram-negative bacteria: *Escherichia coli, Klebsiella, Enterobacter, Proteus, Pseudomonas,* and *Bacteroides;* in the remainder, from gram-positive bacteria: *Streptococcus pneumoniae, Streptococcus pyogenes,* and rarely, *Actinomyces.* Other infections caused by viruses, rickettsiae, chlamydiae, and protozoa may be complicated by shock.

These organisms produce septicemia in persons whose resistance is already compromised by some underlying condition; infection also results from transplantation of these bacteria from other areas of the body through surgery, I.V. therapy, and catheters. A large percentage of septic shock occurs in patients hospitalized for primary infection of the genitourinary, biliary, gastrointestinal, and gynecologic tracts. Other predisposing factors include immunodeficiency, advanced age, trauma, burns, diabetes mellitus, cirrhosis of the liver, and disseminated cancer.

Signs and symptoms

The symptoms of septic shock vary according to the stage of the shock, the organism causing it, and the age of the patient.

• *Early stage:* oliguria, sudden fever (over 101° F. [38.3° C.]), and chills; nausea, vomiting, diarrhea, and prostration.

• *Late stage:* restlessness, apprehension, irritability, thirst from decreased cerebral tissue perfusion, tachycardia, tachypnea. Hypotension, altered consciousness, and hyperventilation may be the *only* signs among infants and the elderly.

Hypothermia and anuria are common late signs. Complications of septic shock include disseminated intravascular coagulation (DIC), renal failure, heart failure, gastrointestinal ulcers, and abnormal hepatic function.

Diagnosis

Observation of one or more typical symptoms (fever, confusion, nausea, vomiting, hyperventilation) in a patient suspected of having an infection suggests septic shock and necessitates immediate treatment.

In early stages, arterial blood gases indicate respiratory alkalosis (low PCO_2, low or normal bicarbonate, high pH);

as shock progresses, metabolic acidosis develops with hypoxemia indicated by decreasing PCO_2 (may increase as respiratory failure ensues), PO_2, HCO_3 −, and pH. The following laboratory tests support the diagnosis and determine the treatment:

• blood cultures to isolate the organism
• decreased platelet count and leukocytosis (15,000 to 30,000/mm^3)
• increased BUN and creatinine, decreased creatinine clearance
• abnormal prothrombin consumption and partial thromboplastin time
• simultaneous measurement of urine and plasma osmolalities for renal failure (urine osmolality below 400 milliosmoles, with a ratio of urine to plasma below 1.5)
• decreased central venous pressure (CVP), pulmonary artery and wedge pressures, decreased cardiac output (in early septic shock, cardiac output increases)
• EKG—S-T segment depression, inverted T waves, and arrhythmias resembling myocardial infarction.

Treatment

The first goal of treatment is to monitor and reverse shock through volume expansion with I.V. fluids, and insertion of a pulmonary artery catheter to check pulmonary circulation and pulmonary wedge pressure (PWP). Administration of whole blood or plasma can then raise pressure to a satisfactory level of 14 to 18mm Hg (PWP). A respirator may be necessary for proper ventilation to overcome hypoxia. Urinary catheterization allows measurement of hourly urine output.

Treatment also requires immediate administration of I.V. antibiotics to control the infection. Depending on the organism, the antibiotic combination usually includes an aminoglycoside, such as gentamicin or tobramycin for gram-negative bacteria, combined with a penicillin, such as carbenicillin or ticarcillin. Sometimes treatment includes a cephalosporin, such as cefazolin, and nafcillin, for suspected staphylococcal infection instead of carbenicillin or ticarcillin. Therapy may include chloramphenicol for nonsporulating anaerobes (*Bacteroides*), although it may cause bone marrow depression, and clindamycin, which may produce pseudomembranous enterocolitis. Appropriate anti-infectives for other causes of septic shock depend on the suspected organism. Other measures to combat infections include surgery to drain and excise abscesses, and debridement.

If shock persists after fluid infusion, treatment with vasopressors, such as dopamine, maintains adequate blood perfusion in the brain, liver, digestive tract, kidneys, and skin. Other treatment includes I.V. bicarbonate to correct acidosis, and I.V. corticosteroids, which may improve blood perfusion and increase cardiac output.

Additional considerations

To prevent septic shock, the hospital staff member should: determine which patients are at high risk of developing septic shock; know the signs of impending septic shock, and not rely solely on technical aids to judge the patient's status; consider any change in mental status and urinary output as significant as a change in CVP; report any such changes promptly.

To care for the patient with septic shock, the staff member should: carefully maintain the pulmonary artery catheter; check blood gases for adequate oxygenation or gas exchange, and report any changes immediately; keep accurate intake and output records; maintain urine output (0.5 to 1 ml/kg/hour) and adequate systolic pressure, avoiding fluid overload; monitor serum gentamicin, and administer drugs, as ordered; watch closely for: DIC (indicated by abnormal bleeding), renal failure (oliguria, increased specific gravity), heart failure (dyspnea, edema, tachycardia, distended neck veins), gastrointestinal ulcers (hematemesis, melena), hepatic abnormality (jaundice, hypoprothrombinemia, and hypoalbuminemia).

OMINOUS SIGN

Hemophilus influenzae Infection

Hemophilus influenzae is a small, gram-negative, pleomorphic aerobic bacillus that appears predominantly as coccobacilli in exudates. It causes diseases in many organ systems but most frequently attacks the respiratory system. It's a common cause of epiglottitis, laryngotracheobronchitis, pneumonia, bronchiolitis, otitis media, and meningitis. Less often, it causes bacterial endocarditis, conjunctivitis, facial cellulitis, septic arthritis, and osteomyelitis. H. influenzae *pneumonia is an increasingly common nosocomial infection. It infects about half of all children before age 1, and virtually all by age 3.*

Signs and symptoms

H. influenzae provokes a characteristic tissue response—acute suppurative inflammation. When it infects the larynx, the trachea, and the bronchial tree, it leads to mucosal edema and thick exudate; when it invades the lungs, it leads to bronchopneumonia. In the pharynx, *H. influenzae* usually produces no remarkable changes, except in epiglottitis, which generally affects both the laryngeal and the pharyngeal surfaces. The pharyngeal mucosa may be reddened, rarely with soft, yellow exudate. More likely, however, it appears normal or shows only slight diffuse redness, even while severe pain makes swallowing difficult or impossible. These infections typically cause high fever and generalized malaise.

Diagnosis

 Isolation of the organism confirms *H. influenzae* infection, usually with a blood culture. Other laboratory findings include:
- polymorphonuclear leukocytosis (15,000 to 30,000/mm³)
- leukopenia (2,000 to 3,000/mm³) in young children with severe infection
- *H. influenzae* bacteremia, found frequently in patients with meningitis.

Treatment

H. influenzae infections usually respond to a 2-week course of chloramphenicol or ampicillin (resistant strains are becoming more common). Tetracycline and sulfonamides are effective alternatives for treatment of patients who are allergic to penicillin.

Additional considerations

Adequate respiration maintenance through proper positioning, humidification (croup tent) in children, and suctioning may be needed. Rate and type of respiration may give indications of cyanosis and dyspnea, which necessitate intubation or tracheotomy. A room humidifier or breathing of moist air from a shower or bath may be used for home treatment.

Patients should be checked for allergies before administration of antibiotics. When therapy includes chloramphenicol, CBC must be monitored for signs of bone marrow depression.

Signs of dehydration, which can present as decreased skin turgor, parched lips, concentrated urine, decreased urine output, or increased pulse can be avoided by monitoring fluid intake and output.

Physical care should be performed as quickly as possible to allow the patient as much rest as possible.

Further spread of infection can be prevented by: maintaining respiratory isolation, using proper handwashing technique, disposing properly of all respiratory secretions, placing soiled tissues in a plastic bag, and decontaminating all equipment used in patient care.

Whooping Cough
(Pertussis)

Whooping cough is a highly contagious respiratory infection usually caused by the nonmotile, gram-negative coccobacillus Bordetella pertussis, *and occasionally, by the related similar bacteria* Bordetella parapertussis *and* Bordetella bronchiseptica. *Characteristically, whooping cough produces an irritating cough that becomes paroxysmal and often ends in a high-pitched inspiratory whoop.*

Since the 1940s, immunization and aggressive diagnosis and treatment have significantly reduced mortality from whooping cough in the United States. Whooping cough mortality in children under age 1 is usually a result of pneumonia and other complications. It's also dangerous in the elderly but tends to be less severe in older children and adults.

Causes

Whooping cough is usually transmitted by the direct inhalation of contaminated droplets from a patient in the acute stage; it may also be spread indirectly through soiled linen and other articles contaminated by the patient.

Whooping cough is endemic throughout the world, and usually occurs in early spring and late winter. About half the time it strikes unimmunized children under the age of 2, probably because women of childbearing age don't usually have high serum levels of *B. pertussis* antibodies to transmit to their offspring.

Microscopic enlargement shows *Bordetella pertussis,* the nonmotile, gram-negative coccobacillus that commonly causes whooping cough. After entering the tracheobronchial tree, *B. pertussis* causes mucus to become increasingly tenacious. Classic 6-week course of whooping cough then follows.

Signs and symptoms

After an incubation period of about 7 to 10 days, *B. pertussis* enters the tracheobronchial mucosa, where it produces progressively tenacious mucus. Whooping cough follows a classic 6-week course that includes three stages, each of which lasts about 2 weeks.

First, the *catarrhal stage* characteristically produces an irritating, hacking, nocturnal cough, anorexia, sneezing, listlessness, infected conjunctiva, and occasionally, a low-grade fever. In this stage, the disease is highly communicable.

After a period of 7 to 14 days, the *paroxysmal stage* produces spasmodic and recurrent coughing that may expel tenacious mucus. Each cough characteristically ends in a loud, crowing inspiratory whoop; subsequent choking on mucus causes vomiting. (Very young infants, however, might not develop the typical whoop.) Paroxysmal coughing may induce complications, such as increased venous pressure, nosebleed, periorbital edema, conjunctival hemorrhage,

hemorrhage of the anterior chamber of the eye, detached retina (and blindness), rectal prolapse, inguinal or umbilical hernia, convulsions, atelectasis, and pneumonitis. In infants, choking spells may cause apnea, anoxia, and disturbed acid-base balance. During this stage, patients are highly vulnerable to fatal, secondary bacterial or viral infections. Since whooping cough itself seldom causes fever, secondary infection (usually otitis media or pneumonia) is likely in any whooping cough patient with a fever.

During the *convalescent stage*, paroxysmal coughing and vomiting gradually subside. However, for months afterward, even a mild upper respiratory infection may trigger the coughing.

Diagnosis
Classical clinical findings, especially during the paroxysmal stage, suggest a diagnosis of whooping cough; laboratory studies confirm it. Nasopharyngeal swabs and sputum cultures show B. pertussis only in the early stages of this disease; fluorescent antibody screening of nasopharyngeal smears provides quicker results than cultures but is less reliable. In addition, the WBC is usually increased, especially early in the paroxysmal stage and in children older than 6 months. Sometimes, the WBC may reach 175,000 to 200,000/mm³, with 60% to 90% lymphocytes.

Treatment
Vigorous supportive therapy requires hospitalization of infants (often in the ICU), and fluid and electrolyte replacement. Other treatment includes adequate nutrition, codeine and mild sedation to decrease coughing, oxygen therapy in apnea, and antibiotics, such as erythromycin and, possibly, tetracycline, to shorten the period of communicability and prevent secondary infections.

Because very young infants are particularly susceptible to whooping cough, immunization is at 2 months, 4 months, and 6 months, and is followed by boosters at 18 months and at 4 to 5 years. Usually, pertussis vaccine is combined with diphtheria and tetanus toxoids (DPT). Fever is a common complication of such immunization, and is so severe in an older child that vaccination is contraindicated in children over age 7.

Additional considerations
Whooping cough calls for aggressive, supportive care and respiratory isolation throughout the illness. The hospital staff member should:
• wear a mask in the patient's room; wash his hands before and after patient contact.
• monitor acid-base, fluid, and electrolyte balance.
• cautiously and properly suction secretions, and monitor oxygen therapy. (Remember that suctioning removes oxygen as well as secretions.)
• establish a quiet environment to decrease coughing stimulation.
• provide small, frequent meals, and watch for and treat constipation and nausea that may result from codeine treatment.
• change soiled linen, empty the suction bottle, and change the trash bag at least once each shift to decrease exposure to organisms.
• offer emotional support to anxious parents of children with this distressing illness.

Plague
(Black death)

Plague is an acute infection caused by the gram-negative, nonmotile, nonsporulating bacillus Yersinia pestis (formerly called Pasteurella pestis).

Plague occurs in several forms. Bubonic plague, *the most common, causes the characteristic swollen, and sometimes suppurating, lymph glands (buboes) that give this infection its name. Other forms include* septicemic plague, *a severe, rapid systemic form, and* pneumonic plague, *which can be primary or secondary to the other two forms.* Primary pneumonic plague *is an acutely fulminant, highly contagious form that causes acute prostration, respiratory distress, and death—often within 2 to 3 days after onset.*

Without treatment, mortality is about 60% in bubonic plague, and approaches 100% in both septicemic and pneumonic plagues. With treatment, reported mortality is approximately 18%, and is related to the delay between onset and treatment and to the patient's age and physical condition.

Causes and incidence
Plague is usually transmitted to a human through the bite of a flea from an infected rodent host, such as a rat, squirrel, prairie dog, or hare. Occasionally, transmission occurs when infected animals or their tissues are handled. Bubonic plague is notorious for the historic pandemics in Europe and Asia during the Middle Ages, which in some areas killed up to two thirds of the population. This form is rarely transmitted from person to person. However, the untreated bubonic form may progress to a secondary pneumonic form, which is transmitted by contaminated respiratory droplets (coughing) and is highly contagious. In the United States, the primary pneumonic form usually occurs after inhalation of *Y. pestis* in a laboratory.

Sylvatic (wild rodent) plague remains endemic to South America, the Near East, central and Southeast Asia, north central and southern Africa, Mexico,

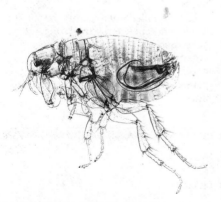

Bubonic plague is transmitted to a human through the bite of a flea—*Xenopsylla cheopis* (bubonic plague flea).

and the western United States and Canada. In the United States, its incidence has been rising, a possible reflection of different bacterial strains or environmental changes that favor rodent growth in certain areas. Plague tends to occur between May and September; between October and February it usually occurs in hunters who skin wild animals. One attack confers permanent immunity.

Signs and symptoms
The incubation period, early symptoms, severity at onset, and clinical course vary in the three forms of plague. In *bubonic plague,* the incubation period is 2 to 6 days. The milder form begins with malaise, fever, and pain or tenderness in regional lymph nodes, possibly associated with swelling. Lymph node damage (usually axillary or inguinal) eventually produces painful, inflamed, and possibly suppurative buboes. The classic sign of plague is an excruciatingly painful bubo. Hemorrhagic areas may become necrotic; in the skin, such areas appear dark—hence the name "black death." This infection can progress extremely rapidly: a seemingly mildly ill person with symptoms limited to fever and adenitis may become moribund within hours. Plague may also begin dramatically, with a sudden high temperature of 103° to 106° F. (39.5° to 41.1° C.), chills, myalgia, headache, prostration, restlessness, disorientation, delirium, toxemia, and staggering gait. Occasionally, it causes abdominal pain, nausea, vomiting, and constipation, followed by diarrhea (frequently bloody), skin mottling, petechiae, and circulatory collapse.

In *primary pneumonic plague,* the incubation period is 2 to 3 days, followed by a typically acute onset, with high fever, chills, severe headache, tachycardia, tachypnea, dyspnea, and a productive cough (first mucoid sputum, later frothy pink or red).

Secondary pneumonic plague, the pulmonary extension of the bubonic form, complicates about 5% of untreated plague. A cough producing bloody sputum signals this complication. Primary and secondary pneumonic plagues rapidly cause severe prostration, respiratory distress, and possibly, death.

Septicemic plague usually develops without overt lymph node enlargement. The patient shows toxicity, hyperpyrexia, convulsions, prostration, shock, and disseminated intravascular coagulation (DIC). Septicemic plague causes widespread nonspecific tissue damage, and is rapidly fatal unless promptly and correctly treated.

Diagnosis

Since plague is rare in the United States, it's often overlooked until after the patient dies or multiple cases develop. Characteristic buboes and a history of exposure to rodents strongly suggest bubonic plague.

 Stained smears and cultures of *Y. pestis* obtained from a needle aspirate of a small amount of fluid from skin lesions confirm this diagnosis.

Postmortem studies of a guinea pig inoculated with a sample of blood or purulent drainage allows isolation of the organism. Other laboratory studies include WBC increased to 20,000 to 40,000, with increased polymorphonuclear leukocytes, and retrospective agglutination (antibody titer) studies. Diagnosis should rule out tularemia, typhus, and typhoid.

In pneumonic plague, diagnosis requires a chest X-ray to show fulminating pneumonia, and stained smears and cultures of sputum to identify *Y. pestis.* Other bacterial pneumonias and psittacosis must be ruled out. Stained smears and blood cultures containing *Y. pestis* are diagnostic in septicemic plague. However, cultures of *Y. pestis* grow slowly; so, in suspected plague (especially pneumonic and septicemic plagues), treatment should begin without laboratory confirmation. The Center for Disease Control performs a fluorescent antibody test on various specimens for a rapid presumptive diagnosis.

Treatment

Antimicrobial treatment of suspected plague must begin immediately after blood specimens have been taken for culture. Generally, treatment consists of large doses of streptomycin, the drug proven most effective against *Y. pestis.* Other effective drugs include tetracycline, chloramphenicol, kanamycin, and sulfadiazine, and possibly, trimethoprim-sulfamethoxazole. Penicillins are ineffective against plague.

In both septicemic and pneumonic plagues, life-saving antimicrobial treatment must begin within 18 hours of onset. Supportive management aims to control fever, shock, and convulsions, and maintain fluid balance. After antimicrobial therapy has begun, glucocorticoids can combat life-threatening toxemia and shock; diazepam will relieve restlessness; and, heparin may be needed for DIC.

Additional considerations

Patients with plague infections require strict isolation, which may be discontinued 48 hours after antimicrobial therapy begins unless respiratory symptoms develop. Anyone coming into contact with a patient with pneumonic plague must always wear a gown, mask, hood, protective goggles, and gloves.

General safety precautions when contacting a plague patient include: carefully disposing of soiled dressings, feces, and sputum; disinfecting soiled linens; handling all exudates, purulent discharges, and laboratory specimens with rubber gloves; and possibly, taking prophylactic antibiotics.

Buboes should be treated with hot,

moist compresses. They must never be excised or drained, since this may spread the infection.

Further injury to necrotic peripheral tissue caused by septicemic plague should be avoided; bedside rails should be padded; restraints and arm boards should not be used.

Individuals contacting the patient during the incubation period must be identified for a quarantine of 6 days of observation, during which time their temperatures will be closely monitored, or they may be given prophylactic tetracycline or sulfadiazine.

Local public health department officials should be immediately notified of suspected cases so they can identify the source of infection.

Measures to help prevent plague include: discouraging contact with wild animals (especially those that are sick or dead); supporting programs aimed at reducing insect and rodent populations; and recommending immunization with plague vaccine to travelers to or residents of endemic areas, even though the effect of immunization is transient.

Tularemia

(Deer fly fever, rabbit fever, Ohara's disease [in Japan])

Tularemia is an acute infection caused by the gram-negative coccobacillus Francisella tularensis. *It occurs in five major forms: ulceroglandular, oculoglandular, typhoidal (enteric), oropharyngeal (pneumonic), and glandular, each with varying symptoms. Because of effective treatment with antibiotics, mortality is about 2% to 3% in typhoidal tularemia and less in all other forms. Initial infection confers lifelong immunity in most people; reinfections are rare and milder.*

Causes and incidence
Transmission of *F. tularensis* occurs by contact with secretions of an infected animal (rabbit, squirrel, rodent); the bite of a tick, a deer fly, or a flea that feeds on these animals; or ingestion of contaminated water or meat. Tularemia occurs throughout North America and parts of Europe and Asia. Most cases of tularemia that occur in the United States each year—fewer than 200 in all—are reported during seasons of peak outdoor activity, especially during the summer and hunting season.

Diagnosis
The initial diagnostic step is a thorough history of the patient's exposure to animals or ticks, since most symptoms are nonspecific. Confirmation requires isolation of *F. tularensis* from nodes, sputum, or gastric washings, or inoculation of laboratory animals with such a specimen. Other reliable tests include:
• *agglutination test:* antibody titers rise from 1:80 during the second week of the illness to a possible high of 1:1,280 in 4 to 6 weeks.
• *skin test:* an antigen challenge with a diluted specimen of *F. tularensis* gives a positive reaction in over 90% of patients within the first week of the disease, but this antigen is not commercially available.
• *blood studies:* may show elevated erythrocyte sedimentation rate, C-reactive protein (usually in typhoidal form), and occasionally, leukocytosis.

Diagnosis must rule out diseases with similar symptoms: cat-scratch fever, infectious mononucleosis, Q fever, sporotrichosis, typhoid fever, rat-bite fever, atypical pneumonia, psittacosis, tuberculosis, histoplasmosis, and coccidioidomycosis.

Treatment
Streptomycin is highly effective against *F. tularensis* and usually reduces fever within 24 to 36 hours. Recent studies

suggest that kanamycin and gentamicin are also effective. However, tetracycline and chloramphenicol, which relieve acute symptoms, are only bacteriostatic and inhibit, but do not eradicate, *F. tularensis*, and so allow relapses.

Additional considerations

The hospital staff member caring for the patient with tularemia should:
• administer antibiotics, as ordered, and provide comfort measures.
• apply wet saline dressings to skin lesions.
• administer codeine for headache, as ordered; not give aspirin or acetaminophen, because they will mask fever, an important diagnostic sign.
• provide a high-calorie, easily digestible diet.

• handle secretions carefully, double-bagging all soiled dressings, and using instruments to change dressings until lesions stop draining.
• advise high-risk persons (hunters, game wardens, lab workers) to be vaccinated. (Vaccine is available through the Center for Disease Control.)
• warn anyone in a tick-infested area to wear protective clothing and to keep trouser legs tucked snugly into boots; teach high-risk persons how to remove ticks; tell them to clean tick bites carefully with 70% alcohol.
• encourage anyone who must handle wild animals to wear rubber gloves and to avoid exposure to animals that appear to be sick.
• stress the need to cook all game thoroughly before eating it.

TYPES OF TULAREMIA

TYPE	CLINICAL FEATURES
Ulceroglandular • Most common type (75% to 85%)	• Macular, erythematous lesions within 48 hours; ulcerations at inoculation sites • Enlarged tender lymph nodes • Sudden persistent fever (104° to 106° F. [40° to 41° C.]) • Hepatomegaly and splenomegaly
Glandular • Occurs in 5% to 10% of cases • Similar to ulceroglandular tularemia	• Lymph node enlargement without detectable skin lesions • Sudden persistent fever (104° to 106° F. [40° to 41° C.]) • Hepatomegaly and splenomegaly
Oculoglandular • Comprises less than 1% of cases • Results from touching eyes with contaminated hands or fingers	• Ocular pain, congestion, lacrimation, itching, chemosis, mucopurulent discharge, photophobia • Regional lymph node enlargement and drainage
Typhoidal (enteric) • Comprises 5% to 15% of cases • Caused by inhalation of contaminated airborne droplets (often released by chewing contaminated meat) that localize in respiratory tract; organisms reach bloodstream through lymphatics, causing bacteremia	• Fever, malaise, myalgia, headache, nonproductive cough
Oropharyngeal (pneumonic) • Most serious form • Occurs in 30% to 80% of typhoidal cases, and 10% to 15% of ulceroglandular cases • Caused by inhalation of minute infected particles, or by systemic spread of other forms of this disease	• Generally nonspecific: dry, hacking cough; mucoid sputum; hemoptysis; pleuritic or retrosternal pain; dyspnea; cyanosis

Brucellosis
(Undulant fever, Bang's disease)

Brucellosis is an acute febrile illness transmitted to humans from animals, and is caused by the nonmotile, nonsporeforming, gram-negative coccobacilli Brucella bacteria, notably Brucella suis (found in swine), Brucella melitensis (in goats), Brucella abortus (in cattle), and Brucella canis (in dogs). Brucellosis causes fever, profuse sweating, anxiety, general aching, and bone, spleen, liver, kidney, or brain abscesses. Prognosis is good. With treatment, brucellosis is rarely fatal, although complications may cause permanent disability.

Causes
Brucellosis is transmitted through the consumption of unpasteurized dairy products, or uncooked or undercooked contaminated meat, and through contact with infected animals or their secretions or excretions. It's most common among farmers, stock handlers, butchers, and veterinarians. Because of such occupational risks, brucellosis infects men six times more often than it does women, especially those between ages 20 and 50; it's less common in children. Since hydrochloric acid in gastric juices kills *Brucella* bacteria, persons with achlorhydria are particularly susceptible to this disease. While brucellosis occurs throughout the world, it's most prevalent in the Middle East, Africa, the Soviet Union, India, South America, and Europe; it is rarely found in the United States. The incubation period is usually from 5 to 21 days but can last for months.

Signs and symptoms
Onset of brucellosis is usually insidious, but the disease course falls into two distinct phases. Characteristically, the acute phase causes fever, chills, profuse sweating, fatigue, headache, backache, enlarged lymph nodes, hepatosplenomegaly, weight loss, and abscess and granuloma formulation in subcutaneous tissues, lymph nodes, the liver, and the spleen. Despite this disease's common name, few patients have a truly intermittent (undulant) fever; in fact, fever is often insignificant.

The chronic phase produces recurrent depression, sleep disturbances, fatigue, headache, sweating, and sexual impotence; hepatosplenomegaly and enlarged lymph nodes persist. In addition, abscesses may form in the testes, ovaries, kidneys, and brain (meningitis and encephalitis). About 10% to 15% of patients with such brain abscesses develop hearing and visual disorders, hemiplegia, and ataxia. Other complications include osteomyelitis, orchitis, and rarely, subacute bacterial endocarditis, which is difficult to treat.

Diagnosis
In persons with characteristic clinical features, a history of exposure to animals suggests brucellosis. Multiple agglutination tests help to confirm the diagnosis.

• Approximately 90% of patients with brucellosis have agglutinin titers of 1:160 or more within 3 weeks of developing this disease. However, elevated agglutinin titers also follow vaccination against tularemia, *Yersinia* infection, or cholera; skin tests; or relapse. Agglutination titers testing can also monitor effectiveness of treatment.

• Multiple (three to six) cultures of blood and bone marrow, and biopsies of infected tissue (for example, the spleen) provide definite diagnosis. Culturing is best done during the acute phase.

• Blood studies indicate increased erythrocyte sedimentation rate (ESR) and normal or reduced WBC.

Diagnosis must rule out infectious diseases that produce similar symptoms, such as typhoid and malaria.

Treatment

Treatment consists of bed rest during the febrile phase; a 3-week course of oral tetracycline, with a 2-week course of streptomycin I.M.; and in severe cases, corticosteroids I.V. for 3 days, followed by oral corticosteroids. Secretion precautions are required until lesions stop draining.

Additional considerations

In suspected brucellosis, a detailed history must be assembled, including whether the patient has traveled recently or eaten unprocessed food, such as goat's milk.

• During the acute phase, the patient's temperature requires monitoring and recording every 4 hours. To evaluate fluctuations reliably, the same route (oral or rectal) must be used every time. The dietary department should provide between-meal milk shakes and other supplemental foods to counter weight loss. Heart murmurs, muscle weakness, vision loss, and joint inflammation may all point to complications.

• During the chronic phase, the patient may exhibit depression and disturbed sleep patterns. Sedatives may be needed. Care should be scheduled to allow for adequate rest.

• Suppurative granulomas and abscesses must be kept dry. All secretions and soiled dressings should be double-bagged and properly disposed of. The patient needs to know that this infection *is* curable.

• Before discharge, the patient must understand the importance of continuing medication for the prescribed duration. To prevent recurrence, patients should cook meat thoroughly and avoid using unpasteurized milk. Meat packers and other persons at risk of occupational exposure must wear protective rubber gloves and goggles.

Rat-bite Fever

Rat-bite fever refers to two distinct gram-negative bacterial infections: streptobacillary rat-bite fever is caused by the aerobic gram-negative bacillus Streptobacillus moniliformis; *spirillary rat-bite fever (spirillar fever, sodoku) by the gram-negative organism* Spirillum minus. *Streptobacillary rat-bite fever is rare but occurs worldwide. Spirillary rat-bite fever is most common in Japan and the Far East. With treatment, prognosis in streptobacillary rat-bite fever is excellent. Untreated, it may cause serious complications, with a mortality rate up to 10%.*

Causes and incidence

Streptobacillary rat-bite fever is transmitted by a bite from an infected rat or mouse. Consequently, it's prevalent in areas of rodent infestation and poor sanitation, and among laboratory personnel who handle infected rodents.

Signs and symptoms

Generally, symptoms of streptobacillary rat-bite fever appear 1 to 3 weeks after the bite. They include inflammation at the bite site; pain and tenderness, caused by regional lymph node infection; chills; fever; malaise; headache; nonsuppurative migrating arthritis of small joints, especially in the hands and feet; and a nonpruritic maculopapular, petechial, or pustular rash on the palms and soles. Usually, the bite itself heals well. Untreated rat-bite fever may lead to endocarditis, abscesses, and pneumonia.

Diagnosis

Typical symptoms and history of a rodent bite suggest streptobacillary rat-bite fever.

 Isolation of *S. moniliformis* from cultured blood, joint fluid, pustules, or bite drainage confirms the diagnosis. Associated laboratory abnormalities include:

• WBC 15,000/mm³, with increased band formation
• false positive serology for syphilis (in about 25% of patients) and rise in titer to 1:80 for agglutination antibodies for *S. moniliformis*, which is diagnostic.

Treatment

Rodent control, sanitation improvement, and safety precautions among lab personnel who work with rodents can prevent rat-bite fever. But when prevention fails, treatment requires:
• cleansing the bite immediately with an antiseptic solution
• antibiotic therapy that consists of a 10-day course of penicillin G procaine I.M., tetracycline P.O., or streptomycin I.M.
• supportive measures and an analgesic-antipyretic to relieve pain and fever
• prompt treatment of complications; for example, in endocarditis, penicillin G potassium I.V. for 3 to 4 weeks, as ordered.

Additional considerations

Care is primarily supportive. Since rat-bite fever isn't transmitted between humans, it doesn't require isolation. But because *S. moniliformis* occurs in pustules, this infection requires careful handling of soiled linens and dressings, and proper handwashing.

When caring for a patient with rat-bite fever, the hospital staff member should:
• thoroughly document symptoms; describe the appearance and distribution of any rash; specify painful joints; record temperature fluctuations.
• administer antibiotics, as ordered; ask the patient about previous allergic reaction before giving penicillin; watch for and treat any hypersensitivity reaction.
• relieve fever and pain with tepid sponge baths and an analgesic-antipyretic; carefully cleanse skin lesions (wear gloves, and properly dispose of contaminated dressings if the lesions are oozing).
• provide gentle, passive range-of-motion exercises for reduced mobility.
• promptly notify local public health authorities if more than one case of rat-bite fever is seen within a short time.

SPIROCHETES

Yaws
(Frambesia tropica)

Yaws is a chronic, relapsing infection caused by the nonsyphilitic spirochete Trepo-nema pertenue. Yaws develops in characteristic primary, secondary, and late phases. The primary phase produces nondestructive skin lesions; after an intervening secondary (sometimes latent) phase, a late stage may develop, producing destructive skin and bone lesions. Yaws is endemic in many tropical zones and in the hot, moist lowlands in Equatorial Africa, Ceylon, South America, and the Philippines. It occurs most often during the rainy season, and abounds in areas where living conditions are crowded, clothing is minimal, and soap and water are used infrequently. Yaws affects more than 1 million people worldwide, but the incidence is decreasing, due to penicillin and improving standards of hygiene and sanitation.

Yaws affects men and women equally. Although it can occur in people of any age, it's primarily a childhood disease. Onset usually occurs between ages 18 months and 15 years. The destructive changes of late-stage yaws usually develop in the third and fourth decades of life. The disease results in poor health and crippling disability but is rarely fatal.

Causes

T. pertenue is a nonsyphilitic spirochete serologically and morphologically indistinguishable from *Treponema pallidum*, the organism that causes syphilis. (Syphilis is rare in populations in which yaws is prevalent, perhaps because of secondary immunity.)

Transmission takes place through skin breaks by inoculation with exudate from open skin lesions. Person-to-person transmission, especially between children and nursing mothers, is common. Some believe that indirect transmission also occurs through flies, but this hasn't been proven.

Signs and symptoms

• *Primary phase (Stage I).* An initial ulcer or granulomatous cutaneous lesion (mother yaw) develops from 2 weeks to 3 months after contact, usually on the leg or foot. This lesion can accompany systemic symptoms, such as joint pain, aching extremities, sporadic fever, and lymph node enlargement. The lesion drains and is highly contagious.

• *Secondary phase (Stage II).* Multiple papules can erupt not only while the initial lesion is still present, but also from a few weeks to 4 months after it appears. These papules can progress to a generalized eruption of papillomas. These small, nondestructive lesions are round, raised, and have a granular surface. They are reddish-yellow and contain a clear yellow fluid. Such papillomas are characteristic of yaws; the papules that don't become papillomas usually disappear spontaneously.

During the secondary phase, patients often have extensive lymphadenopathy and malaise, and also nondestructive, painful bone lesions (for example, periostitis and osteomyelitis), especially in the long bones, and occasionally, in the fingers and paranasal maxillae. If untreated, this phase can continue for 3 to 5 years, with periodic healing and relapses.

• *Late phase (Stage III).* The late stage usually occurs after the patient has been symptomfree for more than 3 years. Plantar and palmar papillomas, called crab yaws (a painful and disabling form), and hyperkeratosis may develop. These papillomas may ulcerate and then heal, leaving areas of scarring and depigmentation. Extensive scarring may cause contractures.

Later, generalized nodules develop on the skin, periosteum, and the bones of the limbs, hands, and head. These nodules appear singly and erupt through the skin. After they heal, a bony thickness becomes evident clinically and on X-rays. Destructive ulceration of the nose and palate (gangosa) may add to the patient's disfigurement.

Diagnosis

 In endemic areas, typical generalized skin eruptions suggest yaws. Demonstration of *T. pertenue* on dark-field examination of lesion exudate and a positive test for syphilis (fluorescent treponemal antibody absorption test or a serologic test for syphilis) confirm it.

In the late stage of the disease, X-rays show hypertrophic periostitis and osteomyelitis. History and scars from healed lesions support the diagnosis.

Treatment

Early-stage yaws responds dramatically to antibiotic therapy with a single I.M. injection of penicillin in aluminum monostearate 2%; the disease disappears totally and skin lesions heal in 1 to 2 weeks. However, penicillin treatment may be repeated if serologic tests remain positive after 6 months. If the patient is allergic to penicillin, oxytetracycline and chlortetracycline are valuable alternatives. The ulcerations of late-stage yaws usually respond to local antiseptic dressings. The close contacts of all patients as well as asymptomatic patients in the latent stage (yaws confirmed by history and serologic testing) also require treatment with penicillin.

Additional considerations

Care of the patient with yaws focuses on supportive measures and patient education.

• Ulcerative lesions must be covered with sterile dressings and kept dry. Analgesics may be used for pain relief.

• The patient will need psychologic support to help cope with disfiguring lesions. If the disease is not advanced, he should know the lesions will heal.

• An accurate history of allergies and past drug reactions must be obtained before administering penicillin.

• To help prevent yaws, all cases should be reported to the World Health Organization. Persons in endemic areas need to know the importance of personal hygiene and good health practices. Patients with unhealed lesions must avoid close contact with others until their lesions heal, and dispose of all exudate-contaminated articles carefully. Epidemics among high-risk populations require mass treatment. Improving sanitation and upgrading social and economic conditions in endemic areas will help minimize the risk of epidemic.

Leptospirosis

Leptospirosis is a disease of lower mammals, transmitted to humans, and caused by spirochetes of the genus Leptospira. *It occurs in two major forms: anicteric, or mild, leptospirosis predominates (90%); a severe icteric leptospirosis with jaundice (Weil's disease) is much less common (10%). Overall, mortality is low but may reach 5% to 10% in severe leptospirosis.*

Causes and incidence

Approximately 150 pathogenic *Leptospira* serotypes cause these diseases worldwide; 17 of them occur in the United States. Each serotype has its own special mammalian host; the most common serotypes are *Leptospira icterohaemorrhagiae,* found in rats; *Leptospira canicola,* in dogs; and *Leptospira pomona,* in cattle and swine.

These spirochetes abound in the convoluted kidney tubules of the animal host. Human infection results from contact with water, soil, food, or vegetation contaminated with the animal host's urine. Inoculation occurs through cuts, abrasions, or contact with mucous membranes of the mouth and nose. Consequently, leptospirosis is a recreational hazard for campers and an occupational hazard for veterinarians, sanitation workers, and farmers, especially those who tend cattle or pigs. Leptospirosis is most common in men aged 20 to 30.

Since *Leptospira* require warmth and moisture for growth, incidence of infection in temperate areas rises in late summer and early fall; incidence of infection in tropical areas is high throughout the year. Incubation period is 7 to 12 days.

Signs and symptoms

Anicteric, or mild, leptospirosis is characterized by abrupt onset of flulike symptoms: fever, chills, headache, myalgia, malaise, abdominal pains, nausea, and vomiting. Conjunctival congestion, mild delirium, and benign meningeal involvement (nuchal rigidity and temporary muscle weakness) may occur later. This form of the disease is rarely fatal. Symptoms usually persist for 4 to 7 days.

In Weil's disease, the symptoms are much more severe. Additional symptoms are azotemia (renal tubular damage), hemorrhage (vasculitis with capillary injury), severe alterations in consciousness, vascular collapse, and jaundice.

Diagnosis

 For both forms of leptospirosis, isolation of the organism in blood during the acute period and its identification under the dark-field microscope confirms this infection. If this isn't possible, inoculation of laboratory animals with suspect blood, CSF, or urine can also identify it.

The indirect hemagglutination (IHA) test can detect increased antibody titers during illness; serologic serum analysis shows antibody rise after 7 to 10 days; subsequent tests show an increasing titer, which is often sufficient for diagnosis. Antibodies peak in 4 to 7 weeks. Another serologic test is a microscopic agglutination test, which determines the antibody titer and tentative identification of serotype. Agglutinins appear in 6 to 12 days (maximum titer in 3 to 4 weeks). Neither test is definitive. With either test, low titers can persist for several years.

Other abnormal laboratory results include the following:
• WBC ranges from normal to slightly elevated; polymorphonuclear leukocytosis may occur from the onset of symptoms.
• Urinalysis shows WBCs, RBCs, and casts.
• Urine culture is positive only inter-

mittently; rarely after the fourth week.
• CSF shows elevated WBC.
• Liver studies are abnormal, especially in Weil's disease, and show increased serum bilirubin, alkaline phosphatase, and urobilinogen.
• Rising serum potassium, BUN, and creatinine suggest nephron damage from Weil's disease.

Treatment

Weil's disease and mild leptospirosis require treatment with antibiotics—penicillin, tetracycline, or erythromycin—for at least 5 days. This therapy *must* begin by the second day of the illness to be of any benefit.

Additional considerations

Health care is supportive and aims to prevent complications.
• Vital signs and temperature should be checked at least every 4 hours.
• Accurate intake and output records, especially if the patient has nausea, vomiting, or diarrhea, are important. He may have an electrolyte imbalance. Decreased urinary output and proteinuria may signal renal damage, as may increased BUN and creatinine.
• Bed rest is essential; the patient should be repositioned often.
• Coughing and deep breathing are important.
• If conjunctiva is irritated, eyestrain can be prevented by instilling soothing eyedrops and keeping room dimly lighted.
• Hypotension and tachycardia, signs of shock due to hemorrhage, must be watched for.

To help prevent recurrence, patients in high-risk occupations (veterinarians, farmers, sewer workers) should wear long rubber boots and gloves while working to reduce the risk of exposure. Campers and travelers should not drink unpurified water.

All outbreaks of leptospirosis must be reported to local public health authorities. Programs to control rats and prevent disease in domestic animals will help prevent this disease.

Relapsing Fever

(Tick, fowl-nest, cabin, or vagabond fever; or bilious typhoid)

An acute infectious disease caused by spirochetes of the genus Borrelia, relapsing fever is transmitted to humans by lice or ticks, and is characterized by relapses and remissions. Rodents and other wild animals serve as the primary reservoirs for the Borrelia spirochetes. Humans can become secondary reservoirs but cannot transmit this infection by ordinary contagion; however, congenital infection and transmission by contaminated blood are possible. Untreated louse-borne relapsing fever normally carries a mortality rate of more than 10%. However, during an epidemic, the mortality rate may rise to as high as 50%. The victims are usually indigent people who are already suffering from other infections and malnutrition. With treatment, however, prognosis for both louse- and tick-borne relapsing fevers is excellent.

Causes and incidence

The body louse *(Pediculus humanis* var. *corporis)* carries louse-borne relapsing fever, which often erupts epidemically during wars, famines, and mass migrations. Cold weather and crowded living conditions also favor the spread of body lice.

Inoculation takes place when the victim crushes the louse, causing its infected blood or body fluid to soak into the victim's bitten or abraded skin, or mucous membranes.

Louse-borne relapsing fever occurs most often in North and Central Africa, Europe, Asia, and South America. No cases of louse-borne relapsing fever have been reported in the United States since 1900.

Tick-borne relapsing fever, however, is found in the United States, and is caused by three species of *Borrelia* most closely identified with tick carriers: hermsii with *Ornithodoros hermsi*, turicatae with *Ornithodoros turicata*, and parkeri with *Ornithodoros parkeri*.

This disease is most prevalent in Texas and in other western states, usually during the summer, when ticks and their hosts (chipmunks, goats, prairie dogs) are most active. However, cold-weather outbreaks sometimes afflict persons, such as campers, who sleep in tick-infested cabins.

Because tick bites are virtually pain-less, and *Ornithodoros* ticks frequently feed at night but do not imbed themselves in the victim's skin, many people are bitten unknowingly.

Signs and symptoms

The incubation period for relapsing fever is 5 to 15 days (the average is 7 days). Clinically, tick- and louse-borne diseases are similar. Both begin suddenly, with a temperature approaching 105° F. (40.5° C.), prostration, headache, severe myalgia, arthralgia, diarrhea, vomiting, coughing, and eye or chest pains. Splenomegaly is common; hepatomegaly and lymphadenopathy are possible. During febrile periods, the victim's pulse rate and respiration rate rises, and a transient, macular rash may develop over his torso.

The first attack usually lasts from 3 to 6 days, then the patient's temperature drops quickly, and is accompanied by profuse sweating. About 5 to 10 days later, a second febrile, symptomatic period begins. In louse-borne infection additional relapses are unusual, but in tick-borne cases a second or third relapse is common. As the afebrile intervals become longer, relapses become shorter and milder because of antibody accumulation. Relapses are possibly due to antigenic changes in the *Borrelia* organism.

Complications from relapsing fever

include nephritis, bronchitis, pneumonia, endocarditis, seizures, cranial nerve lesions, paralysis, and coma.

Death may occur from hyperpyrexia, massive bleeding, circulatory failure, splenic rupture, or a secondary infection.

Diagnosis

Diagnosis requires demonstration of the spirochetes in blood smears during febrile periods, using Wright's or Giemsa stain. *Borrelia* spirochetes may be harder to detect in later relapses, because their number in the blood declines. In such cases, injecting the patient's blood or tissue into a young rat and incubating the organism in the rat's blood for 1 to 10 days often facilitates spirochete identification.

In severe infection, spirochetes are found in the urine and CSF. Other abnormal laboratory results include WBC as high as 25,000/mm³, with increases in lymphocytes and erythrocyte sedimentation rate (ESR); however, WBC may be within normal limits. Because the *Borrelia* organism is a spirochete, relapsing fever may cause a false positive test for syphilis.

Treatment

Oral tetracycline is the treatment of choice; it may be given I.V., if necessary. In cases of tetracycline allergy or resistance, penicillin G may be administered as an alternative. However, neither drug should be given at the height of a severe febrile attack. If they are given, Jarisch-Herxheimer reaction may occur, causing malaise, rigors, leukopenia, flushing, fever, tachycardia, rising respiration rate, and hypotension. This reaction, which is caused by toxic by-products from massive spirochete destruction, can mimic septic shock and may prove fatal. Antimicrobial therapy should be postponed until the fever subsides. Until then, supportive therapy (consisting of parenteral fluids and electrolytes) should be given instead.

When neither tetracycline nor penicillin G controls relapsing fever, chloramphenicol may be given with caution. CBC should be done regularly during treatment with chloramphenicol, because a fatal granulocytopenia, thrombocytopenia, or even aplastic anemia may develop.

Additional considerations

When treating a patient with relapsing fever, the hospital staff member should:
• obtain a complete history of the patient's travels, both in the United States and abroad, during the initial evaluation period.
• monitor vital signs, level of consciousness, and temperature every 4 hours throughout febrile periods; watch for and immediately report any signs of neurologic complications, such as decreasing level of consciousness, or seizures; give tepid sponge baths and antipyretics to reduce fever, as ordered.
• maintain adequate fluid intake to prevent dehydration; provide I.V. fluids as ordered; measure intake and output accurately, especially if the patient is vomiting and has diarrhea.
• administer antibiotics carefully; document and report any hypersensitivity reactions (rash, fever, anaphylaxis), especially a Jarisch-Herxheimer reaction.
• treat flushing, hypotension, or tachycardia with vasopressors or fluids, as ordered.
• look for symptoms of relapsing fever in family members and in others who may have been exposed to ticks or lice along with the victim.
• use proper handwashing technique, and teach it to the patient (isolation is unnecessary because the disease isn't transmitted from person to person).
• report all cases of louse- or tick-borne relapsing fever to local public health authorities, as required by law.
• suggest to anyone traveling to tick-infested areas (Asia, North and Central Africa, South America) that relapsing fever can be prevented by wearing clothing that covers as much skin as possible. Sleeves and collars should be worn snugly and pant legs should be tucked into boots or socks.

MYCOBACTERIA

Extrapulmonary Tuberculosis

Extrapulmonary tuberculosis is caused by Mycobacterium tuberculosis *(tubercle bacillus), an acid-fast bacillus. It can affect any organ but most commonly strikes the lymphatic system, meninges (tuberculous meningitis), genitourinary tract (tuberculous pyelonephritis and tuberculous salpingo-oophoritis), pericardium (tuberculous pericarditis), gastrointestinal tract, peritoneum (tuberculous peritonitis), bones and joints, larynx, and the pleura. In miliary tuberculosis, widespread dissemination through the bloodstream causes septicemia.*

Depending on the patient's immune response, extrapulmonary tuberculosis may develop within weeks after primary tuberculosis or may remain latent for years. Although extrapulmonary tuberculosis can occur at any age, it is most common in the very young or the elderly. It's also more prevalent in Blacks and in American Indians than in the general population.

Early treatment of pulmonary tuberculosis using antitubercular drugs has improved prognosis and has reduced the incidence of extrapulmonary tuberculosis.

Causes
Extrapulmonary tuberculosis usually results from the direct extension of pulmonary tuberculosis to adjacent tissues. In miliary tuberculosis, tubercle bacilli in the lungs form granulomas that become necrotic and release the bacilli into the lymphatics or the bloodstream. Rarely, extrapulmonary tuberculosis results from skin inoculation or ingestion of contaminated food, usually in areas of the world where bovine tuberculosis is prevalent.

Signs and symptoms
Clinical features vary with the site of extrapulmonary infection. Persistent, unexplained fever and patient history suggest extrapulmonary tuberculosis.

Diagnosis
Diagnosis is difficult but may be assisted by:
• positive acid-fast smear for *M. tuberculosis*
• positive tuberculin skin test (usually negative with miliary tuberculosis)
• chest X-ray showing primary pulmonary nodular infiltrates and cavitations (however, chest X-ray is often negative in extrapulmonary tuberculosis)
• culture of appropriate fluid specimens (urine, synovial fluid). Negative fluid cultures with other positive signs may require bone marrow aspiration and biopsy, and liver biopsy.

In *tuberculosis of the lymphatics* (rare in adults), cervical and supraclavicular lymph nodes are usually enlarged; severe infection may cause these nodes to suppurate. Systemic symptoms may be present but are subtle and may go unnoticed.

In *tuberculous meningitis*, early signs include behaviorial changes, headache, stiff neck, projectile vomiting, and cranial nerve deficits (disturbed vision or hearing and facial muscle weakness). Unless treated promptly, this infection may obstruct vascular channels and cause brain infarction, hydrocephalus, and cerebral edema, with resulting neurologic damage, such as quadriplegia, hemiparesis, chronic brain syndrome, and atrophy. CSF analysis and culture show low glucose, elevated protein, elevated WBC, increased pressure, and tubercle bacilli.

Tuberculous pyelonephritis produces recurrent urinary tract infections, pyuria without bacteriuria, unexplained hematuria, and proteinuria; fever and backache are uncommon. Diagnosis requires isolation of tubercle bacilli from a first morning urine specimen. Depending on the severity of renal involvement, intravenous pyelography may show renal damage.

Tuberculous salpingo-oophoritis may cause few symptoms or may cause chronic pelvic inflammatory disease and infertility. Diagnosis requires positive culture of endometrial scrapings, or tissue obtained by biopsy of cervical lesions or laparotomy.

Tuberculous pericarditis, which causes fluid effusion into the pericardial sac, is rare and life-threatening. Slow effusion produces chronic fatigue, weakness, and weight loss; in rare cases, effusion is large enough to produce symptoms of cardiac tamponade: tachycardia, orthopnea, parodoxical pulse (systolic arterial blood pressure decreases 10 mmHg or more during inspiration), and signs of heart failure (enlarged liver and increased jugular venous pulse). Chest X-ray shows cardiac enlargement, and EKG shows low voltage in precordial leads. Diagnosis may require thoracotomy for pericardial tissue biopsy for smear and culture.

Tuberculosis of bones and joints usually affects the ends of long bones, the hips, or the spine. It produces fever, localized pain, arthritis, and osteomyelitis. *Tuberculosis of the spine* (Pott's disease) may also cause neurologic damage through spinal cord compression or paraspinal abscess, and in severe cases, vertebral collapse and spinal deformity. Diagnosis is based on positive smear and culture of bone or abscess fluid.

Gastrointestinal tuberculosis (rare) causes anorexia, weight loss, and symptoms similar to those of gastrointestinal cancer. Positive smear and culture of intestinal tissue confirms diagnosis.

Tuberculous peritonitis causes ascites, fever, and dull cramping abdominal pain. Diagnosis requires positive smear and culture of peritoneal fluid or tissue obtained by peritoneoscopy or laparotomy.

Laryngeal tuberculosis causes hoarseness, dysphagia, pain, and a dry cough. Although rare, it is extremely contagious, because the spray from each cough is loaded with tubercle bacilli. Diagnosis is made on the basis of a positive sputum smear and culture, biopsy, and clinical inspection of the larynx.

Pleural tuberculosis produces pleurisy and pleural effusion, with chest pain, dyspnea on exertion, and a nonproductive cough. Diagnosis requires positive smear and culture of pleural fluid.

Miliary tuberculosis usually causes acute illness (night sweats, chills, high fever, malaise, dyspnea, and headache), which may progress rapidly to death. Occasionally, miliary tuberculosis progresses slowly, and produces only a low-grade fever and chronic debilitation. In the early stages of miliary tuberculosis, the chest X-ray and tuberculin test may both be negative, but culture of the sputum, gastric aspirate, urine, and bone marrow may show tubercle bacilli.

Treatment

In all forms of extrapulmonary tuberculosis, primary treatment is antituberculosis chemotherapy with a combination of isoniazid P.O. or I.M., ethambutol P.O., and rifampin P.O. Drug treatment usually continues for 2 to 3 years, or longer if lesions respond slowly. Other treatment may include glucocorticoids I.V. to decrease intracranial pressure in cerebral edema, pericardiectomy for severe pericardial effusion, and surgical drainage with arthroplasty for necrotic bone in skeletal tuberculosis.

Additional considerations

The health care plan should include supportive measures to relieve symptoms and to ensure adequate rest and nutrition, patient teaching to encourage compliance with long-term therapy, and careful collection of specimens for culture; aseptic technique must be used when handling body fluid contaminants.
• Cool baths and antipyretics, as ordered, will decrease fever, and analgesics will relieve pain.

- After diagnostic biopsy vital signs should be monitored often, with special attention given to signs of bleeding, such as decreased blood pressure and increased pulse.
- In acute miliary tuberculosis, vital signs should be checked every 2 to 4 hours, especially body temperature, urinary output, and level of consciousness.
- In pericardial tuberculosis, paradoxical pulses, distant heart sounds, tachycardia, and signs of decreased cardiac output, such as falling urinary output, may occur. After thoracotomy, chest tubes must be kept patent and drainage recorded.
- In skeletal tuberculosis, after surgical drainage of joints, analgesics, as needed, joint elevation, and hot wet dressings will help decrease inflammation and pain. The patient should try to do mild range-of-motion exercises. In spinal and skeletal tuberculosis, proper patient positioning will help ease discomfort.
- Laryngeal tuberculosis patients must be kept in respiratory isolation.

- Most side effects of antitubercular drugs—such as nausea, vomiting, and constipation—will eventually subside. Regular testing is needed to detect blood dyscrasias (agranulocytosis, hemolytic and aplastic anemia), which may result from these drugs.
- The patient should become responsible for his own care and understand the importance of compliance with long-term treatment.

The best way to prevent extrapulmonary tuberculosis is to prevent primary pulmonary tuberculosis through proper nutrition, sanitation, and avoidance of overcrowding. Routine tuberculin skin tests and chest X-rays are important, especially in a patient with a history of exposure to pulmonary tubercle bacilli. Prompt and effective treatment of primary pulmonary tuberculosis, with long-term follow-up, including chest X-rays, are required to prevent extrapulmonary tuberculosis. All cases should be reported to local public health authorities.

Leprosy
(Hansen's disease)

Leprosy is a chronic, systemic infection characterized by recurring acute illness after prolonged periods of remission. It's caused by Mycobacterium leprae, *an acid-fast bacillus that attacks cutaneous tissue and peripheral nerves, producing skin lesions, anesthesia, infection, and deformities.*

With proper treatment, leprosy has a good prognosis and is rarely fatal. Untreated, however, it can cause severe disability. The lepromatous type may lead to blindness and the dreaded deformities that give this disease its gruesome reputation.

Leprosy occurs in three distinct forms:
- *Lepromatous leprosy*, the most common and most serious type, affects the upper respiratory tract, eyes, and testes, as well as the nerves and skin. Lepromatous leprosy requires continuous treatment if patients fail to build up an immunity to it.
- *Tuberculoid leprosy* affects peripheral nerves and sometimes the surrounding skin, especially on the face, arms, legs, and buttocks. Medication may cure it, or it may subside spontaneously, but treatment should be continued for 1 to 2 years after lesions heal.
- *Borderline (dimorphous) leprosy* has characteristics of both lepromatous and tuberculoid leprosies. Skin lesions in this type are diffuse and poorly defined.

Causes and incidence
Contrary to popular belief, leprosy is not highly contagious; continuous, close contact is needed to transmit it. In fact, 9 out of 10 persons have a natural im-

munity to it. Susceptibility appears highest during childhood and seems to decrease with age. Presumably, transmission occurs through airborne respiratory droplets containing *M. leprae*, or inoculation through skin breaks (with a contaminated hypodermic or tattoo needle, for example). The incubation period is long—6 months to 8 years.

Leprosy is most prevalent in the underdeveloped areas of Asia (especially India and China), Africa, South America, and the islands of the Caribbean and Pacific. About 15 million people worldwide suffer from this disease; approximately 3,000 are in the United States, mostly in the Gulf Coast states and Hawaii.

Signs and symptoms
M. leprae attacks the peripheral nervous system, especially the ulnar, radial, posterior-popliteal, anterior-tibial, and facial nerves. The central nervous system appears highly resistant. If the organism attacks small nerves, it causes skin lesions; if it attacks a large nerve trunk, it causes motor nerve damage, weakness, and pain, followed by peripheral anesthesia, muscle paralysis, or atrophy. In later stages, clawhand, footdrop, and ocular complications—such as corneal insensitivity and ulceration, conjunctivitis, photophobia, and blindness—can occur. Injury, ulceration, infection, and disuse of the deformed parts cause scarring and contracture. Neurologic complications occur in both lepromatous and tuberculoid leprosies but are less extensive and develop more slowly in the lepromatous form. Nevertheless, lepromatous leprosy can cause tissue destruction in virtually every organ of the body, and is thus considered the more serious of the two types.

Lepromatous and tuberculoid leprosies affect the skin in markedly different ways. In lepromatous disease, early lesions are multiple, symmetrical, and erythematous, sometimes appearing as macules or papules with smooth surfaces. Later, they enlarge and form plaques or nodules called lepromas on the earlobes, nose, eyebrows, and forehead, giving the patient a characteristic leonine appearance. In advanced stages, *M. leprae* may infiltrate the entire skin surface. Lepromatous leprosy also causes loss of eyebrows, eyelashes, scalp hair, and sebaceous and sweat gland function; and in advanced stages, conjunctival and scleral nodules. Upper respiratory lesions cause epistaxis, ulceration of the uvula and tonsils, septal perforation, and nasal collapse. Lepromatous leprosy can lead to hepatosplenomegaly, and destruction of the testicles, fingertips, and toes through scarring.

When tuberculoid leprosy affects the skin (sometimes its effect is strictly neural) it produces raised, large, erythematous plaques or macules with clearly defined borders. As they grow, they become rough, hairless, and hypopigmented, and leave anesthetic scars.

In borderline leprosy, skin lesions are numerous, but smaller, less anesthetic, and less sharply defined than tuberculoid lesions. Untreated, borderline leprosy may deteriorate into lepromatous disease.

Complications
Occasionally, acute episodes intensify leprosy's slowly progressing course. It remains a matter of dispute whether such exacerbations are part of the disease process or a reaction to therapy. *Erythema nodosum leprosum* (ENL), seen in lepromatous leprosy, produces fever, malaise, lymphadenopathy, and painful red skin nodules, usually during antimicrobial treatment, although it may occur in untreated persons. In Mexico and other Central American countries, some patients with lepromatous disease develop a *lucio* reaction, which produces acute illness—fever, asthma, tender or painful muscles, and hepatosplenomegaly. Leprosy may also lead to complications, such as tuberculosis, malaria, secondary bacterial infection of skin ulcers, and amyloidosis.

Diagnosis
Early clinical indications of skin lesions and muscular and neurologic deficits are usually sufficiently diagnostic in

patients from endemic areas. Biopsies of skin lesions are also diagnostic. Biopsies of peripheral nerves, or smears of the skin or of ulcerated mucous membranes, help confirm the diagnosis. Blood tests show increased erythrocyte sedimentation rate; decreased albumin, calcium, and cholesterol levels; and possibly, anemia.

Treatment
Treatment consists of antimicrobial therapy using sulfones, primarily oral dapsone and sulfoxone. Hypersensitive reactions are common with these drugs. Hepatitis and exfoliative dermatitis are especially dangerous reactions; if they occur, sulfone therapy should be stopped immediately. Respiratory involvement, other complications, or failure to respond to sulfones calls for the use of streptomycin and isoniazid. In lepromatous disease, therapy must continue until all skin lesions clear, perhaps for as long as 5 years; in tuberculoid disease, for 1 to 2 years after the lesions fade. A positive reaction to a lepromin skin test indicates that the patient has developed sufficient antibodies to warrant discontinuation of treatment. Clawhand and wrist- or footdrop may require surgical correction (tendon transfers or fusions).

Since ENL is often considered a sign that the patient is responding to treatment, antimicrobial therapy should be continued, but cautiously, and perhaps be supplemented by aspirin or glucocorticoids. (ENL has been treated successfully in some countries with thalidomide and clofazimine, but neither drug is available in the United States or Canada.) With lucio reactions, antimicrobial therapy may be changed. In lepromatous disease, corticosteroids or corticotropin (ACTH) may be administered.

A U.S. citizen with confirmed leprosy may be admitted to Carville Hospital in Baton Rouge, La., an international research and educational center for specialized treatment of leprosy. The federal government pays the full cost of medical and nursing care, as well as living expenses.

Additional considerations
Health care is supportive and consists of measures to control acute infection, prevent complications, speed rehabilitation and recovery, and provide psychologic support.

When caring for a leprosy patient, the hospital staff member should:
• give antimicrobials, as ordered, and antipyretics, analgesics, and sedatives, as needed; report ENL or lucio reactions (lucio reactions require significant changes in therapy).
• take precautions against the possible spread of infection, even though leprosy isn't highly contagious; tell patients to cover their mouths with a paper tissue when coughing or sneezing and to dispose of it properly; take infection precautions when handling clothing or articles that have been in contact with any open skin lesions.
• help prevent complications; watch for fatigue, jaundice, and other signs of anemia and hepatitis.
• tell the patient to be careful not to injure an anesthetized leg by putting too much weight on it; advise testing bath water carefully to prevent scalding; suggest the use of sturdy footwear and soaking feet in warm water after any kind of exercise, even a short walk, to prevent ulcerations; advise rubbing the feet with petrolatum, oil, or lanolin.
• help set up an interdisciplinary rehabilitation program, employing a physiotherapist and plastic surgeon, if necessary, for patients with deformities; teach active range-of-motion exercises to minimize stiffness, strengthen weak muscles, and keep fingers and thumbs functional; give passive exercises, if necessary.
• provide emotional support throughout treatment; teach the patient the facts about this feared disease; reassure him that he's not "dirty" or "cursed," despite leprosy's negative connotations.

MYCOSES

Candidiasis
(Candidosis, moniliasis)

Candidiasis is usually a mild, superficial fungal infection caused by the Candida *species. Most often, it infects the nails (paronychial), the skin (diaper rash), or mucous membranes, especially the oropharynx (thrush), vagina (moniliasis), esophagus, and gastrointestinal tract. Rarely, these fungi enter the bloodstream and invade the kidneys, lungs, endocardium, brain, or other structures, and cause serious infections. Such systemic infection is most prevalent among drug addicts and patients already hospitalized, particularly diabetics. Prognosis varies and depends on the patient's resistance.*

Causes

Most cases of *Candida* infection result from *Candida albicans* and *Candida tropicalis*. Other infective strains include *Candida stelladtoidea* (vaginitis), *Candida parapsilosis* (cutaneous, endocarditis), and *Candida guilliermondi* (endocarditis). These fungi are part of the normal flora of the gastrointestinal tract, mouth, vagina, and skin. They cause infection when some change in the body permits their sudden proliferation: rising glucose levels from diabetes mellitus, lowered resistance from a disease such as a carcinoma, immunosuppressive drug, radiation, aging, irritation from dentures, systemic introduction from I.V. or urinary catheters, drug abuse, hyperalimentation, or surgery. However, the most common predisposing factor remains the use of broad-spectrum antibiotics, such as tetracycline, or a combination of drugs that decreases the normal flora and permits an increase of *Candida*. If the mother has vaginal moniliasis, an infant can contract oral thrush while passing through the birth canal. Incidence of candidiasis is rising, particularly because of increasing use of I.V. therapy.

Signs and symptoms

Symptoms of superficial candidiasis correspond to the site of infection:
• Skin: scaly, erythematous papular rash, sometimes covered with exudate, appearing below the breast and between fingers, and at the axillae, groin, and umbilicus. In diaper rash, papules appear at the edges of the rash.
• Nails: red, swollen, darkened nailbed; occasionally, purulent discharge and the separation of a pruritic nail from the nailbed

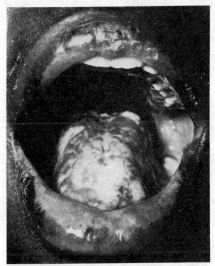

Candidiasis of the oropharyngeal mucosa (thrush) causes cream-colored or bluish-white pseudomembranous patches on the tongue, mouth, or pharynx. Fungal invasion may extend to circumoral tissues.

- Oropharyngeal mucosa (thrush): cream-colored or bluish-white patches of exudate on the tongue, mouth, or pharynx that reveal bloody engorgement when scraped. They may swell, causing respiratory distress in infants. They are only occasionally painful but cause a burning sensation in the throats and mouths of adults.
- Esophageal mucosa: dysphagia, retrosternal pain, regurgitation, and occasionally, scales in the mouth and throat.
- Vaginal mucosa: white or yellow discharge, with pruritus and local excoriation; white or gray raised patches on vaginal walls, with local inflammation; dyspareunia.

Systemic infection produces chills; high, spiking fever; hypotension; prostration; and occasional rash. Specific symptoms depend on the site of infection:
- Pulmonary: hemoptysis, cough, fever
- Renal: fever, flank pain, dysuria, hematuria, pyuria
- Brain: headache, nuchal rigidity, seizures, focal neurologic deficits
- Endocardium: systolic or diastolic murmur, fever, chest pain, embolic phenomena
- Eye: endophthalmitis, blurred vision, orbital or periorbital pain, scotoma, and exudate.

Diagnosis
Diagnosis of superficial candidiasis depends on evidence of *Candida* on a Gram's stain of skin or on vaginal scrapings, pus, or sputum, or on skin scrapings prepared in potassium hydroxide (KOH) solution. Systemic infections require obtaining a specimen for blood or tissue culture.

Treatment
Treatment first aims to improve the underlying condition that predisposes the patient to candidiasis, such as controlling diabetes, and discontinuing antibiotic therapy and catheterization, if possible. Nystatin is an effective antifungal for superficial candidiasis. Topical amphotericin B is effective for candidiasis of the skin and nails; so is gentian violet, which is also effective for thrush and vaginal infections, but is rarely used because it stains the skin. Clotrimazole and miconazole are effective in mucous membrane and vaginal *Candida* infections. Treatment for systemic infection consists of I.V. amphotericin B, flucytosine, or both.

Additional considerations
- A patient using nystatin solution must swish the solution around in his mouth for several minutes before swallowing. Nystatin can be applied to an infant's oral mucosa using a swab. The patient should use a nonirritating mouthwash to loosen tenacious secretions, and a soft toothbrush to avoid irritation. Mouth discomfort can be relieved with a topical anesthetic, such as lidocaine (not to be used within an hour before meals, since it may suppress the gag reflex).
- The patient with severe dysphagia will need a soft diet. The patient with mild dysphagia must chew food thoroughly and be watched while he eats to make sure he doesn't choke.
- Cornstarch or dry padding applied in intertriginous areas of obese patients will absorb perspiration and prevent irritation.
- I.V. catheters must be marked with insertion dates and replaced according to hospital policy to prevent phlebitis.
- The patient with candidiasis should be assessed for underlying systemic causes, such as diabetes mellitus. If the patient is receiving amphotericin B for systemic candidiasis, he may experience severe chills, fever, anorexia, nausea, and vomiting. Severity of side effects may be reduced by premedication with aspirin, antihistamines, or antiemetics.
- Patients with systemic infections require frequent vital signs checks. Patients with renal involvement need to be monitored for intake and output, and urine blood and protein.
- High-risk patients must be checked daily for patchy areas, irritation, sore throat, bleeding of mouth or gums, or other signs of superinfection. Female patients should be checked for vaginal

discharge, and the color and amount of discharge, if present recorded.
- Women in their third trimester of pregnancy should be examined for vaginal candidiasis to protect their infants from infection at birth.

Cryptococcosis
(Torulosis, European blastomycosis)

Cryptococcosis is caused by the fungus Cryptococcus neoformans. *It usually begins as an asymptomatic pulmonary infection but disseminates to extrapulmonary sites, usually to the CNS, but also to the skin, bones, prostate gland, liver, or kidneys.*

With treatment, prognosis in pulmonary cryptococcosis is good. However, untreated pulmonary disease may lead to CNS infection, which is invariably fatal within 3 years of diagnosis. Treatment dramatically reduces mortality but does not always reverse neurologic deficit, such as paralysis and hydrocephalus.

Causes and incidence
Transmission is through inhalation of *C. neoformans* in particles of dust contaminated by pigeon feces that harbor this organism. Therefore, cryptococcosis is primarily an urban infection. It is most prevalent in men, usually those between ages 30 and 60. It's especially likely to develop in immunologically compromised persons, particularly those with Hodgkin's disease, sarcoidosis, leukemia, lymphoma, and those receiving immunosuppressives. In the United States, cryptococcosis is most common in the central and western states.

Signs and symptoms
Typically, pulmonary cryptococcosis is asymptomatic. Onset of CNS involvement is gradual (cryptococcal meningitis), and produces progressively severe frontal and temporal headache, diplopia, blurred vision, dizziness, ataxia, aphasia, vomiting, tinnitus, memory changes, inappropriate behavior, irritability, psychotic symptoms, convulsions, and fever. If untreated, these symptoms progress to coma and death, usually a result of cerebral edema or hydrocephalus. Permanent complications of CNS involvement include optic atrophy, ataxia, hydrocephalus, deafness, paralysis, chronic brain syndrome, and personality changes.

Skin involvement produces red facial papules and other skin abscesses, with or without ulcerations; bone involvement produces painful osseous lesions of the long bones, skull, spine, and joints.

Diagnosis
Although a routine chest X-ray showing a pulmonary lesion may point to pulmonary cryptococcosis, this infection usually escapes diagnosis until it produces symptoms of extrapulmonary dissemination. Firm diagnosis requires identification of *C. neoformans* by culture of sputum, urine, prostatic secretions, bone marrow aspirate or biopsy, or pleural biopsy; and in CNS infection, by an India ink preparation of CSF and culture. Blood cultures are positive only in severe infection.

Supportive values include increased antigen titer in serum and CSF in disseminated infection; increased CSF pressure, protein, and WBC (up to $800/mm^3$) in CNS infection; and moderately decreased CSF glucose in about half these patients. Diagnosis must rule out cancer and tuberculosis.

Treatment
Pulmonary cryptococcosis requires close medical observation for a year after diagnosis. Treatment is unnecessary unless extrapulmonary lesions develop or pulmonary lesions progress.

Treatment of disseminated infection

calls for I.V. amphotericin B (or in CNS infection, intrathecal) for at least 6 weeks and possibly a 6-week course of oral flucytosine. Supportive measures and acetazolamide can decrease CSF pressure.

Additional considerations

Cryptococcosis doesn't necessitate isolation. However, intrathecal administration of amphotericin B requires strict aseptic technique to prevent bacterial contamination.

General hospital care includes: monitoring the patient closely; checking vital functions; noting changes in mental status, orientation, pupillary response, and motor function; and watching for headache, vomiting, and nuchal rigidity.

Treatment with I.V. amphotericin B requires: drawing serum electrolytes to determine baseline renal status; check-ing the I.V. site for phlebitis, diluting the drug as ordered, and infusing it slowly, since rapid infusion may cause circulatory collapse; watching for decreased urinary output, elevated BUN and creatinine, and hypokalemia; monitoring CBC, urinalysis, magnesium, potassium, and hepatic function; and asking the patient to report hearing loss, tinnitus, or dizziness immediately.

Analgesics and antiemetics may be ordered to prevent pain, nausea, and vomiting from this disease, and to relieve side effects of amphotericin B.

The patient and family will need psychological support to help them cope with the long-term hospitalization generally needed. Advising patients to avoid exposure to pigeons, and supporting programs for pigeon control, will help prevent this infection.

Geotrichosis

The term geotrichosis has been applied to several oral, bronchial, pharyngeal, and intestinal disorders existing in patients from whom the fungus Geotrichum candidum can be isolated. However, since this fungus is normally found even in healthy persons, such cultures don't confirm that it's a pathogen in humans. G. candidum grows in soil and is often found in dairy products.

Signs and symptoms

Reportedly, *G. candidum* can cause a bronchopulmonary disorder that produces a cough with viscous, blood-tinged sputum; an allergic asthmatic reaction similar to allergic aspergillosis; and an intestinal disorder that produces abdominal pain, diarrhea, and occasionally, rectal bleeding. Unlike other fungal infections, *G. candidum* has not been linked to CNS involvement. Geotrichosis occurs most often in immunosuppressed patients and in diabetics. The incidence of geotrichosis infection is unclear.

Treatment

Treatment of oral lesions consists of application of a 1:10,000 solution of gentian violet; for intestinal infections, oral administration of gentian violet capsules; and for pulmonary lesions, oral potassium iodide.

Aspergillosis

Aspergillosis is a rare, opportunistic infection caused by fungi of the genus Aspergillus, usually Aspergillus fumigatus, Aspergillus flavus, and Aspergillus niger. It occurs in four major forms: aspergilloma, which produces a fungus ball in the lungs, called mycetoma, caused by A. fumigatus; allergic aspergillosis, *a hypersensitive asthmatic reaction to aspergilli antigens;* aspergillosis endophthalmitis, *an infection of the anterior and posterior chambers of the eye that can lead to blindness; and* disseminated aspergillosis, *a rare, acute, and usually fatal infection that produces septicemia, thrombosis, and infarction of virtually any organ, but especially the heart, lungs, brain, and kidneys.*

Aspergillus *may cause infection of the ear (otomycosis), cornea (mycotic keratitis), and prosthetic heart valves (endocarditis), pneumonia (especially in persons receiving immunosuppressive drugs, such as cyclophosphamide), sinusitis, and brain abscesses. Prognosis varies with each form. Occasionally, aspergilloma causes fatal hemoptysis. Disseminated aspergillosis is almost always fatal.*

Causes
Aspergillus is found worldwide, often in fermenting compost piles and damp hay. It's transmitted through inhalation of fungal spores or, in aspergillosis endophthalmitis, the invasion of spores through a wound or other tissue injury. It's a common laboratory contaminant.

Aspergillus is normally present in the mouth and sputum and only produces clinical infection in persons who become especially vulnerable to it. Such debilitation can result from excessive or prolonged use of antibiotics, and from glucocorticoids or other immunosuppressive therapy; also, from Hodgkin's disease, irradiation, leukemia, azotemia, alcoholism, sarcoidosis, organ transplant, bronchitis, or bronchiectasis; or in aspergilloma, from tuberculosis or some other cavitary lung disease.

Signs and symptoms
The incubation period in aspergillosis ranges from a few days to weeks. In aspergilloma, colonization of the bronchial tree with *Aspergillus* produces plugs and atelectasis, and forms a tangled ball of hyphae (fungal filaments), fibrin, and exudate in a cavity left by a previous illness, such as tuberculosis. Characteristically, aspergilloma either causes no symptoms or mimics tuberculosis, with a productive cough and purulent or blood-tinged sputum, dyspnea, empyema, and lung abscesses.

Allergic aspergillosis causes wheezing, dyspnea, cough with some sputum production, pleural pain, and fever.

Aspergillosis endophthalmitis appears 2 to 3 weeks after an eye injury or surgery, and accounts for half of all cases of endophthalmitis. It causes clouded vision, pain, and reddened conjunctiva. Eventually, *Aspergillus* infects the anterior and posterior chambers, where it produces purulent exudate.

In disseminated aspergillosis, *Aspergillus* invades blood vessels, and causes thrombosis, infarctions, and the typical signs of septicemia (chills, fever, hypotension, delirium), with azotemia, hematuria, urinary tract obstruction, headaches, seizures, bone pain and tenderness, and soft-tissue swelling. It's rapidly fatal.

Diagnosis
Aspergillosis is difficult to diagnose. In patients with aspergilloma, a chest X-ray reveals a crescent-shaped radiolucency surrounding a circular mass, but this is not definitive for aspergillosis. In aspergillosis endophthalmitis, a history of ocular trauma or surgery and a culture or exudate showing *Aspergillus* is diagnostic. In allergic aspergillosis, sputum examination shows eosinophils. Culture of mouth scrapings or sputum showing *Aspergillus* is inconclusive, since even healthy persons harbor this fungus. In disseminated aspergillosis, culture and microscopic examination of affected tissue can confirm diagnosis, but this form is usually diagnosed at autopsy.

Treatment and additional considerations
Aspergillosis doesn't require isolation. Treatment of aspergilloma necessitates

local excision of the lesion and supportive therapy (chest physiotherapy, coughing, deep breathing exercises) to improve pulmonary drainage and function.

Allergic aspergillosis requires desensitization and, possibly, the use of steroids.

Disseminated aspergillosis and aspergillosis endophthalmitis require a 2- to 3-week course of I.V. amphotericin B, prompt discontinuation of immunosuppressive therapy, and possibly flucytosine. However, since the disseminated form is so rapidly progressive, it's often fatal before treatment begins; moreover, it often resists amphotericin B therapy.

Zygomycosis
(Phycomycosis, mucormycosis)

Zygomycosis is a term applied to all infections caused by fungi of the subclass Zygomycetes. Only two orders of Zygomycetes act as pathogens in humans: the Mucorales order, which contains the Mucoraceae family of genera—Rhizopus, Mucor, and Absidia—and causes severe and often fatal mucormycosis; and the Entomophthorales order. All these infections are rare.

Zygomycosis occurs in several forms: rhinocerebral mucormycosis (the most common in the United States), and gastrointestinal, pulmonary, and disseminated mucormycoses. Although antifungal therapy with amphotericin B and surgery have reduced mortality, rhinocerebral and disseminated mucormycoses are usually fatal.

Causes
Zygomycetes are found in decaying vegetable matter and in soil throughout the world, especially in tropical areas. They are also common laboratory contaminants. However, they're not normally a human pathogen, and usually produce mucormycosis only in immunologically compromised hosts—especially persons with diabetic ketoacidosis, renal failure, renal tubular acidosis, leukemias, lymphomas—and those receiving glucosteroids or other immunosuppressants. The incidence of mucormycosis is rising because of the longer survival of patients with diabetic ketoacidosis, renal failure, renal tubular acidosis, leukemia, or other predisposing disorders.

Typically, transmission of rhinocerebral mucormycosis occurs by inhalation of fungi into the paranasal sinuses or nasal turbinates. This fungus then invades the mucous membrane and blood vessel walls. Transmission may also occur through ingestion, trauma, and I.V. catheterization. Because it encourages the overgrowth of nonsusceptible organisms, topical antibacterial treatment of burn patients has increased the incidence of all fungal infections, including mucormycosis.

Signs and symptoms
Rhinocerebral mucormycosis produces ulceration or perforation of the nasal septum and necrosis of the nasal turbinates, with dark, bloody nasal discharge. As this infection progresses, it causes periorbital and perinasal swelling, ptosis and proptosis, ophthalmoplegia, loss of vision, and corneal reflex; also trigeminal anesthesia, facial palsy, headache, nuchal rigidity, hemiplegia, drowsiness, and eventually, coma and death.

Pulmonary mucormycosis causes gradual or sudden onset of chest pain, fever, hemoptysis, and friction rub. Gastrointestinal mucormycosis, which is often associated with malnutrition, causes abdominal pain, bloody diarrhea, and eventually, intestinal perforation and peritonitis. Disseminated mucormycosis usually produces brain and lung abscesses, and less often, liver, spleen, and pancreas abscesses and infarctions. CNS dissemination usually results from paranasal sinus and orbital mucormycosis; it causes drowsiness, headache, stupor, nuchal rigidity, and fever.

Diagnosis

Mucormycosis must be suspected whenever a debilitated patient develops rapidly spreading sinusitis, orbital cellulitis, or ophthalmoplegia. Identification of infecting fungus is extremely difficult (even postmortem) and requires histologic examination of tissue biopsy and culture. A sinus X-ray may show bone destruction, but this finding is nonspecific.

Treatment and additional considerations

Inadequately treated mucormycosis is almost always fatal. Therefore, aggressive treatment must begin promptly, and requires intensive care monitoring, preferably in an ICU. Therapy includes:
• antifungal therapy consisting of a 2- to 3-month course of amphotericin B I.V. (amphotericin B may cause fever, chills, nausea, and vomiting, so antipyretics and antiemetics may be ordered).
• repeated surgical debridement of necrotic tissues (in ocular infection this may require enucleation of the eye and removal of necrotic orbital contents; in pulmonary mucormycosis, removal of the infected lung).
• drainage of infected paranasal sinuses.
• correction of underlying disorders, such as metabolic acidosis.

Mucormycosis doesn't require isola-

ENTOMOPHTHORALES

The order Entomophthorales includes two species that are pathogenic in humans: *Basidiobolus haptosporus*, which causes subcutaneous phycomycosis, and *Entomophthora coronata*, which causes rhinophycomycosis (rhinoentomophthoromycosis). Both infections occur in otherwise healthy persons in tropical and subtropical areas, especially in Africa; both are probably transmitted through puncture wounds or the bites of infected insects.

Subcutaneous phycomycosis produces a solid subcutaneous mass that is fixed to the skin, which may heal spontaneously after months or years. It occurs primarily in boys and in male adolescents, usually remains localized and responsive to oral potassium iodide, and is rarely fatal.

Rhinoentomophthoromycosis causes swelling of the nose and adjacent facial structures, and may also infect the pharynx and the palate. It's extremely rare, usually occurs in adult males, and responds to treatment with potassium iodide or amphotericin B I.V.

---

tion. To help prevent this infection, strict aseptic technique must be maintained, especially when caring for debilitated patients. In addition, signs of inflammation and infection must be watched for, and predisposing disorders prevented or controlled. For instance, by complying with treatment a diabetic can avoid diabetic ketoacidosis.

Histoplasmosis

(Ohio Valley disease, Central Mississippi Valley disease, Appalachian Mountain disease, Darling's disease)

Histoplasmosis is a fungal infection caused by Histoplasma capsulatum. *In the United States, it occurs in three forms: primary acute histoplasmosis, progressive disseminated histoplasmosis (acute disseminated or chronic disseminated disease), and chronic pulmonary (cavitary) histoplasmosis, which produces cavitations in the lung similar to those in pulmonary tuberculosis.*

A fourth form, African histoplasmosis, occurs only in Africa, and is caused by the fungus Histoplasma capsulatum *var.* duboisii.

Prognosis varies with each form. The primary acute disease is benign; the progressive disseminated disease is fatal in 90% of patients; and without proper chemotherapy, chronic pulmonary histoplasmosis is fatal in 50% of patients within 5 years.

Causes

H. *capsulatum* is found in the feces of birds and bats or in soil contaminated by their feces, such as that near roosts, chicken coops, barns, caves, or underneath bridges. Histoplasmosis occurs worldwide, especially in the temperate areas of Asia, Africa, Europe, and North and South America. In the United States, it's most prevalent in the central and eastern states, especially in the Mississippi and Ohio River valleys.

Transmission is through inhalation of *H. capsulatum* or *H. duboisii* spores, or the invasion of spores after minor skin trauma. Probably because of occupational exposure, histoplasmosis is more common in adult males. Fatal disseminated disease, however, is more common in infants and elderly men.

The incubation period is from 5 to 18 days, although chronic pulmonary histoplasmosis may progress slowly for many years.

Signs and symptoms

Symptoms vary with each form of this disease. Primary acute histoplasmosis may be asymptomatic or cause a mild respiratory illness similar to a severe cold or influenza. Clinical effects include fever, malaise, headache, myalgia, anorexia, cough, and chest pain.

Progressive disseminated histoplasmosis causes hepatosplenomegaly, general lymphadenopathy, anorexia, weight loss, fever, and possibly, ulceration of the tongue, palate, epiglottis, and larynx, with resulting pain, hoarseness, and dysphagia. It may also cause endocarditis, meningitis, pericarditis, and adrenal insufficiency.

Chronic pulmonary histoplasmosis mimics pulmonary tuberculosis, and causes a productive cough, dyspnea, and occasional hemoptysis. Eventually, it produces weight loss, extreme weakness, breathlessness, and cyanosis.

African histoplasmosis produces cutaneous nodules, papules, and ulcers; lymphadenopathy; lesions of the skull and long bones; and visceral involvement without pulmonary lesions.

Diagnosis

A history of exposure to contaminated soil in an endemic area, miliary calcification in the lungs or spleen, and a positive histoplasmin skin test indicate exposure to histoplasma. Rising complement fixation and agglutination titers (more than 1:32) strongly suggest histoplasmosis.

The diagnosis of histoplasmosis requires a morphologic examination of tissue biopsy and culture of *H. capsulatum* from sputum, in acute primary and chronic pulmonary histoplasmosis; and from bone marrow, lymph node, blood, and infection sites, in disseminated histoplasmosis. However, cultures take several weeks to grow these organisms. Faster diagnosis is possible with stained biopsies using Gomori's stains (methenamine silver) or the periodic acid-Schiff reaction. Findings must rule out tuberculosis and other diseases that produce similar symptoms.

The diagnosis of histoplasmosis caused by *H. duboisii* necessitates examination of tissue biopsy and culture of the affected site.

Treatment

Treatment consists of chemotherapy, surgery, and supportive care.

• Chemotherapy is most important. Except for asymptomatic primary acute histoplasmosis (which resolves spontaneously) and the African form, histoplasmosis requires high-dose or long-term (10-week) antifungal therapy with amphotericin B.

• Surgery includes lung resection to re-

move pulmonary nodules, a shunt for increased intracranial pressure, and cardiac repair for constrictive pericarditis.
• Supportive care includes oxygen for respiratory distress, glucocorticoids for adrenal insufficiency, and parenteral fluids for dysphagia due to oral or laryngeal ulcerations. Histoplasmosis doesn't require isolation.

Additional considerations
Health care for the patient with histoplasmosis is primarily supportive: giving drugs; teaching him about possible drug side effects; and providing psychologic support. Since amphotericin B may

cause chills, fever, nausea, and vomiting, appropriate antipyretics and antiemetics may be ordered.

Patients with chronic pulmonary or disseminated histoplasmosis need psychologic support because of long-term hospitalization. Parents of children with this disease will need help arranging for a visiting teacher.

To help prevent histoplasmosis, persons in endemic areas should be taught to watch for early signs of this infection and to seek treatment promptly. Persons at risk of occupational exposure to contaminated soil must wear face masks during exposure.

Blastomycosis
(North American blastomycosis, Gilchrist's disease)

Blastomycosis is caused by the fungus Blastomyces dermatitidis, *which usually infects the lungs and produces bronchopneumonia, although it may disseminate through the blood and cause osteomyelitis, and CNS, skin, and genital disorders. Untreated blastomycosis is slowly progressive and usually fatal; however, spontaneous remissions occasionally occur. With treatment, prognosis is good.*

Causes and incidence
Blastomycosis is generally found in North America (where *B. dermatitidis* normally inhabits the soil) and is endemic to the southeastern United States. Sporadic cases have also been reported in Africa. Blastomycosis usually infects men aged 30 to 50, but no occupational link has been found. *B. dermatitidis* is probably inhaled. The incubation period may range from weeks to months.

Signs and symptoms
Initial symptoms of pulmonary blastomycosis mimic those of a viral upper respiratory infection: dry, hacking, or productive cough (occasionally hemoptysis), pleuritic chest pain, fever, shaking, chills, night sweats, malaise, anorexia, and weight loss.

Cutaneous blastomycosis causes small, painless, nonpruritic, and nondistinctive macules or papules on exposed body parts. These lesions become raised and

reddened, and occasionally progress to draining skin abscesses or fistulas.

Dissemination to the bone causes soft-tissue swelling, tenderness, and warmth over bony lesions, which generally occur in the thoracic, lumbar, and sacral regions, long bones of the legs, and in children, the skull.

Genital dissemination produces painful swelling of the testes, the epididymis, or the prostate; deep perineal pain; pyuria; and hematuria. CNS dissemination causes meningitis or cerebral abscesses, and resulting decreased level of consciousness, lethargy, and change in mood or affect. Dissemination to other areas may result in Addison's disease (adrenal insufficiency), pericarditis, and arthritis.

Diagnosis
Diagnosis of blastomycosis requires:
• culture of *B. dermatitidis* from skin lesions, pus, sputum, or pulmonary se-

cretions
• microscopic examination of tissue biopsy from the skin or the lungs, or of bronchial washings, sputum, or pus, as appropriate
• complement fixation testing. While such testing isn't conclusive, a high titer in extrapulmonary disease is a poor prognostic sign.

In addition, suspected pulmonary blastomycosis requires a chest X-ray, which may show pulmonary infiltrates. Other abnormal laboratory findings include increased WBC and erythrocyte sedimentation rate, slightly increased serum globulin, mild normochromic anemia, and with bone lesions, increased alkaline phosphatase.

Treatment and additional considerations

All forms of blastomycosis respond to amphotericin B; primary skin lesions usually respond to hydroxystilbamidine isethionate. Hospital care is primarily supportive.

Hemoptysis may occur in severe pulmonary blastomycosis. The patient will need a cool room and tepid sponge baths, if febrile, and joint elevation and heat, if disseminated blastomycosis causes joint pain or swelling. CNS infection may cause a decreasing level of consciousness and unequal pupillary response. Disseminated disease in men can cause hematuria.

Since too rapid I.V. infusion of amphotericin B may cause circulatory collapse, the infusion must be slow, and the patient's vital signs should be monitored (temperature may rise but should subside within 1 to 2 hours). The patient may experience decreased urinary output, increased BUN and creatinine, and hypokalemia, which may indicate kidney toxicity; also, hearing loss, tinnitus, or dizziness. Amphotericin B's side effects are relieved by antiemetics and antipyretics.

Hydroxystilbamidine isethionate must be protected from light during the infusion.

Mycetoma
(Maduromycosis, Madura foot)

Mycetoma is a chronic infection of skin, subcutaneous tissues, and bone caused by the fungus Allescheria boydii *and at least 20 species of bacteria of the order* Actinomycetales, *especially the genera of the family* Actinomycetaceae—Nocardia *and* Actinomadura. *Usually, mycetoma infects the foot and may produce partially disabling lesions. It's rarely fatal except through secondary bacterial infection.*

Causes and incidence

Because the organisms that cause mycetoma are found in the soil, and because patients usually acquire mycetoma through a break in the skin, mycetoma generally occurs on the feet, especially in tropical and semitropical areas where people commonly go barefoot. This infection occasionally develops on the shoulders, hands, buttocks, or back. Incidence is highest in India and the Sudan; although rare, mycetoma also occurs in the eastern, central, and northern United States.

Signs and symptoms

At onset, mycetoma produces a small swelling, usually on the sole or dorsum of the foot. Over ensuing months, it causes a recurring cycle of swelling, suppuration, and healing, during which nodules and abscesses form and extend through sinus tracts. Despite their disfiguring appearance, these lesions are almost painless until mycetoma destroys deeper tissues and bone. Then, it causes moderate pain, generalized swelling, redness, and sinus drainage (pus often contains characteristic white, yellow, black, or red granules). After this initial stage, mycetoma progresses very slowly over many years.

Diagnosis

 Typical clinical appearance and characteristic granules in sinus discharge strongly suggest mycetoma; histologic tissue examination and culture of fungi and bacteria from tissue biopsy, pus, or sinus drainage confirm it. An X-ray usually shows bone destruction more extensive than pain or external appearance suggests.

Treatment and additional considerations

Drug treatment varies with the causative organism. Sulfonamides are effective against *Nocardia*; penicillin or tetracy-cline against *Actinomyces*. Experimental use of estrogens shows some promise. Surgical debridement of lesions is generally ineffective and is not recommended. Severe secondary bacterial infection or bone and connective tissue involvement may require amputation.

Supportive measures include:
- elevation of feet to relieve edema.
- adequate rest, nutrition, and protection from trauma, to reduce the risk of secondary bacterial infection.
- analgesics for pain.
- emotional support to help patients cope with this disfiguring disease.

Wearing shoes, long pants, long-sleeve shirts and other protective clothing can help prevent this disease in high-risk areas, but climate and economic conditions in these areas often make this an unreachable goal.

Paracoccidioidomycosis
(South American blastomycosis)

Paracoccidioidomycosis is a fungal infection of the skin, lungs, mucous membranes, lymphatics, and viscera, caused by Paracoccidioides brasiliensis. *It occurs in both pulmonary and disseminated forms. Untreated, both forms can be fatal; even with treatment, prognosis in disseminated disease is poor.*

Causes

Paracoccidioidomycosis is seen primarily in the tropical forests of Colombia, Venezuela, and Brazil. It usually strikes men who work as farmers or farm laborers. In these countries, *P. brasiliensis* occurs naturally in the soil, wood, and vegetation; it's presumably transmitted to humans through inhalation.

Signs and symptoms

Characteristically, the pulmonary form causes a productive cough, shortness of breath, fatigue, malaise, and weight loss; complications include pulmonary cavitations and resulting hemoptysis.

The disseminated form produces painful granulomatous lesions that first appear on the mucocutaneous margins of the mouth and nose, but gradually spread to the face, gums, and oropharynx. This dissemination can cause hoarseness, dysphagia, and cervical lymph node enlargement, with sinus formation; such symptoms may be agonizing enough to make eating impossible, which leads to severe weight loss. Possible dissemination to the liver and spleen (signaled by hepatosplenomegaly), and to other organs causes systemic symptoms, such as fever, chills, and weakness.

Diagnosis

 Diagnosis requires microscopic examination of sputum, pus, or tissue biopsy for *P. brasiliensis*. Positive complement fixation test may show high titer levels.

Treatment

Treatment consists of long-term use (possibly 3 to 5 years) of sulfonamides. (Paracoccidioidomycosis is the only systemic fungal disease that responds to sulfonamides.) For disseminated disease, I.V. amphotericin B is preferred in combination with sulfonamides. Cavitary pulmonary disease may also require excision of necrotic pulmonary tissues.

Additional considerations

Care for the patient with paracoccidioidomycosis is primarily supportive.
• If I.V. amphotericin B is ordered, it must be infused slowly, since rapid infusion may cause circulatory collapse. During infusion, vital signs require monitoring (temperature may rise but should subside within 1 to 2 hours).

Possible complications include falling urinary output, increased BUN, elevated creatinine, and hypokalemia. The patient should report hearing loss, tinnitus, or dizziness immediately. To ease side effects of amphotericin B, antiemetics or antipyretics may be given.
• The hospital dietary department should provide a diet of soft, bland, nonirritating foods. After eating, the patient will need thorough mouth care. He should be weighed daily. If the patient can't eat, I.V. fluids will be ordered and the patient monitored for adequate hydration.
• If the patient is on long-term sulfonamide therapy, he must understand the need for compliance to prevent relapses.
• Signs of disseminated disease, such as hepatosplenomegaly, must be monitored and reported.

Coccidioidomycosis

(Valley fever, San Joaquin Valley fever)

Coccidioidomycosis is caused by the fungus Coccidioides immitis, *and occurs primarily as a respiratory infection, although generalized dissemination may occur. The primary pulmonary form is usually self-limiting and rarely fatal. The rare secondary (progressive, disseminated) form produces abscesses throughout the body, and carries a mortality of up to 60%, even with treatment. Such dissemination is more common in dark-skinned men, pregnant women, and patients who are receiving immunosuppressives.*

Causes

Coccidioidomycosis is endemic to the southwestern United States, especially between the San Joaquin Valley in California and southwestern Texas; it also is found in Mexico, Guatemala, Honduras, Venezuela, Colombia, Argentina, and Paraguay. It may result from inhalation of *C. immitis* spores found in the soil in these areas, or from inhalation of spores from dressings or plaster casts of infected persons. It's most prevalent during warm, dry months.

Because of population distribution and an occupational link (it's common in migrant farm laborers), coccidioidomycosis generally strikes Philippine Americans, Mexican Americans, Ameri-

can Indians, and Blacks. In primary infection, the incubation period is from 1 to 4 weeks.

Signs and symptoms

Primary coccidioidomycosis usually produces acute or subacute respiratory symptoms (dry cough, pleuritic chest pain, pleural effusion), fever, sore throat, chills, malaise, headache, and an itchy macular rash. Occasionally, the sole symptom is a fever that persists for weeks. From 3 days to several weeks after onset, some patients, particularly Caucasian women, may develop tender red nodules (erythema nodosum) on their legs, especially the shins, with joint pain in the knees and ankles. Generally, primary disease heals spontaneously within a few weeks.

In rare cases, coccidioidomycosis disseminates to other organs several weeks or months after the primary infection. Disseminated coccidioidomycosis causes fever and abscesses throughout the body, especially in skeletal, CNS, splenic, hepatic, renal, and subcutaneous tissues. Depending on the location of these abscesses, disseminated coccidioidomycosis may cause bone pain and meningitis. Chronic pulmonary cavitation, which can occur in both the primary and the disseminated form, causes hemoptysis with or without chest pain.

Diagnosis

Typical clinical features, and skin and serologic studies confirm this diagnosis. The primary form—and sometimes the disseminated form— produces a positive coccidioidin skin test. In the first week of illness, complement fixation for IgG antibodies, or in the first month, positive serum precipitins (immunoglobulins) also establish this diagnosis. Examination or, more recently, immunodiffusion testing of sputum, pus from lesions, and a tissue biopsy may show *C. immitis* spores. Presence of antibodies in pleural and joint fluid, and a rising serum or body fluid antibody titer indicate dissemination.

Other abnormal laboratory results include increased WBC, eosinophilia, increased erythrocyte sedimentation rate, and a chest X-ray showing bilateral diffuse infiltrates.

In coccidioidal meningitis, examination of CSF shows WBC increased to more than 500/mm³ (due primarily to mononuclear leukocytes), increased protein, and decreased glucose. Ventricular fluid obtained from the brain may contain complement fixation antibodies.

After diagnosis, the results of serial skin tests, blood cultures, and serologic testing may document the effectiveness of therapy.

Treatment

Usually, mild primary coccidioidomycosis requires only bed rest and relief of symptoms. Severe primary disease and dissemination, however, also require long-term I.V. infusion, or in CNS dissemination, intrathecal administration of amphotericin B, and possibly, excision or drainage of lesions. Severe pulmonary lesions may require lobectomy. Investigational use of miconazole shows some promise.

Additional considerations

• The circle drawn on the skin for serial skin tests must not be washed off, since this aids in reading test results.

• In mild primary disease, the patient needs bed rest and adequate fluid intake. The amount and color of sputum must be recorded. Shortness of breath should be watched for. It may point to pleural effusion. Patients with arthralgia may need analgesics.

• Coccidioidomycosis requires strict secretion precautions if the patient has draining lesions. "No touch" dressing technique and careful handwashing are essential.

• In CNS dissemination, decreased level of consciousness or change in mood or affect must be monitored and reported.

• Before intrathecal administration of amphotericin B, the patient should know the procedure and be reassured that he'll receive analgesics before a lumbar puncture. If the patient is to receive amphotericin B intravenously, it must be infused slowly. This is important because rapid infusion may cause circulatory collapse. During infusion, vital signs require close monitoring. Although the patient's temperature may rise, it should return to normal within 1 to 2 hours. The hospital staff member needs to watch for decreased urinary output, elevated BUN, elevated creatinine, and hypokalemia.

• The patient must immediately report hearing loss, tinnitus, dizziness, and all signs of toxicity.

• Antiemetics and antipyretics may ease side effects of amphotericin B.

Sporotrichosis

Sporotrichosis is a chronic disease caused by the fungus Sporotrix schenckii. *It occurs in three forms:* cutaneous lymphatic, *which produces nodular erythematous primary lesions and secondary lesions along lymphatic channels;* pulmonary, *a rare form that produces a productive cough and pulmonary lesions; and* disseminated, *another rare form, which may cause arthritis or osteomyelitis. The course of sporotrichosis is slow, prognosis is good, and fatalities are rare. However, untreated skin lesions may cause secondary bacterial infection.*

Causes
S. schenckii is found in soil, wood, sphagnum moss, and decaying vegetation throughout the world. Since this fungus usually enters through broken skin (the pulmonary form through inhalation), sporotrichosis is more common in horticulturalists, agricultural workers, and home gardeners. Perhaps because of occupational exposure, it's more prevalent in adult men than in women and children. The incubation period is from 1 week to 3 months.

Signs and symptoms
Cutaneous lymphatic sporotrichosis produces characteristic skin lesions, usually on the hands or fingers. Each lesion begins as a small, painless, movable subcutaneous nodule, but progressively grows larger, discolors, and eventually ulcer-

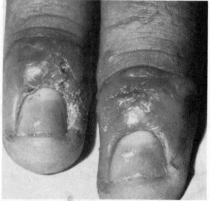

Ulceration, swelling, and crusting of nodules on fingers is characteristic of cutaneous-lymphatic sporotrichosis.

ates. Later, additional lesions form along the adjacent lymph node chain.

Pulmonary sporotrichosis causes a productive cough, lung cavities and nodules, hilar adenopathy, pleural effusion, fibrosis, and the formation of a fungus ball. It's often associated with sarcoidosis and tuberculosis.

Disseminated sporotrichosis produces multifocal lesions that spread from the primary lesion in the skin or lungs. Onset is insidious. Characteristically, it causes weight loss, anorexia, synovial or bony lesions, and possibly, arthritis or osteomyelitis.

Diagnosis

Typical clinical findings and culture of *S. schenckii* in sputum, pus, or bone drainage confirm this diagnosis. Histologic identification is difficult. Diagnosis must rule out tuberculosis and sarcoidosis, and in patients with the disseminated form, bacterial osteomyelitis and neoplasm.

Treatment
Sporotrichosis doesn't require isolation. The cutaneous lymphatic form usually responds to application of saturated solution of potassium iodide, generally continued for 1 to 2 months after lesions heal. Occasionally, cutaneous lesions must be excised or drained. The disseminated form responds to intravenous amphotericin B but may require several weeks of treatment. Local heat application relieves pain. Cavitary pulmonary lesions may require surgical excision.

Additional considerations

Supportive care includes keeping lesions clean, making the patient as comfortable as possible, and carefully disposing of contaminated dressings.

Patients should understand about possible adverse effects of drugs. Because amphotericin B may cause fever, chills, nausea, and vomiting, antipyretics and antiemetics may be ordered.

To help prevent sporotrichosis, horticulturists and home gardeners (especially those who use sphagnum moss) should wear gloves while working.

Rhinosporidiosis

Rhinosporidiosis is a fungal infection caused by Rhinosporidium seeberi. *It produces painless, vascularized, friable, and often large, tumorlike lesions; they usually appear on the nose, nasopharynx, and larynx, but occasionally on the outer ear, bronchi, penis, and vagina. An ocular form of this illness also occurs in Texas and in other dry, dusty areas where it's probably spread by dust storms.*

Causes and incidence

Rhinosporidiosis is most common in Ceylon and in India, where it usually infects boys and young men; it's probably transmitted by bathing or swimming in contaminated water.

Signs and symptoms

Nasal rhinosporidiosis causes rhinitis, nosebleed, and nasal obstruction; the laryngeal form, occasional hoarseness; and the ocular form, unilateral conjunctivitis. Although rhinosporidiosis isn't fatal in itself, it may lead to fatal secondary infection.

Diagnosis and treatment

In addition to characteristic clinical findings, diagnosis requires microscopic examination of smear or biopsy material. *R. seeberi* can't be cultured.

Treatment consists of electrocauterization or, if this isn't available, surgical excision of lesions, followed by appropriate treatment of secondary infection, as ordered.

Chromomycosis
(Chromoblastomycosis)

Chromomycosis is a rare, slowly spreading, opportunistic fungal infection of the skin and subcutaneous tissues caused by Phialophora verrucosa, Fonsecaea pedrosoi, *and* Cladosporium carrioni. *It usually appears on the legs but may also appear on the buttocks or arms. Occasionally, it spreads by the lymphatic system to the brain, where it produces abscesses.*

Despite its disfiguring cauliflowerlike lesions, chromomycosis doesn't interfere with limb function. It's rarely fatal unless it causes brain abscesses.

Causes

Chromomycosis occurs worldwide. It's most common in barefoot male agricultural workers in the Caribbean, Central and South America, South Africa, the Orient, the South Pacific, and other tropical and subtropical areas. Most patients are between ages 30 and 50. Chromomycosis can occur in otherwise healthy persons but usually causes brain abscesses only in debilitated persons.

Chromomycosis is transmitted from

soil and vegetation through a break in the skin. Incubation time is unknown but may be several months.

Signs and symptoms
In early stages, chromomycosis causes violet, warty, unilateral cutaneous papules on the arms and legs, and along areas of lymphatic drainage. These early lesions are painless but may itch. Without treatment, they gradually multiply, grow larger, become hard and cauliflower-shaped, and eventually cover the entire extremity. When chromomycosis spreads to the brain, it produces CNS symptoms typical of other brain abscesses.

Diagnosis
In early stages, a potassium hydroxide 10% (KOH) preparation of scrapings or pus from lesions or a lesion biopsy reveals hyphae (fungal filaments) and septate bodies. Culture of lesion biopsies or crusts may identify fungi, but such cultures grow very slowly. In late stages, diagnosis rests on typical, cauliflower-shaped lesions.

Treatment and additional considerations
Early-stage treatment removes the lesion with liquid nitrogen, electrocoagulation, or surgical excision. Subsequent intralesional injections of amphotericin B combined with procaine, given at weekly intervals with daily oral doses of flucytosine, may slow progression of this disease. A saturated solution of potassium iodide P.O. may also inhibit progression when combined with weekly injections of calciferol. In late stages, chromomycosis resists treatment.

To help prevent chromomycosis, people living in high-risk areas must thoroughly flush and bandage even small cuts and abrasions. As a protective measure, they should wear pants, shirts, socks, and shoes. This precautionary step, however, may be unrealistic, given climate and economic conditions in endemic areas.

RESPIRATORY VIRUSES

Common Cold

The common cold is an acute, usually afebrile viral infection that causes inflammation of the upper respiratory tract. It accounts for more time lost from school or work than any other cause, and is the most common infectious disease among people of all ages. Although the common cold is benign and self-limiting, it can lead to secondary bacterial infections.

Causes and incidence
The common cold shows certain traits: it's more prevalent in children than in adults; it affects more boys than girls among adolescents and more women among adults. In temperate zones, it occurs more often in the colder months; in the Tropics, during the rainy season.

About 90% of colds stem from a viral infection of the upper respiratory passages and consequent mucous membrane inflammation; occasionally, colds result from mycoplasma. Since any one of over a hundred different viruses may be responsible for the common cold, development of an effective vaccine is highly unlikely. Approximately 25% of adult colds and 10% of children's colds are caused by some form of rhinovirus. Other responsible viruses include coronaviruses, myxoviruses, adenoviruses, coxsackieviruses, and echoviruses.

Usually, transmission occurs through airborne respiratory droplets; occasionally, from objects contaminated with respiratory droplets. Recent studies indicate that hand-to-hand transmission of viruses occurs. Children serve as the main reservoir for respiratory viruses; they commonly acquire new strains from their schoolmates and pass them on to family members. Fatigue or exposure to drafts doesn't increase susceptibility.

Signs and symptoms
After a 1- to 4-day incubation period, the common cold produces pharyngitis, nasal congestion, coryza, headache, and burning, watery eyes; there may be fever (more common in children), chills, myalgia and arthralgia, malaise, and lethargy. It may also cause a hacking, nonproductive, or nocturnal cough.

As the cold progresses, clinical features develop more fully. After a day, symptoms include copious nasal discharge and a feeling of fullness from the nasopharyngeal and upper bronchial inflammation. Nasal discharge often irritates the nose, adding to discomfort. About 3 days after onset, major signs diminish, but the residual "stuffed up" feeling often persists for a week. Reinfection (with productive cough) is common, but complications (sinusitis, otitis media, pharyngitis, lower respiratory tract infection) are rare. A cold is communicable for 2 to 3 days after the onset of symptoms.

Diagnosis
No explicit diagnostic test exists to isolate the specific organism responsible for the common cold. Consequently, diagnosis rests on the typically mild, localized and afebrile upper respiratory symptoms. Despite infection, WBC and differential are within normal limits. Diagnosis must rule out allergic rhinitis, measles, rubella, and other disorders that produce similar early symptoms. A temperature higher than 100° F. (37.8° C.), severe malaise, anorexia, tachycardia, exudate on the tonsils or throat, petechiae, and tender lymph glands may point to more serious disorders and require additional diagnostic tests.

Treatment
The primary treatment—aspirin, fluids, and rest—is purely symptomatic, as the common cold has no cure. Aspirin eases myalgia and headache; fluids help loosen accumulated respiratory secretions and maintain hydration; and rest is the logical response to the fatigue and weakness that inevitably accompany a cold.

Decongestants can relieve congestion. Throat lozenges relieve soreness. Steam, either cold or hot, encourages expectoration. Nasal douching and sinus drainage aren't necessary except in sinus complications; antibiotics aren't needed except in complications or chronic illness. Pure antitussives (codeine, dextromethorphan) relieve severe coughs but are contraindicated with productive coughs, when cough suppression is harmful. The role of vitamin C remains controversial. In infants, saline nose drops and mucus aspiration with a bulb syringe may be beneficial.

Currently, no known measure can prevent the common cold. Vitamin therapy and ultraviolet irradiation are under investigation. Research using interferon, a protein produced by body cells in response to viral invasion, appears most promising. So far, however, this substance is available only in minute quantities. Mass production is not yet feasible, since interferon can't be synthesized and is species-specific (only human interferon works against human infection).

Additional considerations
• Antibiotics are not effective against the common cold, since most colds result from viruses.
• Symptomatic treatment includes: maintaining bed rest during the first few days (when the cold is communicable); using a lubricant on nostrils to decrease irritation; relieving throat irritation with hard candy or cough drops; increasing fluid intake (tea, soft drinks, fruit juice); and eating light meals (gelatin, toast, cooked cereal).
• Warm baths or heating pads can reduce aches and pains but won't hasten a cure.

- Hot steam or cold mist vaporizers may help congestion. Commercial expectorants are available, but their effectiveness is questionable.
- Overuse of nose drops or sprays may cause rebound congestion.

- To help prevent colds, the patient should minimize contact with people who have colds. To avoid spreading colds, the patient should wash hands often, cover coughs and sneezes, and avoid sharing towels and drinking glasses.

Respiratory Syncytial Virus Infection

Respiratory syncytial virus (RSV) infection results from a subgroup of the myxoviruses resembling paramyxovirus. RSV is the leading cause of lower respiratory tract infections in infants and young children; it's the major cause of pneumonia, tracheobronchitis, and bronchiolitis in this age-group, and a suspected cause of the fatal respiratory diseases of infancy.

Causes and incidence
Antibody titers seem to indicate that few children under age 4 escape contracting some form of RSV, even if it's mild. In fact, RSV is the only viral disease that has its maximum impact during the first few months of life (incidence of RSV bronchiolitis peaks at age 2 months).

This virus creates annual epidemics that occur during the late winter and early spring in temperate climates, and during the rainy season in the Tropics. The organism is transmitted from person to person by respiratory secretions, and has an incubation period of 4 to 5 days.

Reinfection is common, producing milder symptoms than the primary infection. School-age children, adolescents, and young adults with mild reinfections are probably the source of infection for infants and young children.

Signs and symptoms
Clinical features of RSV infection vary in severity, ranging from mild coldlike symptoms to bronchiolitis or bronchopneumonia, and in a few patients, severe, life-threatening lower respiratory tract infections. Generally, symptoms include coughing, wheezing, malaise, pharyngitis, dyspnea, and inflamed mucous membranes in the nose and throat.

Otitis media is a common complication of RSV in infants. RSV has also been identified in patients with a variety of CNS disorders, such as meningitis and myelitis.

Diagnosis
Diagnosis is usually made on the basis of clinical findings and epidemiologic information.
- Cultures of nasal and pharyngeal secretions may show RSV; however, the virus is very labile, so cultures aren't always reliable.
- Serum antibody titers may be elevated, but before 6 months of age, maternal antibodies may impair test results.
- Two recently developed serologic techniques are the indirect immunofluorescent and the enzyme-linked immunosorbent assay (ELISA) methods.
- Chest X-rays help detect pneumonia.

Treatment
Treatment aims to support respiratory function, maintain fluid balance, and relieve symptoms.

Additional considerations
A health care plan must provide support and relief of symptoms. The hospital staff member should:
- monitor respiratory status; observe the rate and pattern of respiration; watch for nasal flaring or retraction, cyanosis, pallor, and dyspnea; listen for or auscultate for wheezing, rhonchi, or other signs of respiratory distress; monitor ar-

terial blood gases.
- maintain a patent airway, and be especially watchful when the patient has periods of acute dyspnea; perform percussion, and provide drainage and suction when necessary; use a croup tent to provide a high-humidity atmosphere; use the semi-Fowler's position to help prevent aspiration of secretions.
- monitor intake and output carefully; watch for signs of dehydration, such as decreased skin turgor; encourage the patient to drink plenty of high-calorie fluids; administer I.V. fluids, as needed.
- promote bed rest; plan care to allow uninterrupted rest.
- hold and cuddle infants; talk to and play with toddlers; offer diversional activities suitable to the child's condition and age; foster parental visits and cuddling; restrain the child only as necessary.
- impose oral secretion precautions; enforce strict handwashing, since RSV may be transmitted from fomites.

Staff members with respiratory illnesses should not care for infants.

Parainfluenza

Parainfluenza refers to any of a group of respiratory illnesses caused by paramyxoviruses, a subgroup of the myxoviruses. Affecting both the upper and lower respiratory tracts, these self-limiting diseases resemble influenza but are milder and seldom fatal. Parainfluenza is rare among adults, but it's widespread among children. Incidence of parainfluenza in children rises in the winter and spring.

Causes
Parainfluenza is transmitted by direct contact or by inhalation of contaminated airborne droplets. Paramyxoviruses occur in four forms—Para 1 to 4—that are linked to several diseases: croup (Para 1, 2, 3), acute febrile respiratory illnesses (1, 2, 3), the common cold (1, 3, 4), pharyngitis (1, 3, 4), bronchitis (1, 3), and bronchopneumonia (1, 3). Para 3 ranks second to respiratory syncytial viruses (RSV) as the most common infecting organism in childhood lower respiratory tract infections. Para 4 rarely causes symptomatic infections in humans.

By age 8, most children demonstrate antibodies to Para 1 and Para 3. Most adults have antibodies to all four types as a result of childhood infections and subsequent multiple exposures. Reinfection is usually less severe and affects only the upper respiratory tract.

Signs and symptoms
After a short incubation period (usually 3 to 6 days), symptoms emerge that are similar to those of other respiratory diseases: sudden fever, nasal discharge, reddened throat (with little or no exudate), chills, and muscle pain. Bacterial complications are uncommon, but in infants and very young children, parainfluenza may lead to croup or laryngotracheobronchitis.

Diagnosis
Parainfluenza infections are usually clinically indistinguishable from similar viral infections. Isolation of the virus and serum antibody titers differentiate parainfluenza from other respiratory illness but are rarely done.

Treatment and additional considerations
Parainfluenza infection may require no treatment, or may require bed rest, antipyretics, analgesics, and antitussives, depending on the severity of the symptoms. Complications, such as croup and pneumonia, require appropriate treatment. No vaccine is effective against parainfluenza. Throughout this illness, respiratory status and temperature should be monitored. The patient should take adequate fluids and rest.

Adenovirus Infection

Adenoviruses cause acute self-limiting febrile infections, with inflammation of the respiratory or the ocular mucous membranes, or both.

Causes and incidence

Adenovirus has 35 known serotypes; it causes five major infections, all of which occur in epidemics. These organisms are common and can remain latent for years; they infect almost everyone early in life (though maternal antibodies offer some protection during the first 6 months of life).

Transmission of adenovirus can occur by direct inoculation into the eye, by the fecal-oral route (adenovirus may persist in the GI tract for years after infection), or by inhalation of an infected droplet. The incubation period is usually less than 1 week; acute illness lasts less than 5 days and can be followed by prolonged asymptomatic reinfection.

Signs and symptoms

Clinical features vary. (See chart below.)

Diagnosis

Definitive diagnosis requires isolation of the virus from respiratory or ocular secretions, or fecal smears; during epidemics, however, typical symptoms alone can confirm diagnosis. Since adenoviral illnesses resolve rapidly, serum antibody titers aren't useful for diagnosis. Adenoviral diseases cause lymphocytosis in children. When they cause respiratory disease, chest X-ray may show pneumonitis.

Treatment

Supportive treatment includes bed rest,

MAJOR ADENOVIRAL INFECTIONS

DISEASE	AGE-GROUP	CLINICAL FEATURES
Acute febrile respiratory illness (AFRI)	Children	Nonspecific coldlike symptoms, similar to other viral respiratory illness: fever, pharyngitis, tracheitis, bronchitis, pneumonitis
Acute respiratory disease (ARD)	Adults (usually military recruits)	Malaise, fever, chills, headache, pharyngitis, hoarseness, and dry cough
Viral pneumonia	Children and adults	Sudden onset of high fever, rapid infection of upper and lower respiratory tracts, skin rash, diarrhea, intestinal intussusception
Acute pharyngoconjunctival fever (APC)	Children (particularly after swimming in pools or lakes)	Spiking fever lasting several days, headache, pharyngitis, conjunctivitis, rhinitis, cervical adenitis
Acute follicular conjunctivitis	Adults	Unilateral tearing and mucoid discharge; later, milder symptoms in other eye
Epidemic keratoconjunctivitis (EKC)	Adults	Unilateral or bilateral ocular redness and edema, preorbital swelling, local discomfort, superficial opacity of the cornea without ulceration
Hemorrhagic cystitis	Children (boys)	Adenoviruria, hematuria, dysuria, urinary frequency

antipyretics, and analgesics. Ocular infections may require corticosteroids and direct supervision by an ophthalmologist. Hospitalization is required in cases of pneumonia (in infants) to prevent death and in epidemic keratoconjunctivitis (EKC) to prevent blindness.

Additional considerations
During the acute illness, respiratory status, and intake and output should be monitored. Analgesics and antipyretics may be needed. Bed rest is important.

To help minimize further spread of the adenoviral disease, all patients should follow proper handwashing techniques to reduce fecal-oral transmission. EKC can be prevented by sterilization of ophthalmic instruments, adequate chlorination in swimming pools, and avoidance of swimming pools during EKC epidemics. Killed virus vaccine (not widely available) and a live oral virus vaccine can prevent adenoviral infection and are recommended for high-risk groups.

Influenza

(Grippe, flu)

Influenza, an acute, highly contagious infection of the respiratory tract, results from three different types of Myxovirus influenzae. It occurs sporadically or in epidemics (usually during the colder months). Epidemics tend to peak within 2 to 3 weeks after initial cases and subside within a month.

Although influenza affects all age-groups, it is particularly prevalent among schoolchildren (aged 6 to 14) and people over age 40. Influenza may be fatal, especially in the elderly and in persons with chronic cardiac, pulmonary, renal, or metabolic diseases. The catastrophic pandemic of 1918 was responsible for an estimated 20 million deaths. The most recent pandemics—in 1957, 1968, and 1977—began in mainland China.

Causes
Transmission of influenza occurs through inhalation of a respiratory droplet from an infected person or by indirect contact, such as the use of a contaminated drinking glass. The influenza virus then invades the epithelium of the respiratory tract, causing inflammation and desquamation.

One of the remarkable features of the influenza virus is its capacity for antigenic variation. Such variation leads to infection by strains of the virus to which little or no immunologic resistance is present in the population at risk. Antigenic variation is characterized as *antigenic drift* (minor changes that occur yearly or every few years) and *antigenic shift* (major changes that lead to pandemics). Influenza viruses are classified into three groups:
• Type A, the most lethal, strikes every

2 to 3 years, with a major new strain occurring every 10 to 15 years.
• Type B strikes every 4 to 6 years, causing epidemics.
• Type C is endemic and causes only sporadic cases.

Signs and symptoms
Following an incubation period of from 24 to 48 hours, flu symptoms begin to appear: sudden onset of chills, temperature of 101° to 104° F. (38.5° to 40° C.), headache, malaise, myalgia (particularly in the back and limbs), a nonproductive cough, and occasionally, laryngitis, hoarseness, conjunctivitis, rhinitis, and rhinorrhea. These symptoms usually subside in 3 to 5 days, but cough and weakness may persist. Fever is usually higher in children than in adults. Also, cervical adenopathy and croup are likely to be associated with

influenza in children. In some patients (especially the elderly), lack of energy and easy fatigability may persist for several weeks.

Fever that persists longer than 3 to 5 days signals the onset of complications. The most common complication is pneumonia, which can be primary influenzal viral pneumonia or secondary to bacterial infection. Influenza may also cause myositis, exacerbation of chronic obstructive pulmonary disease (COPD), Reye's syndrome, and rarely, myocarditis, pericarditis, transverse myelitis, and encephalitis.

Diagnosis

At the beginning of an influenza epidemic, early cases are usually mistaken for other respiratory disorders. Since signs and symptoms are not pathognomonic, isolation of *M. influenzae* through inoculation of chicken embryos (with nasal secretions from infected patients) is essential at the first sign of an epidemic. Nose and throat cultures, and increased serum antibody titers help confirm this diagnosis.

After these measures confirm an influenza epidemic, diagnosis requires only observation of clinical symptoms. Uncomplicated cases show decreased WBCs with an increase in lymphocytes.

Treatment

Treatment of uncomplicated influenza includes bed rest, adequate fluid intake, aspirin or another analgesic-antipyretic to relieve fever and muscle pain, and guaifenesin or another expectorant to relieve nonproductive coughing. Prophylactic antibiotics aren't recommended, because they have no effect on the virus.

Amantadine (an antiviral agent) has proven to be effective in reducing the duration of signs and symptoms in influenza A infection. In influenza complicated by pneumonia, supportive care (fluid and electrolyte supplements, oxygen, assisted ventilation) and treatment of bacterial superinfection with appropriate antibiotics are necessary. No specific therapy exists for cardiac, CNS, or other complications.

Additional considerations

Unless complications occur, influenza doesn't require hospitalization. Like medical treatment, supportive care focuses on relief of symptoms.

• The patient should use mouthwashes and increase his fluid intake. Warm baths or heating pads may relieve myalgia. Nonnarcotic analgesics-antipyretics may be ordered.

• The patient's visitors must be screened as a precautionary measure to protect the patient from bacterial infection and the visitor from influenza.

• The patient must properly dispose of tissues and follow proper handwashing techniques.

• The patient and family should know the signs of developing pneumonia, which include rales, another temperature rise, and coughing accompanied by purulent or bloody sputum.

• The patient will have to return to his normal activities gradually.

Patient education about influenza immunizations, which usually provide protection for 3 to 6 months, is important. High-risk patients and health-care personnel should consider annual inoculations at the start of the flu season (late autumn). However, since these vaccines are made from chicken embryos, they must not be taken by persons who are hypersensitive to eggs, feathers, or chickens. The vaccine administered is based on the previous year's virus and is usually about 75% effective.

All persons receiving the vaccine should be made aware of possible side effects (discomfort at the vaccination site, fever, malaise, and rarely, Guillain-Barré syndrome). Although the vaccine has not been proven harmful to the fetus, it is not recommended for pregnant women, except those who are highly susceptible to influenza, such as those with chronic diseases. For people who are hypersensitive to eggs, amantadine is an effective alternative to the vaccine.

RASH-PRODUCING VIRUSES

Varicella
(Chickenpox)

Varicella is a common, acute, and highly contagious infection caused by the herpesvirus varicella-zoster (V-Z), the same virus that in its latent stage causes herpes zoster (shingles).

Causes and incidence

Chickenpox can occur at any age, but it's most common in 2- to 8-year-olds. Neonatal infection is rare, probably due to transient maternal immunity. Second attacks are also rare. This infection is transmitted by direct contact (primarily, with secretions from the respiratory tract; less often, with skin lesions).

The incubation period lasts from 13 to 17 days. Chickenpox is probably communicable from 1 day before lesions erupt to 6 days after vesicles form (it's most contagious in the early stages of eruption of skin lesions).

Chickenpox has worldwide distribution and is endemic in large cities. Outbreaks occur sporadically, usually in areas with large groups of susceptible children. It affects all races and both sexes equally. Seasonal distribution varies; in temperate areas, incidence is higher during late autumn, winter, and spring.

Most children recover completely. The few who are susceptible to potentially fatal complications include children receiving corticosteroids, antimetabolites, or other immunosuppressives, and those with leukemia, other neoplasms, or immunodeficiency disorders.

Signs and symptoms

Chickenpox produces distinctive signs and symptoms, notably a pruritic rash. During the prodromal phase, the patient has slight fever, malaise, and anorexia. Within 24 hours, the rash typically begins as crops of small, erythematous macules on the trunk or scalp that progress to papules and then clear vesicles

on an erythematous base (the so-called "dewdrop on a rose petal"). The vesicles become cloudy and break easily; then scabs form. The rash spreads to the face and, rarely, to the extremities. New vesicles continue to appear for 3 or 4 days, so the rash contains a combination of red papules, vesicles, and scabs in various stages. Occasionally, chickenpox also produces shallow ulcers on mucous membranes of the mouth, conjunctivae, and genitalia.

The severe pruritus that accompanies this rash may provoke persistent scratching, which can lead to superinfection, and consequent scarring, impetigo, furuncles, and cellulitis. Rare complications include pneumonia, myocarditis, encephalitis, fulminating encephalitis associated with fatty liver (Reye's syndrome), Guillain-Barré syndrome, bleeding disorders, arthritis, nephritis, hepatitis, and acute myositis.

Diagnosis

Diagnosis rests on the characteristic clinical signs, and usually doesn't require laboratory tests. However, the virus can be isolated from vesicular fluid within the first 3 or 4 days of the rash. Giemsa stain distinguishes between V-Z and vaccinia-variola viruses. Serum contains antibodies as early as 7 days after onset.

Treatment

Chickenpox calls for strict isolation until all the vesicles and most of the scabs disappear (usually, for 1 week after the onset of the rash). Children can go back to school, however, if just a few scabs remain, since at this stage, chickenpox is no longer contagious.

Generally, the only treatment required for chickenpox is local or systemic antipruritics: cool bicarbonate of soda baths, calamine lotion, diphenhydramine or another antihistamine. Antibiotics are unnecessary unless bacterial infection develops.

Additional considerations

Health care is supportive and primarily emphasizes patient and family teaching and preventive measures.

The child and his family should be taught how to apply topical antipruritics properly, with stress placed on the importance of good hygiene.

The patient should not scratch the lesions. However, because the need to scratch may be overwhelming, parents should trim the child's fingernails to minimize injury and tie mittens on a very young child. Parents should report signs of complications immediately.

To help prevent chickenpox and its complications, a child exposed to chickenpox should not be admitted to a hospital unit that contains children who receive immunosuppressives or who have leukemia or immunodeficiency disorders. An immunologically vulnerable child who has been exposed to chickenpox should receive V-Z immunoglobulin. This treatment won't prevent the chickenpox, but will lessen the disease's severity.

Rubella

(German measles)

Rubella is an acute, mildly contagious, viral disease that produces a distinctive, 3-day rash and lymphadenopathy. Often considered an early childhood disease, rubella is actually rare in infants and uncommon in preschool children. It occurs most often among children aged 5 to 9, adolescents, and young adults (especially college students and military personnel). Worldwide in distribution, rubella flourishes during the spring, particularly in big cities. Epidemics occur sporadically, as in 1964, when rubella struck more than 12 million people in the United States. This disease is self-limiting, and the prognosis is excellent.

Causes

The rubella virus is transmitted through contact with the blood, urine, stools, or nasopharyngeal secretions of infected persons, and possibly, by means of contact with contaminated articles of clothing. Transplacental transmission, especially during the first trimester of pregnancy, can cause serious birth defects. Humans are the only known hosts for the rubella virus. The period of communicability lasts from approximately 10 days before until 5 days after the rash appears.

Signs and symptoms

In children, after an incubation period of from 16 to 18 days, an exanthematous,

maculopapular rash erupts abruptly. In adolescents and adults, prodromal symptoms—headache, malaise, anorexia, low-grade fever, coryza, lymphadenopathy, and sometimes, conjunctivitis—appear first. Suboccipital, postauricular, and postcervical lymph node enlargement is a hallmark of rubella but is not pathognomonic.

Typically, the rubella rash begins on the face. This maculopapular eruption spreads rapidly, often covering the trunk and extremities within hours. Small, red, petechial macules on the soft palate (Forcheimer spots) may precede or accompany the rash. By the end of the second day, the facial rash begins to fade, but the rash on the trunk may be confluent, and may be mistaken for scarlet fever. The rash continues to fade in the downward order in which it appeared. The rash generally disappears on the third day, but it may persist for 4 or 5 days—sometimes accompanied by mild coryza and conjunctivitis. The rapid appearance and disappearance of the rubella rash distinguishes it from rubeola. Rubella can occur without a rash, but this is rare. Low-grade fever may accompany the rash (99° to 101° F. [37.5° to 38.7° C.]), but it usually doesn't persist after the first day of the rash; rarely, temperature may reach 104° F. (40° C.).

Complications seldom occur in children with rubella, but when they do, they often appear as hemorrhagic problems, such as thrombocytopenia. Young women, however, often experience transient joint pain or arthritis, usually just as the rash is fading. Fever may then recur. These complications usually subside spontaneously within 5 to 30 days.

Diagnosis
The rubella rash, lymphadenopathy, other characteristic signs, and a history of exposure to infected persons usually make the clinical diagnosis. Convalescent serum that shows a fourfold rise in antibody titers confirms it.

Treatment
Since the rubella rash is self-limiting and only mildly pruritic, it doesn't require topical or systemic medication. Treatment consists of aspirin for fever and joint pain. Bed rest isn't necessary, but the patient should be isolated until the rash disappears.

Immunization with the live virus vaccine RA27/3, the only rubella vaccine available in the United States, is necessary for prevention and appears to be more immunogenic than previous vaccines.

Additional considerations
Good health care of the rubella patient includes:
• making the patient as comfortable as possible; giving children books to read or games to play to keep them occupied.

EXPANDED RUBELLA SYNDROME

Congenital rubella is by far the most serious form of the disease. Intrauterine rubella infection, especially during the first trimester, can lead to spontaneous abortion or stillbirth, as well as single or multiple birth defects. (As a rule, the earlier the infection occurs during pregnancy, the greater the damage to the fetus.) The combination of cataracts, deafness, and cardiac disease comprises the classic rubella syndrome. Low birth weight, microcephaly, and mental retardation are other common manifestations. However, researchers now believe that congenital rubella can cause several more disorders, many of which don't appear until later in life. These include dental abnormalities, thrombocytopenic purpura, hemolytic and hypoplastic anemia, encephalitis, giant-cell hepatitis, seborrheic dermatitis, and diabetes mellitus. Indeed, it now appears that congenital rubella may be a lifelong disease. This theory is supported by the fact that the rubella virus has been isolated from urine 15 years after its acquisition in the uterus.

Infants born with congenital rubella should be isolated immediately, because they excrete the virus for a period of from several months to a year after birth. Cataracts and cardiac defects may require surgery. Prognosis depends on the particular malformations that occur. The overall mortality for rubella infants is 6%, but it's higher for babies born with thrombocytopenic purpura, congenital cardiac disease, or encephalitis. Parents of affected children need emotional support and guidance in finding help from community resources and organizations.

• explaining why respiratory isolation is necessary; making sure the patient understands how important it is to avoid exposing pregnant women to this disease.
• reporting confirmed cases of rubella to local public health officials.

Proper administration of rubella vaccine includes:
• obtaining a history of allergies, es-

pecially to neomycin; checking with the doctor before administering the vaccine if the patient has this allergy or if he's had an adverse reaction to an immunization in the past.

• asking women of childbearing age if they're pregnant, and not giving the vaccine if they are or think they may be pregnant; warning women who receive rubella vaccine to use an effective means of birth control for at least 3 months after immunization.

• observing the patient for at least 30 minutes for signs of anaphylaxis after giving the vaccine; keeping epinephrine 1:1,000 handy.

• warning about possible mild fever, slight rash, transient arthralgia (in adolescents), and arthritis (in the elderly).

• suggesting aspirin or acetaminophen for fever.

• advising the patient to apply heat to the injection site for 24 hours after immunization (to help the body absorb the vaccine); suggesting a cold compress to promote vasoconstriction and prevent antigenic cyst formation if swelling persists after the initial 24 hours.

Rubeola

(Measles, morbilli)

Rubeola is an acute, highly contagious paramyxovirus infection that may be one of the most common and the most serious of all communicable childhood diseases. Before the widespread use of measles vaccine, incidence was highest in young children. Use of the vaccine has reduced the occurrence of measles during childhood; as a result, measles is becoming more prevalent in adolescents and adults.

In the United States, prognosis is usually excellent. However, measles is a major cause of death in children in underdeveloped countries, where malnutrition and poor health care are widespread.

Causes and incidence

Measles is spread by direct contact or by contaminated airborne respiratory droplets. The portal of entry is the upper respiratory tract. In temperate zones, incidence is highest in late winter and early spring. Before the availability of measles vaccine, epidemics occurred every 2 to 5 years in large urban areas.

Signs and symptoms

Incubation is from 10 to 14 days. Initial symptoms begin and greatest communicability occurs during a prodromal phase, about 11 days after exposure to the virus. This phase lasts from 4 to 5 days; symptoms include fever, photophobia, malaise, anorexia, conjunctivitis, coryza, hoarseness, and hacking cough.

At the end of the prodrome, Koplik's spots, the hallmark of the disease, appear. These spots look like tiny, bluish-gray specks surrounded by a red halo. They appear on the oral mucosa opposite the molars and occasionally bleed. About 5 days after Koplik's spots appear, temperature rises sharply, spots slough off, and a slightly pruritic rash appears. This characteristic rash starts as faint macules behind the ears, and on the neck and cheeks. These macules become papular and erythematous, rapidly spreading over the entire face, neck, eyelids, arms, chest, back, abdomen, and thighs. When the rash reaches the feet (2 to 3 days later), it begins to fade in the same sequence it appeared, leaving a brownish discoloration that disappears in 7 to 10 days.

The disease climax occurs 2 to 3 days after the rash appears, and is marked by a temperature of 103° to 105° F. (39.5° to 40.5° C.), severe cough, puffy red eyes, and rhinorrhea. About 5 days after the rash appears, other symptoms disappear and communicability ends. Symptoms are usually mild in patients with partial immunity (conferred by administration of gamma globulin) or infants with transplacental antibodies.

Severe infection may lead to secondary bacterial infection and to autoimmune reaction or organ invasion by the virus, resulting in otitis media, pneumonia, and encephalitis. Subacute sclerosing panencephalitis (SSPE), a rare and invariably fatal complication, may develop several years after measles.

Diagnosis

Diagnosis rests on distinctive clinical features, especially the pathognomonic Koplik's spots. Mild measles may resemble rubella, roseola infantum, enterovirus infection, toxoplasmosis, and drug eruptions; laboratory tests are required for a differential diagnosis. If necessary, measles virus may be isolated from the blood, nasopharyngeal secretions, and urine during the febrile period. Serum antibodies appear within 3 days after onset of the rash, and reach peak titers 2 to 4 weeks later.

Treatment and additional considerations

Treatment for measles requires bed rest, relief of symptoms, and respiratory isolation throughout the communicable period (although measles often spreads widely before it's diagnosed). Vaporizers help reduce respiratory irritation. Cough preparations and antibiotics are generally ineffective. Antipyretics can reduce fever. Therapy must also appropriately combat complications.

Parents should be instructed about appropriate supportive measures, especially their child's need for isolation, plenty of rest, and increased fluid intake to avoid dehydration. The discomfort of photophobia may be eased by darkening the room or providing sunglasses. Fever may be reduced with antipyretics and tepid sponge baths.

Parents should watch for and report signs of complications, such as encephalitis, otitis media, and pneumonia.

ADMINISTERING MEASLES VACCINE

The administration procedure includes:
- warning the patient or his parents that possible side effects include anorexia, malaise, rash, mild thrombocytopenia or leukopenia, and fever, which may appear in mild forms, usually within 10 days.
- asking the patient about known allergies, especially to neomycin, since each dose contains a small amount. (However, a patient who's allergic to eggs may receive the vaccine, because it contains only minimal amounts of albumin and yolk components.)
- not giving the vaccine to a pregnant woman (the date of last menstrual period is important) and warning female patients to avoid pregnancy for at least 3 months following vaccination.
- not vaccinating children with untreated tuberculosis, immunodeficiencies, leukemia, lymphoma, or those receiving immunosuppressives. If such children are exposed to the virus, they should receive gamma globulin, which won't prevent measles but will lessen its severity.
- delaying vaccination for 8 to 12 weeks after administration of whole blood, plasma, or gamma globulin, since measles antibodies in these components may neutralize the vaccine.
- watching for signs of anaphylaxis for 30 minutes after vaccination and keeping epinephrine 1:1,000 handy.
- advising application of a warm compress to the vaccination site to facilitate absorption of the vaccine. If swelling occurs within 24 hours after vaccination, the patient should apply cold compresses to promote vasoconstriction and to prevent antigenic cyst formation.

Generally, one bout of measles renders immunity (a second infection is extremely rare and may represent misdiagnosis); infants under 4 months of age may be immune because of circulating maternal antibodies. Measles vaccine isn't administered to children younger than 15 months, except during an epidemic, when infants as young as 6 months may be vaccinated (and reimmunized at 15 months).

Herpes Simplex

Herpes simplex, a recurrent viral infection, is caused by herpesvirus hominis (HVH), one of the most widespread infectious agents. In its most common nongenital form, herpes causes cold sores or fever blisters on the mouth and face. As a genital infection, it's transmitted venereally and is becoming more prevalent. Rarely, herpes infects the eye (herpetic keratoconjunctivitis).

Causes and incidence

Primary HVH is the leading cause of childhood gingivostomatitis. Up to 95% of all herpes simplex infections occur in children under age 5; many infections are overlooked because symptoms are often subclinical. Herpes is equally common in males and in females. Worldwide in distribution, it is most prevalent among children from lower socioeconomic groups who live in crowded environments. Saliva, stools, skin lesions, purulent eye exudate, and urine are potential sources of infection.

Signs and symptoms

Primary infection in childhood may be generalized or localized. After an incubation period of from 2 to 12 days, onset of generalized infection begins with fever and pharyngitis with erythema and edema. After causing brief prodromal discomfort (tingling and itching), typical primary lesions erupt as vesicles on an erythematous base, eventually rupturing and leaving a painful ulcer, followed by a yellowish crust. Healing begins 7 to 10 days after initial onset, and is complete within 3 weeks. Vesicles may form on any part of the oral mucosa, especially the tongue, gingiva, and cheeks. In generalized infection, the vesicles are accompanied by submaxillary lymphadenopathy, increased salivation, halitosis, anorexia, and fever of up to 105° F. (40.5° C.). Herpetic stomatitis may lead to severe dehydration in children. A generalized infection usually runs its course in 4 to 10 days.

Herpetic keratoconjunctivitis is generally unilateral and causes only local symptoms: conjunctivitis with regional adenopathy and blepharitis, and vesicles on the lid. Other ocular symptoms may include excessive lacrimation, edema, chemosis, photophobia, and purulent exudate. Fever and other systemic symptoms are possible but uncommon.

After a primary infection, despite antibody formation, a person becomes a lifelong carrier of the virus, susceptible to recurrent infections. Fever, menses, emotional strain, and overexposure to heat and cold can provoke recurrence and its characteristic vesicular eruptions on the lips (fever blisters) or buccal mucosa. Reinfection doesn't usually progress to generalized symptoms.

Diagnosis

Typical lesions suggest this diagnosis. However, confirmation requires isolation of the virus from local lesions, histologic biopsy, and also serologic tests showing a rise in the level of neutralizing antibodies during convalescence.

Treatment

Generalized primary infection requires an analgesic-antipyretic to reduce fever and relieve oral pain, and perhaps anesthetic mouthwash or lidocaine viscous. (Lidocaine's effect lasts only a few minutes, so it carries a possible risk of overdose.)

Treatment of recurrent infections includes tincture of benzoin for prodromal stages, and later on, petrolatum or any other soothing ointment to prevent cracking and discomfort. Topical antiviral agents aren't usually effective enough to justify their expense, although topical idoxuridine is occasionally useful for eye infections.

Additional considerations

In certain situations, the hospital staff member may be given total responsibility for the management of herpes simplex infection. This includes providing supportive care and being familiar with the medical treatment. Since oral lesions can be quite painful during the acute period, frequent sips of cool liquids or ice pops, a soft, nonirritating diet that requires little chewing, and avoiding irritating acidic drinks like orange juice will increase patient comfort. Analgesics and antipyretics may be needed. Parents of children with this infection should be reassured that starvation or dehydration are unlikely during this brief illness and that recurrent lesions aren't serious. They can apply topical ointments, wearing gloves to avoid direct contact with lesions. In some cases, a 1-hour application of an ice cube within 24 hours of the lesion's appearance will promote rapid healing.

Herpes Zoster
(Shingles)

Herpes zoster is an acute unilateral and segmental inflammation of the dorsal root ganglia caused by infection with the herpesvirus varicella (varicella-zoster, V-Z), which also causes chickenpox. This infection usually occurs in adults; it produces localized vesicular skin lesions confined to a dermatome, and severe neuralgic pain in peripheral areas innervated by the nerves arising in the inflamed root ganglia.

Prognosis is good unless the infection spreads to the brain. Eventually, most patients recover completely, except for possible scarring and, in corneal damage, visual impairment. Occasionally, postherpetic neuralgia may persist for months or years.

Causes

Herpes zoster results from reactivation of varicella virus that has lain dormant in the cerebral ganglia (extramedullary ganglia of the cranial nerves) or the ganglia of posterior nerve roots since a previous episode of chickenpox. Such reactivation may follow trauma, malignancy (especially of the reticuloendothelial system), and local radiation; it provokes acute ganglionitis. Exactly how or why this reactivation occurs isn't clear. Occasionally, herpes zoster arises without any identifiable provocation.

Herpes zoster is found primarily in adults, especially those past age 50. It seldom recurs.

Signs and symptoms

Onset of herpes zoster is characterized by fever and malaise. Within 2 to 4 days, severe deep pain, pruritus, and paresthesia or hyperesthesia develop, usually on the trunk and occasionally on the arms and legs. Such pain may be continuous or intermittent and usually lasts from 1 to 4 weeks. Up to 2 weeks after

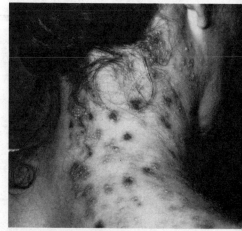

Characteristic skin lesions in herpes zoster are fluid-filled vesicles that dry and form scabs after about 10 days.

the first symptoms, small red nodular skin lesions erupt on the painful areas (commonly, such lesions spread unilaterally around the thorax or vertically over the arms or legs). Sometimes nodules don't appear at all, but when they do, they quickly become vesicles filled with clear fluid or pus. About 10 days after they appear, the vesicles dry and form scabs. When ruptured, such lesions often become infected and, in severe cases, may lead to enlargement of regional lymph nodes; lesions may even become gangrenous.

Occasionally, herpes zoster involves the cranial nerves, especially the trigeminal and geniculate ganglia or the oculomotor nerve. Geniculate zoster may cause vesicle formation in the external auditory canal, ipsilateral facial palsy, hearing loss, dizziness, and loss of taste. Trigeminal ganglion involvement causes eye pain and, possibly, corneal and scleral damage and impaired vision. Rarely, oculomotor involvement causes conjunctivitis, extraocular weakness, ptosis, and paralytic mydriasis.

In rare cases, herpes zoster leads to generalized CNS infection, muscle atrophy, motor paralysis (usually transient), acute transverse myelitis, and ascending myelitis. More often, generalized infection causes acute retention of urine and unilateral paralysis of the diaphragm. In postherpetic neuralgia, a complication most common in the elderly, intractable neurologic pain may persist for years.

Diagnosis
Diagnosis of herpes zoster usually isn't possible until the characteristic unilateral skin lesions develop. Before then, the pain may mimic appendicitis, pleurisy, or other conditions. Examination of vesicular fluid and infected tissue shows eosinophilic intranuclear inclusions and varicella virus. In general, a lumbar puncture shows increased pressure; examination of CSF shows increased protein levels and, possibly, pleocytosis. Differentiation of herpes zoster from localized herpes simplex (which may cause similar lesions) requires staining antibodies obtained from vesicular fluid and identification under fluorescent light.

Treatment
The primary goal of treatment is to relieve itching and neuralgic pain with calamine lotion or another antipruritic; aspirin, possibly with codeine or another analgesic; and occasionally, application of collodion or tincture of benzoin to unbroken lesions. If bacteria have infected ruptured vesicles, treatment includes an appropriate systemic antibiotic.

Trigeminal zoster with corneal involvement calls for application of idoxuridine ointment or another antiviral agent. To help a patient cope with the intractable pain of postherpetic neuralgia, the doctor may order a systemic corticosteroid—such as cortisone or, possibly, corticotropin—to reduce inflammation, tranquillizers, sedatives, or tricyclic antidepressants with phenothiazines. Vidarabine given I.V. also appears to relieve pain. As a last resort, consideration may also be given to transcutaneous peripheral nerve stimulation, cordotomy (used with limited success in "suicidal pain"), or a small dose of radiotherapy.

Additional considerations
The health care plan should emphasize keeping the patient as comfortable as possible and preventing infection. During the acute phase, adequate rest and supportive care can promote proper healing of lesions and reduce the risk of infection.

If calamine lotion has been ordered, it should be applied liberally to the lesions. If lesions are severe and widespread, a wet dressing can provide relief.

If vesicles rupture, a cold compress may be ordered. The patient should avoid scratching the lesions.

To minimize neuralgic pain, analgesics must never be delayed or withheld. They should be given exactly on schedule, because the pain of herpes zoster can be distressingly severe. In postherpetic neuralgia, narcotic analgesics should be avoided because of the danger of addiction with long-term use.

Reassuring the patient that herpetic pain will eventually subside and providing diversionary activity to take his mind off the pain and pruritus will lessen his distress.

Variola
(Smallpox)

Variola was an acute, highly contagious infectious disease caused by the Poxvirus variola. *After a global eradication program, begun in 1967, the World Health Organization pronounced smallpox eradicated on October 26, 1979, 2 years after the last naturally occurring case was reported in Somalia. The last known case of smallpox in the United States was reported in 1949. Although naturally occurring smallpox has been eradicated, variola virus preserved in laboratories remains a possible though unlikely source of infection.*

Smallpox developed in three major forms: variola major *(classic smallpox), which carried a high mortality;* variola minor, *a mild form that occurred in nonvaccinated persons and resulted from a less virulent strain; and* varioloid, *a mild variant of smallpox that occurred in previously vaccinated persons who had only partial immunity.*

Causes

Smallpox affected people of all ages. In temperate zones, incidence was highest during the winter; in the Tropics, during the hot, dry months. Smallpox was transmitted directly by respiratory droplets or dried scales of virus-containing lesions, or indirectly through contact with contaminated linens or other objects. Variola major was contagious from onset until after the last scab was shed.

Signs and symptoms

Characteristically, after an incubation period of from 10 to 14 days, smallpox caused an abrupt onset of chills (and possible convulsive seizures in children), high fever (temperature rose above 104° F. [40° C.]), headache, backache, severe malaise, vomiting (especially in children), marked prostration, and occasionally, violent delirium, stupor, or coma. Two days after onset, symptoms became more severe, but by the third day, the patient began to feel better.

However, he soon developed a sore throat and cough, and lesions appeared on the mucous membranes of the mouth, throat, and respiratory tract. Within days, skin lesions also appeared, and progressed from macular to papular, vesicular, and pustular (pustules were as large as ⅓" [8 mm] in diameter). During the pustular stage, the patient's temperature again rose, and early symptoms returned. By day 10, the pustules began to rupture, and eventually dried and formed scabs. Symptoms finally subsided about 14 days after onset. Desquamation of the scabs took another 1 to 2 weeks, caused intense pruritus, and often left permanently disfiguring scars. In fatal cases, a diffuse dusky appearance came over the patient's face and upper chest. Death was the result of encephalitic manifestations, extensive bleeding from any or all orifices, or from secondary bacterial infections.

Diagnosis

Smallpox was readily recognizable, especially during an epidemic or after known contact.

 The most conclusive laboratory test was a culture of variola virus isolated from an aspirate of vesicles and pustules. Other laboratory tests included microscopic examination of smears from lesion scrapings, and complement fixation to detect virus or antibodies to the virus in the patient's blood.

Treatment and additional considerations
Treatment required hospitalization, with strict isolation, antimicrobial therapy to treat bacterial complications, vigorous supportive measures, and symptomatic treatment of lesions with antipruritics, starting during the pustular stage. Aspirin, codeine, or as needed, morphine relieved pain; I.V. infusions and gastric tube feedings helped meet fluid, electrolyte, and caloric requirements, since pharyngeal lesions often made swallowing difficult. Eye care involved careful cleansing with normal saline.

Roseola Infantum
(Exanthema subitum)

Roseola infantum, an acute, benign, presumably viral infection, usually affects infants and young children (ages 6 months to 3 years). Characteristically, it first causes a high fever and then a rash that accompanies an abrupt drop to normal temperature.

Causes and incidence
Roseola affects boys and girls equally. It occurs year-round but is most prevalent in the spring and fall. Overt roseola, the most common exanthem in infants under age 2, affects 30% of all children; inapparent roseola (febrile illness without a rash) may affect the rest. The mode of transmission isn't known. Only rarely does an infected child transmit roseola to a sibling.

Signs and symptoms
After a 10- to 15-day incubation period, the infant with roseola develops an abruptly rising, unexplainable fever and, sometimes, seizures. Temperature peaks at 103° to 105° F. (39.5° to 40.5° C.) for 3 to 5 days, then drops suddenly. In the early febrile period, the infant may be anorexic, irritable, and listless but doesn't seem particularly ill. Simultaneously with an abrupt drop in temperature, a maculopapular, nonpruritic rash develops, which blanches on pressure. The rash is profuse on the infant's trunk, arms, and neck, and is mild on the face and legs. It fades within 24 hours. Complications are extremely rare.

Diagnosis
Diagnosis requires observation of the typical rash that appears about 48 hours after fever subsides.

INCUBATION AND DURATION OF COMMON RASH-PRODUCING INFECTIONS

INFECTION	INCUBATION (DAYS)	DURATION (DAYS)
Roseola	10-15	3-6
Varicella	10-14	7-14
Rubeola	13-17	5
Rubella	16-18	3
Herpes simplex	2-12	7-21

Treatment and additional considerations

Because roseola is self-limiting, treatment is supportive and symptomatic: antipyretics to lower fever and, if necessary, anticonvulsants to relieve seizures.

Parents should be taught how to lower their infant's fever by giving tepid baths, keeping him in lightweight clothes, and maintaining normal room temperature.

Adequate fluid intake to avoid dehydration is necessary but strict bed rest and isolation are not.

Parents should know that roseola is usually benign, that a short febrile convulsion will not cause brain damage, and that convulsions will cease after fever subsides. Phenobarbital, which may be ordered to prevent convulsions, is likely to cause drowsiness; if it causes stupor, parents should call their doctor immediately.

ENTEROVIRUSES

Herpangina

Herpangina is an acute infection caused by group A coxsackieviruses (usually types 1 through 6, 8, 10, 16, 22, and 23) and, less commonly, by group B coxsackieviruses and echoviruses. The disease characteristically produces vesicular lesions on the mucous membranes of the soft palate, tonsillar pillars, and throat.

Causes

Fecal-oral transfer is the primary mode of transmission. Because of this, herpangina usually affects children under age 10 (except newborns, because of maternal antibodies). It occurs slightly more often in late summer and fall, and can be sporadic, endemic, or epidemic. Herpangina generally subsides spontaneously within 4 to 7 days.

Signs and symptoms

After a 2- to 9-day incubation period, herpangina begins abruptly with a sore throat; pain on swallowing; a temperature of 100° to 104° F. (37.8° to 40° C.) that persists for 1 to 4 days and may cause convulsions; headache; anorexia; vomiting (common in infants); malaise; diarrhea; and pain in the stomach, back of the neck, legs, and arms. After this prodromal stage, 10 to 20 grayish-white papulovesicles appear on the soft palate and, less frequently, on the tonsils, uvula, tongue, and larynx. At first these lesions are only 1 to 2 mm in diameter, but evolve into large, punched out ulcers surrounded by small, inflamed margins.

Diagnosis

 Characteristic lesions in the anterior oral cavity suggest this diagnosis; isolation of the virus from mouth washings or feces, and elevated specific antibody titer confirm it. Other routine laboratory results are normal

---

ENTEROVIRUS FACTS

Enteroviruses (polioviruses, coxsackieviruses, echoviruses) inhabit the gastrointestinal tract. These viruses, among the smallest viruses that affect humans, include 3 known polioviruses, 23 group A coxsackieviruses, 6 group B coxsackieviruses, and 34 echoviruses. They usually infect humans as a result of ingestion of fecally contaminated material, causing a wide range of diseases (hand, foot, and mouth disease; aseptic meningitis; myocarditis; pericarditis; gastroenteritis; poliomyelitis). They can show up in the pharynx, feces, blood, CSF, and CNS tissue. Enterovirus infections are more prevalent in the summer and fall.

except for slight leukocytosis.

Diagnosis requires distinguishing the mouth lesions in herpangina from those in streptococcal tonsillitis (no ulcers; lesions confined to tonsils).

Treatment and additional considerations

Because herpangina subsides spontaneously, treatment is entirely symptomatic, emphasizing measures to reduce fever and prevent convulsions and possible dehydration. Herpangina doesn't require isolation or hospitalization but those caring for the patient must observe careful handwashing techniques and sanitary disposal of excretions.

Parents can treat their child at home by encouraging adequate fluid intake, enforcing bed rest, and administering tepid sponge baths and antipyretics to control fever.

Poliomyelitis
(Polio, infantile paralysis)

Poliomyelitis is an acute communicable disease caused by the poliovirus, and ranges in severity from inapparent infection to fatal paralytic illness. First recognized in 1840, poliomyelitis became epidemic in Norway and Sweden in 1905. Outbreaks reached pandemic proportions in Europe, North America, Australia, and New Zealand during the first half of this century. Incidence peaked during the 1940s and early 1950s, and led to the development of the Salk vaccine.

Minor polio outbreaks still occur, usually among nonimmunized groups, as among the Amish of Pennsylvania in 1979. The disease strikes most often during the summer and fall. Once confined mainly to infants and children—hence the synonym infantile paralysis—poliomyelitis occurs more often today in people over age 15. Among children, it paralyzes boys most often; adults and girls are at greater risk of infection but not of paralysis.

Prognosis depends largely on the site affected. If the central nervous system (CNS) is spared, prognosis is excellent. However, CNS infection can cause paralysis and death. The mortality for all types of poliomyelitis is 5% to 10%.

Causes

The poliovirus has three antigenically distinct serotypes—types I, II, and III—all of which cause poliomyelitis. These polioviruses are found worldwide and are transmitted from person to person by direct contact with infected oropharyngeal secretions or feces. The incubation period ranges from 5 to 35 days—7 to 14 days on the average. The virus usually enters the body through the alimentary tract, multiplies in the oropharynx and lower intestinal tract, then spreads to regional lymph nodes and the blood. Factors that increase the probability of paralysis include pregnancy; old age; localized trauma, such as a recent tonsillectomy, tooth extraction, or inoculation (such as DPT injection); and unusual physical exertion at or just before clinical onset of the disease.

Signs and symptoms

Manifestations of poliomyelitis follow three basic patterns. Inapparent (subclinical) infections comprise 95% of all poliovirus infections. Abortive poliomyelitis (minor illness), which makes up between 4% and 8% of all cases, causes slight fever, malaise, headache, sore throat, inflamed pharynx, and vomiting. The patient usually recovers within 72 hours. Most inapparent and abortive cases of poliomyelitis go unnoticed.

Major poliomyelitis, however, involves the CNS, and takes two forms: nonparalytic and paralytic. Children often show a biphasic course, in which the onset of major illness occurs after recovery from the minor illness stage. Nonparalytic poliomyelitis produces moderate fever, headache, vomiting, lethargy, irritability, and pains in the neck, back, arms, legs, and abdomen. It also causes muscle tenderness and spasms in the extensors of the neck and back, and sometimes in the hamstring and other muscles. (These spasms may be observed during maximum range-of-motion exercises.) Nonparalytic polio usually lasts about a week, with meningeal irritation persisting for about 2 weeks.

Paralytic poliomyelitis usually develops within 5 to 7 days of the onset of fever. The patient displays symptoms similar to nonparalytic poliomyelitis, with asymmetrical weakness of various muscles, loss of superficial and deep reflexes, paresthesia, hypersensitivity to touch, urine retention, constipation, and abdominal distention. The extent of paralysis depends on the level of the spinal cord lesions, which may be cervical, thoracic, or lumbar.

Resistance to neck flexion is a characteristic sign in nonparalytic and paralytic poliomyelitis. The patient will "tripod"—extend his arms behind him for support—when he sits up. He'll also display Hoyne's sign—his head will fall back when he is supine and his shoulders are elevated. From a supine position, he won't be able to raise his legs a full 90°. Paralytic poliomyelitis also causes positive Kernig's and Brudzinski's (contralateral) signs.

When the disease affects the medulla of the brain, it's called bulbar paralytic poliomyelitis, which is the most perilous type. Bulbar paralytic poliomyelitis weakens the muscles supplied by the cranial nerves (particularly the ninth and tenth) and produces symptoms of encephalitis. Other symptoms include facial weakness, dysphasia, difficulty in chewing, inability to swallow or expel saliva, regurgitation of food through the nasal passages, and dyspnea, as well as abnormal respiratory rate, depth, and rhythm, which may lead to respiratory arrest. Fatal pulmonary edema and shock

POLIO PROTECTION

Dr. Jonas Salk's poliomyelitis vaccine, which became available in 1955, has been rightly called one of the miracle drugs of modern medicine. The vaccine contains dead (formalin-inactivated) polioviruses that stimulate production of circulating antibodies in the human body. This vaccine so effectively eliminated poliomyelitis that today it's hard to appreciate how feared the disease once was.

However, even miracle drugs can be improved. Today, the Sabin vaccine, which can be taken orally and is more than 90% effective, is the vaccine of choice in preventing poliomyelitis. The Sabin vaccine is available in trivalent and monovalent forms. The trivalent form (TOPV) contains live but weakened organisms of all three poliovirus serotypes in one solution. TOPV is generally preferred to the monovalent form (MOPV), which contains only one viral type and is useful only when the particular serotype is known.

All infants should be immunized with the Sabin vaccine; pregnant women may be vaccinated without risk. However, because of the risk of contracting poliomyelitis from the vaccine, it's contraindicated in patients with immunodeficiency diseases, leukemia, or lymphoma, and in those receiving corticosteroids, antimetabolites, other immunosuppressives, or radiation therapy. These patients are usually immunized with the Salk vaccine. When possible, immunodeficient patients should avoid contact with family members who are receiving the Sabin vaccine for at least 2 weeks after vaccination. Sabin vaccine is no longer routinely advised for adults unless they're apt to be exposed to this disease or plan travel to endemic areas.

are possible.

Complications—many of which result from prolonged immobility and respiratory muscle failure—include hypertension, urinary tract infection, urolithiasis, atelectasis, pneumonia, myocarditis, cor pulmonale, skeletal and soft-tissue deformities, and paralytic ileus.

Diagnosis

Diagnosis requires isolation of the poliovirus from throat washings early in the disease, from stools throughout the disease, and from CSF cultures in CNS infection. Coxsackievirus and echovirus infections must be ruled out. Convalescent serum antibody titers four times greater than acute titers support a diagnosis of poliomyelitis. Routine laboratory tests are usually within normal limits, though CSF pressure and protein levels may be slightly increased and WBC elevated initially, mostly due to polymorphonuclear leukocytes, which constitute 50% to 90% of the total count. Thereafter normal, the CBC will consist mostly of mononuclear cells.

Treatment

Treatment is supportive, and includes giving analgesics to ease headache, back pain, and leg spasms; morphine is contraindicated because of the danger of additional respiratory suppression. Moist heat applications may also reduce muscle spasm and pain. Bed rest is necessary only until extreme discomfort subsides; in paralytic poliomyelitis, this may take a long time. Paralytic polio also requires long-term rehabilitation using physical therapy, braces, corrective shoes, and in some cases, orthopedic surgery.

Additional considerations

The health care plan must be comprehensive to help prevent complications and to assist polio patients during prolonged convalescence.

During this time the hospital staff member should:
• observe the patient carefully for signs of paralysis and other neurologic damage, which can occur rapidly.
• maintain a patent airway, and watch for respiratory weakness and difficulty in swallowing; perform a tracheotomy, if necessary, to ease respiratory distress and then place the patient on a mechanical ventilator; reassure the patient that his breathing is being supported.
• practice strict aseptic technique during suctioning; use only sterile solutions

to nebulize medications.
• perform a brief neurologic assessment at least once a day, but avoid any vigorous muscle activity; encourage a return to mild activity as soon as the patient is able.
• check blood pressure frequently, especially with bulbar poliomyelitis, which can cause hypertension or shock, due to its effect on the brain stem.
• watch for signs of fecal impaction (due to dehydration and intestinal inactivity); give sufficient fluids to prevent this and to ensure an adequate daily output of low specific gravity urine (1.5 to 2 liters/day for adults).
• monitor the bedridden patient's food intake for an adequate, well-balanced diet; give liquid baby foods, juices, lactose, and vitamins if tube feedings are required.
• give good skin care, reposition the patient often, and keep the bed dry to prevent pressure sores, since muscle paralysis may cause bladder weakness or transient bladder paralysis.
• apply high-top sneakers, or use a footboard to prevent footdrop; use foam rubber pads and sandbags to alleviate discomfort, as needed, and light splints, as ordered.
• wash hands thoroughly after contact with the patient, especially after contact with excretions, to control the spread of the disease; instruct the ambulatory patient to do the same. (Caution: Only hospital personnel who have been vaccinated against poliomyelitis should have direct contact with the patient.)
• provide emotional support; reassure the nonparalytic patient that his chances for recovery are good (long-term support and encouragement are essential for maximum rehabilitation).
• help set up an interdisciplinary rehabilitation program when caring for a paralytic patient.

Such a program should include physical and occupational therapists, doctors, and if necessary, a psychiatrist to help manage the emotional problems that develop in a patient suddenly facing severe physical disabilities.

ARBOVIRUSES

Yellow Fever

Yellow fever is an arbovirus infection that causes sudden illness accompanied by fever, a slow pulse rate, and headache. Although it's endemic in tropical Africa and Central and South America, summer epidemics also occur in temperate zones. However, no outbreaks of yellow fever have occurred in United States cities since 1942. Yellow fever attacks people of all ages and races and of both sexes. Its mortality is usually less than 5%, except during epidemics, when it can be as high as 50%. Recovery confers permanent immunity. Infants born to mothers who have had yellow fever have passive immunity up to age 6 months.

Causes
The transmission of this arbovirus occurs through an insect vector, the *Aedes* mosquito. The incubation period is from 3 to 6 days. The human host then becomes a reservoir for the infection within 3 to 5 days after the original bite.

Signs and symptoms
Symptoms of yellow fever vary and may even be absent. However, the typical presenting symptoms include fever (102.2° to 104° F. [39° to 40° C.]), tachycardia, and conjunctival and facial erythema (with either the mild or severe form of the disease). On the third day, the fever subsides, and if the patient has the mild form, he recovers. Otherwise, the fever continues, and the patient begins to experience severe body pains, extreme prostration, bradycardia, and hemorrhages of varying severity. Such hemorrhaging may occur subcutaneously, through the mucosa of the gastrointestinal tract, mouth, nose, and bladder; it results in oliguria, jaundice, hypotension, delirium, coma, and possibly, death. Hiccups, copious black vomitus, and melena are ominous signs and point to a poor prognosis. Oozing around I.V. sites or vaginal bleeding signals development of disseminated intravascular coagulation (DIC), the most frequent complication of severe yellow fever. This form of yellow fever is usually fatal within 6 to 9 days of clinical onset.

Diagnosis
Abnormal laboratory findings include decreased leukocyte (WBC) count, albuminuria (in 90% of patients), mild hyperbilirubinemia, and bilirubinuria (if patient is jaundiced). Liver biopsy is not recommended because of the high risk of complications. Isolation of the arbovirus from blood or an elevated antibody titer reliably confirms yellow fever.

Treatment and additional considerations
In general, patients with yellow fever need a high-protein, high-carbohydrate

---

PREVENTING YELLOW FEVER

The key to prevention lies in international support of mosquito control programs. Live virus vaccines are very effective (vaccination with the 17-D strain confers immunity for up to 10 years) and are recommended for anyone living in or traveling to endemic areas. The United States requires immunization of all travelers to South America and sub-Sahara Africa. People allergic to eggs or chicken proteins can be vaccinated by scarification.

Hospitalized patients with yellow fever don't require isolation but do need protection from mosquitoes to prevent the spread of the disease.

liquid diet to counter dehydration from vomiting; analgesics and sedatives for headache and myalgia; antipyretics, sponge baths, and bed rest for fever; and saline enemas for constipation.

If yellow fever is severe, I.V. fluid intake and electrolyte balance should be strictly monitored, with careful checks for oliguria, anuria, and hematuria.

Signs of hemorrhage, such as abdom-inal distension, epistaxis, increased lethargy, and decreased level of con-sciousness, should be reported imme-diately. Close monitoring of the results of daily coagulation studies may prevent this development. Blood and blood com-ponents should be readily available if hemorrhage and DIC develop.

All cases of yellow fever must be re-ported to local public health authorities.

Dengue
(Breakbone or dandy fever)

Dengue is an acute, febrile disease caused by group B arboviruses of four distinct serotypes. It occurs endemically during the warmer months in the Tropics and subtropics, especially in Southeast Asia, Polynesia, Micronesia, Tahiti, the Carib-bean, and Central and South America. In the United States, it usually occurs only in travelers returning from endemic areas. While it may cause epidemics, dengue is rarely fatal unless it progresses to dengue hemorrhagic shock syndrome, which has an 8% mortality in children.

Causes and incidence
Dengue is transmitted by the female *Aedes* mosquito, usually *Aedes aegypti*. Within 2 to 15 days of feeding on an infected person, the mosquito vector be-comes permanently infective. Dengue is most common in children under age 14 and in migrant workers.

Signs and symptoms
Immediately after being bitten by an in-fected mosquito, the host may develop a nonspecific fever that lasts from 1 to 3 days. Then, after an incubation period of from 5 to 8 days, typical symptoms include fever, anorexia, headache, flushed face, conjunctival infection, and severe eye, bone, and muscle pain. The fever persists for 5 to 7 days. On the second to sixth day after onset of these symp-toms, itchy, maculopapular scarlatini-form rash may develop on the chest, palms, and soles, with lymphadenopa-thy and loss of taste. On the last day of fever, a petechial rash develops on the arms, legs, axillae, or mucous mem-branes. Remission follows, but residual fatigue may persist for several weeks.

Although dengue is often milder in children, in those under age 10 it some-times leads to hemorrhagic shock syn-drome that begins 2 to 6 days after onset of fever. This causes widespread bleed-ing, with petechiae, ecchymoses, me-lena, nosebleed, bleeding from gums, and hematemesis, accompanied by hypotension, shortness of breath, cya-nosis, vomiting, and hepatomegaly.

Diagnosis
 If patient history does not in-dicate exposure to group B ar-boviruses, serologic tests (complement fixation, hemag-glutination-inhibition, neu-tralization) confirm dengue if they show seroconversion or a fourfold rise in titer. Attempts to isolate the virus—which ne-cessitate inoculating tissue culture with blood, throat washings, urine, and CSF— are usually impractical. Other diagnostic tests show the following:

• *CBC:* leukopenia, granulocytopenia, and mild thrombocytopenia, with increased immature polymorphonuclear cells
• *skin biopsy:* endothelial swelling and

perivascular edema with infiltrates. The characteristic maculopapular rash rules out diseases with similar clinical features, such as malaria, yellow fever, and influenza.

Treatment and additional considerations

Treatment includes nonaspirin analgesics for the relief of severe headache, ocular pain, and myalgia, and I.V. fluid replacement to combat dehydration due to high fever, anorexia, and vomiting. If hemorrhagic shock syndrome develops, patients require close observation and infusion of plasma expanders to relieve hypotension and hemoconcentration. They need blood transfusion only after major hemorrhage or progressively falling hematocrit.

Proper hospital care includes:
• monitoring fluid and electrolyte balance and watching for signs of dehydration (dry mucous membranes, sunken eyeballs).
• reducing fever and preventing convulsions by placing the patient on a hypothermia blanket or by administering a tepid sponge bath (aspirin should not be given, since it aggravates bleeding).
• covering the patient with mosquito netting or making sure the room has screens, to prevent further transmission (if in an area where dengue is endemic).

Travelers to endemic areas should use mosquito netting while sleeping and regularly spray themselves liberally with insect repellent.

Colorado Tick Fever

Colorado tick fever is a benign infection that results from the Colorado tick fever virus, an arbovirus, and is transmitted to humans by a hard-shelled wood tick called Dermacentor andersoni. *The adult tick acquires the virus when it bites infected rodents, and remains permanently infective. Colorado tick fever occurs in the Rocky Mountain region of the United States, mostly in April and May at lower altitudes and in June and July at higher altitudes. Because of occupational or recreational exposure, it's more common in men than in women. Colorado tick fever apparently confers long-lasting immunity against reinfection.*

Signs and symptoms

After a 4- to 5-day incubation period, Colorado tick fever begins abruptly with chills; temperature up to 104° F. (40° C.); severe aching of back, arms, and legs; anorexia; and nausea. Rare clinical effects include vomiting, petechial or maculopapular rashes, and CNS involvement. After several days, symptoms subside but return within 2 to 3 days and continue for an additional 3 days before gradually disappearing.

Diagnosis

Diagnosis requires a history of recent exposure to ticks, an increased antibody titer in convalescent serum as compared with acute serum, and moderate to severe leukopenia.

Treatment and additional considerations

The tick may be removed by grasping it with forceps or gloved fingers and pulling gently. Care should be taken not to crush the tick so it may be positively identified. The wound should then be washed with soap and water. However, if the tick's head remains embedded, immediate surgical removal and tetanus prophylaxis are necessary.

After correct removal of the tick, supportive treatment relieves symptoms, combats secondary infection, and maintains fluid balance. The hospital staff member should:
• be alert for secondary infection.
• monitor fluid and electrolyte balance, and provide replacement accordingly.

- reduce fever with antipyretics and tepid sponge baths.

People working in infested areas may prevent tick-borne infection by wearing protective clothing (long pants tucked into boots, a long-sleeved shirt) and carefully checking their body and scalp for ticks several times a day.

MISCELLANEOUS VIRUSES

Mumps
(Infectious or epidemic parotitis)

Mumps is an acute viral disease caused by a paramyxovirus. It is most prevalent in children older than age 5 but younger than 15. Infants less than 1 year old seldom get this disease because of passive immunity from maternal antibodies. Peak incidence occurs during late winter and early spring. Prognosis for complete recovery is good, although mumps sometimes causes complications.

Causes
The mumps paramyxovirus is found in the saliva of an infected person and is transmitted by droplets or by direct contact. The virus is present in the saliva 6 days before to 9 days after onset of parotid gland swelling; the 48-hour period immediately preceding onset of swelling is probably the time of highest communicability. The incubation period ranges from 14 to 25 days (the average is 18). One attack of mumps (even if unilateral) almost always confers lifelong immunity.

Signs and symptoms
The clinical features of mumps vary widely. An estimated 30% of susceptible

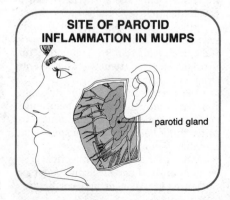

SITE OF PAROTID INFLAMMATION IN MUMPS

parotid gland

people have subclinical illnesses.

Mumps usually begins with prodromal symptoms that last for 24 hours and include myalgia, anorexia, malaise, headache, and low-grade fever, followed by an earache that's aggravated by chewing, parotid gland tenderness and swelling, a temperature of 101° to 104° F. (38.3° to 40° C.), and pain when chewing or when drinking sour or acidic liquids. Simultaneously with the swelling of the parotid gland or several days later, one or more of the other salivary glands may become swollen.

Complications include epididymo-orchitis and mumps meningitis. Epididymo-orchitis occurs in approximately 25% of postpubertal males who contract mumps, and produces abrupt onset of testicular swelling and tenderness, scrotal erythema, lower abdominal pain, nausea, vomiting, fever, and chills. Swelling and tenderness may last for several weeks; epididymitis may precede or accompany orchitis. In 50% of men with mumps-induced orchitis, the testicles show some atrophy, but *sterility after mumps epididymo-orchitis is extremely rare.*

Mumps meningitis complicates mumps in 10% of patients and affects males three to five times more often than females. Symptoms include fever, signs of meningeal irritation (nuchal rigidity, headache, and irritability), vomiting, drowsiness, and a CSF lymphocyte count ranging from 500 to 2,000/mm³. Recovery is almost always complete.

Less common complications include pancreatitis, deafness, arthritis, myocarditis, encephalitis, pericarditis, oophoritis, and nephritis.

Diagnosis
Diagnosis usually rests on typical clinical features, especially parotid gland enlargement and a history of exposure to mumps. Serologic antibody testing can verify the diagnosis when parotid or other salivary gland enlargement is absent. If comparison between a blood specimen obtained during the acute phase of illness and another specimen obtained 3 weeks later shows a fourfold rise in antibody titer, the patient most likely had mumps.

Treatment
Treatment includes analgesics for pain, antipyretics for fever, and adequate fluid intake for dehydration from fever and anorexia. If the patient can't swallow, I.V. fluid replacement should be considered.

Additional considerations
Bed rest until parotid gland swelling subsides is important. Analgesics and warm or cool compresses to the neck may help relieve pain. Antipyretics and tepid sponge baths will help reduce fever. To prevent dehydration, the patient should drink plenty of fluids; to minimize pain and anorexia, he should avoid spicy, irritating foods and those that require a lot of chewing. During the acute phase, the patient should be observed closely for signs of CNS involvement, such as altered level of consciousness and nuchal rigidity.

Because the mumps virus is present in the saliva throughout the course of the disease, respiratory isolation is recommended until symptoms subside.

Live attenuated mumps virus (paramyxovirus) vaccine should be given to patients over age 15 months and to susceptible patients (especially males) who are approaching or are past puberty. Immunization within 24 hours of exposure may prevent or attenuate the actual disease. Immunity lasts at least 9½ years.

All cases of mumps should be reported to local public health authorities.

Infectious Mononucleosis

Infectious mononucleosis is an acute infectious disease caused by the Epstein-Barr virus (EBV), a member of the herpes group. It primarily affects young adults and children, although in children it's usually so mild that it's often overlooked. Characteristically, infectious mononucleosis produces fever, sore throat, and cervical lymphadenopathy (the hallmarks of the disease), as well as hepatic dysfunction, increased lymphocytes and monocytes, and development and persistence of heterophil antibodies. Prognosis is excellent, and major complications are uncommon.

Causes and incidence
Apparently, the reservoir of EBV is limited to humans. Infectious mononucleosis probably spreads by the oral-pharyngeal route, since about 80% of patients carry EBV in the throat during the acute infection and for an indefinite period afterward. It can also be transmitted by blood transfusion, and has

been reported after cardiac surgery as the "post-pump perfusion" syndrome. Infectious mononucleosis is probably contagious from before symptoms develop until the fever subsides and oral-pharyngeal lesions disappear.

Infectious mononucleosis is fairly common in the United States, Canada, and Europe, and both sexes are affected equally. Incidence varies seasonally among college students (most common in the early spring and early fall) but not among the general population.

Signs and symptoms

The symptoms of mononucleosis mimic those of many other infectious diseases including hepatitis, rubella, and toxoplasmosis. Typically, after an incubation period of about 10 days in children and from 30 to 50 days in adults, infectious mononucleosis produces prodromal symptoms, such as headache, malaise, and fatigue. After 3 to 5 days, patients typically develop a triad of symptoms: sore throat, cervical lymphadenopathy, and temperature fluctuations, with an evening peak of 101° to 102° F. (38.3° to 38.9° C.). Splenomegaly, hepatomegaly, stomatitis, exudative tonsillitis, or pharyngitis may also develops.

Sometimes, early in the illness, a maculopapular rash that resembles rubella develops; also, jaundice occurs in about 5% of patients. Major complications are rare but may include splenic rupture, aseptic meningitis, encephalitis, hemolytic anemia, and Guillain-Barré syndrome. Symptoms usually subside about 6 to 10 days after onset of the disease but may persist for weeks.

Diagnosis

Physical examination demonstrating the clinical triad suggests infectious mononucleosis. The following abnormal laboratory results confirm it:
• Leukocyte count increases 10,000 to 20,000/mm³ during the second and third weeks of illness. Lymphocytes and monocytes account for 50% to 70% of the total white cell count; 10% of the lymphocytes are atypical.
• Heterophil antibodies (agglutinins for sheep RBC) in serum drawn during the acute illness and at 3- to 4-week intervals rise to four times normal.
• Indirect immunofluorescence shows antibodies to EBV and cellular antigens. Such testing is usually more definitive than heterophil antibodies.
• Liver function studies are abnormal.

Treatment

Infectious mononucleosis resists preventive and antimicrobial treatment. Consequently, therapy is essentially supportive: relief of symptoms, bed rest during the acute febrile period, and aspirin or another salicylate for headache and sore throat. When throat inflammation is severe, steroids can relieve airway obstruction and prevent tracheotomy. Splenic rupture, an uncommon complication, is marked by abrupt onset of abdominal pain, and requires splenectomy.

Additional considerations

Since uncomplicated infectious mononucleosis doesn't require hospitalization, patient understanding of the disease is essential. Convalescence may take several weeks, usually until WBC returns to normal.
• During the acute illness, bed rest is important. If the patient is a student, he may continue with less demanding school assignments and keep in contact with his friends but should avoid long, difficult projects until after recovery.
• Throat discomfort can be minimized by drinking milk shakes, fruit juices, and broths, and also by eating cool, bland foods. Saline gargles and aspirin should be used, as needed.

Rabies

(Hydrophobia)

Rabies, usually transmitted by an animal bite, is an acute CNS infection caused by an RNA virus. If symptoms occur, rabies is almost always fatal. Treatment soon after a bite, however, may prevent fatal CNS invasion.

Causes and incidence

Generally, the rabies virus is transmitted to a human through the bite of an infected animal that implants virus-containing saliva in or near nerve tissues. Occasionally, it's transmitted through the mucous membrane or the conjunctiva following contact with an infected animal's saliva.

If the bite is on the trunk or an extremity, the virus spreads from the bite site, along sensory nerve pathways to the posterior column of the spinal cord; if the bite is on the face or neck, the virus travels through the cranial nerves, to the brain stem. Because of the density of sensory nerve endings in these areas, a bite on the head, face, neck, or fingers is especially dangerous; so is an extensive and severe wound that exposes a large area of nerve tissue to infected saliva.

In the United States, the vaccination of most dogs has effectively reduced transmission of rabies to humans. Wild animals such as skunks, foxes, bobcats, bats, badgers, and coyotes are now the major vectors.

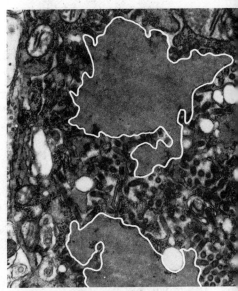

Negri bodies (outlined above) in the brain tissue of an animal suspected to be rabid conclusively confirm rabies. This electron micrograph also shows the rabies virus. Negri bodies are the areas of viral inclusion.

Signs and symptoms

Typically, after an incubation period of from 1 to 3 months, rabies produces local or radiating pain or burning, a sensation of cold, pruritus, and tingling at the bite site. It also produces prodromal symptoms, such as a slight fever (100° to 102° F. [37.8° to 38.9° C.]), malaise, headache, anorexia, nausea, sore throat, persistent loose cough, nervousness, anxiety, irritability, hyperesthesia, photophobia, increased sensitivity to loud noises, pupillary dilation, tachycardia, shallow respirations, and excessive salivation, lacrimation, and perspiration.

About 2 to 10 days after onset of prodromal symptoms, a phase of excitation begins. This phase is characterized by agitation, marked restlessness, anxiety, apprehension, and cranial nerve dysfunction that causes ocular palsies, strabismus, asymmetrical pupillary dilation or constriction, absence of corneal reflexes, weakness of facial muscles, and hoarseness. Severe systemic symptoms include tachycardia or bradycardia, cyclic respirations, urinary retention, and a temperature of about 103° F. (39.4° C.).

About 50% of affected patients exhibit hydrophobia (literally, "fear of water"), during which forceful, painful pharyngeal muscle spasms expel liquids from the mouth and cause dehydration and, possibly, apnea, cyanosis, and death. Difficulty swallowing causes frothy saliva to drool from the patient's mouth. Eventually, even the sight, mention, or thought of water causes uncontrollable pharyngeal muscle spasms and excessive salivation. Between episodes of excitation and hydrophobia, the patient commonly is cooperative and lucid. After about 3 days, excitation and hydrophobia subside and the progressively paralytic, terminal phase of this illness begins.

OMINOUS SIGN

The patient experiences progressive, generalized, flaccid paralysis that ultimately leads to peripheral vascular collapse, coma, and death.

FIRST AID IN ANIMAL BITES

The wound must be washed vigorously with soap and water for at least 10 minutes to remove the animal's saliva. As soon as possible, the wound should be flushed with a viricidal agent, and rinsed with water. After cleansing the wound, a sterile dressing is applied. If possible, the bleeding should not be stopped immediately (unless it's massive), since blood flow helps to cleanse the wound. Also the wound should not be sutured.

Circumstances surrounding the bite are important. If the animal was provoked, it's probably not rabid. The animal should be identified since it may need to be confined for observation.

Diagnosis

Because rabies is fatal unless treated promptly, it should always be suspected in any person who suffers an unprovoked animal bite, unless the animal can be shown to be free of the virus.

 Isolation of the virus from the patient's saliva or throat and examination of his blood for fluorescent rabies antibody (FRA) are considered the most diagnostic tests. Other results typical of rabies include elevated WBC, with increased polymorphonuclear and large mononuclear cells; elevated urinary glucose and protein; and ketonuria.

Confinement of the suspected animal for 10 days of observation by a veterinarian is necessary. If the animal appears rabid, it should be killed and its brain tissue tested for FRA and Negri bodies (oval or round masses that conclusively confirm rabies).

Treatment

Treatment consists of local wound cleansing to reduce the amount of possible rabies virus in the wound and, if diagnosis points to rabies, injection of rabies (duck embryo) vaccine for 14 consecutive days, with boosters 10 to 20 days after the last consecutive injection. A human diploid cell strain (HDCS) rabies vaccine is now available for persons who have reactions to duck embryo vaccine or who have been bitten by animals proven to be rabid. The patient may also require immediate tetanus prophylaxis. Severe or multiple bites, or bites to the head and neck, also require administration of human rabies immune globulin (HRIG). HRIG is preferred to rabies antiserum, because it is less likely to cause allergic reactions.

Additional considerations

Public health authorities will have to determine the vaccination status of the animal in question. If the animal is proven rabid, they will have to identify other people at risk.

Injection sites on the abdomen for the rabies vaccine should be rotated. Any reaction at the injection site should be treated symptomatically.

If rabies develops, aggressive supportive care (even after onset of coma) can make probable death less agonizing. This care includes:
• monitoring cardiac and pulmonary function continuously.
• isolating the patient; wearing a gown and gloves when handling saliva and articles contaminated with saliva; taking precautions to avoid being bitten by the patient during the excitation phase.
• keeping the room dark and quiet.
• establishing communication with the patient and his family; providing psychologic support to help them cope with the patient's agonizing symptoms and probable death.

Various measures may help prevent this disease. Household pets that may be exposed to rabid wild animals should be vaccinated. Persons should not try to touch wild animals, especially if they appear ill or overly docile (a possible sign of rabies). Prophylactic administration of rabies vaccine should be given to high-risk persons, such as farm workers, forest rangers, spelunkers (cave explorers), and veterinarians.

Cytomegalovirus Infection
(Generalized salivary gland disease, cytomegalic inclusion disease [CID])

Cytomegalovirus (CMV) infection is a mild illness caused by the cytomegalovirus, which is a DNA, ether-sensitive virus belonging to the herpes family. The disease occurs worldwide and is transmitted by human contact. About four out of five people over age 35 have been infected with cytomegalovirus, usually during childhood or early adulthood. In most people, the disease is so mild that it's overlooked. However, CMV infection during pregnancy can be severly hazardous to the fetus, possibly leading to stillbirth, brain damage and other birth defects, or severe neonatal illness.

Causes
Cytomegalovirus has been found in the saliva, urine, semen, breast milk, feces, and blood of infected persons. Transmission usually takes place through contact with these infected secretions, which harbor the virus for months or even years. Outbreaks of CMV infection often occur in children's boarding schools and other crowded places. Immunodeficient patients, especially those who have received transplanted organs, run a 90% chance of contracting CMV infection. Recipients of blood transfusions from donors with positive CMV antibodies are also likely victims.

Signs and symptoms
Cytomegalovirus probably spreads through the body in lymphocytes or mononuclear cells to the lungs, liver, and CNS, where it often produces inflammatory reactions. Most patients with CMV infection, however, exhibit mild, nonspecific clinical symptoms, or none at all, even though antibody titers show they have been infected. In these patients, the disease usually runs a benign, self-limiting course. However, immunodeficient patients and those receiving immunosuppressives may develop pneumonia or other secondary infections. Infected infants aged 3 to 6 months usually appear asymptomatic but may develop hepatic dysfunction, hepatosplenomegaly, spider angiomas, pneumonitis, and lymphadenopathy.

Congenital CMV infection is often not apparent at birth, although the infant's urine contains the cytomegalovirus. About 1% of all newborns have CMV infection. The virus can cause serious brain damage that may not show up for weeks or months after birth. It can also produce a rapidly fatal neonatal illness characterized by jaundice, petechial rash, hepatosplenomegaly, thrombocytopenia, hemolytic anemia, microcephaly, psychomotor retardation, mental deficiency, and hearing loss.

CMV can also cause a febrile illness with symptoms that mimic mononucleosis—hepatosplenomegaly, skin rash, lymphadenopathy, and immunologic reactions—in patients who have received multiple blood transfusions (during cardiopulmonary bypass, for example). Immunodeficient patients have a 50% chance of developing such infection, while patients with healthy defenses have only a 5% chance.

Diagnosis
Since an apparently healthy person can excrete the cytomegalovirus in urine, only the discovery of persistent or rising antibody titers, or the isolation of the virus in tissues that were formerly uninfected (through lung or liver biopsies, or blood cultures) justifies a diagnosis of active CMV infection. Increased lymphocytes (with 10% to 20% being atypical) and abnormal liver function tests further support the diagnosis.

Treatment and additional considerations

Treatment aims to relieve symptoms and prevent complications. Most important, parents of children with severe congenital infection need emotional support and counseling to help them accept the possibility of brain damage or even death.

Measures to help prevent CMV infection include: warning immunodeficient patients and pregnant women to avoid persons with confirmed or suspected CMV infection, and urging patients with CMV infection to wash their hands thoroughly to prevent spreading it. This is especially important with young children, who are usually unconcerned with personal hygiene.

Care is needed when handling urine and saliva, or articles contaminated with these or other body secretions. These articles must be disposed of properly. Contaminated linens should be marked for special handling.

Lassa Fever

Lassa fever is an epidemic hemorrhagic fever caused by the Lassa virus, an arenavirus. As many as 100 cases occur annually in western Africa; the disease is rare in the United States. Lassa fever kills up to 50% of its victims, but those who survive its early stages usually recover and acquire immunity to secondary attacks.

Causes

A chronic infection in rodents, Lassa virus is transmitted to humans by contact with infected rodent urine, feces, and saliva (therefore, Lassa fever sometimes strikes laboratory workers). The virus enters the bloodstream, lymph vessels, and respiratory and digestive tracts; it multiplies in cells of the reticuloendothelial system. In the early stages of illness, when the virus is in the throat, human transmission may occur through inhalation of infected droplets.

Signs and symptoms

After a 7- to 15-day incubation period, this disease produces a fever that persists for 2 to 3 weeks, exudative pharyngitis, oral ulcers, lymphadenopathy with swelling of the face and neck, purpura, conjunctivitis, and bradycardia. Severe infection may also cause hepatitis, myocarditis, pleural infection, encephalitis, and permanent unilateral or bilateral deafness. Virus multiplication in reticuloendothelial cells causes capillary lesions that lead to erythrocyte and platelet loss, mild to moderate thrombocytopenia (with a tendency to bleeding), and secondary bacterial infection. Capillary lesions also cause focal hemorrhage in the stomach, small intestine, kidneys, lungs, and brain, and possibly, hemorrhagic shock and peripheral vascular collapse.

Diagnosis

 Isolation of the Lassa virus from throat washings, pleural fluid, or blood confirms the diagnosis. Recent travel to an endemic area and specific antibody titer support this diagnosis.

Treatment and additional considerations

Treatment includes administration of antibiotics (depending on the organism cultured) for secondary bacterial infection, I.V. colloids for shock, analgesics for pain, and antipyretics for fever.

• Fluid and electrolytes, vital signs, and intake and output should be carefully monitored. Signs of infection or shock must be reported immediately.

• Strict isolation is necessary for at least 3 weeks, until throat washings and urine are free of virus. To prevent spread of this contagious disease, all materials contaminated with urine, feces, respiratory secretions, or exudates must be

carefully disposed of or disinfected.
• Good mouth care is important. A soft-bristled brush should be used to avoid irritating mouth ulcers. The hospital dietary department should supply a soft, bland, nonirritating diet.
• All cases of Lassa fever must be reported immediately to local public health authorities.
• According to the Center for Disease Control (CDC) recommendations, the patient should be transferred as soon as possible to one of the few hospitals specially equipped to treat this infection. The CDC can supply the names of these hospitals.

RICKETTSIA

Rocky Mountain Spotted Fever

Rocky Mountain spotted fever (RMSF) is a febrile, rash-producing illness caused by Rickettsia rickettsii *and is transmitted through a tick bite. Endemic throughout the continental United States, RMSF is particularly prevalent in the Southeast and Southwest. RMSF is on the rise because of the increasing popularity of outdoor activities, such as camping and backpacking. Because it's associated with such activities, the incidence is usually higher in the spring and summer.*

RMSF is fatal in about 5% of patients. Mortality rises when treatment is delayed; it also increases in older patients.

Causes
R. rickettsii is transmitted by the wood tick (*Dermacentor andersoni*) in the West and by the dog tick (*Dermacentor variabilis*) in the East. RMSF is transmitted to a human or small animal by a prolonged bite (4 to 6 hours) of an adult tick. Occasionally, this disease is acquired through inhalation or through contact of abraded skin with tick excreta. In most tick-infested areas, 1% to 5% of the ticks harbor R. rickettsii.

Signs and symptoms
The incubation period is usually about 7 days, but it can range anywhere from 2 to 14 days. Generally, the shorter the incubation time, the more severe the infection. Onset of symptoms is usually abrupt, producing a persistent temperature of 102° to 104° F. (38.9° to 40° C.); a generalized, excruciating headache; and aching in the bones, muscles, joints, and back. In addition, the tongue is covered with a thick white coating that gradually turns brown as the fever persists and rises.

Initially, the skin may simply appear flushed. But between days 2 and 5, eruptions begin about the wrists, ankles, or forehead, and within 2 days cover the entire body, including the scalp, palms, and soles. The rash consists of erythematous macules 1 to 5 mm in diameter that blanch on pressure; if untreated, the rash may become petechial and maculopapular. By the third week, the skin peels off and may become gangrenous over the elbows, fingers, and toes.

At onset, the pulse is strong but grad-

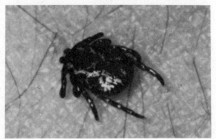

Rocky Mountain spotted fever is transmitted by the prolonged bite of an adult tick.

PATIENT TEACHING AID

How to Prevent Rocky Mountain Spotted Fever

You can prevent Rocky Mountain spotted fever by taking the following precautions:
• Avoid tick-infested areas, if possible. If you must go to a tick-infested area, check your entire body, including scalp, every 3 to 4 hours for attached ticks. Wear protective clothing, such as a long-sleeved shirt, and slacks tucked into firmly laced boots.
• Apply insect repellent to clothes and exposed skin.

• If you find a tick attached to your body, don't crush it, as this may contaminate the bite wound. To detach the tick, place a drop of oil, alcohol, gasoline, or kerosene on it or hold a lighted cigarette near it.
• If you're at high risk (for instance, if you work in a laboratory with rickettsiae, or if you're planning an extended camping trip and will be far from adequate medical facilities), you should receive vaccination against this disease.

This patient teaching aid is intended for distribution to patients by doctors and nurses. It should not be used without a doctor's approval.

---

ually becomes rapid (possibly reaching 150 bpm) and thready.

Rapid pulse and hypotension (less than 90 mmHg systolic) herald imminent death from vascular collapse.

OMINOUS SIGN

Other clinical manifestations include a bronchial cough, rapid respirations (as many as 60/min), anorexia, nausea, vomiting, constipation, abdominal pain, hepatosplenomegaly, insomnia, restlessness, and in extreme cases, delirium. Urinary output falls to half or less of the normal level, and the urine is dark and contains albumin. Complications, though uncommon, include lobar pneumonia, disseminated intravascular coagulation (DIC), and possibly, renal failure.

Diagnosis

Diagnosis generally rests on a history of a tick bite or travel to a tick-infested area and a positive complement fixation test. This test is positive when it shows a fourfold increase in convalescent antibody titer compared with acute titers. Another antibody titer test commonly in use, although not as reliable, is the Weil-Felix reaction, which also shows a fourfold increase between the acute and convalescent sera titer levels. This reaction usually becomes positive after 10 to 14 days; increased titers persist for several months. Blood cultures should also be performed to isolate the organism.

Additional laboratory results consist of a thrombocytopenic platelet count (12,000 to 150,000/mm³) and WBC elevation to 11,000 to 33,000/mm³ during the second week of illness.

Treatment

Treatment requires careful removal of the tick and administration of antibiotics, such as chloramphenicol or tetracycline, until 3 days after the fever subsides. Treatment also includes symptomatic measures, and in DIC, heparin and platelet transfusion.

Additional considerations

• Vital signs should be monitored closely, with special attention given to signs of hypotension and shock. Oxygen therapy and assisted ventilation may be required for pulmonary complications.
• Intake and output must be measured carefully. Decreased urinary output is a possible indicator of renal failure. Antipyretics will help reduce fever, and tepid sponse baths will help reduce dehydration.
• The patient should be turned fre-

quently to prevent decubitus ulcers and pneumonia.
- The patient's nutritional status needs

close attention, as vomiting may necessitate I.V. nutrition or frequent small meals.

Q Fever

An acute systemic disease caused by Coxiella burnetii *(formerly* Rickettsia burnetii*), Q fever was discovered in 1937 during an outbreak of febrile disease among Australian slaughterhouse workers. The "Q" stands for "query." The first case of Q fever in the United States occurred in Montana in 1938; later C.* burnetii *was found in wood ticks in that area. Epidemics broke out during World War II. Q fever usually strikes people exposed to cattle, sheep, or goats, so it's common among laboratory, slaughterhouse, and dairy workers. Prognosis is good and complications are rare; mortality is less than 1%. One attack usually confers lifelong immunity.*

Causes

Ticks carry *C. burnetii*, which resembles other rickettsial organisms but is more resistant to treatment. Humans contract Q fever by inhaling dust contaminated with tick feces (on animal hides, for example), drinking unpasteurized milk from an infected cow, handling infected animal tissues (as in laboratories), and rarely, from tick bites. Person-to-person transmission of *C. burnetii* has not been reported.

Signs and symptoms

After an incubation period of 18 to 21 days, Q fever begins suddenly with severe frontal headache, temperature of 101° to 104° F. (38.3° to 40° C.), chills, pneumonitis, myalgia, malaise, anorexia, nausea, and vomiting. It affects the eyes in various ways—retro-orbital pain, burning, lacrimation, and conjunctival infection. Significantly, Q fever doesn't cause a rash as do other rickettsial infections. It does cause a dry cough, with mild coryza, around the fifth day. Other clinical effects include extreme and persistent disorientation or confusion, neck and back stiffness, chest pain, sore throat, profuse sweating, and marked weight loss. Complications of Q fever include endocarditis (most common in the elderly), hepatitis, pericarditis, meningitis, and optic neuritis.

Diagnosis

Characteristic clinical features and a history of possible exposure to ticks and infected animal tissues or livestock may suggest Q fever. Isolation of *C. burnetii* from guinea pigs inoculated with the patient's serum, sputum, or urine during the febrile phase confirms it, but this is seldom done because an isolated sample of *C. burnetii* is so pathogenic it is difficult to handle safely. A complement fixation test demonstrating a fourfold rise in convalescent serum antibody titers is a safer, more specific way to confirm Q fever. In addition, agglutinins appear early in the disease; half are positive during the first week, more than 90% the second week, and 100% by the fourth week of illness. Chest X-rays may show segmental or lobar infiltrations, much like pneumococcal pneumonia. Differential diagnosis must rule out brucellosis, typhoid, paratyphoid, hepatitis, leptospirosis, and other rickettsial diseases.

Treatment

Tetracycline is the treatment of choice; chloramphenicol is an alternative. However, Q fever tends to resist these medications more than other rickettsial infections do. Antibiotic therapy should continue for at least 5 days after the fever subsides. Complications, such as endocarditis, require appropriate treatment.

Additional considerations

Analgesics should be given for myalgia. Plenty of fluids, aspirin, and tepid sponge baths will help to relieve fever.

Extreme care should be taken when handling sputum and blood, or any articles soiled with them. All contaminated articles must be disposed of properly and promptly.

Patients should be watched closely and complications reported immediately.

To prevent this disease, laboratory, slaughterhouse, and dairy workers, and others who risk exposure to Q fever should be immunized with a vaccine made from formalin-killed *C. burnetii.* They should carefully disinfect and properly dispose of potentially infected placentas, feces, and urine.

All cases of Q fever should be immediately reported to local public health authorities.

Epidemic Typhus

(European, classic, or louse-borne typhus)

The source of epidemic typhus is a small, gram-negative, pleomorphic organism, Rickettsia prowazekii. Typhus occurs worldwide but is more common in cool climates and in areas with poor hygiene and louse infestation. Historically, epidemic typhus is associated with war and famine, and hasn't occurred in the United States since 1921. Mortality may reach 60% in patients older than age 60, and 10% in those between ages 10 and 30. It's seldom fatal in children younger than 10. Death is usually due to renal failure during the second week of illness. With treatment, prognosis is excellent.

Causes

Transmission usually occurs by a body louse vector that feeds on an infected,

---

BRILL-ZINSSER DISEASE

While typhus confers permanent immunity against reinfection, relapses can occur for years after the primary attack. Such relapse is known as Brill-Zinsser disease and results from persistence of latent *Rickettsia prowasekii* in body tissues. Brill-Zinsser disease is a brief illness and seldom produces a rash. Otherwise, it's clinically similar to epidemic typhus and requires the same treatment. An important diagnostic difference is that Brill-Zinsser disease doesn't cause a positive Weil-Felix reaction unless relapse occurs more than 10 years after the primary attack. However, the complement fixation test is usually positive within 4 to 6 days after the onset of symptoms. Like endemic typhus, Brill-Zinsser disease must be reported to local public health authorities.

---

febrile human, and then, itself infected, passes on *R. prowazekii* to its next host. Sometimes inhalation of dried louse feces also causes typhus infection. Direct transmission from human to human doesn't occur.

Signs and symptoms

Generally, the incubation period is from 7 to 14 days—usually 12. Onset is variable but often abrupt. Some patients can pinpoint the exact hour when the illness began. Epidemic typhus produces a severe, intense, intractable headache; nervousness; frightful dreams; potentially fatal hypotension; conjunctival suffusion; deafness; marked stupor (on day 3 or day 4); delirium; and in severe infection, coma (on day 6 or day 7). It also causes facial flushing and a macular rash that erupts on shoulders and axillae between day 4 and day 7 and spreads to the abdomen, chest, back, arms, and legs (rarely to palms and soles). At first, the rash consists of numerous rose spots that blanch under pressure; later, the rash becomes dull red. About 10 days after it appears, the rash becomes brownish-red and fades.

Other symptoms include a slight nonproductive cough; increased respiratory rate; signs of bronchitis, often followed by bronchopneumonia, pleurisy, or empyema; muscular pains that are especially severe in the back and legs; pronounced toxemia; chills; and a temperature up to 104° F. (40° C.) for about 12 to 13 days, followed by a rapid drop.

 Profound stupor, hypotension (blood pressure as low as 80/50) with peripheral vascular collapse, and renal failure herald imminent death.

OMINOUS SIGN

Diagnosis
The Weil-Felix reaction with Proteus OX-19 showing a fourfold rise in agglutination titer is diagnostic and usually occurs between days 8 and 12. This test is positive in 90% of patients with typhus; however, it is also positive in other rickettsial diseases. Complement fixation for group-specific typhus antigens is also usually positive between days 8 and 12; rising antibody titer indicates active infection.

Other laboratory findings include decreased WBC (2,000 to 8,000/mm³), and RBC (3.5 million/mm³) during the second and third weeks.

Treatment
Typhus responds readily to antibiotic therapy with tetracycline, doxycycline, or chloramphenicol. Analgesics and antipyretics can help relieve symptoms. Treatment also includes laundering, delousing, and disinfecting the patient's and his family's clothing, bedding, and home with an insecticide (usually 10% DDT). It also requires delousing the patient and his family with a pediculicide, such as lindane.

Additional considerations
During the acute illness, the hospital staff member should:
• carefully monitor intake and output;

ENDEMIC TYPHUS
Endemic (murine, rat, or flea) typhus is a milder form caused by *Rickettsia typhi* (formerly *Rickettsia mooseri*). Unlike epidemic typhus, the endemic form infects animals, especially rats and mice. It is transmitted to humans by the bites of infected fleas or lice, or by inhalation of contaminated flea feces. Also, unlike epidemic typhus, endemic typhus does occur in the United States, although fewer than 50 cases are reported annually. Mortality averages 2% but is higher in patients over age 50.

Endemic typhus produces a fever, rash, headache, cough, and muscle aches, but these symptoms are less severe than in epidemic typhus. Diagnostic and treatment methods are the same as for epidemic typhus.

A vaccine is not available for endemic typhus, but rat control can prevent it. Endemic typhus must be reported to local public health authorities.

---

keep fluids at a level sufficient to maintain urine output of at least 1,000 ml/day.
• closely monitor vital signs; be especially alert for ominous signs, such as stupor and profound hypotension (moderate hypotension, however, is common in this disease).
• observe safety precautions; use padded side rails to prevent the stuporous patient from harming himself.
• reposition the patient often to avoid skin breakdown.
• give good mouth care.
• warn the patient receiving tetracycline or doxycycline that these drugs may cause candidal overgrowth and photosensitivity; use tetracycline cautiously in patients with impaired renal or hepatic function, since another side effect of this antibiotic is raised BUN; watch for signs of thrombocytopenia, granulocytopenia, and aplastic anemia, if the patient receives chloramphenicol.
• relieve pain with analgesics, as needed; reduce fever with antipyretics and tepid sponge baths.

An attack of epidemic typhus usually

confers permanent immunity. However, to control spread of the disease, the staff member should:
• delouse the patient thoroughly, wearing a gown and gloves; advise the patient and family to launder bedding and clothing, and spray them with insecticide.

• report all cases and also persons who may have been exposed to the local public health department.
• advise persons who risk louse exposure or plan travel to endemic areas to receive two subcutaneous typhus vaccine injections, given at least 4 weeks apart.

Rickettsialpox

Rickettsialpox is a mild, self-limiting disease caused by Rickettsia akari. *It was discovered in 1946 in New York City, then later appeared in New England, Philadelphia, and Cleveland. During that year, approximately 200 cases were reported in New York City alone; incidence has since declined to only a few cases a year, most of them in crowded urban areas. Even without treatment, persons with rickettsialpox usually recover, without complications, in 1 to 2 weeks.*

Causes
The reservoir of *R. akari* is a species of mites called *Allodermanyssus sanguineus* and the common house mouse (*Mus musculi*). The mites acquire this infection from infected house mice and spread it to uninfected house mice through bites. Transmission to humans is through mite bites. Thus, the mite is both reservoir and vector.

Signs and symptoms
Rickettsialpox begins abruptly with severe headache, photophobia, backache, general muscle aches, fever, malaise, and regional lymph node enlargement and tenderness.

Seven to ten days after the patient is bitten by an infected mite, a firm, red, but painless papule appears at the bite site and may at first be overlooked. Eventually, the papule enlarges to 1 to 1.5 cm; about 2 days later, the surrounding area becomes erythematous, vesiculates, dries, and forms a black eschar. About 1 week later, a low-grade fever develops, raising the patient's temperature to 103° to 104° F. (39.4° to 40° C.) and lasting for a week. At the same time, discrete maculopapular erythematous lesions appear randomly distributed over the body (except on palms or soles). Within 1 to 2 days, these lesions vesiculate, then dry, forming black crusts which ultimately fall off, leaving no scars. In mild cases, the rash persists for 2 to 3 days; in severe cases, for 10 days.

Diagnosis
Diagnosis is usually based on characteristic clinical features, especially the presence of an eschar before onset of fever, and a history of exposure to mites.

A complement fixation test confirms this diagnosis: complement-fixing antibodies in convalescent serum increase during the weeks following the illness. This test also rules out chickenpox and other rickettsial diseases.

Treatment and additional considerations
For most patients, treatment consists of antipyretics and tepid sponge baths for fever, analgesics for headache and myalgia, and increased fluid intake to prevent dehydration. For severe infection, treatment includes tetracycline or, if this is ineffective, chloramphenicol. Rodent control programs, prompt garbage collection and incineration, and use of insecticides can prevent this disease.

Scrub Typhus
(Japanese river disease, tsutsugamushi fever)

Scrub typhus is an acute infection caused by Rickettsia tsutsugamushi *and transmitted to humans by mite larvae. Occurring almost exclusively in the western Pacific, Japan, and Southeast Asia, this rickettsial disease infected many soldiers during World War II. Untreated scrub typhus carries a mortality rate as high as 40%; mortality is even higher among the elderly.*

Causes
The primary reservoir for infection includes small rodents such as voles, rats, or bandicoots. Human transmission of *R. tsutsugamushi* (also known as *Rickettsia orientalis*) is through the bite of red mites (during the larval stage) that have fed on infected rodents or acquired the disease transovarially. Human-to-human transmission doesn't occur.

Signs and symptoms
After an incubation period of from 6 to 18 days, symptoms appear suddenly and include a small necrotic ulcer at the bite site in 50% of the patients and severe, intractable headache, delirium, lymphadenopathy (especially of the groin, axillae, and neck), and fever of 104° to 105° F. (40° to 40.6° C.). In 20% of patients, some hearing loss and tinnitus occur.

About 5 to 8 days after onset, a red macular rash appears on the trunk and extends to the arms and legs. This rash may become maculopapular and generally persists for several days but sometimes disappears within a few hours.

During the second week of illness, scrub typhus produces conjunctival congestion, palpable spleen, cough, and chills.

The pulse rate rises to 120 to 140 bpm, while systolic blood pressure falls below 100 mm Hg. Stupor and muscular twitching appear late in this disease and herald impending death unless treatment begins immediately. Complications include secondary bacterial pneumonia, encephalitis, interstitial myocarditis, and circulatory collapse.

Diagnosis

Isolation of *R. tsutsugamushi* confirms scrub typhus. Intraperitoneal inoculation of mice with the patient's blood during the first 10 days of the

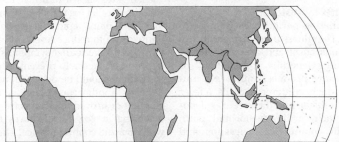

GEOGRAPHIC INCIDENCE OF SCRUB TYPHUS

Brown areas of map show the nearly exclusive incidence of scrub typhus in that part of the world bounded by Pakistan, Australia, and Japan, including the western Pacific islands, India, and most of Southeast Asia.

disease is the most effective means of identifying this organism; in addition, the Weil-Felix reaction is positive (shows a fourfold rise in antibody titer) in 50% to 70% of patients with this disease. Chest X-ray may show pneumonitis.

Treatment and additional considerations

Treatment with chloramphenicol or tetracycline P.O. usually controls fever and alleviates symptoms within 24 to 48 hours. Symptoms may recur if antibiotic therapy is instituted within the first 3 days of illness, but a second course of drug therapy rapidly controls the recurring symptoms.

Adequate fluid and dietary intake should be carefully maintained. Signs of complications, such as pneumonia, should be reported immediately. Fever may be reduced with sponge baths and antipyretics, as ordered. Bed rest is recommended during the acute febrile stage. Mite repellents should be used by individuals likely to be exposed.

Trench Fever

(Wolhynia fever, shin bone fever, His-Werner disease, quintana fever)

Trench fever is a self-limiting illness caused by Rickettsia quintana. *This disease was first recognized during World War I, when over a million men contracted it in the trenches. While a major epidemic hasn't occurred since the 1940s, trench fever still occurs sporadically in Eastern Europe, Asia, North Africa, and Mexico. About 80% of patients recover in 5 to 6 weeks, but elderly and debilitated patients may remain ill for as long as 2 years.*

Causes

Transmission occurs through a body louse (*Pediculus humanus* var. *corporis*) that feeds on an infected human, and then, itself infected (within 5 to 10 days), feeds on a healthy human and excretes *R. quintana* in its feces at the feeding site. When the host rubs the bite, actual infection occurs. Feces containing *R. quintana* enter the wound and infect the bloodstream.

Signs and symptoms

The incubation period lasts from 14 to 30 days. The illness may have an abrupt or insidious onset and may be mild or debilitating. Generally, it lasts for 2 or 3 weeks, and produces multiple symptoms: headache, dizziness, chills, a fever that may subside and then recur, splenomegaly, tachycardia, postorbital pain, nystagmus, conjunctival congestion, and severe pain in the back and legs, especially the shins; also, macules or papules transiently appear on the chest, abdomen, and back.

Diagnosis

In trench fever, blood culture shows *R. quintana,* complement fixation shows elevated antibody titers, and WBC varies between 4,000 and 27,000/mm^3.

Treatment and additional considerations

Trench fever is self-limiting, so therapy consists of relieving symptoms: analgesics to relieve pain, tepid sponge baths and antipyretics to reduce fever, and bed rest for at least 1 week after symptoms subside to prevent relapse. To prevent recurrence, the patient should be deloused, using lindane or another pediculicide, and his clothing destroyed or disinfected. During delousing, a gown and gloves must be worn to avoid contracting lice. The patient must subsequently practice proper hygiene to prevent recurrence.

All cases should be reported to local public health authorities.

PROTOZOA

Malaria

Malaria, an acute infectious disease, is caused by protozoa of the genus Plasmodium: Plasmodium falciparum, Plasmodium vivax, Plasmodium malariae, *and* Plasmodium ovale, *all of which are transmitted to humans by mosquito vectors. Falciparum malaria is the most severe form of the disease. When treated, malaria is rarely fatal; untreated, it's fatal in 10% of victims, usually as a result of complications, such as disseminated intravascular coagulation (DIC). Untreated primary attacks last from a week to a month, or longer. Relapses are common and can recur sporadically for several years. Susceptibility to the disease is universal.*

Malaria is a tropical as well as a subtropical disease, and is most prevalent in Asia, Africa, and Latin America. Incidence in the United States during the last 10 years has ranged from a high of 4,230 cases in 1970 (mainly among military personnel returning from Vietnam) to a low of 222 cases in 1973. Only 10 cases of malaria have actually been contracted in the United States within the last 15 years, resulting from blood transfusions or the use of contaminated needles by drug addicts.

Causes
Malaria literally means "bad air" and for centuries was thought to result from the inhalation of swamp vapors. It is now known that malaria is transmitted by the bite of female *Anopheles* mosquitoes, which abound in humid, swampy areas. When an infected mosquito bites, she injects *Plasmodium* sporozoites into the wound. The infective sporozoites migrate by blood circulation to parenchymal cells of the liver; there they form cystlike structures containing thousands of merozoites. Upon release, each merozoite invades an erythrocyte and feeds on hemoglobin. Eventually, the erythrocyte ruptures, releasing heme (malaria pigment), cell debris, and more merozoites that, unless destroyed by phagocytes, enter other erythrocytes. At this point, the infected person becomes a reservoir of malaria who infects any

mosquito that feeds on him, thus beginning a new cycle of transmission. Hepatic parasites (*P. vivax, P. ovale,* and *P. malariae*) may persist for years in the liver and are responsible for the chronic carrier state. Since blood transfusions and street-drug paraphernalia can also spread malaria, drug addicts have a higher incidence of the disease.

Signs and symptoms
After an incubation period of 12 to 30 days, malaria produces chills, fever, headache, and myalgia, interspersed with

---

HOW TO PREVENT MALARIA

• Drain, fill, and permanently eliminate breeding areas of the *Anopheles* mosquito.
• Install screens in living and sleeping quarters in endemic areas.
• Use a residual insecticide on clothing and exposed skin to prevent mosquito bites.
• Seek treatment for known cases of acute and chronic malaria.
• Do not donate blood if you have a history of malaria or possible exposure to malaria. You may donate blood *following* antimalarial drug treatment and if you are symptomfree for 6 months outside an endemic area.
• Seek suppressive or prophylactic drug therapy before traveling to an endemic area.

periods of well-being (the hallmark of the benign form of malaria). Acute attacks (paroxysms) occur when erythrocytes rupture, and have three stages:

• *cold stage,* lasting 1 to 2 hours, ranging from chills to extreme shaking
• *hot stage,* lasting 3 to 4 hours, characterized by a high fever (temperature up to 107° F. [41.6° C.])
• *wet stage,* lasting 2 to 4 hours, characterized by profuse sweating.

Paroxysms occur every 48 to 72 hours when caused by *P. malariae,* and every 42 to 50 hours with *P. vivax* and *P. ovale.* All three types have low levels of parasitosis and are self-limiting, due to early acquired immunity. Vivax and ovale malaria also produce hepatosplenomegaly. Hemolytic anemia is present in all but the mildest infections.

The most severe form of malaria is caused by *P. falciparum,* the only life-threatening strain. This species produces persistent high fever, orthostatic hypotension, and massive erythrocytosis that leads to capillary obstruction at various sites:

• *cerebral:* hemiplegia, convulsions, delirium, coma
• *pulmonary:* coughing, hemoptysis
• *splanchnic:* vomiting, abdominal pain, diarrhea, melena
• *renal:* oliguria, anuria, uremia.

Because it produces these severe systemic complications, falciparum malaria prevents the respites of well-being common to other malarial infections. During blackwater fever (a complication of *P. falciparum* infection), massive intravascular hemolysis causes jaundice, hemoglobinuria, a tender and enlarged spleen, acute renal failure, and uremia. This dreaded complication is fatal in about 20% of patients.

Diagnosis

A history showing travel to endemic areas, recent blood transfusion, or drug abuse in a person with high fever of unknown origin strongly suggests malaria. But because symptoms of malaria mimic other diseases, unequivocal diagnosis depends on laboratory identification of the parasites in RBCs of multiple peripheral blood smears. The Center for Disease Control can identify infected donors responsible for transfusion malaria through indirect fluorescent serum antibody tests. These tests are unreliable in the acute phase, because antibodies can remain undetectable for 2 weeks after onset of acute malaria.

Supplementary laboratory values that support this diagnosis include decreased hemoglobin, normal to decreased leukocyte count (as low as 3,000/mm³), and protein and leukocytes in urine sediment. In falciparum malaria, serum values reflect DIC: reduced number of platelets (20,000 to 50,000/mm³), prolonged prothrombin time (18 to 20 seconds), prolonged partial thromboplastin time (60 to 100 seconds), and decreased plasma fibrinogen.

Treatment

Malaria is best treated with chloroquine P.O. in all but chloroquine-resistant *P. falciparum.* Within 24 hours after such therapy begins, both symptoms and parasitosis decrease, and the patient usually recovers within 3 to 4 days. If the patient is comatose or vomiting frequently, chloroquine is given I.M. instead. Although rare, toxic reactions include gastrointestinal upset, pruritus, headache, and visual disturbances.

Malaria due to *P. falciparum,* which is resistant to chloroquine, requires treatment with quinine P.O. for 10 days, given concurrently with pyrimethamine and a sulfonamide, such as sulfadiazine. Relapses require the same treatment, or quinine alone, followed by tetracycline.

The only drug effective against the hepatic stage of the disease that is available in the United States is primaquine phosphate, given daily for 14 days. This medication can induce DIC from increased hemolysis of RBCs; consequently, it's contraindicated during an acute attack.

Additional considerations

Hospital care for the malaria patient includes:

• obtaining a detailed patient history, paying particular attention to possible recent travel, foreign residence, blood transfusion, or drug addiction; recording symptom pattern, fever, type of malaria, and any systemic signs.

• assessing the patient upon admission and daily thereafter for fatigue, fever, orthostatic hypotension, disorientation, myalgia, and arthralgia—and planning care with these symptoms in mind; enforcing bed rest during periods of acute illness.

• protecting the patient from secondary bacterial infection by following proper handwashing and aseptic techniques; wearing gloves when handling blood or body fluids containing blood; and wearing a gown and gloves while in contact with the patient, if DIC occurs; discarding needles and syringes in an impervious container designated for incineration; double-bagging all contaminated linen and sending it to the laundry as an isolation item.

• reducing fever by administering antipyretics, as ordered; documenting onset of fever, its duration, and symptoms before and after episodes.

• keeping a strict record of intake and output; monitoring I.V. fluids closely; taking care to avoid fluid overload (especially with *P. falciparum*), since it can lead to pulmonary edema and the aggravation of cerebral symptoms; observing blood chemistry levels for hyponatremia, increased BUN, creatinine, and bilirubin; monitoring urine output hourly, and maintaining it at 40 to 60 ml/hr for an adult and at 15 to 30 ml/hr for a child; immediately reporting any decrease in urine output or onset of hematuria as a possible sign of renal failure (peritoneal dialysis for uremia caused by renal failure may be necessary); administering furosemide or mannitol I.V., as ordered, for oliguria.

• slowly administering packed RBCs or whole blood, while checking for rales, tachycardia, and shortness of breath.

• noting the patient's response if humidified oxygen is ordered because of anemia, particularly any changes in rate

---

ANTIMALARIAL DRUG CONSIDERATIONS

Chloroquine and amodiaquine
• Baseline and periodic ophthalmologic examinations should be performed to detect such side effects as blurred vision, increased sensitivity to light, and muscle weakness.
• Therapy should be altered if muscle weakness appears in a patient on long-term therapy.
• Audiometric examinations should be given before, during, and after therapy, particularly in long-term therapy.
• Excessive exposure to the sun should be avoided to prevent exacerbation of drug-induced dermatoses.

Primaquine
• To be given with meals or antacids.
• Administration should be discontinued if there is a sudden fall in hemoglobin concentration or in erythrocyte or leukocyte count, or marked darkening of the urine, suggesting impending hemolytic reaction.

Pyrimethamine
• To be administered with meals to minimize gastrointestinal distress.
• Blood counts (including platelets) should be checked twice a week. If signs of folic or folinic acid deficiency develop, dosage should be reduced or discontinued while patient receives parenteral folinic acid until blood counts become normal.

Quinine
• To be used with caution in patients with cardiovascular condition. Dosage should be discontinued upon signs of idiosyncrasy or toxicity, such as headache, epigastric distress, diarrhea, rashes, and pruritus, in a mild reaction; or delirium, convulsions, blindness, cardiovascular collapse, asthma, hemolytic anemia, and granulocytosis, in a severe reaction.
• Blood pressure should be monitored frequently during administation of quinine I.V. Rapid administration causes marked hypotension.

---

or character of respirations, or improvement in mucous membrane color.

• watching for and immediately reporting signs of internal bleeding, such as tachycardia, hypotension, and pallor.

• encouraging frequent coughing and

deep breathing, especially if the patient is on bed rest or has pulmonary complications; recording the amount and color of sputum.
• watching for side effects of drug therapy, and taking measures to relieve them.
• making frequent, gentle changes in the patient's position, if he's comatose, and giving passive range-of-motion exercises every 3 to 4 hours. If the patient is unconscious or disoriented, restraints and an artificial airway or padded tongue blade may be needed.
• providing emotional support, especially in critical illness; explaining procedures and treatment to the patient and his family; listening sympathetically, and answering questions; suggesting that other family members be tested for malaria; stressing the need for follow-up care to check the effectiveness of treatment and to manage residual problems.
• reporting all cases of malaria to the local public health authorities.

Amebiasis
(Amebic dysentery)

Amebiasis is an acute or chronic protozoal infection caused by Entamoeba histolytica. *This infection produces varying degrees of illness from no symptoms at all or mild diarrhea, to fulminating dysentery. Extraintestinal amebiasis can induce hepatic abscess, and infections of the lungs, pleural cavity, pericardium, peritoneum, and rarely, the brain.*

Amebiasis occurs worldwide, but is most common in the Tropics, subtropics, and other areas with poor sanitation and health practices. Incidence in the United States averages between 3% and 5%, but may be higher among institutionalized groups in whom fecal-oral contamination is common.

Prognosis is generally good, although complications—such as ameboma, intestinal stricture, hemorrhage or perforation, intussusception, or abscess—increase mortality. Brain abscess, a rare complication, is usually fatal.

Causes
E. histolytica exists in two forms: a cyst (which can survive outside the body) and a trophozoite (which can't survive outside the body). Transmission occurs through ingesting feces-contaminated food or water. The ingested cysts pass through the intestine, where digestive secretions break down the cysts and liberate the motile trophozoites within. The trophozoites multiply, and either invade and ulcerate the mucosa of the large intestine, or simply feed on intestinal bacteria. As the trophozoites are carried slowly toward the rectum, they are encysted and then excreted in feces. Man is the principal reservoir of infection.

Signs and symptoms
The clinical effects of amebiasis vary with the severity of the infestation. *Acute amebic dysentery* causes a sudden high fever of 104° to 105° F. (40° to 40.5° C.) accompanied by chills and abdominal cramping; profuse, bloody diarrhea with tenesmus; and diffuse abdominal tenderness due to extensive rectosigmoid ulcers. *Chronic amebic dysentery* produces intermittent diarrhea that lasts for 1 to 4 weeks and recurs several times a year. Such diarrhea produces 4 to 8 (or, in severe diarrhea, up to 18) foul-smelling mucus- and blood-tinged stools daily in a patient with a mild fever, vague abdominal cramps, possible weight loss, tenderness over the cecum and ascending colon, and occasionally hepatomegaly. Amebic granuloma (ameboma), often mistaken for cancer, can be a complication of the chronic infection. Amebic granuloma produces blood and mucus in the stool and, when granulomatous

tissue covers the entire circumference of the bowel, causes partial or complete obstruction.

Parasitic and bacterial invasion of the appendix may produce typical signs of subacute appendicitis (abdominal pain, tenderness). Occasionally, *E. histolytica* perforates the intestinal wall and spreads to the liver. When it perforates the liver and diaphragm, it spreads to the lungs, pleural cavity, peritoneum, and rarely, the brain.

Diagnosis

 Isolating *E. histolytica* (cysts and trophozoites) in fresh feces or aspirates from abscesses, ulcers, or tissue confirms acute amebic dysentery.

Diagnosis also must distinguish between cancer and ameboma with X-rays, sigmoidoscopy, and stool examination for amebae and palpation of the cecum. In patients with amebiasis, exploratory surgery is hazardous because it can lead to peritonitis, perforation, and pericecal abscess.

Other lab tests that support the diagnosis of amebiasis include:
• indirect hemagglutination test—positive with current or previous infection
• complement fixation—usually positive only during active disease
• barium studies—rule out nonamebic

causes of diarrhea, such as polyps and cancer
• sigmoidoscopy—detects rectosigmoid ulceration; a biopsy may be helpful.

Patients with amebiasis shouldn't have preparatory enemas, since these may remove exudates and destroy the trophozoites, thus interfering with test results.

Treatment and additional considerations

Drugs used to treat amebic dysentery include metronidazole, an amebicide at intestinal and extraintestinal sites; emetine hydrochloride, also an amebicide at intestinal and extraintestinal sites, including the liver and lungs; diiodohydroxyquin, an effective amebicide for asymptomatic carriers; chloroquine, for liver abscesses, not intestinal infections; and tetracycline (in combination with emetine hydrochloride, metronidazole, or paromomycin), which supports the antiamebic effect by destroying intestinal bacteria on which the amebae normally feed.

Patients with amebiasis should:
• avoid drinking alcohol when taking metroxidazole; the combination may produce a serious disulfiram-like reaction.
• avoid metronidazole entirely if they're pregnant; it crosses the placenta and may have an adverse effect on the fetus.

African Trypanosomiasis
(Sleeping sickness)

African trypanosomiasis is a febrile illness caused by protozoa of the genus Trypanosoma, *and transmitted by the bite of the tsetse fly. It occurs in two forms:* Gambian trypanosomiasis, *which is found most often in west and central Africa, and* Rhodesian trypanosomiasis, *a more virulent type that prevails in the drier areas of east Africa. Both types usually affect young men. With prompt and adequate treatment, prognosis is good. Untreated sleeping sickness, however, especially the Rhodesian type, is invariably fatal.*

Causes

The tsetse fly found in tropical west and central Africa, especially along the Congo River and its tributaries, transmits Gam-

bian trypanosomiasis. These flies breed in and around rivers and water holes, and infect humans, the only known reservoirs for this form of the disease. *Glos-*

sina morsitans, a tsetse fly of South Africa, found on savannahs and near bush areas, transmits Rhodesian trypanosomiasis. Along with humans, antelopes, bushbucks, other wild animals, and domestic cattle serve as reservoirs for this form of the disease.

Signs and symptoms

In both forms of trypanosomiasis, a local chancre appears 2 to 3 weeks after the painful bite of the tsetse fly. As the chancre develops, the surrounding area becomes red, swollen, and indurated. The trypanosomes multiply locally, then spread to nearby lymph glands, causing lymph tenderness and enlargement. The posterior cervical lymph nodes become especially prominent (Winterbottom's sign), a hallmark of trypanosomiasis. Other early symptoms include a persistent high temperature (106° F. [41.1° C.]) that lasts for weeks, severe headache, insomnia, inability to concentrate, emaciation, debilitation, and transient, painful edema (especially of the eyes, hands, and feet).

In Rhodesian trypanosomiasis, the trypanosomes invade the CNS, and may induce sudden convulsions, deep coma, and death within a few days. More often, trypanosomiasis produces classic sleeping sickness syndrome—apathy, sleepiness, melancholy, lethargy, and anorexia. This syndrome causes the patient to become progressively obtunded, lethargic, and unresponsive; speech becomes slurred, gait is unsteady, and hands and tongue are tremulous. Finally, he is plunged into a deep sleep from which he can't be aroused. Coma follows, then death—usually from heart failure, meningitis, infection, or malnutrition.

In Gambian trypanosomiasis, systemic symptoms may be delayed from several months to years after the tsetse fly bite; when they finally occur, the patient becomes progressively sleepy and lethargic, with lymphatic tenderness and increasing CNS manifestations. With early treatment, Gambian trypanosomiasis has a 90% cure rate. The Rhodesian form of trypanosomiasis is more often fatal.

Diagnosis

It's important to diagnose African trypanosomiasis early, before the parasites invade the CNS. As a rule, African trypanosomiasis should be suspected in any resident of or visitor to equatorial Africa who shows inexplicable personality changes and general debilitation. Diagnosis of Gambian trypanosomiasis requires identification of trypanosomes in aspirated lymph; in the Rhodesian form, in peripheral blood smears. In both forms, serum contains high IgM antibody titers. In advanced Gambian trypanosomiasis, examination of CSF shows trypanosomes with high IgM antibody titers, mononuclear pleocytosis, and increased protein levels. Diagnosis also must rule out syphilis, tuberculosis, Hodgkin's disease, mononucleosis, and other disorders that produce similar symptoms.

Treatment

In patients without CNS involvement, therapy consists of suramin I.V. at 4-day intervals, until a total dose of 10 g is achieved. This drug is contraindicated in patients with renal disease; in such patients, pentamidine is an effective alternative for use against Gambian trypanosomiasis. In patients with signs of CNS involvement, treatment consists of three courses of melarsoprol given I.V. for 3 days, with 7-day rest periods in between. (In the United States, these drugs are available only from the Center for Disease Control.) Close medical follow-up is required for early detection and treatment of relapses. In Gambian trypanosomiasis, follow-up includes CSF analysis for trypanosomes every 6 months for 2 years; since relapses occur sooner in Rhodesian trypanosomiasis, follow-up should be performed more often.

Additional considerations

A care plan should emphasize a detailed patient history, cautious antibiotic therapy, and supportive care.

• In suspected African trypanosomiasis, a patient history of recent travels is neccessary. The patient's family can tell if his behavior has been out of character lately, or if he's displayed other unusual symptoms.

• Before suramin treatment, a detailed medical history should be obtained. This drug is contraindicated if there is a history of renal disease. Even if there is no such history, a test dose should be given first. Side effects of suramin treatment, which can occur throughout therapy, include papular eruptions, peripheral neuritis, agranulocytosis, and severe renal damage (as evidenced by casts, hematuria, and proteinuria). Severe reactions to melarsoprol therapy, which may also be seen throughout therapy, include exfoliative dermatitis, toxic hepatitis, nephritis, agranulocytosis, and severe encephalopathy, as a result of massive trypanosomal death in the brain. With both suramin and melarsoprol, the I.V. line should be monitored closely, especially for phlebitis and extravasation at the I.V. site.

• Chills and fever may occur. WBC count can document response to therapy and detect relapse.

• Adequate nutrition must be maintained. Keeping a calorie count is helpful.

• Hands should be washed thoroughly, and aseptic technique used to prevent secondary infection.

• To help prevent African trypanosomiasis, visitors to and residents of endemic areas should wear protective clothing and use insect netting and repellents, if possible. Short-term chemoprophylaxis is not recommended for brief visits to such areas.

Giardiasis
(Giardia *enteritis, lambliasis*)

Giardiasis is an infection of the small bowel caused by the symmetrical flagellate protozoan Giardia lamblia. *A mild infection may not produce intestinal symptoms. In untreated giardiasis, symptoms wax and wane; with treatment, recovery is complete.*

Causes
G. lamblia has both cystic and trophozoite stages. Ingestion of *G. lamblia* cysts in fecally contaminated water, or the fecal-oral transfer of cysts by an infected person results in giardiasis. When cysts enter the small bowel, they become trophozoites, and attach themselves with their sucking disks to the bowel's epithelial surface. These trophozoites encyst again, travel down the colon, and are excreted. Unformed feces that pass quickly through the intestine may contain trophozoites as well as cysts.

Humans are the only known hosts for *G. lamblia.* Giardiasis occurs worldwide but is most common in developing countries and other areas where sanitation and hygiene are poor. In the United States, giardiasis is most common in travelers who've recently returned from endemic areas, and in campers who drink unpurified water from contaminated streams. Probably because of frequent hand-to-mouth activity, children are more likely to become infected than adults; hypogammaglobulinemia also appears to predispose persons to this disorder. Giardiasis doesn't confer immunity, so reinfections may occur.

Signs and symptoms
Attachment of *G. lamblia* to the intestinal lumen causes superficial mucosal invasion and destruction, inflammation, and irritation, all of which decrease food transit time through the small intestine and result in malabsorption. Such malabsorption produces chronic gastrointestinal complaints—such as abdominal cramps—and pale, loose, greasy, malodorous, and frequent stools (from 2 to 10 daily), with concurrent nausea. Stools may contain mucus but not pus or blood.

Chronic giardiasis may also cause fatigue and weight loss.

Diagnosis

Suspect giardiasis when travelers to endemic areas or campers who may have drunk unpurified water develop symptoms. Diagnosis requires laboratory examination of a fresh stool specimen for cysts, or examination of duodenal aspirate for trophozoites. A barium X-ray of the small bowel may show mucosal edema and barium segmentation Diagnosis must also rule out other causes of diarrhea and malabsorption.

Treatment

Giardiasis responds readily to a 10-day course of metronidazole. Severe diarrhea may require parenteral fluid replacement to prevent dehydration, if oral fluid intake is inadequate.

Additional considerations

• The patient receiving metronidazole must know the expected side effects of this drug: commonly, headache, anorexia, and nausea; less commonly, vomiting, diarrhea, and abdominal cramps.

He must not drink any alcoholic beverages, since these may provoke a disulfiramlike reaction. If the patient is pregnant, she must not take metronidazole.

• Family members and other suspected contacts must have their stools examined for cysts.

• Hospitalization may be required, although strict isolation is not necessary. However, the patient should have a private room if he's incontinent. When caring for such a patient, handwashing is important, particularly after handling stool specimens. The patient must practice good personal hygiene, particularly proper handwashing technique. Fecal material should be disposed of immediately.

• To help prevent giardiasis, travelers to endemic areas must not drink water or eat uncooked and unpeeled fruits or vegetables (they may have been rinsed in contaminated water). Prophylactic drug therapy isn't recommended. Campers should purify all stream water before drinking it. Epidemic situations must be reported to local public health authorities.

Leishmaniasis

Leishmaniasis refers to a group of illnesses caused by flagellate protozoa of the genus Leishmania. *Types of leishmaniasis include* kala-azar *(visceral leishmaniasis, dumdum fever, black fever),* Old World cutaneous leishmaniasis *(oriental sore, Bagdad boil, Delhi boil, Salek, Penjdeh sore),* New World cutaneous leishmaniasis *(chicle ulcer, forest yaws, bay sore, diffuse cutaneous disease) and* New World mucocutaneous leishmaniasis *(espundia, uta). Old World and New World cutaneous leishmaniases are self-limiting diseases; kala-azar and New World mucocutaneous leishmaniasis are sometimes fatal.*

Causes and incidence

Generally, transmission to a human occurs through the bite of a sandfly that has fed on a canine, a rodent, or rarely, a human infected with *Leishmania*. The organism moves into the skin and bloodstream, localizes in the reticuloendothelial system, and spreads from there.

Kala-azar results from infection by *Leishmania donovani*. It occurs in the Mediterranean area, Russia, China, India, Latin America, and eastern Africa, and is most common in children. The infecting organism in Old World cutaneous leishmaniasis is *Leishmania tropica*. This form is most common near the Mediterranean and in India, Central Asia, and Ethiopia, and primarily affects children. New World cutaneous leish-maniasis results from infection by *L. mexicana* and other species. It is found in Mexico, Central America, and South America, and primarily affects men. *L. braziliensis* causes New World muco-cutaneous leishmaniasis. It occurs in Central America and South America, and is also most prevalent among men.

Signs and symptoms

Kala-azar begins with abdominal swell-ing (due to hepatosplenomegaly) with-out apparent illness. Other clinical features include characteristic darken-ing of skin on forehead, temples, hands, nails, mouth, and abdomen; fever, with temperature rarely over 102° F. (38.9° C.), and with peaks and remissions twice a day; profuse sweating; diarrhea; pur-pura; gingivitis; stomatitis; trophic hair changes; and emaciation.

Old World cutaneous leishmaniasis typically produces a small pruritic pap-ule (or papules), with a crust that even-tually ulcerates. These papules spread through erosion.

New World cutaneous leishmaniasis most commonly produces a chronic, de-structive lesion on the ear. New World mucocutaneous leishmaniasis begins as an ulcer, usually on the oral or nasal mucosa, and may lead to destruction of the soft palate. Overwhelming, second-ary bacterial infection may occur.

Diagnosis

Diagnosis depends on identification of the particular species of *Leishmania* in stained smears from scrapings of edges of lesion. Confirmation may also result from a positive leishmanin skin test. Other tests for kala-azar include flu-orescent antibody test, hemagglutina-tion, or complement fixation.

Treatment and additional considerations

In Old World cutaneous, New World cu-taneous, and New World mucocutaneous leishmaniases, treatment consists of an-timony sodium gluconate I.V. or I.M., cycloguanil pamoate I.M., or as an al-ternative, amphotericin B I.V. Treatment for kala-azar also consists of antimony sodium gluconate I.V. or, if it's ineffec-tive, neostibosan I.V. or pentamidine I.M. (all these drugs, except amphoter-icin B, are available only from the Center for Disease Control). Sometimes treat-ment requires as many as three courses of drug therapy.

The patient must be informed about possible drug side effects. Antimony so-dium gluconate may cause thrombocy-topenia, hypotension, syncope, bradycardia, nausea, vomiting, diar-rhea, colic, dyspnea, severe arthralgia, fever, and dermatitis. Amphotericin B may cause bone marrow depression and renal damage.

The patient should understand how transmission occurs, and what he can do to prevent it, such as routinely spray-ing insecticide on stone walls, dog-houses, and other places where sandflies breed; immediately eliminating trash heaps (also breeding places); and spray-ing the inside and outside of buildings where infection has occurred.

Leishmaniasis must be reported to public health authorities.

South American Trypanosomiasis
(Chagas' disease)

South American trypanosomiasis is caused by the protozoa Trypanosoma cruzi and is most prevalent in Mexico, Central America, and especially, South America, where it's a major health problem. This disease rarely occurs in the United States. Characteristically, South American trypanosomiasis produces an acute stage, with fever, diarrhea, and edema, and a chronic stage, with cardiomyopathy, megaesoph-

*agus, and megacolon. Although caused by a trypanosome, as is African trypano-
somiasis, this disease more closely resembles leishmaniasis (kala-azar). In adults,
acute South American trypanosomiasis is often benign, although chronic cardiomyopathy may develop in men between ages 25 and 44. In children (who make up
most of its victims), it can be severe.*

Causes

This disease usually affects persons who
live in houses made of wood or mud.
These materials are excellent breeding
ground for the reduviid beetle, or cone-
nose bug, which is the vector of South
American trypanosomiasis. The reduviid beetle usually bites humans at night,
near a mucocutaneous junction on the
face, most often on the lip (for which it
has earned the nickname "kissing bug")
or the outer canthus of the eye. This insect habitually deposits feces containing
T. cruzi in or near the bite; rubbing or
scratching the bite introduces the protozoa into the wound. The parasites then
multiply intracellularly in a leishmanial
form, spread to nearby lymph nodes, and
assume trypanosomal form in the bloodstream. Transmission can also occur
transplacentally and through blood
transfusions from an infected person. In
addition to humans, armadillos, opos-
sums, raccoons, and domestic animals
serve as reservoirs for *T. cruzi*.

Signs and symptoms

The incubation period for South American trypanosomiasis is 8 to 14 days. The
insect bite may not leave any identifying
mark, or it may produce an erythematous nodule called a chagoma. Unilateral
eyelid edema and conjunctivitis (Ro-
maña's sign) are hallmarks of this disease. Other early symptoms include fever,
malaise, irritability, anorexia, and diarrhea. Severe infections may cause hypothermia. If meningoencephalitis develops,
death usually follows. However, up to
90% of patients experience spontaneous
remission before the disease reaches this
life-threatening stage.

The chronic stage of South American
trypanosomiasis is characterized by signs
of cardiomyopathy—syncope, irregular
pulse, cardiomegaly, and congestive heart
failure. Ventricular tachycardia or pul-

monary emboli may cause sudden death.
Dysphagia from megaesophagus develops insidiously; the patient has difficulty
drinking liquids and regurgitates what
little he can swallow. Persistent constipation signals megacolon. Congenital
infection by *T. cruzi* may cause stillbirth
or spontaneous abortion in the first
trimester.

Diagnosis

In acute South American trypanosomiasis, diagnosis is based on microscopic
examination of peripheral blood smears
or lymph node fluid for trypanosomes,
preferably during the early febrile period, when they're most numerous. Within
30 days after onset, indirect immunofluorescence and complement fixation tests
are positive for *T. cruzi* antibodies. In
addition, X-rays show a narrowed
esophagogastric junction and proximal
dilation (in extreme dilation, it can even
extend into the right hemithorax). A flat
plate of the abdomen may show dilated
colon filled with feces.

Another way to diagnose this disease
is through xenodiagnosis, in which
laboratory-bred insects, known to be
parasitefree, feed on the patient for 15 to
30 minutes. (A 1% hydrocortisone solution applied to the site of the bite prevents local inflammation.) The feces and
gut contents of these insects are then examined for parasites at 30- to 60-day intervals.

Treatment

Nifurtimox is the drug of choice for treatment of South American trypanosomiasis. This drug is available through the
Center for Disease Control. In chronic
disease, treatment is symptomatic and
essentially the same as for heart failure.
However, diuretics, potassium salts, and
digitalis must be used cautiously because of extreme cardiac irritability.

Megaesophagus and megacolon require surgical intervention.

Additional considerations
• To help detect South American trypanosomiasis, a detailed history, including recent travel, place of birth, and socioeconomic background, should be obtained. Family members may also be infected.

• Signs of cerebral infection which require prompt intervention include nuchal rigidity, obtundation, and rising pulse or respiration rate.

• Accurate intake and output records are important, especially if the patient is taking diuretics or shows signs of congestive heart failure. The patient's pulse should be taken apically.
• If the patient has cardiomyopathy, a low-sodium diet and, before discharge, instruction about how to restrict salt intake are necessary.
• To help prevent this disease in endemic areas, blood donors should be screened, and 0.5% gentian violet should be added to blood products 24 hours before transfusion.

Toxoplasmosis

Toxoplasmosis, one of the most common infectious diseases, results from the protozoa Toxoplasma gondii. *Distributed worldwide, it's less common in cold or hot, arid climates and at high elevations. It usually causes localized infection but may produce significant generalized infection, especially in immunodeficient patients or newborns. Congenital toxoplasmosis may result in stillbirth or serious birth defects.*

Causes
T. gondii exists in trophozoite forms in the acute stages of infection and in cystic forms (tissue cysts and oocysts) in the latent stages. Ingestion of tissue cysts in raw or uncooked meat (heating, drying, or freezing destroys these cysts) or fecal-oral contamination from infected cats transmits toxoplasmosis. However, toxoplasmosis also occurs in vegetarians who aren't exposed to cats, so other means of transmission may possibly exist. Congenital toxoplasmosis follows transplacental transmission from a chronically infected mother or one who acquired toxoplasmosis shortly before or during pregnancy.

Signs and symptoms
Toxoplasmosis acquired late in pregnancy often results in stillbirth or prematurity, and about one third of infants who survive have congenital toxoplasmosis. The later maternal infection occurs in pregnancy, the greater the risk of congenital infection in the infant. Obvious signs of congenital toxoplasmosis include retinochoroiditis, hydrocephalus or microcephalus, cerebral calcification, convulsions, lymphadenopathy, fever, hepatosplenomegaly, jaundice, and rash. Other defects, which may become apparent months or years later, include strabismus, blindness, epilepsy, and mental retardation.

OCULAR TOXOPLASMOSIS

Ocular toxoplasmosis (active retinochoroiditis), characterized by focal necrotizing retinitis, accounts for about 25% of all granulomatous uveitis. It is usually the result of congenital infection, but may not appear until adolescence or young adulthood, when infection is reactivated. Symptoms include blurred vision, scotoma, pain, photophobia, and impairment or loss of central vision. Vision improves as inflammation subsides but usually without recovery of lost visual acuity. Ocular toxoplasmosis may subside after treatment with prednisone.

Acquired toxoplasmosis may cause localized (mild lymphatic) or generalized (fulminating, disseminated) infection. Localized infection produces fever and a mononucleosislike syndrome (malaise, myalgia, headache, fatigue, sore throat) and lymphadenopathy. Generalized infection produces encephalitis, fever, headache, vomiting, delirium, convulsions, and a diffuse maculopapular rash (except on the palms, soles, and scalp). Generalized infection may lead to myocarditis, pneumonitis, hepatitis, and polymyositis.

Diagnosis

 Isolation of *T. gondii* in mice after their inoculation with specimens of body fluids, blood, and tissue, or *T. gondii* antibodies in such specimens confirms toxoplasmosis.

Treatment

Treatment is most effective during the acute stage and consists of drug therapy with sulfonamides and pyrimethamine for approximately 4 weeks and, possibly, folinic acid to control pyrimethamine side effects. No safe, effective treatment exists for chronic toxoplasmosis or toxoplasmosis occurring during the first trimester.

Additional considerations

When caring for patients with toxoplasmosis, careful monitoring during drug therapy and teaching patients measures to prevent complications and control spread of the disease are important.

• Since sulfonamides cause blood dyscrasias, and pyrimethamine depresses bone marrow, hematologic values must be followed closely. Patients should understand the need for regularly scheduled follow-up care.

• All persons should be taught to wash their hands after working with soil (since it may be contaminated with cat oocysts); to cook meat thoroughly or freeze it promptly if it's not for immediate use; to change cat litter daily (cat oocysts become infective 1 to 4 days after excretion); to cover children's sand boxes; and to keep flies away from food (flies transport oocysts).

• All cases of toxoplasmosis should be reported to local public health officials.

HELMINTHS

Trichinosis

(Trichiniasis, trichinellosis)

Trichinosis is an infection caused by larvae of the intestinal roundworm Trichinella spiralis. *It occurs worldwide, especially in populations that eat pork or bear meat. Trichinosis may produce multiple symptoms; respiratory, CNS, and cardiovascular complications; and rarely, death.*

Causes

Transmission is through ingestion of uncooked or undercooked meat that contains *T. spiralis* cysts. Such cysts are found primarily in swine, less often in dogs, cats, bears, foxes, wolves, and marine animals. These cysts result from the animals' ingestion of similarly contaminated flesh. In swine, such infection results from eating table scraps or raw garbage.

After gastric juices free the worm from the cyst capsule, it reaches sexual maturity in a few days. The female roundworm burrows into the intestinal mucosa, and reproduces. Larvae are then transported through the lymphatic system and the bloodstream. They become embedded as cysts in striated muscle, especially in the diaphragm, chest, arms, and legs. Human-to-human transmission does not take place.

Signs and symptoms

In the United States, trichinosis is usually mild and seldom produces symptoms. When symptoms do occur, they vary with the stage and degree of infection:

• *Stage 1*—Invasion: Occurs 1 week after ingestion. Release of larvae and reproduction of adult *T. spiralis* cause anorexia, nausea, vomiting, diarrhea, abdominal pain, and cramps.

• *Stage 2*—Dissemination: Occurs 7 to 10 days after ingestion. *T. spiralis* penetrates the intestinal mucosa and begins to migrate to striated muscle. Symptoms include edema, especially of the eyelids or face; muscle pain, particularly in extremities; and occasionally, itching and burning skin, sweating, skin lesions, a temperature of 102° to 104° F. (38.9° to 40° C.), and delirium; and in severe respiratory, cardiovascular, or CNS infections, palpitations and lethargy.

• *Stage 3*—Encystment: Occurs during convalescence—generally 1 week later. *T. spiralis* larvae invade muscle fiber and become encysted.

Diagnosis

A history of ingestion of raw or improperly cooked pork or pork products, with typical clinical features, suggests trichinosis, but infection may be difficult to prove. Stools may contain mature worms and larvae during the invasion stage. Skeletal muscle biopsies can show encysted larvae 10 days after ingestion; and, if available, analyses of contaminated meat also show larvae.

Skin testing may show a positive histamine-like reactivity 15 minutes after intradermal injection of the antigen (within 17 to 20 days after ingestion). However, such a result may remain positive for up to 5 years after exposure. Elevated acute and convalescent antibody titers (determined by flocculation tests 3 to 4 weeks after infection) confirm this diagnosis.

Other abnormal results include elevated serum glutamic oxalic transaminase (SGOT), serum glutamic pyruvic transaminase (SGPT), creatinine phosphokinase, and lactic dehydrogenase during the acute stages, and elevated eosinophil count (up to 15,000/mm³). Normal or increased CSF lymphocyte level (to 300/mm³) and increased protein levels indicate CNS involvement.

Treatment and additional considerations

Thiabendazole effectively combats this parasite during the intestinal stage; severe infection (especially CNS invasion) may warrant glucocorticoids to combat inflammation.

• A patient history should include information about recent ingestion of pork products and the methods used to store and cook them.

• Fever can be reduced with alcohol rubs, tepid baths, cooling blankets, or antipyretics. Muscular pain can be relieved with analgesics, enforced bed rest, and proper body alignment. Affected muscle areas should not be touched, since this may cause pain.

• Decubitus ulcers can be prevented by frequently repositioning the patient and gently massaging bony prominences.

• Possible side effects of thiabendazole are nausea, vomiting, dizziness, dermatitis, and fever.

• Bed rest is important. Sudden death from cardiac involvement may occur in a patient with moderate to severe infection who has resumed activity too soon. The patient should continue bed rest into the convalescent stage to avoid a serious relapse and possible death.

Trichinosis can be prevented by properly cooking and storing susceptible meats (pork and meat from carnivores); internal meat temperatures should reach 131° F. (55.0° C.) unless the meat has been cured or frozen.

Travelers to foreign countries or to very poor areas in the United States should avoid eating pork.

All cases of trichinosis should be reported to local public health authorities.

Toxocariasis
(Visceral larva migrans, [VLM])

Toxocariasis is a chronic, frequently mild syndrome common in children that is caused by the ingestion of Toxocara (roundworm) larvae and their migration from the intestine to various organs and tissues. This syndrome primarily affects preschool children (boys twice as often as girls), but also, on occasion, adult gardeners and mentally retarded persons. Toxocariasis probably occurs worldwide.

Causes
Toxocariasis follows the ingestion of soil that contains infective ova of *Toxocara canis* (common roundworm in dogs) or, less often, *Toxocara cati* (feline roundworm). No known method exists to destroy *Toxocara* ova in the soil. Carrier animals may be infected in utero and can begin to pass ova in feces as early as 3 weeks after birth; at age 6 months they harbor mature roundworms. From several weeks to months after ingestion, the ova hatch in the intestine and become first-stage larvae. After they mature to second-stage larvae, they migrate through lymphatic and vascular channels to all parts of the body, continuing to live as larvae in tissue for several years.

Signs and symptoms
Most often, toxocariasis produces fever, cough, rales, and wheezing in pulmonary infestation, and hepatomegaly and hepatic granuloma formation in hepatic infestation; less often it produces nausea, vomiting, weight loss, and malnutrition. Invasion of additional body systems produces lymphadenopathy, splenomegaly, ataxia, seizures, convulsions, and hemiparesis. Ocular lesions, strabismus, or vision loss may develop several years after infection.

Diagnosis
Persistent pulmonary symptoms or hepatomegaly suggests toxocariasis in any young child who has a dog, a history of pica, or eosinophilia. The following abnormal test results confirm it:
- massive leukocytosis ($\geq$100,000/mm^3), with hypereosinophilia ($\geq$3,000/mm^3)
- precipitating serum antibody to *T. canis*
- liver biopsy shows *T. canis* larvae
- bentonite flocculation, hemagglutination, and skin tests may further support the diagnosis.

Siblings of a child with confirmed toxocariasis should also be checked for *T. canis* infection.

Treatment
Toxocariasis is self-limiting; treatment usually necessitates no more than the relief of symptoms.

Thiabendazole and diethylcarbamazine citrate may decrease the number of viable larvae in tissues, but do not completely eliminate them. In ocular infections, such drugs should be given cautiously, if at all, since the destruction of the larvae produces an inflammatory reaction in the host (conjunctivitis, uveitis) that may further damage ocular function. The concomitant administration of corticosteroids minimizes such reactions. Bronchodilators like theophylline effectively alleviate respiratory distress and wheezing.

Additional considerations
Isolation of patients is not required. When examining a patient for toxocariasis, the hospital staff member should:
- obtain a thorough history of the patient's habits, especially pica.
- explain the disease and how it's transmitted to both patient and family; stress the importance of washing hands before eating to the patient.

If the patient is hospitalized, the staff member should:
- monitor vital signs for deterioration,

especially in a patient with respiratory, ocular, or CNS infection.
• if a patient is having seizures, keep the side rails up at all times, keep an airway or padded tongue blade available, and report changes in level of consciousness.

To prevent this disease:
• pet owners should worm their dogs and cats during the first 6 months of life; after that, they should establish regular worming schedules.
• children's play areas should be protected from animal feces.

Hookworm Disease
(Uncinariasis)

Hookworm disease is an infection of the upper intestine caused by Ancylostoma duodenale—*Old World form, found in the eastern hemisphere*—or Necator americanus—*New World form, found in the western hemisphere. Sandy soil, high humidity, a warm climate, and failure to wear shoes all favor transmission of this disease. In the United States, hookworm disease is most common in the Southeast.*

Although hookworm infection can cause respiratory and cardiac complications, it's rarely fatal, except in debilitated persons or infants under age 1.

Causes
Both forms of hookworm disease are transmitted to humans through direct skin penetration (usually in the foot) by hookworm larvae in soil contaminated with feces containing hookworm ova. These ova develop into infectious larvae in 7 to 10 days. Larvae travel through the lymphatics to the pulmonary capillaries, where they penetrate alveoli and move up the bronchial tree to the trachea and epiglottis. There they are swallowed. When they reach the small intestine, they mature, attach to the jejunal mucosa, and suck blood, oxygen, and glucose from the intestinal wall. These mature worms then deposit ova, which are excreted in the stool, starting the cycle anew. Hookworm larvae mature in approximately 5 to 6 weeks.

Signs and symptoms
Most cases of hookworm disease produce few symptoms and may be overlooked until worms are passed in the stool. The earliest signs include irritation, pruritus, and edema at the site of entry, sometimes accompanied by secondary bacterial infection, with pustule formation. When the larvae reach the lungs, they may cause pneumonitis and hemorrhage, with

fever, sore throat, rales, and cough. Finally, intestinal infection may cause fatigue, nausea, weight loss, dizziness, melena, and uncontrolled diarrhea. In severe and chronic infection, anemia from blood loss may lead to cardiomegaly (a result of increased oxygen demands), heart failure, and generalized massive edema.

Diagnosis
 Identification of hookworm ova in the stool confirms the diagnosis. Anemia suggests severe chronic infection. In infected patients, blood studies show:
• hemoglobin 5 to 9 g (in severe case)
• leukocyte count as high as 47,000/mm^3
• eosinophil count of 500 to 700/mm^3.

Treatment
Treatment for hookworm infection includes administering mebendazole or pyrantel, and providing an iron-rich diet or iron supplements to prevent or correct anemia.

Additional considerations
If a patient is suspected of having a hookworm infection, the hospital staff mem-

ber should:

• obtain a complete history, with special attention to travel or residency in endemic areas; note the sequence and onset of symptoms; interview the family and other close contacts to see if they have any symptoms.

• carefully assess the patient, noting signs of entry, lymphedema, and respiratory status.

If the patient has confirmed hookworm infestation, the staff member should:

• segregate the incontinent patient.

• wash hands thoroughly after every patient contact.

• administer oxygen for severe anemia (the oxygen should be humidified, because the patient may already have upper airway irritation from the parasites); encourage coughing and deep breathing to stimulate removal of blood or secretions from involved lung areas and to

prevent secondary infection; plan care to allow frequent rest periods, since the patient may tire easily; reposition the patient often to prevent skin breakdown, if anemia causes immobility.

• closely monitor intake and output; note quantity and frequency of diarrheal stools; dispose of feces promptly, and wear gloves when doing so.

• weigh the patient daily to help assess nutritional status; emphasize the importance of good nutrition, with particular attention to foods high in iron and protein; explain that, if ordered, iron supplements will darken stools; administer anthelmintics on an empty stomach but without a purgative.

• educate the patient in proper handwashing technique and sanitary disposal of feces to help prevent reinfection; stress the need to wear shoes in endemic areas.

Ascariasis

(Roundworm infection)

Ascariasis, an infection caused by Ascaris lumbricoides, *occurs worldwide, but is most common in tropical areas with poor sanitation and in the Orient, where farmers use human feces as fertilizer. In the United States, it's more prevalent in the South, particularly among 4- to 12-year-olds.*

Causes and incidence

A. lumbricoides is a large roundworm resembling the common earthworm. Its transmission to humans occurs through ingestion of soil contaminated with human feces that harbor A. lumbricoides ova. Such ingestion may occur directly (in children who eat contaminated soil) or indirectly (by eating improperly washed raw vegetables grown in contaminated soil). Ascariasis never passes directly from person to person.

After ingestion of A. lumbricoides ova, the ova hatch and release larvae, which penetrate the intestinal wall and eventually reach the lungs through the bloodstream. After remaining about 10 days in pulmonary capillaries and alveoli, the larvae migrate to the bronchioles, bron-

chi, trachea, and epiglottis. There they are swallowed, and return to the small intestine, to mature into adult worms.

Signs and symptoms

Ascariasis produces two phases: early pulmonary and prolonged intestinal. Mild intestinal infection may cause only vague stomach discomfort. Often the first clue of ascariasis infection is vomiting a worm or passing a worm in the stool. Severe infection, however, causes stomach pain, vomiting, restlessness, disturbed sleep, and in extreme cases, intestinal obstruction. Larvae migrating by the lymphatic and the circulatory systems cause symptoms that vary with location; for instance, when they invade the lungs, pneumonitis may result.

Diagnosis

 Identifying ova or adult worms in a patient's stool or mouth is the key to diagnosis. When migrating larvae invade alveoli, other conclusive tests include X-rays that show characteristic bronchovascular markings: infiltrates, patchy areas of pneumonitis, and widening of hilar shadows. These findings usually accompany a CBC that shows eosinophilia.

Treatment

Anti-ascaris drug therapy, the primary treatment, uses pyrantel (the drug of choice) or piperazine to temporarily paralyze the worms, permitting peristalsis to expel them. Mebendazole is also used to block helminth nutrition. These drugs are up to 95% effective, even after a single dose. In multiple helminth infection, one of these three anti-ascaris drugs should always be the first treatment; using some other anthelmintic first may stimulate *A. lumbricoides* perforation into other organs. No specific treatment exists for migratory infection, as anthelmintics only affect mature worms.

In intestinal obstruction, nasogastric suctioning controls vomiting. When suctioning can be discontinued, piperazine is instilled and the tube clamped. If vomiting does not occur, a second dose of piperazine is given orally 24 hours later. If this is ineffective, treatment probably requires surgery.

Additional considerations

• Although isolation is unnecessary, properly disposing of feces and soiled linen, and careful handwashing after patient contact are important.
• Good mouth care should be followed if the patient is receiving nasogastric suction.
• The patient can prevent reinfection by washing hands and cleaning fingernails thoroughly, and by bathing and changing underwear and bed linens daily.
• All the drugs used in ascariasis treatment have possible side effects. Piperazine may cause stomach upset, dizziness, and urticaria; this drug is contraindicated in convulsive disorders. Pyrantel may cause stomach upset, headache, dizziness, and skin rash. Mebendazole may cause abdominal pain and diarrhea.
• All cases of ascariasis should be reported to local public health authorities for investigation of environmental sources.

Trichuriasis

(Whipworm disease)

Trichuriasis is a nematode infection of the cecum and the anterior portions of the large intestine. It occurs worldwide, especially in tropical countries, where poverty and unsanitary conditions favor its spread, and is most prevalent in children aged 5 to 15. Generally, prognosis is good, but massive infections can cause potentially fatal anemia and abdominal complications.

Causes

Whipworms—so named because of their distinctive whiplike shape—enter the human body in food contaminated with soil containing embryonated ova. After these ova attach to the small bowel, they mature and then migrate to the cecum and the large intestine. Embedding most of their length in the intestinal mucosa, they take up residence in the bowel for perhaps as long as 15 to 20 years. About 90 days after ingestion, female whipworms start producing ova—as many as 3,000 to 10,000 a day. The ova are then excreted in feces. After about 3 weeks in warm, moist soil, they become infective, and if ingested, start a new cycle of infection.

Signs and symptoms

The severity of symptoms depends on the degree of infection. Mild trichuriasis may be asymptomatic, but extensive infection can cause intermittent abdominal pain, localized tenderness, nausea, vomiting, constipation, bloody or mucoid diarrhea, weight loss, weakness, anemia (each whipworm ingests a small amount of blood), and in children, rectal prolapse. Appendiceal lumen obstruction produces signs of appendicitis. Complications include secondary infection of the colon.

Diagnosis

Diagnosis hinges on identification of whipworm ova in stool. Eosinophil count is moderately elevated; in chronic trichuriasis, the hemoglobin count is significantly lowered, reflecting anemia. Unfortunately, trichuriasis often eludes diagnosis until surgery is performed for suspected appendicitis.

Treatment and additional considerations

Trichuriasis usually responds to a 3-day course of mebendazole; severe cases may require a second course of therapy, as well as blood transfusions for anemia. Isolation is not necessary.

When treating a patient with trichuriasis, the hospital staff member should:
• obtain a complete patient history; ask about living conditions and eating habits; check family members and playmates for signs of infection.
• monitor vital signs and record weight loss after diagnosis; check skin for cyanosis from anemia, or loss of turgor from dehydration.
• observe stools for blood loss; be sure fresh stool specimens are taken to the laboratory immediately.
• wash hands thoroughly before and after patient contact, especially after handling urine or feces; instruct the patient to wash his hands carefully, particularly after using the bathroom and before eating; wear a gown and gloves when handling the patient, bedpans, or soiled linen in suspected secondary bacterial enteritis.
• report rectal prolapse; apply a moist sterile gauze sponge to the prolapsed mucosa to prevent drying; document and report observed whipworms.
• reposition the patient often, and give good skin care to prevent decubitus ulcers in the cachectic patient.
• encourage the patient to eat a balanced diet, high in protein and iron, and to get plenty of rest.
• tell the patient to report for periodic stool specimen examinations before stopping treatment.
• instruct residents of endemic areas to wash their hands carefully before eating, especially after handling soil, and to avoid contaminating soil with human feces, to help prevent this disease.

Taeniasis

(Tapeworm disease, cestodiasis)

Taeniasis is a parasitic infestation by Taenia saginata *(beef tapeworm),* Taenia solium *(pork tapeworm),* Diphyllobothrium latum *(fish tapeworm), or* Hymenolepis nana *(dwarf tapeworm). Taeniasis is usually a chronic, benign intestinal disease; however, infestation with* T. solium *may cause dangerous systemic and CNS symptoms if larvae invade the brain and striated muscle of vital organs.*

Causes

T. saginata, T. solium, and D. latum are transmitted to humans by ingestion of beef, pork, or fish that contains tapeworm cysts. Gastric acids break down these cysts in the stomach, liberating them to mature, fasten to the intestinal wall, and form ova that are passed in

COMMON TAPEWORM INFESTATION

TYPE	SOURCE OF INFECTION	INCIDENCE	CLINICAL FEATURES
Taenia saginata (beef tapeworm)	Uncooked or undercooked infected beef	Worldwide but prevalent in Europe and East Africa	Crawling sensation in the perianal area caused by worm segments that have been passed rectally; intestinal obstruction and appendicitis due to long worm segments that have twisted or curled in the intestinal lumen
Taenia solium (pork tapeworm)	Uncooked or undercooked infected pork	Highest in Mexico, Latin America; lowest among Muslims and Jews	Seizures, headaches, personality changes; often overlooked in adults
Diphyllobothrium latum (fish tapeworm)	Uncooked or undercooked infected fresh water fish, such as pike, trout, salmon, and turbot	Finland, northern U.S.S.R., Japan, Alaska, Australia, the Great Lakes region of the United States, Switzerland, Chile, and Argentina	Anemia (hemoglobin as low as 6 to 8 g)
Hymenolepis nana (dwarf tapeworm)	No intermediate host; parasite passes directly from person to person via ova passed in stool. Inadequate handwashing facilitates its spread.	Most common tapeworm in humans; particularly prevalent among institutionalized mentally retarded children and in underdeveloped countries.	Dependent on patient's nutritional status and number of parasites; often no symptoms with mild infestation; with severe infestation, anorexia, diarrhea, restlessness, dizziness, and apathy.

the feces. Transmission of *H. nana* occurs directly from person to person and doesn't require an intermediate host; this parasite fully matures and completes its life cycle in the intestine.

Diagnosis

In all types of tapeworm infestation, diagnosis requires laboratory observation of tapeworm ova or body segments in feces. Since ova aren't excreted continuously, confirmation may require multiple specimens. A supporting dietary or travel history helps confirm this diagnosis.

Treatment

Treatment with niclosamide offers a cure in up to 95% of patients. In beef, pork, and fish tapeworm infestation, the drug is given once; in dwarf tapeworm infestation, for 5 to 7 days. (This drug is available from the Center for Disease Control.)

In beef tapeworm disease, absence of strobila (multiple tapeworm segments) in feces within 2 to 3 hours after such treatment necessitates administration of a laxative. During treatment for pork tapeworm, a laxative or induced vomiting is contraindicated because of the danger of autoinfection and systemic disease.

After drug treatment, all types of tapeworm infestation require follow-up stool specimens during the next 3 to 5 weeks to check for remaining ova or worm segments. Persistent tapeworm infestation often requires a second course of medication.

Additional considerations

When treating a patient with tapeworm infection, the hospital staff member should:

• obtain a complete history, including recent travel to endemic areas, dietary habits, and physical symptoms.

• wear gloves when giving personal care and handling fecal excretions, bedpans, and bed linens; wash hands thoroughly and instruct the patient to do the same.

• instruct the patient not to eat or drink anything after midnight on the day therapy is to start, as niclosamide must be given on an empty stomach; document passage of strobila after giving the drug.

• use enteric and secretion precautions in pork tapeworm infestation; avoid pro-

cedures and drugs that may cause vomiting or gagging; provide a private room if the patient is a child or is incontinent; obtain a list of contacts who may also harbor this disease.

• document level of consciousness, and report any changes immediately; if pork tapeworm infestation causes CNS symptoms, keep an artificial airway or padded tongue blade close at hand, raise the side rails, keep the bed low, and assist with walking, as required.

• teach proper handwashing technique and the importance of cooking meat and fish thoroughly to prevent reinfection; stress the need for follow-up medical evaluations to monitor the success of therapy and to detect possible reinfection.

Enterobiasis

(Pinworm disease, oxyuriasis, seatworm or threadworm infection)

Enterobiasis is a benign intestinal disease caused by the nematode Enterobius vermicularis. *Found worldwide, it's common even in temperate regions with good sanitation. It's the most prevalent helminthic infection in the United States, and may infect up to 15% of the population.*

Causes

Adult pinworms live in the intestine; female worms migrate to the perianal region to deposit their ova. Hand-to-mouth transmission occurs after contact with contaminated bed linens, clothing, or toilet seats. Enterobiasis occurs most often in children between ages 5 and 14 and in certain institutionalized groups because of poor hygiene and frequent hand-to-mouth activity. For the same reason, continual reinfection is also common in these groups. Since crowded living conditions enhance its spread, enterobiasis often affects several members of a family.

Signs and symptoms

Enterobiasis is often overlooked if no symptoms are present. It may, however, produce intense perianal pruritus, especially at night, when the female worm

crawls out of the anus to deposit her ova. Such pruritus disturbs sleep and causes irritability, scratching, skin irritation, and sometimes, vaginitis. Complications are rare but include appendicitis, salpingitis, and pelvic granuloma.

Diagnosis

 A history of pruritus ani suggests enterobiasis; identification of *Enterobius* ova recovered from the perianal area with a cellophane tape swab (Grahan Scotch tape test) confirms it. In this test, cellophane tape is placed sticky side out on the base end of a test tube, and the tube is rolled around the perianal region. The tape is then examined under a microscope. This test should be done first thing in the morning, before the patient bathes and defecates. A stool sample is generally ova-

and wormfree, because these worms deposit the ova outside the intestine and die after migration to the anus.

Treatment and additional considerations

Drug therapy with pyrantel, piperazine, or mebendazole destroys these parasites. Effective eradication requires simultaneous treatment of family members and, in institutions, other patients.

Possible side effects of pyrantel, which the patient and family should be aware of, are bright red stools and vomiting (vomitus will also be red). The tablet form of this drug is coated with aspirin and shouldn't be given to aspirin-sensitive patients.

Before giving a patient piperazine, a history of convulsive disorders should be obtained. Piperazine may aggravate these disorders and is contraindicated in a patient with such a history.

To help prevent this disease, parents should bathe children daily (showers are preferable to tub baths) and also change underwear and bed linens daily. Children should know proper personal hygiene rules and must understand the need for handwashing after defecation and before handling food. If children bite their nails and can't stop, wearing gloves until the infection clears may prevent reinfection. *All* outbreaks of enterobiasis should be immediately reported to school authorities.

Schistosomiasis

(Bilharziasis)

Schistosomiasis is a slowly progressive disease caused by blood flukes of the class Trematoda. These parasites are of three major types: Schistosoma mansoni *and* Schistosoma japonicum *infect the intestinal tract;* Schistosoma haematobium *infects the urinary tract.*

The degree of infection determines the intensity of illness. Complications—such as portal hypertension, pulmonary hypertension, heart failure, ascites, hematemesis from ruptured esophageal varices (in intestinal form), and renal failure (in urinary form)—can be fatal.

Causes

The mode of transmission is bathing, swimming, wading, or working in water contaminated with *Schistosoma* larvae, known (in their infective stage) as cercariae. The cercariae penetrate the skin or mucous membranes, and work their way to the liver's venous portal circulation. There, they mature in one to three months. The adults then migrate to other parts of the body.

After copulation, the female cercariae lay spiny eggs in blood vessels surrounding the large intestine or bladder. After penetrating the mucosa of these organs, the eggs are excreted in feces or urine. If the eggs hatch in fresh water, the first-stage larvae (miracidia) penetrate freshwater snails, which act as passive intermediate hosts. Cercariae produced in snails escape into water, and begin a new life cycle.

SCHISTOSOMAL DERMATITIS

This form of dermatitis, also known as swimmer's itch or clam digger's itch, affects those who bathe in and camp along the freshwater lakes of both eastern and western United States. It's caused by a type of schistosomal cercariae that is harbored by migratory birds and can penetrate the skin, causing a pruritic papular rash. Initially mild, the reaction becomes more severe with repeated exposure. Antipruritic treatment consists of topical calamine lotion, menthol, and an antihistamine, such as diphenhydramine.

TYPES OF SCHISTOSOMES

SPECIES AND INCIDENCE	SIGNS AND SYMPTOMS	TREATMENT	SIDE EFFECTS
S. mansoni Western hemisphere, particularly Puerto Rico, Lesser Antilles, Brazil, and Venezuela; also Nile delta, Sudan, and central Africa	Irregular fever, malaise, weakness, abdominal distress, weight loss, diarrhea, ascites, hepatosplenomegaly, portal hypertension, fistulas, intestinal stricture	Niridazole P.O. (available from Center for Disease Control); antimony sodium dimercapto succinate I.M. once a week for 5 weeks	Vomiting, abdominal pain, anorexia, weakness, diarrhea, headache, lassitude, myalgia
S. japonicum Affects men more than women; particularly prevalent among farmers in Japan, China, and the Philippines	Irregular fever, malaise, weakness, abdominal distress, weight loss, diarrhea, ascites, hepatosplenomegaly, portal hypertension, fistulas, intestinal stricture	Antimony potassium tartrate by slow I.V.; usually for 15 doses	Thrombocytopenia, hypotension, syncope, bradycardia, EKG changes, nausea, vomiting, diarrhea, colic, hepatic necrosis, dyspnea, severe arthralgia, albuminuria, fever, dermatitis
S. haematobium Africa, Cyprus, Greece, India	Terminal hematuria, dysuria, ureteral colic; with secondary infection—colicky pain, intermittent flank pain, vague GI complaints, total renal failure	Metrifonate P.O.; niridazole P.O. (available from Center for Disease Control)	Nausea, vomiting, diarrhea, anorexia, dizziness, headache, abdominal pain, insomnia, cardiac arrhythmia, anxiety, confusion, hallucinations, convulsions

Signs and symptoms

Symptoms of schistosomiasis depend on the site of infection and the stage of the disease. Initially, a transient, pruritic rash develops at the site of penetration; other early effects include fever, myalgia, and cough. Aberrant worm migration and egg deposition may result in such bizarre complications as flaccid paralysis, seizures, and skin abscesses.

Diagnosis

 Characteristic symptoms and a history of travel to endemic areas suggest the diagnosis; ova in the patient's urine or stool, or a biopsy of a mucosal lesion confirms it. White blood count shows eosinophilia.

Treatment

Drugs effective against schistosomiasis are highly toxic, and are available only from the Center for Disease Control. Patients must be monitored for signs of toxicity and side effects.

Three to six months after treatment, the patient should be examined again. If living eggs are found, treatment may be resumed.

Additional considerations

To prevent schistosomiasis, persons in endemic areas should try to avoid entering contaminated water. If they must enter contaminated water, they should wear protective clothing. Then, they should thoroughly clean their clothing and dry themselves promptly afterward.

Strongyloidiasis
(Threadworm infection)

Strongyloidiasis is a parasitic intestinal infection caused by the helminth Strongyloides stercoralis. Occurring worldwide, this infection is endemic in the Tropics and subtropics. Susceptibility to strongyloidiasis is universal; infection doesn't confer immunity. Since the reproduction cycle of the threadworm may continue in the untreated host for as long as 45 years after the initial infection, autoinfection is highly probable. Most patients with strongyloidiasis recover completely, but debilitation from protein loss is occasionally fatal.

Causes

Transmission to humans usually occurs through contact with soil that contains infective *S. stercoralis* filariform larvae; such larvae develop from noninfective rhabdoid (rod-shaped) larvae in human feces. The filariform larvae penetrate the human skin, usually at the feet, then migrate by way of the lymphatic system to the bloodstream and the lungs. Once into pulmonary circulation, the larvae break through the alveoli and migrate upward to the pharynx, where they are swallowed. Then, they lodge in the small intestine, where they deposit eggs that mature into noninfectious rhabdoid larvae. Next, these larvae migrate into the large intestine, and are excreted in feces, starting the cycle again. The threadworm life cycle—from penetration of the skin to excretion of rhabdoid larvae—takes 17 days.

In autoinfection, rhabdoid larvae mature within the intestine to become infective filariform larvae.

Signs and symptoms

The patient's resistance and the extent of infection determine the severity of symptoms. Some patients have no symptoms, but many develop an erythematous maculopapular rash at the site of penetration that produces swelling and pruritus, and that may be confused with an insect bite. As the larvae migrate to the lungs, pulmonary signs develop, including minor hemorrhage, pneumonitis, and pneumonia; later, intestinal infection produces frequent, watery, and bloody diarrhea, accompanied by intermittent abdominal pain. Severe infection can cause malnutrition from substantial fat and protein loss, anemia, and lesions resembling ulcerative colitis, all of which invite secondary bacterial infection. Ulcerated intestinal mucosa may lead to perforation and, possibly, potentially fatal dissemination. Such dissemination occurs most often in patients with malignancy or immunodeficiency diseases, or in patients who are receiving immunosuppressives.

Diagnosis

Diagnosis of strongyloidiasis requires observation of *S. stercoralis* larvae in a fresh stool specimen (2 hours after excretion, rhabdoid larvae appear identical to hookworm larvae). During the pulmonary phase, sputum may show large numbers of eosinophils and larvae; marked eosinophilia also occurs in disseminated strongyloidiasis.

Other helpful tests include:
• *chest X-ray* (positive during pulmonary phase of infection)
• *hemoglobin* (as low as 6 to 10g/100 ml)
• *WBC with differential* (eosinophils 450 to 700/mm³).

Treatment

Because of potential autoinfection, treatment with thiabendazole is required for 2 to 3 days (total dose not to exceed 3 g). Patients also need protein replacement, blood transfusions, and I.V. fluids. Repetition of treatment is necessary if stools aren't free of *S. stercoralis* after therapy.

Treatment should not include glucocorticoids, because they increase the risk of autoinfection and dissemination.

Additional considerations
• Accurate intake and output records must be kept, especially if treatment includes administration of blood transfusions and I.V. fluids. The hospital dietary department should provide a high-protein diet. The patient may need tube feedings to increase caloric intake.
• Gloves should be worn when handling bedpans or giving perineal care, and feces must be disposed of promptly.
• Since direct person-to-person transmission doesn't occur, isolation is not required. Stool specimens for laboratory tests are considered contaminated.
• Thiabendazole may cause mild nausea and vomiting.
• In pulmonary infection, the patient should be repositioned frequently, encouraged to cough and breathe deeply, and administered oxygen, as ordered.
• To prevent reinfection, the patient should follow proper handwashing techniques, especially before eating and after defecating. Wearing shoes when in endemic areas can also help prevent reinfection. The patient's family and close contacts should be examined for signs of infection. Follow-up stool examinations continuing for several weeks after treatment are necessary to check for residual parasites.

MISCELLANEOUS INFECTIONS

Ornithosis
(Psittacosis, parrot fever)

Ornithosis is caused by the gram-negative intracellular parasite Chlamydia psittaci and is transmitted by infected birds. This disease occurs worldwide, and is mainly associated with occupational exposure to birds (such as poultry farming). Incidence is higher in women and in persons aged 20 to 50 years. With adequate antimicrobial therapy, ornithosis is fatal in less than 4% of patients.

Causes
Psittacine birds (parrots, parakeets, cockatoos), pigeons, and turkeys may harbor *C. psittaci*; this organism is found in the blood, feathers, tissues, nasal secretions, liver, spleen, and feces of infected birds. Transmission to humans primarily occurs through inhalation of dust containing *C. psittaci* from bird droppings; less often, through direct contact with infected secretions or body tissues, as in laboratory personnel who work with birds. Person-to-person transmission is rare, but in such cases, the disease is usually more severe.

Signs and symptoms
After an incubation period ranging from 7 to 15 days (average 10 days), onset of symptoms may be insidious or sudden. Clinical effects include chills and a low-grade fever that increases to 103° to 105° F. (39.4° to 40.6° C.) for 7 to 10 days, then, with treatment, declines during the second or third week. Other signs include headache, myalgia, sore throat, cough (may be dry, hacking, and nonproductive, or may produce blood-tinged sputum), abdominal distention and tenderness, nausea, vomiting, photophobia, decreased pulse rate, normal or slightly increased respirations, secondary purulent lung infection, and a faint macular rash. Severe infection also produces delirium, stupor, and in extensive pulmonary infiltration, cyanosis. Ornithosis may recur, but reinfections are usually milder.

Diagnosis

These symptoms and a recent history of exposure to birds suggest ornithosis.

 Firm diagnosis requires recovery of *C. psittaci* from mice, eggs, or tissue culture inoculated with the patient's blood or sputum. Comparison of acute and convalescent serum shows a fourfold rise in *Chlamydia* antibody titers; the blood contains antibodies by the fourth day of this illness. (However, if the patient is receiving antibiotics, antibody titer won't rise until 3 to 5 weeks after antibiotic treatment ends.) In addition, a patchy lobar infiltrate appears on chest X-rays during the first week of illness, but it's often hard to distinguish from viral pneumonia.

Treatment

Ornithosis calls for rigorous treatment with tetracycline. If the infection is severe, tetracycline may be given I.V. until the fever subsides. Fever and other symptoms should begin to subside 48 to 72 hours after antibiotic treatment begins; nevertheless, treatment must continue for 2 weeks after temperature returns to normal.

If the patient can't tolerate tetracycline, penicillin G procaine or chloramphenicol is an effective alternative.

Additional considerations

During treatment of an ornithosis patient, the hospital staff member should:
• give I.V. fluids, as needed, to maintain adequate hydration.
• watch for lethargy, drowsiness, and stupor—signs of overwhelming infection.
• reduce fever with tepid alcohol or sponge baths and a cooling blanket.
• reposition the patient often to minimize muscle discomfort.
• observe secretion precautions; wear a face mask when giving patient care and wash hands carefully afterward, if the patient has a cough during the acute febrile stage; instruct the patient to use tissues when he coughs and to dispose of them in a closed plastic bag.

To help prevent ornithosis, persons who raise birds for sale should feed them tetracycline-treated birdseed and closely follow regulations on importation of birds. They should segregate infected or possibly infected birds from those known to be diseasefree, and disinfect structures that housed infected birds.

All cases of ornithosis must be reported to public health authorities.

Cat-scratch Fever

(Cat-scratch disease [CSD], nonbacterial regional lymphadenitis, benign lymphoreticulosis)

Cat-scratch fever is a subacute, self-limiting disease of the regional lymph nodes caused by an unknown agent. Complications are rare.

Causes and incidence

As its name suggests, cat-scratch fever is transmitted from cats to humans. In fact, two thirds of patients have a history of being scratched by cats, while 90% admit some contact with cats. Sometimes contact with cat saliva or excreta is sufficient to produce cat-scratch fever. Cats that transmit this disease show no evidence of illness themselves.

Occurring worldwide, this disease most frequently affects children, probably because they're more likely to tease or play with cats. Often more than one family member has the disease. Whether a single attack of cat-scratch fever confers permanent immunity is unknown.

Signs and symptoms

Cat-scratch fever produces a primary local lesion—a papule, vesicle, or pustule—within 2 weeks of contact, usually at the site of the scratch or injury. Within 1 to 10 weeks after the scratch, regional lymphadenopathy usually develops in a single node; such a node is moderately tender and freely movable, and becomes suppurative in up to 50% of patients. Generalized lymphadenopathy is rare.

In one third of patients, such lymphadenopathy is the only symptom of cat-scratch fever; other possible clinical effects include malaise, mild fever (99.4° to 100.8° F. [37.4° to 38.2° C.]), chills, general aching, nausea, and occasionally, conjunctivitis (probably implicating the eye as the portal of entry).

Diagnosis

A history of contact with a cat in a person with regional lymphadenopathy suggests cat-scratch fever. Confirmation requires an individually prepared skin test. This test uses antigen diluted and processed from purulent material from the involved lymph node. Within 36 to 48 hours, a positive test shows induration of 5 mm or more, erythema of 10 mm or more, or both. Diagnosis must rule out tularemia, toxoplasmosis, infectious mononucleosis, and tumors.

Treatment and additional considerations

Treatment and health care are entirely symptomatic. Cat-scratch fever doesn't require isolation, since person-to-person transmission doesn't occur.

• Hygiene must be maintained. Hands should be washed thoroughly before and after changing soiled dressings, especially if drainage is purulent. Soiled dressings should be placed in a sealed bag and disposed of promptly.

• Antibiotics are ineffective. Because the disease is self-limiting, complications are uncommon. Encephalitis one or more weeks after onset has been reported.

• Patients will need emotional support while waiting for results of tests to rule out serious illnesses.

• Family members (especially siblings) or close contacts of the patient should be examined for signs of cat-scratch fever.

• Since the cat isn't sick, it doesn't need to be destroyed.

Fish Poisoning

(Ichthyosarcotoxism)

The most common types of fish poisoning, scombroid and ciguatera, result from ingestion of normally edible fish (such as tuna, grouper, pompano, snapper, sea bass, and perch) or inedible fish (such as puffers, parrot fish, and moray eels). Although both produce severe symptoms, ciguatera poisoning is more serious, possibly causing death from respiratory arrest. Mortality is higher from the ingestion of inedible fish and may range as high as 50%.

Causes

Scombroid poisoning results from the ingestion of dark fish meat infected with heat-resistant, toxin-producing bacteria. Ciguatera poisoning results from eating tropical fish that have fed on certain marine organisms.

Symptoms and diagnosis

Symptoms of fish poisoning appear within 1 to 4 hours after ingestion. Scombroid poisoning typically produces facial flushing, a bitter taste in the mouth, nausea, vomiting, abdominal cramps, and diarrhea. Ciguatera poisoning produces perioral numbness and tingling, nausea, muscle weakness, abdominal pain, and in severe infection, dyspnea, convulsions, foaming at the mouth, paralysis, and respiratory distress.

Laboratory examination of the fish may reveal increased histamine levels, but other laboratory findings are not contributory.

**Treatment and
additional considerations**
Severe ciguatera poisoning requires emergency measures, such as maintaining respiratory function by mechanical ventilation, injecting epinephrine 1:1,000, and performing cardiopulmonary resuscitation. Other treatment for fish poisoning includes gastric lavage to remove undigested fish and supportive measures such as fluid and electrolyte replacement. Antihistamines may be ordered.

Toxic Shock Syndrome

Toxic shock syndrome (TSS) is an acute bacterial infection caused by penicillin-resistant Staphylococcus aureus, *generally in association with continuous use of tampons during the menstrual period. This condition usually affects menstruating women under age 30. Of the approximately 300 cases reported to the Center for Disease Control from January to September 1980, 95% (285) were in women; among these, 25 deaths were reported. However, about 5% of cases occurred in men. Incidence is rising, and the recurrence rate is about 30%.**

Causes
Although tampons are clearly implicated in TSS, their exact role is uncertain. Theoretically, tampons may contribute to development of TSS by:
● introducing *S. aureus* into the vagina during insertion.
● absorbing toxin from the vagina.
● traumatizing the vaginal mucosa during insertion, leading to infection.
● providing a favorable environment for the growth of *S. aureus.*

When TSS is not associated with menstruation, *S. aureus* seems to originate in bone, skin lesions, or lungs.

Signs and symptoms
Typically, TSS produces a sudden onset of high fever in previously healthy women (usually a temperature of about 102° F. [38.9° C.]); myalgia; vomiting; diarrhea; sudden hypotension, which sometimes

*Center for Disease Control: "Morbidity and Mortality Report," September 19, 1980.

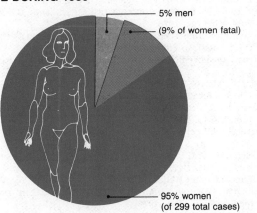

TOXIC SHOCK SYNDROME DURING 1980

During the first 8 months of 1980, the Center for Disease Control received 299 confirmed reports of toxic shock syndrome. Of these, 95% involved women, nearly all of whom experienced symptoms during menses. The remaining 5% of all cases involved men. About 9% of the total number of cases involving women proved fatal.

5% men
(9% of women fatal)

95% women
(of 299 total cases)

leads to shock; and a macular erythematous rash, followed by desquamation 1 to 2 weeks after onset, especially on the fingers and toes. Other possible signs include vaginal, oropharyngeal, or conjunctival hyperemia, and disorientation or changes in level of consciousness.

Diagnosis

Clinical signs of acute infection in a patient with negative blood, throat, or CSF culture, and a history of tampon use strongly suggest TSS; identification of *S. aureus* in cervical or vaginal culture confirms it. Supportive laboratory test results include:

- elevated WBC (more than five white blood cells per high-power field), BUN, and creatinine level
- elevated bilirubin and hepatic enzymes (SGOT, SGPT)
- decreased platelets (less than 100,000/mm³). Diagnosis must also rule out other febrile illnesses, especially leptospirosis and Rocky Mountain spotted fever.

Treatment and additional considerations

Treatment consists of penicillinase-resistant antibiotics, such as methicillin, and vigorous I.V. fluid replacement. Other therapy is supportive and depends on associated symptoms.

- Vital signs, especially blood pressure, must be carefully monitored; the patient must also be closely observed for signs of shock.
- All cases must be reported to local public health authorities.
- Patients treated for TSS should avoid using tampons until cultures show eradication of *S. aureus* from the vaginal tract.

To prevent TSS, patients should use tampons intermittently (wear sanitary napkins at night); change them frequently; discontinue use and notify their doctors immediately if they develop nausea, vomiting, diarrhea, or fever; and avoid using tampons if they have local infections, such as boils. Women who use tampons should choose tampons made entirely of cotton and avoid the superabsorbent types that hold a great deal of fluid and encourage prolonged use. Hands should be washed thoroughly before tampon insertion, since *S. aureus* is commonly found on the hands.

Selected References

American Academy of Pediatrics. REPORT OF THE COMMITTEE ON INFECTIOUS DISEASES. Evanston, Ill.: American Academy of Pediatrics, 1977.

Aronson, Sara P. COMMUNICABLE DISEASE NURSING. Garden City, N.Y.: Medical Examination Publishing Co., 1978.

Benenson, Abram S., ed. CONTROL OF COMMUNICABLE DISEASES IN MAN, 12th ed. Washington, D.C.: American Public Health Association, 1975.

Bloom, Arnold, ed. TOOHEY'S MEDICINE FOR NURSES, 12th ed. New York: Churchill Livingstone, 1978.

Conrad, Marcel E. *Hematologic Manifestations of Parasitic Infections*, SEMINARS IN HEMATOLOGY. 8:267-302, July 1979.

D'Angelo, L.J., et al. *Q Fever in the United States, 1948-1977*, JOURNAL OF INFECTIOUS DISEASES. 139:613-615, 1979.

D'Angelo, L.J., et al. *Rocky Mountain Spotted Fever in the United States, 1975-1977*, JOURNAL OF INFECTIOUS DISEASES. 138:273-276, 1978.

Diefenbach, W.C.L. *The Tick in All Seasons*, CONSULTANT. 43-51, December 1977.

Dixon, R. ISOLATION TECHNIQUES FOR USE IN HOSPITALS. Washington, D.C.: Dept. of Health, Education and Welfare, 1978.

Edington, G.M., and H.M. Gilles. PATHOLOGY IN THE TROPICS, 2nd ed. Chicago: Year Book Medical Pubs., Inc., 1976.

Evans, Alfred. VIRAL INFECTIONS OF HUMAN EPIDEMIOLOGY AND CONTROL. New York: Plenum Publishing Corp., 1976.

Fahlberg, W.J., and D. Groschal, ed. HANDBOOK ON HOSPITAL-ASSOCIATED INFECTIONS VOLUME I AND II. New York: Marcel Dekker, Inc., 1979.

Gardner, Pierce, and Harriet T. Provine. MANUAL OF ACUTE BACTERIAL INFECTIONS: EARLY DIAGNOSIS AND TREATMENT. Boston, Mass.: Little, Brown & Co., 1975.

Harbor General Hospital. *Amebiasis—a Symposium,* CALIFORNIA MEDICINE. March 1971.

Hattwick, M.A.W., et al. *Fatal Rocky Mountain Spotted Fever,* JOURNAL OF AMERICAN MEDICAL ASSOCIATION. 240:1499-1503, 1978.

Hoeprich, Paul D., ed. INFECTIOUS DISEASES, 2nd ed. New York: Harper & Row Pubs., 1977.

Hook, E., et al, eds. CURRENT CONCEPTS OF INFECTIOUS DISEASES. New York: John Wiley & Sons, Inc., 1977.

Hunter, George W., and J. Clyde Swartzwelder. TROPICAL MEDICINE, 5th ed. Philadelphia: W.B. Saunders Co., 1976.

ISOLATION TECHNIQUES FOR USE IN HOSPITALS. Washington, D.C.: Department of Health, Education and Welfare, 1975.

Kavaler, Lucy. STREPTOCOCCAL DISEASE. Kalamazoo, Mich.: Upjohn Co., 1973.

Kenyon, R.H., et al. *Prophylactic Treatment of Rocky Mountain Spotted Fever,* JOURNAL OF CLINICAL MICROBIOLOGY. 8:102-104, 1978.

Kolff, Cornelis A., and Ramon C. Sanchez. HANDBOOK FOR INFECTIOUS DISEASE MANAGEMENT. Reading, Mass.: Addison-Wesley Publishing Co., 1979.

Krugman, Saul. INFECTIOUS DISEASES OF CHILDREN, 6th ed. St. Louis: C.V. Mosby Co., 1977.

Ledger, J. *Nursing Care in Leprosy,* NURSING MIRROR. March 4, 1976.

Lennette, E.H., *Rocky Mountain Spotted Fever,* NEW ENGLAND JOURNAL OF MEDICINE. 297:884-885, 1977.

McInnes, Mary E., ed. ESSENTIALS OF COMMUNICABLE DISEASE, 2nd ed. St. Louis: C.V. Mosby Co., 1975.

Maegraith, Brian. ADAMS AND MAEGRAITH: CLINICAL TROPICAL DISEASES, 6th ed. London: Blackwell Scientific Publications, 1976.

Magnarelli, L.A., et al. *Rocky Mountain Spotted Fever in Connecticut: Human Cases, Spotted Fever, Group Rickettsine in Ticks, and Antibodies in Mammals,* AMERICAN JOURNAL OF EPIDEMIOLOGY. 110:148-155, 1979.

Mandell, G., et al, eds. PRINCIPLES AND PRACTICE OF INFECTIOUS DISEASES. New York: John Wiley & Sons, Inc., 1979.

Marcial-Rojas. PATHOLOGY OF PROTOZOAL AND HELMINTHIC DISEASES. Huntington, N.Y.: Robert E. Krieger Publishing Co., 1975.

Markell, Edward K., and Marietta Voge. MEDICAL PARASITOLOGY, 4th ed. Philadelphia: W.B. Saunders Co., 1976.

Melnick, J.L., ed. PROGRESS IN MEDICAL VIROLOGY, Vol. 24. New York: S. Karger, 1978.

Mikat, D.M., and K.W. Mikat. A CLINICIAN'S DICTIONARY GUIDE TO BACTERIA AND FUNGI, 3rd ed. Indianapolis, Ind.: Eli Lilly and Co., 1977.

Morbidity and Mortality Weekly Report, TYPHUS VACCINE. June 2, 1978.

Neva, F.A., et al. *Malaria: Host-defense Mechanisms and Complications,* ANNALS OF INTERNAL MEDICINE. 73:295-306, 1970.

Nursing79, in consultation with Rosemary Hutchinson. *The Common Cold Primer,* NURSING79. 9:57-61, March 1979.

Sartwell, Philip E. MAXCY-ROSENAU PREVENTIVE MEDICINE AND PUBLIC HEALTH, 10th ed. New York: Appleton-Century-Crofts, 1973.

Spincer, H.C., et al. *Imported African Trypanosomiasis in the United States,* ANNALS OF INTERNAL MEDICINE. 82:633-638, 1975.

Taylor, Carol Margaret. *When to Anticipate Septic Shock,* NURSING75. 5:34-38, April 1975.

Top, Franklin H., Sr., and Paul F. Wehrle. COMMUNICABLE AND INFECTIOUS DISEASES, 8th ed. St. Louis: C.V. Mosby Co., 1976.

Wallach, Jacques B. INTERPRETATION OF DIAGNOSTIC TESTS: A HANDBOOK SYNOPSIS OF LABORATORY MEDICINE, 2nd ed. Boston: Little, Brown & Co., 1974.

Wilcocks, Charles, and P.E. Manson-Bahr. MANSON'S TROPICAL DISEASES, 17th ed. Baltimore: Williams & Wilkins Co., 1972.

Winterbauer, R.H., and K.G. Kramer. *The Infectious Complications of Sarcoidosis,* ARCHIVES OF INTERNAL MEDICINE. 136:1356-1362, 1976.

Youmans, G., et al. THE BIOLOGIC AND CLINICAL BASIS OF INFECTIOUS DISEASES. Philadelphia: W.B. Saunders Co., 1980.

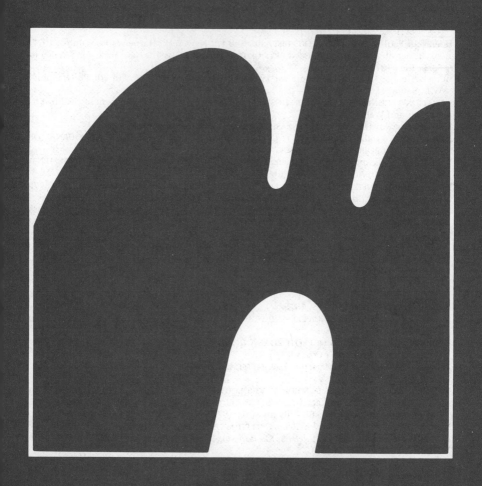

7 Respiratory Disorders

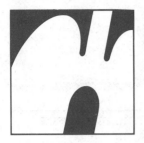

Respiratory Disorders

Introduction

The respiratory system distributes air to the alveoli, where gas exchange—the addition of oxygen (O_2) and the removal of carbon dioxide (CO_2) from pulmonary capillary blood—takes place. Certain specialized structures within this system play a vital role in preparing air for use by the body. The nose, for example, contains vestibular hairs that filter the air and an extensive vascular network that warms it. The nose also contains a layer of goblet cells and a moist mucosal surface; water vapor enters the airstream from this mucosal surface to fully saturate inspired air as it's warmed in the upper airways. Ciliated mucosa in the posterior portion of the nose and nasopharynx, as well as major portions of the tracheobronchial tree, propels particles deposited by impaction or gravity to the oropharynx, where the particles are swallowed. In addition to carbon dioxide, gases such as carbon monoxide may diffuse from pulmonary capillary blood to alveoli, where they are excreted by the lungs.

External respiration

The external component of respiration—ventilation or breathing—delivers inspired gas to the lower respiratory tract and alveoli. Expansion and contraction of the respiratory muscles move air into and out of the lungs. Ventilation begins with the contraction of the inspiratory muscles: the diaphragm—the major muscle of respiration—descends, while external intercostal muscles move the rib cage upward and outward. The accessory muscles of inspiration, which include the scalene and sternocleidomastoid muscles, raise the clavicles, upper ribs, and sternum. The accessory muscles are not used in normal inspiration but are used in certain disease states. As the diaphragm descends and the rib cage expands, pressure in the pleural space becomes more negative, and the lungs adhere to the chest wall. As the thorax expands, the pressure in the lungs falls below atmospheric pressure, and the lungs expand. Air then enters the lungs in response to the pressure gradient between the atmosphere and the lungs.

Normal expiration is passive; the inspiratory muscles cease to contract, and the elastic recoil of the lungs pushes air out. These actions raise the pressure within the lungs above atmospheric pressure, moving air from the lungs to the atmosphere. Active expiration causes the pleural pressure to become less negative.

An adult lung contains an estimated 300 million alveoli; each alveolus is supplied by many capillaries. To reach the capillary lumen, O_2 must cross the alveolar-capillary membrane, which consists of an alveolar epithelial cell, a thin interstitial space, the capillary basement membrane, and the capillary endothelial cell membrane. The oxygen tension of air entering the respiratory tract is approximately 160 mmHg. In the alveoli, inspired air mixes with CO_2 and water vapor, lowering its pressure to approximately 100 mmHg. Since alveolar partial pressure of O_2 (PO_2) is higher than that present in mixed venous blood entering the pulmonary capillaries (approximately 40 mmHg), O_2 diffuses across the alveolar-capillary membrane into the blood.

O_2 and CO_2 transport and internal (cellular) respiration

Circulating blood delivers O_2 to the cells of the body for metabolism, and transports metabolic wastes and CO_2 from the tissues back to the lungs. When oxygenated arterial blood reaches tissue capillaries, O_2 diffuses from the blood into the cells again because of an oxygen tension gradient. The amount of O_2 available is determined by the concentration of hemoglobin (the principal carrier of O_2), regional blood flow, arterial oxygen tension, and carboxyhemoglobin tension.

Internal (cellular) respiration occurs as a part of cellular metabolism, which can take place with O_2 (aerobic) or without it (anaerobic). The most efficient method for providing fuel (high-energy compounds such as adenosine triphosphate [ATP]) for cellular reactions is aerobic metabolism, which produces CO_2 and water in addition to ATP. Anaerobic metabolism is less efficient, because a cell produces only a limited amount of ATP and yields lactic acid as well as CO_2 as a metabolic by-product.

Because circulation is continuous, CO_2 does not normally accumulate in tissues. CO_2 produced during cellular respiration diffuses from tissues to regional capillaries and is transported by systemic venous circulation. When CO_2 reaches the alveolar capillaries, it diffuses into the alveoli, where the partial pressure of CO_2 is lower; CO_2 is removed from the alveoli during exhalation.

Mechanisms of control

The central nervous system's control of respiration lies in the respiratory center, located in the lateral medulla oblongata of the brain stem. Impulses travel down the phrenic nerves to the diaphragm, and then down the intercostal nerves to the intercostal muscles, where the impulses change the rate and depth of respiration. The inspiratory and expiratory centers, located in the posterior medulla, establish the involuntary rhythm of the breathing pattern.

Apneustic and pneumotaxic centers in the pons influence the pattern of breathing. Stimulation of the midpontine apneustic center (by trauma, tumor, or cerebrovascular accident, for example)

EXTERNAL RESPIRATION

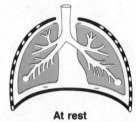

At rest
- resting inspiratory muscles
- atmospheric pressure in tracheo-bronchial tree
- no airflow

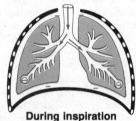

During inspiration
- contraction of inspiratory muscles and chest expansion
- negative alveolar pressure
- airflow into lungs

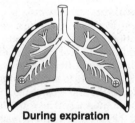

During expiration
- relaxation of inspiratory muscles causes lung recoil
- positive alveolar pressure
- airflow from lungs

KEYS
- − negative intrapleural pressure
- ⊖ negative alveolar pressure
- ⊕ positive alveolar pressure

produces forceful inspiratory gasps alternating with weak expiration. This pattern does not occur if the vagi are intact. The pneumotaxic center stimulates the medullary control center to inhibit inspiratory efforts. The tonically active pontine apneustic center continually excites the medullary inspiratory center and thus facilitates inspiration. Signals from the periodically active pneumotaxic center, as well as afferent impulses from the vagus nerve, actuate the expiratory center and cause it to "turn off" inspiration.

Arterial Po_2 and pH, as well as pH of cerebrospinal fluid (CSF), influence output from the respiratory center. When CO_2 enters the CSF, the pH of CSF falls, stimulating central chemoreceptors to increase ventilation.

The respiratory center also receives information from peripheral chemoreceptors in the carotid and aortic bodies, which respond primarily to decreased arterial Po_2 but also to decreased pH. Either change results in increased ventilatory drive within minutes.

Several other factors can alter the respiratory pattern. During exercise, when the volume of inspired air with each breath may exceed 1 liter, stretch receptors in lung tissue and the diaphragm prevent overdistention of the lungs. During eating and drinking, the cortex can interrupt automatic control of ventilation. External sensations, such as pain, temperature, and fear, can also alter the respiratory pattern; so can drugs, chronic hypercapnia, and increased or decreased body heat.

Diagnostic tests

A host of diagnostic tests are available to evaluate physiologic characteristics and pathologic states within the respiratory tract.

Noninvasive tests:
- *Chest X-ray* shows conditions such as atelectasis, pleural effusion, infiltrates, pneumothorax, lesions, mediastinal shifts, pulmonary edema.
- *Analysis of sputum specimen* permits study of sputum quantity, color, viscos-

ity, and odor; microbiologic stains and culture of sputum can identify infectious organisms; cytologic preparations can detect respiratory tract malignancy.

• *Pulmonary function tests* measure lung volumes, flow rates, and compliance. Normal values are individualized by body stature and age, and are reported in percentage of the normal predicted value. *Static measurements* are volume measurements, and include tidal volume (VT), volume of air contained in a normal breath; functional residual capacity (FRC), volume of air remaining in the lungs at the end of normal expiration; vital capacity (VC), volume of air that can be exhaled after a maximal inspiration; residual volume (RV), air remaining in the lungs after maximal expiration; and total lung capacity (TLC), volume of air in the lungs after maximal inspiration. *Dynamic measurements* characterize the movement of air into and out of the lungs, and show changes in lung mechanics. They include: measurement of forced expiratory volume in one second (FEV_1), maximum volume of air that can be expired in 1 second from total lung capacity; maximal voluntary ventilation (MVV), volume of air that can be expired in 1 minute with the patient's maximum voluntary effort; and forced vital capacity (FVC), maximal volume of air that the patient can exhale from TLC.

Invasive tests:

• *Bronchoscopy:* direct visualization of the trachea, and mainstem, lobar, segmental, and subsegmental bronchi. May be used to localize the site of lung hemorrhage, visualize masses in these airways, and collect respiratory tract secretions. Brush biopsy may be used to obtain specimens from the lungs for microbiologic stains, culture, and cytology. Lesion biopsies may be performed by using small forceps under direct visualization (when present in the proximal airways) or with the aid of fluoroscopy (when present distal to regions of direct visualization). Bronchoscopy can also be used for therapeutic purposes, such as removal of a foreign body.

• *Thoracentesis:* needle insertion into the pleural space under local anesthetic. Permits removal of fluid for analysis.

• *Pleural biopsy:* insertion of biopsy apparatus into the pleural space. Obtains pleural tissue for histologic examination and culture. This test can show neoplasms or granulomatous infections of the pleural space.

• *Lung scan* (scintiphotography): I.V. injection and inhalation of radioisotope. Demonstrates ventilation and perfusion patterns, and is used primarily to evaluate pulmonary embolus.

• *Transtracheal aspiration:* obtains secretions from trachea and proximal bronchi for microbiologic analysis.

• *Arterial blood gas (ABG) measurements:* assess gas exchange. Decreased arterial PO_2 may indicate hypoventilation, ventilation-perfusion mismatching, or shunting of blood away from gas exchange sites. Increased PCO_2 reflects hypoventilation or marked ventilation-perfusion mismatching; decreased PCO_2 reflects increased alveolar ventilation. Changes in pH may reflect metabolic or respiratory dysfunction.

Assessment

Complete assessment of the respiratory system helps explore present and potential respiratory problems. Such assessment always begins with a thorough patient *history.* This includes asking the patient to describe his respiratory problem or difficulty. How long has he had it? How long does each attack last? Does one attack differ from another? Does any activity in particular bring on an attack or make it worse? What relieves the symptoms? The patient must also be asked if he was or is a smoker, what and how often he smoked or smokes, and how long he smoked or has been smoking. This information is recorded in "pack-years"—the number of packs of cigarettes per day multiplied by the number of smoking years. Nicotine stains on fingers or teeth point to a chronic habit. Occupation, hobbies, and travel are also important; some involve exposure to toxic or allergenic substances.

NONDISPOSABLE UNDERWATER-SEAL CHEST DRAINAGE

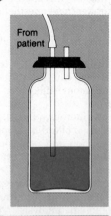

From patient

- *One-bottle setup:* used for water-seal and drainage; acts as a one-way valve, permitting air and fluid to escape from pleural space and preventing transmission of atmospheric pressure to the pleural space.

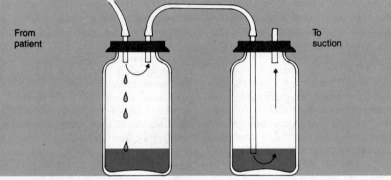

From patient

To suction

- *Two-bottle setup:* one bottle collects fluid draining from pleural cavity, for easy measurement; the other is the water-seal bottle.

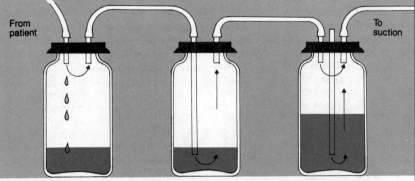

From patient

To suction

- *Three-bottle setup:* controls amount of suction. The first bottle is the drainage collection bottle; the second, the underwater-seal bottle; the third bottle, attached to the wall suction or portable suction apparatus, maintains negative pressure throughout the closed drainage setup and in the pleural space. The amount of suction (or negative pressure) is regulated by the difference between the water surface and the submerged end of the long glass straw, usually ⅝" to ¾" (10 to 20 cm).

If the patient has dyspnea, he should be asked if it occurs during activity or at rest. What position is he in when dyspnea occurs? How far can he walk? How many flights of stairs can he climb? Can he relate dyspnea to allergies or environmental conditions? Does it occur only at night, during sleep? If the patient has a cough, the following should be determined: its severity, persistence, and duration; if it produces sputum and, if so, what kind. Have the patient's cough and sputum habits changed recently?

The next step is looking for telltale clues to respiratory disease. The patient's general appearance can give many clues. If he's frail or cachectic, he may have a chronic disease that has impaired his appetite. If he's diaphoretic, restless, irritable, or protective of a painful body part, he may be in acute distress. Also, behavior changes may indicate hypoxia or hypercapnia. Confusion, lethargy, bizarre behavior, or quiet sleep from which he can't be aroused may point to hypercapnia. Marked cyanosis, indicated by bluish or ashen skin (usually best seen on the lips, tongue, earlobes, and nail beds), may be due to hypoxemia or poor tissue perfusion.

Chest configuration should be checked at rest and during ventilation. Increased anteroposterior diameter ("barrel chest") characterizes emphysema. Kyphoscoliosis also alters chest configuration, which in turn restricts breathing. To assess the muscles used on inspiration, the patient is placed in semi-Fowler's or a flat position and observed. If the epigastric area rises during inspiration, he's using his diaphragm. Use of upper chest and neck muscles is normal only during physical stress.

The rate and pattern of breathing are important. Certain disorders produce characteristic changes in breathing patterns. An acute respiratory disorder, for example, can produce tachypnea (rapid, shallow breathing) or hyperpnea (increased rate and depth of breathing); intracranial lesions—Cheyne-Stokes and Biot's respirations; increased intracranial pressure—central hyperventilation,

and apneustic or ataxic breathing; metabolic disorders—Kussmaul's respirations; and airway obstruction—prolonged forceful expiration and pursed lip breathing. Posture and carriage are also important. A patient with chronic obstructive disease, for example, usually supports rib cage movement by placing his arms on the sides of a chair to increase expansion, and leans forward during exhalation to help expel air.

Physical examination

Palpation of the chest wall detects masses, areas of tenderness, changes in fremitus (palpable vocal vibrations), or crepitus (air in subcutaneous tissues). To assess chest excursion and symmetry, hands are placed in a horizontal position, bilaterally on the posterior chest, with thumbs pressed lightly against the spine, creating folds in the skin. As the patient takes a deep breath, thumbs should move quickly and equally away from the spine. This is repeated with hands placed anteriorly, at the costal margins (lower lobes) and clavicles (apices). Unequal movement indicates differences in expansion, seen in atelectasis, diaphragm or chest wall muscle disease, or splinting with pain.

Percussion should detect resonance over lung fields that are not covered by bony structures or the heart. A dull sound on percussion may mean consolidation or pleural disease.

Auscultation normally detects soft, vesicular breath sounds throughout most of the lung fields. Absent or adventitious breath sounds may indicate fluid in small airways or interstitial lung disease (rales), secretions in moderate and large airways (rhonchi), and airflow obstruction (wheezes).

Special respiratory care

The hospitalized patient with respiratory disease may require an artificial upper airway, chest tubes, chest physiotherapy, and supervision of mechanical ventilation. In cardiopulmonary arrest, establishing an airway always takes precedence. In a patient with this condition, airway obstruction usually results when the tongue slides back and blocks the posterior pharynx. The head-tilt method or, in suspected or confirmed cervical fracture or arthritis, the jaw-thrust maneuver can immediately push the tongue forward and relieve such obstruction. Endotracheal intubation and, sometimes, a tracheotomy may be necessary.

Chest tubes

An important procedure in patients with respiratory disease is chest tube drainage, which removes air or fluid from the pleural space, allowing the collapsed lung to reexpand to fill the evacuated pleural space. Chest drainage also allows removal of pleural fluid for culture. Chest tubes are commonly used after thoracic surgery, penetrating chest wounds, pleural effusion, and empyema, and for evacuation of pneumo-, hydro-, or hemothorax. Sometimes, chest tubes are used to instill sclerosing drugs into the pleural space to prevent recurrent malignant pleural effusions.

Commonly, the chest tube is placed in the eighth or ninth intercostal space in the axillary region. Occasionally, in pneumothorax, the tube is placed in the second or third intercostal space, in the midclavicular region.

Hospital care for a patient with chest tubes includes:
• monitoring changes in suction pressure.
• maintaining tube patency by milking and stripping the tubes every 1 to 2 hours.
• ensuring that all connections in the system are tightly connected and secured with tape over insertion sites.
• checking for air leaks, and adding water to the suction bottle, as needed.
• recording the amount, color, and consistency of drainage.
• watching for signs of shock if drainage is excessive.
• keeping two hemostats at the bedside at all times in case the tube is disconnected.
• telling the patient to cough once an hour, and having him take several deep breaths to enhance drainage and lung function.

Ventilator methods

Mechanical ventilators are used when the normal bellows action usually provided by the diaphragm and rib cage fails. Pressure-cycled ventilators deliver gas until they reach a predetermined airway pressure; they provide no specified tidal volume. Volume-cycled ventilators deliver a preset volume of gas. The tidal volume is set at 10 to 15 ml/kg of body weight. Positive end-expiratory pressure (PEEP) can be applied to trap a certain volume of air in the lungs at the end of expiration, increasing functional residual capacity. PEEP is especially beneficial for patients with adult respiratory distress syndrome.

Several methods can be used to wean a patient from a ventilator. In conventional weaning, the patient is disconnected from the ventilator and put on a T piece (endotracheal tube oxygen adapter) that provides supplemental O_2 and humidification. The patient is allowed to breathe spontaneously without the ventilator for gradually increasing periods of time. With intermittent mandatory ventilation (IMV)—another method of weaning—the ventilator provides a specific number of breaths, and the patient is able to breathe spontaneously between ventilator breaths. The frequency of ventilator breaths is gradually decreased, so that the patient takes over the task of ventilation. This process is continued until the patient is able to breathe entirely on his own. Vital signs and arterial blood gases should be monitored periodically during weaning, to assess the patient's status.

Chest physiotherapy

In respiratory conditions marked by excessive accumulation of secretions in the lungs, chest physiotherapy may enhance removal of secretions. Chest physiotherapy includes chest assessment, breathing and coughing exercises, postural drainage, percussion, vibration, and evaluation of the therapy's effectiveness. Before starting treatment, X-rays are reviewed to de-

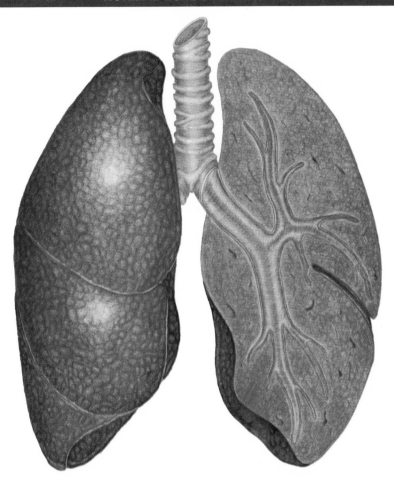

Microscopic cross section of alveoli

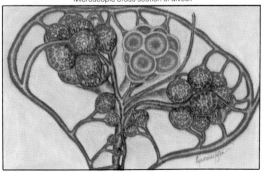

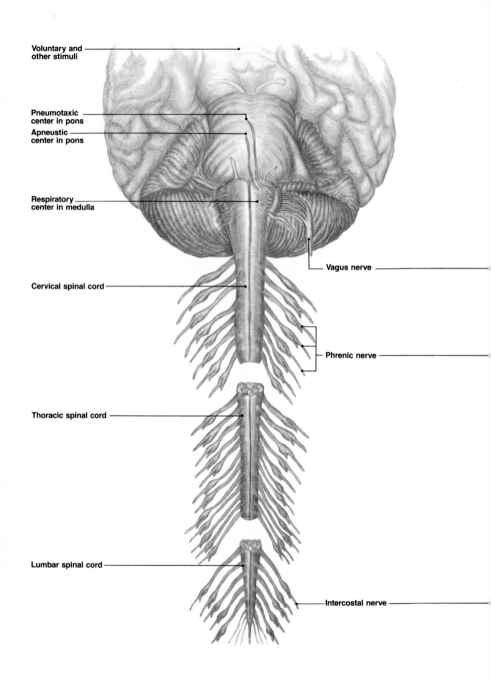

Voluntary and other stimuli

Pneumotaxic center in pons

Apneustic center in pons

Respiratory center in medulla

Vagus nerve

Cervical spinal cord

Phrenic nerve

Thoracic spinal cord

Lumbar spinal cord

Intercostal nerve

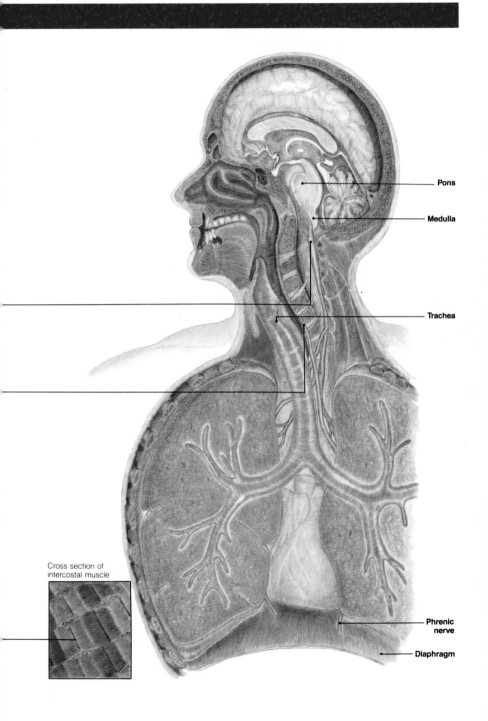

Pons

Medulla

Trachea

Phrenic
nerve

Diaphragm

Cross section of
intercostal muscle

PATHOLOGY IN FOUR COMMON LUNG DISEASES

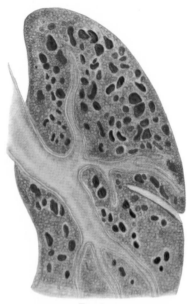

Emphysema

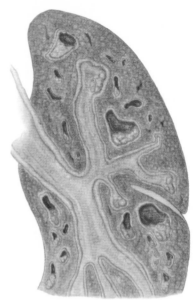

Bronchiectasis

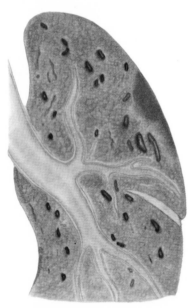

Pulmonary emboli and infarction

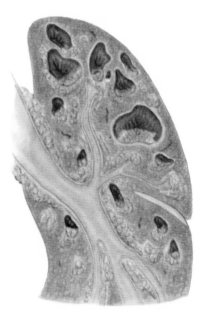

Tuberculosis

termine areas of consolidation.

• *Deep breathing* maintains use of diaphragm, increases negative intrathoracic pressure, and promotes venous return; it is important when pain or dressings restrict chest movement. An incentive spirometer can provide positive visual reinforcement to promote deep breathing.

• *Pursed lip breathing* is used primarily in obstructive disease to slow expiration and prevent large airway collapse. Such breathing funnels air through a narrow opening, creating a positive back pressure on airways to keep them open.

• *Segmental breathing or lateral costal breathing* is used after lung resection and for basilar disorders. A hand is placed over the lung area on the affected side. The patient then tries to push that portion of his chest against the hand on deep inspiration. This movement should be discernible.

• *Coughing* that is controlled and staged gradually increases intrathoracic pressure, reducing pain and bronchospasm of explosive coughing. When wound pain prevents effective coughing, the wound should be splinted with a pillow, towel, or hand during coughing exercises.

• *Postural drainage* uses gravity to drain secretions into larger airways, where they can be expectorated. This technique is used in patients with copious or tenacious secretions. Before performing postural drainage, the patient's chest is auscultated and chest X-rays reviewed to determine the best position for maximum drainage. Postural drainage should be scheduled at least 1 hour after meals, to prevent vomiting.

• *Percussion* augments effectiveness of postural drainage by loosening lung secretions. This technique impacts air against the chest wall, using a cupped hand. Percussion is contraindicated in severe pain, extreme obesity (prevents effective contact with chest wall), cancer that has metastasized to the ribs, crushing chest injuries, bleeding disorders, spontaneous pneumothorax, and spinal compression fractures.

• *Vibration* can be used alone or with percussion.

• *Auscultation* of the patient's lung fields before and after chest physiotherapy is used to evaluate the effectiveness of the therapy.

CONGENITAL & PEDIATRIC DISORDERS

Hyaline Membrane Disease
(Respiratory distress syndrome [RDS])

Hyaline membrane disease (HMD) is the most common cause of neonatal mortality. In the United States alone, it causes the death of 40,000 newborns every year. Hyaline membrane disease occurs in premature infants and, if untreated, is fatal within 72 hours of birth in up to 14% of infants weighing less than 5.5 lb (2,500 g). Aggressive management using mechanical ventilation can improve prognosis, but a few infants who survive have bronchopulmonary dysplasia.

Causes and incidence
HMD occurs almost exclusively in infants born before the 37th week of gestation (in 60% of those born before the 28th week). It occurs more often in infants of diabetic mothers, those delivered by cesarean section, and those delivered suddenly after antepartum hemorrhage. Although airways and alveoli of an infant's respiratory system are present by the 27th week of gestation, the intercostal muscles are weak and the alveoli and

capillary blood supply immature. In HMD, the premature infant develops widespread alveolar collapse because of lack of surfactant, a lipoprotein present in alveoli and respiratory bronchioles which lowers surface tension and aids in maintaining alveolar patency, preventing collapse, particularly at end expiration. This surfactant deficiency results in widespread atelectasis, which in turn leads to inadequate alveolar ventilation with shunting of blood through collapsed areas of lung, causing hypoxia and acidosis.

Signs and symptoms
While a HMD infant may breathe normally at first, he usually develops rapid, shallow respirations within minutes or hours of birth, with intercostal, subcostal, or sternal retractions, nasal flaring, and audible expiratory grunting. This grunting is a natural compensatory mechanism designed to produce positive end-expiratory pressure (PEEP) and prevent further alveolar collapse. The infant may also display hypotension, peripheral edema, and oliguria; in severe disease, apnea, bradycardia, and cyanosis (from hypoxemia, left-to-right shunting through the foramen ovale, or right-to-left shunting through atelectatic regions of the lung). Other clinical features include pallor, frothy sputum, and low body temperature as a result of an immature nervous system and the absence of subcutaneous fat.

Diagnosis
While signs of respiratory distress in a premature infant during the first few hours of life strongly suggest HMD, chest X-ray and arterial blood gases are necessary to confirm the diagnosis.
• *Chest X-ray* may be normal for the first 6 to 12 hours (in 50% of newborns with HMD), but later shows a fine reticulo-nodular pattern.
• *Arterial blood gases* show decreased PO_2, with normal, decreased, or increased PCO_2 and decreased pH (a combination of respiratory and metabolic acidosis).

• *Chest auscultation* reveals normal or diminished air entry and rales (rare in early stages).

When a cesarean section is necessary before the 30th week of gestation, amniocentesis enables determination of the lecithin/sphingomyelin (L/S) ratio, which helps to assess prenatal lung development and the risk of HMD.

Treatment
Treatment requires vigorous respiratory support. Warm, humidified, oxygen-enriched gases are administered by oxygen hood (the treatment of choice) or, if such treatment fails, by mechanical ventilation. Severe cases may require mechanical ventilation with PEEP or continuous positive airway pressure (CPAP), administered by tightly fitting face mask or, when absolutely necessary, endotracheal intubation. Treatment also includes:
• a radiant infant warmer or isolette to control hypothermia
• sodium bicarbonate I.V. to control severe acidosis and I.V. fluids to maintain fluid and electrolyte balance
• tube feedings or hyperalimentation to maintain adequate nutrition if the infant is too weak to eat.

Additional considerations
Infants with HMD require continual assessment and monitoring in an intensive care nursery.
• Close attention should be paid to blood gases (by umbilical catheter or other indwelling arterial line), as well as fluid intake and output. If the infant has an umbilical catheter (arterial and venous), arterial hypotension or abnormal central venous pressure must be avoided. Possible complications include infection, thrombosis, and decreased circulation to the legs. If the infant has a transcutaneous PO_2 monitor (an accurate method for determining PO_2), the site of the lead placement must be changed every 2 to 4 hours to prevent burning the skin.
• The infant should be weighed once or twice daily. His progress can be evaluated by assessing skin color, rate and

depth of respirations, severity of retractions, nostril flaring, frequency of expiratory grunting, frothing at the lips, and restlessness.

• The effectiveness of oxygen or ventilator therapy should be assessed. Every FIO_2 and PEEP or CPAP change must be evaluated by drawing blood 20 minutes after each change for arterial blood gas (ABG) studies. PEEP or CPAP are then adjusted as indicated by the ABGs.

• When the infant is on mechanical ventilation, possible complications include barotrauma (increase in respiratory distress, subcutaneous emphysema) and accidental disconnection from the ventilator. Ventilator settings should be checked frequently. Signs of complications of PEEP or CPAP therapy include decreased cardiac output, pneumothorax, and pneumomediastinum. Mechanical ventilation increases the risk of infection in premature infants, so preventive measures are essential.

• The doctor may request a follow-up visit with a neonatal ophthalmologist to check for retinal damage.

• Parents should understand their infant's condition and, if possible, participate in his care (using aseptic technique). They should know that full recovery may take up to 12 months. When prognosis is poor, they must be prepared for the infant's death.

• Mortality in HMD can be reduced by early detection of respiratory distress and by immediate treatment. Signs of HMD that should be recognized, especially in a premature infant, are intercostal retractions and grunting.

Sudden Infant Death Syndrome
(Crib death, cot death)

Sudden infant death syndrome (SIDS) kills apparently healthy infants, usually between ages 4 weeks and 7 months, for reasons that are not fully understood. Typically, parents put the infant to bed and later find him dead, often with no indications of a struggle or distress of any kind. Some infants may have had signs of a cold, but such symptoms are usually absent. SIDS has occurred throughout history, all over the world, and in all climates. Research on SIDS has shown that it may have several different causes.

Causes and incidence
SIDS accounts for 6,000 to 7,000 deaths annually in the United States, making it one of the leading causes of infant death. Most of these deaths occur during the winter, in poor families, and among underweight babies and those born to mothers under age 20. Although infants who die from SIDS often appear healthy, research suggests that many may have had undetected abnormalities such as an immature respiratory system and respiratory dysfunction. In fact, the current thinking is that SIDS may result from an abnormality in the control of ventilation, which causes prolonged apneic periods with profound hypoxemia and serious cardiac arrhythmias. Bottle feeding, instead of breast feeding, and advanced parental age *don't* cause SIDS.

Signs and symptoms
Unfortunately, at risk babies are usually not detected until their death. Typically, SIDS babies don't cry out and show no signs of having been disturbed in their sleep, although their positions or tangled blankets may suggest movement just before death, perhaps due to terminal muscle spasm.

Depending on how long the infant has been dead, a SIDS baby may have a mottled complexion with extreme cyanosis of the lips and fingertips, or pooling of blood in the legs and feet that may be mistaken for bruises. Pulse and respirations are absent, and the infant's diaper is wet and full of stool.

Some babies have been found in the middle of an apneic episode ("infantile apnea"), while they can still be resuscitated. If resuscitation is successful, the infant is said to have experienced an aborted SIDS. These episodes may be more common than realized, but have not been associated with SIDS until recently. Testing has shown that many of these babies undergo the prolonged apneic episodes that are thought to be one of the risk factors for SIDS.

Diagnosis

Diagnosis of SIDS after death requires an autopsy to rule out other causes of death. Characteristic histologic findings on autopsy include small or normal adrenal glands and petechiae over the visceral surfaces of the pleura, within the thymus (which is enlarged), and in the epicardium. Autopsy also reveals extremely well-preserved lymphoid structures and certain pathologic characteristics which suggest chronic hypoxemia, such as increased pulmonary artery smooth muscle.

Children at risk may now be tested for apnea in specialized hospital laboratories. Any child who has had an apneic episode (no breathing, dusky or blue color) or had a sibling who died of SIDS, should be tested for apnea. If testing reveals apneic episodes, a home monitoring system may be recommended. This system may monitor the child's breathing, heart rate, or both. An alarm sounds when the child's heart rate or respiration falls below a predetermined level. If the alarm does not wake the child, the parent follows progressive steps from gentle prodding to resuscitation.

Treatment and additional considerations

If the parents bring the infant to the emergency room, the doctor will decide whether or not resuscitation should be tried. Since most infants cannot be resuscitated, however, treatment focuses on emotional support for the grief-stricken family.

• Both parents should be present when the child's death is announced. The parents may lash out at emergency room personnel, the babysitter, grandparents, or anyone else involved in the child's care—even at each other. They will need reassurance that they were not to blame.

• The parents should be allowed to see the baby in a private room and to express their grief in their own way. They may want to call clergy, friends, or relatives.

• After the parents and family have recovered from their initial shock, they must understand the necessity for an autopsy to confirm the diagnosis of SIDS (in some states, this is mandatory). At this time, they should be given some basic facts about SIDS and encouraged to give their consent for the autopsy.

• The parents should be referred to a local counseling and information program for SIDS parents. Participants in such a program will contact the parents, put them in touch with a professional counselor, and maintain supportive telephone contact. They may also want to be referred to a local SIDS group made up of other parents whose babies died from the syndrome; such a group can provide significant emotional support. Both groups can also help parents cope with a monitoring system if one is recommended. The National Sudden Infant Death Foundation can provide more information about such local groups.

Croup

Croup is a severe inflammation and obstruction of the upper airway, occurring as acute laryngotracheobronchitis (most common), laryngitis, and acute spasmodic laryngitis, and must always be distinguished from epiglottitis. Croup is a childhood disease affecting boys more often than girls (typically between ages 3 months and 3 years), that usually occurs during the winter. Up to 15% of patients have a strong family history of croup. Recovery is usually complete.

Causes

Croup usually results from a viral infection. Parainfluenza viruses cause two thirds of such infections; adenoviruses, respiratory syncytial virus (RSV), influenza and measles viruses, and bacteria (pertussis and diphtheria) account for the rest.

Signs and symptoms

The onset of croup usually follows an upper respiratory tract infection. Clinical features include inspiratory stridor, hoarse or muffled vocal sounds, varying degrees of laryngeal obstruction and respiratory distress, and a characteristic sharp, barklike cough. These symptoms may last only a few hours or persist for a day or two. As it progresses, croup causes inflammatory edema and, possibly, spasm, which can obstruct the upper airway and severely compromise ventilation.

Each form of croup has additional characteristics:

In *laryngotracheobronchitis* (LTB), the symptoms seem to worsen at night. Inflammation causes edema of the bronchi and bronchioles and increasingly difficult expiration which frightens the child. Other characteristic features include fever, diffusely decreased breath sounds, expiratory rhonchi, and scattered rales.

Laryngitis, which results from vocal cord edema, is usually mild and produces no respiratory distress except in infants. Early signs include a sore throat and cough which, rarely, may progress to marked hoarseness, suprasternal and intercostal retractions, inspiratory stridor, dyspnea, diminished breath sounds, restlessness, and in later stages, severe dyspnea and exhaustion.

Acute spasmodic laryngitis affects children between ages 1 and 3, particularly those with allergies and a family history of croup. It typically begins with mild to moderate hoarseness and nasal discharge, followed by the characteristic cough and noisy inspiration (which often awaken the child at night), labored breathing with retractions, rapid pulse, and clammy skin. The child understandably becomes anxious, which may lead to increasing dyspnea and transient cyanosis. These severe symptoms diminish after several hours but reappear in a milder form on the next one or two nights.

Diagnosis

When bacterial infection is the cause, throat cultures may identify organisms and their sensitivity to antibiotics, and also rule out diphtheria. A neck X-ray may show areas of upper airway narrowing and edema in subglottic folds, while laryngoscopy may reveal inflammation and obstruction in epiglottal and laryngeal areas. In evaluating the patient, it is necessary to consider foreign body obstruction (a common cause of croupy cough in young children) as well as masses and cysts.

Treatment

For most children with croup, home care with rest, cool humidification during sleep, and antipyretics, such as aspirin or acetaminophen, relieve symptoms. However, respiratory distress that interferes with oral hydration requires hospitalization and parenteral fluid replacement to prevent dehydration. If bacterial infection is the cause, antibiotic therapy is necessary. Oxygen therapy may also be required.

Additional considerations

Care consists of monitoring and supporting respiration and controlling fever. Because croup is so frightening to the child and his family, they'll need support and reassurance.

• The patient must be monitored for cough and breath sounds, hoarseness, severity of retractions, inspiratory stridor, cyanosis, respiratory rate and character (especially prolonged and labored respirations), restlessness, fever, and cardiac rate.

• The child must be kept as quiet as possible, but shouldn't be sedated, since this may depress respiration. If the patient is an infant, he should be put in an infant seat or propped up with a pillow; an older child should be placed in Fowler's position. An older child may require a cool mist tent to help him breathe.

• Patients suspected of having RSV and parainfluenza infections require isolation, if possible. Hands must be washed carefully before leaving the room to avoid transmission to other children, particularly infants. This precaution must be observed by parents and everyone involved in the care of these children.

• Fever can be controlled with sponge baths and antipyretics. A hypothermia blanket may help patients with temperatures above 102° F. (38.9° C.). In infants and young children with high fevers, seizures are a potential problem. I.V. antibiotics may be ordered.

• Sore throat can be soothed with water-based ices such as fruit sherbet and popsicles. Thicker, milk-based fluids should not be given if the child is producing heavy mucus or has great difficulty in swallowing. Petrolatum jelly or another ointment applied around the nose and lips will soothe irritation from nasal discharge and mouth breathing.

• The patient should be told about all procedures. Any questions the family has should be answered candidly.

When croup doesn't require hospitalization:

• The patient and family need thorough teaching for effective home care. They may want to use a cool humidifier (vaporizer). To relieve croupy spells, parents should carry the child into the bathroom, shut the door, and turn on the hot water. Breathing in warm, moist air quickly eases an acute spell of croup.

• Parents must know that ear infections and pneumonia are complications of croup which may appear about 5 days after recovery. They should report earache, productive cough, high fever, or increased shortness of breath immediately.

Epiglottitis

Acute epiglottitis is an acute inflammation of the epiglottis that tends to cause airway obstruction. It occurs in children between ages 2 and 12. A critical emergency, it can prove fatal in 8% to 12% of victims unless it is recognized and treated promptly.

Causes
Epiglottitis usually results from infection with the bacteria *Hemophilus influenzae* type B and, occasionally, pneumococci and group A streptococci.

Signs and symptoms
Sometimes preceded by an upper respiratory infection, epiglottitis may rapidly progress to complete upper airway obstruction within 2 to 5 hours. Laryngeal obstruction occurs due to inflammation and edema of the epiglottis. Accompanying symptoms include high fever, stridor, sore throat, dysphagia, ir-

ritability, restlessness, and drooling. To relieve severe respiratory distress, the child with epiglottitis may hyperextend his neck, sit up, and lean forward with his mouth open, his tongue protruding, and nostrils flaring as he tries to breathe. He may develop inspiratory retractions and rhonchi.

Diagnosis
In acute epiglottitis, throat examination reveals a large, edematous, bright red epiglottis. Such examination should follow neck X-rays and, generally, should not be performed if suspected degree of

obstruction is great; special equipment (laryngoscope and endotracheal tubes) should be available, since a tongue depressor can cause sudden complete airway obstruction. Trained personnel (such as an anesthesiologist) should be on hand during throat examination to secure an emergency airway.

Treatment
A child with acute epiglottitis and airway obstruction requires emergency hospitalization; he may need emergency endotracheal intubation or a tracheotomy, and should be carefully monitored in an ICU. Respiratory distress that interferes with swallowing necessitates parenteral fluid administration to prevent dehydration. A patient with acute epiglottitis should always receive a 10-day course of parenteral antibiotics— usually ampicillin (if the child is allergic to penicillin or if there is a significant incidence of ampicillin-resistant endemic *H. influenzae,* chloramphenicol or another antibiotic may be substi-

tuted). Oxygen therapy and blood gas monitoring may also be desirable.

Additional considerations
The following must be available in case of sudden complete airway obstruction: a tracheotomy tray, endotracheal tubes, AMBU bag, oxygen equipment, and a laryngoscope, with blades of various sizes. Blood gases require monitoring for hypoxia and hypercapnia.

Signs and symptoms include increasing restlessness, rising cardiac rate, fever, dyspnea, and retractions, which may indicate a need for a tracheotomy. After tracheotomy, the child will need as much attention as possible, since he won't be able to cry or call out. He'll also need emotional support. The patient and family should be reassured that the tracheotomy is short-term (usually from 4 to 7 days). Rising temperature and pulse rate, and hypotension— signs of secondary infection—must be watched for and reported.

ACUTE DISORDERS

Acute Respiratory Failure in COPD

In patients with essentially normal lung tissue, acute respiratory failure (ARF) usually means PCO_2 above 50 mmHg and PO_2 below 50 mmHg. These limits, however, don't apply to patients with chronic obstructive lung disease (COPD), who often have consistently high PCO_2 and low PO_2 values. In patients with COPD, only acute deterioration in blood gas values, with corresponding clinical deterioration, indicates ARF.

Causes
ARF may develop in COPD patients as a result of any condition that increases the work of breathing and decreases the respiratory drive. Such conditions include respiratory tract infection (such as bronchitis or pneumonia)—the most common precipitating factor—bronchospasm, or accumulating secretions secondary to cough suppression. Other causes of ARF in COPD include:

• *CNS depression*—injudicious use of sedatives, narcotics, tranquilizers, or oxygen, or from head trauma
• *cardiovascular disorders*—myocardial infarction, congestive heart failure, or pulmonary emboli
• *airway irritants*—smoke, fumes, or air pollution
• *endocrine and metabolic disorders*—myxedema or metabolic alkalosis
• *thoracic abnormalities*—chest trauma,

pneumothorax, or thoracic or abdominal surgery.

Signs and symptoms

In COPD patients with ARF, increased ventilation-perfusion mismatching and reduced alveolar ventilation decrease arterial PO_2 (hypoxemia) and increase arterial PCO_2 (hypercapnia). This rise in carbon dioxide tension lowers the pH. The resulting hypoxemia and acidemia affect all body organs, especially the central nervous, respiratory, and cardiovascular systems. Specific symptoms vary with the underlying cause of ARF, but may include:

• *Respiratory*—Rate may be increased, decreased, or normal depending on the cause; respirations may be shallow, deep, or alternate between the two; air hunger may occur. Cyanosis may or may not be present, depending on the hemoglobin level and arterial oxygenation. Auscultation of the chest may reveal rales, rhonchi, wheezes, or diminished breath sounds.

• *CNS*—There is evidence of restlessness, confusion, loss of concentration, irritability, tremulousness, diminished tendon reflexes, papilledema, coma.

• *Cardiovascular*—Tachycardia with increased cardiac output and mildly elevated blood pressure secondary to adrenal release of catecholamine, occurs early in response to low PO_2. With myocardial hypoxia, arrhythmias may develop. Pulmonary hypertension also occurs.

Diagnosis

Progressive deterioration in blood gas values and pH, when compared to the patient's "normal" values, strongly suggests ARF in COPD. (In patients with essentially normal lung tissue, pH above 7.35 usually indicates ARF, but COPD patients display an even greater deviation from this normal value, as they do with blood PCO_2 and PO_2.) Other laboratory findings supporting the diagnosis include:

• HCO_3—Increased levels indicate metabolic alkalosis, or reflect metabolic compensation for chronic respiratory acidosis.

• *Hematocrit and hemoglobin*—Abnormally low levels may be due to blood loss, indicating decreased oxygen-carrying capacity.

• *Serum electrolytes*—Hypokalemia may result from compensatory hyperventilation—an attempt to correct alkalosis; hypochloremia often occurs in metabolic alkalosis.

• *WBC*—Count is elevated if ARF is due to bacterial infection; Gram's stain and culture of sputum can identify causative organisms.

• *Chest X-ray*—Findings identify pulmonary pathology, such as emphysema, atelectasis, lesions, pneumothorax, infiltrates, or effusions.

• *EKG*—Arrhythmias characteristic of cor pulmonale and myocardial hypoxia are common.

Treatment

ARF in COPD patients is an emergency which requires cautious oxygen therapy (using nasal prongs or venturi mask) to raise the patient's PO_2 to an acceptable level. If significant respiratory acidosis persists after correction of severe hypoxemia, mechanical ventilation through an endotracheal or a tracheostomy tube may be necessary. Treatment routinely includes antibiotics for infection and bronchodilators.

Additional considerations

• Since most ARF patients are treated in an ICU, they should be oriented to the environment, procedures, and routines to minimize anxiety.

• To reverse hypoxemia, oxygen should be administered at appropriate concentrations to maintain PO_2 at a minimum of 50 to 60 mmHg. Patients with COPD usually require only small amounts of supplemental oxygen. Positive responses include improvement in the patient's breathing and color and in arterial blood gas results.

• A patent airway must be maintained. If the patient is retaining CO_2, he should try to cough and to breathe deeply with "pursed lips." While awake, he should be turned every hour. Regular postural drainage and chest physiotherapy will facilitate expectoration of secretions.

• An intubated patient will need hourly tracheal suction after hyperoxygenation. Any change in quantity, consistency, and color of sputum should be noted. Humidification adequate to liquefy secretions should be provided.

• The patient must be watched closely for respiratory arrest. Changes in arterial blood gases should be reported immediately.

• Serum electrolytes must be monitored and imbalances corrected; fluid balance should be monitored by recording intake and output or daily weights.

• Any arrhythmias will be apparent on the cardiac monitor.

If the patient requires mechanical ventilation:

• Ventilator settings and arterial blood gas values must be checked frequently, since FIO_2 setting will depend on the results of the blood gases. Specimens to monitor them should be drawn 20 to 30 minutes after every FIO_2 change.

• Infection can be avoided by using sterile suctioning technique and by changing ventilator circuits every 24 hours.

• Since stress ulcers are common in intubated ICU patients, gastric secretions should be checked for evidence of bleeding if the patient has a nasogastric tube or complains of epigastric tenderness, nausea, or vomiting. Also, any changes in hemoglobin or hematocrit levels should be reported, all stools checked for occult blood, and antacids or cimetidine administered, as ordered.

• Tracheal erosion can result from artificial airway cuff overinflation, which compresses tracheal wall vasculature. This can be prevented by using minimal leak technique and a cuffed tube with high residual volume (low pressure cuff), foam cuff, or pressure regulating valve on cuff.

• The nasotracheal tube must be kept clean and midline within the nostrils, to prevent nasal necrosis. Tape can be loosened periodically to prevent skin breakdown. The ventilator tubing interface should be adequately supported, and excessive movement of tubes avoided.

Adult Respiratory Distress Syndrome
(Shock, stiff, white, wet, or Da Nang lung)

A form of pulmonary edema that causes acute respiratory failure, adult respiratory distress syndrome (ARDS) results from increased permeability of the alveolar capillary membrane. Fluid accumulates in the lung interstitium, alveolar spaces, and small airways, causing the lung to stiffen. Effective ventilation is thus impaired, prohibiting adequate oxygenation of pulmonary capillary blood. Severe ARDS can cause intractable and fatal hypoxia; however, patients who recover usually have little or no permanent lung damage.

Causes
ARDS results from a variety of respiratory and nonrespiratory insults such as:
• aspiration of gastric contents
• sepsis (primarily gram-negative), trauma (lung contusion, head injury, long bone fracture with fat emboli), or oxygen toxicity
• viral, bacterial, or fungal pneumonia or microemboli (fat or air emboli, or disseminated intravascular coagulation [DIC])
• drug overdose (barbiturates, glutethimide, narcotics) or blood transfusion
• smoke or chemical inhalation (nitrous oxide, chlorine, ammonia)
• hydrocarbon and paraquat ingestion
• pancreatitis, uremia, or miliary tuberculosis (rare)
• near-drowning.

Altered permeability of the alveolar capillary membranes causes fluid to accumulate in the interstitial space. If the pulmonary lymphatics can't remove this fluid, interstitial edema develops. The fluid collects in the peribronchial and peribronchiolar spaces, producing bronchiolar narrowing. Hypoxia occurs as a result of fluid accumulation in alveoli and subsequent alveolar collapse, causing the shunting of blood through nonventilated lung regions. Also, regional differences in compliance and airway narrowing cause regions of low ventilation and inadequate perfusion, which lead to hypoxemia.

Signs and symptoms
ARDS initially produces rapid, shallow breathing and dyspnea within hours to days of the initial injury (sometimes after the patient's condition appears to have stabilized). Hypoxia develops, causing an increased drive for ventilation. Because of the effort required to expand the stiff lung, intercostal and suprasternal retractions result. Fluid accumulation produces rales and rhonchi, and worsening hypoxia causes restlessness, apprehension, mental sluggishness, motor dysfunction, and tachycardia (possibly with transient increased arterial blood pressure). Severe ARDS causes overwhelming hypoxemia which, if uncorrected, results in hypotension, decreasing urinary output, respiratory and metabolic acidosis, and eventually, ventricular fibrillation or standstill.

Diagnosis
On room air, arterial blood gases (ABG) initially show decreased Po_2 (less than 60 mmHg) and Pco_2 (less than 35 mmHg). The resulting pH usually reflects respiratory alkalosis. As ARDS becomes more severe, ABGs show respiratory acidosis (increasing Pco_2 [more than 45 mmHg]) and metabolic acidosis (decreasing HCO_3 [less than 22 mEq/liter]) and a decreasing Po_2 despite oxygen therapy.

Other diagnostic tests include:
• *Pulmonary artery catheterization* helps identify the cause of pulmonary edema by evaluating capillary wedge pressure (PCWP); allows collection of pulmonary artery blood which shows decreased oxygen saturation, reflecting tissue hypoxia; measures pulmonary artery pressure; and measures cardiac output by thermodilution techniques.
• *Serial chest X-rays* initially show bilateral infiltrates; in later stages, ground-glass appearance, and eventually (as hypoxia becomes irreversible), "whiteouts" of both lung fields.

Differential diagnosis must rule out cardiogenic pulmonary edema, pulmonary vasculitis, and diffuse pulmonary hemorrhage. To establish etiology, laboratory work should include sputum, Gram's stain, culture, and sensitivity; blood cultures to detect infections; toxicology screen for drug ingestion; and when pancreatitis is a consideration, a serum amylase determination.

Treatment
When possible, treatment is designed to correct the underlying cause of ARDS and to prevent progression and potentially fatal complications of hypoxia and respiratory acidosis. Supportive medical care consists of administering humidified oxygen by a tight-fitting mask, which allows for use of continuous positive airway pressure (CPAP). Hypoxia that doesn't respond adequately to these measures requires ventilatory support with intubation, volume ventilation, and positive end-expiratory pressure (PEEP). Other supportive measures include fluid restriction, diuretics, and correction of electrolyte and acid-base abnormalities.

When ARDS requires mechanical ventilation, sedatives, narcotics, or neuromuscular blocking agents, such as tubocurarine or pancuronium bromide, may be ordered to minimize restlessness and, thereby, oxygen consumption and carbon dioxide production, and to facilitate ventilation. When ARDS results from fat emboli or chemical injuries to the lungs, a short course of high-dose steroids may help if given early. Treatment to reverse severe metabolic acidosis with sodium bicarbonate may be necessary, and use of fluids and vasopressors may be required to maintain blood pressure. Nonviral infections require antimicrobial drugs.

Additional considerations
ARDS requires careful monitoring and supportive care, which includes:
• frequently assessing the patient's respiratory status and being alert for retractions on inspiration; noting rate, rhythm, and depth of respirations; watching for dyspnea and the use of accessory muscles of respiration; listening for adventitious or diminished breath sounds while auscultating all lobes; checking for clear, frothy sputum that may indicate pulmonary edema.
• observing and documenting the hypoxic patient's neurologic status (level of consciousness, mental sluggishness).
• maintaining a patent airway by suctioning, using sterile, nontraumatic technique; instilling saline solution to help liquefy tenacious secretions when necessary.
• closely monitoring heart rate and blood pressure; watching for arrhythmias that may result from hypoxemia, acid-base disturbances, or electrolyte imbalance; being aware of the desired PCWP level with pulmonary artery catheterization; checking readings frequently and watching for a decrease in mixed venous oxygen saturation.
• monitoring serum electrolytes carefully, and correcting imbalances; measuring intake and output, and weighing patient daily.

• checking ventilator settings frequently, and emptying condensation from tubing promptly to assure maximum oxygen delivery; monitoring ABG studies; checking for metabolic and respiratory acidosis and PO_2 changes; controlling mechanical ventilation with positive airway pressure, for the patient with severe hypoxia; giving sedatives, as needed, to reduce restlessness; checking for hypotension, tachycardia, and decreased urinary output in the patient receiving PEEP; suctioning only as needed to maintain PEEP; repositioning often and recording any increase in secretions, temperature, or hypotension that may indicate a deteriorating condition.
• monitoring nutrition, maintaining joint mobility, and preventing skin breakdown; recording calorie intake; giving tube feedings and hyperalimentation, as ordered; performing passive range-of-motion exercises or helping the patient perform active exercises, if possible; providing meticulous skin care; planning patient care to allow periods of uninterrupted sleep.
• providing emotional support, especially for the ventilated patient; warning the patient who is recovering from ARDS that recovery will take time and he will feel weak for a while.
• watching for and immediately reporting all respiratory changes in the patient who has suffered injuries that may adversely affect the lung, especially during 2- to 3-day period after the injury, when the patient may appear to be improving.

Pulmonary Edema

Pulmonary edema is the accumulation of fluid in the extravascular spaces of the lung. In cardiogenic pulmonary edema, fluid accumulation results from elevations in pulmonary venous and capillary hydrostatic pressures. A common complication of cardiac disorders, pulmonary edema can occur as a chronic condition or develop quickly and rapidly become fatal.

Causes
Pulmonary edema usually results from left ventricular failure due to arterio- sclerotic, hypertensive, cardiomyopathic, or valvular cardiac disease. In such disorders, the compromised left

ventricle requires increased filling pressures to maintain adequate output; these pressures are transmitted to the left atrium, pulmonary veins, and pulmonary capillary bed. This increased pulmonary capillary hydrostatic force promotes transudation of intravascular fluids into the pulmonary interstitium, decreasing lung compliance and interfering with gas exchange. Other factors which may predispose to pulmonary edema include:
• infusion of excessive volumes of I.V. fluids
• decreased serum colloid osmotic pressure as a result of nephrosis, protein-loosing enteropathy, extensive burns, hepatic disease, or nutritional deficiency
• impaired lung lymphatic drainage from Hodgkin's disease or obliterative lymphangitis after radiation
• mitral stenosis and left atrial myxoma which impair left atrial emptying
• pulmonary veno-occlusive disease.

Signs and symptoms

The early symptoms of pulmonary edema reflect interstitial fluid accumulation and diminished lung compliance: dyspnea on exertion, paroxysmal nocturnal dyspnea, orthopnea, and coughing. Clinical features include tachycardia, tachypnea, dependent rales, and a diastolic (S_3) gallop on auscultation. With severe pulmonary edema, the alveoli and bronchioles may fill with fluid and intensify the early symptoms. Respiration becomes labored and rapid, with more diffuse rales and coughing productive of frothy, bloody sputum. Tachycardia increases and arrhythmias may appear. Skin becomes cold, clammy, and cyanotic. Blood pressure falls and pulse becomes thready as cardiac output falls.

Symptoms of severe heart failure with pulmonary edema may also include depressed level of consciousness and confusion.

Diagnosis

Clinical features of pulmonary edema permit a working diagnosis. Arterial blood gases usually show hypoxia; Pco_2 is variable. Both profound respiratory alkalosis and acidosis may occur. Metabolic acidosis occurs when cardiac output is low. Chest X-ray shows diffuse haziness of the lung fields and, often, cardiomegaly and pleural effusions. Pulmonary artery catheterization helps identify left ventricular failure by showing elevated pulmonary wedge pressures. This helps to rule out adult respiratory distress syndrome (ARDS)—in which pulmonary wedge pressure is usually normal.

Treatment

Treatment of pulmonary edema is designed to reduce extravascular fluid, improve gas exchange and myocardial function, and if possible, to correct underlying pathology. Administration of high concentrations of oxygen by cannula, mask, and if necessary, assisted ventilation, improves oxygen delivery to the tissues and often improves acid-base disturbances. A bronchodilator, such as aminophylline, may decrease bronchospasm and enhance myocardial contractility. Diuretics, such as furosemide and ethacrynic acid, promote diuresis, thereby assisting in the mobilization of extravascular fluid.

Treatment of myocardial dysfunction includes digitalis or pressor agents to increase cardiac contractility, antiarrhythmics (particularly when arrhythmias are associated with decreased cardiac output), and occasionally, arterial vasodilators, such as nitroprusside, which decrease peripheral vascular resistance and thereby decrease left ventricular workload. Other therapy includes morphine to reduce anxiety and dyspnea and to dilate the systemic venous bed. Rotating tourniquets may be used as an emergency measure to reduce venous return to the heart from the extremities. tremities.

Additional considerations

When caring for the vulnerable patient, the hospital staff member should:
• watch for early signs of pulmonary edema, especially tachypnea, tachycardia,

and abnormal breath sounds; report any abnormalities; check for peripheral edema, which may also indicate that fluid is accumulating in pulmonary tissue.
• administer oxygen, as ordered.
• monitor vital signs every 15 to 30 minutes while administering nitroprusside in 5% dextrose in water by I.V. drip; discard unused nitroprusside solution after 4 hours, and protect it from light by wrapping the bottle or bag with aluminum foil; watch for arrhythmias in patients receiving digitalis and for marked respiratory depression in those receiving morphine.

• assess the patient's condition frequently, and record response to treatment; monitor arterial blood gases, oral and I.V. fluid intake, urinary output, and, if he has a pulmonary artery catheter, pulmonary end diastolic and wedge pressures; check cardiac monitor often and report changes immediately.
• record the sequence and time of rotating tourniquets.
• reassure the patient, who will be frightened by decreased respiratory capability, in a calm voice and explain all procedures to him; provide emotional support to his family as well.

Cor Pulmonale

The World Health Organization defines chronic cor pulmonale as "hypertrophy of the right ventricle resulting from diseases affecting the function and/or the structure of the lungs, except when these pulmonary alterations are the result of diseases that primarily affect the left side of the heart or of congenital heart disease." Invariably, cor pulmonale follows some disorder of the lungs, pulmonary vessels, chest wall, or respiratory control center. For instance, chronic obstructive pulmonary disease (COPD) produces pulmonary hypertension, which leads to right ventricular hypertrophy and failure. Since cor pulmonale generally occurs late during the course of COPD and other irreversible diseases, prognosis is generally poor.

Causes and incidence

Approximately 85% of patients with cor pulmonale have COPD, and 25% of patients with emphysema eventually develop cor pulmonale. Other respiratory disorders that produce cor pulmonale include:
• obstructive lung diseases such as chronic bronchitis
• restrictive lung diseases such as pneumoconiosis, cystic fibrosis, interstitial pneumonitis, bronchiectasis, scleroderma, and sarcoidosis
• loss of lung tissue after extensive lung surgery
• pulmonary vascular diseases such as recurrent thromboembolism, primary pulmonary hypertension, schistosomiasis, and pulmonary vasculitis
• respiratory insufficiency without pulmonary disease, as seen in chest wall disorders such as kyphoscoliosis, neu-

romuscular incompetence due to muscular dystrophy and amyotrophic lateral sclerosis, polymyositis, and spinal cord lesions above C6
• obesity hypoventilation syndrome (pickwickian syndrome) and upper airway obstruction
• living at high altitudes (chronic mountain sickness).

Pulmonary capillary destruction and pulmonary vasoconstriction (usually secondary to hypoxia) reduce the cross sectional area of the pulmonary vascular bed, thus increasing pulmonary vascular resistance and causing pulmonary hypertension. To compensate for the extra work needed to force blood through the lungs, the right ventricle dilates and hypertrophies. In response to low oxygen content, the bone marrow produces more red blood cells, causing erythrocytosis. When the hematocrit exceeds

55%, blood viscosity increases, which further aggravates pulmonary hypertension and increases the hemodynamic load on the right ventricle. Right ventricular failure is the result.

Cor pulmonale accounts for about 25% of all types of heart failure. It's most common in areas of the world where the incidence of cigarette smoking and COPD is high; cor pulmonale affects middle-aged to elderly men more often than women, but incidence in women is increasing. In children, cor pulmonale may be a complication of cystic fibrosis, hemosiderosis, upper airway obstruction, scleroderma, extensive bronchiectasis, neurologic diseases affecting respiratory muscles, or abnormalities of the respiratory control center.

Signs and symptoms

As long as the heart can compensate for the increased pulmonary vascular resistance, clinical features reflect the underlying disorder and occur mostly in the respiratory system. They include chronic productive cough, exertional dyspnea, wheezing respirations, fatigue, and weakness. Progression of cor pulmonale is associated with dyspnea (even at rest) that worsens on exertion, tachypnea, orthopnea, edema, weakness, and right upper quadrant discomfort. Examination of the chest reveals findings that are characteristic of the underlying lung disease.

Signs of cor pulmonale and right ventricular failure include dependent edema; distended neck veins; enlarged, tender liver; prominent parasternal or epigastric cardiac impulse; hepatojugular reflux; and tachycardia. Decreased cardiac output may cause a weak pulse and hypotension. Chest examination yields various findings, depending on the underlying cause of cor pulmonale. In COPD, auscultation reveals rales, rhonchi, and diminished breath sounds. When the disease is secondary to upper airway obstruction or damage to CNS respiratory centers, chest examination may be normal except for a right ventricular lift, gallop rhythm, and loud pulmonic component of S_2. Tricuspid insufficiency produces a pansystolic murmur heard at the lower left sternal border; its intensity increases on inspiration, distinguishing it from a murmur due to mitral valve disease. A right ventricular early diastolic rhythm which increases on inspiration can be heard at the left sternal border or over the epigastrium. A systolic pulmonic ejection click may also be heard. Drowsiness and alterations in consciousness may also occur.

Diagnosis

Pulmonary artery pressure measurements (by pulmonary artery catheter) show increased right ventricular and pulmonary artery pressures as a result of increased pulmonary vascular resistance. Both right ventricular systolic and pulmonary artery systolic pressures will be more than 30 mmHg. Pulmonary artery diastolic pressure will be more than 15 mmHg.

• *Echocardiography* or *angiography* indicates right ventricular enlargement.

• *Chest X-ray* shows large central pulmonary arteries and suggests right ventricular enlargement by rightward enlargement of cardiac silhouette on an anterior chest film.

• *Arterial blood gases* show decreased Po_2 (often less than 70 mmHg and never more than 90 mmHg).

• *EKG* frequently shows arrhythmias such as premature atrial and ventricular contractions and atrial fibrillation during severe hypoxia; may also show right bundle branch block, right axis deviation, prominent P waves and inverted T wave in right precordial leads, and right ventricular hypertrophy.

• *Pulmonary function tests* are consistent with underlying pulmonary disease.

• *Hematocrit* is often greater than 50%.

Treatment

Treatment of cor pulmonale is designed to reduce hypoxia, increase the patient's exercise tolerance, and when possible, correct the underlying condition. In addition to bed rest, treatment includes:

• *digitalis glycoside* (digoxin)

• *antibiotics* when respiratory infection is present; culture and sensitivity of sputum specimen aid in selection of antibiotics

• *potent pulmonary artery vasodilators* (such as phentolamine, diazoxide, nitroprusside, or hydralazine) in primary pulmonary hypertension

• *oxygen* by mask or cannula in concentrations ranging from 24% to 40%, depending on arterial PO_2, as necessary. In acute cases, therapy may also include mechanical ventilation. Patients with COPD generally shouldn't receive high concentrations of oxygen because of possible subsequent respiratory depression.

• *low-salt diet, restricted fluid intake,* and *diuretics* such as furosemide to reduce edema. Occasionally, cor pulmonale may require phlebotomy to reduce red cell mass.

• *anticoagulation* with small doses of heparin may be used, since these patients probably are at increased risk of thromboembolism.

Depending on the underlying cause, some variations in treatment may be indicated. A tracheotomy, for example, may be necessary if the patient has an upper airway obstruction, and steroids may be used in patients with polymyositis.

Additional considerations

• The patient's diet should be carefully planned by a dietitian. Since the patient may lack energy and tire easily when eating, he will need small, frequent feedings rather than three heavy meals.

• Fluid retention can be prevented by limiting the patient's fluid intake to 1,000 to 2,000 ml/day and by providing a low-sodium diet. The patient with cor pulmonale must understand the need for this restriction, since patients with COPD probably have been encouraged to drink up to 10 glasses of water a day.

• Serum potassium levels require close monitoring if the patient is receiving diuretics. Low serum potassium levels can potentiate the risk of arrhythmias associated with digitalis.

• Signs of digitalis toxicity include anorexia, nausea, vomiting, and yellow halos around visual images. The patient should be monitored for cardiac arrhythmias. He'll need to be taught how to check his radial pulse before taking digoxin or any digitalis glycoside and notify the doctor of changes in pulse rate.

• The bedridden patient will require frequent repositioning to prevent atelectasis.

• Meticulous respiratory care, including oxygen therapy and, for COPD patients, pursed-lip breathing exercises are important. Arterial blood gases should be measured periodically, and the patient watched for signs of respiratory failure: change in pulse rate; deep, labored respirations; and increased fatigue produced by less exertion.

Before discharge:

• The patient must understand the importance of maintaining a low-salt diet, weighing himself daily, and watching for and immediately reporting edema. To detect edema, he can press the skin over his shins with one finger, hold it for a second or two, then check for a finger impression.

• He should allow himself frequent rest periods and do his breathing exercises regularly. Adequate rest is very important.

• If the patient needs suctioning or supplemental oxygen at home, he should be referred to a social service agency which can help him obtain the necessary equipment, and arrange for follow-up examinations by a visiting nurse.

• Since pulmonary infection often exacerbates COPD and cor pulmonale, the patient must watch for and immediately report early signs and symptoms of infection such as increased sputum production, change in sputum color from clear white, increased coughing or wheezing, chest pain, fever, and tightness in the chest. He should avoid crowds, especially during the flu season.

• The cor pulmonale patient must not use nonprescribed medications, especially sedatives which may depress the ventilatory drive.

Legionnaires' Disease

Legionnaires' disease is an acute bronchopneumonia produced by a fastidious, gram-negative bacillus. It derives its name and notoriety from the peculiar, highly publicized disease that struck 182 people (29 of whom died) at an American Legion convention in Philadelphia in July 1976. This disease may occur epidemically or sporadically, usually in late summer or early fall. Its severity ranges from a mild illness, with or without pneumonitis, to multilobar pneumonia, with a mortality as high as 15%. A milder, self-limiting form (Pontiac syndrome) subsides within a few days but leaves the patient fatigued for several weeks; this form mimics Legionnaires' disease but produces few or no respiratory symptoms, no pneumonia, and no fatalities.

Causes and incidence

Legionnaires' disease bacterium (LDB), recently named *Legionella pneumophila*, is an aerobic, gram-negative bacillus that probably is transmitted by an airborne route. In past epidemics, it has spread through cooling towers or evaporation condensers in air-conditioning systems. However, LDB also flourishes in soil and excavation sites. It does not spread from person to person.

Legionnaires' disease occurs more often in men than in women and is most likely to affect:
• persons in the middle-aged to elderly age-group.
• immunocompromised patients (particularly those receiving corticosteroids, for example, after a transplant), or those with lymphoma or other disorders associated with delayed hypersensitivity.
• patients with a chronic underlying disease, such as diabetes, chronic renal failure, or chronic obstructive pulmonary disease (COPD).
• alcoholics.
• cigarette smokers (three to four times more likely to develop Legionnaires' disease than nonsmokers).

Signs and symptoms

The multisystem clinical features of Legionnaires' disease follow a predictable sequence, although onset of the disease may be gradual or sudden. After a 2- to 10-day incubation period, nonspecific, prodromal signs and symptoms appear, including diarrhea, anorexia, malaise, diffuse myalgias and generalized weakness, headache, recurrent chills, and an unremitting fever, which develops within 12 to 48 hours with a temperature that may reach 105° F. (40.5° C.). A cough then develops that, initially, is nonproductive but eventually may produce grayish, nonpurulent, and occasionally, blood-streaked sputum.

Other characteristic features of LDB are nausea, vomiting, disorientation, mental sluggishness, confusion, mild temporary amnesia, pleuritic chest pain, tachypnea, dyspnea, fine rales, and in 50% of patients, bradycardia. Patients who develop pneumonia may also experience hypoxia. Other complications include hypotension, delirium, congestive heart failure, arrhythmias, acute respiratory failure, renal failure, and shock (usually fatal).

Diagnosis

Patient history focuses on possible sources of infection and predisposing conditions. In addition:
• *Chest X-ray* shows patchy, localized infiltration, which progresses to multilobar consolidation (usually involving the lower lobes), pleural effusion, and in fulminant disease, opacification of the entire lung.
• *Auscultation* reveals fine rales, progressing to coarse rales as the disease advances.
• *Abnormal test results* include leuko-

cytosis, increased ESR, moderate increase in liver enzymes (SGOT, SGPT, alkaline phosphatase), decreased Po_2, and initially, decreased Pco_2. Bronchial washings, blood and pleural fluid cultures, and transtracheal aspirates rule out other pulmonary infections.

 Definitive tests include direct immunofluorescence of respiratory tract secretions and tissue, culture of *L. pneumophila,* and indirect fluorescent antibody testing of serum comparing acute samples with convalescent samples drawn at least 3 weeks later. A convalescent serum showing a fourfold or greater rise in antibody titer for LDB confirms this diagnosis.

Treatment

Antibiotic treatment begins as soon as Legionnaires' disease is suspected and diagnostic material is collected, and shouldn't await laboratory confirmation. Erythromycin is the drug of choice; if erythromycin is contraindicated, rifampin or rifampin with tetracycline may be used. Supportive therapy includes administration of antipyretics, fluid replacement, circulatory support with pressor drugs, if necessary, and oxygen administration by mask or cannula, or by mechanical ventilation with positive end-expiratory pressure (PEEP).

Additional considerations

• The patient's respiratory rate is important. Chest wall expansion, ease of ventilation, depth and pattern of respirations, cough, and chest pain should be noted. Restlessness may indicate that the patient is hypoxic, requiring suctioning, change of position, or more aggressive oxygen therapy.

• Vital signs, arterial blood gases, level of consciousness, orientation, and dryness and color of lips and mucous membranes must be continually monitored. Signs of shock (decreased blood pressure, thready pulse, diaphoresis, clammy skin) require immediate intervention.

• The patient should be kept comfortable and away from drafts. Good mouth care is important. Soothing cream on the nostrils may ease discomfort.

• Fluid and electrolytes should be replaced, as needed, to correct imbalances. The patient with renal failure may require dialysis.

• Mechanical ventilation and other respiratory therapy may be needed. The patient must learn how to cough effectively and do deep breathing exercises. Coughing and deep breathing exercises should continue until recovery is complete.

• If antibiotics are ordered, the patient must be observed carefully for side effects.

Atelectasis

Atelectasis is incomplete expansion of lobules (clusters of alveoli) or lung segments which may result in partial or complete lung collapse. This causes the loss of regions of the lung for gas exchange; unoxygenated blood passes through these areas unchanged, thereby producing hypoxia. Atelectasis may be chronic or acute, and occurs to some degree in many patients undergoing upper abdominal or thoracic surgery. Prognosis depends on prompt removal of any airway obstruction, relief of hypoxia, and reexpansion of collapsed lung.

Causes

Atelectasis often results from bronchial occlusion by mucous plugs (a special problem in persons with chronic obstructive pulmonary disease), bronchiectasis, cystic fibrosis, and prolonged heavy smoking (smoking increases mucus production and also damages cilia). Atelectasis may also result from occlusion by foreign bodies, bronchogenic carcinoma, and inflammatory lung disease.

Other causes include idiopathic respiratory distress syndrome of the newborn (hyaline membrane disease), oxygen toxicity, and pulmonary edema, in which alveolar surfactant changes increase surface tension and permit complete alveolar deflation.

External compression which inhibits full lung expansion or any condition that makes deep breathing painful may also cause atelectasis. Such compression or pain may result from upper abdominal surgical incisions, rib fractures, pleuritic chest pain, tight dressings around the chest, or obesity (which elevates the diaphragm and reduces tidal volume). Atelectasis may also result from prolonged immobility, since this causes preferential ventilation of one area of the lung over another, or mechanical ventilation using constant small tidal volumes without intermittent deep breaths. CNS depression (as in drug overdose) eliminates periodic sighing and is a predisposing factor of progressive atelectasis.

Signs and symptoms

Clinical effects vary with the cause of collapse, the degree of hypoxia, and any underlying disease, but generally include some dyspnea. Atelectasis of a small area of the lung may produce only minimal symptoms which subside without specific treatment. However, massive collapse can produce severe dyspnea, anxiety, cyanosis, diaphoresis, peripheral circulatory collapse, tachycardia, and substernal or intercostal retraction. Also, atelectasis may result in compensatory hyperinflation of unaffected areas of the lung, mediastinal shift to the affected side, and elevation of the ipsilateral hemidiaphragm.

Diagnosis

Diagnosis requires an accurate patient history, physical examination, and most importantly, a chest X-ray. Auscultation reveals decreased breath sounds. When a large portion of the lung is collapsed,

percussion is dull. However, extensive areas of "microatelectasis" may exist without abnormalities on chest X-ray. Chest X-ray shows characteristic horizontal lines in the lower lung zones and, with segmental or lobar collapse, characteristic dense shadows often associated with hyperinflation of neighboring lung zones. If the cause is unknown, diagnostic procedures may include bronchoscopy to rule out obstructing neoplasm or foreign body.

Treatment

Treatment includes incentive spirometry, chest percussion, postural drainage, frequent coughing and deep breathing exercises, or intermittent positive pressure breathing (IPPB). If these measures fail, bronchoscopy may be helpful in removing secretions. Humidity and bronchodilators can improve mucociliary clearance and dilate airways; they are sometimes used with IPPB. Atelectasis secondary to an obstructing neoplasm may require surgery or radiation therapy. Postoperative thoracic and abdominal surgery patients require analgesics to facilitate deep breathing—to minimize the risk of atelectasis.

Additional considerations

• To prevent atelectasis, postoperative and other high-risk patients should be encouraged to cough and deep breathe every 1 to 2 hours. A pillow held tightly over the incision will minimize pain during coughing exercises in postoperative patients. These patients must be repositioned *gently* and helped to walk as soon as possible. They will need analgesics adequate to control pain.
• During mechanical ventilation, tidal volume should be set at 10 to 15 ml/kg of body weight to ensure adequate expansion of lungs. If appropriate, the sigh mechanism on the ventilator can be used to intermittently increase tidal volume at the rate of three to four sighs per hour.
• Use of an incentive spirometer will encourage deep inspiration. The patient should use the spirometer every 1 to 2 hours.

• In patients who receive IPPB, abdominal distention may result from swallowing air. Signs of pneumothorax, such as sudden onset of dyspnea and cyanosis, should be reported immediately. Response to IPPB and development of a productive cough should be noted.

• Chest percussion and postural drainage will help mobilization and clearance of secretions; if the patient is intubated or uncooperative, suctioning may be needed. Sedatives should be used with discretion, since they depress the cough reflex and suppress sighing. However, the patient will not cooperate with treatment if he is in pain. Humidified air and adequate fluid intake will help mobilize secretions.

• Breath sounds should be assessed frequently and any change reported immediately.

• The patient must understand all aspects of respiratory care, including postural drainage, coughing, and deep breathing. He should stop smoking and lose weight, if needed. He must be given reassurance and emotional support, as he will undoubtedly be frightened by limited breathing capacity and difficulty in speaking.

Respiratory Acidosis

An acid-base disturbance characterized by reduced alveolar ventilation and manifested by hypercapnia (PCO_2 greater than 45 mmHg), respiratory acidosis can be acute (due to a sudden failure in ventilation) or chronic (as in long-term pulmonary disease). Prognosis depends on severity of the underlying disturbance, as well as the patient's general clinical condition.

Causes

Some predisposing factors in respiratory acidosis:

• *Drugs:* Narcotics, anesthetics, hypnotics, and sedatives decrease the sensitivity of the respiratory center.

• *CNS trauma:* Medullary injury may impair ventilatory drive.

• *Chronic metabolic alkalosis:* Respiratory compensatory mechanisms attempt to normalize pH by decreasing alveolar ventilation.

• *Neuromuscular disease* (such as myasthenia gravis, Guillain-Barré syndrome, and poliomyelitis): Failure of respiratory muscles to respond properly to respiratory drive reduces alveolar ventilation.

In addition, respiratory acidosis can result from airway obstruction or parenchymal lung disease which interferes with alveolar ventilation. Chronic obstructive pulmonary disease (COPD), asthma, severe adult respiratory distress syndrome (ARDS), chronic bronchitis, large pneumothorax, extensive pneumonia, and pulmonary edema may lead to respiratory acidosis.

Hypoventilation compromises excretion of CO_2 produced through metabolism. The retained CO_2 then combines with H_2O to form an excess of carbonic acid (H_2CO_3), decreasing the blood pH. As a result, concentration of hydrogen ions in body fluids, which directly reflects acidity, increases.

Signs and symptoms

Acute respiratory acidosis produces CNS disturbances which reflect changes in the pH of CSF rather than increased CO_2 levels, and cause the patient to become restless, confused and apprehensive, or somnolent and to develop a fine or flapping tremor (asterixis), or to slip into a coma. He may complain of headaches and exhibit dyspnea and tachypnea with papilledema and depressed reflexes. Unless the patient is receiving oxygen, hypoxemia accompanies respiratory acidosis. This disorder may also cause cardiovascular abnormalities, such as tachycardia, hypertension, atrial and ventricular arrhythmias, and in severe acidosis, hypotension with vasodilation (bounding pulses and warm periphery).

Diagnosis

Arterial blood gases confirm respiratory acidosis: PCO_2 over the normal 45 mmHg; pH usually below the normal range of 7.35 to 7.45; and HCO_3 normal in the acute stage, but elevated in the chronic stage.

Treatment

Effective treatment for respiratory acidosis is designed to correct the underlying source of alveolar hypoventilation.

Significantly reduced alveolar ventilation may require mechanical ventilation until the underlying condition can be effectively treated. In COPD this includes bronchodilators, oxygen, and antibiotics; drug therapy for conditions such as myasthenia gravis; removal of foreign bodies from the airway; antibiotics for pneumonia; dialysis to remove toxic drugs; and correction of metabolic alkalosis.

Dangerously low blood pH levels (less than 7.15) can produce profound CNS and cardiovascular deterioration and may require administration of sodium bicarbonate I.V. In chronic lung disease, elevated CO_2 may persist despite optimal treatment.

Additional considerations

With a patient with respiratory acidosis, the hospital staff member should:
• be alert for critical changes in the patient's respiratory, CNS, and cardiovascular functions; report any such changes immediately, as well as any variations in arterial blood gases and electrolyte status; maintain adequate hydration.
• maintain a patent airway and provide adequate humidification if acidosis requires mechanical ventilation; perform tracheal suctioning regularly and vigorous chest physiotherapy, if ordered; continuously monitor ventilator settings and respiratory status.
• closely monitor patients with COPD and chronic CO_2 retention for signs of acidosis; administer oxygen at low flow rates; closely monitor all patients who receive narcotics and sedatives; instruct the patient who has received a general anesthetic to turn, cough, and perform deep-breathing exercises frequently to prevent the onset of respiratory acidosis.

Respiratory Alkalosis

Respiratory alkalosis is a condition marked by a decrease in PCO_2 to less than 35 mmHg, which is due to alveolar hyperventilation. Uncomplicated respiratory alkalosis leads to a decrease in hydrogen ion concentration, which causes elevated blood pH. Hypocapnia occurs when the elimination of CO_2 by the lungs exceeds the production of CO_2 at the cellular level.

Causes

Causes of respiratory alkalosis fall into two categories:
• *pulmonary*—pneumonia, interstitial lung disease, pulmonary vascular disease, and acute asthma
• *nonpulmonary*—anxiety, fever, aspirin toxicity, metabolic acidosis, CNS disease (inflammation or tumor), gram-negative septicemia, and hepatic failure.

Signs and symptoms

The cardinal sign of respiratory alkalosis is deep, rapid breathing, possibly above 40 respirations a minute and much like the Kussmaul breathing of diabetic acidosis. Such hyperventilation usually leads to CNS and neuromuscular disturbances, causing lightheadedness or dizziness (subnormal CO_2 levels decrease cerebral blood flow), agitation, circumoral and peripheral paresthesias, carpopedal spasms, twitching (possibly progressing to tetany), and muscle weakness. Characteristic effects of severe respiratory alkalosis include hyperpnea and cardiac arrhythmias (that may fail to respond to conventional treatment).

Diagnosis

 Arterial blood gases confirm respiratory alkalosis and rule out respiratory compensation for metabolic acidosis: PCO_2 below 35 mmHg; pH elevated in proportion to fall in PCO_2 in the acute stage, but falling toward normal in the chronic stage; HCO_3 normal in the acute stage, but below normal in the chronic stage.

Treatment

Treatment is designed to eradicate the underlying condition—for example, removal of ingested toxins, treatment of fever or sepsis, and treatment of CNS disease. In severe respiratory alkalosis, the patient may be instructed to breathe into a paper bag, which helps relieve acute anxiety and increases CO_2 levels.
• Prevention of hyperventilation in patients receiving mechanical ventilation requires monitoring arterial blood gases and adjusting dead space or minute ventilation volume.

Additional considerations

With a patient with respiratory alkalosis, the hospital staff member should:
• observe the patient carefully for subtle changes in neurologic, neuromuscular, or cardiovascular functions; report any such changes immediately.
• remember that twitching and cardiac arrhythmias may be associated with alkalemia and electrolyte imbalances; monitor arterial blood gases and serum electrolytes closely.
• explain all diagnostic tests and procedures to reduce anxiety.

Pneumothorax

Pneumothorax is an accumulation of air or gas between the parietal and visceral pleurae. The amount of air or gas trapped in the intrapleural space determines the degree of lung collapse. In a tension pneumothorax, the air in the pleural space is under higher pressure than air in adjacent lung and vascular structures. Without prompt treatment, a tension or a large pneumothorax results in fatal pulmonary and circulatory impairment.

Causes and incidence

Spontaneous pneumothorax usually occurs in otherwise healthy adults aged 20 to 40. Air leakage from ruptured congenital blebs adjacent to the visceral pleural surface, near the apex of the lung, causes this form of pneumothorax. Less often, it results from underlying pulmonary disease—for instance, an emphysematous bulla that ruptures during exercise or coughing, or tubercular or malignant lesions that erode into the pleural space. Spontaneous pneumothorax may also occur in interstitial lung disease, such as eosinophilic granuloma.

Traumatic pneumothorax may result from insertion of a central venous pressure line, thoracic surgery, or a penetrating chest injury, such as a gunshot or knife wound, or it may follow a transbronchial biopsy. It may also occur during thoracentesis or a closed pleural biopsy. When traumatic pneumothorax follows a penetrating chest injury, it often coexists with hemothorax (blood in pleural space).

In *tension pneumothorax*, positive pleural pressure develops as a result of any of the causes of traumatic pneumothorax. When air enters the pleural space through a tear in lung tissue and is unable to leave by the same vent, each inspiration traps air in the pleural space, resulting in positive pleural pressure. This in turn causes collapse of the ipsilateral lung and marked impairment of venous return, which can severely compromise cardiac output, and may cause a mediastinal shift. Decreased filling of the great veins of the chest results in diminished cardiac output and lowered blood pressure.

Pneumothorax can also be classified as open or closed. In *open pneumothorax* (usually the result of trauma), air flows between the pleural space and the outside of the body. In *closed pneumothorax,* air reaches the pleural space directly from the lung.

Signs and symptoms

The cardinal features of pneumothorax are sudden, sharp, pleuritic pain (exacerbated by movement of the chest, breathing, and coughing); asymmetric chest wall movement; shortness of breath; and cyanosis. In moderate to severe pneumothorax, profound respiratory distress may develop, with signs of tension pneumothorax: weak and rapid pulse, pallor, neck vein distention, anxiety. Tension pneumothorax produces the most severe respiratory symptoms; a spontaneous pneumothorax that releases only a small amount of air into the pleural space may cause no symptoms.

Diagnosis

Sudden, sharp chest pain and shortness of breath suggest pneumothorax.

 Chest X-ray showing air in the pleural space and, possibly, mediastinal shift confirms this diagnosis. In the absence of a definitive chest X-ray, physical examination occasionally reveals:

• *on inspection:* overexpansion and rigidity of the affected chest side; in tension pneumothorax, neck vein distention with hypotension and tachycardia.

• *on palpation:* crackling beneath the skin, indicating subcutaneous emphysema (air in tissue) and decreased vocal fremitus.

• *on percussion:* hyperresonance on the affected side.

• *on auscultation:* decreased or absent breath sounds over the collapsed lung.

If the pneumothorax is significant, arterial blood gas findings include pH less than 7.35, Po_2 less than 80 mmHg, and Pco_2 above 45 mmHg.

Treatment

Treatment is conservative for spontaneous pneumothorax in which no signs of increased pleural pressure (indicating tension pneumothorax) appear, lung collapse is less than 30%, and the patient shows no signs of dyspnea or other indications of physiologic compromise. Such treatment consists of bed rest; careful monitoring of blood pressure, pulse rate, and respirations; oxygen administration; and possibly, needle aspiration of air with a large-bore needle attached to a syringe. If more than 30% of lung is collapsed, treatment to reexpand the lung includes placing a thoracostomy tube in the second or third intercostal space in the midclavicular line, connected to an underwater seal or low suction pressures.

Recurring spontaneous pneumothorax requires thoracotomy and pleurectomy; these procedures prevent recurrence by causing the lung to adhere to the parietal pleura. Traumatic and tension pneumothoraces require chest tube drainage; traumatic pneumothorax may also require surgical repair.

Additional considerations

• The patient should be watched for pallor, gasping respirations, and sudden chest pain; and vital signs should be monitored at least every hour for indications of shock, increasing respiratory distress, or mediastinal shift. Breath sounds should be present over both lungs. Falling blood pressure, and rising pulse and respiration rates, may indicate tension pneumothorax, which can be fatal without prompt treatment.

• The patient should try to control coughing and gasping during thoracotomy. After the chest tube is in place, coughing and breathing deeply (at least once an hour) will facilitate lung expansion.

• In the patient undergoing chest tube drainage, continuing air leakage (bubbling) may indicate that the lung defect has failed to close; this may require surgery. Also, increasing subcutaneous emphysema will cause crackling beneath the skin around the neck or at the tube insertion site. The patient on a ventilator should be watched for difficulty in breathing in time with the ventilator, as well as pressure changes on ventilator gauges.

• Dressings around the chest tube insertion site should be changed, as necessary, with care taken to avoid repositioning or dislodging the tube. If the tube dislodges, a petrolatum gauze dressing over the opening will prevent rapid lung collapse.

• Vital signs must be monitored frequently after thoracotomy. Also, for the first 24 hours, respiratory status should be assessed hourly by checking breath sounds. The amount and color of leakage around the chest tube site, if any, should be noted. Walking, as ordered (usually on the first postoperative day), will facilitate deep inspiration and lung expansion.

• The patient should be told what pneumothorax is and what causes it, and about all diagnostic tests and procedures. He should be made as comfortable as possible. (The patient with pneumothorax is usually most comfortable sitting upright.)

Pneumonia

Pneumonia is an acute infection of the lung parenchyma which often impairs gas exchange. Prognosis is generally good for people who have normal lungs and adequate host defenses before the onset of pneumonia; however, bacterial pneumonia is the fifth leading cause of death in debilitated patients.

Causes

Pneumonia can be classified in several ways:

• *Microbiologic etiology*—Pneumonia can be viral, bacterial, fungal, protozoal, mycobacterial, mycoplasmal, or rickettsial in origin.

• *Location*—Bronchopneumonia involves distal airways and alveoli; lobular pneumonia, part of a lobe; and lobar pneumonia, an entire lobe.

• *Type*—Primary pneumonia results from inhalation or aspiration of a pathogen; it includes pneumococcal and viral pneumonia. Secondary pneumonia may follow initial lung damage from a noxious chemical or other insult (superinfection), or may result from hematogenous spread of bacteria from a distant focus.

Predisposing factors to bacterial and viral pneumonia include chronic illness and debilitation, cancer (particularly lung cancer), abdominal and thoracic surgery, atelectasis, common colds or other viral respiratory infections, chronic respiratory disease (COPD, asthma, bronchiectasis, cystic fibrosis), influenza, smoking, malnutrition, alcoholism, sickle cell disease, tracheostomy, exposure to noxious gases, aspiration, and immunosuppressive therapy. Predisposing factors to aspiration pneumonia include old age, debilitation, nasogastric tube feedings, impaired gag reflex, poor oral hygiene, and decreased level of consciousness.

Signs and symptoms

The five cardinal symptoms of early bacterial pneumonia are coughing, sputum production, pleuritic chest pain, shaking chills, and fever. Physical signs vary widely, ranging from diffuse, fine rales to signs of localized or extensive consolidation and pleural effusion.

Complications include hypoxemia,

TYPES OF PNEUMONIA

TYPE	SIGNS AND SYMPTOMS
VIRAL	
Influenza (prognosis poor even with treatment; 50% mortality)	• Cough (initially nonproductive; later, purulent sputum), marked cyanosis, dyspnea, high fever, chills, substernal pain and discomfort, moist rales, frontal headache, myalgia • Death results from cardiopulmonary collapse.
Adenovirus (insidious onset; generally affects young adults)	• Sore throat, fever, cough, chills, malaise, small amounts of mucoid sputum, retrosternal chest pain, anorexia, rhinitis, adenopathy, scattered rales, and rhonchi
Respiratory syncytial virus/RSV (most prevalent in infants and children)	• Listlessness, irritability, tachypnea with retraction of intercostal muscles, slight sputum production, fine moist rales, fever, severe malaise, and possibly, cough or croup
Measles/rubeola	• Fever, dyspnea, cough, small amounts of sputum, coryza, skin rash, and cervical adenopathy
Chickenpox/varicella (uncommon in children, but present in 30% of adults with varicella)	• Cough, dyspnea, cyanosis, tachypnea, pleuritic chest pain, hemoptysis and rhonchi 1 to 6 days after onset of rash
Cytomegalovirus/CMV	• Difficult to distinguish from other nonbacterial pneumonias • Fever, cough, shaking chills, dyspnea, cyanosis, weakness, and diffuse rales • Occurs in neonates as devastating multisystemic infection; in normal adults resembles mononucleosis; in immunocompromised hosts, varies from clinically inapparent to devastating infection
BACTERIAL	
Streptococcus (Diplococcus pneumoniae)	• Sudden onset of a single, shaking chill, and sustained temperature of 102° to 104° F. (38.9° to 40° C.); often preceded by upper respiratory tract infection
Klebsiella	• Fever and recurrent chills; cough producing rusty, bloody, viscous sputum (currant jelly); cyanosis of lips and nail beds due to hypoxemia; shallow, grunting respirations • Likely in patients with chronic alcoholism, pulmonary disease, and diabetes
Staphylococcus	• Temperature of 102° to 104° F. (38.9° to 40° C.), recurrent shaking chills, bloody sputum, dyspnea, tachypnea, and hypoxemia • Should be suspected with viral illness, such as influenza or measles, and in patients with cystic fibrosis
ASPIRATION	
Results from vomiting and aspiration of gastric or oropharyngeal contents into trachea and lungs.	• Noncardiogenic pulmonary edema may follow damage to respiratory epithelium from contact with stomach acid. • Rales, dyspnea, cyanosis, hypotension, and tachycardia • May be subacute pneumonia with cavity formation, or lung abscess may occur if foreign body is present

DIAGNOSIS	TREATMENT
• *Chest X-ray:* diffuse bilateral bronchopneumonia radiating from hilus • *WBC:* normal to slightly elevated • *Sputum smears:* no specific organisms	*Supportive:* for respiratory failure, endotracheal intubation and ventilator assistance; for fever, hypothermia blanket or antipyretics; for influenza A, amantadine
• *Chest X-ray:* patchy distribution of pneumonia, more severe than indicated by physical examination • *WBC:* normal to slightly elevated	• Treat symptoms only. • Mortality low; usually clears with no residual effects
• *Chest X-ray:* patchy bilateral consolidation • *WBC:* normal to slightly elevated	• *Supportive:* humidified air, oxygen, antimicrobials often given until viral etiology confirmed • Complete recovery in 1 to 3 weeks
• *Chest X-ray:* reticular infiltrates, sometimes with hilar lymph node enlargement • *Lung tissue specimen:* characteristic giant cells	• *Supportive:* bed rest, adequate hydration, antimicrobials; assisted ventilation, if necessary
• *Chest X-ray:* shows more extensive pneumonia than indicated by physical examination, and bilateral, patchy, diffuse, nodular infiltrates • *Sputum analysis:* predominant mononuclear cells and characteristic intranuclear inclusion bodies, with characteristic skin rash confirm diagnosis	• *Supportive:* adequate hydration, oxygen therapy in critically ill patients
• *Chest X-ray:* in early stages, variable patchy infiltrates; later, bilateral, nodular, and more predominant in lower lobes • *Percutaneous aspiration of lung tissue, transbronchial biopsy or open lung biopsy:* microscopic examination shows typical intranuclear and cytoplasmic inclusions; the virus can be cultured from lung tissue	• Generally, benign and self-limiting in mononucleosis-like form • *Supportive:* adequate hydration and nutrition, oxygen therapy, bed rest • In immunosuppressed patients, disease is more severe and may be fatal
• *Chest X-ray:* areas of consolidation, often lobar • *WBC:* elevated • *Sputum culture:* may show gram-positive *S. pneumoniae;* this organism not always recovered	• *Antimicrobial therapy:* penicillin G or a cephalosporin for 7 to 10 days. Such therapy begins after obtaining culture specimen but without waiting for results.
• *Chest X-ray:* typically, but not always, consolidation in the upper lobe that causes bulging of fissures • *WBC:* elevated • *Sputum culture and Gram's stain:* may show gram-positive cocci *Klebsiella*	• *Antimicrobial therapy:* gentamicin, tobramycin, kanamycin, or a cephalosporin
• *Chest X-ray:* multiple abscesses and infiltrates; high incidence of empyema • *WBC:* elevated • *Sputum culture and Gram's stain:* may show gram-positive staphylococci	• *Antimicrobial therapy:* nafcillin or oxacillin for 14 days • Chest tube drainage of empyema
• *Chest X-ray:* locates areas of infiltrates, which suggest diagnosis	• *Antimicrobial therapy:* penicillin G or clindamycin • *Supportive:* oxygen therapy, suctioning, coughing, deep breathing, adequate hydration, and I.V. steroids

respiratory failure, pleural effusion, empyema, lung abscess, and bacteremia, with spread of infection to other parts of the body resulting in meningitis, endocarditis, and pericarditis.

Diagnosis

Clinical features, chest X-ray showing infiltrates, and sputum smear demonstrating acute inflammatory cells support this diagnosis. Positive blood cultures in patients with pulmonary infiltrates strongly suggest pneumonia produced by the organisms isolated from the blood cultures. Pleural effusions, if present, should be tapped and fluid analyzed for evidence of infection in the pleural space. Occasionally, a transtracheal aspirate of tracheobronchial secretions or pneumocentesis of the involved area may be done to obtain material for smear and culture. The patient's response to antimicrobial therapy also provides important evidence of the presence of pneumonia.

Treatment

Antimicrobial therapy varies with the causative agent. Therapy should be re-evaluated early in the course of treatment. Supportive measures include humidified oxygen therapy for hypoxia, mechanical ventilation for respiratory failure, a high-calorie diet and adequate fluid intake, bed rest, and an analgesic to relieve pleuritic chest pain. Patients with severe pneumonia on mechanical ventilation may require positive end-expiratory pressure (PEEP) to facilitate adequate oxygenation.

Additional considerations

Correct supportive care can increase patient comfort, avoid complications, and speed recovery.

Throughout the illness, the hospital staff member should:
• maintain patent airway and adequate oxygenation; measure arterial blood gases, especially in hypoxic patients; administer supplemental oxygen if PO_2 is less than 55 to 60 mmHg—patients with underlying chronic lung disease should be given oxygen cautiously.
• teach the patient how to cough and perform deep breathing exercises to clear secretions, and encourage him to do so often; provide thorough respiratory care and frequent suctioning, using sterile technique, to remove secretions in severe pneumonia that requires endotracheal intubation or tracheostomy with or without mechanical ventilation.
• obtain sputum specimens as needed (by suction if the patient can't produce specimens independently); collect specimens in a sterile container and deliver them promptly to the microbiology laboratory.
• administer antibiotics, as ordered, and pain medication, as needed; record the patient's response to medications; give I.V. fluids and electrolyte replacement for fever and dehydration as required.
• maintain adequate nutrition to offset high caloric utilization secondary to infection; ask the dietary department to provide a high-calorie, high-protein diet consisting of soft, easy-to-eat foods; encourage the patient to eat; supplement oral feedings with nasogastric tube feedings or parenteral nutrition, as necessary; monitor fluid intake and output.
• provide a quiet, calm environment for the patient, with frequent rest periods.
• give emotional support by explaining all procedures (especially intubation and suctioning) to the patient and his family; encourage family visits; provide diversionary activities.
• dispose of secretions properly, to control the spread of infection; tell the patient to sneeze and cough into a disposable tissue; tape a waxed bag to the side of the bed for used tissues.

Various measures can be taken to prevent pneumonia:
• A patient should avoid using antibiotics indiscriminately during minor viral infections—this may cause upper airway colonization with antibiotic-resistant bacteria. If the patient then develops pneumonia, the organisms producing the pneumonia may require treatment with more toxic antibiotics.
• Annual influenza vaccination and pneumovax are recommended for high-

risk patients, such as those with COPD, chronic heart disease, and sickle cell disease.
• All bedridden and postoperative patients should perform deep breathing and coughing exercises frequently. Proper patient position will promote full aeration and drainage of secretions.
• To prevent aspiration during naso-

gastric tube feedings, the patient's head should be elevated, the position of the tube checked, and the feeding administered slowly. Large volumes must not be given at one time, since this could cause vomiting. The patient's head should be elevated for at least a half hour after feeding. If he has an endotracheal tube, the tube cuff must be inflated.

Pulmonary Embolism and Infarction

The most common pulmonary complication in hospitalized patients, pulmonary embolism is an obstruction of the pulmonary arterial bed by a dislodged thrombus or foreign substance. It strikes an estimated 6 million adults each year in the United States, resulting in 100,000 deaths. Although pulmonary infarction may be so mild as to be asymptomatic, massive embolism (more than 50% obstruction of pulmonary arterial circulation) and infarction can be rapidly fatal.

Causes
Pulmonary embolism generally results from dislodged thrombi originating in the leg veins. More than half of such thrombi arise in the deep veins of the legs and are usually multiple. Other less common sources of thrombi are the pelvic veins, renal veins, hepatic vein, right heart, and upper extremities. Such thrombus formation results directly from vascular wall damage, venostasis, or hypercoagulability of the blood.

Rarely, the emboli contain air, fat, amniotic fluid, talc (from drugs intended for oral administration which are injected intravenously by addicts), or tumor cells. Thrombi may embolize spontaneously during clot dissolution or may be dislodged during trauma, sudden muscular action, or a change in peripheral blood flow.

Rarely, pulmonary infarction (tissue death) may evolve from pulmonary embolism. Pulmonary infarction develops more frequently when pulmonary embolism occurs in patients with chronic cardiac or pulmonary disease. If the embolus obstructs a large vessel, bronchial circulation may provide an adequate oxygen supply to the lung supplied by the occluded vessel.

Predisposing factors to pulmonary embolism include long-term immobility, chronic pulmonary disease, congestive heart failure or atrial fibrillation, thrombophlebitis, polycythemia vera, thrombocytosis, autoimmune hemolytic anemia, sickle cell disease, varicose veins, recent surgery, advanced age, pregnancy, lower extremity fractures or surgery, burns, obesity, vascular injury, malignancy, or oral contraceptives.

Signs and symptoms
Total occlusion of the main pulmonary artery is rapidly fatal; smaller or fragmented emboli produce symptoms that vary with the size, number, and location of the emboli. Usually, the first symptom of pulmonary embolism is dyspnea, which may be accompanied by anginal or pleuritic chest pain. Other clinical features include tachycardia, productive cough (sputum may be blood-tinged), low-grade fever, and pleural effusion. Less common signs include massive hemoptysis, splinting of the chest, leg edema, and with a large embolus, cyanosis, syncope, and distended neck veins.

In addition, pulmonary embolism may cause pleural friction rub and signs of circulatory collapse (weak, rapid pulse;

hypotension), signs of cerebral ischemia (syncope, coma, convulsions, and transient unconsciousness), signs of hypoxia (restlessness), and particularly in elderly patients, hemiplegia and other focal neurologic abnormalities.

Diagnosis

History reveals any predisposing conditions for pulmonary embolism.

• *Chest X-ray* helps to rule out other pulmonary diseases; shows areas of atelectasis, elevated diaphragm and pleural effusion, prominent pulmonary artery, and occasionally, the characteristic wedge-shaped infiltrate suggestive of pulmonary embolism.

• *Lung scan* shows perfusion defects in areas beyond occluded vessels; normal lung scan rules out pulmonary embolism.

• *Pulmonary angiography* is the most definitive test but requires a skilled angiographer and radiologic equipment; it also poses some risk to the patient. Its use depends on the uncertainty of the diagnosis and the need to avoid unnecessary anticoagulant therapy in high-risk patients.

• *EKG* is inconclusive but helps distinguish pulmonary embolism from myocardial infarction. In extensive embolism, EKG may show right axis deviation, right bundle branch block, tall peaked P waves, depression of S-T segments and T wave inversions (indicative of right heart strain), and supraventricular tachyarrhythmias.

• *Auscultation* occasionally reveals a right ventricular S_3 gallop and increased intensity of a pulmonic component of S_2. Also, rales and a pleural rub may be heard at the site of embolism.

• *Arterial blood gas measurements* showing decreased Po_2 and Pco_2 are characteristic but do not always occur.

If pleural effusion is present, thoracentesis may rule out empyema, which indicates pneumonia.

Treatment

Treatment is designed to maintain adequate cardiovascular and pulmonary functions during resolution of the obstruction and to prevent recurrence of embolic episodes. Since most emboli largely resolve within 10 to 14 days, treatment consists of oxygen therapy, as needed, and anticoagulation with heparin to inhibit new thrombus formation. Heparin therapy is monitored by daily coagulation studies (partial thromboplastin time [PTT]). Patients with massive pulmonary embolism and shock may require fibrinolytic therapy with urokinase or streptokinase to enhance fibrinolysis of the pulmonary emboli and remaining thrombi. Emboli that cause hypotension may require the use of vasopressors. Treatment for septic emboli requires antibiotic therapy, not anticoagulants, and careful evaluation for the source of infection, particularly endocarditis.

Surgery to interrupt the inferior vena cava is reserved for patients who can't take anticoagulants or who have recurrent emboli during anticoagulant therapy. Surgery should not be undertaken without angiographic demonstrations of pulmonary embolism. Surgery consists of vena caval ligation, plication, or insertion of an "umbrella" filter to filter the blood returning to the heart and lungs.

Additional considerations

When treating a patient with pulmonary embolism or infarction, the hospital staff member should:

• give oxygen by nasal cannula or mask; check arterial blood gases in the event of fresh emboli or worsening dyspnea; be prepared to provide endotracheal intubation with assisted ventilation if breathing is severely compromised.

• administer heparin, as ordered, through I.V. push or continuous drip; monitor coagulation studies daily—effective heparin therapy raises PTT to approximately 2½ times normal; watch closely for nosebleed, petechiae, and other signs of abnormal bleeding; check stools for occult blood; tell the patient to prevent bleeding by using an electric razor instead of a safety razor and to brush his teeth with a soft toothbrush.

• encourage the patient to move about often, after he is stable, and assist with isometric and range-of-motion exercises; check pedal pulses, temperature, and color of feet to detect venostasis; *never* vigorously massage the patient's legs; offer diversional activities to promote rest and relieve restlessness.

• walk the patient as soon as possible after surgery to prevent venostasis.

• report frequent pleuritic chest pain, so analgesics can be prescribed (also, incentive spirometry can assist in deep breathing); provide tissues and a bag for easy disposal of expectorations.

• warn the patient not to cross his legs—this promotes thrombus formation.

• explain procedures and treatments, to relieve anxiety; encourage the patient's family to participate in his care.

Most patients need treatment with an oral anticoagulant (warfarin) for 4 to 6 months after a pulmonary embolism. These patients should be advised to watch for signs of bleeding (bloody stools, blood in urine, large ecchymoses), to take the prescribed medication exactly as ordered, and to avoid taking any additional medication (even for headaches or colds) or changing doses of medication without consulting their doctors. They must also understand the importance of follow-up laboratory tests (prothrombin time [PT]) to monitor anticoagulant therapy.

To prevent pulmonary emboli, early ambulation is recommended for patients predisposed to this condition. With close medical supervision, low-dose heparin may be useful prophylactically.

Sarcoidosis

Sarcoidosis is a multisystemic, granulomatous disorder that characteristically produces lymphadenopathy, pulmonary infiltration, and skeletal, liver, eye, or skin lesions. It occurs most often in young adults (aged 20 to 40). In the United States, sarcoidosis occurs predominantly among Blacks, affecting twice as many women as men. Acute sarcoidosis usually resolves within 2 years. Chronic, progressive sarcoidosis, which is uncommon, is associated with pulmonary fibrosis and progressive pulmonary disability.

Causes and incidence

The cause of sarcoidosis is unknown, but the following possible causes have been considered:

• *hypersensitivity response* (possibly from T cell imbalance) to such agents as atypical mycobacteria, fungi, and pine pollen

• *genetic predisposition* (suggested by a slightly higher incidence of sarcoidosis within the same family)

• *chemicals* such as zirconium or beryllium can lead to illnesses resembling sarcoidosis, suggesting an extrinsic cause for this disease.

Signs and symptoms

Initial symptoms of sarcoidosis include arthralgia (in the wrists, ankles, and elbows), fatigue, malaise, and weight loss. Other clinical features vary according to the extent and location of the fibrosis:

• *respiratory*—breathlessness, cough (usually nonproductive), substernal pain; complications in advanced pulmonary disease include pulmonary hypertension and cor pulmonale

• *cutaneous*—erythema nodosum, subcutaneous skin nodules with maculopapular eruptions, extensive nasal mucosal lesions.

• *ophthalmic*—anterior uveitis (common); glaucoma, blindness (rare)

• *lymphatic*—bilateral hilar and right paratracheal lymphadenopathy, and splenomegaly

• *musculoskeletal*—muscle weakness,

polyarthralgia, pain, punched-out lesions on phalanges
- *hepatic*—granulomatous hepatitis, usually asymptomatic
- *genitourinary*—hypercalciuria
- *cardiovascular*—arrhythmias (premature beats, bundle branch or complete heart block) and, rarely, cardiomyopathy
- *CNS*—cranial or peripheral nerve palsies, basilar meningitis, convulsions, pituitary and hypothalamic lesions producing diabetes insipidus.

Diagnosis
Typical clinical features with appropriate laboratory data and X-ray findings suggest sarcoidosis. A positive Kveim-Siltzbach skin test supports the diagnosis. In this test, the patient receives an intradermal injection of an antigen prepared from human sarcoidal spleen or lymph nodes from patients with sarcoidosis. If the patient has active sarcoidosis, granuloma develops at the injection site in 2 to 6 weeks. This reaction is considered positive when a biopsy of the skin at the injection site shows discrete epitheloid cell granuloma. Other relevant findings include:
- *chest X-ray*—bilateral hilar and right paratracheal adenopathy with or without diffuse interstitial infiltrates; occasionally large nodular lesions are present in lung parenchyma
- *lymph node, skin, or lung biopsy*—noncaseating granulomas with negative cultures for mycobacteria and fungi
- *other laboratory data*—rarely, increased serum calcium, mild anemia, leukocytosis, hyperglobulinemia
- *pulmonary function tests*—decreased total lung capacity and compliance, and decreased diffusing capacity
- *arterial blood gases*—decreased arterial oxygen tension.

Negative tuberculin skin test, fungal serologies, and sputum cultures for mycobacteria and fungi, as well as negative biopsy cultures, help rule out infection.

Treatment
Asymptomatic sarcoidosis requires no treatment. However, sarcoidosis that causes ocular, respiratory, CNS, cardiac, or systemic symptoms (such as fever and weight loss) requires treatment with systemic or topical steroids; as does sarcoidosis that produces hypercalcemia or destructive skin lesions. Such therapy is usually continued for 1 to 2 years, but some patients may need lifelong therapy. Other treatment includes a low-calcium diet and avoidance of direct exposure to sunlight in patients with hypercalcemia.

Additional considerations
Care for the sarcoidosis patient includes:
- watching for and reporting any complications; noting any abnormal lab results (anemia, for example) which could alter patient care.
- giving analgesics to the patient with arthralgia, as ordered; noting signs of progressive muscle weakness.
- providing a nutritious, high-calorie diet and plenty of fluids; giving the patient with hypercalcemia a low-calcium diet; weighing the patient regularly.
- monitoring respiratory function; checking chest X-rays for extent of lung involvement; noting and recording any bloody sputum or increase in sputum; if the patient has pulmonary hypertension or end-stage cor pulmonale, checking arterial blood gases, watching for arrhythmias, and administering oxygen, as needed.
- testing urine for glucose and acetone at least every 12 hours at the beginning of steroid therapy, since steroids may induce or worsen diabetes mellitus, and watching for other steroid side effects, including: fluid retention, electrolyte imbalance (especially hypokalemia), moonface, hypertension, and personality change; watching for and reporting vomiting, orthostatic hypotension, hypoglycemia, restlessness, anorexia, malaise, and fatigue during or after steroid withdrawal; being aware that the patient on long-term or high-dose steroid therapy is vulnerable to infection.
- preparing the patient for discharge by stressing the need for compliance with prescribed steroid therapy and regular,

careful follow-up examinations and treatment; supporting and advising the patient with failing vision, and referring the blind patient to community support and resource groups or the American Foundation for the Blind, if necessary.

Lung Abscess

Lung abscess is a lung infection accompanied by pus accumulation and tissue destruction. The abscess may be putrid (due to anaerobic bacteria) or nonputrid (due to anaerobes or aerobes), and often has a well-defined border. The availability of effective antibiotics has made lung abscess much less common than it was in the past.

Causes

Lung abscess is a manifestation of necrotizing pneumonia, often the result of aspiration of oropharyngeal contents. Poor oral hygiene with dental or gingival (gum) disease is strongly associated with putrid lung abscess. Septic pulmonary emboli commonly produce cavitary lesions. Infected cystic lung lesions and cavitating bronchial carcinoma must be distinguished from lung abscesses.

Signs and symptoms

The clinical effects of lung abscess include a cough that may produce bloody, purulent, or foul-smelling sputum, pleuritic chest pain, dyspnea, excessive sweating, chills, fever, headache, malaise, diaphoresis, and weight loss. Complications include rupture into the pleural space, which results in empyema and, rarely, massive hemorrhage. Chronic lung abscess may cause localized bronchiectasis. Failure of an abscess to improve with antibiotic treatment suggests possible underlying neoplasm or other causes of obstruction.

Diagnosis

• Auscultation of the chest may reveal rales and decreased breath sounds.
• Chest X-ray shows a localized infiltrate with one or more clear spaces, usually containing air-fluid levels.
• Percutaneous aspiration of an abscess may be attempted or bronchoscopy used to obtain cultures to identify the causative organism. Bronchoscopy is only used if abscess resolution is achieved and the patient's condition permits it.
• Blood cultures, Gram's stain, and culture of sputum are also used to detect the organism; leukocytosis (white blood cell count more than $10,000/mm^3$) is commonly present.

Treatment

Treatment consists of prolonged antibiotic therapy, which may have to continue for months, until radiographic resolution or definite stability occurs. Symptoms usually disappear in a few weeks. Postural drainage may facilitate discharge of necrotic material into upper airways where expectoration is possible; oxygen therapy may relieve hypoxemia. Poor patient response to therapy requires resection of the lesion or removal of the diseased section of the lung. All patients need rigorous follow-up and serial chest X-rays.

Additional considerations

Health care emphasizes aiding the patient with chest physiotherapy (including coughing and deep breathing), increasing fluid intake to loosen secretions, and providing a quiet, restful atmosphere.

To prevent lung abscess, secretions must be suctioned in unconscious patients and patients with seizures. Positioning patients to promote drainage of secretions also helps. The patient must understand the importance of practicing good oral hygiene.

Hemothorax

In hemothorax, blood from damaged intercostal, pleural, mediastinal, and (infrequently) lung parenchymal vessels enters the pleural cavity. Depending on the amount of bleeding and the underlying cause, hemothorax may be associated with varying degrees of lung collapse and mediastinal shift. Pneumothorax—air in the pleural cavity—often accompanies hemothorax.

Causes

Hemothorax usually results from blunt or penetrating chest trauma; in fact, about 25% of patients with such trauma have hemothorax. Less often, it results from thoracic surgery, pulmonary infarction, neoplasm, dissecting thoracic aneurysm, or anticoagulant therapy.

Signs and symptoms

The patient with hemothorax may experience chest pain, tachypnea, and mild to severe dyspnea, depending on the amount of blood in the pleural cavity and associated pathology. If respiratory failure results, the patient may appear anxious, restless, possibly stuporous, and cyanotic; marked blood loss produces hypotension and shock. The affected side of the chest expands and stiffens, while the unaffected side rises and falls with the patient's gasping respirations.

Diagnosis

Characteristic clinical signs with a history of trauma strongly suggest hemothorax. Percussion reveals dullness and, on auscultation, decreased to absent breath sounds over the affected side. Thoracentesis yields blood or serosanguineous fluid; chest X-rays show pleural fluid with or without mediastinal shift. Blood gases may document respiratory failure; hemoglobin may be decreased, depending on blood loss.

Treatment

Treatment is designed to stabilize the patient's condition, stop the bleeding, evacuate blood from the pleural space, and re-expand the underlying lung. Mild hemothorax usually clears rapidly in 10 to 14 days, requiring only observation for further bleeding. In severe hemothorax, thoracentesis serves not only as a diagnostic tool but also to remove fluid from the pleural cavity.

After diagnosis is confirmed, a chest tube is inserted quickly into the sixth intercostal space in the posterior axillary line. Suction may be used; a large-bore tube is used to prevent clot blockage. If the chest tube doesn't improve the patient's condition, he may need thoracotomy to evacuate blood and clots and control bleeding.

Additional considerations

When treating hemothorax, the hospital staff member should:

• give oxygen by face mask or nasal cannula.

• give I.V. fluids and blood transfusions, as needed, to treat shock; monitor blood gases often.

• explain all procedures to the patient to allay his fears; assist with thoracentesis; warn the patient not to cough during this procedure.

• observe chest tube drainage carefully and record volume drained at least every hour; milk the chest tube every hour to keep it open and free of clots; report to the doctor immediately if the tube is warm and full of blood, and the bloody fluid level in the water-seal bottle is rising rapidly, since the patient may need immediate surgery.

• watch the patient closely for pallor and gasping respirations; monitor his vital signs diligently. Falling blood pressure, rising pulse rate, and rising respiration rate may indicate shock or massive bleeding.

Pulmonary Hypertension

In adults, pulmonary hypertension is indicated by a resting systolic pulmonary artery pressure above 30mmHg and a mean pulmonary artery pressure above 18mmHg. It may be primary (rare) or secondary (far more common). Primary, or idiopathic, pulmonary hypertension *occurs most often in women between ages 20 and 40, usually is fatal within 3 to 4 years, and shows the highest mortality among pregnant women.* Secondary pulmonary hypertension *results from existing cardiac and/or pulmonary disease. Prognosis depends on the severity of the underlying disorder.*

Causes

Primary pulmonary hypertension begins as hypertrophy of the small pulmonary arteries. The medial and intimal muscle layers of these vessels thicken, decreasing distensibility and increasing resistance. This disorder then progresses to vascular sclerosis and obliteration of small vessels. Because this form of pulmonary hypertension occurs in association with collagen diseases, it is thought to result from altered immune mechanisms.

Usually, pulmonary hypertension is secondary to hypoxemia from an underlying disease process, including:

• *alveolar hypoventilation* from chronic obstructive pulmonary disease (most common cause in the United States), sarcoidosis, diffuse interstitial pneumonia, malignant metastases, and certain diseases, such as scleroderma. These diseases may cause pulmonary hypertension through alveolar destruction and increased pulmonary vascular resistance. Other disorders that cause alveolar hypoventilation without lung tissue damage include obesity and kyphoscoliosis.

• *vascular obstruction* from pulmonary embolism, vasculitis, and disorders that cause obstructions of small or large pulmonary veins, such as left atrial myxoma, idiopathic veno-occlusive disease, fibrosing mediastinitis, and mediastinal neoplasm.

• *primary cardiac disease,* which may be congenital or acquired. Congenital defects that cause left-to-right shunting of blood—such as patent ductus arteriosus, or atrial or ventricular septal defect—increase blood flow into the lungs and, consequently, raise pulmonary vascular pressure. Acquired cardiac disease, such as rheumatic valvular disease and mitral stenosis, increases pulmonary venous pressure by restricting blood flow returning to the heart.

Signs and symptoms

Most patients complain of increasing dyspnea on exertion, weakness, syncope, and fatigability. Many also show signs of right heart failure, including peripheral edema, ascites, neck vein distention, and hepatomegaly. Other clinical effects vary according to the underlying disorder.

Diagnosis

Characteristic diagnostic findings in patients with pulmonary hypertension include the following:

• *auscultation:* abnormalities associated with the underlying disorder

• *arterial blood gases:* hypoxemia (decreased P_{O_2})

• *EKG:* in right ventricular hypertrophy, shows right axis deviation and tall or peaked P waves in inferior leads

• *cardiac catheterization:* increased pulmonary artery pressures (PAP)—pulmonary systolic pressure above 30 mmHg; pulmonary capillary wedge pressure (PCWP) increases if the underlying cause is left atrial myxoma, mitral stenosis, or left ventricular failure—otherwise, PCWP is normal

• *pulmonary angiography:* detects filling defects in pulmonary vasculature such as develop in patients with pulmonary emboli

• *pulmonary function tests:* in underlying obstructive disease, may show decreased flow rates and increased residual volume; in underlying restrictive disease, total lung capacity may decrease.

Treatment

Treatment usually includes oxygen therapy to decrease hypoxemia and resulting pulmonary vascular resistance. For patients with right ventricular failure, treatment also includes fluid restriction, digitalis to increase cardiac output, and diuretics to decrease intravascular volume and extravascular fluid accumulation. Of course, an important goal of treatment is correction of the underlying cause.

Additional considerations

Pulmonary hypertension requires keen observation and careful monitoring, as well as skilled supportive care.

• Response to oxygen therapy is important. Signs of increasing dyspnea indicate the need to adjust treatment.

• Arterial blood gases should be monitored for signs of acidosis and hypoxemia. Any change in level of consciousness must be reported immediately.

• With a patient who has right heart failure, especially one receiving diuretics, daily weight, and intake and output, must be monitored. Increasing neck vein distention can indicate fluid overload.

• Vital signs, especially blood pressure and heart rate, should be closely watched. Hypotension and tachycardia should be noted and reported. If the patient has a pulmonary artery catheter, PAP and PCWP must be checked, as ordered, and any changes reported.

• Before discharge, the patient should understand the limitations imposed by this disorder. He must avoid overexertion and take rest periods between activities. If special equipment, such as oxygen equipment, is needed for home use, the patient will have to be referred to a social services agency. The patient must know that following the prescribed diet and taking the medications will help relieve and prevent symptoms associated with pulmonary hypertension.

Pleural Effusion and Empyema

Pleural effusion is an excess of fluid in the pleural space. Normally, this space contains a small amount of extracellular fluid that lubricates the pleural surfaces. Increased production or inadequate removal of this fluid results in pleural effusion. Empyema is the accumulation of pus and necrotic tissue in the pleural space. Blood (hemothorax) and chyle (chylothorax) may also collect in this space.

Causes

The balance of osmotic and hydrostatic pressures in parietal pleural capillaries normally results in fluid movement into the pleural space. Balanced pressures in visceral pleural capillaries promote reabsorption of this fluid. Excessive hydrostatic pressure or decreased osmotic pressure can cause excessive amounts of fluid to pass across intact capillaries. The result is a transudative pleural effusion, an ultrafiltrate of plasma containing low concentrations of protein. Such effusions frequently result from congestive heart failure, hepatic disease with ascites, peritoneal dialysis, hypoalbuminemia, and disorders resulting in overexpanded intravascular volume.

Exudative pleural effusions result when capillaries exhibit increased permeability with or without changes in hydrostatic and colloid osmotic pressures, allowing protein-rich fluid to leak into the pleural space. Exudative pleural effusions occur with tuberculosis, subphrenic abscess, pancreatitis, bacterial or fungal pneumonitis or empyema, malignancy, pulmonary embolism with or without infarction, collagen disease (lupus erythematosus and rheumatoid arthritis), myxedema, and chest trauma.

Empyema is usually associated with infection in the pleural space. Such infection may be idiopathic, or may be related to pneumonitis, carcinoma, perforation, or esophageal rupture.

Signs and symptoms

Patients with pleural effusion characteristically display symptoms relating to the underlying pathology. Most patients with large effusions, particularly those with underlying pulmonary disease, complain of dyspnea. Those with effusions associated with pleurisy complain of pleuritic chest pain. Other clinical features depend on the cause of the effusion. Patients with empyema also develop fever and malaise.

Diagnosis

Chest X-ray shows radiopaque fluid in dependent regions. Auscultation of the chest reveals decreased breath sounds; percussion detects dullness over the effused area, which doesn't change with respiration. These tests verify pleural effusion. However, diagnosis also requires other tests to distinguish transudative from exudative effusions and to help pinpoint the underlying disorder. The most useful test is thoracentesis, in which analysis of aspirated pleural fluid shows:

• *transudative effusions:* specific gravity usually <1.015 and protein <3 g/dl
• *exudative effusions:* ratio of protein in pleural fluid to serum ≥0.5, pleural fluid lactic dehydrogenase (LDH) ≥ 200 IU, and ratio of LDH in pleural fluid to LDH in serum ≥0.6
• *empyema:* acute inflammatory WBCs and microorganisms
• *empyema or rheumatoid arthritis:* extremely decreased pleural fluid glucose levels.

In addition, if a pleural effusion results from esophageal rupture or pancreatitis, fluid amylase levels are usually higher than serum levels. Aspirated fluid may be tested for LE cells, antinuclear antibodies, and neoplastic cells. It may also be analyzed for color and consistency; acid-fast bacillus, fungal, and bacterial cultures; and triglycerides (in chylothorax). Cell analysis shows leukocytosis in empyema. Negative tuberculin skin test strongly rules against tuberculosis as the cause. In exudative pleural effusions in which thoracentesis is not definitive, pleural biopsy may be done; it is particularly useful for confirming tuberculosis or malignancy.

Treatment

Depending on the amount of fluid present, symptomatic effusion may require thoracentesis to remove fluid, or careful monitoring of the patient's own reabsorption of the fluid. Hemothorax requires drainage to prevent fibrothorax formation. Treatment of empyema requires insertion of one or more chest tubes after thoracentesis, to allow drainage of purulent material, and possibly, decortication (surgical removal of the thick coating over the lung) or rib resection to allow open drainage and lung expansion. Empyema also requires parenteral antibiotics. Associated hypoxia requires oxygen administration.

Additional considerations

• The patient undergoing thoracentesis should understand the procedure. He can expect a stinging sensation from the local anesthetic and a feeling of pressure when the needle is inserted. If he feels uncomfortable or has trouble breathing during the procedure, he should tell a hospital staff member immediately.
• The patient will need reassurance during thoracentesis. He must remember to breathe normally and avoid sudden movements, such as coughing or sighing. He should be watched for signs of syncope. If fluid is removed too quickly, he may suffer bradycardia, hypotension, pain, pulmonary edema, or even cardiac arrest. Respiratory distress or pneumo-

thorax (sudden onset of dyspnea, cyanosis) may occur after thoracentesis.

• Oxygen and, in empyema, antibiotics may be ordered.

• The patient should try to do deep breathing exercises to promote lung expansion. A spirometer may help promote deep breathing.

• Meticulous chest tube care and aseptic technique when changing dressings around the tube insertion site are necessary in empyema. Bubbles in the underwater seal chamber indicate tube patency. The amount, color, and consistency of any tube drainage require monitoring.

• If the patient has open drainage through a rib resection or intercostal tube, hand and dressing precautions are important. Since weeks of such drainage are usually necessary to obliterate the space, any patient who will be discharged with the tube in place will need a visiting nurse.

• If pleural effusion was a complication of pneumonia or influenza, the patient should seek prompt medical attention for chest colds.

Pleurisy
(Pleuritis)

Pleurisy is inflammation of the visceral and parietal pleurae that line the inside of the thoracic cage and envelop the lungs.

Causes

Pleurisy develops as a complication of pneumonia, tuberculosis, viruses, systemic lupus erythematosus, rheumatoid arthritis, uremia, Dressler's syndrome, malignancy, pulmonary infarction, and chest trauma. Pleuritic pain is caused by the inflammation or irritation of sensory nerve endings in the parietal pleura. As the lungs inflate and deflate, the visceral pleura covering the lungs moves against the fixed parietal pleura lining the pleural space, causing pain. This disorder usually begins suddenly.

Signs and symptoms

Sharp, stabbing pain that increases with respiration may be so severe that it limits movement on the affected side during breathing. Dyspnea also occurs. Other symptoms vary according to the underlying pathologic process.

Diagnosis

Auscultation of the chest reveals a characteristic *pleural friction rub*—a coarse, creaky sound heard during late inspiration and early expiration, directly over the area of pleural inflammation. Palpation over the affected area may reveal coarse vibration.

Treatment

Treatment is generally symptomatic and includes anti-inflammatory agents, analgesics, and bed rest. Severe pain may require an intercostal nerve block of two or three intercostal nerves. Pleurisy with pleural effusion calls for thoracentesis as both a therapeutic and diagnostic measure.

Additional considerations

• Bed rest is very important. The patient should be allowed to get as much uninterrupted rest as possible.

• Antitussives and pain medication may be ordered. Dosage must be controlled carefully, to avoid overmedication. If the pain requires a narcotic analgesic, the patient about to be discharged should be warned to avoid overuse of the drug, because of the possibility of addiction, and because such medication depresses coughing and respiration.

• Coughing is helpful. To minimize pain, firm pressure may be applied at the site of the pain during coughing exercises.

CHRONIC DISORDERS

Chronic Obstructive Pulmonary Disease
(Chronic obstructive lung disease [COLD])

Chronic obstructive pulmonary disease (COPD) is chronic airway obstruction that results from emphysema, chronic bronchitis, asthma, or any combination of these disorders. Usually, more than one of these underlying conditions coexist; most often, bronchitis and emphysema occur together. The most common chronic lung disease, COPD affects an estimated 17 million Americans, and its incidence is rising. It affects males more often than females, probably because until recently men were more likely to smoke heavily. It doesn't always produce symptoms and causes only minimal disability in many patients. However, COPD tends to worsen with time.

Causes
Predisposing factors to COPD include cigarette smoking, recurrent or chronic respiratory infections, and allergies. Smoking is by far the most important of these factors; it impairs ciliary action and macrophage function, and causes inflammation in airways, increased mucus production, destruction of alveolar septae, and peribronchiolar fibrosis. Early inflammatory changes may reverse if the patient stops smoking before lung destruction is extensive. Familial and hereditary factors (such as deficiency of $alpha_1$-antitrypsin) may also predispose to the development of COPD.

Signs and symptoms
The typical patient, a long-term cigarette smoker, has no symptoms until middle age, when his ability to exercise or do strenuous work gradually starts to decline, and he begins to develop a productive cough. While subtle at first, these signs become more pronounced as the patient gets older and the disease progresses. Eventually the patient develops dyspnea on minimal exertion, frequent respiratory infections, intermittent or continuous hypoxemia, and grossly abnormal pulmonary function studies. In its advanced form, COPD may cause thoracic deformities, overwhelming disability, cor pulmonale, severe respiratory failure, and death.

Treatment and additional considerations
Treatment is designed to relieve symptoms and prevent complications. Because most COPD patients receive outpatient treatment, they need comprehensive patient teaching to help them comply with therapy and understand the nature of this chronic, progressive, debilitating disease. If programs in pulmonary rehabilitation are available, the patient should try to enroll in one.

• He must try to stop smoking and avoid other respiratory irritants. At home, an air conditioner with an air filter may prove helpful.

• Bronchodilators alleviate bronchospasm and enhance mucociliary clearance of secretions. The patient should be familiar with any bronchodilators prescribed.

• Antibiotics may be ordered to treat respiratory infections. The patient must understand the need to complete the prescribed course of antibiotic therapy. He and his family need to know early signs of infection; he should try to avoid contact with persons with respiratory infections. Good oral hygiene will help prevent infection. Pneumococcal vaccination every 3 years and annual influenza vaccinations are important preventive measures against infection.

• To strengthen the muscles of respiration, the patient should take slow, deep

CHRONIC OBSTRUCTIVE PULMONARY DISEASE

DISEASE	CAUSES AND PATHOPHYSIOLOGY	CLINICAL FEATURES
Emphysema • Abnormal irreversible enlargement of air spaces distal to terminal bronchioles due to destruction of alveolar walls, resulting in decreased elastic recoil properties of lungs • Most common cause of death from respiratory disease in the United States	• Cigarette smoking, deficiency of alpha-antitrypsin • Recurrent inflammation associated with release of proteolytic enzymes from cells in lungs causes bronchiolar and alveolar wall damage and, ultimately, destruction. Loss of lung supporting structure results in decreased elastic recoil and airway collapse on expiration. Destruction of alveolar walls decreases surface area for gas exchange.	• Insidious onset, with dyspnea the predominant symptom • *Other signs and symptoms of long-term disease:* chronic cough, anorexia, weight loss, malaise, "barrel chest," use of accessory muscles of respiration, prolonged expiratory period with grunting, pursed-lip breathing and tachypnea, peripheral cyanosis, and digital clubbing • *Complications* include recurrent respiratory tract infections, cor pulmonale, and respiratory failure.
Chronic bronchitis • Excessive mucus production with productive cough for at least 3 months a year for 2 successive years • Only a minority of patients with the clinical syndrome of chronic bronchitis develop significant airway obstruction	• Severity of disease related to amount and duration of smoking; respiratory infection exacerbates symptoms • Hypertrophy and hyperplasia of bronchial mucous glands, increased goblet cells, damage to cilia, squamous metaplasia of columnar epithelium, and chronic leukocytic and lymphocytic infiltration of bronchial walls; widespread inflammation, distortion, narrowing of airways, and mucus within the airways produce resistance in small airways and cause severe ventilation-perfusion imbalance	• Insidious onset, with productive cough and exertional dyspnea predominant symptoms • *Other signs and symptoms:* colds associated with increased sputum production and worsening dyspnea which take progressively longer to resolve; copious sputum (gray, white, or yellow); weight gain due to edema; cyanosis; tachypnea; wheezing; prolonged expiratory time, use of accessory muscles of respiration
Asthma • Increased bronchial reactivity to a variety of stimuli, which produces episodic bronchospasm and airway obstruction • Asthma with onset in adulthood: often without distinct allergies; asthma with onset in childhood: often associated with definite allergens. Status asthmaticus is an acute asthma attack with severe bronchospasm that fails to clear with bronchodilator therapy. • *Prognosis:* More than half of asthmatic children become asymptomatic as adults; more than half of asthmatics with onset after age 15 have persistent disease, with occasional severe attacks.	• Possible mechanisms include allergy (family tendency, seasonal occurrence); allergic reaction results in release of mast cell vasoactive and bronchospastic mediators • Upper airway infection, exercise, anxiety, and rarely, coughing or laughing can precipitate an asthma attack. • Paroxysmal airway obstruction associated with nasal polyps may be seen in response to aspirin or indomethacin ingestion. • Airway obstruction from spasm of bronchial smooth muscle narrows airways; inflammatory edema of the bronchial wall and inspissation of tenacious mucoid secretions are also important, particularly in status asthmaticus.	• History of intermittent attacks of dyspnea and wheezing • Mild wheezing progresses to severe dyspnea, audible wheezing, chest tightness (a feeling of not being able to breathe), and cough productive of thick mucus. • *Other signs:* prolonged expiration, intercostal and supraclavicular retraction on inspiration, use of accessory muscles of respiration, flaring nostrils, tachypnea, tachycardia, perspiration, and flushing; patients often have symptoms of eczema and allergic rhinitis ("hay fever"). • Status asthmaticus, unless treated promptly, can progress to respiratory failure.

CONFIRMING DIAGNOSTIC MEASURES	MANAGEMENT

- *Physical examination:* hyperresonance on percussion, decreased breath sounds, expiratory prolongation, quiet heart sounds
- *Chest X-ray:* in advanced disease, flattened diaphragm, reduced vascular markings at lung periphery, over-aeration of lungs, vertical heart, enlarged anteroposterior chest diameter, large retrosternal air space
- *Pulmonary function tests:* increased residual volume, total lung capacity, and compliance; decreased vital capacity, diffusing capacity, and expiratory volumes
- *Arterial blood gases:* reduced Po_2 with normal Pco_2 until late in disease
- *EKG:* tall, symmetric P waves in leads II, III, and AVF; vertical QRS axis; signs of right ventricular hypertrophy late in disease
- *RBC:* increased hemoglobin late in disease when persistent severe hypoxia is present

- Bronchodilators, such as aminophylline, to reverse bronchospasm and promote mucociliary clearance
- Antibiotics to treat respiratory infection; flu vaccine to prevent influenza; and pneumovax to prevent pneumococcal pneumonia
- Adequate fluid intake and, in selected patients, chest physiotherapy to mobilize secretions
- O_2 at low-flow settings to treat hypoxia
- Avoidance of smoking and air pollutants

- *Physical examination:* rhonchi and wheezes on auscultation, expiratory elongation; neck vein distention, pedal edema
- *Chest X-ray:* may show hyperinflation and increased bronchovascular markings
- *Pulmonary function tests:* increased residual volume, decreased vital capacity and forced expiratory volumes, normal static compliance and diffusing capacity
- *Arterial blood gases:* decreased Po_2; normal or increased Pco_2
- *Sputum:* contains many organisms and neutrophils
- *EKG:* may show atrial arrhythmias; peaked P waves in leads II, III, and AVF; and occasionally, right ventricular hypertrophy

- Antibiotics for infections
- Avoidance of smoking and air pollutants
- Bronchodilators to relieve bronchospasm and facilitate mucociliary clearance
- Adequate fluid intake and chest physiotherapy to mobilize secretions
- Ultrasonic or mechanical nebulizer treatments to loosen secretions and aid in mobilization
- Occasionally, patients respond to corticosteroids.
- Diuretics for edema
- Oxygen for hypoxia

- *Physical examination:* usually normal between attacks; auscultation shows rhonchi and wheezing throughout lung fields on expiration and, at times, inspiration; absent or diminished breath sounds during severe obstruction. Loud bilateral wheezes may be grossly audible; chest is hyperinflated
- *Chest X-ray:* hyperinflated lungs with air trapping during attack; normal during remission
- *Sputum:* presence of Curschmann's spirals (casts of airways), Charcot-Leyden crystals, and eosinophils
- *Pulmonary function tests:* during attacks, decreased forced expiratory volumes which improve significantly after inhaled bronchodilator; increased residual volume and, occasionally, total lung capacity; may be normal between attacks
- *Arterial blood gases:* decreased Po_2; decreased, normal, or increased Pco_2 (in severe attack)
- *EKG:* sinus tachycardia during an attack; severe attack may produce signs of cor pulmonale (right axis deviation, peaked P wave) which resolve after the attack
- *Skin tests:* may identify allergens

- Aerosol containing beta-adrenergic agents such as isoproterenol or isoetharine; also, oral beta-adrenergic agents (terbutaline) and oral methylxanthines (aminophylline). Occasionally, patients require inhaled or oral corticosteroids.
- *Emergency treatment:* O_2 therapy, corticosteroids, and bronchodilators such as subcutaneous epinephrine, intravenous aminophylline, and inhaled agents such as isoproterenol.
- Monitor for deteriorating respiratory status and note sputum characteristics; provide adequate fluid intake and oxygen, as ordered.
- *Prevention:* Tell the patient to avoid possible allergens and to use antihistamines, decongestants, inhalation of cromolyn powder, and oral or aerosol bronchodilators, as ordered. Explain the influence of stress and anxiety on asthma and frequent association with exercise (particularly running) and cold air.

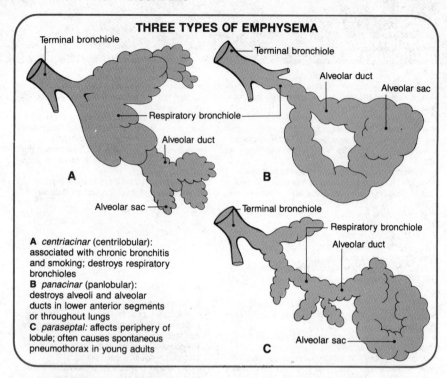

THREE TYPES OF EMPHYSEMA

Terminal bronchiole

Respiratory bronchiole

Alveolar duct

Alveolar sac

A

Terminal bronchiole

Alveolar duct

Alveolar sac

B

Terminal bronchiole

Respiratory bronchiole

Alveolar duct

Alveolar sac

C

A *centriacinar* (centrilobular): associated with chronic bronchitis and smoking; destroys respiratory bronchioles
B *panacinar* (panlobular): destroys alveoli and alveolar ducts in lower anterior segments or throughout lungs
C *paraseptal*: affects periphery of lobule; often causes spontaneous pneumothorax in young adults

breaths and exhale through pursed lips.
• To help mobilize secretions, the patient must know how to cough effectively. If the patient with copious secretions has difficulty mobilizing secretions, his family has to know how to perform postural drainage and chest physiotherapy. If secretions are thick, the patient should drink 12 to 15 glasses of fluid a day. A home humidifier may be beneficial, particularly in the winter.
• Oxygen, in low concentrations, may be ordered. Blood gas analysis will help determine O_2 need and help avoid CO_2 narcosis. If the patient is to continue O_2 therapy at home, he must know how to use the equipment correctly. Patients with COPD rarely require more than 2 to 3 liters per minute to maintain adequate oxygenation. Higher flow rates will further increase PO_2, but patients whose ventilatory drive is largely based on hypoxemia will often develop markedly increased PCO_2 tensions. In these patients, chemoreceptors in the brain are rela-

tively insensitive to the increase in CO_2. Patients and family have to understand that excessive O_2 therapy may eliminate the hypoxic respiratory drive, causing confusion and drowsiness, signs of CO_2 narcosis.
• A balanced diet is very important. Since the patient may tire easily when eating, he might take frequent, small meals and consider using oxygen, administered by nasal cannula, during meals.
• The patient and his family will need help adjusting their life-styles to accommodate the limitations imposed by this debilitating chronic disease. The patient must make time for daily rest and exercise periods as his doctor directs.
• As COPD progresses, the patient should be encouraged to discuss his fears concerning the illness.
• Not smoking will help prevent COPD, especially in people with a family history of COPD or in those in the early stages of the disease.

- Early detection of COPD can be achieved by having periodic physical examinations, including spirometry and medical evaluation of a chronic cough, and by seeking treatment for recurring respiratory infections promptly.
- Parents should set a good example by not smoking.

Bronchiectasis

A condition marked by chronic abnormal dilation of bronchi and destruction of bronchial walls, bronchiectasis can occur throughout the tracheobronchial tree or can be confined to one segment or lobe. However, it is usually bilateral and involves the basilar segments of the lower lobes. This disease has three forms: cylindrical (fusiform), varicose, and saccular (cystic). It affects people of both sexes and all ages. Because of the availability of antibiotics to treat acute respiratory tract infections, the incidence of bronchiectasis has dramatically decreased in the past 20 years. Its incidence is highest among Eskimos and the Maoris of New Zealand. Bronchiectasis is irreversible.

Causes

The different forms of bronchiectasis may occur separately or simultaneously. In *cylindrical bronchiectasis*, the bronchi expand unevenly, with little change in diameter, and end suddenly in a squared-off fashion. In *varicose bronchiectasis*, abnormal, irregular dilation and narrowing of the bronchi give the appearance of varicose veins. In *saccular bronchiectasis*, many large dilations end in sacs.

This disease results from conditions associated with repeated damage to bronchial walls, and abnormal mucociliary clearance, which cause a breakdown of supporting tissue adjacent to airways. Such conditions include:
- mucoviscidosis (cystic fibrosis of the pancreas)
- immunologic disorder (agammaglobulinemia, for example)
- recurrent, inadequately treated bacterial respiratory tract infections, such as tuberculosis, and as a complication of measles, pneumonia, pertussis, or influenza
- obstruction (by a foreign body, tumor, or stenosis) in association with recurrent infection
- inhalation of corrosive gas or repeated aspiration of gastric juices into the lungs
- congenital anomalies (uncommon), such as bronchomalacia, congenital bronchiectasis, and Kartagener's syndrome (bronchiectasis, sinusitis, and dextrocardia), and a variety of rare disorders, such as immotile-cilia syndrome.

In bronchiectasis, hyperplastic squamous epithelium denuded of cilia replaces ulcerated columnar epithelium. Abscess formation involving all layers of the bronchial wall produces inflammatory cells and fibrous tissue, resulting in both dilation and narrowing of the airways. Mucous plugs or fibrous tissue obliterates smaller bronchioles, while peribronchial lymphoid tissue becomes hyperplastic. Extensive vascular proliferation of bronchial circulation occurs and produces frequent hemoptysis.

Signs and symptoms

Initially, bronchiectasis may be asymptomatic. When symptoms do arise, they're often attributed to other illnesses. The patient usually complains of frequent bouts of pneumonia or hemoptysis. The classic symptom, however, is a chronic cough that produces copious, foul-smelling, mucopurulent secretions, possibly totaling several cupfuls daily. Characteristic findings include coarse rales during inspiration over involved lobes or segments, occasional wheezes, dyspnea, sinusitis, weight loss, anemia,

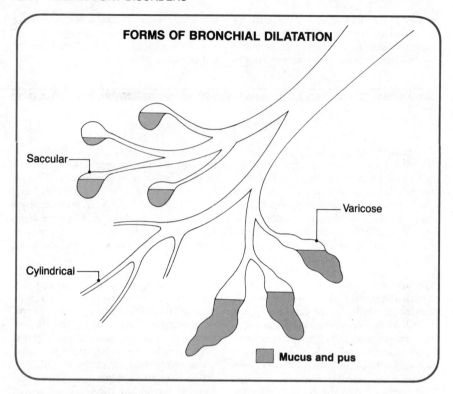

FORMS OF BRONCHIAL DILATATION

Saccular

Varicose

Cylindrical

Mucus and pus

malaise, clubbing, recurrent fever, chills, and other signs of infection.

Advanced bronchiectasis may produce chronic malnutrition and amyloidosis, as well as right heart failure and cor pulmonale due to hypoxic pulmonary vasoconstriction.

Diagnosis
History of recurrent bronchial infections, pneumonia, and hemoptysis in a patient whose chest X-rays show peribronchial thickening, areas of atelectasis, and scattered cystic changes suggests bronchiectasis. Bronchography, however, is the most reliable diagnostic tool. Although this test is not done routinely, it should be considered for patients being evaluated for possible surgery or those with recurrent or severe hemoptysis. In bronchography, a radiopaque dye outlines the bronchial walls, revealing the location and extent of the disease. Bronchoscopy does not establish this diag-

nosis, but helps identify the source of secretions or the site of bleeding in hemoptysis.

Other helpful laboratory tests include:
• *sputum culture and Gram's stain* to identify predominant organisms
• *blood count* for possible anemia and leukocytosis
• *pulmonary function studies* to detect decreased vital capacity, expiratory flow, and hypoxemia; these tests also help determine the physiologic severity of the disease and the effects of therapy, and help evaluate patients for surgery. If symptoms warrant, evaluation may include urinalysis and EKG (the latter is normal unless cor pulmonale develops). When cystic fibrosis is suspected as the underlying cause of bronchiectasis, a sweat electrolyte test is useful.

Treatment
Treatment includes antibiotics, given P.O. or I.V., for 7 to 10 days or until sputum

production decreases. Bronchodilators, with postural drainage and chest percussion, help remove secretions if the patient has bronchospasm and thick, tenacious sputum. Bronchoscopy may occasionally be used to aid mobilization of secretions. Hypoxia requires oxygen therapy; severe hemoptysis often requires lobectomy or segmental resection.

Additional considerations
Throughout this illness, the patient will need supportive care and help in adjusting to the permanent changes in lifestyle that irreversible lung damage necessitates. Thorough teaching is vital.
• Antibiotics and various diagnostic tests may be ordered. Chest physiotherapy, including postural drainage and chest percussion designed for involved lobes should be performed several times a day. The best times for these procedures are early morning and just before bedtime. The patient maintains each position for 10 minutes, then percussion is performed and the patient coughs. Family members must know how to do postural drainage and chest percussion. Coughing and deep breathing techniques will also help promote good ventilation and the removal of secretions.
• The patient should stop smoking, since it stimulates secretions and irritates the airways. He should go to a local self-help group, if necessary.
• A warm, quiet, comfortable environment will allow the patient to rest as much as possible. Balanced, high-protein meals will promote good health and tissue healing, and plenty of fluids will aid expectoration. Frequent mouth care is necessary to remove foul-smelling sputum. The patient should dispose of all secretions properly to prevent spreading infection.
• The patient should also avoid air pollutants and people with upper respiratory infections, and he should take his medications (especially antibiotics) exactly as ordered.
• Measures that will help prevent this disease include vigorous treatment of bacterial pneumonia, and immunization to prevent childhood diseases.

Tuberculosis

An acute or chronic infection caused by Mycobacterium tuberculosis *and, sometimes, other strains of* Mycobacteria, *tuberculosis (TB) is characterized by pulmonary infiltrates, formation of granulomas with caseation, fibrosis, and cavitation. The American Lung Association estimates that active disease afflicts nearly 14 out of every 100,000 people. Those living in crowded, poorly-ventilated conditions are most likely to become infected. Prognosis is excellent with correct treatment.*

Causes
After exposure to *M. tuberculosis*, roughly 5% of infected persons develop active tuberculosis within 1 year; in the remainder, microorganisms cause a latent infection. The host's immunologic defense system usually controls the tubercle bacillus by killing it or walling it up in a tiny nodule (tubercle). However, the bacillus may lie dormant within the tubercle for years and later reactivate and spread, causing active infection.

Although the primary focus of infection is in the lungs, mycobacteria commonly exist in other parts of the body, such as the kidneys and the lymph nodes. A number of factors increase the likelihood of reactivation of infection: gastrectomy, uncontrolled diabetes mellitus, Hodgkin's disease, leukemia, treatment with corticosteroids and immunosuppressives, and silicosis.

Transmission is by droplet nuclei produced when infected persons cough or sneeze. After inhalation, if a tubercle bacillus settles in an alveolus, infection occurs, with alveolar capillary dilation and endothelial cell swelling. Alveolitis results, with replication of tubercle bacilli and influx of polymorphonuclear leukocytes. These organisms disseminate through the lymph system to the circulatory system and then throughout the body. Cell-mediated immunity to the mycobacteria, which develops about 3 to 6 weeks later, usually contains the infection and arrests the disease. If the infection reactivates, the body's response characteristically leads to caseation—the conversion of necrotic tissue to a cheeselike material. The caseum may localize, undergo fibrosis, or excavate and form cavities, the walls of which are studded with multiplying tubercle bacilli. If this happens, infected caseous debris may spread throughout the lungs by the tracheobronchial tree. Sites of extrapulmonary TB include pleura, meninges, joints, lymph nodes, peritoneum, genitourinary tract, or bowel.

Signs and symptoms
In primary infection, after an incubation period of from 4 to 8 weeks, tuberculosis is usually asymptomatic but may produce nonspecific symptoms, such as fatigue, weakness, anorexia, weight loss, night sweats, and low-grade fever. In reactivation, symptoms may include a cough that produces mucopurulent sputum, occasional hemoptysis, and chest pains.

Diagnosis
Diagnostic tests include physical examination, chest X-ray, tuberculin skin test, and sputum smears and cultures to identify tubercle bacilli. Diagnosis must be precise, since several other diseases (lung carcinoma, lung abscess, pneumoconiosis, bronchiectasis) may mimic tuberculosis. The following procedures permit diagnosis:
• *Auscultation* detects crepitant rales, bronchial breath sounds, wheezes, and whispered pectoriloquy.
• *Chest percussion* detects a dullness over the affected area, indicating consolidation or pleural fluid.

• *Chest X-ray* shows nodular lesions, as well as patchy infiltrates (especially in the upper lobes), cavity formation, scar tissue, and calcium deposits; although a valuable diagnostic tool, chest X-rays may not be able to distinguish active from inactive TB.
• *Tuberculin skin test* detects infection with tuberculosis but doesn't distinguish the disease from uncomplicated infection. In this test, intermediate-strength purified protein derivative (PPD) or 5 tuberculin units (0.1 ml) are injected intracutaneously on the forearm and read in 48 to 72 hours; a positive reaction (equal to or more than 10 mm induration) develops within 2 to 10 weeks after infection with the tubercle bacillus in both active and inactive TB.

 • *Stains and cultures* (of sputum, CSF, urine, drainage from abscess, or pleural fluid) show heat-sensitive, nonmotile, aerobic, acid-fast bacilli.

Treatment
Chemotherapy with daily oral doses of isoniazid and ethambutol or rifampin for 9 to 18 months or longer usually cures tuberculosis. After 2 to 4 weeks the disease is generally no longer infectious, and the patient can resume his normal life-style while continuing to take medication. Patients with atypical mycobacterial disease or drug-resistant TB may require second-line drugs, such as apremycin, para-aminosalicylic acid, pyrazinamide, cycloserine, and ethionamide.

Additional considerations
During hospital care of a tuberculosis patient, the staff member should:
• isolate the infectious patient in a quiet, well-ventilated room until he's no longer contagious; teach the patient to cough and sneeze into tissues and to dispose of all secretions properly; place a covered trash can nearby or tape a waxed bag to the side of the bed for used tissues; instruct the patient to wear a mask when outside of his room; make sure visitors and other hospital personnel also wear masks when in the patient's room.

• remind the patient to get plenty of rest; stress the importance of eating balanced meals to promote recovery; urge the patient, if he is anorexic, to eat small meals throughout the day; record weight weekly.
• watch for drug side effects; monitor SGOT and SGPT levels, since isoniazid can cause hepatitis or peripheral neuritis; give pyridoxine (vitamin B_6), as ordered, to prevent or treat peripheral neuritis; watch for optic neuritis if the patient receives ethambutol and discontinue the drug if it develops; watch for hepatitis and purpura if the patient receives rifampin; observe the patient for other complications, such as hemoptysis.
• teach the patient, before discharge, to watch for side effects, and warn him to report them immediately; emphasize the importance of regular follow-up examinations, and instruct the patient and his family concerning the signs and symptoms of recurring tuberculosis; stress the need to follow long-term treatment.
• advise persons who have been exposed to infected patients to receive tuberculin tests and, if ordered, chest X-rays and prophylactic isoniazid.

PNEUMOCONIOSES

Silicosis

Silicosis is a progressive lung disease characterized by nodular lesions, which frequently progress to fibrosis. It is the most common form of pneumoconiosis. Silicosis can be classified according to the severity of pulmonary disease and the rapidity of its onset and progression; it usually occurs as a simple asymptomatic illness. Acute silicosis develops after 1 to 3 years in workers (sand blasters, tunnel workers) exposed to very high concentrations of respirable silica. Accelerated silicosis appears after an average of 10 years of exposure to lower concentrations of free silica. Chronic silicosis develops after 20 or more years of exposure to lower concentrations of free silica. Prognosis is good, unless the disease progresses into the complicated fibrotic form, which causes respiratory insufficiency and cor pulmonale, and is associated with pulmonary tuberculosis.

Causes
Silicosis results from the inhalation and pulmonary deposition of respirable crystalline silica dust, mostly from quartz. The danger to the worker depends on the concentration of dust in the atmosphere, the percentage of respirable free silica particles in the dust, and the duration of exposure. Respirable particles are less than 10 microns in diameter, but the disease-causing particles deposited in the alveolar space are usually 1 to 3 microns in diameter.

Industrial sources of silica in its pure form include the manufacture of ceramics (flint) and building materials (sandstone). It occurs in mixed form in the production of construction materials (cement); it's found in powder form (silica flour) in paints, porcelain, scouring soaps, and wood fillers, and in the mining of gold, coal, lead, zinc, and iron. Foundry workers, boiler scalers, and stonecutters are all exposed to silica dust and, therefore, are at high risk of developing silicosis.

Nodules result when alveolar macrophages ingest silica particles, which they are unable to process. As a result, the macrophages die and release proteolytic enzymes into the surrounding tissue. The subsequent inflammation attracts other macrophages and fibroblasts into the region to produce fibrous tissue and wall off the reaction. The resulting nodule has an onionskin appearance when viewed under a microscope. Nodules develop adjacent to terminal and respiratory bronchioles, concentrate in the upper lobes, and are frequently accompanied by bullous changes in both lobes. If the disease process does not progress, minimal physiologic disturbances and no disability occur. Occasionally, however, the fibrotic response accelerates, engulfing and destroying large areas of the lung (progressive massive fibrosis [PMF] or conglomerate lesions). Fibrosis may continue despite termination of exposure to dust.

Signs and symptoms

Silicosis initially may be asymptomatic, or it may produce dyspnea on exertion, often attributed to being "out of shape" or "slowing down." If the disease progresses to the chronic and complicated stage, dyspnea on exertion worsens, and other symptoms—usually tachypnea and an insidious dry cough, which is most pronounced in the morning—appear. Progression to the advanced stage causes dyspnea on minimal exertion, worsening cough, and pulmonary hypertension, which in turn leads to right ventricular failure and cor pulmonale. Patients with silicosis have a high incidence of active tuberculosis, which should be considered when evaluating a patient with this disease. CNS changes—confusion, lethargy, decrease in the rate and depth of respiration as PCO_2 increases—also occur in advanced silicosis. Other clinical features include malaise, disturbed sleep, and hoarseness. (*Note:* The severity of these symptoms may not correlate with chest X-ray findings or the results of pulmonary function studies.)

Diagnosis

Patient history reveals occupational exposure to silica dust. Physical examination is normal in *simple silicosis;* in *chronic silicosis* with conglomerate lesions, it may reveal decreased chest expansion, diminished intensity of breath sounds, areas of hypo- and hyperreso-

nance, fine to medium rales, and tachypnea. In *simple silicosis,* chest X-rays show small, discrete, nodular lesions distributed throughout both lung fields but typically concentrated in the upper lung zones; the hilar lung nodes may be enlarged and exhibit "eggshell" calcification. In *complicated silicosis,* X-rays show one or more conglomerate masses of dense tissue.

Pulmonary function studies yield the following results:
• *FVC:* reduced in complicated silicosis
• *FEV$_1$:* reduced in obstructive disease (emphysematous areas of silicosis); reduced in complicated silicosis, but ratio of FEV_1 to FVC is normal or high
• *MVV:* reduced in both restrictive and obstructive diseases
• *DLCO:* reduced when fibrosis destroys alveolar walls and obliterates pulmonary capillaries, or when fibrosis thickens alveolar capillary membrane.

In addition, arterial blood gas studies show:
• PO_2: normal in simple silicosis; may be significantly decreased in the late stages of chronic or complicated disease, when the patient breathes room air
• PCO_2: normal in early stages but may decrease due to hyperventilation; may increase as restrictive pattern develops, particularly if the patient is hypoxic and has severe impairment of alveolar ventilation.

Treatment and additional considerations

The goal of treatment is to relieve respiratory symptoms, to manage hypoxia and cor pulmonale, and to prevent respiratory tract irritation and infections. Treatment also includes careful observation for the development of tuberculosis. Respiratory symptoms may be relieved through daily use of bronchodilating aerosols and increased fluid intake (at least 3 liters daily). Steam inhalation and chest physical therapy techniques, such as controlled coughing and segmental bronchial drainage, with chest percussion and vibration, help clear secretions. In severe cases, it may be necessary to administer oxygen by cannula or mask (1 to 2 liters/min) for the patient with chronic hypoxia, or by mechanical ventilation if arterial oxygen cannot be maintained above 40 mmHg. Respiratory infections require that antibiotics be administered to the patient promptly.

• To prevent infections, the patient should avoid crowds and persons with respiratory infections, and receive influenza and pneumococcal vaccines.

• Regular activity will increase the patient's exercise tolerance. He should plan his daily activities to decrease the work of breathing; he should pace himself, rest often, and generally move slowly through his daily routine.

Asbestosis

Asbestosis is a form of pneumoconiosis characterized by diffuse interstitial fibrosis. It can develop as long as 15 to 20 years after regular exposure to asbestos has ended. Asbestos also causes pleural plaques and mesotheliomas of pleura and the peritoneum; a potent co-carcinogen, it aggravates the risk of lung cancer in cigarette smokers.

Causes

Asbestosis results from the inhalation of respirable asbestos fibers (50 microns or more in length, 0.5 microns or less in diameter), which assume a longitudinal orientation in the airway, move in the direction of airflow, and penetrate respiratory bronchioles and alveolar walls. Sources include the mining and milling of asbestos, the construction industry (where asbestos is used in a prefabricated form), and the fireproofing and textile industries; asbestos is also used in the production of paints, plastics, and brake and clutch linings.

Asbestos-related diseases develop in families of asbestos workers as a result of exposure to fibrous dust shaken off workers' clothing at home. Such diseases develop in the general public as a result of exposure to fibrous dust or waste piles from nearby asbestos plants.

Inhaled fibers become encased in a brown, proteinlike sheath rich in iron (ferruginous bodies or asbestos bodies), found in sputum and lung tissue. Interstitial fibrosis develops in lower lung zones, causing obliterative changes in lung parenchyma and pleurae. Raised hyaline plaques may form in parietal pleura, diaphragm, and pleura contiguous with the pericardium.

Signs and symptoms

Clinical features may appear before chest X-ray changes. The first symptom is usually dyspnea on exertion, typically after 10 years' exposure. As fibrosis extends, dyspnea on exertion increases, until eventually, dyspnea occurs even at rest; advanced disease also causes a dry cough (may be productive in smokers), chest pain (often pleuritic), recurrent respiratory infections, and tachypnea.

Cardiovascular complications include pulmonary hypertension, right ventricular hypertrophy, and cor pulmonale. Finger clubbing commonly occurs.

Diagnosis

Patient history reveals occupational, family, or neighborhood exposure to asbestos fibers. Physical examination reveals characteristic dry, crackling rales at bases of the lungs. Chest X-rays show fine, irregular, and linear diffuse infiltrates; extensive fibrosis results in a "honeycomb" or "ground glass" appearance. X-rays may also show pleural thickening and pleural calcification, with bilateral obliteration of costophrenic angles and, in later stages, an enlarged heart with a classic "shaggy" heart border.

Pulmonary function studies show:

- *VC, FVC, and TLC:* decreased
- FEV_1: decreased or normal
- $DLCO$: reduced when fibrosis destroys alveolar walls and thickens alveolar capillary membrane.

Arterial blood gas analysis reveals:
- PO_2: decreased
- PCO_2: low due to hyperventilation.

Treatment and additional considerations

The goal of treatment is to relieve respiratory symptoms and, in advanced disease, manage hypoxia and cor pulmonale. Respiratory symptoms may be relieved by chest physical therapy techniques, such as controlled coughing and segmental bronchial drainage, with chest percussion and vibration. Aerosol therapy, inhaled mucolytics, and increased fluid intake (at least 3 liters daily) may also help relieve respiratory symptoms. Diuretics, digitalis preparations, and salt restriction may be indicated for patients with cor pulmonale. Hypoxia requires oxygen administration by cannula or mask (1 to 2 liters/min), or by mechanical ventilation if arterial oxygen cannot be maintained above 40 mmHg. Respiratory infections require prompt administration of antibiotics and patient isolation.

Infections can be prevented if the patient tries to avoid crowds and persons with infections, and receives influenza and pneumococcal vaccines.

The efficiency of the patient's ventilation can be improved by physical reconditioning, energy conservation in daily activities, and relaxation techniques.

Berylliosis

(Beryllium poisoning, beryllium disease)

Berylliosis, a form of pneumoconiosis, is a systemic granulomatous disorder with dominant pulmonary manifestations. It occurs in two forms: acute nonspecific pneumonitis and chronic noncaseating granulomatous disease with interstitial fibrosis, which may cause death from respiratory failure and cor pulmonale. Most patients with chronic interstitial disease become only slightly to moderately disabled by impaired lung function and other symptoms, but with each acute exacerbation the prognosis worsens.

Causes

Berylliosis is caused by the inhalation of beryllium dusts, fumes, and mists, with the pattern of disease related to the "dose" inhaled. Beryllium may also be absorbed through the skin. This disease occurs among beryllium alloy workers, cathode ray tube makers, gas mantle makers, missile technicians, and nuclear reactor workers; it's generally associated with the milling and use of beryllium, not with the mining of beryl ore. Berylliosis may also affect the families of workers as a result of dust shaken off workers' clothing at home, and people who live near plants where beryllium alloy is used. The mechanism by which beryllium exerts its toxic effect is unknown.

Signs and symptoms

Absorption of beryllium through broken skin produces an itchy rash, which usually subsides within 2 weeks after exposure. A "beryllium ulcer" results from accidental implantation of beryllium metal in the skin. Respiratory symptoms of acute berylliosis include swelling and ulceration of nasal mucosa, which may progress to septal perforation, tracheitis, and bronchitis (dry cough). Acute pulmonary disease may develop rapidly (within 3 days) or weeks later, producing a progressive dry cough, tightness in the chest, substernal pain, tachycardia, and signs of bronchitis. This disease has a significant mortality related to respiratory failure.

About 10% of patients with acute berylliosis develop chronic disease 10 to 15 years after exposure. The chronic form causes increasing dyspnea that becomes progressively unremitting, mild chest pain, dry unproductive cough, and tachypnea. Pneumothorax may occur, with pulmonary scarring and bleb formation.

Cardiovascular complications include pulmonary hypertension, right ventricular hypertrophy, and cor pulmonale. Other clinical features include hepatosplenomegaly, renal calculi, lymphadenopathy, anorexia, weight loss, and fatigue.

Diagnosis

Patient history reveals occupational, family, or neighborhood exposure to beryllium dust, fumes, or mists. Physical examination reveals basal rales and rhonchi and shallow breathing; liver and spleen may be palpable. In *acute berylliosis*, chest X-rays may be suggestive of pulmonary edema, showing acute miliary process or a patchy acinous filling, and diffuse infiltrates with prominent peribronchial markings. In *chronic berylliosis*, X-rays show reticulonodular infiltrates and hilar adenopathy, and large coalescent infiltrates in both lungs.

Pulmonary function studies show decreased VC, FVC, RV/TLC, and DLco, and compliance as lungs stiffen from fibrosis. Arterial blood gas analysis shows decreased Po_2 and Pco_2.

Positive beryllium patch test establishes only hypersensitivity to beryllium, not the presence of disease. Tissue biopsy and spectrographic analysis are positive for most exposed workers but not absolutely diagnostic. In addition, urinalysis may show beryllium in urine, but this indicates only that beryllium has been deposited in the body at some time. Differential diagnosis must rule out sarcoidosis and granulomatous infections.

Treatment and additional considerations

Beryllium ulcer requires excision or curettage. Acute berylliosis requires prompt corticosteroid therapy. Hypoxia may require oxygen administration by nasal cannula or mask (1 to 2 liters/min). Severe respiratory failure requires mechanical ventilation if arterial oxygen cannot be maintained above 40 mmHg.

Chronic berylliosis is usually treated with corticosteroids, although it's not certain that steroids alter the progression of the disease. A lifelong maintenance dose may be necessary.

Respiratory symptoms may be treated with bronchodilators, increased fluid intake (at least 3 liters daily), and chest physical therapy techniques. Diuretics, digitalis preparations, and salt restriction may be useful in patients with cor pulmonale.

Infections can be prevented if the patient makes an attempt to avoid crowds and persons with an infection, and receives influenza and pneumococcal vaccines.

The patient should be encouraged to practice physical reconditioning, energy conservation in daily activities, and relaxation techniques.

Coal Worker's Pneumoconiosis

(Black lung disease, coal miner's disease, miner's asthma, anthracosis, anthracosilicosis)

A progressive nodular pulmonary disease, coal worker's pneumoconiosis (CWP) occurs in two forms. Simple CWP is characterized by small lung opacities; in complicated CWP, also known as progressive massive fibrosis (PMF), masses of fibrous tissue occasionally develop in the lungs of patients with simple CWP. The risk of developing CWP depends upon the duration of exposure to coal dust (usually

15 years or longer), intensity of exposure (dust count, particle size), location of the mine, silica content of the coal (anthracite coal has the highest silica content), and the worker's susceptibility. Incidence of CWP is highest among anthracite coal miners in the eastern United States. Prognosis varies. Simple asymptomatic disease is self-limiting, although progression to complicated CWP is more likely if CWP begins after a relatively short period of exposure. Complicated CWP may be disabling, resulting in severe ventilatory failure and right heart failure secondary to pulmonary hypertension.

Causes

CWP is caused by the inhalation and prolonged retention of respirable coal dust particles (less than 5 microns in diameter). *Simple CWP* results in the formation of macules (accumulations of macrophages laden with coal dust) around the terminal and respiratory bronchioles, surrounded by a halo of dilated alveoli. Macule formation leads to atrophy of supporting tissue, causing permanent dilation of small airways (focal emphysema). Simple disease may progress to *complicated CWP*, involving one or both lungs. In this form of the disease, fibrous tissue masses enlarge and coalesce, causing gross distortion of pulmonary structures (destruction of vasculature, alveoli, and airways).

Signs and symptoms

Simple CWP is asymptomatic, especially in nonsmokers. Symptoms appear if PMF develops and include exertional dyspnea and a cough that is occasionally productive of inky-black sputum, when fibrotic changes undergo avascular necrosis and their centers cavitate. Other clinical features of CWP include increasing dyspnea and a cough that produces milky, gray, clear, or coal-flecked sputum. Recurrent bronchial and pulmonary infections produce yellow, green, or thick sputum.

Complications include pulmonary hypertension, right ventricular hypertrophy and cor pulmonale, and pulmonary tuberculosis. In cigarette smokers, chronic bronchitis and emphysema may also complicate the disease.

Diagnosis

Patient history reveals exposure to coal dust. Physical examination shows barrel chest, hyperresonant lungs with areas of dullness, diminished breath sounds, rales, rhonchi, and wheezes. In *simple CWP*, chest X-rays show small opacities (less than 10 mm in diameter), which may be present in all lung zones but are more prominent in the upper lung zones; in *complicated CWP*, one or more large opacities (1 to 5 cm in diameter), possibly exhibiting cavitation, are seen.

The results of pulmonary function studies include:

- *VC:* normal in simple CWP, but decreased with PMF
- *FEV_1:* decreased in complicated disease
- *RV/TLC:* normal in simple CWP; decreased in PMF
- *DLCO:* significantly decreased in complicated CWP as alveolar septae are destroyed and pulmonary capillaries obliterated.

In addition, arterial blood gas studies show:

- Po_2: normal in simple CWP, but decreased in complicated disease
- Pco_2: normal in simple CWP, but may be decreased due to hyperventilation; may also be increased if the patient is hypoxic and has severe impairment of alveolar ventilation.

Treatment and additional considerations

The goal of treatment is to relieve respiratory symptoms, to manage hypoxia and cor pulmonale, and to avoid respiratory tract irritants and infections. Treatment also includes careful observation for the development of tuberculosis. Respiratory symptoms may be relieved through bronchodilator therapy with theophylline or aminophylline (if bronchospasm is reversible), oral or inhaled sympathomimetic amines (metaproterenol), corticosteroids (oral prednisone or an aerosol form of beclomethasone), or cromolyn sodium aerosol. Chest physical therapy techniques, such as controlled coughing and segmental bronchial drainage, with chest percussion and vibration, help remove secretions.

Other measures include increased fluid intake (at least 3 liters daily) and respiratory therapy techniques, such as aerosol therapy, inhaled mucolytics, and intermittent positive pressure breathing (IPPB). Diuretics, digitalis preparations, and salt restriction may be indicated in cor pulmonale. In severe cases,

it may be necessary to administer oxygen for hypoxia by cannula or mask (1 to 2 liters/min) if the patient has chronic hypoxia, or by mechanical ventilation if arterial oxygen cannot be maintained above 40 mmHg. Respiratory infections require prompt administration of antibiotics.

The patient can help prevent infections by avoiding crowds and persons with respiratory infections, and by receiving influenza and pneumococcal vaccines.

The patient should stay active to avoid a deterioration in his physical condition, but should pace his activities and practice relaxation techniques.

Selected References

Abels, Linda, ed. *Acute Respiratory Failure*, CRITICAL CARE QUARTERLY, March 1979.

Beaty, Harry N., et al. *When You Suspect Legionnaires' Disease*, PATIENT CARE. 13:12, January 15, 1979.

Burton, George C., and Glen N. Gee. RESPIRATORY CARE: A GUIDE TO CLINICAL PRACTICE. Philadelphia: J.B. Lippincott Co., 1976.

Committee on Mineral Resources and the Environment, National Research Council. COAL WORKERS' PNEUMOCONIOSIS—MEDICAL CONSIDERATIONS, SOME SOCIAL IMPLICATIONS: MINERAL RESOURCES AND THE ENVIRONMENT SUPPLEMENTARY REPORT. Washington, D.C.: National Academy of Sciences, 1976.

Comroe, Julius H., Jr. PHYSIOLOGY OF RESPIRATION, 2nd ed. Chicago: Year Book Medical Publishers, 1974.

Glover, Dennis W., and Margaret M. Glover. RESPIRATORY THERAPY: BASICS FOR NURSING AND ALLIED HEALTH PROFESSIONS. St. Louis: C.V. Mosby Co., 1978.

Guenter, Clarence A., and Martin H. Welsh, eds. PULMONARY MEDICINE. Philadelphia: J.B. Lippincott Co., 1977

Hinshaw, H. Corwin. DISEASES OF THE CHEST, 4th ed. Philadelphia: W.B. Saunders Co., 1980.

Hopewell, P.C., and J.F. Murray. *The Adult Respiratory Distress Syndrome*, ANNUAL REVIEW OF MEDICINE. 27:343-356, 1976.

Kirby, B., et al. *Legionnaires' Disease: Clinical Features of 24 Cases*, ANNALS OF INTERNAL MEDICINE. 89:297, September 1978.

Lee, J.A. THE NEW NURSE IN INDUSTRY. Washington, D.C.: Dept. of Health, Education and Welfare, 1979.

Legionnaires, CENTER FOR DISEASE CONTROL LABORATORY MANUAL. Washington, D.C.: Dept. of Health, Education and Welfare, 1978.

Levine, R.J. ASBESTOS—AN INFORMATION SOURCE. Washington, D.C.: Dept. of Health, Education and Welfare, May 1978.

Levy, M. and J. Stubbs. *Nursing Implications in the Care of Patients with Assisted Mechanical Ventilation Modified with Positive End-Expiratory Pressure*, HEART & LUNG. 7:299, March-April 1978.

Ohman, K.H. *Prevention of Silica Exposure and Elimination of Silicosis*, AMERICAN INDUSTRIAL HYGIENE ASSOCIATION JOURNAL. November 1978, pp. 847-859.

Shapiro, Barry A., et al. CLINICAL APPLICATIONS OF RESPIRATORY CARE, 2nd ed. Chicago: Year Book Medical Publishers, 1979.

Ziment, I., RESPIRATORY PHARMACOLOGY AND THERAPEUTICS. Philadelphia: W.B. Saunders Co., 1978.

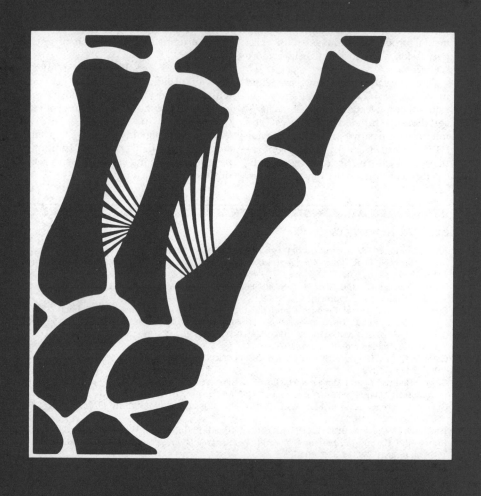

8 Musculoskeletal Disorders

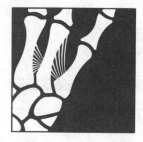

Musculoskeletal Disorders

Introduction

A complex system of bones, muscles, ligaments, tendons, and other connective tissue, the musculoskeletal system gives the body form and shape. It also protects vital organs, makes movement possible, stores calcium and other minerals, and provides the site for hematopoiesis.

The human skeleton contains 206 bones, which are composed of inorganic salts, such as calcium and phosphate, imbedded in a framework of collagen fibers. Bones are classified by shape: long, short, flat, or irregular.

Long bones

Long bones are found in the extremities, and include the humerus, radius, and ulna of the arm; the femur, tibia, and fibula of the leg; the phalanges and metatarsals. These bones have a long shaft, or diaphysis, and widened, bulbous ends, called epiphyses. A long bone is made up mainly of compact bone, which surrounds the medullary cavity (also called the yellow bone marrow cavity), a storage site for fat. The lining of the medullary cavity (the endosteum) is a thin layer of connective tissue.

In children and young adults, epiphyseal cartilage separates the diaphysis and epiphysis, allowing the bone to grow longer. In adults, in whom bone growth is complete, this cartilage is ossified and forms the epiphyseal line. The epiphysis also has a surface layer made up of compact bone, but its center is made of spongy or cancellous bone. Cancellous bone contains many open spaces between thin threads of bone, called trabeculae, which are arranged in various directions to correspond with the lines of maximum stress or pressure. This arrangement gives the bone added structural strength.

Unlike cancellous bone, adult compact bone is composed of numerous orderly networks of interconnecting canals. Each of these networks is called a haversian system and is comprised of a central haversian canal surrounded by layers (lamellae) of bone. Between adjacent lamellae are small openings called lacunae, which contain bone cells or osteocytes. All lacunae are joined by an interconnecting network of tiny canals called canaliculi, each of which contains one or more capillaries and provides a route for tissue fluids. The haversian system runs parallel to the bone's long axis and is responsible for carrying blood to the bone through blood vessels that enter the system through Volkmann's canal.

Short, flat, or irregular bones

Short bones include the tarsal and carpal bones; flat bones, the frontal and parietal bones of the cranium, the ribs, sternum, scapulae, ilium, and pubis; and irregular bones, the bones of the spine (vertebrae, sacrum, coccyx) and certain bones of the skull—the sphenoid, ethmoid, and mandible.

A short, flat, or irregular bone has an outer layer of compact bone and an inner portion of spongy bone, which in some bones—the sternum and certain areas in the flat bones of the skull—contain red marrow.

All bones are covered by a fibrous layer called the periosteum except at joints, where they're covered by articular cartilage.

Joints

The tissues connecting two bones comprise a joint, which allows for motion between the bones and provides stability. Joints, like bones, have varying forms.

• *Fibrous joints,* called synarthroses, have only minute motion and provide stability when tight union is necessary, as in the sutures that join the cranial bones.

• *Cartilaginous joints,* called amphiarthroses, allow limited motion, as between vertebrae.

• *Synovial joints,* called diarthroses, are the most common and allow the greatest degree of movement. Such joints include the elbows and knees. Synovial joints have special characteristics: the bones' two articulating surfaces have a smooth hyaline covering (articular cartilage), which is resilient to pressure; their opposing surfaces are congruous and glide smoothly on each other; a fibrous (articular) capsule holds them together. Beneath the capsule, lining the joint cavity, is the synovial membrane, which secretes a clear viscous fluid called synovial fluid. This fluid lubricates the two opposing surfaces during motion and also nourishes the articular cartilage. Surrounding a synovial joint are ligaments, muscles, and tendons, which strengthen and stabilize the joint but allow free movement.

In some synovial joints, the synovial membrane forms two additional structures—bursae and tendon sheaths—which reduce friction that normally accompanies movement. Bursae are small, cushionlike sacs lined with synovial membranes and filled with synovial fluid; most are located between tendons and bones. Tendon sheaths wrap around the tendon and cushion it as it crosses the joint.

There are two types of synovial joint movements: angular and circular. Angular movements include *flexion* (decrease in joint angle), *extension* (increase in the joint angle), and *hyperextension* (increase in the angle of extension beyond the usual arc). Joints of the knees, elbows, and phalanges permit such movement. Other angular movements are *abduction* (movement away from the body's midline) and *adduction* (movement toward the body's midline).

Circular movements include *rotation* (motion around a central axis), as in the ball and socket joints of the hips and shoulders; *pronation* (wrist motion to place palmar surface of the hand down, with the thumb toward the body); *supination* (begging position, with palm up). Other kinds of movement are *inversion* (movement facing inward), *eversion* (movement facing outward), *protraction* (as in forward motion of mandible), and *retraction* (returning protracted part into place).

Muscles make motion possible

Muscle tissues' most specialized feature—contractility—makes movement of bones and joints possible. Muscles also pump blood through the body, move food through the intestines, and make breathing possible. Muscular activity produces heat, making it an important component in temperature regulation. Muscles maintain body positions, such as sitting and standing. Muscle mass accounts for about 40% of a man's weight.

Muscles are classified in many ways. *Skeletal* muscles are attached to bone; *visceral* muscles permit function of internal organs; and *cardiac* muscles comprise the heart wall. Also, muscles may be striated or nonstriated (smooth), depending on their cellular configuration.

When muscles are classified according to activity, they are voluntary or involuntary. *Voluntary* muscles can be controlled at will and are under the influence of the somatic nervous system; these are the skeletal muscles. *Involuntary* muscles, controlled by the autonomic nervous system, include the cardiac and visceral muscles.

Each skeletal muscle is composed of many elongated muscle cells, called *muscle fibers,* through which run slender threads of protein, called myofibrils. Muscle fibers are held together in bundles by sheaths of fibrous tissue, called fascia. Blood vessels and nerves pass into muscles through the fascia to reach the individual muscle fibers.

Skeletal muscles are attached to bone directly or indirectly by fibrous cords

known as tendons. The least movable end of the muscle attachment (generally proximal) is called the point of origin; the most movable end (generally distal) is the point of insertion.

Mechanism of contraction

To stimulate muscle contraction and movement, the brain sends motor impulses by the peripheral motor nerves to the voluntary muscle, which contains motor nerve fibers. These fibers reach membranes of skeletal muscle cells at neuromuscular (myoneural) junctions. When an impulse reaches the myoneural junction, the neurochemical acetylcholine is released. This triggers the transient release of calcium from the sarcoplasmic reticulum, a membranous network in the muscle fiber, which, in turn, triggers muscle contraction. The energy source for such contraction is adenosine triphosphate (ATP). ATP release is also triggered by the impulse at the myoneural junction. Relaxation of a muscle is believed to take place by reversal of the above mechanisms.

Musculoskeletal assessment

Patients with musculoskeletal disorders are often elderly, have other concurrent medical conditions, or are victims of trauma. Generally, they face prolonged immobilization. These factors make thorough assessment essential. Assessment should include a complete history and a careful physical examination.

The patient is interviewed to obtain a complete medical, social, and personal history. This includes general activity (does he jog daily, or is he sedentary?), which may be significantly altered by musculoskeletal disease or trauma. Also needed is information about occupation, diet, sexual activity, and elimination habits, and an assessment of how the problem will affect body image. Also, how does the patient function at home? Can he perform daily activities? Does he have trouble getting around? Are there stairs where he lives? Where are the bathroom and bedroom? Does he use any prosthetic devices? Can other family

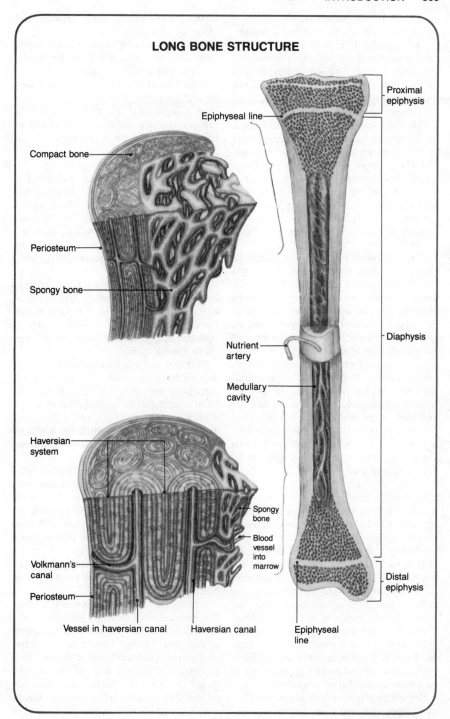

LONG BONE STRUCTURE

members help with his care?

An accurate account of the musculoskeletal problem is necessary. Has the problem caused the patient to change his everyday routine? When did symptoms begin? Did they progress and/or limit function? Has he previously received treatment for this problem?

The level of pain must be determined. Is the patient in pain at the moment? Are ordinary methods of pain relief successful? What was past response to treatment? For instance, if the patient has arthritis and uses corticosteroids, how effective are they? Does he require more or less medication than before? Did he comply with all the prescribed treatments?

The physical examination helps to determine diagnosis and records the patient's disabilities for evaluating the effects of treatment. What is the patient's general appearance? Is there localized edema, reddening of pressure points, point tenderness, and other deformities (kyphosis, for example)? This information is important in planning health care. Mobility and gait should be noted. To check range of motion, the patient should try to abduct, adduct, or flex the muscles in question. What is his neurovascular status, including motion sensation and circulation? Discrepancies in muscle circumference or leg length should be measured and recorded.

Diagnostic tools

• *X-ray* is probably the most useful diagnostic tool for evaluating musculoskeletal diseases.

• *Myelography* is an invasive procedure that is especially helpful for evaluating abnormalities of the spinal canal and cord. Myelography entails injection of a radiopaque contrast medium into the subarachnoid space of the spine. Then, serial X-rays visualize progress of the contrast medium through the subarachnoid space. Displacement of the medium indicates a space-occupying lesion, such as a herniated disc or a tumor.

• *Arthrography* similarly is an injection of opaque contrast material to give in-

formation regarding shape, outline, and integrity of a joint capsule.

• *Bone scan* identifies areas of increased bone activity or active bone formation by injection of radioisotopes.

Other useful tests include bone and muscle biopsies, microscopic examination of synovial fluid, and multiple laboratory studies of urine and blood to identify systemic abnormalities.

Health care

Each patient with musculoskeletal disease needs an individual health care plan formulated early in his hospital stay. This will be developed by the doctor, nurse, physical therapist, and occupational therapist. The plan will have short- and long-term goals, during and after hospitalization.

Caring for the patient with a musculoskeletal disease usually includes managing at least one of the following: traction, casts, braces, splints, crutches, and prolonged immobilization. All require special care.

Traction is the application of a steady pulling force, by manual or mechanical means, to reduce a fracture, minimize muscle spasms, or immobilize or align a joint.

• *Skin traction* is the indirect application of traction to the skeletal system through skin and soft tissues.

• *Skeletal traction* is the direct application of traction to bones by transversing the affected bone with a pin (Steinmann's pin) or wire (Kirschner wire), or by gripping the bone with calipers or a tonglike device (Crutchfield tongs).

• *Manual traction,* for emergency use, is the direct application of traction to a body part by hand.

During the use of all types of traction, the hospital staff member should:

• explain to the patient how traction works, and advise how much activity and elevation of the head of the bed are permissible; inform him of the anticipated duration of traction and whether or not the traction is removable; teach active range-of-motion exercises.

• check neurovascular status to prevent nerve damage; make sure the mattress is firm, that the traction ropes aren't frayed, that they're on the center track of the pulley, and that traction weights are hanging free; thoroughly investigate any patient complaint.

• check for signs of infection (odor, local inflammation and drainage, fever) at pin sites if the patient is in skeletal traction; check with the doctor regarding pin site care, such as use of peroxide or povidone-iodine.

Ideally, a cast immobilizes without adding too much weight. It's snug-fitting but doesn't constrict, and has a smooth inner surface and smooth edges to prevent pressure or skin irritation. Casts require comprehensive patient teaching.

• A wet cast takes 24 to 48 hours to dry. To prevent indentations, the patient should not: squeeze the cast with his fingers; cover or walk on the cast until it has dried; bump a damp cast on hard surfaces, since dents can cause pressure areas. The patient must know that while the cast is drying he'll feel a transient sensation of heat under the cast.

• The patient must keep the cast above heart level for *24 hours* following its application, to reduce swelling in the extremity.

• While the cast is drying and after drying is complete, the patient should watch for and immediately report persistent pain in the extremity inside or distal to the cast, as well as edema, changes in skin color, coldness, or tingling or numbness in this area. If any of these signs occur, the patient should position the casted body part above heart level and notify his doctor.

• The patient should also report drainage through the cast, or an odor that may indicate infection. He should not insert foreign objects under the cast, get it wet, pull out its padding, or scratch inside it. A broken cast requires immediate attention.

• The patient must exercise the joints above and below the cast to prevent stiffness and contracture.

Braces, splints, and slings also provide alignment, immobilization, and pain relief for musculoskeletal diseases. Slings and splints are usually used for short-term immobilization. The patient and his family must understand why these appliances are necessary, and be shown how to properly apply the sling, splint, or brace for optimal benefit. Other necessary information which they will need is how long the appliance will have to be worn, and any activity limitations that must be observed. If the patient has a brace, his orthotist can instruct him in proper care. The patient should refer additional questions to his doctor. If necessary, he should be taught proper crutch-walking.

Coping with immobility

Immobilized patients require meticulous care to prevent complications. Without constant care, the bedridden patient becomes susceptible to decubitus ulcers, caused by the increased pressure on tissue over bony prominences, and is especially vulnerable to cardiopulmonary complications.

• Decubitus ulcers can be prevented by turning the patient regularly, massaging areas over bony prominences, and placing a flotation pad, a sheepskin pad, or an alternating–air-current, egg crate, or foam mattress under bony prominences. If needed, the patient should be instructed in the use of a Balkan frame with a trapeze to enable him to move about in bed.

• Increased fluid intake will minimize the risk of renal calculi.

• Passive range-of-motion exercises should be performed on the affected side, as ordered, to prevent contractures, and the patient instructed in active range-of-motion exercises on the unaffected side. Footboards or high-topped sneakers will help prevent footdrop.

• Since most bedridden patients involuntarily perform a Valsalva maneuver when using the upper arms and trunk to move, the patient must exhale (instead of holding his breath) as he turns. This will prevent possible cardiac complica-

tions that result from increased intrathoracic pressure.
• Coughing and deep breathing are important. A spirometer may be ordered to act as an incentive when the patient performs these exercises.
• A bowel program (fluids, roughage, laxatives, stool softeners) should be established, as needed, to prevent constipation.

Rehabilitation
Restoring the patient to his former state of health is not always possible. When it is not, the patient will have to adjust to a modified life-style. Allowing the patient time to finish difficult tasks by himself will promote independence. If necessary, he should be referred to an appropriate community facility for continued rehabilitation.

CONGENITAL DISORDERS

Clubfoot
(Talipes)

Clubfoot, the most common congenital disorder of the lower extremities, is marked primarily by a deformed talus and shortened Achilles tendon, which give the foot a characteristic clublike appearance. In talipes equinovarus, the foot points downward (equinus) and turns inward (varus), while the front of the foot curls toward the heel (forefoot adduction).

Clubfoot, which has an incidence of approximately 1 per 1,000 live births, usually occurs bilaterally and is twice as common in boys as in girls. It may be associated with other birth defects, such as myelomeningocele, spina bifida, and arthrogryposis. Clubfoot is correctable with prompt treatment.

Causes
A combination of genetic and environmental factors in utero appears to cause clubfoot. Heredity is a definite factor in some cases, although the mechanism of transmission is undetermined. If a child is born with clubfoot, his sibling has a 1 in 35 chance of being born with the same anomaly. Children of a parent with clubfoot have 1 chance in 10. In children without a family history of clubfoot, this anomaly seems linked to arrested development during the ninth and tenth weeks of embryonic life, when the feet are formed. Researchers also suspect muscle abnormalities, leading to variations in length and tendon insertions, as possible causes of clubfoot.

Signs and symptoms
Talipes equinovarus varies greatly in severity. Deformity may be so extreme that the toes touch the inside of the ankle, or it may be only vaguely apparent. In every case, the talus is deformed, the Achilles tendon shortened, and the calcaneus somewhat shortened and flattened. Depending on the degree of the varus deformity, the calf muscles are shortened and underdeveloped, with soft-tissue contractures at the site of the deformity. The foot is tight in its deformed position and resists manual efforts to push it back into normal position. Clubfoot is painless, except in elderly, arthritic patients. In older children, clubfoot may be associated with paralysis, poliomyelitis, and cerebral palsy, in which case treatment is different than for clubfoot alone.

Diagnosis
Early diagnosis of clubfoot is extremely important. This is usually no problem, because the deformity is obvious. In sub-

tle deformity, however, true clubfoot must be distinguished from apparent clubfoot (metatarsus varus or "pigeontoe"). Apparent clubfoot results when a fetus maintains a position in utero that gives his feet a clubfoot appearance at birth. Unlike true clubfoot, apparent clubfoot can usually be corrected manually. Another form of apparent clubfoot is inversion of the feet, resulting from the peroneal type of progressive muscular atrophy and progressive muscular dystrophy. In the child with true clubfoot, X-rays show the talus and the calcaneus superimposed.

Treatment

Treatment for clubfoot is administered in three stages: correcting the deformity, maintaining the correction until the foot regains normal muscle balance, and observing the foot closely for several years to prevent the deformity from recurring. In newborns, corrective treatment for true clubfoot should begin at once; this point can't be overemphasized. An infant's foot contains large amounts of cartilage; the muscles, ligaments, and tendons are supple. The ideal time to begin treatment is during the first few days and weeks of life—when the foot is most malleable.

Clubfoot deformities are usually corrected in sequential order: forefoot adduction first, then varus (or inversion), then equinus (or plantar flexion). Trying to correct all three deformities at once only results in a misshapen, rocker-bottomed foot. Forefoot adduction is corrected by uncurling the front of the foot away from the heel (forefoot abduction); the varus deformity, by turning the foot so the sole faces outward (eversion); and finally, equinus is corrected by casting the foot with the toes pointing up (dorsiflexion). This last correction may have to be supplemented with a subcutaneous tenotomy of the Achilles tendon and posterior capsulotomy of the ankle joint.

Several therapeutic methods have been tested and found effective in correcting clubfoot. The first is simple manipulation and casting, whereby the foot is gently manipulated into a partially corrected position, then held there in a cast for several days or weeks. (The skin should be painted with a nonirritating adhesive liquid beforehand to prevent the cast from slipping.) After the cast is removed, the foot is manipulated into an even better position and casted again. This procedure is repeated as many times as necessary. In some cases, the shape of the cast can be transformed through a series of wedging maneuvers (Kite method), instead of changing the cast each time.

After correction of clubfoot, proper foot alignment should be maintained through exercise, night splints, and orthopedic shoes. With manipulating and casting, correction usually takes about 3 months. The Denis Browne splint, a device that consists of two padded, metal footplates connected by a flat, horizontal bar, is sometimes used as a follow-up measure. This splint helps promote bilateral correction and strengthen the foot muscles.

Resistant clubfoot may require surgery. Older children, for example, with recurrent or neglected clubfoot usually need surgery. Tenotomy, tendon transfer, stripping of the plantar fascia, and capsulotomy are some of the surgical procedures that may be used. In severe cases, bone surgery (wedge resections, osteotomy, or astragalectomy) may be appropriate. After surgery, a cast preserves the correction. Whenever clubfoot is severe enough to require surgery, it's rarely totally correctable; however, surgery can usually ameliorate the deformity.

Additional considerations

The hospital staff member's primary concern is to recognize clubfoot as early as possible, preferably in newborn infants. He should:
• look for any exaggerated attitudes in an infant's feet; know the difference between true clubfoot and apparent clubfoot; avoid using excessive force in trying to manipulate a clubfoot—the foot with apparent clubfoot moves easily.
• stress the importance of prompt treat-

ment to parents; make sure they understand that clubfoot, perhaps more than any other bone or joint disorder, demands immediate therapy and orthopedic supervision until growth is completed.

• elevate the child's feet with pillows after casting; check the toes every 1 to 2 hours for temperature, color, sensation, motion, and capillary refill (blanch test); watch for signs of edema; teach parents how to recognize circulatory impairment before a child in a clubfoot cast is discharged.

• insert plastic petals over the top edges of a new cast while it's still wet, to keep urine from soaking and softening the cast; petal the edges with adhesive tape, when the cast is dry, to keep out plaster crumbs and prevent skin irritation; perform good skin care under the cast edges every 4 hours; rub the skin with alcohol after washing and drying (oils or powders shouldn't be used—they tend to macerate the skin).

• warn parents of an older child not to let the foot part of the cast get soft and thin from wear—if it does, much of the correction may be lost.

• when the Kite method is being used, check circulation frequently because of increased pressure on tissues and blood vessels (the equinus correction especially places considerable strain on ligaments, blood vessels, and tendons).

• elevate the child's feet with pillows after surgery to decrease swelling and pain; report any signs of discomfort or pain immediately; try to locate the source of pain—it may result from cast pressure, not the incision; circle the location of any bleeding that occurs and mark the time on the cast; report any spread in bleeding.

• make sure the older child and his parents don't expect too much from surgery; explain that surgery in older children can improve clubfoot but can't cure it.

• emphasize the need for long-term orthopedic care to maintain correction; teach parents the prescribed exercises that the child can do at home; urge them to make the child wear the corrective shoes ordered, and splints during naps and at night; make sure they understand that clubfoot isn't a condition that is corrected immediately, that correcting this defect permanently takes time and patience.

Congenital Hip Dysplasia

Congenital dysplasia, an abnormality of the hip joint present from birth, is the most common disorder that affects the hip joints of children under age 3. It can be unilateral or bilateral. This abnormality occurs in three forms of varying severity: unstable hip dysplasia, *in which the hip is positioned normally but can be dislocated by manipulation;* subluxation or incomplete dislocation, *in which the femoral head rides on the edge of the acetabulum; and* complete dislocation, *in which the femoral head is totally outside the acetabulum.*

Congenital hip subluxation or dislocation can cause abnormal acetabular development and permanent disability. About 85% of affected infants are females.

Causes
Two theories exist concerning the cause of congenital hip dysplasia, although neither has been proven.

• Hormones that relax maternal ligaments in preparation for labor may also cause laxity of infant ligaments around the capsule of the hip joint.

• Dislocation is 10 times more common after breech delivery (malpositioning in utero) than after cephalic delivery.

Signs and symptoms
Clinical effects of hip dysplasia vary with age. In newborns, dysplasia produces no gross deformity or pain. However, in

complete dysplasia, the hip rides above the acetabulum, causing the leg on the affected side to appear shorter, or the affected hip to appear more prominent. As the child grows older and begins to walk, uncorrected bilateral dysplasia may cause him to sway from side to side, a condition known as "duck waddle"; unilateral dysplasia may produce a limp. If corrective treatment doesn't begin until after age 2, congenital hip dysplasia may cause degenerative hip changes, lordosis, joint malformation, and soft-tissue damage.

Diagnosis

Several observations during physical examination strongly suggest congenital hip dysplasia. First, the child is placed on his back, and the folds of skin over his thighs inspected. Usually, a child in this position has an equal number of thigh folds on each side, but a child with subluxation or dislocation may have an extra fold on the affected side (this extra fold is also apparent when the child lies prone). Next, with the child lying prone, the alignment of the buttock fold is checked. In a child with dysplasia, the buttock fold on the affected side is higher. In addition, abduction of the affected hip is restricted.

 A positive Ortolani or Trendelenburg's sign confirms congenital hip dysplasia. To test for the Ortolani sign, the infant is placed on his back, with his hip flexed and in abduction. The hip is then adducted while the femur is pressed downward. This will dislocate the hip. Then, the hip is abducted while the femur is moved upward. A click or a jerk (produced by the femoral head moving over the acetabular rim) indicates subluxation in an infant younger than 1 month; this sign indicates subluxation or complete dislocation in an older infant.

To elicit Trendelenburg's sign, the child rests his weight on the side of the dislocation and lifts his other knee. His pelvis drops on the normal side because of weak abductor muscles in the affected hip. However, when the child stands with his weight on the normal side and lifts the other knee, the pelvis remains horizontal; these phenomena make up a positive Trendelenburg's sign.

X-rays show the location of the femur head and a shallow acetabulum; X-rays can also monitor the progress of the disease or treatment.

Treatment

The earlier the infant receives treatment, the better his chances are for normal development. Treatment varies with the patient's age. In infants younger than 3 months, treatment includes *gentle* manipulation to reduce the dislocation, followed by holding the hips in a flexed and abducted position with a splint-brace, to maintain the reduction. The infant must wear this apparatus continuously for 2 to 3 months and then use a night splint for another month, so the joint capsule can tighten and stabilize in correct alignment.

If treatment doesn't begin until the infant is between ages 3 months and 2 years, then bilateral skin traction (in infants) or skeletal traction (in older children who have started walking) will be needed. Such traction attempts to reduce the dislocation by gradually abducting the hips. If traction fails, gentle closed reduction under general anesthesia can further abduct the hips; the child is then placed in a spica cast for 4 to 6 months. If closed treatment fails, open reduction,

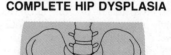

COMPLETE HIP DYSPLASIA

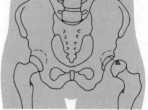

In complete dislocation, the femoral head (right) is totally displaced outside the acetabulum.

followed by immobilization in a spica cast for an average of 6 months, or osteotomy may be considered. In the child aged 2 to 5 years, treatment is difficult, and includes skeletal traction and subcutaneous adductor tenotomy; in the child older than age 5, restoration of satisfactory hip function is rare.

Additional considerations
The child who must wear a splint, brace, or body cast needs special personal care, requiring parent teaching.
• Parents must be taught how to correctly splint or brace the hips, as ordered. Frequent checkups are mandatory.
• Parents will be anxious and fearful. Explaining possible causes of congenital hip dislocation, and giving reassurance that prompt treatment will probably result in complete correction, will help calm them.
• During the child's first few days in a cast or splint-brace, parents should stay with the child as much as possible to calm and reassure him, since restricted movement will make him irritable. They should be assured that the child will adjust to this restriction and return to normal sleeping, eating, and playing behavior in a few days.
• Parents will have to remove braces and splints while bathing the infant, and replace them immediately afterward. Good hygiene is very important. Parents should bathe and change the child frequently and wash his perineum with warm water and soap at each diaper change.
If treatment requires a spica cast:
• When transferring the child immediately after casting, palms should be used to avoid making dents in the cast. Such dents predispose the patient to pressure sores. The cast will need 24 to 48 hours to dry naturally. Heat shouldn't be used to make it dry faster, since heat also makes it more fragile.
• Immediately after the cast is applied, a plastic sheet must be used to protect it from moisture around the perineum and buttocks. This is done by cutting the sheet in strips long enough to cover the outside of the cast, and tucking them about a fin-

ger length beneath the cast edges. Then, using overlapping strips of tape, the corner of each petal is tacked to the outside of the cast. The plastic under the cast must be removed every 4 hours, then washed, dried, and retucked. Disposable diapers folded lengthwise over the perineum may also be used.
• The child should be positioned either on a Bradford frame elevated on blocks, with a bedpan under the frame, or on pillows to support the child's legs. The cast must be kept dry, and diapers changed often.
• The skin under the cast edges should be washed and dried every 2 to 4 hours, then rubbed with alcohol. Oils or powders shouldn't be used.
• The child will need to be turned every 2 hours during the day, and every 4 hours at night, at which time color, sensation, and motion of the infant's legs and feet, and toes should be checked.
• A flashlight is used to check for objects and crumbs under the cast every 4 hours. Daily checks are done for odors, to detect infection.
• If the child complains of itching, he may benefit from diphenhydramine. Persistent itching requires investigation.
• Renal calculi and constipation, both complications of inactivity, can be avoided through adequate nutrition and fluid intake.
• If the child is very restless, a jacket restraint will keep him from falling out of bed or off the frame.
• The child will need adequate stimuli to promote growth and development. If the child's hips are abducted in a frog-legs position, he may be able to fit on a kiddy car. So that he may play at a table, parents may seat him on top of pillows on a chair. Parents should be encouraged to put him on the floor for short periods of play and to let him play with other children his age.
• Parents must watch for signs of outgrowing the cast (cyanosis, cool extremities, pain).
• The parents need to know that effective treatment is apt to be prolonged and requires patience.

Legg-Calvé-Perthes Disease
(Coxa plana)

A self-limiting disease, Legg-Calvé-Perthes disease is ischemic necrosis leading to eventual flattening of the head of the femur due to vascular interruption. This usually unilateral condition occurs most frequently in boys aged 4 to 10 and tends to occur in families.

Although this disease usually runs its course in 3 to 4 years, it may lead to joint problems later in life from misalignment of the acetabulum and the flattened femoral head.

Causes
The vascular changes that initiate Legg-Calvé-Perthes disease may result from injury or disease. The disease occurs in four stages:
• spontaneous vascular interruption causes necrosis of the femoral head: 1 to 3 weeks
• new blood supply causes bone resorption and deposition of new bone cells; deformity may result from pressure on weakened area: 6 months to 1 year
• new bone replaces necrotic bone: 2 to 3 years
• completion of healing or regeneration fixes shape of the joint: residual stage.

Signs and symptoms
The first indication of Legg-Calvé-Perthes disease is a persistent limp that becomes progressively severe. This symptom appears during the second stage, when bone resorption and deformity begin. Other clinical effects may include mild pain (in the hip or knee) that is aggravated by activity and relieved by rest, muscle spasm, atrophy of muscles in the upper thigh, slight shortening of the leg, and severely restricted abduction and rotation of the hip.

Diagnosis
A thorough physical examination and clinical history suggest Legg-Calvé-Perthes disease. Hip X-rays taken every 3 to 4 months confirm the diagnosis, with findings that vary according to the stage of the disease. Diagnostic evaluation must also differentiate between Legg-Calvé-Perthes disease (restriction of only the abduction and rotation of the hip) and infection or arthritis (restriction of all motion). Aspiration and culture of synovial fluid rule out joint sepsis.

Treatment
The aim of treatment is to protect the femoral head from further stress and damage by containing it within the acetabulum. Therapy may include reduced weight-bearing through bed rest in bilateral split counterpoised traction to reduce muscle spasm, then application of hip abduction cast, or weight-bearing while a cast or brace holds the leg in abduction. Analgesics help relieve pain.

For a young child in the early stages of the disease, osteotomy and subtrochanteric derotation provide maximum confinement of the epiphysis within the acetabulum to allow return of the femoral head to normal shape and full range of motion. Proper placement of the epiphysis thus allows remolding with ambulation. Postoperatively, the patient requires a spica cast for about 2 months.

Additional considerations
When caring for a child with Legg-Calvé-Perthes disease the hospital staff member should:
• monitor fluid intake and output; maintain sufficient fluid balance; provide a diet sufficient for growth but one that doesn't cause excessive weight gain, which might necessitate cast change with ultimate loss of the corrective position.

• provide good cast care; always turn a child in a wet cast with the palms, since depressions in the plaster may lead to pressure sores; turn the child every 2 to 3 hours to expose the cast to air; "petal" the cast, after it dries, with pieces of adhesive tape or moleskin, changing them as they become soiled; protect the cast with a plastic covering during each bowel movement.

• watch for complications; check toes for color, temperature, swelling, sensation, and motion; report dusky, cool, numb toes immediately; check the skin under the cast with a flashlight every 4 hours while the patient is awake; follow a consistent plan of washing, drying (alcohol may be used), and rubbing the skin under cast edges to improve circulation and prevent skin breakdown; *never* use oils or powders under the cast, since they increase skin breakdown and soften the cast; check under the cast daily for odors, particularly after surgery, to detect skin breakdown or wound problems; report any persistent complaints of soreness.

• administer analgesics, as ordered.

• relieve itching by using a hair dryer (set on cool) at the cast edges—this also decreases dampness from perspiration; get an order for an antipruritic if itching becomes excessive; *never* insert an object under the cast to scratch.

• provide emotional support; explain all procedures and the need for bed rest, cast, or braces to the child; encourage him to verbalize his fears and anxiety.

• encourage parents to participate in their child's care; teach them proper cast care and how to recognize signs of skin breakdown (reddened or blanched areas); offer practical tips for making home management of the bedridden child easier; tell them what special supplies are needed: pajamas (and later, trousers) a size larger (the side seam should be opened, and Velcro fasteners attached to close it), bedpan, adhesive tape, moleskin, and possibly a hospital bed.

• after removal of the cast, debride dry, scaly skin *gradually* by applying lotion after bathing.

• stress the need for follow-up care to monitor rehabilitation.

Muscular Dystrophy

Muscular dystrophy is actually a group of congenital disorders characterized by progressive symmetric wasting of skeletal muscles without neural or sensory defects. Paradoxically, these wasted muscles tend to enlarge because of connective tissue and fat deposits, giving an erroneous impression of muscle strength. Four main types of muscular dystrophy occur: pseudohypertrophic (Duchenne's) *muscular dystrophy, which accounts for 50% of all cases;* facioscapulohumeral (Landouzy-Déjerine) *dystrophy;* limb-girdle (juvenile, Erb's) *dystrophy; and a* mixed *type.*

Prognosis varies. Duchenne's muscular dystrophy generally strikes during early childhood and results in death within 10 to 15 years of onset. Facioscapulohumeral and limb-girdle dystrophies usually don't shorten life expectancy. The mixed type progresses rapidly and is usually fatal within 5 years after onset.

Causes and incidence

Duchenne's muscular dystrophy is an X-linked recessive disorder, affecting males exclusively; incidence is approximately 4 per 100,000. Facioscapulohumeral dystrophy is an autosomal dominant disorder that is transmitted to both sexes. Limb-girdle muscular dys-

trophy may be inherited in several ways, but is usually an autosomal recessive disorder that affects both sexes. The mixed type doesn't appear to be inherited and strikes both sexes.

Exactly how these inherited and acquired defects cause progressive muscle weakness isn't clear. They may cause an abnormality in muscle fiber intracellular metabolism, possibly related to an enzyme deficiency or dysfunction, or to an inability to synthesize, absorb, or metabolize some unknown substance vital to muscle function. Vitamin E deficiency has been suggested as a possible cause, but this hypothesis has not been confirmed.

Signs and symptoms

Although the four types of muscular dystrophy all cause progressive muscular deterioration, degree of severity and age at onset vary.

Duchenne's muscular dystrophy begins insidiously, between ages 3 and 5. Initially, it affects leg and pelvic muscles, but eventually spreads to the involuntary muscles. Muscle weakness produces a waddling gait, toe-walking, and lordosis. Children with this disorder have difficulty climbing stairs, fall down often, can't run properly, and their scapulae flare out (or "wing") when they raise their arms. Calf muscles especially become enlarged and firm. Muscle deterioration progresses rapidly, and contractures develop. Usually, these children are confined to wheelchairs by ages 9 to 12. Late in the disease, progressive weakening of cardiac muscle causes tachycardia, EKG abnormalities, and pulmonary complications. Death commonly results from sudden heart failure, respiratory failure, or infection.

Facioscapulohumeral dystrophy is a slowly progressive and relatively benign form of muscular dystrophy that usually occurs before age 10, but may develop during adolescence. Initially, it weakens the muscles of the face, shoulders, and upper arms but eventually spreads to all voluntary muscles, producing a pendulous lower lip and absence of the nasolabial fold. Early symptoms include inability to pucker the mouth or whistle, abnormal facial movements, and absence of facial movements when laughing or crying. Other signs consist of diffuse facial flattening that leads to a masklike expression, winging of the scapulae, inability to raise the arms above the head, and in infants, inability to suckle.

Limb-girdle dystrophy follows a similarly slow course and often causes only slight disability. Usually, it begins between ages 6 and 10; less often, in early adulthood. Muscle weakness first appears in the upper arm and pelvic muscles. Other symptoms include winging of the scapulae, lordosis with abdominal protrusion, waddling gait, poor balance, and inability to raise the arms.

Mixed dystrophy generally begins between ages 30 and 50, affects all voluntary muscles, and causes rapidly progressive deterioration.

Diagnosis

Characteristic abnormalities of gait and other voluntary movements, with a typical medical and family history, suggest this diagnosis.

 A muscle biopsy showing fat and connective tissue deposits confirms it. Electromyography often shows short, weak bursts of electrical activity in affected muscles, but this isn't conclusive. However, with a positive muscle biopsy, electromyography can help rule out neurogenic muscle atrophy by showing intact muscle innervation.

Other relevant laboratory results in Duchenne's muscular dystrophy include increased urinary creatinine excretion and elevated serum levels of creatinine phosphokinase (CPK), lactic dehydrogenase (LDH), and transaminase. Usually, CPK level rises before muscle weakness becomes severe and is a good early indicator of Duchenne's muscular dystrophy. These diagnostic tests are also useful for genetic screening, since unaffected carriers of Duchenne's muscular dystrophy also show elevated CPK and other enzyme levels.

Treatment

No treatment can stop the progressive muscle impairment of muscular dystrophy, but orthopedic appliances, exercise, physical therapy, and surgery to correct contractures can help preserve mobility and independence. Family members who are carriers of muscular dystrophy should receive genetic counseling regarding the risk of transmitting this disease. Amniocentesis can't detect muscular dystrophy, but it can reveal the fetus' sex, so it's often recommended for known carriers of Duchenne's muscular dystrophy who are pregnant.

Additional considerations
Comprehensive long-term care, follow-up patient and family teaching, and psychological support can help the patient and family deal with this disorder.
• When respiratory involvement occurs in Duchenne's muscular dystrophy, coughing, deep breathing exercises, and diaphragmatic breathing will help slow deterioration. Parents should be taught to recognize early signs of respiratory complications.
• Active and passive range-of-motion exercises will help preserve joint mobility and prevent muscle atrophy. The patient must avoid long periods of bed rest and inactivity; if necessary, TV viewing and other sedentary activities should be limited. The patient will need special physical therapy. Splints, braces, surgery to correct contractures, grab bars, overhead slings, and a wheelchair can help preserve mobility. A footboard or high-topped sneakers and a foot cradle in-crease comfort and prevent footdrop.
• Because inactivity may cause constipation, adequate fluid intake, increased dietary bulk, and possibly a stool softener are needed to prevent this. Since such a patient is prone to obesity because of reduced physical activity, he and his family will need help planning a low-calorie, high-protein, high-fiber diet.
• The patient will need time to perform even simple physical tasks, since he's apt to be slow and awkward.
• Communication between family members must be encouraged, to help them deal with the emotional strain this disorder produces. The patient will need emotional support to help him cope with continual changes in his body image.
• The child with Duchenne's muscular dystrophy should be helped to maintain peer relationships and to realize his intellectual potential. Encouraging his parents to keep him in a regular school as long as possible will help.
• If necessary, adult patients should be referred for sexual counseling. Some patients may need to learn new job skills for vocational rehabilitation. (The state Department of Labor and Industry can provide more information.) These patients and their families can obtain information on social services and financial assistance from the Muscular Dystrophy Association, Inc.

JOINTS

Septic Arthritis
(Infectious arthritis)

A medical emergency, septic arthritis is caused by bacterial invasion of a joint, resulting in inflammation of the synovial lining. If the organisms enter the joint cavity, effusion and pyogenesis follow, with eventual destruction of bone and cartilage. Septic arthritis can lead to ankylosis and even fatal septicemia. However, prompt antibiotic therapy cures most patients.

Causes
In most cases of septic arthritis, bacteria spread from a primary site of infection, usually in adjacent bone or soft tissue, through the bloodstream to the joint. Common infecting organisms include

four strains of gram-positive cocci: *Staphylococcus aureus, Streptococcus pyogenes, Streptococcus pneumoniae,* and *Streptococcus viridans;* two strains of gram-negative cocci: *Neisseria gonorrhoeae* and *Hemophilus influenzae;* and various gram-negative bacilli: *Escherichia coli, Salmonella, Pseudomonas,* and so forth. Anaerobic organisms such as gram-positive cocci usually infect adults, and children over age 2. *H. influenzae* most often infects children under age 2; *N. gonorrhoeae* is especially prevalent among sexually active adults.

Various factors can predispose to septic arthritis. Any concurrent bacterial infection (of the genitourinary or the upper respiratory tract, for example) or serious chronic illness (malignancy, renal failure, diabetes, or cirrhosis) heightens susceptibility. Consequently, alcoholics and the elderly run a higher risk of developing septic arthritis. Of course, susceptibility increases with diseases that depress the autoimmune system or with prior immunosuppressive therapy. Prolonged use of I.V. drugs (by heroin addicts, for example) can also cause septic arthritis. Other predisposing factors include recent articular trauma, joint surgery, and intra-articular injections.

Signs and symptoms

Acute septic arthritis begins abruptly, causing intense pain, inflammation, and swelling of the affected joint, with accompanying fever and chills. It usually affects a single joint. It most often develops in the large joints but can strike any joint, including the spine and small peripheral joints. Overt signs of inflammation may not appear in some patients. Migratory polyarthritis sometimes precedes localization of the infection. Muscle spasms are common. If the bacteria invade the hip, pain usually occurs in the groin, upper thigh, or buttock, or may be referred to the knee.

Diagnosis

Identifying the causative organism in a Gram's stain or culture of synovial fluid suggests septic arthritis. Joint fluid analysis shows gross pus or watery, cloudy fluid of decreased viscosity with 50,000/mm³ or more white cells, containing many neutrophils. When synovial fluid culture is negative, positive blood culture may confirm the diagnosis. Synovial fluid glucose is often low as compared to a simultaneous 6-hour postprandial blood sugar.

Other diagnostic measures:

• *X-rays* can show characteristic changes as early as 1 to 2 weeks after the initial infection—distention of joint capsules, for example, followed by narrowing of joint space (indicating cartilage damage) and erosions of the bone.

• *Radioisotope joint scan* for less accessible joints (such as spinal articulations) may help detect infection or inflammation but isn't itself diagnostic.

• *WBC* may be elevated, with many polymorphonuclear cells; ESR increased.

 • *Culture and Gram's stain smears* of skin exudates, sputum, urethral discharge, or stools. Two sets of positive cultures confirm septic arthritis.

Treatment

Antibiotic therapy should begin as soon as culture specimens have been taken; this treatment may be modified later, when sensitivity results become available. Penicillin G is effective against infections caused by *S. aureus, S. pyogenes, S. pneumoniae, S. viridans,* and *N. gonorrhoeae.* Methicillin is recommended for penicillin G—resistant strains of *S. aureus;* ampicillin, for *H. influenzae;* gentamicin or tobramycin, for gram-negative bacilli. Definitive medication selection requires drug sensitivity studies of the infecting organism. If doubt exists as to the effectiveness of antibiotic therapy, bioassays or bactericidal assays of synovial fluid may confirm clearing of the infection.

Treatment of septic arthritis requires close monitoring of progress through frequent analysis of joint fluid cultures, synovial fluid leukocyte counts, and glucose determinations. Plain codeine or propoxyphene can be given for pain, if needed. Aspirin causes a misleading reduction in swelling and interferes with accurate monitoring of the patient's progress. The affected joint can be immobilized with a splint or put into traction until motion and exercise can be tolerated.

Needle aspiration (arthrocentesis) to remove grossly purulent joint fluid may be used as an adjunct and repeated daily until fluid appears normal. If fluid accumulates rapidly, the procedure can be performed more frequently. Open surgical drainage (usually arthrotomy with lavage of the joint) may be necessary for resistant infection or chronic septic arthritis. A biopsy of the synovial membrane may be done for culture and histologic examination.

Late reconstructive surgery is warranted only for severe joint damage and only after all signs of active infection have disappeared, which usually takes several months. In some cases, the recommended procedure may be arthroplasty or joint fusion. Prosthetic replacement remains controversial, since it may exacerbate the infection, but has helped patients with damaged femoral heads or acetabula.

Additional considerations

Management of septic arthritis demands meticulous supportive care, close observation, and control of infection.

• All procedures must be done using strict aseptic technique. This includes washing hands carefully before and after giving care, and disposing of soiled linens and dressings properly. Contact between immunosuppressed patients and infected patients must be prevented.

• Signs of joint inflammation include: heat, redness, swelling, pain, or drainage. Vital signs and fever pattern require monitoring. Note that corticosteroids mask signs of infection.

• Splints or traction must be checked regularly. The joint requires continuous proper alignment, but prolonged immobilization must be avoided. The patient should begin passive range-of-motion exercises immediately, and progress to active exercises as soon as he can move the affected joint and put weight on it.

• Pain levels must be monitored and the patient medicated accordingly, especially before exercise, remembering that the pain of septic arthritis shouldn't be underestimated. Analgesics and narcotics may be used for acute pain, and heat or ice packs for moderate pain.

• The patient's condition must be carefully evaluated after joint aspiration or intra-articular injection. The patient will need emotional support throughout the diagnostic tests and procedures, including a warning before the first injection that it will be *extremely* painful.

• The patient should learn about all prescribed medications—what they are for and why they must be taken on schedule.

• Septic arthritis can be prevented through good aseptic technique (especially in immunosuppressed patients) and health education, primarily regarding complications of gonorrhea.

Gout
(Gouty arthritis)

Gout is a metabolic disease marked by urate deposits, which cause painfully arthritic joints. It can strike any joint but favors those in the feet and legs. Primary gout usually occurs in men older than age 30 and in postmenopausal women; secondary gout occurs in the elderly. Gout follows an intermittent course and often leaves patients totally free of symptoms for years between attacks. Gout can lead to chronic disability or incapacitation, and rarely, severe hypertension and progressive renal disease. Prognosis is good with treatment.

Causes

The word gout comes from the Latin *gutta,* meaning "drop." The ancients believed this condition was caused by a poison "dropping" into weakened joints. Although the exact cause of primary gout remains unknown, it seems linked to a genetic defect in purine metabolism, which causes overproduction of uric acid (hyperuricemia), retention of uric acid, or both. In secondary gout, which develops during the course of another disease (such as polycythemia vera, granulocytic leukemia, or multiple myeloma), hyperuricemia results from the breakdown of nucleic acid. Secondary gout can also follow drug therapy, especially after hydrochlorothiazide or pyrazinamide, which interferes with urate excretion. Increased concentration of uric acid leads to urate deposits, called *tophi,* in joints or tissues, causing local necrosis or fibrosis.

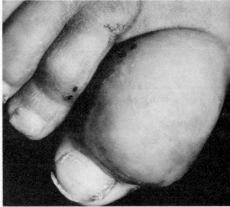

The final stage of gouty arthritis (chronic or tophaceous gout) is marked by painful polyarthritis, with large, subcutaneous, tophaceous deposits in cartilage, synovial membranes, tendons, and soft tissue. The skin over the tophus is shiny, thin, and taut.

Signs and symptoms

Gout develops in four stages: asymptomatic, acute, intercritical, and chronic. In asymptomatic gout, serum urate levels rise but produce no symptoms. As the disease progresses, it may cause hypertension or nephrolithiasis, with severe back pain. The first acute attack strikes suddenly and peaks quickly. Although it generally involves only one or a few joints, this initial attack is extremely painful. Affected joints appear hot, tender, inflamed, dusky-red, or cyanotic. The metatarsophalangeal joint of the great toe usually becomes inflamed first (podagra), then the instep, ankle, heel, knee, or wrist joints. Sometimes a low-grade fever is present. Mild acute attacks often subside quickly but tend to recur at irregular intervals. Severe attacks may persist for days or weeks.

Intercritical periods are the symptom-free intervals between gout attacks. Most patients have a second attack within 6 months to 2 years, but in some the second attack is delayed for 5 to 10 years. Delayed attacks are more common in those who are untreated, and tend to be longer and more severe than initial attacks. Such attacks are also polyarticular, invariably affecting joints in the feet and legs, and are sometimes accompanied by fever. A migratory attack sequentially strikes various joints and the Achilles tendon, and is associated with either subdeltoid or olecranon bursitis.

Eventually, chronic polyarticular gout sets in. This final, unremitting stage of the disease (chronic or tophaceous gout) is marked by persistent painful polyarthritis, with large, subcutaneous, tophaceous deposits in cartilage, synovial membranes, tendons, and soft tissue. The classic site is the helix of the ear (above the earlobe), but urate deposits also form in fingers, hands, knees, feet, ulnar sides of the forearms, Achilles tendons, and rarely, in internal organs, such as the kidneys. The skin over the tophus may ulcerate and release a chalky, white exudate or pus. Chronic inflammation and tophaceous deposits precipitate secondary joint degeneration, with eventual deformity and disability. Kidney involvement, with associated tubular damage, leads to chronic renal dysfunction. Hypertension and albuminuria occur in some patients; urolithiasis is common.

SYDENHAM'S DESCRIPTION OF GOUT

For clarity and vividness, few passages in medical literature can rival the following classic description of an acute gout attack written by Thomas Sydenham, the famous 17th-century British doctor who suffered from gout for 34 years:

"The victim goes to bed and sleeps in good health. About two o'clock in the morning he is awakened by a severe pain in the great toe; more rarely in the heel, ankle, or instep. This pain is like that of a dislocation, and yet the parts feel as if cold water were poured over them. Then follow chills and shivers, and a little fever. The pain, which was at first moderate, becomes more intense. With its intensity the chills and shivers increase. After a time this comes to its height, accommodating itself to the bones and ligaments of the tarsus and metatarsus. Now it is a violent stretching and tearing of the ligaments—now it is a gnawing pain and now a pressure and tightening. So exquisite and lively meanwhile is the feeling of the part affected, that it cannot bear the weight of bedclothes nor the jar of a person walking in the room. The night is passed in torture, sleeplessness, turning of the part affected, and perpetual change of posture; the tossing about of the body being as incessant as the pain of the tortured joint, and being worse as the fit comes on. Hence the vain effort by change of posture, both in the body and the limb affected, to obtain an abatement of the pain."*

* THE WORKS OF THOMAS SYDENHAM, translated by R.G. Latham (London: Sydenham Society 1850), Vol. II, p. 214.

Diagnosis

Urate deposits in or near the affected joints or bursae, or soft-tissue deposits in the helixes of the ears, fingertips, Achilles tendons, or elsewhere strongly suggest chronic gout. Aspiration of synovial fluid (arthrocentesis) or of tophaceous material reveals needlelike intracellular crystals of sodium urate.

Serum uric acid is above normal; urinary uric acid values are usually higher in secondary gout than in idiopathic primary gout.

X-rays show clearly defined, punched out areas of bone lysis. Similar erosions occur in other diseases (rheumatoid arthritis, degenerative joint disease, tuberculosis, sarcoidosis, syphilis, leprosy, yaws), but only gout manifests outward displacement of the overhanging margin from the bone contour. Positive test for rheumatoid factor distinguishes rheumatoid arthritis from gout.

Treatment

Correct management seeks to terminate an acute attack, correct hyperuricemia, and prevent recurrence, complications, and the formation of kidney stones. Treatment for acute gout consists of bed rest; immobilization of the inflamed, painful joints; and local application of heat or cold. Simple analgesics like aspirin or acetaminophen relieve the pain of mild attacks, but acute inflammation requires concomitant treatment with colchicine (P.O. or I.V.) every hour for 8 hours, until the pain subsides or nausea, vomiting, cramping, or diarrhea develops. Phenylbutazone or indomethacin in therapeutic doses may be used instead but is less specific. Resistant inflammation may require corticosteroids or corticotropin (I.V. drip or I.M.), or joint aspiration and an intra-articular corticosteroid injection.

Treatment for chronic gout aims to decrease serum uric acid level. Continuing maintenance dosage of allopurinol is often given to suppress uric acid formation or control uric acid levels, preventing further attacks. However, this powerful drug should be used cautiously in patients with renal failure. Colchicine prevents recurrent acute attacks until uric acid returns to its normal level but doesn't affect the acid level. Uricosuric agents—probenecid and sulfinpyrazone—promote uric acid excretion and inhibit accumulation of uric acid, but their value is limited in patients with renal impairment; they should not be given to patients with urinary stones.

Adjunctive therapy emphasizes a few dietary restrictions, primarily the avoidance of alcohol and purine-rich foods. Obese patients should try to lose weight, because obesity puts additional stress on painful joints. In some cases, surgery may be necessary to improve joint function or correct deformities. Tophi must be excised and drained if they become infected or ulcerated. They can also be excised to prevent ulceration, improve the patient's appearance, or make it easier for him to wear shoes or gloves.

Additional considerations

Health care for the patient with gout includes:

• encouraging bed rest, but using a bed cradle to keep bedcovers off extremely sensitive, inflamed joints.

• giving pain medication, as needed, especially during acute attacks; applying hot or cold packs to inflamed joints; administering anti-inflammatory medication and other drugs, as ordered; watching for side effects (see also RHEUMATOID ARTHRITIS) and, with colchicine for gastrointestinal disturbances.

• urging the patient to drink plenty of fluids (up to 2 liters a day) to prevent formation of kidney stones; recording intake and output accurately; monitoring serum uric acid levels regularly; alkalinizing urine with sodium bicarbonate or other agent, if ordered.

• watching for acute gout attacks 24 to 96 hours after surgery, since even minor surgery can precipitate an attack.

• making sure the patient understands the importance of checking serum uric acid levels periodically; telling him to avoid high-purine foods, such as anchovies, liver, sardines, kidneys, sweetbreads, lentils, and alcoholic beverages—especially beer and wine—which raise the urate level; explaining to obese patients the principles of a gradual weight reduction diet, which features foods containing moderate amounts of protein and very little fat.

• advising the patient receiving allopurinol, probenecid, and other drugs to report any side effects immediately; warning the patient taking probenecid or sulfinpyrazone to avoid aspirin or any other salicylate, since their combined effect causes urate retention.

• informing the patient that long-term colchicine therapy is essential during the first 3 to 6 months of treatment with uricosuric drugs or allopurinol.

Juvenile Rheumatoid Arthritis

Juvenile rheumatoid arthritis (JRA) is a systemic disorder of the connective tissues that encompasses several arthritis-like syndromes and accompanies extra-articular manifestations. This disease affects children under age 16 and is marked by remissions, exacerbations, and chronic synovitis. JRA can occur at a very young age—as early as 6 weeks, although rarely before 6 months—with peaks of onset between ages 1 and 3, and 8 and 12. Considered the major chronic rheumatic disorder of childhood, this disease affects as many as 250,000 children (mostly girls) in the United States.

Causes

Like adult rheumatoid arthritis (RA), the juvenile form of the disease has no known cause. Research continues to test several theories, particularly those linking JRA to infection or to an abnormal immune response. Upper respiratory infection, trauma, and emotional stress may be precipitating factors, but their relationship to JRA remains unclear.

Signs and symptoms

There are three major types of JRA: systemic (Still's disease or acute febrile type), polyarticular, and pauciarticular. In systemic JRA, arthralgia or transient arthritis during fever is the primary musculoskeletal symptom. Most patients develop polyarthritis; about 25%, chronic polyarthritis. Joint involvement may not be evident at first, but an affected child's behavior may clearly suggest joint pain. Such a child may want to constantly sit in a flexed position to minimize pain, may not walk much, or may refuse to walk at all. Young children with JRA look irritable and listless; older children may look healthy.

Fever in systemic JRA occurs suddenly and spikes to a temperature of 103° F. (39.4° C.) or higher once or twice a day, usually in the evening, then rapidly returns to normal or below normal. Shaking chills occasionally accompany fever, which can persist for weeks or even months. When fever spikes, an evanescent rheumatoid rash often appears as small, pale, or red macules on the face, trunk, and extremities, particularly on the palms and soles. Massaging or applying heat intensifies this rash, which is usually most conspicuous where the skin has been rubbed or subjected to pressure, such as that from underclothing. Lightly scratching the skin at a susceptible site will cause the macules to appear. They last for a day or two and are sometimes pruritic. Growth disturbances adjacent to inflamed joints may result in overgrowth or undergrowth of that part.

Other signs of systemic JRA include dramatic splenomegaly, hepatomegaly, or lymphadenopathy; pleuritis, pericarditis, or myocarditis; and unexplained progressive dyspnea and rising heart rate. Abdominal pain can mimic acute abdomen.

Polyarticular JRA presents in two forms, according to whether the patient is seronegative (90%) or seropositive (10%).

The seronegative subtype involves four or more joints, including small joints of the hands, which can swell suddenly or slowly; this can occur anytime during childhood and usually affects females. Symmetric polyarthritis of the small joints in the wrists, knees, ankles, elbows, and feet is common. These joints become swollen, tender, and stiff. Polyarticular JRA, which is usually mild, can also confine itself to larger joints, most often the cervical spine, hips, and shoulders. The patient usually runs a mild to low-grade fever with daily peaks. Tachycardia, listlessness, and weight loss can occur, with lymphadenopathy and hepatosplenomegaly. Other signs of polyarticular JRA include subcutaneous nodules on the elbows or heels and noticeable developmental retardation.

Seropositive polyarticular JRA, which is the more severe type and usually occurs late in childhood, can cause destructive arthritis, mimicking severe adult RA. Most patients (75%) are positive for antinuclear antibody (ANA) and do not carry HLA-B27, the specific antigen found in the blood of RA patients, suggesting an autoimmune etiology. Prognosis is poor with this subtype.

Pauciarticular JRA involves few joints (most commonly large joints and usually no more than four), and most often affects the knees. Two subtypes exist. The first strikes girls under age 6 (usually about age 4), primarily affects knees, elbows, and ankles, and is not associated with HLA-B27. About half of all patients have positive ANA but negative RF, and half of these in turn will develop chronic iridocyclitis. Such inflammation of the iris and ciliary body is often asymptomatic, but may produce pain, redness, and photophobia. The second subtype usually strikes boys over age 8, who tend to test positive for HLA-B27. This type affects large joints, especially in the legs, producing hip, heel, and foot pain, and Achilles tendinitis. These patients are likely to later develop ankylosing spondylitis. Some experience acute iritis in addition to hip girdle involvement and sacroiliitis.

Diagnosis

Characteristic joint inflammation, rash, and fever clearly point to JRA. Laboratory tests are useful mainly for monitoring disease activity.

• *Blood studies* often show leukocytosis,

particularly neutrophilia, especially in systemic JRA. Hypochromic anemia is often present; erythrocyte sedimentation rate is usually elevated.

• *ANA test* is positive, except in systemic JRA, seronegative polyarticular JRA, and pauciarticular JRA that develops in late childhood. This test may identify children with pauciarticular JRA who run a risk of developing chronic iridocyclitis, but this aspect of the test remains controversial. RF is present in serum in no more than 15% of cases.

• *Positive HLA-B27* may forecast later development of ankylosing spondylitis.

• *Protein in urine* may signify secondary amyloidosis.

• *X-rays* are generally not diagnostic in JRA. Early changes tend to be nonspecific. In later stages, however, X-rays may show erosion of cartilage and bone.

Treatment and additional considerations
Therapy and nursing care for JRA are essentially the same as for adult RA (see RHEUMATOID ARTHRITIS) and include daily administration of aspirin, with dosage based on the child's weight. However, hydroxychloroquine and indomethacin are not used. Growth disturbances may

require braces or splints; iridocyclitis, precautions against photosensitivity, such as the wearing of sunglasses. The treatment program usually includes physical therapy.

Long-range management should be tailored to individual needs. It's imperative that the child and parents be involved in all aspects of therapy. Because parents often experience guilt and anxiety when their child develops JRA, they may need professional counseling to help them overcome these feelings. Parents and health care professionals should encourage the child to develop a positive attitude toward school and social development. Regular eye examinations are necessary, especially in pauciarticular JRA. Mydriatic drops and corticosteroids are commonly used for treatment of iridocyclitis.

Generally, the prognosis for JRA is good, although disabilities can occur in acute cases. Surgery is usually limited to early synovectomy, although the long-term benefits of this procedure remain a matter of dispute. Corrective or reconstructive surgery is usually delayed until the child has matured physically and is able to undertake a vigorous rehabilitation program.

Rheumatoid Arthritis

A chronic, systemic, inflammatory disease, rheumatoid arthritis (RA) primarily attacks peripheral joints and surrounding muscles, tendons, ligaments, and blood vessels. Spontaneous remissions and unpredictable exacerbations mark the course of this potentially crippling disease. Rheumatoid arthritis usually requires lifelong treatment and, sometimes, surgery. In most patients the disease follows an intermittent course and allows normal activity, while 10% suffer total disability from severe articular deformity or associated extra-articular symptoms. Prognosis worsens with the development of nodules, vasculitis, and high titers of rheumatoid factor.

Causes and incidence
RA occurs worldwide, striking females three times more often than males. Although RA can occur at any age, most patients are women between ages 20 and 60 (peak onset period, 35 to 45). It affects

more than 6.5 million people in the United States alone.

Recent studies suggest susceptibility to RA results from genetic defects that impair the autoimmune system. Theoretically, impaired autoimmune defenses

WHEN ARTHRITIS REQUIRES SURGERY

Arthritis severe enough to necessitate total knee or total hip arthroplasty calls for comprehensive preoperative teaching and postoperative care, such as:

• explaining preoperative procedures (skin scrubs, prophylactic antibiotics); explaining surgical procedures and showing the patient the prosthesis to be used, if available.

• teaching the patient postoperative exercises (such as isometrics), and supervising his practice; also, teaching deep-breathing and coughing exercises.

• explaining that total hip or knee arthroplasty requires frequent range-of-motion exercises of the leg after surgery; also, that total knee arthroplasty requires frequent leg-lift exercises.

• showing the patient how to use a trapeze to move himself about in bed after surgery, and making sure he has a fracture bedpan handy.

• telling the patient what kind of dressings to expect after surgery. After total knee arthroplasty, he may have a cast, compression dressing, or dressing with a posterior splint. After total hip arthroplasty, he'll have an abduction pillow between his legs to help keep the hip prosthesis in place.

• closely monitoring and recording vital signs; watching for complications, such as steroid crisis and shock in patients receiving steroids; measuring distal leg pulses often, marking them with a waterproof marker to make them easier to find.

• having the patient do active dorsiflex-ion exercises; reporting any inability to do this; supervising isometrics every 2 hours; checking traction after total hip arthroplasty for pressure areas, and keeping the head of the bed raised between 30° and 45°.

• changing or reinforcing dressings, as needed, using aseptic technique; checking wounds for hematoma, excessive drainage, color changes, or foul odor—all possible signs of infection (wounds on RA patients may heal slowly); avoiding contaminating dressings while helping the patient use the urinal or bedpan.

• administering blood replacement products, antibiotics, and pain medication, as ordered; monitoring serum electrolytes, hemoglobin, and hematocrit.

• having the patient turn, cough, and deep breathe every 2 hours; then, percussing his chest.

• after total knee arthroplasty, keeping the patient's leg extended and slightly elevated.

• after total hip arthroplasty, keeping the patient's hip in abduction to prevent dislocation; watching for and immediately reporting any inability to rotate the hip or bear weight on it, increased pain, or a leg that appears shorter—all may indicate dislocation.

• helping the patient, as soon as allowed, to get out of bed and sit in a chair, keeping his weight on the unaffected side; consulting with the physical therapist, when the patient's ready to walk, for walking instruction and aids.

lead to the creation of antigen-antibody complexes, which activate a complement sequence that attracts polymorphonuclear leukocytes to the affected joint. These leukocytes ingest the complexes and release destructive enzymes.

Another theory proposes that bacteria or viruses cause RA, as it often follows infection; however, although vigorous research continues, a specific agent has not been identified. Environmental factors are also under investigation, since onset of RA often occurs in the spring, and certain environmental conditions (such as damp weather) exacerbate the symptoms. Also, since RA frequently follows stress, trauma, menopause, childbirth, or surgery, researchers are investigating endocrine, nutritional, and metabolic factors, as well as occupational and psychosocial influences.

Much more is known about the pathogenesis of RA. If unarrested, the inflammatory process within the joints occurs in four stages. First, synovitis develops from congestion and edema of the synovial membrane and joint capsule. Formation of pannus, thickened layers of granulation tissue, marks the onset of the second stage. Pannus covers and invades cartilage, and eventually destroys the joint capsule and bone. Progression to the third stage is characterized by fibrous ankylosis, fibrous invasion of the pannus and scar formation that occludes the joint space. Bone atrophy and malalignment cause visible deformities and disrupt the articulation of opposing bones, causing muscle atrophy and imbalance, and possibly, partial dislocations or subluxations. In the fourth stage, fibrous tissue calcifies, and bony ankylosis results, causing total immobility.

Signs and symptoms

RA usually develops insidiously, and initially produces nonspecific symptoms, such as fatigue, malaise, anorexia, persistent low-grade fever, weight loss, lymphadenopathy, and vague articular symptoms. Then, more specific localized articular symptoms develop, frequently in the fingers at the proximal interphalangeal (PIP), metacarpophalangeal (MCP), and metatarsophalangeal (MTP) joints. These symptoms usually occur bilaterally and symmetrically, and may extend to the wrists, knees, elbows, and ankles. The affected joints stiffen after inactivity, especially upon rising in the morning. The fingers may assume a spindle shape from marked edema and congestion in the joints. The joints become tender and painful, at first only when the patient moves them, but eventually even at rest. They often feel hot to the patient, a sure sign of active disease. Ultimately, joint function is diminished.

Deformities are inevitable if active disease progresses. PIP joints may develop flexion deformities or become hyperextended. MCP joints may swell dorsally, and volar subluxation and stretching of tendons may pull the fingers to the ulnar side ("ulnar drift"). The fingers may become fixed in a characteristic "swan's neck" appearance, or "boutonnière" de-

formity. The hands appear foreshortened, the wrists boggy; carpal tunnel syndrome from synovial pressure on the median nerve causes tingling paresthesias in the fingers.

The most common extra-articular symptom is the gradual appearance of rheumatoid nodules—subcutaneous, round or oval, nontender masses—usually on the elbows. Vasculitis can lead to skin lesions, leg ulcers, and multiple systemic complications. Peripheral neuropathy may produce numbness or tingling in the feet or weakness and loss of sensation in the fingers. Stiff, weak, or painful muscles are common. Other extra-articular effects include pericarditis, pulmonary nodules or fibrosis, pleuritis, scleritis, and episcleritis.

A less common complication is degeneration of the ondontoid process, part of the second cervical vertebra. Rarely, cord compression may occur, particularly in patients with longstanding deforming RA. Upper motor neuron signs, such as a positive Babinski sign, and weakness, may also develop. RA can also cause temporomandibular disease, which impairs chewing and causes earaches. Other potential complications include infec-

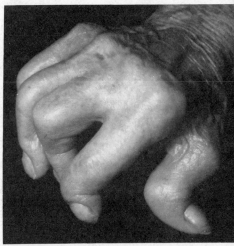

In advanced rheumatoid arthritis, marked edema and congestion cause spindle-shaped interphalangeal joints and severe flexion deformities.

DRUG THERAPY FOR ARTHRITIS

DRUG AND SIDE EFFECTS	CLINICAL CONSIDERATIONS
Aspirin • Prolonged bleeding time; GI disturbances including nausea, dyspepsia, anorexia, ulcer; and hemorrhage; hypersensitivity reactions ranging from urticaria to anaphylaxis; salicylism (mild toxicity: tinnitus, dizziness; moderate toxicity: restlessness, hyperpnea, delirium, marked lethargy; and severe toxicity: coma, convulsions, severe hyperpnea)	• Not used in GI ulcer, bleeding, hypersensitivity, or newborns. • Given with food, milk, antacid, or large glass of water to reduce GI side effects. • May cause toxicity to develop rapidly in febrile, dehydrated children. • Salicylate level monitored. • Patient taught to reduce dose, one tablet at a time, if tinnitus occurs, and to watch for signs or indications of bleeding, such as bruising, melena, and petechiae.
Fenoprofen, ibuprofen, and naproxen • Prolonged bleeding time, CNS abnormalities (headache, drowsiness, restlessness, dizziness, tremor), GI disturbances including hemorrhage and peptic ulcer, increased BUN and liver enzymes	• Not used for patients with renal disease, asthmatics with nasal polyps, or children. • Used cautiously in GI disorders, cardiac disease, or when patient is allergic to other noncorticosteroid, anti-inflammatory drugs. • Given with milk or meals to reduce GI side effects. • May have a delayed therapeutic effect 2 to 3 weeks after administration. • Kidney, liver, and auditory functions checked periodically in long-term therapy. Drug stopped if abnormalities develop.
Indomethacin • Blood dyscrasias; hemolytic, aplastic, and iron deficiency anemia; blurred vision; corneal and retinal damage; hearing loss; tinnitus; GI disturbances including GI ulcer, hematuria	• Not used for children under age 14 or for patients with aspirin allergy or GI disorders. • A single dose at bedtime may be prescribed to alleviate morning stiffness. • Always given with food or milk. • May cause severe headache within 1 hour. Drug stopped if headache persists. • Patient should report any visual changes immediately. Regular eye examinations needed during long-term therapy.
Gold • Dermatitis, pruritus, rash, stomatitis, nephrotoxicity, blood dyscrasias	• To avoid local nerve irritation, drug mixed well and given deep I.M. in buttock. • Side effects watched for and reported, especially nitritoid reaction (flushing, fainting, sweating). • Urine checked for blood and albumin before each dose. If positive, drug witheld and doctor notified. Regular follow-up examinations, including blood and urine testing, must be given. • Patient advised not to expect improvement for 3 to 6 months.
Penicillamine • Blood dyscrasias, glomerulonephropathy	• Given on empty stomach, before meals, and separately from other drugs or milk. • Urine (for protein and blood), liver function, and CBC monitored. • Patient should report fever, sore throat, chills, bruising, or bleeding.

Other drugs that may be used include tolmetin, phenylbutazone, prednisone, chloroquine, azathioprine, and cyclophosphamide.

tion, osteoporosis, amyloidosis, and Sjögren's syndrome.

Diagnosis

Typical clinical features suggest rheumatoid arthritis, but firm diagnosis relies on laboratory and other test results:
• X-rays: in early stages, show bone demineralization and soft-tissue swelling; later, loss of cartilage and narrowing of joint spaces; finally, cartilage and bone destruction, and erosion, subluxations, and deformities
• rheumatoid factor (RF) test: positive in 75% to 80% of patients, as indicated by a titer of 1:160 or higher
• antinuclear antibody (ANA) and lupus erythematosus (LE) cell tests: also positive, but in fewer patients
• synovial fluid analysis: increased volume and turbidity, but decreased viscosity and complement (C3 and C4) levels; WBC often more than 10,000/mm³
• serum protein electrophoresis: may show elevated serum globulins
• erythrocyte sedimentation rate (ESR): elevated in 85% to 90% of patients (useful to monitor response to therapy, since elevation parallels disease activity)
• CBC: usually moderate anemia and slight leukocytosis.

A C-reactive protein test can monitor response to therapy.

Treatment

Salicylates, particularly aspirin, are the mainstay of RA therapy, since they decrease inflammation and relieve joint pain. Other useful medications include nonsteroidal, anti-inflammatory agents (such as indomethacin, fenoprofen, and ibuprofen), antimalarials (chloroquine and hydroxychloroquine), gold salts, penicillamine, and corticosteroids (prednisone). Immunosuppressives, such as cyclophosphamide and azathioprine, are also therapeutic.

Supportive measures include 8 to 10 hours of sleep every night, frequent rest periods between daily activities, and splinting or traction to rest inflamed joints. Frequent range-of-motion exercises and carefully individualized therapeutic exercises forestall loss of joint function; application of heat relaxes muscles and relieves pain. Moist heat (hot soaks, paraffin baths, whirlpool) usually works best for patients with chronic disease. Ice packs are effective during acute episodes.

Advanced disease may require surgical repair, often including total hip and knee arthroplasty.

Other useful surgical procedures in RA include metatarsal head and distal ulnar resectional arthroplasty; insertion of a Silastic prosthesis between MCP and PIP joints to free and stabilize them; and arthrodesis (joint fusion), usually in wrists feet, or spine. Arthrodesis sacrifices joint mobility for stability and relief of pain.

Several investigative procedures are being evaluated. Synovectomy (removal of destructive, proliferating synovium, usually in the wrists, knees, and fingers) is under investigation as a means to halt or delay the course of this disease. Osteotomy (the cutting of bone or excision of a wedge of bone) can realign joint surfaces and redistribute stresses. Tendon transfers may prevent deformities or relieve contractures.

Additional considerations

When treating an RA patient, the hospital staff member should:
• assess all joints carefully; look for deformities, contractures, immobility, and inability to perform everyday activities.
• monitor vital signs often, and note weight changes, sensory disturbances, and level of pain; administer analgesics, as ordered, and watch closely for side effects.
• give meticulous skin care; check for rheumatoid nodules, as well as pressure areas and breakdowns due to immobility, vascular impairment, corticosteroid treatment, or improper splinting; use lotion or cleansing oil, not soap, for dry skin.
• explain all diagnostic tests and procedures; tell the patient to expect the need for multiple blood samples to allow firm diagnosis and accurate monitoring of therapy.

• monitor the duration, not the intensity, of morning stiffness, because duration more accurately reflects the severity of the disease; encourage the patient to take hot showers or baths at bedtime or in the morning to reduce the need for pain medication.

• apply splints carefully and correctly; observe for pressure sores if the patient is in traction or wearing splints.

• encourage a balanced diet, but make sure the patient understands that special diets won't cure RA; stress the need for weight control, since obesity adds further stress to joints.

• urge the patient to perform activities of daily living, such as dressing and feeding himself (supply easy-to-open cartons, lightweight cups, and unpackaged silverware); allow the patient enough time to calmly perform these tasks.

• provide emotional support, knowing that the patient with chronic illness easily becomes depressed, discouraged, and irritable; encourage the RA patient to discuss his fears concerning dependency, sexuality, body image, and self-esteem; refer him to an appropriate social service agency, as needed.

• before discharge, make sure the patient knows how and when to take prescribed medication and how to recognize possible side effects.

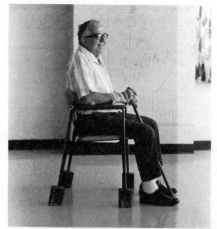

Wooden blocks secured to chair legs make sitting easier for the arthritic patient.

• explain the nature of RA; make sure the patient and his family understand that RA is a chronic disease that requires major changes in their life-styles; emphasize that there are no miracle cures, despite irresponsible claims to the contrary.

• teach the patient how to stand, walk, and sit correctly: upright and erect; tell the patient to sit in chairs with high seats and armrests—he'll find it easier to get up from a chair if his knees are lower than his hips; recommend putting blocks of wood under the legs of a favorite chair if the patient doesn't own a chair with a high seat; suggest an elevated toilet seat.

The patient must carefully pace daily activities, resting for 5 to 10 minutes out of each hour and alternating sitting and standing tasks. Adequate sleep is important, and so is correct sleeping posture. The patient should sleep on his back on a firm mattress, using a small pillow. He should avoid placing a pillow under his knees; this encourages flexion deformity.

The patient will have to be taught: to avoid putting undue stress on joints and to use the largest joint available for a given task; to support weak or painful joints as much as possible; to avoid positions of flexion and promote positions of extension; to hold objects parallel to the knuckles as briefly as possible; to always use his hands toward the center of his body and to slide—not lift—objects, whenever possible. The patient should obtain shoes with proper support. An occupational therapist can teach him how to simplify activities and protect arthritic joints.

Various dressing aids (long-handled shoehorn, reacher, elastic shoelaces, zipper-pull, and buttonhook) and helpful household items (easy-to-open drawers, hand shower nozzle, hand rails, and grab bars) will make the patient's day-to-day life easier. He should dress in a sitting position as much as possible.

For more information on coping with RA, the patient should be referred to the Arthritis Foundation.

Neurogenic Arthropathy
(Charcot's arthropathy)

Neurogenic arthropathy, most common in men over age 40, is a progressively degenerative disease of peripheral and axial joints, resulting from impaired sensory innervation. The loss of sensation in the joints permits further deterioration, resulting from trauma or primary disease, which leads to laxity of supporting ligaments and eventual disintegration of the affected joints.

Causes and incidence

In adults, the most common cause of neurogenic arthropathy is diabetes mellitus. Other causes include tabes dorsalis (especially among patients aged 40 to 60), syringomyelia (progresses to neurogenic arthropathy in about 25% of patients), myelopathy of pernicious anemia, spinal cord trauma, paraplegia, hereditary sensory neuropathy, Charcot-Marie-Tooth disease, peripheral nerve injury, myelomeningocele (in children), and leprosy.

A rare cause is the intra-articular injection of corticosteroids. The analgesic effect of the corticosteroids may mask symptoms and allow continuous damaging stress to accelerate rheumatoid arthritis and osteoarthritis.

Signs and symptoms

Neurogenic arthropathy begins insidiously with swelling, warmth, increased mobility, and instability in a single joint or in many joints. The first clue to vertebral neuroarthropathy, which progresses to gross spinal deformity, may be nothing more than a mild, persistent backache. Characteristically, pain is minimal despite obvious deformity.

The specific joint affected varies. Diabetes usually attacks the joints and bones of the feet; tabes dorsalis attacks the large weight-bearing joints, such as the knee, hip, ankle, or lumbar and dorsal vertebrae (Charcot spine); syringomyelia, the shoulder, elbow, or cervical intervertebral joint. Neurogenic arthropathy related to intra-articular injection of corticosteroids usually develops in the hip or knee joint.

Diagnosis

Patient history of painless joint deformity and underlying primary disease suggests neurogenic arthropathy. Physical examination may reveal bone fragmentation in advanced disease. X-rays confirm diagnosis and assess severity of joint damage. In the early stage of the disease, soft-tissue swelling may be the only overt effect; in the advanced stage, articular fracture, subluxation, erosion of articular cartilage, periosteal new bone formation, and excessive growth of marginal loose bodies (osteophytosis) may be revealed.

Other helpful diagnostic measures include:
- *vertebral examination:* narrowing of disk spaces, deterioration of vertebrae, and osteophyte formation, leading to ankylosis and deforming kyphoscoliosis
- *synovial biopsy:* bony fragments and bits of calcified cartilage.

Treatment

Effective management relieves pain with analgesics and immobilization, using crutches, splints, braces, and restriction of weight-bearing.

In severe disease, surgery may include arthrodesis or, in severe diabetic neuropathy, amputation. However, surgery risks further damage through nonunion and infection.

Additional considerations

- The patient should be checked frequently for severity of pain, sensory perception, range of motion, joint swelling, and the status of underlying disease.
- The patient can take various preven-

tive measures. He should: pace daily activities; rest, even when he doesn't feel pain; avoid physically stressful actions that may cause pathologic fractures; and take safety precautions, such as removing throw rugs and clutter that may cause falls.
• The patient must report joint pain, swelling, or instability. Warm compresses may be applied to relieve local pain and tenderness.

• The patient should know the proper technique for crutches or other orthopedic devices, and understand the importance of proper fitting and regular professional readjustment of such devices, since impaired sensation might allow damage from these aids without discomfort.
• The patient must appreciate the need to continue regular treatment of the underlying disease.

Reiter's Syndrome

A self-limiting syndrome associated with arthritis (dominant feature), urethritis, conjunctivitis, and mucocutaneous lesions, Reiter's syndrome appears to be related to infection and is probably transmitted venereally. This disease usually affects young men (aged 20 to 40); it's rare in women and children.

Causes
While the exact cause of Reiter's syndrome is unknown, most cases seem to result from infection and closely follow sexual contact. Since 85% of patients with Reiter's syndrome display histocompatibility for the lymphocytic antigen HLA-B27, research suggests that an unknown infectious agent transmitted through sexual intercourse causes this disease in a genetically susceptible host. Reiter's syndrome has followed infections caused by *Mycoplasma*, *Shigella*, and *Salmonella* organisms.

Signs and symptoms
Reiter's syndrome produces acute urethritis. The patient complains of dysuria, urgent and frequent urination, and mucopurulent penile discharge, with swelling and reddening of the urethral meatus. He may also experience suprapubic pain, fever, and anorexia with weight loss. This disorder may also cause other genitourinary complications, such as prostatitis and hemorrhagic cystitis.

Within a few days to 4 weeks, arthritic symptoms usually appear, often lasting from 2 to 4 months. Asymmetric and extremely variable polyarticular arthritis occurs most often and tends to develop

in weight-bearing joints of the legs, and sometimes in the low back or sacroiliac. The arthritis is usually acute, with warm, erythematous, and painful joints; it may be mild, with minimal synovitis.

Ocular symptoms include mild bilateral conjunctivitis, possibly complicated by keratitis, iritis, retinitis, or optic neuritis. In severe cases, burning, itching, and profuse mucopurulent discharge are possible.

Skin lesions usually develop several weeks after onset of other symptoms and may last for several weeks. These lesions, often closely resembling those of psoriasis, occur most commonly on the palms and soles but can develop anywhere on the trunk, extremities, or scalp. Nails become thick, opaque, and brittle; keratic debris accumulates under the nails. Mucocutaneous lesions also appear in most patients. In many patients, painless, transient ulcerations erupt in the buccal mucosa, palate, and tongue; superficial lesions may erupt on the glans penis (balanitis).

Diagnosis
Nearly all patients with Reiter's syndrome show histocompatibility for the HLA-B27 antigen, and elevated WBC

and ESR. Anemia may develop. Urethral discharge and synovial fluid contain many WBCs, mostly polymorphonuclear leukocytes; synovial fluid is high in complement and protein, and grossly purulent. Cultures of any drainage are negative for gonococci.

During the first few weeks, X-rays are normal and may remain so, but some patients may show osteoporosis in inflamed areas, often several weeks after onset of symptoms. If inflammation persists, X-rays may also show erosions of the small joints, periosteal proliferation (new bone formation) of involved joints, and calcaneal spurs.

Treatment

No specific treatment exists for Reiter's syndrome. Most patients recover in 2 to 16 weeks. Lesions heal without a trace, and many patients regain full joint function. However, about 50% of patients have recurring acute attacks, while the rest follow a chronic course, experiencing continued synovitis, elevated ESR, and sacroiliitis. In acute stages, limited weight-bearing or complete bed rest may be necessary.

Anti-inflammatory agents, including salicylates, can be given for relief of discomfort and fever. More resistant cases may require indomethacin. Phenylbutazone may be effective but is recommended only for patients whose blood counts can be closely monitored for possible bone marrow depression. Physical therapy includes range-of-motion exercises, and the use of padded or supportive shoes to correct contractures and deformities of the feet.

Additional considerations

• The patient may be embarrassed if attacks are associated with sexual activity, so the hospital staff must communicate an accepting, nonjudgmental attitude.
• The patient should understand Reiter's syndrome and the recommended medications and their possible side effects. He must take medications with meals or milk to prevent gastrointestinal bleeding.
• The patient's independence can be promoted through the encouragement of normal daily activity and moderate exercise. He must not immobilize an affected joint.
• Occupational counseling may be necessary if the patient has severe or chronic joint impairment.

Osgood-Schlatter Disease
(Osteochondrosis)

Osgood-Schlatter disease is a painful, incomplete separation of the epiphysis of the tibial tubercle from the tibial shaft. It's common in active adolescent boys, frequently affecting both knees. Severe disease may cause permanent tubercle enlargement.

Causes

Osgood-Schlatter disease probably results from trauma, before the complete fusion of the epiphysis to the main bone has occurred (between ages 10 and 15). Such trauma may be a single violent action, or repeated knee flexion against tight quadriceps muscle as occurs when riding a bicycle. Other possible causes include locally deficient blood supply and genetic factors.

Signs and symptoms

The patient complains of aching—that continues even when he is at rest—and pain and tenderness below the kneecap which worsens during any activity that causes forceful contraction of the patellar tendon on the tubercle, such as ascending or descending stairs. Such pain may be associated with some obvious soft-tissue swelling, localized heat, and local tenderness.

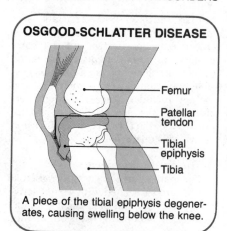

OSGOOD-SCHLATTER DISEASE

Femur

Patellar tendon

Tibial epiphysis

Tibia

A piece of the tibial epiphysis degenerates, causing swelling below the knee.

Diagnosis

Physical examination supports the diagnosis: the examiner forces the tibia into internal rotation while slowly extending the patient's knee from 90° of flexion; at about 30° such flexion produces pain that subsides immediately with external rotation of the tibia.

X-rays may be normal or show epiphyseal separation and soft-tissue swelling for up to 6 months after onset; eventually, they may show bone fragmentation.

Treatment

Treatment usually consists of immobilization for 6 to 8 weeks, and supportive measures. Leg immobilization through reinforced elastic knee support, plaster cast, or splint allows revascularization and reossification of the tubercle and minimizes the pull of the quadriceps. Supportive measures include bed rest, activity restrictions, and possibly, cortisone injections into the joint to relieve tenderness. In very mild cases, simple restriction of predisposing activities (bicycling, running) may be adequate.

Rarely, conservative measures fail, and surgery may be necessary. Such surgery includes removal or fixation of the epiphysis or drilling holes through the tubercle to the main bone to form channels for rapid revascularization.

Additional considerations

• The patient's circulation, sensation, and pain must be monitored, with special attention paid to excessive bleeding after surgery.
• Motion limitation should be assessed daily, and analgesics administered.
• The patient must understand the importance of bed rest.
• Knee support or splint shouldn't be too tight. The cast must be kept dry and clean, and petaled around the top and bottom margins to avoid skin irritation.
• The patient must be taught proper use of crutches. He should protect the injured knee with padding, and avoid trauma and repeated flexion (running, contact sports).
• Reassurance and emotional support will be needed, since disruption of normal activities is difficult for an active teenager. Emphasizing that the restrictions are temporary will help.

Psoriatic Arthritis

Psoriatic arthritis is a syndrome of rheumatoid-like joint disease associated with psoriasis of nearby skin and nails. Although the arthritis component of this syndrome may be clinically indistinguishable from rheumatoid arthritis, the rheumatoid nodules are absent, and serologic tests for rheumatoid factor are negative. Psoriatic arthritis usually is mild, with intermittent flare-ups, but rarely may progress to crippling arthritis mutilans. This disease affects both men and women equally; usually, onset occurs between ages 30 and 35.

Causes

Evidence suggests that predisposition to psoriatic arthritis is hereditary. However, onset is usually precipitated by streptococcal infection, or trauma.

Signs and symptoms

Psoriatic lesions usually, though not invariably, precede the arthritic component. However, once the full syndrome is established, joint and skin lesions recur simultaneously. Arthritis (swelling, tenderness, warmth, and restricted movement) varies from involvement of a single joint to a symmetric involvement of several joints. It can develop in any peripheral joint but is most common in the distal interphalangeal joints of the hands, almost always associated with psoriasis of the nails. Low back pain and spondylitis are usually late manifestations. Psoriatic lesions are usually present on the skin and nails adjacent to the affected joint; less often, small lesions are hidden on the scalp, intergluteal fold, or navel. Characteristic nail changes include pitting, transverse ridging, onycholysis, keratosis, yellow discoloration, and destruction of the entire nail. Psoriatic arthritis may also produce general malaise and, occasionally, fever.

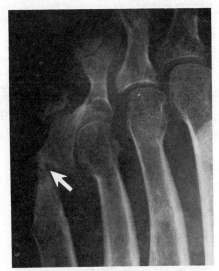

X-ray of toes shows "pencil-in-cup deformity" in psoriatic arthritis. The area marked by an arrow shows erosion of the distal end of the fifth metatarsal and the proximal phalanx of the fifth toe, and other changes at the interphalangeal joint.

Diagnosis

Inflammatory arthritis in a patient with psoriatic skin lesions suggests psoriatic arthritis.

X-rays confirm arthritic involvement and show: erosion of terminal phalangeal tufts; "whittling" of the distal end of the terminal phalanges; "pencil-in-cup" deformity of the distal interphalangeal joints; relative absence of osteoporosis; sacroiliitis; and spondylitis, with paravertebral ossification, bony overgrowth, and vertebral fusion with disk calcification.

Typical serum values include negative rheumatoid factor and elevated ESR. Diagnostic evaluation must rule out gout (by examining synovial fluid for white crystals) and septic arthritis (by culturing synovial fluid for microorganisms).

Treatment

In mild psoriatic arthritis, treatment is supportive, and consists of immobilization through bed rest or splints, isometric exercises, paraffin baths, heat therapy, and anti-inflammatory drugs. In severe psoriatic arthritis, treatment may also include methotrexate and synovectomy. Antimalarials are contraindicated in patients with psoriatic arthritis, because these drugs can provoke exfoliative dermatitis.

Additional considerations

• The patient and his family should receive formal instruction to explain the disease and its treatment.
• The patient with psoriatic plaques must know they aren't contagious. Those around the patient must avoid showing any revulsion to unsightly psoriatic patches—doing so will only reinforce the patient's fear of rejection.
• The patient must know how to apply skin care products and medications correctly and how to identify their side effects.
• Adequate rest and protection of affected joints are important for recovery.
• The patient should get regular, moderate exposure to the sun.

Osteoarthritis

The most common form of arthritis, osteoarthritis is a chronic, progressive disorder causing deterioration of the joint cartilage and formation of reactive new bone at the margins and subchondral areas of the joints. This degeneration results from a breakdown of chondrocytes, most often in the hips and knees.

Osteoarthritis is widespread, with incidence rising among the elderly. Its earliest symptoms generally begin in middle age and become progressively severe with advancing age. Osteoarthritis occurs equally in both sexes.

Prognosis depends on the site and severity of involvement, and can range from minor limitation of the fingers to severe disability in persons with hip or knee involvement. Rate of progression varies, and joints may remain stable for years in an early stage of deterioration.

Causes

Primary osteoarthritis, a normal part of aging, results from genetic predisposition. Secondary osteoarthritis, an acquired form, is brought about by joint damage from trauma, infection, stress, excessive "wear and tear," metabolic disorders (Wilson's disease), or underlying joint disease (chondrocalcinosis).

Signs and symptoms

The most common symptom of osteoarthritis is joint pain, particularly after exercise or weight bearing, that is usually relieved by rest. Other common symptoms include: stiffness in the morning and after exercise (relieved by rest), aching during changes in weather, "grating" of the joint during motion, limited movement, and fluid accumulation in the joint. The severity of these effects increases with poor posture, obesity, and occupational stress.

Osteoarthritis of the interphalangeal joints produces irreversible changes in the distal joints (Heberden's nodes) and proximal joints (Bouchard's nodes). These nodes may be painless at first but eventually become red, swollen, and tender,

causing numbness and loss of dexterity.

Diagnosis

After a thorough physical examination confirms typical symptoms, diagnosis of osteoarthritis depends on X-rays of the affected joint. Appropriate X-rays may require posterior, anterior, lateral, and oblique views (with spinal involvement), and characteristically show:
- narrowing of joint space or margin.
- cystlike bony deposits in joint space and margins.
- joint deformity due to degeneration or articular damage.
- bony growths at weight-bearing areas (hips, knees).
No laboratory test is specific for osteoarthritis.

Treatment

Treatment is primarily palliative, through medication and surgery. Medications for relief of pain and joint inflammation include aspirin (or other nonnarcotic analgesics), phenylbutazone, indomethacin, fenoprofen, ibuprofen, propoxyphene, and in severe cases, intra-articular injections of corticosteroids. Such injections can delay the irreversible development of nodes in the hands. The combined use of quinine and aminophylline may relieve leg cramps.

Effective treatment also reduces stress by taking weight off the joint with crutches, braces, cane, walker, cervical collar, or traction. Other supportive measures include massage, moist heat, paraffin dips for hands, protective techniques for preventing undue stress on the joints, and adequate rest, particularly after activity.

The following surgical procedures are

reserved for severe osteoarthritis with disability or uncontrollable pain:

• *arthroplasty* (partial or total): replacement of deteriorated part of joint with prosthetic appliance

• *arthrodesis:* surgical fusion of bones; used primarily in spine (laminectomy)

• *osteoplasty:* scraping of deteriorated bone from joint

• *osteotomy:* change in alignment of bone to relieve stress by excision of wedge of bone or cutting of bone.

Additional considerations

The patient with osteoarthritis must get adequate rest, particularly after activity. He'll need rest periods during the day, and adequate sleep at night. Moderation is the key—the patient should be taught to "pace" daily activities.

If he needs surgery, the patient should get appropriate preoperative and postoperative health care (see RHEUMATOID ARTHRITIS).

He'll also need emotional support and reassurance to help cope with limited mobility. He should know that osteoarthritis is *not* a systemic disease, so joint problems won't spread to other areas.

Specific care depends on the affected joint:

• *Hand:* Application of hot soaks and paraffin dips, as ordered, will help relieve pain.

• *Spine* (lumbar and sacral): A firm mattress (or bed board) will help decrease the patient's morning pain.

• *Spine* (cervical): The patient's neck should be checked for signs of constriction and redness (with prolonged use).

• *Hip:* Moist heat pads will help relieve pain, and antispasmodic drugs, as ordered, should be administered. The patient will need assistance with range-of-motion and strengthening exercises, and must get proper rest afterward. Crutches, cane, braces, and walker should be inspected for proper fit, and the patient must be shown how to use them correctly. (For example, the patient with unilateral joint involvement should use an orthopedic appliance on the normal side. He should use cushions when sitting, and an elevated toilet seat.)

• *Knee:* The patient will need assistance, twice daily, with prescribed range-of-motion exercises, exercises to maintain muscle tone, and progressive resistance exercises to increase muscle strength. Elastic supports or laced-up knee braces may be needed to provide the patient with extra support.

To minimize the long-term effects of osteoarthritis, the patient must:

• plan for adequate rest during the day, after mild to moderate exertion, and at night.

• take medication exactly as prescribed, and report side effects immediately.

• avoid overexertion, taking care to stand and walk correctly, to minimize weight-bearing activities, and to be especially careful when stooping or picking up objects.

• always wear well-fitting supportive shoes; avoid allowing the heels to become too worn down.

• install safety measures at home, if necessary, such as guard rails in the bathroom.

• do gentle range-of-motion exercises.

• maintain proper body weight to lessen strain on joints.

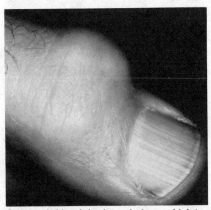

Osteoarthritis of the interphalangeal joints produces irreversible changes in the distal joints (Heberden's nodes). These nodes can be initially painless, with gradual progression or sudden flare-up of redness, swelling, tenderness, and impairment of sensation and dexterity.

Ankylosing Spondylitis
(Rheumatoid spondylitis, Marie-Strümpell disease)

A chronic, usually progressive inflammatory disease, ankylosing spondylitis primarily affects the sacroiliac, apophyseal, and costovertebral joints and adjacent soft tissue. Generally, it begins in the sacroiliac joints and gradually progresses to the lumbar, thoracic, and cervical regions of the spine. Deterioration of bone and cartilage can lead to fibrous tissue formation and eventual fusion of the spine.

Ankylosing spondylitis occurs almost exclusively (90%) in young men; incidence is slightly higher in Caucasians. Age at onset ranges from 10 to 30 years.

Causes

Recent evidence suggests a relationship to the histocompatibility antigen HLA-B27 that is positive in over 90% of patients with this disease. Although this predisposing factor is inherited, the disease itself is not.

Signs and symptoms

The first indication of ankylosing spondylitis is intermittent low back pain. This pain is usually most severe in the morning or after a period of inactivity, and is not relieved by rest. Other symptoms depend on the stage of the disease and may include:

• stiffness and limited motion of the lumbar spine.
• pain and limited expansion of the chest due to involvement of the thoracic spine.
• peripheral arthritis involving shoulders, hips, and knees.
• kyphosis in advanced stages, caused

CLINICAL EXAMINATION FOR ANKYLOSING SPONDYLITIS

TEST	METHOD	RESULT
Occiput to wall (*fleche*)	Patient places heels and back against wall and tries to touch wall with back of head. Distance from occiput to wall is measured.	Inability to touch head to wall suggests cervical involvement.
Fingers to floor (*forward flexion*)	Patient bends forward with knees straight, and distance from fingertips to floor is measured.	Inability to touch toes is evidence of early lumbar disease.
Schober test	Examiner marks spine at level of L5 and, again, about 4" (10 cm) above it while patient stands erect. Patient bends forward maximally, and distance between the marks is measured.	An increase of less than 2" (5 cm) indicates early lumbar involvement.
Chest expansion	Measure maximum chest expansion at nipple line.	Chest expansion less than 2" (5 cm) suggests early costovertebral involvement.
Sacroiliac compression	Exert direct compression over sacroiliac joints.	Tenderness or pain suggests sacroiliac involvement.
Gaenslen's sign	Maneuver to stress sacroiliacs.	Evokes sacroiliac pain.

Adapted with permission from B.L. Bluestone, "Ankylosing Spondylitis" in ARTHRITIS AND ALLIED CONDITIONS (Philadelphia: Lea & Febiger, 1979).

PATIENT TEACHING AID

Exercises for Ankylosing Spondylitis

You have ankylosing spondylitis, but the following exercises can help maintain muscle strength and prevent deformity:

Spine extension exercises

• *Pelvic tilt:* Stand with your legs slightly apart and your back against the wall. Take a deep breath and pull your abdomen in and up, flattening the small of your back against the wall. Hold for four counts and exhale.

• *Bridging:* Lie on your back, with your knees bent and your soles on the floor. Keeping your arms at your sides, arch your back and place weight on your forearms, shoulders, and soles. Hold for six counts.

• Stand with your arms tightly against your sides. Bend your elbows, bringing your forearms to the front of your body. Take a deep breath, and rotate your forearms toward the back, keeping your elbows tightly against your body. Hold for four counts and exhale.

• Stand and face the corner of the room. Place one hand on each wall at shoulder level. Bend your elbows slightly, and pull your abdomen in slowly, while leaning forward and forcing your chest toward the corner. Hold for six counts, and return to starting position. Repeat 10 to 20 times.

• Lie on your stomach, and stretch your arms out at shoulder level. Lift your head, chest, shoulders, and arms off the bed as far as possible. Hold for six counts, and then return to starting position (recommended only for early stage).

Chest-expanding exercises

• While lying on your back, clasp your hands behind your head, pulling your elbows toward each other. Push your elbows to the bed, while breathing in deeply. Hold that breath for 10 counts; then exhale and relax.

• Lie on your back with your arms at your sides. Take a deep breath while raising your arms over your head. As you let the breath out slowly with a hissing noise, bring your arms back to your sides.

• Stand with your hands clasped behind your head. While keeping your head erect, extend your elbows as far as possible toward your back.

• Stand with your feet slightly apart. Hold your left arm at your side, and extend your right arm over your head. Bend your body to the left. Repeat this exercise on the opposite side.

Breathing exercise (for diaphragm)

• Lie on your back, and rest your hands on your abdomen. On inspiration you'll feel your abdomen swell, and on expiration you'll feel it flatten. Repeat this exercise while standing and sitting.

This patient teaching aid is intended for distribution to patients by doctors and nurses. It should not be used without a doctor's approval.

---

by chronic stooping to relieve symptoms.
• hip damage.
• tenderness over site of inflammation.
• mild fatigue, fever, anorexia, or loss of weight.
• occasional iritis.

These symptoms progress unpredictably, and the disease can go into sudden remission, exacerbation, or arrest at any stage.

Diagnosis

Typical symptoms and demonstration of positive HLA-B27 histocompatibility antigen strongly suggest ankylosing spondylitis. However, confirmation requires characteristic X-ray findings:

• blurring of the bony margins of the joints in the early stage
• bilateral sacroiliac involvement
• patchy sclerosis
• eventual squaring of vertebral bodies
• "bamboo spine" and completely ankylosed sacroiliac joints.

ESR may be slightly elevated. A negative rheumatoid factor rules out rheumatoid arthritis, which produces similar symptoms.

Treatment

No treatment reliably stops progression of this disease, so management aims to delay further deformity by good posture, stretching and deep-breathing exercises, and in some patients, braces and light-weight supports. Anti-inflammatory analgesics, such as aspirin, indomethacin, and phenylbutazone, control pain.

Severe hip involvement usually necessitates surgical replacement of the hip. Severe spinal involvement requires a spinal wedge osteotomy to separate and reposition the bones in the spine. This surgery is a treatment of last resort because of the high risk of spinal cord damage and the long convalescence involved.

Additional considerations

Ankylosing spondylitis is an extremely painful and crippling disease, so a health care professional's main responsibility is to promote the patient's comfort. He must keep in mind when dealing with such a patient that limited range of motion makes simple tasks difficult. The patient will need support and reassurance.

A hospital staff member should: administer medication, as ordered; apply local heat and provide massage to relieve pain; assess mobility and degree of discomfort frequently; assist with daily exercises, as needed; stress the importance of maintaining good posture.

If treatment includes surgery, good postoperative health care is essential. Since ankylosing spondylitis is a chronic, progressively crippling condition, a comprehensive treatment plan should also reflect counsel from a social worker, visiting nurse, and dietitian. To minimize deformities, the patient should:
• avoid any physical activity that places undue stress on the back, such as lifting heavy objects.
• stand upright; sit upright in a high, straight chair; and avoid leaning over a desk.
• sleep in a prone position on a firm mattress and avoid using pillows under neck or knees.
• avoid prolonged walking, standing, sitting, or driving.
• perform regular stretching and deep breathing exercises, and swim regularly, if possible.
• have height measured every 3 to 4 months to detect any tendency to lean forward.
• seek vocational counseling if work requires standing or prolonged sitting at a desk.

Carpal Tunnel Syndrome

The most common of the nerve entrapment syndromes, carpal tunnel syndrome results from compression of the median nerve at the wrist, within the carpal tunnel, through which important nerves, blood vessels, and flexor tendons to the fingers and thumb pass from the forearm to the hand. This compression neuropathy causes sensory and motor changes in the median distribution of the hand. Carpal tunnel syndrome usually occurs in women between ages 30 and 60, and poses a serious occupational health problem. Assembly-line workers and packers, and persons who repeatedly use poorly designed tools are most likely to develop this disorder. Any strenuous use of the hands—sustained grasping, or twisting or turning—aggravates this condition.

Causes

The carpal tunnel is formed by the carpal bones and the transverse carpal ligament. Inflammation or fibrosis of the tendon sheaths that pass through the carpal tunnel often causes edema and compression of the median nerve. Many conditions can cause the contents or structure of the carpal tunnel to swell and press the median nerve against the transverse carpal ligament. Such conditions include flexor tenosynovitis (often associated with rheumatic disease), nerve compression, pregnancy, renal failure, menopause, diabetes mellitus, acromegaly, edema following Colles' fracture, hypothyroidism, amyloidosis, myxedema, benign tumors, Raynaud's disease, tuberculosis, and other granulomatous diseases. Another source of damage to the median nerve is dislocation or acute sprain of the wrist.

Signs and symptoms

The patient with carpal tunnel syndrome usually complains of weakness, pain, burning, numbness, or tingling in one or both hands. This paresthesia affects the thumb, forefinger, and middle finger but not the fourth or fifth finger. The patient is unable to clench his hand into a fist; the nails may be atrophic, the skin dry and shiny. Because of vasodilatation and venous stasis, symptoms are often worse at night and in the morning. The pain may spread to the forearm and, in severe cases, as far as the shoulder. The patient can usually relieve such pain by shaking his hands vigorously or dangling his arms at his side.

Diagnosis

Physical examination reveals decreased sensation to light touch or pinpricks in the affected fingers. Thenar muscle atrophy occurs in about half of all cases of carpal tunnel syndrome. The patient exhibits a positive Tinel's sign (tingling over the median nerve on light percussion) and responds positively to Phalen's wrist-flexion test (holding the forearms vertically and allowing both hands to drop into complete flexion at the wrists for 1 minute reproduces symptoms of carpal tunnel syndrome). A compression test supports this diagnosis: a blood pressure cuff inflated above systolic pressure on the forearm for 1 to 2 minutes provokes pain and paresthesia along the distribution of the median nerve.

X-rays reveal bony abnormalities such as osteophytes. Electromyography detects a median nerve motor conduction

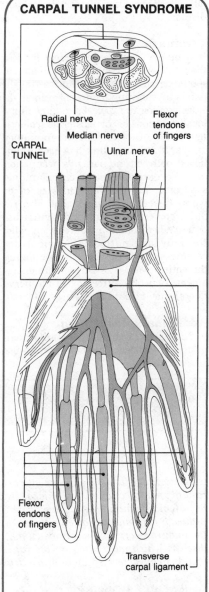

CARPAL TUNNEL SYNDROME

Radial nerve

Median nerve

CARPAL TUNNEL

Ulnar nerve

Flexor tendons of fingers

Flexor tendons of fingers

Transverse carpal ligament

The carpal tunnel is clearly visible in this palmar view and cross section of a right hand. Note the median nerve, flexor tendons of fingers, and blood vessels passing through the tunnel on their way from the forearm to the hand.

delay of more than 5 milliseconds. Other laboratory tests may identify underlying disease.

Treatment

If symptoms have been present for less than 2 months, conservative treatment should be tried first, including resting the hands by splinting the forearm in slight extension for 1 to 2 weeks, night splints, local injections of corticosteroids, or systemic use of other anti-inflammatory agents. If a definite link has been established between the patient's occupation and the development of carpal tunnel syndrome, he may have to seek other work. Effective treatment may also require correction of an underlying disorder. When conservative treatment fails, the only alternative is surgical decompression of the nerve by sectioning the entire transverse carpal tunnel ligament. Neurolysis (freeing of the nerve fibers) may also be necessary.

Additional considerations

• The patient may be given mild analgesics, as needed. He should try to use his hands as much as possible; however, if the condition has impaired the dominant hand, he may need help with eating and bathing.

• The patient must know how to apply a splint. He shouldn't make it too tight, and should report any discomfort. He must also know how to remove the splint to perform gentle range-of-motion exercises, which should be done daily. The patient must know how to do these exercises before he's discharged.

• The patient's vital signs will require monitoring. The affected hand must be checked regularly for color, sensation, and motion.

• The discharged patient must exercise his hands occasionally in warm water. If he's still wearing a surgical dressing, he should put on rubber gloves before immersing his hands. If the arm is in a sling, he should remove the sling several times a day to exercise his elbow and shoulder.

• Occupational counseling may be appropriate for the patient who has to change jobs because of carpal tunnel syndrome.

BONES

Osteomyelitis

Osteomyelitis is a pyogenic bone infection that may be chronic or acute. It commonly results from a combination of local trauma—usually quite trivial but resulting in hematoma formation—and an acute infection originating elsewhere in the body. Although osteomyelitis often remains localized, it can spread through the bone to the marrow, cortex, and periosteum. Acute osteomyelitis is usually a blood-borne disease, which most often affects rapidly growing children. Chronic osteomyelitis (rare) is characterized by multiple draining sinus tracts and metastatic lesions.

Causes and incidence

Osteomyelitis occurs more often in children than in adults—and particularly in boys—usually as a complication of an acute localized infection. The most common sites in children are the lower end of the femur and the upper end of the tibia, humerus, and radius. In adults,

the most common sites are the pelvis and vertebrae, generally the result of contamination associated with surgery or trauma. The incidence of both chronic and acute osteomyelitis is declining, except in drug abusers. With prompt treatment, prognosis for acute osteomyelitis is very good; for chronic osteomyelitis, which is more prevalent in adults, prognosis is still poor.

The most common pyogenic organism in osteomyelitis is *Staphylococcus aureus;* others include *Streptococcus pyogenes, Pneumococcus, Pseudomonas aeruginosa, Escherichia coli,* and *Proteus vulgaris.* Typically, these organisms find a culture site in a hematoma from recent trauma or in a weakened area, such as the site of local infection (for example, furunculosis), and spread directly to bone. As the organisms grow and form pus within the bone, tension builds within the rigid medullary cavity, forcing pus through the haversian canals. This forms a subperiosteal abscess that deprives the bone of its blood supply. If this condition persists, it eventually causes necrosis. In turn, necrosis stimulates the periosteum to create new bone (involucrum); the old bone (sequestrum) detaches and works its way out through an abscess or the sinuses. By the time sequestrum forms, osteomyelitis is chronic.

Signs and symptoms

Onset of *acute* osteomyelitis is usually rapid, with sudden pain in the affected bone, and tenderness, heat, swelling, and restricted movement over it. Associated systemic symptoms may include tachycardia, sudden fever, nausea, and malaise. Generally, the clinical features of both chronic and acute osteomyelitis are the same, except that chronic infection can persist intermittently for years, flaring up spontaneously after minor trauma. Sometimes, however, the only symptom of chronic infection is the persistent drainage of pus from an old pocket in a sinus tract.

Diagnosis

Patient history, physical examination, and blood tests help to confirm osteomyelitis:

• *WBC* shows leukocytosis.
• *ESR* is elevated.
• *Blood cultures* identify causative organism.

X-rays may not show bone involvement until disease has been active for some time, usually 2 to 3 weeks. Diagnosis must rule out poliomyelitis, rheumatic fever, myositis, and bone fractures.

Treatment

To prevent further bone damage, treatment for acute osteomyelitis should begin before definitive diagnosis.

• Large doses of antibiotics are given I.V. (usually a penicillinase-resistant penicillin, such as nafcillin or oxacillin) after blood cultures are taken to determine infecting organism.
• Early surgical drainage is done to relieve pressure buildup and sequestrum formation.
• Affected bone is immobilized by plaster cast, traction, or bed rest.
• Patient is given supportive measures, such as analgesics and I.V. fluids.

If an abscess forms, treatment includes incision and drainage, followed by a culture of the drainage. Antibiotic therapy to control infection may include administration of systemic antibiotics; intracavitary instillation of antibiotics through closed-system continuous irrigation with low intermittent suction; limited irrigation with blood drainage system with suction (Hemovac); or local application of packed, wet, antibiotic-soaked dressings.

In addition to antibiotics and immobilization, chronic osteomyelitis usually requires surgery to remove dead bone (sequestrectomy) and to promote drainage (saucerization). Prognosis is poor even after surgery. Patients are often in great pain and require prolonged hospitalization. Resistant chronic osteomyelitis in an arm or leg may require amputation.

Additional considerations

Health care concerns are to control infection, protect the bone from injury, and offer supportive care, including:

• maintaining strict aseptic technique when changing dressings and irrigating wounds; washing hands before and after giving care; if the patient is in skeletal traction for compound fractures, covering insertion points of pin tracks with small, dry dressings, and warning the patient not to touch the skin around the pins and wires; always starting at the center of the wound when cleaning, and working outward.

• administering I.V. fluids to maintain adequate hydration, as necessary; providing a diet high in protein and vitamin C.

• assessing once a day vital signs, wound appearance, and new pain, which may indicate secondary infection.

• carefully monitoring suctioning equipment; not letting containers of solution being instilled become empty, which allows air into the system; monitoring the amount of solution instilled and suctioned.

• supporting the affected limb with firm pillows; keeping the limb level with the body—it must not sag; providing good skin care, since the patient will be immobile and hesitant to move because of pain; turning him gently every 2 hours; watching for signs of developing decubitus ulcers.

• providing good cast care; supporting the cast with firm pillows and "petaling" the edges with pieces of adhesive tape or moleskin to smooth rough edges; checking circulation and drainage; circling any wet spots that appear on the cast with a marking pen and noting (on the cast) the time of appearance; being aware of how much drainage is expected; checking the circled spot at least every 4 hours, and reporting any enlargement immediately.

• protecting the patient from jerky movements and falls, which may threaten bone integrity; reporting sudden pain, crepitus, or deformity immediately; watching for sudden malposition of the limb, which may indicate fracture.

• teaching the patient, before discharge, how to protect and clean the wound, and how to recognize signs of recurring infection (increased temperature, redness, localized heat, and swelling); stressing the need for follow-up examinations; instructing him to seek prompt treatment for possible sources of recurrence—blisters, boils, styes, and impetigo.

Osteoporosis

Osteoporosis is a metabolic bone disorder in which the rate of bone resorption accelerates while the rate of bone formation slows down, causing a loss of bone mass. Bones affected by this disease lose calcium and phosphate salts, and thus become porous, brittle, and abnormally vulnerable to fracture. Osteoporosis may be primary or secondary to an underlying disease. Primary osteoporosis is often called senile or postmenopausal osteoporosis because it most commonly develops in elderly, postmenopausal women.

Causes
The cause of primary osteoporosis is unknown; however, a mild but prolonged negative calcium balance, resulting from an inadequate dietary intake of calcium, may be an important contributing factor—so may declining gonadal adrenal function, faulty protein metabolism due to estrogen deficiency, and sedentary life-style. Causes of secondary osteoporosis are many: prolonged therapy with steroids or heparin, total immobilization or disuse of a bone

(as with hemiplegia, for example), alcoholism, malnutrition, malabsorption, scurvy, lactose intolerance, hyperthyroidism, osteogenesis imperfecta, and Sudeck's atrophy (localized to hands and feet, with recurring attacks).

Signs and symptoms
Osteoporosis is usually discovered when an elderly person bends to lift something, hears a snapping sound, then feels a sudden pain in the lower back. Vertebral collapse, producing a backache

with pain that radiates around the trunk, is the most common presenting feature. Any movement or jarring aggravates the backache.

In another common pattern, osteoporosis can develop insidiously, with increasing deformity, kyphosis, loss of height, and a markedly aged appearance. As vertebral bodies weaken, spontaneous wedge fractures, pathologic fractures of the neck and femur, Colles' fractures following a minor fall, and hip fractures are all common.

Osteoporosis primarily affects the weight-bearing vertebrae. Only when the condition is advanced or severe, as in Cushing's syndrome or hyperthyroidism, do comparable changes occur in the skull, ribs, and long bones.

Diagnosis

Differential diagnosis must exclude other causes of rarefying bone disease, especially those affecting the spine, such as metastatic carcinoma and advanced multiple myeloma. Initial evaluation attempts to identify the specific cause of osteoporosis through patient history.

• X-rays show typical degeneration in the lower thoracic and lumbar vertebrae. As the spongy trabeculae become progressively fewer and more delicate, the cortical rims stand out by contrast. The involved bone has a ground-glass appearance because the trabeculae have lost definition. The vertebral bodies may appear flattened, with varying degrees of collapse and wedging, and may look denser than normal. Loss of bone mineral becomes evident in later stages.

• Serum calcium, phosphorus, and alkaline phosphatase are all within normal limits, but parathyroid hormone may be elevated.

• Bone biopsy shows thin, porous, but otherwise normal-looking bone.

Treatment

Treatment is basically symptomatic, and aims to prevent additional fractures and control pain. A physical therapy program, emphasizing gentle exercise and activity, is an important part of the treatment. Estrogen may be given to decrease the rate of bone resorption; fluoride, to stimulate bone formation; and calcium and vitamin D, to support normal bone metabolism. However, drug therapy merely arrests osteoporosis and doesn't cure it. Weakened vertebrae should be supported, usually with a back brace. Surgery can correct pathologic fractures of the femur by open reduction and internal fixation. Colles' fracture requires reduction with plaster immobilization for 4 to 6 weeks.

The incidence of senile osteoporosis may be reduced through adequate intake of dietary calcium and regular exercise. Hormonal and fluoride treatments may also offer some preventive benefit and are sometimes used this way. Secondary osteoporosis can be prevented through effective treatment of the underlying disease, as well as through judicious use of steroid therapy, early mobilization after surgery or trauma, decreased alcohol consumption, careful observation for signs of malabsorption, and prompt treatment of hyperthyroidism.

Additional considerations

The health care plan should focus on the patient's fragility, stressing careful positioning, ambulation, and prescribed exercises.

• The patient's skin should be checked daily for redness, warmth, and new sites of pain, which may indicate new fractures. Activity should be encouraged; the patient should walk several times daily. As appropriate, passive range-of-motion exercises or active exercises will help rehabilitation. The patient should regularly attend scheduled physical therapy sessions.

• Safety precautions are necessary. Side rails must be kept up to prevent the patient from falling out of bed. The patient has to be moved gently and carefully at all times. The patient's family and ancillary hospital personnel must understand how easily an osteoporotic patient's bones can fracture.

• A balanced diet must be provided that is high in nutrients that support skeletal

metabolism: vitamin D, calcium, and protein. Analgesics may be needed. Heat can relieve pain.
• Before discharge, the patient and his family must clearly understand the prescribed drug regimen. They must be able to recognize significant side effects and should report them immediately. The patient should also report any new pain sites immediately, especially after trauma, no matter how slight. The patient should sleep on a firm mattress and avoid excessive bed rest. He must know how to wear his back brace. If a female patient is taking estrogen, she must understand the need for routine gynecologic check-ups, including Pap smears, and should report any abnormal bleeding.
• The patient and family will need a good explanation of osteoporosis. If the patient and family don't understand the nature of this disease, they may feel guilty, thinking that the fractures could have been prevented if they had been more careful.
• The patient should be taught good body mechanics—to stoop before lifting anything, and to avoid twisting movements and prolonged bending.
• The female patient taking estrogen must know the proper technique for self-examination of the breasts. She should perform this examination at least once a month and report any lumps immediately.

Paget's Disease
(Osteitis deformans)

Paget's disease is a slowly progressive metabolic bone disease characterized by an initial phase of excessive bone resorption (osteoclastic phase), followed by a reactive phase of excessive abnormal bone formation (osteoblastic phase). The new bone structure, which is chaotic, fragile, and weak, causes painful deformities of both external contour and internal structure. Paget's disease usually localizes in one or several areas of the skeleton (most frequently the lower torso), but occasionally, skeletal deformity is widely distributed. It can be fatal, particularly when it is associated with congestive heart failure (widespread disease creates a continuous need for high cardiac output), bone sarcoma, or benign or malignant giant cell tumors.

Causes and incidence
Paget's disease occurs worldwide but is extremely rare in Asia, the Middle East, Africa, and Scandinavia. In the United States, it affects approximately 2.5 million people over age 40 (mostly men). Although its exact cause is unknown, one theory holds that early viral infection (possibly with mumps virus) causes a dormant skeletal infection that erupts many years later as Paget's disease.

Signs and symptoms
Clinical effects of Paget's disease vary. Early stages may be asymptomatic, but when pain does develop, it is usually severe and persistent, and may coexist with impaired movement resulting from impingement of abnormal bone on the spinal cord or sensory nerve root. Such pain intensifies with weight-bearing.

The patient with skull involvement shows characteristic cranial enlargement over frontal and occipital areas (hat size may increase), and may complain of headaches. Other deformities include kyphosis (spinal curvature due to compression fractures of pagetic vertebrae), accompanied by a barrel-shaped chest and asymmetric bowing of the tibia and femur, which often reduces height. Pagetic sites are warm and tender, and are susceptible to pathologic fractures after minor trauma. Pagetic fractures heal slowly and often incompletely.

Bony impingement on the cranial nerves

may cause blindness, and hearing loss with tinnitus and vertigo. Other complications include hypertension, renal calculi, hypercalcemia, gout, congestive heart failure, and a waddling gait (from softening of pelvic bones).

Diagnosis

X-rays taken before overt symptoms develop show increased bone expansion and density. A bone scan, which is more sensitive than X-rays, clearly shows early pagetic lesions (radioisotope concentrates in areas of active disease). Bone biopsy reveals characteristic mosaic pattern. Other laboratory findings include:
• anemia
• elevated serum alkaline phosphatase (an index of osteoblastic activity and bone formation)
• elevated 24-hour urine levels for hydroxyproline (amino acid excreted by kidneys and an index of osteoclastic hyperactivity). Increasing use of routine chemistry screens—which include serum alkaline phosphatase—is making early diagnosis more common.

Treatment

Primary treatment consists of drug therapy and includes one of the following:
• *calcitonin* (a hormone, given subcutaneously or I.M.) and *etidronate* (P.O.) to retard bone resorption (which relieves bone lesions) and reduce serum alkaline phosphate and urinary hydroxyproline secretion. Although calcitonin requires long-term maintenance therapy, there is noticeable improvement after the first few weeks of treatment; etidronate produces improvement after 1 to 3 months.
• *mithramycin*, a cytotoxic antibiotic, to decrease calcium, urinary hydroxyproline, and serum alkaline phosphatase. This medication produces remission of symptoms within 2 weeks and biochemical improvement in 1 to 2 months. However, mithramycin may destroy platelets or compromise renal function.

Self-administration of calcitonin and etidronate helps patients with Paget's disease lead near-normal lives. Nevertheless, these patients may need surgery to reduce or prevent pathologic fractures, correct secondary deformities, and relieve neurologic impairment. To decrease the risk of excessive bleeding due to hypervascular bone, drug therapy with calcitonin and etidronate or mithramycin must precede surgery. Joint replacement is difficult because bonding material (methylmethacrylate) doesn't set properly on pagetic bone.

Other treatment is symptomatic and supportive, and varies according to symptoms. Aspirin, indomethacin, or ibuprofen usually controls pain.

Additional considerations

The health care professional caring for the patient with Paget's disease should:
• evaluate the effectiveness of analgesics by assessing level of pain daily; watch for new areas of pain or restricted movements—which may indicate new fracture sites—and sensory or motor disturbances, such as difficulty in hearing, seeing, or walking.
• monitor serum calcium and alkaline phosphatase levels.
• prevent decubitus ulcers with the patient on bed rest by providing good skin care; reposition the patient frequently, and use a flotation mattress; provide high-topped sneakers to prevent footdrop.
• monitor intake and output; encourage adequate fluid intake to minimize renal calculi formation.
• demonstrate how to inject calcitonin properly and rotate injection sites; warn the patient that side effects may occur (nausea, vomiting, local inflammatory reaction at injection site, facial flushing, itching of hands, and fever); give reassurance that these side effects are usually mild and infrequent.
• help the patient adjust to the changes in life-style imposed by this disease by teaching him how to pace activities and, if necessary, how to use assistive devices; encourage him to follow a recommended exercise program—avoiding both immobilization and excessive activity; suggest a firm mattress or a bedboard to minimize spinal deformities; warn

against imprudent use of analgesics; prevent falls at home by advising removal of throw rugs and other small obstacles.
• emphasize the importance of regular checkups, including the eyes and ears.
• tell the patient receiving etidronate to take this medication with fruit juice 2 hours before or after meals (milk or other high-calcium fluids impair absorption), to divide daily dosage to minimize side effects, and to watch for and

report stomach cramps, diarrhea, fractures, and increasing or new bone pain.
• tell the patient receiving mithramycin to watch for signs of infection, easy bruising, bleeding, and temperature elevation, and to report for regular follow-up laboratory tests.
• help the patient and his family make use of available community support resources, such as a visiting nurse or home health agency.

Achilles Tendon Contracture

Achilles tendon contracture is a shortening of the Achilles tendon (tendo calcaneus or heel cord), which causes foot pain and strain, with limited ankle dorsiflexion.

Causes
Achilles tendon contracture may reflect a congenital structural anomaly or a muscular reflex to poor posture, especially in women who wear high-heeled shoes or joggers who land on the balls of their feet instead of their heels. Other causes include paralytic conditions of the legs, such as poliomyelitis or cerebral palsy.

Signs and symptoms
Sharp, spasmodic pain during dorsiflexion of the foot characterizes the reflex type of Achilles tendon contracture. In footdrop (fixed equinus), contracture of the flexor foot muscle prevents placing the heel on the ground.

Diagnosis

A simple test confirms Achilles tendon contracture: while the patient keeps his knee flexed, the examiner places the foot in dorsiflexion; gradual knee extension forces the foot into plantar flexion.

Treatment
Conservative treatment aims to correct Achilles tendon contracture by raising the inside heel of the shoe in the reflex type; gradually lowering the heels of

shoes (sudden lowering can aggravate the problem), and stretching exercises, if the cause is high heels; or using support braces or casting to prevent footdrop in a paralyzed patient. Alternative therapy includes using wedged plaster casts or stretching the tendon by manipulation. Analgesics may be given to relieve pain.

With fixed footdrop, treatment may include surgery (z-tenotomy), although this procedure may weaken the tendon. Z-tenotomy allows further stretching by cutting the tendon. After surgery, a short leg cast maintains the foot in 90° dorsiflexion for 6 weeks. Some surgeons allow partial weight-bearing on a walking cast after 2 weeks.

Additional considerations
After surgery to lengthen the tendon, the health care professional should:
• elevate the casted foot to decrease venous pressure and edema by raising the foot of the bed or supporting the foot with pillows.
• record the neurovascular status of the toes (temperature, color, sensation, blanching sign, ability to move toes) every hour for the first 24 hours, then every 4 hours; increase the elevation of the patient's legs, and notify the surgeon immediately if any changes in the neuro-

vascular status are detected.

• prepare the patient for ambulation by having him dangle his foot over the side of the bed for short periods (5 to 15 minutes) before he gets out of bed, allowing for gradual increase of venous pressure; assist the patient in walking, as ordered (usually within 24 hours of surgery), using crutches and a non-weight–bearing or touch-down gait.

• protect the patient's skin with mole-skin or by petaling the edges of the cast; teach the patient before discharge how to care for the cast, and advise him to elevate his foot regularly when sitting or whenever the foot throbs or becomes edematous; make sure the patient understands how much exercise and walking are recommended after discharge.

• to prevent Achilles tendon contracture in paralyzed patients, apply support braces, universal splints, casts, or high-topped sneakers; make sure the weight of the sheets doesn't keep paralyzed feet in plantar flexion; teach other patients good foot care and urge them to seek immediate medical care for foot problems; warn women against wearing high heels constantly, and suggest regular foot (dorsiflexion) exercises.

Hallux Valgus

Hallux valgus is a lateral deviation of the great toe at the metatarsophalangeal joint. It occurs with medial enlargement of the first metatarsal head and bunion formation (bursa and callus formation at the bony prominence).

Causes and incidence
Hallux valgus may be congenital (usually familial as well), but is more often acquired from degenerative arthritis or prolonged pressure on the foot, especially from narrow-toed, high-heeled shoes that compress the forefoot. Consequently, hallux valgus is more common in women.

In congenital hallux valgus, abnormal bony alignment (increased space between first and second metatarsal [metatarsus primus varus]) causes bunion formation. In acquired hallux valgus, bony alignment is normal at the outset of the disorder.

Signs and symptoms
Hallux valgus characteristically begins as a tender bunion covered by deformed, hard, erythematous skin and palpable bursa, often distended with fluid. The first indication of hallux valgus may be pain over the bunion from shoe pressure. Pain can also stem from traumatic arthritis, bursitis, or abnormal stresses on the foot, since hallux valgus changes the body's weight-bearing pattern. In an advanced stage, a flat, splayed forefoot occurs, with severely curled toes (hammer toes).

Diagnosis

A red, tender bunion makes hallux valgus obvious. X-rays confirm diagnosis by showing medial deviation of first metatarsal and lateral deviation of the great toe.

Treatment
In the very early stages of acquired hallux valgus, good foot care and proper shoes may eliminate the need for further treatment. Other useful measures for early management include felt pads to protect the bunion, foam pads or other devices to separate the first and second toes at night, and a supportive pad and exercises to strengthen the metatarsal arch. Early treatment is vital in patients predisposed to foot problems, such as those with rheumatoid arthritis or diabetes mellitus. If the disease progresses to severe deformity with disabling pain, bunionectomy is necessary.

HAMMER TOE

In hammer toe (claw toe), the toe assumes a clawlike pose from the extension of the proximal phalanx of the toe (usually the second toe) while the second distal phalanx flexes, usually under pressure from hallux valgus displacement. This causes a painful corn on the back of the interphalangeal joint and on the bone end, and a callus on the sole of the foot, both of which make walking painful. Hammer toe may be mild or severe, and can affect one toe or all five, as in clawfoot (which also causes a very high arch).

Hammer toe can be congenital (and familial), or acquired from constantly wearing short, narrow shoes, which put pressure on the end of the long toe. Acquired hammer toe is commonly bilateral and often develops in children who rapidly outgrow shoes and socks.

In young children, or adults with early deformity, repeated foot manipulation and splinting of the affected toe relieve discomfort and may correct the deformity. Other treatment includes protection of protruding joints with felt pads, corrective footwear (open-toed shoes and sandals, or special shoes that conform to the shape of the foot), the use of a metatarsal arch support, and exercises, such as passive manual stretching of the tight proximal interphalangeal joint. Severe deformity requires surgical fusion of the flexed proximal interphalangeal joint in a straight position.

After surgery, the toe is immobilized in its corrected position one of two ways: with a soft compression dressing (which may cover the entire foot or just the great toe and the second toe, which serves as a splint); or with a short cast (such as a light slipper spica cast).

The patient may need crutches or controlled weight-bearing. Depending on their doctors' orders, some patients walk on their heels a few days after surgery; others must wait 4 to 6 weeks to bear weight on the affected foot. Supportive treatment may include physical therapy, such as warm compresses, soaks, and exercises, and analgesics to relieve pain and stiffness.

Additional considerations

Before surgery, the hospital staff member must obtain a patient history and assess the neurovascular status of the foot (temperature, color, sensation, blanching sign). If necessary, the patient should be taught how to walk with crutches.

After bunionectomy, the staff member should:
• apply ice to reduce swelling, and increase negative venous pressure and reduce edema by supporting the foot with pillows, elevating the foot of the bed, or putting it in a Trendelenburg position.
• record the neurovascular status of the toes, including the patient's ability to move the toes (dressing may inhibit movement), every hour for the first 24 hours, then every 4 hours; report any change in neurovascular status to the surgeon immediately.
• prepare the patient for walking by having him dangle his foot over the side of the bed for a short time before he gets up, allowing a gradual increase in venous pressure; supervise the patient in using crutches, if appropriate, and make sure this skill is mastered before discharge; make sure the patient has a proper cast shoe or boot to protect the cast or dressing.
• before discharge, instruct the patient to limit activities, to rest frequently with feet elevated, to elevate his feet whenever he feels pain or has edema, and to wear wide-toed shoes and sandals after the dressings are removed.
• teach proper foot care, such as cleanliness, massages, and cutting toenails straight across to prevent ingrown nails and infection.
• suggest exercises to do at home to strengthen foot muscles, such as standing at the edge of a step on the heel, then raising and inverting the top of the foot.
• stress the importance of follow-up care and prompt medical attention for painful bunions, corns, and calluses.

Kyphosis
(Roundback)

Kyphosis is an anteroposterior curving of the spine that causes a bowing of the back, commonly at the thoracic, but sometimes at the sacral, level. Normally, the spine displays some convexity, but excessive thoracic kyphosis is pathologic. Kyphosis occurs in children and adults.

Causes and incidence

Congenital kyphosis is rare but usually severe, with resultant cosmetic deformity, reduced pulmonary function, and paraplegia.

Adolescent kyphosis (Scheuermann's disease, juvenile kyphosis, vertebral epiphysitis), the most common form of this disorder, may result from growth retardation or a vascular disturbance in the vertebral epiphysis (usually at the thoracic level) during periods of rapid growth, or from congenital deficiency in the thickness of the vertebral plates. Other causes include infection, inflammation, aseptic necrosis, and disk degeneration. The subsequent stress of weight-bearing on the compromised vertebrae may result in the thoracic hump often seen in adolescents with kyphosis. Symptomatic adolescent kyphosis is more prevalent in girls than in boys, and occurs most often between ages 12 and 16.

Adult kyphosis (adult roundback) may result from aging and associated degeneration of intervertebral disks, atrophy, and osteoporotic collapse of the vertebrae; from endocrine disorders, such as hyperparathyroidism, Cushing's disease, and prolonged steroid therapy. Adult kyphosis may also result from conditions such as arthritis, Paget's disease, polio, compression fracture of the thoracic vertebrae, metastatic tumor, plasma cell myeloma, or tuberculosis. In both children and adults, kyphosis may also result from poor posture.

Disk lesions called Schmorl's nodes may develop in anteroposterior curving of the spine and are localized protrusions of nuclear material through the cartilage plates and into the spongy bone of the vertebral bodies. If the anterior portions of the cartilage are destroyed, bridges of new bone may transverse the intervertebral space, causing ankylosis.

Signs and symptoms

Development of adolescent kyphosis is usually insidious, often occurring after a history of excessive sports activity, and may be asymptomatic except for the obvious curving of the back (sometimes more than 70°). In some adolescents, kyphosis may produce mild pain at the apex of the curve (about 50% of patients), fatigue, tenderness or stiffness in the involved area or along the entire spine, and prominent vertebral spinous processes at the lower dorsal and upper lumbar levels, with compensatory increased lumbar lordosis, and hamstring tightness. Rarely, kyphosis may induce neurologic damage: spastic paraparesis secondary to spinal cord compression or herniated nucleus pulposus. In both adolescent and adult forms of kyphosis that is not due to poor posture alone, the spine will not straighten out when the patient assumes a recumbent position.

Adult kyphosis produces a characteristic roundback appearance, possibly associated with pain, weakness of the back, and generalized fatigue. Unlike the adolescent form, adult kyphosis rarely produces local tenderness, except in senile osteoporosis with recent compression fracture.

Diagnosis

Physical examination reveals curvature of the thoracic spine in varying degrees of severity. X-rays may show vertebral wedging, Schmorl's nodes, irregular end plates, and possibly, mild scoliosis of 10° to 20°. Adolescent kyphosis must be distinguished from tuberculosis and other inflammatory or neoplastic diseases that cause vertebral collapse; the severe pain, bone destruction, or systemic symptoms associated with these diseases rule out a diagnosis of kyphosis. Other sites of bone disease, primary sites of malignancy, and infection must also be evaluated, possibly through vertebral biopsy.

Treatment

For kyphosis caused by poor posture alone, treatment may consist of therapeutic exercises, bed rest on a firm mattress (with or without traction), and a Milwaukee brace to straighten the kyphotic curve until spinal growth is complete. Corrective exercises include pelvic tilt to decrease lumbar lordosis, hamstring stretch to overcome muscle contractures, and thoracic hyperextension to flatten the kyphotic curve. These exercises may be performed in or out of the brace. Lateral X-rays taken every 4 months evaluate correction. Gradual weaning from the brace can begin after maximum correction of the kyphotic curve, vertebral wedging has decreased, and the spine has reached full skeletal maturity. Loss of correction indicates that weaning from the brace has been too rapid, and time out of the brace is decreased accordingly.

Treatment for both adolescent and adult kyphosis also includes appropriate measures for the underlying cause and, possibly, spinal arthrodesis for relief of symptoms. Although rarely necessary, surgery may be recommended when kyphosis causes neurologic damage or intractable and disabling back pain in a patient with full skeletal maturity. Preoperative measures may include halofemoral traction. Corrective surgery includes a posterior spinal fusion with Harrington rod instrumentation, iliac bone grafting, and plaster immobilization. Anterior spinal fusion followed by immobilization in plaster may be necessary when kyphosis produces a spinal curve greater than 70°.

Additional considerations

Effective management of kyphosis necessitates first-rate supportive care for patients in traction or a Milwaukee brace, skillful patient teaching, and sensitive emotional support.

• The adolescent with kyphosis caused by poor posture alone must know the prescribed therapeutic exercises and the fundamentals of good posture. Bed rest may help when pain is severe, as will use of a firm mattress, preferably with a bed board. If the patient needs a brace, he should understand its purpose and how and when to wear it. He should also know good skin care, including not using lotions, ointments, or powders where the brace contacts the skin. Only the doctor or orthotist should adjust the brace.

• If corrective surgery is needed, the patient must understand all preoperative tests thoroughly, as well as the need for postoperative traction or casting, if applicable. After surgery, neurovascular status must be checked every 2 to 4 hours for the first 48 hours, with any changes reported immediately. The patient requires frequent turning, using the logrolling technique.

• The patient may need pain medication every 3 or 4 hours for the first 48 hours. Blood product replacement may be ordered. Fluid intake and output requires accurate monitoring, including urine specific gravity. A nasogastric tube and a Foley catheter may be inserted; a rectal tube may also be necessary if paralytic ileus causes abdominal distention.

• The patient will need meticulous skin care. The skin at the cast edges should be checked several times a day; heel and elbow protectors can help prevent skin breakdown. Antiembolism stockings should be removed at least three times a day for at least 30 minutes and dressings changed as ordered.

• The adolescent patient is likely to exhibit mood changes and periods of depression. Hospital staff members should maintain communication, and offer frequent encouragement and reassurance about progress.

• Removal of sutures and application of

a new cast is usually done about 10 days after surgery. The patient should engage in gradual ambulation (often with the use of a tilt-table in the physical therapy department). At discharge, the patient will need detailed, written cast care instructions. He should immediately report pain, burning, skin breakdown, loss of feeling, tingling, numbness, or cast odor, and any illness (especially abdominal pain or vomiting). He must drink plenty of liquids to avoid constipation. Home visits by a social worker or home care nurse may be needed.

Herniated Disk

(Ruptured or slipped disk, herniated nucleus pulposus)

Herniated disk occurs when all or part of the nucleus pulposus—the soft, mucoid, central portion of an intervertebral disk—is forced through the disk's weakened or torn outer ring (anulus fibrosus). When this happens, the extruded disk may impinge on spinal nerve roots as they exit from the spinal canal or on the spinal cord itself, resulting in back pain and other signs of nerve root irritation. Herniated disk usually occurs in adults (mostly men) under age 45.

Causes
Herniated disks may result from severe trauma or strain, or may be related to intervertebral joint degeneration. In the elderly, whose disks have begun to degenerate from aging, even minor trauma may cause herniation. Herniation usually occurs in the lumbar and lumbosacral regions, but may occur anywhere along the spine. Patients with a congenitally small lumbar spinal canal or with osteophyte formation along the vertebrae may be more susceptible to nerve root compression with a herniated disk and thus more likely to develop acute neurologic symptoms.

Signs and symptoms
The overriding symptom of herniated disk is severe low back pain, which may radiate to the buttocks, legs, and feet, usually unilaterally. When herniation follows trauma, the pain may begin suddenly, subside in a few days, then recur at shorter intervals and with progressive intensity. Sciatic pain follows, beginning as a dull pain in the buttocks. Valsalva's maneuver, coughing, sneezing, or bending intensifies the pain, which is often accompanied by muscle spasms. Herniated disk may also cause sensory and motor loss in the area innervated by the compressed spinal nerve root, and in later stages, weakness and atrophy of leg muscles.

Diagnosis
Obtaining a careful patient history is vital, since the mechanisms that intensify disk pain are diagnostically significant. The straight-leg–raising test and its variants are perhaps the best tests for herniated disk. For the straight-leg–raising test, the patient lies supine while the examiner places one hand on the patient's ilium, to stabilize the pelvis, and the other hand under the ankle, then slowly raises the patient's leg. The test is positive only if the patient complains of posterior leg (sciatic) pain, not back pain. In LeSegue's test, the patient lies flat while the thigh and knee are flexed to a 90° angle. Resistance and pain, as well as loss of ankle or knee-jerk reflex, indicate spinal root compression.

X-rays of the spine are essential but may not diagnose herniated disk, since marked disk prolapse can be present despite a normal X-ray. CAT scan may diagnose herniated disk in a patient who has not had previous back surgery. A thorough check of the patient's peripheral vascular status—including posterior tibial and dorsalis pedis pulses, and skin temperature of extremities—helps rule out ischemic disease, another cause of leg pain or numbness. After physical examination and X-rays, myelography provides the most specific diagnostic information, showing spinal compression by herniated disk material.

Treatment

If the patient's neurologic status permits, treatment is initially conservative, and consists of several weeks of bed rest (possibly with pelvic traction if the pain is severe), heat applications, and an exercise program. Aspirin reduces inflammation and edema at the site of injury; rarely, corticosteroids, such as dexamethasone, may be prescribed for the same purpose. Muscle relaxants, especially diazepam or methocarbamol, also may be beneficial.

A herniated disk that fails to respond to conservative treatment may necessitate surgery. The most common procedure, laminectomy, involves excision of a portion of the lamina and removal of the protruding disk (nucleus pulposus). If laminectomy doesn't alleviate pain and disability, a spinal fusion may be necessary to overcome segmental instability. Laminectomy and spinal fusion are sometimes performed concurrently to stabilize the spine.

Although still under investigation, chemonucleolysis—injection of the enzyme chymopapin directly into the disk to dissolve prolapsed tissue—is a possible alternative to laminectomy.

Additional considerations

Herniated disk requires supportive care, careful patient teaching, and strong emotional support to help the patient cope with the discomfort and frustration of chronic low back pain. The health care professional should:

• question the patient carefully, if he requires myelography, about allergies to iodides, iodine-containing substances, or seafood, since such allergies may indicate sensitivity to the test's radiopaque dye; reinforce the doctor's explanation of the need for this test, and tell the patient to expect some pain; assure him that he'll receive a sedative before the test, if needed, to keep him as calm and comfortable as possible; urge the patient after the test to remain supine in bed and drink plenty of fluids; monitor intake and output; watch for allergic reaction to the dye.

• watch for any deterioration in neurologic status during conservative treatment (especially during the first 24 hours after admission), which may indicate an urgent need for surgery; use antiembolism stockings, as prescribed, and encourage the patient to move his legs, as allowed; provide high-topped sneakers to prevent footdrop; work closely with the physical therapy department to ensure a consistent regimen of leg- and back-strengthening exercises; give plenty of fluids to prevent renal stasis, and remind the patient to cough, deep breathe, and use blow bottles or an incentive spirometer to preclude pulmonary complications; provide good skin care; assess for bowel function; use a fracture bedpan for the patient on complete bed rest.

• enforce bed rest, after laminectomy or spinal fusion, as ordered; check the blood drainage system (Hemovac) tubing frequently, if applicable, for kinks and a secure vacuum; empty the Hemovac at the end of each shift, and record the amount and color of drainage; report colorless moisture on dressings (possible CSF leakage) or excessive drainage immediately; observe neurovascular status of legs (color, motion, temperature, sensation).

• urge the patient during the immediate postoperative period to remain supine to prevent any pressure on the involved vertebrae; check for bowel sounds and abdominal distention; use logrolling technique to turn the patient; administer analgesics, as ordered, especially 30 minutes before initial attempts at sitting or walking; give the patient assistance—preferably with a coworker—during his first attempt to walk; provide a straight-backed chair for prolonged sitting.

• teach the patient who has undergone spinal fusion how to wear a brace; assist with straight-leg–raising and toe-pointing exercises, as ordered; teach proper body mechanics before discharge—bending at the knees and hips (never at the waist), standing straight, carrying objects close to the body; advise the patient to lie down when tired and to sleep on his side (never on the abdomen) on an extra-firm mattress or a bed board; urge maintenance of proper weight to prevent lordosis caused by obesity.

• make sure, before chemonucleolysis, that the patient is not allergic to meat tenderizers (chymopapain is a similar substance) or radiopaque dyes (such allergies contraindicate the use of this enzyme, and severe anaphylaxis may result from its administration to a sensitive patient); after chemonucleolysis, enforce bed rest, as ordered; administer analgesics and apply heat, as needed; urge the patient to cough and deep breathe; assist with special exercises, and tell the patient to continue these exercises after discharge.

• tell the patient who must receive a muscle relaxant of possible side effects, especially drowsiness; warn him to avoid activities that require alertness until he has built up a tolerance to the drug's sedative effects.

• provide emotional support; try to cheer the patient during periods of frustration and depression; assure him of his progress, and offer encouragement.

Scoliosis

Scoliosis is a lateral curvature of the spine that may be found in the thoracic, lumbar, or thoracolumbar spinal segment. The curve may be convex to the right (more common in thoracic curves) or to the left (more common in lumbar curves). Rotation of the vertebral column around its axis occurs and may cause rib cage deformity. Scoliosis is often associated with kyphosis (humpback) and lordosis (swayback).

Causes
Scoliosis may be functional or structural. *Functional (postural) scoliosis* usually results from poor posture or a discrepancy in leg lengths, not fixed deformity of the spinal column. In *structural scoliosis,* curvature results from a deformity of the vertebral bodies. Structural scoliosis may be:

• *congenital:* usually related to a congenital defect, such as wedge vertebrae, fused ribs or vertebrae, or hemivertebrae

• *paralytic or musculoskeletal:* develops several months after asymmetric paralysis of the trunk muscles due to polio, cerebral palsy, or muscular dystrophy

• *idiopathic (the most common form):* may be transmitted as an autosomal dominant or multifactoral trait. This form appears in a previously straight spine, during the growing years.

Idiopathic scoliosis can be classified as *infantile,* which affects mostly male infants between birth and age 3, and causes left thoracic and right lumbar curves; *juvenile,* which affects both sexes between ages 4 and 10, and causes varying types of curvature; or *adolescent,* which generally affects girls between age 10 and achievement of skeletal maturity, and causes varying types of curvature.

Signs and symptoms
The most common curve in functional or structural scoliosis arises in the thoracic segment, with convexity to the right, and compensatory curves in the cervical segment above and the lumbar segment below, both with convexity to the left. As the spine curves laterally, compensatory curves (S curves) develop to maintain body balance and mark the deformity. Scoliosis rarely produces subjective symptoms until it's well estab-

---

PARENT TEACHING AID

How to Detect Scoliosis

To check your child for scoliosis—abnormal curvature of the spine—perform this simple test. First, have your child remove her shirt and stand up straight. Then look at her back, and answer these questions:

• Is one shoulder higher than the other, or is one shoulder blade more prominent?
• When the child's arms hang loosely at her sides, does one arm swing away from the body more than the other?
• Is one hip higher or more prominent than the other?
• Does the child seem to tilt to one side?

Then, ask your child to bend forward, with arms hanging down and palms together at knee level. Can you see a hump on the back at the ribs or near the waist?

If your answer to any of these questions is "yes," notify your doctor. Your child needs careful evaluation for scoliosis.

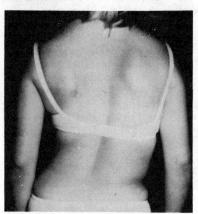

Patient shown above demonstrates the obvious effects of scoliosis. Notice this patient tilts to the right; her left hip is higher than her right hip; her right shoulder is higher than her left shoulder; and she holds her right arm further from her body than her left arm.

This parent teaching aid is intended for distribution to patients by doctors and nurses.
It should not be used without a doctor's approval.

---

lished; when symptoms do occur, they include backache, fatigue, and dyspnea. Since many teenagers are shy about their bodies, their parents suspect that something is wrong only after they notice uneven hemlines, pantlegs that appear unequal in length, or subtle physical signs like one hip appearing higher than the other. Untreated scoliosis may result in pulmonary insufficiency (curvature may decrease lung capacity), back pain, degenerative arthritis of the spine, disk disease, and sciatica.

Diagnosis

Anterior, posterior, and lateral spinal X-rays, taken with the patient standing upright and bending, confirm scoliosis and determine the degree of curvature (Cobb method) and

flexibility of the spine. Physical examination reveals unequal shoulder heights, elbow levels, and heights of the iliac crests. Muscles on the convex side of the curve may be rounded; those on the concave side, flattened, producing asymmetry of paraspinal muscles.

Treatment

The severity of the deformity and potential spine growth determine appropriate treatment, which may include close observation, exercise, a brace (for example, Milwaukee brace), surgery, or a combination of these. To be most effective, treatment should begin early, when spinal deformity is still subtle.

A curve of less than 25° is considered mild and is monitored by spinal X-rays and a physical examination every 3 months. An exercise program that includes sit-up pelvic tilts, hyperextension of the spine, pushups, and breathing exercises may strengthen the torso muscles and prevent progression of the curve. A heel lift may be helpful.

A curve of 30° to 50° requires spinal exercises and a brace. Usually, a brace halts progression in about 90% of patients but doesn't reverse established curvature. The Milwaukee brace consists of a leather or plastic pelvic girdle that holds one anterior and two posterior metal uprights connected to a neck ring. This brace can be adjusted as the patient grows and is worn until bone growth is complete (usually 1 to 4 years, depending on when treatment begins).

A curve of 60° or more requires surgery (spinal fusion), since a lateral curve continues to progress at the rate of 1° a year even after skeletal maturity.

Most spinal fusions require preoperative immobilization in a localizer cast (Risser cast) for 3 to 6 months. However, some surgeons prescribe Cotrel dynamic traction for 7 to 10 days for preoperative preparation. This traction consists of a belt-pulley-weight system. While in traction, the patient should exercise for 10 minutes every hour, increasing muscle strength while keeping the vertebral column immobile. Such exercise helps prevent cast syndrome.

Surgery corrects lateral curvature by posterior spinal fusion and internal stabilization with a Harrington rod. A distraction rod on the concave side of the curve "jacks" the spine into a straight position and provides an internal splint. An alternative procedure, anterior spinal fusion with Dwyer instrumentation, corrects curvature with vertebral staples and an anterior stabilizing cable. Postoperatively, periodic checkups are required for several months to monitor stability of the correction.

Additional considerations

Scoliosis often affects adolescent girls, who are likely to find limitations on their activities and treatment with orthopedic appliances distressing. Therefore, they need special emotional support, along

CAST SYNDROME

Cast syndrome is a serious complication that sometimes follows spinal surgery and application of a body cast. Characterized by nausea, abdominal pressure, and vague abdominal pain, cast syndrome probably results from hyperextension of the spine. Hyperextension of the spine accentuates lumbar lordosis, with compression of the third portion of the duodenum between the superior mesenteric artery anteriorly, and the aorta and vertebral column posteriorly. High intestinal obstruction produces nausea, vomiting, and ischemic infarction of the mesentery.

After removal of the cast, treatment includes decompression and removal of gastric contents with a nasogastric tube and suction. The patient is given I.V. fluids and nothing by mouth. Antiemetics should be given sparingly, since they may mask symptoms of cast syndrome. Surgery may be required to release the ligament of Treitz, which attaches to the fourth portion of the duodenum. Untreated cast syndrome may be fatal.

Patients who are discharged in body jackets, localized casts, or high hip spica casts must be taught to recognize and immediately report cast syndrome, which may develop as late as several weeks or months after application of the cast.

with meticulous skin and cast care, and patient teaching. Many hospital staffs include a physical therapist, a social worker, and an orthotist (orthopedic appliance specialist) who will help in that care.

If the patient needs a Milwaukee brace, she should:
• know what the brace does and how to care for it (how to check the screws for tightness and pad the uprights to prevent excessive wear on clothing); wear loose-fitting, oversized clothes for greater comfort.
• wear the brace 23 hours a day and remove it only for bathing and exercise; lie down and rest several times a day, while she's still adjusting to the brace.

COBB METHOD FOR MEASURING ANGLE OF CURVATURE

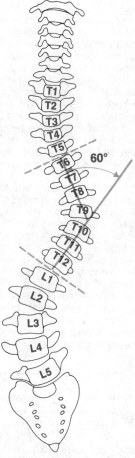

60°

The Cobb method measures the angle of curvature in scoliosis. The top vertebra in the curve (T6 in the illustration) is the uppermost vertebra whose upper face tilts toward the curve's concave side. The bottom vertebra in the curve (T12) is the lowest vertebra whose lower face tilts toward the curve's concave side. The angle at which perpendicular lines drawn from the upper face of the top vertebra and the lower face of the bottom vertebra intersect is the angle of the curve.

• use a soft mattress if a firm one is uncomfortable.

• prevent skin breakdown by not using lotions, ointments, or powders on areas where the brace contacts the skin, and instead, using rubbing alcohol or tincture of benzoin to toughen the skin; know proper care techniques to keep the skin dry and clean; wear a snug T-shirt under the brace.

• increase activities gradually and avoid vigorous sports; know the importance of conscientiously performing prescribed exercises; swim during the 1 hour out of the brace but *never* dive.

• learn to turn her whole body, instead of just her head, when looking to the side; make reading easier by holding the book at eye level so she can look straight ahead at it instead of down (if she finds this difficult, she should get prism glasses).

If the patient needs traction or a cast before surgery, the hospital staff member caring for her should:

• explain the procedures to the patient and family, knowing that application of a body cast can be traumatic, since it's done on a special frame and the patient's head and face are covered throughout the procedure.

• check the skin around the cast edge daily; keep the cast clean and dry, and edges of the cast petaled (padded); warn the patient not to insert or let anything get under the cast or allow it to get wet, and to immediately report cracks in the cast, pain, burning, skin breakdown, numbness, or odor.

• assure the patient and family that she'll receive adequate medication to control pain postoperatively; check sensation, movement, color, and blood supply in all extremities to detect neurovascular deficit, a serious complication following spinal surgery.

After corrective surgery, the hospital staffer should:

• check neurovascular status every 2 to 4 hours for the first 48 hours; then several times a day; logroll the patient often to provide stimulation.

• measure intake, output, and urine

specific gravity to monitor effects of blood loss, which is often substantial.

• monitor abdominal distention and bowel sounds.

• encourage deep-breathing exercises to avoid pulmonary complications.

• medicate for pain, especially before any activity.

• promote active range-of-motion arm exercises to help maintain muscle strength, knowing that any exercise, even brushing the hair or teeth, is helpful; encourage the patient to perform quadriceps-setting, calf-pumping, and active range-of-motion exercises of ankles and feet.

• watch for skin breakdown and signs of cast syndrome; teach the patient how to recognize these signs.

• remove antiembolism stockings for at least 30 minutes daily.

• offer emotional support to help prevent depression that may result from altered body image and immobility; encourage the patient to wear her own clothes, wash her hair, and use makeup. If the patient is being discharged with a Harrington rod and cast and must have bed rest, a social worker and a visiting nurse should provide home care. Before discharge, the patient needs to know about activity limitations and understand the importance of following them. In schools children should be screened routinely for scoliosis during physical examinations.

MUSCLE & CONNECTIVE TISSUE

Lupus Erythematosus

A chronic inflammatory disorder of the connective tissues, lupus erythematosus appears in two forms: discoid lupus erythematosus *(DLE), which affects only the skin, and* systemic lupus erythematosus *(SLE), which usually affects multiple organ systems, as well as the skin, and can be fatal. Like rheumatoid arthritis, SLE is characterized by recurring remissions and exacerbations. The annual incidence of SLE averages 75 cases per 1 million people. It strikes women 8 times as often as men, increasing to 15 times as often during childbearing years. SLE occurs worldwide but is most prevalent among Asians and Black Americans. Exacerbations are more common during the spring and summer. Prognosis improves with early detection and treatment but remains poor for patients who develop cardiovascular, renal, or neurologic complications, or severe bacterial infections.*

Causes

The exact cause of SLE remains a mystery, but three theories have been postulated. The first holds that SLE is an abnormal reaction of the body to its own tissues, caused by a breakdown in the autoimmune system. According to this theory, the body produces antibodies, such as antinuclear antibody (ANA), which form antigen-antibody complexes that "poison" cells, suppressing the body's normal immunity.

The second theory suggests that certain predisposing factors make a person susceptible to SLE. Physical or mental stress, streptococcal or viral infections, exposure to sunlight or ultraviolet light, immunization, and pregnancy may all affect the development of this disease. Because SLE has been found in certain families for several generations, genetic predisposition is also suspected.

The third theory proposes that SLE may be triggered or aggravated by certain drugs—procainamide, hydralazine, anticonvulsants, and less frequently, penicillins, sulfa drugs, and oral contraceptives.

SIGNS OF SYSTEMIC LUPUS ERYTHEMATOSUS

Diagnosing systemic lupus erythematosus is far from easy, because SLE often mimics other diseases; symptoms may be vague and vary greatly from patient to patient. For these reasons, the American Rheumatism Association has issued a list of criteria for classification of SLE, to be used primarily for consistency in epidemiologic surveys. Usually, four or more of these symptoms are present some time during the course of the disease:

• nondeforming arthritis
• facial erythema (butterfly rash)
• photosensitivity
• oral or nasopharyngeal ulcerations
• alopecia
• discoid lupus erythematosus (DLE)
• pleuritis or pericarditis
• Raynaud's phenomenon
• convulsions or psychoses
• hemolytic anemia, leukopenia, or thrombocytopenia
• positive ANA or LE cell test
• chronic false positive serologic test for syphilis
• profuse proteinuria (3.5 g/day)
• excessive cellular casts in the urine.

Permission to quote the Fourteen Preliminary Criteria for the Diagnosis of Systemic Lupus Erythematosus from *Primer on the Rheumatic Diseases*, pp. 139-140 granted by the American Rheumatism Association.

Signs and symptoms

Primary clinical features include nondeforming arthritis, a characteristic "butterfly rash," and photosensitivity. The first and most common symptom is joint pain and stiffness, which is rarely deforming and usually involves the hands, feet, and large joints. Joints may show redness, warmth, tenderness, and synovial effusions, with associated muscle weakness and tenderness.

Perhaps the most distinctive feature of SLE is the "butterfly rash" that appears in a malar distribution across the nose and cheeks (in about 40% of patients). This rash may range from malar erythema to discoid lesions (plaques), most commonly on the face, neck, and scalp. Similar rashes may appear on other body surfaces, especially exposed areas. Ultraviolet rays often provoke or aggravate skin eruptions. Vasculitis can occur (especially in the digits), possibly leading to infarctive lesions, necrotic leg ulcers, or digital gangrene. Raynaud's phenomenon appears in about 20% of patients. Patchy alopecia and ulcers of the mucous membranes are common.

Constitutional symptoms of SLE include aching, malaise, fatigue, low-grade or spiking fever, chills, anorexia, and weight loss. Lymph node enlargement (diffuse or local, and nontender), abdominal pain, nausea, vomiting, diarrhea, and constipation may occur. Women may experience irregular menstrual periods or amenorrhea, particularly during the active phase of this disease.

About 50% of SLE patients develop signs of cardiopulmonary abnormalities, such as pleuritis, pericarditis, and dyspnea. Myocarditis, endocarditis, tachycardia, parenchymal infiltrates, and pneumonitis may occur. Renal effects that may progress to total kidney failure include hematuria, proteinuria, urine sediment, and cellular casts. Urinary tract infections may result from heightened susceptibility to infection. Convulsive disorders and mental dysfunction may indicate neurologic damage. CNS involvement may produce emotional instability, psychosis, and organic brain syndrome. Headaches, irritability, and depression are especially common.

Diagnosis

Appropriate diagnostic tests for patients with SLE include a CBC with differential, which may show anemia and decreased WBC; platelet count, which may be decreased; ESR, which is often elevated; and serum electrophoresis, which may show hypergammaglobulinemia.

Specific tests for SLE include:
• ANA, anti-DNA, and lupus erythematosus (LE) cell tests: positive in most patients with active SLE; since the anti-DNA test is rarely positive in other conditions, it's the most specific test for SLE.

However, if the patient is in remission, anti-DNA may be reduced or absent. (This test correlates well with disease activity, especially with renal involvement, and helps monitor response to therapy.)

• *urine studies:* may show RBCs and WBCs, urine casts and sediment, and significant protein loss (more than 3.5 g/24 hours). Decreased serum complement (C3 and C4) levels indicate active disease.

• *chest X-ray:* may show abnormalities with pulmonary involvement.

• *EKG:* may show conduction defect if there is cardiac involvement.

• *kidney biopsy:* determines the extent of renal involvement and stage of the disease.

Treatment

Patients with mild disease require little or no medication. Nonsteroidal, anti-inflammatory compounds, including aspirin, often control arthritic symptoms. Skin lesions need topical treatment. Corticosteroid creams, such as flurandrenolide, are recommended for early plaques; fluorinated steroids are recommended for acute lesions; nonfluorinated, for prolonged use.

Refractory skin lesions are treated with intralesional corticosteroids or antimalarials, such as hydroxychloroquine and chloroquine. Because hydroxychloroquine and chloroquine can cause retinal damage, such treatment requires ophthalmologic examination every 6 months.

Corticosteroids remain the treatment of choice for systemic symptoms of SLE, for acute generalized exacerbations, or for serious disease related to vital organ systems, such as pleuritis, pericarditis, lupus nephritis, vasculitis, and CNS involvement. Initial doses equivalent to 60 mg or more of prednisone often bring noticeable improvement within 48 hours. As soon as symptoms are under control, steroid dosage is tapered down slowly. (Rising serum complement levels and decreasing anti-DNA titers indicate patient response.) Diffuse proliferative glomerulonephritis, a major cause of death

in patients with SLE, requires treatment with large doses of steroids. If renal failure occurs, dialysis or kidney transplant may be necessary.

The photosensitive patient should wear protective clothing (hat, sunglasses, long sleeves, slacks) when out in the sun and use a screening agent containing para-aminobenzoic acid (PABA). Since SLE usually strikes women of childbearing age, questions associated with pregnancy often arise. The best evidence available indicates that a woman with SLE can have a safe, successful pregnancy if she has no renal or neurologic impairment.

Additional considerations

Careful assessment, supportive measures, emotional support, and patient teaching are all important in the health care plan for treating patients with SLE.

• These constitutional symptoms must be watched for: pain or stiffness in the joints, weakness, fever, fatigue, and chills. General patient monitoring includes: watching for dyspnea, chest pain, and any edema of the extremities; noting the size, type, and location of skin lesions; checking urine for

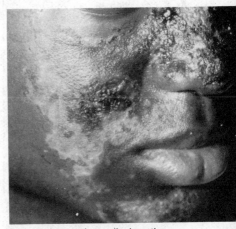

Patient shown above displays the characteristic "butterfly rash" of SLE. Notice the malar distribution, across the nose and cheeks. (This occurs in about 40% of patients.) This rash may vary in severity from malar erythema to discoid lesions (plaques).

DISCOID LUPUS ERYTHEMATOSUS

Discoid lupus erythematosus (DLE) is a benign form of systemic lupus erythematosus (SLE) marked by chronic skin eruptions, which can lead to scarring and permanent disfigurement. About 1 out of 20 patients with DLE later develops SLE. The exact cause of DLE is unknown, but some evidence suggests an autoimmune defect. An estimated 60% of patients with DLE are women in their late 20s or older. This disease is rare in children.

DLE lesions are raised, red, scaling plaques, with follicular plugging and central atrophy. The raised edges and sunken centers give them a coin-like appearance. Although these lesions can appear anywhere on the body, they usually erupt on the face, scalp, ears, neck, and arms, or any part of the body that's exposed to sunlight. Such lesions can resolve completely or may cause hypo- or hyperpigmentation, atrophy, and scarring. Facial plaques sometimes assume the butterfly pattern characteristic of SLE. Hair tends to become brittle or may fall out in patches.

As a rule, patient history and the appearance of the rash itself are diagnostic. LE cell test is positive in less than 10% of patients. Skin biopsy reveals immunoglobulins or complement components. SLE must be ruled out.

Patients with DLE should avoid prolonged exposure to the sun, fluorescent lighting, or reflected sunlight. They should wear protective clothing, use sunscreening agents, engage in outdoor activities only in the early morning or late afternoon, (before 10 a.m. or after 2 p.m.) and report any changes in the lesions. Drug treatment consists of topical, intralesional, or systemic medication, as in SLE.

• The patient will need a balanced diet. Renal involvement may mandate a low-sodium, low-protein diet.

• The patient must get plenty of rest. Diagnostic tests and procedures should be scheduled to allow this. The patient should understand all tests and procedures. She should know that several blood samples are needed initially, then periodically, to monitor progress.

• Heat packs will help relieve joint pain and stiffness. Also, regular exercise will help maintain full range of motion and prevent contractures. The patient should be taught range-of-motion exercises, as well as body alignment and postural techniques. She may need physical therapy and occupational counseling.

During hospitalization, the hospital staff member should:

• explain the expected benefit of prescribed medications, and watch for side effects, especially when the patient is taking high doses of corticosteroids.

• monitor vital signs, intake and output, weight, and laboratory reports closely; check pulse rates regularly; observe for orthopnea; check stools and gastrointestinal secretions for blood; note and report any nosebleed.

• watch for hypertension, weight gain, and other signs of renal involvement.

• note signs of neurologic damage: personality change, paranoid or psychotic behavior, ptosis, or diplopia; take seizure precautions; if Raynaud's phenomenon is present, warm and protect the patient's hands and feet.

• support the female patient's self-image by offering helpful cosmetic tips, such as using of hypoallergenic makeup, and by referring her to a hairdresser who specializes in scalp disorders; encourage her to take an interest in her appearance.

• advise the patient to purchase medications in quantity, if possible; warn against miracle drugs for relief of arthritic symptoms.

Help and counseling are available from the Lupus Foundation of America and the Arthritis Foundation.

hematuria, scalp for hair loss, and skin and mucous membranes for petechiae, bleeding, ulceration, pallor, and bruising. All symptoms must be reported promptly.

Tendinitis and Bursitis

Tendinitis is a painful inflammation of tendons and of tendon-muscle attachments to bone, usually in the shoulder rotator cuff, hip, Achilles tendon, or hamstring. Bursitis is a painful inflammation of one or more of the bursae—closed sacs that are lubricated with small amounts of synovial fluid which facilitate the motion of muscles and tendons over bony prominences. Bursitis usually occurs in the subdeltoid, olecranon, trochanteric, calcaneal, or prepatellar bursae.

Causes and incidence

Tendinitis commonly results from trauma (such as strain during sports activity), another musculoskeletal disorder (rheumatic diseases, congenital defects), postural misalignment, abnormal body development, or hypermobility.

Bursitis usually occurs in middle age, and results from recurring trauma that stresses or pressures a joint or from an inflammatory joint disease (rheumatoid arthritis, gout). Chronic bursitis follows attacks of acute bursitis or repeated trauma and infection. Septic bursitis may result from wound infection or from bacterial invasion of skin overlying the bursa.

Signs and symptoms

The patient with tendinitis of the shoulder complains of restricted shoulder movement, especially abduction, and localized pain, which is most severe at night and often interferes with sleep. The pain extends from the acromion (the shoulder's highest point) to the deltoid muscle insertion, predominately in the so-called painful arc—that is, when the patient abducts his arm between 50° and 130°. Fluid accumulation causes swelling. In calcific tendinitis, calcium deposits in the tendon cause proximal weakness and, if calcium erodes into adjacent bursae, acute calcific bursitis.

In bursitis, fluid accumulation in the bursae causes irritation, inflammation, sudden or gradual pain, and limited movement. Other symptoms vary according to the affected site. Subdeltoid bursitis impairs arm abduction; prepatellar bursitis (housemaid's knee) produces pain when the patient climbs stairs; hip bursitis makes crossing the legs painful.

Diagnosis

In tendinitis, X-rays may be normal at first but later show bony fragments, osteophyte sclerosis, or calcium deposits. Arthrography is usually normal, with occasional small irregularities on the undersurface of the tendon. Diagnosis of tendinitis must rule out other causes of shoulder pain, such as myocardial infarction, cervical spondylosis, and tendon rupture. Significantly, in tendinitis, heat aggravates shoulder pain; in other painful joint disorders, heat usually provides relief.

Localized pain and inflammation, and a history of unusual strain or injury 2 to 3 days before onset of pain are the bases for diagnosing bursitis. During early stages, X-rays are usually normal, except in calcific bursitis, where X-rays show calcium deposits.

Treatment

Treatment to relieve pain includes resting the joint (by immobilization with a sling, splint, or cast), systemic analgesics, or local injection of an anesthetic and corticosteroids to reduce inflammation. A mixture of a corticosteroid and an anesthetic, such as lidocaine, generally provides immediate pain relief. Extended-release injections of a corticosteroid, such as triamcinolone or prednisolone, offer longer pain relief. Until the patient is free of pain and able to perform range-of-motion exercises easily, treatment also includes oral anti-

PATIENT TEACHING AID

Exercises for Shoulder Pain

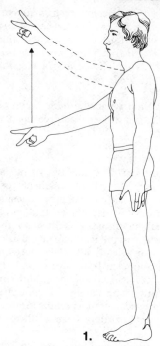

1.

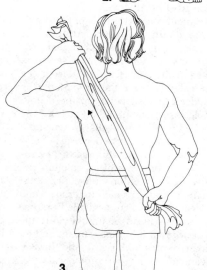

2.

1. Stand facing a wall an arm's length away. Slowly, walk your fingers up the wall as high as you can. Then walk your fingers back down.

2. Then stand at a right angle to the wall and repeat the exercise. As your hand gets higher, step closer to the wall to allow your shoulder the maximum range of motion.

3. Grasp the ends of a large bath towel behind your back. Then simulate the motion of drying your back, reaching and pulling as far as possible. Reverse the position of your arms and repeat the exercise.

3.

inflammatory agents, such as phenylbutazone and indomethacin. Short-term analgesics include codeine, propoxyphene, acetaminophen with codeine, and occasionally, oxycodone or pentazocine.

Supplementary treatment includes fluid removal by aspiration, physical therapy to preserve motion and prevent frozen joints (improvement usually follows in 1 to 4 weeks), and heat therapy, or for calcific tendinitis, ice packs. Rarely, calcific tendinitis requires surgical removal of calcium deposits. Long-term control of chronic bursitis and tendinitis may require changes in life-style to prevent recurring joint irritation.

Additional considerations

The severity of pain and the range of motion should be determined to allow assessment of subsequent treatment.

The patient should be asked about drug allergies before he is given injections of corticosteroids or local anesthetics.

Prior to intra-articular injection, the patient's skin is scrubbed thoroughly with poloxamer iodine or a comparable solution, and the injection site is shaved, if necessary. After the injection, the area is massaged to ensure penetration through the tissue and joint space. Ice is applied intermittently for about 4 hours to minimize pain. Heat should not be applied to the area for 2 days.

Patient teaching is essential. The patient should be told to:
• take anti-inflammatory agents with milk to minimize gastrointestinal distress, and report any such distress immediately.
• avoid excessive exercise or physical work that stresses the painful joint.
• wear a triangular sling, particularly at night, during the first few days of an attack of subdeltoid bursitis or tendinitis. This will support the arm and protect the shoulder. The sling should be worn so that it doesn't put too much weight on the shoulder. The patient's family will have to know how to pin the sling or how to tie a square knot that will lie flat on the back of the patient's neck. To protect the shoulder during sleep, a splint may be worn instead of a sling. The patient should remove the splint during the day.

To maintain joint mobility and prevent muscle atrophy, the patient should perform exercises or participate in physical therapy when he is free of pain.

Polymyositis and Dermatomyositis

A diffuse, inflammatory myopathy of unknown cause, polymyositis produces symmetrical weakness of striated muscle. This disease usually progresses slowly, with frequent exacerbations and remissions. It's twice as common in women as in men and usually occurs between ages 30 and 60. Prognosis is related to age; the younger the patient, the better the prognosis.

Dermatomyositis occurs when such muscle weakness is accompanied by cutaneous involvement. Although death may result from respiratory infection, heart failure, debilitation due to concurrent malignancy, or side effects of therapy (corticosteroids or immunosuppressives), dermatomyositis—like polymyositis—is usually not fatal. When dermatomyositis is diagnosed in a man over age 40, concurrent malignancy is possible. In dermatomyositis with malignancy, treatment of the malignancy can induce remission of both conditions. Childhood dermatomyositis often progresses rapidly to disabling contractures and muscular atrophy.

Causes and incidence

Polymyositis causes diffuse or focal degeneration of muscle fibers, which are invaded by inflammatory cells (lymphocytes). Regeneration of new cells (basophils, myofibrils) follows invasion.

Predisposing factors include allergic reactions; connective tissue diseases (systemic lupus erythematosus [SLE], scleroderma, rheumatoid arthritis); carcinoma of the lungs, breasts, or other organs; penicillamine administration; or systemic viral infection.

Signs and symptoms

Polymyositis begins acutely or insidiously with muscle weakness, tenderness, and discomfort. It affects proximal muscles (shoulder, pelvic girdle) more often than distal muscles. Muscle weakness makes performance of ordinary activities difficult. The patient has trouble getting up from a chair, combing his hair, reaching into a high cupboard, climbing stairs, or even raising his head from a pillow. Other muscular symptoms include inability to move against resistance, proximal dysphagia (regurgitation of fluid through nose), and dysphonia (nasal voice).

In dermatomyositis, an erythematous rash usually erupts on the face, neck, upper back, chest, arms, and around nail beds. A characteristic heliotropic rash appears on the eyelids, along with periorbital edema. Grotton's papules (violet, flat-topped lesions) may appear on the interphalangeal joints.

Diagnosis

Diagnosis requires muscle biopsy that shows necrosis, degeneration, regeneration, and interstitial chronic lymphocytic infiltration. Appropriate laboratory tests differentiate polymyositis from diseases that cause similar muscular or cutaneous symptoms, such as muscular dystrophy, advanced trichinosis, psoriasis, seborrheic dermatitis, and SLE.

Typical laboratory results in polymyositis include: elevated ESR; elevated WBC; elevated muscle enzymes (CPK, aldolase, SGOT) not attributable to hemolysis of RBCs, or hepatic or other diseases; increased urine creatine (more than 150 mg/24 hours); decreased creatinine; electromyography showing polyphasic, short-duration potentials, fibrillation (positive spike waves), and bizarre, high-frequency, repetitive changes; and positive antinuclear antibodies (ANA).

Treatment

High-dose corticosteroid therapy relieves inflammation and lowers muscle enzyme levels. Within 2 to 6 weeks following treatment, serum muscle enzyme levels return to normal and muscle strength improves, permitting a gradual tapering down of corticosteroid dosage. If the patient responds poorly to corticosteroids, treatment may include cytotoxic or immunosuppressive drugs, such as cyclophosphamide intermittent I.V. or daily P.O. Supportive therapy includes bed rest during the acute phase, range-of-motion exercises to prevent contractures, analgesics and application of heat to relieve painful muscle spasms, and diphenhydramine to relieve dermal itching. Older men with dermatomyositis need thorough assessment for coexisting malignancies.

Additional considerations

• Level of pain, muscular weakness, and range of motion should be assessed daily. Analgesics may be needed.

• If the patient is confined to bed, good skin care can prevent decubitus ulcers. High-topped sneakers and passive range-of-motion exercises at least four times daily will help prevent footdrop and contractures. The patient's family should be taught how to perform these exercises.

• If 24-hour urine collection for creatine/creatinine is necessary, all hospital staff involved must be acquainted with the procedure. They should also know that muscle biopsies must not be taken from an area of recent needle insertion, such as an injection or electromyography site.

• If the patient has a skin rash, scratching it may cause infection. If antipruritic medication, such as diphenhydramine, doesn't relieve severe itching, tepid sponges or compresses may help.

• The patient should be encouraged to feed and dress himself to the best of his

ability, but to ask for help when needed. He should pace his activities to counteract muscle weakness. He will probably be anxious about this. His fear of dependence may be eased if he is given reassurance that any muscle weakness is probably temporary.
• The patient and family will need to understand the disease. They should be prepared for diagnostic procedures and possible side effects of corticosteroid therapy (weight gain, hirsutism, cervicodorsal fat, hypertension, edema, amenorrhea, purplish striae, glycosuria, girdle obesity, moonface, acne, easy bruising). A low-sodium diet will be needed to prevent fluid retention. The steroid-induced weight gain will diminish when the drug is discontinued. The patient must know that he *must not* abruptly discontinue the corticosteroids. Because his own adrenals are suppressed, discontinuance can have serious results.

Epicondylitis
(Tennis elbow, epitrochlear bursitis)

Epicondylitis is inflammation of the forearm extensor supinator tendon fibers at their common attachment to the lateral humeral epicondyle, which produces acute or subacute pain.

Causes and incidence
Epicondylitis probably begins as a partial tear and is common among tennis players or persons whose activities require a forceful grasp, wrist extension against resistance, or frequent rotation of the forearm. Untreated epicondylitis may become disabling.

Signs and symptoms
The initial symptom is elbow pain that gradually worsens and often radiates to the forearm and back of the hand when the patient grasps an object or twists his elbow. Other effects include tenderness over the lateral epicondyle or over the head of the radius, and a weak grasp. Epicondylitis rarely causes local heat, swelling, or restricted range of motion.

Diagnosis
Since X-rays are almost always negative, diagnosis depends on clinical symptoms and a patient history of playing tennis or engaging in similar activities.

Treatment
Treatment aims to relieve pain, usually by local injection of corticosteroid and a local anesthetic, and systemic anti-inflammatory therapy with aspirin or indomethacin. Supportive treatment includes an immobilizing splint from the distal forearm to the elbow, which generally relieves pain in 2 to 3 weeks; heat therapy, such as warm compresses, short wave diathermy, and ultrasound (alone or in combination with diathermy); and physical therapy, such as manipulation and massage to detach the tendon from the chronically inflamed periosteum. A "tennis elbow strap" has helped many patients. If these conservative measures prove ineffective or if the condition recurs, surgical excision of the tendon at the epicondyle may be necessary.

Additional considerations
The health care professional caring for the patient with epicondylitis should: assess the patient's level of pain, range of motion, and sensory function; monitor heat therapy to prevent burns, and evaluate its effectiveness; and advise the patient to take anti-inflammatory drugs with milk to avoid gastrointestinal irritation.
  The health care professional can help insure proper healing of the arm by:
• instructing the patient to get sufficient

rest.
* removing the splint daily, and gently moving the arm to prevent stiffness and contracture.
* suggesting that the patient exercise every 2 to 4 hours while wearing the splint (he should stretch his arm and flex his wrist to the maximum, then press the back of his hand against a wall until he can feel a pull in his forearm, and hold this position for 1 minute).
* advising the patient to warm up for 15 to 20 minutes before sports activity.
* urging the patient to wear an elastic support or splint during any activity that stresses the forearm or elbow.

Progressive Systemic Sclerosis
(Scleroderma)

Progressive systemic sclerosis (PSS) is a diffuse connective tissue disease characterized by fibrotic, degenerative, and occasionally, inflammatory changes in skin, blood vessels, synovium, skeletal muscles, and internal organs. It affects women more frequently than men, especially between ages 30 and 50.

Causes
The cause of PSS is unknown. This disease occurs in two distinctive forms:
* *CREST syndrome:* the more benign form, characterized by calcinosis, Raynaud's phenomenon, esophageal dysfunction, sclerodactyly, and telangiectasia
* *progressively fatal form:* characterized by generalized skin thickening and invasion of internal organ systems.

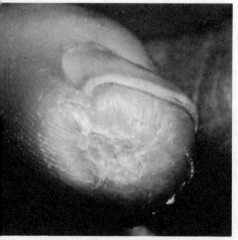

Ulceration of the fingertip occurs as part of Raynaud's phenomenon in the more benign form of progressive systemic sclerosis.

Signs and symptoms
PSS typically begins with Raynaud's phenomenon—blanching, cyanosis, and erythema of the fingers and toes in response to exposure to cold or stress. Progressive resorption of the ends of the phalanges may shorten the fingers. Compromised circulation may cause ulcerations on the tips of the fingers or toes that are difficult to heal and may lead to gangrene. This compromised circulation results from thickening of the intima. In scleroderma, the arterial intima thickens from the normal 1- to 2-cell thickness to many cells, compromising blood flow. Raynaud's phenomenon may precede diagnosis of PSS by months or years.

Later symptoms include pain, stiffness, and swelling of fingers (which appear sausagelike) and joints. Thickening of the skin progresses to taut, shiny skin over the entire hand and forearm. Facial skin also becomes tight and inelastic, causing a masklike appearance (no wrinkles) and "pinching" of the mouth. As tightening progresses, contractures may develop.

Gastrointestinal dysfunction causes frequent reflux, heartburn, the sensation of food sticking behind the breastbone, and bloating after meals, all of which may cause the patient to decrease food intake and lose weight. Other common gastrointestinal complaints include abdominal distention, diarrhea, constipation, and malodorous floating stools.

In advanced disease, cardiac and pulmonary involvement may produce arrhythmia, dyspnea, and pulmonary fibrosis. Renal involvement is usually accompanied by malignant hypertension and renal failure.

Diagnosis
Typical cutaneous and visceral involvement is the basis for diagnosis. Other test results include:
• *blood studies:* mildly elevated ESR and hypergammaglobulinemia
• *urinalysis:* proteinuria, microscopic hematuria, and casts (with renal involvement)
• *positive antinuclear antibody (ANA):* low titer, speckled pattern
• *hand X-rays:* terminal phalangeal tuft resorption, subcutaneous calcification, joint space narrowing and erosion
• *chest X-rays:* bilateral basilar pulmonary fibrosis
• *gastrointestinal X-rays:* distal esophageal hypomotility and stricture, duodenal loop dilation and hypomobility, small bowel malabsorption pattern, and large diverticuli
• *pulmonary function studies:* decreased diffusion and vital capacity
• *EKG:* possible nonspecific abnormalities
• *skin biopsy:* may show changes consistent with the progress of the disease, such as marked thickening of the dermis and occlusive vessel changes.

Treatment
Primary treatment—chemotherapy with immunosuppressives, such as chlorambucil—is merely palliative. Treatment aims to preserve normal body functions. Corticosteroids and colchicine have been used experimentally and seem to stabilize symptoms; D-penicillamine may also be helpful. Blood platelet levels need to be monitored throughout drug and immunosuppressive therapy. Other treatment varies according to symptoms:

PATIENT TEACHING AID

Managing Progressive Systemic Sclerosis
You can minimize the effects of progressive systemic sclerosis by doing the following:
• Report any abnormal bruising, non-healing abrasions or cuts immediately. They may indicate bleeding problems.
• Keep regular appointments with the doctor for periodic laboratory testing to monitor the effects of immunosuppressives.
• Wear warm socks and gloves, and avoid exposure to cold to lessen hand and foot debilitation.
• Minimize digital ulcerations by avoiding burns and cuts, and treating any local infections immediately.
• Use skin-softening lotions, soaps, and bath oils to prevent skin dryness and cracking.
• Eat small, frequent meals. Drink liquids with meals. Chew food slowly and carefully to minimize dysphagia.
• To control heartburn, take an antacid and sit upright for 30 to 45 minutes after each meal.
• Prevent nocturnal esophageal reflux by using additional pillows or raising the head of your bed.

This patient teaching aid is intended for distribution to patients by doctors and nurses. It should not be used without a doctor's approval.

• *Raynaud's phenomenon:* various vasodilators and antihypertensive agents (such as methyldopa, reserpine), intermittent cervical sympathetic blockade, or rarely, thoracic sympathectomy
• *chronic digital ulcerations:* debridement after soaking in half-strength hydrogen peroxide solution. A digital plaster cast immobilizes the affected area, minimizes trauma, and maintains cleanliness
• *esophagitis with stricture:* antacids, a soft, bland diet, and periodic esophageal dilation
• *small-bowel involvement* (diarrhea, malabsorption, weight loss): broad-spectrum antibiotics, such as erythro-

mycin or tetracycline, to counteract bacterial overgrowth in the duodenum and jejunum
• *scleroderma kidney* (with malignant hypertension and impending renal failure): dialysis, antihypertensives, and transplant (rare, because disease may invade new kidney)
• *hand debilitation:* physical therapy to maintain function and promote muscle strength, heat therapy to relieve joint stiffness, and patient teaching to make performance of daily activities easier.

Additional considerations
• Limitation of motion, pain, vital signs, fluid intake and output, respiratory function, and weight should be assessed daily.
• Because of compromised circulation, finger-stick blood tests are contraindicated.

• Air conditioning may aggravate Raynaud's phenomenon.
• The patient and family will need help adjusting to the patient's new body image, and the severe limitations and dependence these changes cause. The patient should avoid fatigue by pacing activities and organizing work schedules to include necessary rest. The patient and family have to accept the fact that this condition is incurable. They should be encouraged to express their feelings, and assisted in setting realistic goals. Getting information about the disease, its treatment, and relevant diagnostic tests will help them cope with their fears and frustrations. Whenever possible, the patient should be encouraged to participate in treatment by measuring his own fluid intake and output, planning his own diet, assisting in dialysis, giving himself heat therapy, and doing prescribed exercises.

Torticollis
(Wryneck)

This neck deformity, in which the sternocleidomastoid neck muscles are spastic or shortened, causes bending of the head to the affected side and rotation of the chin to the opposite side. This disorder may be congenital or acquired. Incidence of congenital (muscular) torticollis is highest in infants after difficult delivery (breech presentation), in firstborn infants, and in girls. Acquired torticollis usually develops during the first 10 years of life.

Causes
Possible causes of congenital torticollis include malposition of the head in utero, prenatal injury, fibroma, interruption of blood supply, or fibrotic rupture of the sternocleidomastoid muscle, with hematoma and scar formation.

The three types of acquired torticollis—acute, spasmodic, and hysterical—have differing causes. The acute form results from muscular damage caused by inflammatory diseases, such as myositis, lymphadenitis, and tuberculosis, and from cervical spinal injuries that produce scar tissue contracture. The spasmodic form results from rhythmic muscle spasms caused by an organic

CNS disorder (probably due to irritation of the nerve root by arthritis or osteomyelitis). Hysterical torticollis is due to a psychogenic inability to control neck muscles.

Signs and symptoms
The first sign of congenital torticollis is often a firm, nontender, palpable enlargement of the sternocleidomastoid muscle that is visible at birth and for several weeks afterward. It slowly regresses during a period of 6 months, although incomplete regression can cause permanent contracture. If the deformity is severe, the infant's face and head flatten from sleeping on the affected side;

this asymmetry gradually worsens. The infant's chin turns away from the side of the shortened muscle, and his head tilts to the shortened side. His shoulder may elevate on the affected side, restricting neck movement.

The first sign of acquired torticollis is usually recurring unilateral stiffness of neck muscles, followed by a drawing sensation and a momentary twitching or contraction that pulls the head to the affected side. This type of torticollis often produces severe neuralgic pain throughout the head and neck.

Diagnosis

A history of painless neck deformity from birth suggests congenital torticollis; gradual onset of painful neck deformity suggests acquired torticollis. However, diagnosis must rule out tuberculosis of the cervical spine, pharyngeal or tonsillar inflammations, subdural hematoma, dislocations and fractures, scoliosis, congenital abnormalities of the cervical spine, rheumatoid arthritis, and osteomyelitis. In acquired torticollis, cervical spine X-rays are negative for bone or joint disease but may reveal an associated disorder (such as tuberculosis, scar tissue formation, or arthritis).

Treatment

Treatment of congenital torticollis aims to stretch the shortened muscle. Nonsurgical treatment includes, for the infant, passive neck stretching and proper positioning during sleep and, for the older child, active stretching exercises. One such exercise would be touching the ear opposite the affected side to the shoulder and touching the chin to the same shoulder.

Surgical correction involves sectioning the sternocleidomastoid muscle; this should be done during preschool years and only if other therapies fail.

Treatment of acquired torticollis aims to correct the underlying cause of the disease. In the acute form, application of heat, cervical traction, and gentle massage may help relieve pain. Psycho-therapy, stretching exercises, and a neck brace may relieve symptoms of the spasmodic and hysterical forms.

Additional considerations

To aid early diagnosis, especially of the congenital type, any suspect infant should be watched for limited movement and his degree of discomfort assessed.

Parents must be taught how to perform stretching exercises with the child. Placing toys or hanging mobiles on the side of the crib opposite the affected side will force the child to move his head and stretch his neck.

• If surgery is necessary, preparation of the patient will include shaving the neck up to the hairline on the affected side.

• After corrective surgery, the patient should be monitored closely for nausea or signs of respiratory complications, especially if he's in cervical traction. Suction equipment must be available to prevent aspiration.

• The patient may be in a cast or in traction day and night or at night only. Meticulous cast care will be necessary. This care includes: monitoring the patient's circulation, sensation, and color around the cast; protecting the cast around the patient's chin and mouth with waterproof material; and checking for skin irritation, pressure areas, or softening of cast pad.

• The patient will need emotional support to relieve his anxiety due to fear, pain, limitations from the brace or traction, and an altered body image. The patient's family will also need help adjusting to these changes.

• Stretching exercises to regain mobility, such as those outlined above, should begin as soon as the patient can tolerate them.

• Before discharge, the patient or parents must be told the importance of continuing daily heat applications, massages, and stretching exercises, as prescribed, and of keeping the cast clean and dry. Physical therapy will be essential for successful rehabilitation once the cast is removed.

Sjögren's Syndrome

Sjögren's syndrome is a benign chronic inflammation of unknown cause that diminishes lacrimal and salivary gland secretion (sicca complex). It occurs mainly in women (90% of patients) whose mean age is 50 and often accompanies connective tissue disorders.

Causes and incidence

Because Sjögren's syndrome is associated with high levels of abnormal serum factors (rheumatoid and antinuclear) and circulating antibodies, it may be an immunologic disorder. Arthritis usually precedes or accompanies the sicca complex. If arthritis doesn't develop within 1 year of the sicca complex, it probably won't appear later. About 50% of patients with Sjögren's syndrome have rheumatoid arthritis; 10% to 20% have Raynaud's phenomenon (spasm of small arteries and arterioles, especially in the digits, with intermittent pallor or cyanosis); and some have systemic lupus erythematosus (SLE), polyarteritis, or polymyositis.

Signs and symptoms

Patients with Sjögren's syndrome usually have confirmed rheumatoid arthritis and a history of slowly developing sicca complex. However, some have no associated disease but seek medical help solely for rapidly progressive and severe oral, ocular, vaginal, and skin dryness, accompanied in 50% of patients by parotid gland enlargement, with fluctuation in glandular size.

Dryness of the nose, mouth, larynx, pharynx, and tracheobronchial tree leads to difficulty in chewing, swallowing, and talking; ulcers of the lips, tongue, and oral mucous membranes; abnormal taste sensation, thirst, cracked lips (especially at the corners of the mouth); and severe dental cavities. Nasal crusting, nosebleed, sinus inflammation, hoarseness, cough, and recurrent otitis media may also occur. Ocular dryness leads to foreign body sensation (gritty, sandy eye), burning, redness, photosensitivity, inability to cry, poor vision, mucoid discharge, itching, and eye fatigue. Rarely, Sjögren's syndrome causes renal and pulmonary involvement.

Diagnosis

In patients with salivary gland enlargement, diagnosis must rule out other disorders, such as lymphoma, leukemia, tuberculosis, sarcoidosis, hepatic cirrhosis, and malnutrition. Ruling out malignancy is especially important when lymphoid infiltration and proliferation are severe.

Laboratory studies in patients with Sjögren's syndrome often show nonspecific anemia, leukopenia (WBC less than 4,000/mm^3), elevated ESR, and hypergammaglobulinemia, as well as a variety of autoantibodies. Typically, 90% of patients have high rheumatoid factor titers, 70% have high antinuclear factor titers, and most also have antisalivary duct antibody (apparently a specific antibody for Sjögren's syndrome).

Other tests support this diagnosis:
• In *Schirmer's filter paper test,* rose bengal dye and biomicroscopy of the eye are used to measure lacrimal and parotid gland involvement.
• *Salivary scintigraphy* can determine uptake, concentration, and excretion of radioactive material by the salivary glands.
• *Lower lip biopsy* shows salivary gland infiltration by lymphocytes.

Treatment and additional considerations

Treatment is usually symptomatic and includes conservative measures to control ocular or oral dryness. Mouth dryness can be relieved by using a methylcellulose swab or spray, chewing sugarless gum or candy, and drinking plenty of fluids. Frequent dental checkups can control cavities.

Tracheobronchial hyposecretion may require antibiotics to fight infection; pseudolymphoma with renal and pulmonary involvement may require corticosteroids and immunosuppressives; accompanying malignancies may require a combination of chemotherapy, surgery, or radiotherapy.

• If mouth lesions make eating painful, high-protein, high-calorie supplements will help prevent malnutrition.

• Methylcellulose (0.5%) eyedrops (artificial tears) may be needed as often as every half hour to prevent eye damage (corneal ulcerations, corneal opacifications) from insufficient tear secretion. The patient may benefit from the instillation of an antibiotic eye ointment just before sleeping.

• Sunglasses may be used to protect the patient's eyes from dust and strong light.

• Humidifying home and work environments will help prevent respiratory complications for the patient.

Selected References

Anthony, Catherine Parker. TEXTBOOK OF ANATOMY AND PHYSIOLOGY, 10th ed. St. Louis: C.V. Mosby Co., 1979.

Brashear, H. Robert, and Beverly R. Raney. SHANDS' HANDBOOK OF ORTHOPAEDIC SURGERY, 9th ed. St. Louis: C.V. Mosby Co., 1978.

Dubois, Edmund L., and Mavis B. Cox, eds. LUPUS ERYTHEMATOSUS. Torrance, Calif.: American Lupus Society, pp. 1-14.

Erlich, G. REHABILITATION MANAGEMENT OF RHEUMATIC CONDITIONS (Rehabilitation Medicine Library Series). Baltimore: Williams & Wilkins Co., 1980.

Farrell, Jane. ILLUSTRATED GUIDE TO ORTHOPEDIC NURSING. Philadelphia: J.B. Lippincott Co., 1977.

Gartland, John J. FUNDAMENTALS OF ORTHOPEDICS. Philadelphia: W.B. Saunders Co., 1979.

Hilt, Nancy E., and Shirly B. Cogburn. MANUAL OF ORTHOPEDICS. St. Louis: C.V. Mosby Co., 1980.

Kay, Marguerite, et al., eds. AGING, IMMUNITY, AND ARTHRITIC DISEASES, Vol. 13. New York: Raven Press, 1980.

Khairi, M.R.A., et al. Sodium Etidronate in the Treatment of Paget's Disease of Bone, ANNALS OF INTERNAL MEDICINE. 87:656-663, December 1977.

Larson, Carroll, and Marjorie Gould. ORTHOPEDIC NURSING. St. Louis: C.V. Mosby Co., 1978.

Lovell, Wood, and Robert Winter, eds. PEDIATRIC ORTHOPEDICS. Philadelphia: J.B. Lippincott Co., 1978.

McCarthy, Daniel J. ARTHRITIS AND ALLIED CONDITIONS. Philadelphia: Lea & Febiger, 1979.

Price, Sylvia, and Lorraine McCarty Wilson. PATHOPHYSIOLOGY: CLINICAL CONCEPTS OF DISEASE PROCESSES. New York: McGraw-Hill Book Co., 1978.

Rowe, Joyce, and Lois Dyer, eds. CARE OF THE ORTHOPEDIC PATIENT. Philadelphia: J.B. Lippincott Co., 1977.

Wallace, Roberta, et al. STAFF MANUAL FOR TEACHING PATIENTS ABOUT RHEUMATOID ARTHRITIS. Chicago: American Hospital Association, 1979.

Wallach, Stanley. PAGET'S DISEASE OF BONE. Phoenix, Ariz.: Armour Pharmaceutical Co., 1977.

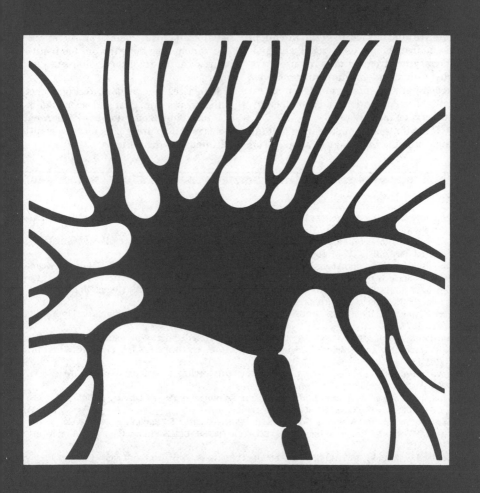

9 Neurologic Disorders

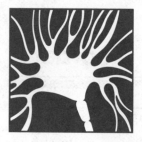

Neurologic Disorders

Introduction

The neurologic system, the body's communications network, coordinates and organizes the functions of all body systems. This intricate network has three main divisions:

• *central nervous system (CNS),* the control center, made up of the brain and the spinal cord

• *peripheral nervous system,* which includes nerves that connect the CNS to remote body parts and relay and receive messages from them

• *autonomic nervous system,* which regulates involuntary functioning of internal organs.

Fundamental unit

The fundamental unit of the nervous system is the neuron, a highly specialized conductor cell that receives and transmits electrochemical nerve impulses. It has a special, distinguishing structure. Delicate, threadlike nerve fibers extend from the central cell body and transmit signals: *axons* carry impulses away from the cell body; *dendrites* carry impulses to it. Most neurons have multiple dendrites but only one axon. *Sensory (afferent) neurons* transmit impulses from special receptors to the spinal cord or the brain; *motor (efferent) neurons* transmit impulses from the CNS to regulate activity of muscles or glands; and *interneurons (connecting or association neurons)* shuttle signals through complex pathways between sensory and motor neurons. Interneurons account for 99% of all the neurons in the nervous system and include most of the neurons in the brain itself.

Intricate control system

This intricate network of interlocking receptors and transmitters, with the brain and spinal cord, forms a dynamic control system—a living computer—that controls and regulates every mental and physical function. From birth to death, this astonishing system efficiently organizes the body's affairs—controlling the smallest action, thought, or feeling; monitoring communication and instinct for survival; and allowing introspection, wonder, abstract thought, and—unique to humans—awareness of one's own intelligence. The brain, the primary center of this central system, is the large soft mass of nervous tissue housed within the cranium, and protected and supported by the meninges.

The fragile brain and spinal cord are protected by bone (the skull and vertebrae), cushioning cerebrospinal fluid (CSF), and three membranes:

• The *dura mater,* or outer sheath, is made of tough white fibrous tissue.

• The *arachnoid membrane,* the middle layer, is delicate and lacelike.

• The *pia mater,* the inner meningeal layer, is made of fine blood vessels held together by connective tissue. It's thin and transparent, and clings to the brain and spinal cord surfaces, carrying branches of the cerebral arteries deep into the brain's fissures and sulci.

Between the dura mater and the arachnoid membrane is the *subdural space;* between the pia mater and the arachnoid membrane is the *subarachnoid space.* Circulating within the subarachnoid space and the brain's four ventricles is *cerebrospinal fluid,* a liquid containing water and traces of organic materials (particularly protein) and minerals.

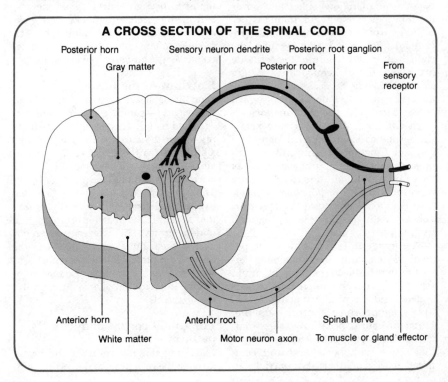

A CROSS SECTION OF THE SPINAL CORD

Posterior horn
Gray matter
Sensory neuron dendrite
Posterior root ganglion
Posterior root
From sensory receptor
Anterior horn
White matter
Anterior root
Motor neuron axon
Spinal nerve
To muscle or gland effector

CSF is formed from blood in capillary networks called *choroid plexi,* which are located primarily in the brain's lateral ventricles. CSF is eventually reabsorbed into the venous blood through the *arachnoid villi,* in dural sinuses on the brain's surface.

The *cerebrum,* the largest portion of the brain, houses the nerve center that controls sensory and motor activities, and intelligence. The outer layer of the cerebrum, the *cerebral cortex,* consists of neuron cell bodies, or gray matter; the inner layers consist of axons, or white matter, plus basal ganglia, which control motor coordination and steadiness. The cerebral surface is deeply convoluted, furrowed with elevations (gyri) and depressions (sulci). The *longitudinal fissure* divides the cerebrum into two hemispheres connected by a wide band of nerve fibers called the *corpus callosum,* which allows the hemispheres to share learning and intellect. Both hemispheres don't share equally—one always dominates, giving one side control over the other. Because motor impulses descending from the brain through the pyramidal tract cross in the medulla, the right hemisphere controls the left side of the body; the left hemisphere, the right side of the body. Several fissures divide the cerebrum into lobes, each of which is associated with specific functions.

The *thalamus,* a relay center below the corpus callosum, further organizes cerebral function by transmitting impulses to and from appropriate areas of the cerebrum. In addition to its primary relay function, it's responsible for primitive emotional response, such as fear, and for distinguishing pleasant stimuli from unpleasant ones.

The *hypothalamus,* which lies beneath the thalamus, is an autonomic center that has connections with the brain, the spinal cord, the autonomic nervous system, and the pituitary gland. It regulates temperature control, appetite, blood pressure, breathing, sleep patterns, and peripheral nerve discharges that occur with behavioral and emotional expression. It also has partial control of pituitary gland secretion and stress reaction.

The base of the brain

Beneath the cerebrum, at the base of the brain, is the *cerebellum,* also called the hindbrain. It's responsible for smooth muscle movements, coordinating sensory impulses with muscle activity, and maintaining muscle tone and equilibrium.

The *brain stem* houses cell bodies for most of the cranial nerves and includes the *midbrain,* the *pons,* and the *medulla oblongata.* With the thalamus and the hypothalamus, it makes up a nerve network called the *reticular formation,* which acts as an arousal mechanism. It also relays nerve impulses between the spinal cord and other parts of the brain. The midbrain is the reflex center for the third and fourth cranial nerves, and mediates pupillary reflexes and eye movements. The pons helps regulate respirations. It's also the reflex center for the fifth through eighth cranial nerves, and mediates chewing, taste, saliva secretion, hearing, and equilibrium. The medulla oblongata influences cardiac, respiratory, and vasomotor functions.

Bloodline to the brain

Four major arteries—two *vertebral* and two *carotid*—supply the brain with oxygenated blood. These arteries originate in or near the aortic arch. The two vertebral arteries (branches of the subclavians) converge to become the basilar artery, which supplies the posterior brain. The common carotids branch into the two internal carotids, which divide further to supply the anterior brain and the middle brain. These arteries interconnect through the *circle of Willis,* at the base of the brain. This anastomosis ensures continual circulation to the brain, despite interruption of any of the brain's major vessels.

The spinal cord: Conductor pathway

Extending downward from the brain, through the vertebrae, to the second lum-

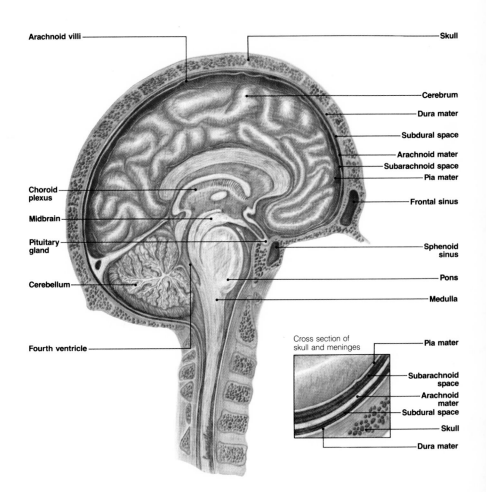

Arachnoid villi

Skull

Cerebrum

Dura mater

Subdural space

Arachnoid mater

Subarachnoid space

Pia mater

Choroid plexus

Midbrain

Pituitary gland

Cerebellum

Frontal sinus

Sphenoid sinus

Pons

Medulla

Fourth ventricle

Cross section of skull and meninges

Pia mater

Subarachnoid space

Arachnoid mater

Subdural space

Skull

Dura mater

Nerve origin

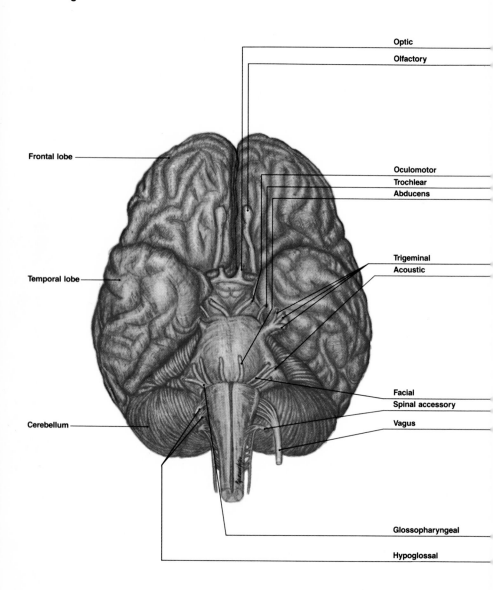

Optic

Olfactory

Frontal lobe

Oculomotor

Trochlear

Abducens

Trigeminal

Acoustic

Temporal lobe

Facial

Spinal accessory

Cerebellum

Vagus

Glossopharyngeal

Hypoglossal

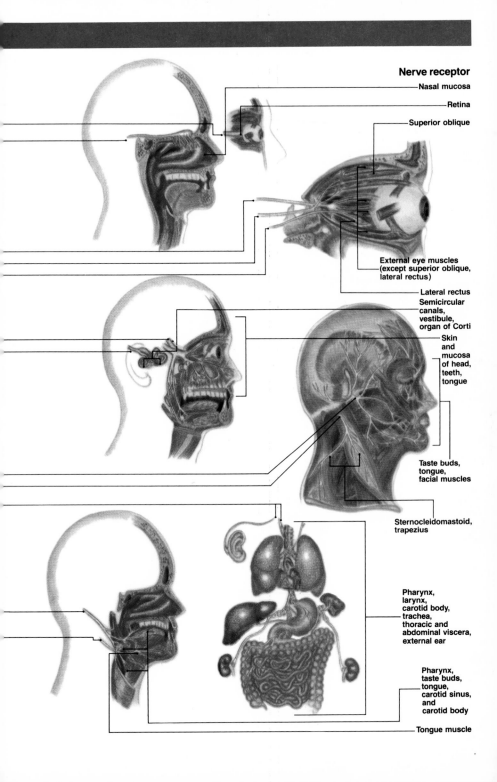

Nerve receptor

Nasal mucosa

Retina

Superior oblique

External eye muscles
(except superior oblique,
lateral rectus)

Lateral rectus

Semicircular
canals,
vestibule,
organ of Corti

Skin
and
mucosa
of head,
teeth,
tongue

Taste buds,
tongue,
facial muscles

Sternocleidomastoid,
trapezius

Pharynx,
larynx,
carotid body,
trachea,
thoracic and
abdominal viscera,
external ear

Pharynx,
taste buds,
tongue,
carotid sinus,
and
carotid body

Tongue muscle

AUTONOMIC NERVOUS SYSTEM

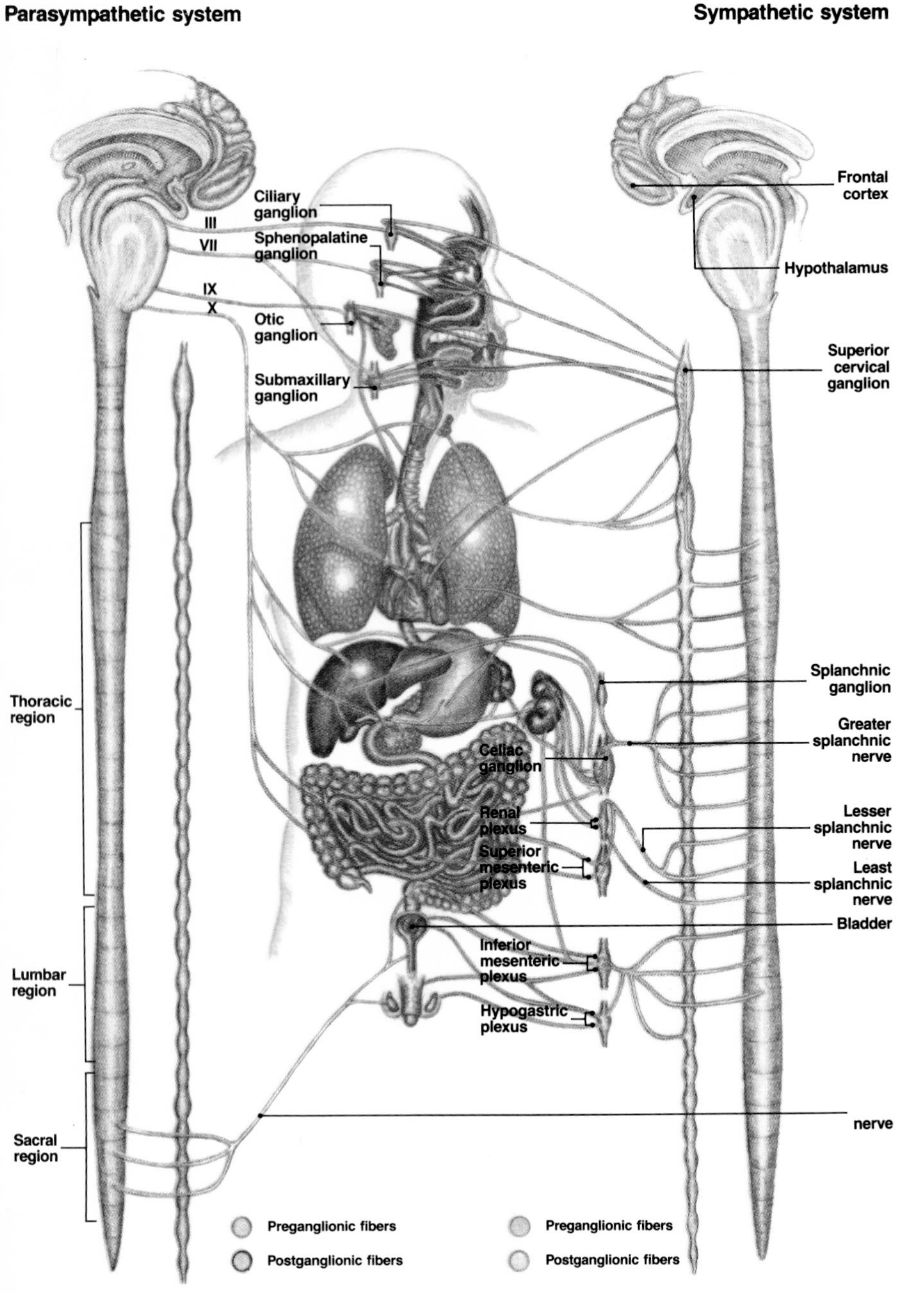

Parasympathetic system

Sympathetic system

Ciliary ganglion

Sphenopalatine ganglion

III
VII

IX
X

Otic ganglion

Submaxillary ganglion

Frontal cortex

Hypothalamus

Superior cervical ganglion

Thoracic region

Celiac ganglion

Renal plexus

Superior mesenteric plexus

Splanchnic ganglion

Greater splanchnic nerve

Lesser splanchnic nerve

Least splanchnic nerve

Bladder

Lumbar region

Inferior mesenteric plexus

Hypogastric plexus

Sacral region

nerve

Preganglionic fibers

Postganglionic fibers

Preganglionic fibers

Postganglionic fibers

bar vertebra is the *spinal cord,* a two-way conductor pathway between the brain stem and the peripheral nervous system. The spinal cord is also the reflex center for activities that don't require brain control, such as a knee-jerk reaction to a reflex hammer.

A cross section of the spinal cord shows an internal H-shaped mass of gray matter divided into horns, which consist primarily of neuron cell bodies. Cell bodies in the *posterior,* or *dorsal, horn* primarily relay sensations; those in the *anterior,* or *ventral, horn* are needed for voluntary or reflex motor activity. The white matter surrounding the outer part of these horns consists of myelinated nerve fibers grouped functionally in vertical columns called *tracts.*

The *sensory,* or *ascending, tracts* carry sensory impulses up the spinal cord to the brain, while *motor,* or *descending, tracts* carry motor impulses down the spinal cord. The brain's motor impulses reach a descending tract and continue through the peripheral nervous system by *upper motor neurons.* These neurons originate in the brain and form two major systems:

• The *pyramidal system* (corticospinal tract) is responsible for fine, skilled movements of skeletal muscle. An impulse in this system originates in the frontal lobe's motor cortex, and travels downward to the pyramids of the medulla, where it crosses to the opposite side of the spinal cord.

• The *extrapyramidal system* (extra-corticospinal tract) controls gross motor movements. An impulse traveling in this system originates in the frontal lobe's motor cortex, and is mediated by basal ganglia, the thalamus, cerebellum, and reticular formation before descending to the spinal cord.

Reaching outlying areas

Messages transmitted through the spinal cord reach outlying areas through the *peripheral nervous system,* which originates in 31 pairs of segmentally arranged spinal nerves attached to the spinal cord. Spinal nerves are numbered

A LOOK AT THE LOBES

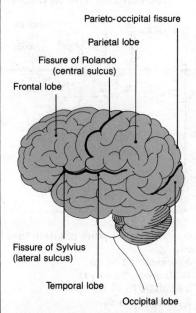

Parieto-occipital fissure

Parietal lobe

Fissure of Rolando
(central sulcus)

Frontal lobe

Fissure of Sylvius
(lateral sulcus)

Temporal lobe

Occipital lobe

Several fissures divide the cerebrum into hemispheres and lobes; each lobe has a specific function. The *fissure of Sylvius* (lateral sulcus) separates the temporal lobe from the frontal and parietal lobes. The *fissure of Rolando* (central sulcus) separates the frontal lobes from the parietal lobe. The *parieto-occipital fissure* separates the occipital lobe from the two parietal lobes.

• The *frontal lobe* controls voluntary muscle movements and contains motor areas (including the motor area for speech, or Broca's area). It's the center for personality, behavioral, and intellectual functions, such as judgment, memory, and problem-solving; for autonomic functions; and for cardiac and emotional resonses.

• The *temporal lobe* is the center for taste, hearing, and smell, and in the brain's dominant hemisphere, interprets spoken language.

• The *parietal lobe* coordinates and interprets sensory information from the opposite side of the body.

• The *occipital lobe* interprets visual stimuli.

STRUCTURE OF THE NEURON

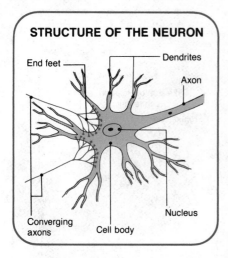

End feet

Dendrites

Axon

Nucleus

Converging axons

Cell body

according to their point of origin in the cord:

- 8 cervical: C1 to C8
- 12 thoracic: T1 to T12
- 5 lumbar: L1 to L5
- 5 sacral: S1 to S5
- 1 coccygeal.

The cross section of the spinal cord shows that these spinal nerves are attached to the spinal cord by two roots:
- The *anterior,* or *ventral, root* consists of motor fibers that relay impulses from the cord to glands and muscles.
- The *posterior,* or *dorsal, root* consists of sensory fibers that relay sensory information from receptors to the cord. The posterior root has a swelling on it— the posterior root ganglion—which is made up of sensory neuron cell bodies.

After leaving the vertebral column, each spinal nerve separates into *rami* (branches), which distribute peripherally, with extensive but organized overlapping. This overlapping reduces the chance of lost sensory or motor function from interruption of a single spinal nerve.

Two functional systems
- The *somatic (voluntary) nervous system* is activated by will but can also function independently. It's responsible for all conscious and higher mental processes and for subconscious and reflex actions, such as shivering.

- The *autonomic (involuntary) nervous system* regulates functions of the unconscious level to control involuntary body functions, such as digestion, respiration, and cardiovascular function. It's usually divided into two antagonistic systems. The *sympathetic nervous system* controls energy expenditure, especially in stressful situations, by releasing the adrenergic catecholamine *norepinephrine.* The *parasympathetic nervous system* helps conserve energy by releasing the cholinergic neurohormone *acetylcholine.* These antagonistic systems balance each other to support homeostasis.

Assessing neurologic function
A complete neurologic assessment helps confirm the diagnosis in a suspected neurologic disorder. It establishes a clinical baseline and can offer lifesaving clues to rapid deterioration. Neurologic assessment includes:
- *Patient history:* In addition to the usual information, the history should cover the patient's and his family's perception of the disorder. The patient interview is a good time to make observations that will help evaluate mental status and behavior.
- *Physical examination:* Particular attention must be paid to obvious abnormalities that may signal serious neurologic problems, for example, fluid draining from the nose or ears.
- *Neurologic examination:* Cerebral, cerebellar, motor, sensory, and cranial nerve function must be determined.

Obviously, there isn't always time for a complete neurologic examination during bedside assessment. Therefore, priorities must be set. For example, typical ongoing bedside assessment focuses on level of consciousness, pupillary response, motor function, reflexes, and vital signs. However, when time permits, a complete neurologic examination can provide valuable information regarding total neurologic function.

Mental status, intellect, and behavior
Mental status and behavior are good indi-

cators of cerebral function, and they're easy to assess. This includes: noting the patient's appearance, mannerisms, posture, facial expression, grooming, and tone of voice; checking for orientation to time, place, and person, and for memory of recent and past events; asking the patient to count backward from 100 by 7s, to read aloud, or to interpret a common proverb, and see how well he understands and follows commands. If such checks are done frequently, questions should be varied to avoid a programmed response.

Level of consciousness

Level of consciousness is the single most valuable indicator of neurologic function. It can vary from alertness (response to verbal stimulus) to coma (failure to respond even to painful stimulus). The patient's exact response to the stimulus should be documented; for example, "patient pulled away in response to nail bed pressure" rather than just "stuporous."

The Glasgow Coma Scale (GCS), which assesses eye opening as well as verbal and motor responses, provides a quick standardized account of neurologic status and is becoming widely used. In this test, each response receives a numerical value. For instance, if the patient readily responds verbally, and is oriented to time, place, and person, he scores a 5; if he's totally unable to respond verbally, he scores a 1. A score of 15 for all three parts is normal; 7 or less indicates coma; 3—the lowest score possible—generally (but not always) points to brain death. Although the GCS is useful, it's not a substitute for a complete neurologic assessment.

Assessing motor function

Inability to perform the following simple tests, or observation of tics, tremors, or other abnormalities during such testing, suggests cerebellar dysfunction.
• Can the patient touch his nose with each index finger, alternating hands? Can he repeat this test with his eyes closed?
• Can the patient tap the index finger and thumb of each hand together rapidly?

• Can the patient draw a figure eight in the air with his foot?
• Can the patient walk heel to toe in a straight line?
• Can the patient perform the Romberg test (standing with feet together, eyes closed, and arms outstretched without losing balance)?

Motor function is a good indicator of level of consciousness and can also point to central or peripheral nervous system damage. During all tests of motor function, watch for differences between right and left side functions.
• To check gait: the patient walks while he is observed for posture, balance, and coordination of leg movement and arm swing.
• To check muscle tone: the patient's muscles are palpated at rest and in response to passive flexion. They may exhibit flaccidity, spasticity, and rigidity, or involuntary movements, such as rapid jerks, tremors or contractions. Muscle size is also measured.
• To evaluate muscle strength: the patient grips the evaluator's hands and squeezes. Then he pushes against the evaluator's palm with his foot. Muscle strength is compared on each side, using a 5-point scale (5 is normal strength, 0 is complete paralysis). The evaluator must also test the patient's ability to extend and flex the neck, elbows, wrists, fingers, toes (especially the great toe), hips, and knees; to extend the spine; to contract and relax the abdominal muscles; and to rotate the shoulders.
• To evaluate reflexes: a 4-point scale is used (4 is hyperactive reflex, 0 is absent reflex). Before reflex testing, the patient should be comfortable and relaxed. Then, for superficial reflex testing, the skin of the abdominal, gluteal, plantar, and scrotal regions is stroked with a moderately sharp object (such as a key) that won't puncture the skin. A normal reflex is flexion in response to this stimulus. For deep reflex testing, a reflex hammer is used to briskly tap the biceps, the triceps, and the brachioradialis (wrist), patellar (knee), and Achilles tendon regions. Normal response is rapid muscle

extension and contraction.

Assessing sensory function

Impaired or absent sensation in the trunk or extremities can point to brain, spinal cord, or peripheral nerve damage. The extent of sensory dysfunction must be determined, since this helps locate neurologic damage. For instance, localized dysfunction indicates local peripheral nerve damage; dysfunction over a single dermatome (an area served by 1 of the 31 pairs of spinal nerves) indicates damage to the nerve's dorsal root; and dysfunction extending over more than one dermatome suggests brain or spinal cord damage.

In assessing sensory function, both sides of symmetric areas must be tested; for instance, both arms, not just one. The patient should know that the test won't be painful.

• *Superficial pain perception:* The point of an open safety pin is pressed against the patient's skin, lighly enough so it doesn't scratch or puncture the skin.

• *Thermal sensitivity:* The patient says what he feels when two test tubes, one filled with hot water and one filled with cold water, are placed against his skin.

• *Tactile sensitivity:* The patient closes his eyes and says what he feels when touched lightly with a wisp of cotton on hands, wrists, arms, thighs, lower legs, feet, and trunk.

• *Sensitivity to vibration:* The base of a vibrating tuning fork is placed against the patient's wrists, elbows, knees, or other bony prominences. It is held in place, and the patient says when it stops vibrating.

• *Position sense:* The patient's toes or fingers are moved up, down, and to the side. The patient identifies the direction of movement.

• *Discriminatory sensation:* The patient closes his eyes and identifies familiar textures (velvet, burlap) or objects placed in his hand, or numbers and letters traced on his palm.

• *Two-point discrimination:* The patient is touched with calipers or other sharp objects in two different places simultaneously. He says if he can feel one or two points.

Localizing cranial nerve function

The simple tests that follow can reliably localize cranial nerve dysfunction.

• *Olfactory nerve (I):* The patient closes his eyes and, using each nostril separately, tries to identify common nonirritating smells, such as cinnamon, coffee, or peppermint.

• *Optic nerve (II):* The patient's eyes are examined with an ophthalmoscope, and he reads a Snellen eye chart or a newspaper. To test peripheral vision, he covers one eye and fixes his other eye on a point directly in front of him. Then he says if he can see the examiner's finger being wiggled to his far right or left.

• *Oculomotor nerve (III):* The size and shape of the patient's pupils are compared, as are the equality of pupillary response to a small light in a darkened room.

• *Trochlear nerve (IV) and abducens nerve (VI):* To assess for conjugate and lateral eye movement, the patient follows the examiner's finger with his eyes, as it slowly moves from his far left to his far right.

• *Trigeminal nerve (V):* To test facial sensory response, the patient's jaws, cheeks, and forehead are stroked with a cotton applicator, the point of a pin, or test tubes filled with hot or cold water. Since testing for a blink reflex is irritating to the patient, it's not commonly done. If testing for this response must be done (it may be decreased in patients who wear contact lenses), the cornea is touched lightly with a wisp of cotton or tissue. If possible, the test is not repeated. To test for jaw jerk, the patient holds his mouth slightly open, then the middle of his chin is tapped with a reflex hammer. The jaw should jerk closed.

• *Facial nerve (VII):* To test upper and lower facial motor function, the patient is asked to raise his eyebrows, wrinkle his forehead, or show his teeth. To test sense of taste, well-known salty, sour, sweet, and bitter substances are placed on his tongue and he is asked to identify them.

• *Acoustic nerve (VIII):* The patient iden-

ASSESSING RESPIRATORY FUNCTION

In an unconscious patient, these patterns of respiration indicate neurologic abnormalities.

PATTERN OF RESPIRATION	CHARACTERISTICS	SIGNIFICANCE
Cheyne-Stokes	• Rhythmic waxing and waning of both rate and depth of respirations, alternating regularly with briefer periods of apnea	• May indicate deep cerebral or cerebellar lesions, usually bilateral; may occur with upper brain stem involvement
Central neurogenic hyperventilation	• Sustained, regular, rapid respirations with forced inspiration and expiration	• May indicate a lesion of the low midbrain, or upper pons areas of the brain stem
Apneustic	• Prolonged inspiratory cramp with a pause at full inspiration; there may also be expiratory pauses	• May indicate a lesion of the mid- or low pons
Cluster breathing	• Clusters of irregular respirations alternating with longer periods of apnea	• May indicate a lesion of the low pons or upper medulla
Ataxic breathing	• A completely irregular pattern with random deep and shallow respirations; irregular pauses may also appear	• May indicate a lesion of the medulla

tifies common sounds, such as a ticking clock. He is also tested, with a tuning fork, for air and bone conduction.

• *Glossopharyngeal nerve (IX):* To test gag reflex, a tongue depressor is touched to each side of the patient's pharynx.

• *Vagus nerve (X):* The patient's ability to swallow is observed. Then the patient is asked to say, "Ah" and his soft palate is observed for symmetrical movement.

• *Spinal accessory nerve (XI):* To test shoulder muscle strength, the patient's shoulders are palpated and he is asked to shrug against a resistance.

• *Hypoglossal nerve (XII):* To test tongue movement, the patient sticks out his tongue. It is inspected for tremor, atrophy, or lateral deviation. To test for strength, the patient moves his tongue from side to side while a tongue depressor is held against it.

Testing for a firm diagnosis

A firm diagnosis of many neurologic

disorders often requires more than neurologic assessment—it requires a wide range of relevant diagnostic tests. If possible, noninvasive tests are done first, since they're less dangerous for the patient, and may include the following:

• A *skull X-ray* identifies skull malformations, fractures, erosion, or thickening that may indicate tumors or increased intracranial pressure (ICP).

• *Computerized axial tomography (CAT scan)* is a series of X-rays of "slices" of the brain, which produces a three-dimensional effect. It's used to identify intracranial tumor, hemorrhage, or malformation, and cerebral atrophy, calcification, edema, and infarction. If a contrast medium is used, this is an invasive procedure.

• *Electroencephalography* detects abnormal electrical activity in the brain, which may result from a seizure disorder, tumor, metabolic disease, mental retardation, drug overdose, or a psychological disorder.

• *Echoencephalography* determines if the midline structures in the brain have shifted, indicating a lesion.

Invasive tests may include:

• *Lumbar puncture:* A needle is inserted into the subarachnoid space of the spinal cord, usually between L3 and L4 (or L4 and L5), allowing aspiration of cerebrospinal fluid (CSF) for examination. This specimen is used to detect infection (culture and Gram's stain) or hemorrhage; to determine cell count, and glucose, protein, and globulin levels; and to measure CSF pressure. Lumbar puncture is usually contraindicated in hydrocephalus and in known increased ICP, since quick reduction in pressure may cause brain herniation.

• *Myelography:* Following a lumbar puncture and CSF removal, a radiologic dye is instilled. X-rays determine spinal cord compression related to back pain or extremity weakness, and show spinal abnormalities.

• *Pneumoencephalography:* This test is seldom used now that CAT scans are available. After lumbar puncture, a small amount of air is introduced into the sub-arachnoid space. Subsequent X-ray visualizes tumors and lesions in the brain stem and the ventricles.

• *Arteriography (cerebral angiography):* A catheter is inserted into an artery—usually the femoral artery—and is indirectly threaded up to the carotid artery. Then, a radiopaque dye is injected, which allows X-ray visualization of the cerebral vasculature. Sometimes the catheter is threaded directly into the brachial or carotid artery, rather than indirectly through the femoral artery. This test can show cerebral vascular abnormalities and spasms, plus arterial changes due to tumor, arteriosclerosis, hemorrhage, aneurysm, or blockage from a cerebrovascular accident.

• *Ventriculography:* Air is introduced into the lateral ventricle through an opening in the skull, usually in the occipital region. X-rays are then taken and are used to identify tumors or anomalies that affect the ventricular system.

• *Brain scan:* A special scanner is used to measure gamma rays produced by a small amount of radioisotope injected I.V. Uptake and distribution of isotope in the brain can detect intracranial masses or vascular lesions.

• *Intracranial pressure (ICP) monitoring:* A screw-type device with a sensor tip is inserted into a burr hole, usually in the parietal region. A transducer attached to the screw converts CSF pressure measurements into electric impulses, which are visualized by an oscilloscope and recorded on a printout. An alternate way to measure CSF pressure is by using an intraventricular catheter with a three-way stopcock, flushing solution, and a manometer. ICP monitoring is performed when even a slight rise in ICP is an emergency or when a precipitous rise is possible, as in a ruptured cerebral aneurysm or cerebral edema.

• *Electromyography:* A needle inserted into selected muscles at rest and during voluntary contraction picks up nerve impulses and measures nerve conduction time. This test is used to detect lower motor neuron disorders, neuromuscular disorders, and nerve damage.

CONGENITAL ANOMALIES

Cerebral Palsy

The most common cause of crippling in children, cerebral palsy comprises a group of neuromuscular disorders resulting from prenatal, perinatal, or postnatal CNS damage. Although nonprogressive, these disorders may become more obvious as an affected infant grows older. Three major types of cerebral palsy occur—spastic, athetoid, and ataxic—sometimes in mixed forms. Motor impairment may be minimal (sometimes apparent only during physical activities such as running) or severely disabling. Associated defects, such as seizures, speech disorders, and mental retardation, are common. Prognosis varies. In mild impairment, proper treatment may make a near-normal life possible.

Cerebral palsy occurs in an estimated 15,000 live births every year. Incidence is highest in premature infants (25% of newborns with cerebral palsy weigh less than 5½ lb [2.5 kg] at birth) and in those who are small for their gestational age. Cerebral palsy is slightly more common in males than in females, and occurs more often in Caucasians.

Signs and symptoms

The *spastic* form of cerebral palsy predominates, affecting about 70% of the patients. This form is characterized by hyperactive deep tendon reflexes, increased stretch reflexes, rapid alternating muscle contraction and relaxation, muscle weakness, underdevelopment of affected limbs, muscle contraction in response to manipulation, and a tendency toward contractures. Typically, a child with spastic cerebral palsy walks on his toes with a scissors gait, crossing one foot in front of the other.

In *athetoid cerebral palsy,* which affects approximately 20% of patients, involuntary movements—grimacing, wormlike writhing, dystonia, and sharp jerks—impair voluntary movement. These involuntary movements usually affect the arms more severely than the legs; involuntary facial movements may make speech difficult. These movements become more severe during stress, decrease with relaxation, and disappear entirely during sleep.

Ataxic cerebral palsy accounts for about 10% of patients. Its characteristics include disturbed balance, incoordination (especially of the arms), hypoactive reflexes, nystagmus, muscle weakness, tremor, lack of leg movement during infancy, and a wide gait as the child begins to walk. Ataxia makes sudden or fine movements almost impossible.

Some children with cerebral palsy display a combination of these clinical features. In most, impaired motor function makes eating, especially swallowing, difficult, and retards growth and development. Up to 40% of these children are mentally retarded, about 25% have seizure disorders, and about 80% have impaired speech. Many also have dental abnormalities, vision and hearing defects, and reading disabilities.

Diagnosis

Early diagnosis is essential for effective treatment and requires careful clinical observation during infancy and precise neurologic assessment. Suspect cerebral palsy whenever an infant:

- has difficulty sucking or keeping the nipple or food in his mouth
- seldom moves voluntarily, or has arm or leg tremors with voluntary movement
- crosses his legs when lifted from behind rather than pulling them up or "bicycling" like a normal infant

CAUSES OF CEREBRAL PALSY

Conditions that result in cerebral anoxia, hemorrhage, or other damage are probably responsible for cerebral palsy.
• *Prenatal causes:* maternal infection (especially rubella), radiation, anoxia, toxemia, maternal diabetes, abnormal placental attachment, malnutrition, and isoimmunization
• *Perinatal and birth difficulties:* forceps delivery, breech presentation, placenta previa, abruptio placentae, depressed maternal vital signs from general or spinal anesthetic, prolapsed cord with delay in delivery of head, premature birth, prolonged or unusually rapid labor, multiple birth (especially infants born last in a multiple birth)
• *Infection or trauma during infancy:* kernicterus resulting from erythroblastosis fetalis, brain infection, head trauma, prolonged anoxia, brain tumor, cerebral circulatory anomalies causing blood vessel rupture, and systemic disease resulting in cerebral thrombosis or embolus.

• has legs that are hard to separate, making diaper changing difficult
• persistently uses only one hand or, as he gets older, uses his hands well but not his legs.

Careful follow-up is especially important for infants who are premature or who have had a difficult birth. However, all infants should have a screening test for cerebral palsy as part of their 6-month checkup. One test consists of placing a blanket or a diaper over the infant's face. Normally, an infant will pull it off with both hands; an infant with cerebral palsy will use only one hand or won't be able to pull the blanket off at all.

Treatment
Cerebral palsy can't be cured, but proper treatment can help affected children reach their full potential within the limits set by this disorder. Such treatment requires a comprehensive and cooperative effort involving doctors, nurses, teachers, psychologists, the child's family, and occupational, physical, and speech therapists. Home care is often possible. Treatment usually includes:
• braces or splints and special appliances, such as adapted eating utensils and a low toilet seat with arms, to help these children independently perform activities they would otherwise find impossible.
• range-of-motion exercises to minimize contractures.
• orthopedic surgery to correct contractures.
• phenytoin, phenobarbital, or another anticonvulsant to control seizures.
• sometimes muscle relaxants or neurosurgery to decrease spasticity.

Children with milder forms of cerebral palsy should attend a regular school; severely afflicted children need special education classes.

Additional considerations
A child with cerebral palsy may be hospitalized for orthopedic surgery to correct contractures and for treatment of other complications. The hospital staff member caring for him should:
• assign the child a room with children in the same age-group.
• speak slowly and distinctly; encourage the child to ask for things he wants; listen patiently and don't rush him.
• during meals, maintain a quiet, unhurried atmosphere with as few distractions as possible; provide the child with special utensils and a chair with a solid footrest, if necessary; teach him to place food far back in his mouth to facilitate swallowing.
• encourage the child to chew food thoroughly, drink through a straw, and suck on a lollipop between meals to develop the muscle control needed to minimize drooling.
• allow the child to wash and dress himself independently, assisting only as needed.
• give all care in an unhurried manner—otherwise, muscle spasticity may increase.

- encourage the child and his family to participate in the care plan so they can continue it at home.
- minimize muscle spasms that increase postoperative pain by moving and turning the child carefully after surgery.
- give good cast care after orthopedic surgery; wash and dry the skin at the edge of the cast frequently, and rub it with alcohol; reposition the child often, check for foul odor, and ventilate under the cast with a blow-dryer; use a flashlight to check for skin breakdown beneath the cast; help the child relax, perhaps by giving a warm bath, before reapplying a bivalved cast.

The hospital staffer can help parents deal with their child's handicap by:
- giving them a good understanding of normal growth and development so they can set realistic goals.
- assisting in planning crafts and other activities.
- stressing the child's need to develop peer relationships; warning against being overprotective.
- identifying and dealing with family stress; minimizing the parents' feeling of guilt about their child's handicap.
- making a referral to supportive community organizations; telling parents to contact the United Cerebral Palsy Association, Inc., or their local cerebral palsy agency for more information.

Hydrocephalus

Hydrocephalus is an excessive accumulation of cerebrospinal fluid (CSF) within the ventricular spaces of the brain. It occurs most often in newborns, but it can also occur in adults as a result of injury or disease. In infants, hydrocephalus enlarges the head; and in both infants and adults, resulting compression can damage brain tissue. With early detection and surgical intervention, prognosis improves but remains guarded. Even after surgery, complications, such as mental retardation, impaired motor function, and vision loss, can persist. Without surgery, prognosis is poor: mortality may result from increased intracranial pressure in persons of all ages; infants may also die prematurely of infection and malnutrition.

Causes

Hydrocephalus may result from an obstruction in CSF flow (noncommunicating hydrocephalus) or from faulty absorption of CSF (communicating hydrocephalus).

In noncommunicating hydrocephalus, the obstruction occurs most frequently between the third and fourth ventricles, at the aqueduct of Sylvius, but it can also occur at the outlets of the fourth ventricle (foramina of Luschka and Magendie) or, rarely, at the foramen of Monro. This obstruction may result from faulty fetal development, infection (syphilis, granulomatous diseases, meningitis), a tumor, cerebral aneurysm, or a blood clot (after intracranial hemorrhage).

In communicating hydrocephalus, faulty absorption of CSF may result from

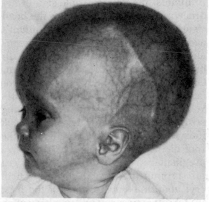

In infants, characteristic changes of hydrocephalus include marked enlargement of the head; distended scalp veins; thin, shiny, and fragile-looking scalp skin; and underdeveloped neck muscles.

NORMAL CIRCULATION OF CSF

CSF is produced from blood in a capillary network (choroid plexus) in the brain's lateral ventricles. From the lateral ventricles, CSF flows through the interventricular foramen (foramen of Monro) to the third ventricle. From there, it flows through the aqueduct of Sylvius to the fourth ventricle and through the foramina of Luschka and Magendie to the cisterna of the subarachnoid space.

Then, the fluid passes under the base of the brain, upward over the brain's upper surfaces, and down around the spinal cord. Eventually, CSF reaches the arachnoid villi, where it's reabsorbed into venous blood at the venous sinuses.

Normally, the amount of fluid produced (about 500 ml/day) equals the amount absorbed. The average amount circulated at one time is 150 to 175 ml.

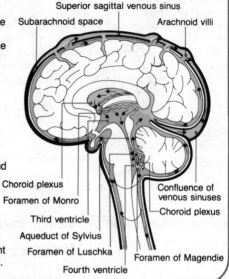

Superior sagittal venous sinus
Subarachnoid space
Arachnoid villi
Choroid plexus
Foramen of Monro
Third ventricle
Aqueduct of Sylvius
Foramen of Luschka
Fourth ventricle
Confluence of venous sinuses
Choroid plexus
Foramen of Magendie

surgery to repair a myelomeningocele, adhesions between meninges at the base of the brain, or meningeal hemorrhage. Rarely, a tumor in the choroid plexus causes overproduction of CSF, producing hydrocephalus.

Signs and symptoms

In infants, the unmistakable sign of hydrocephalus is enlargement of the head clearly disproportionate to the infant's age. Only in communicating hydrocephalus does head size remain normal, with bulging fontanelles the only visible sign. Other characteristic changes in hydrocephalic infants include distended scalp veins; thin, fragile- and shiny-looking scalp skin; and underdeveloped neck muscles. In severe hydrocephalus, the roof of the orbit is depressed, the eyes are displaced downward, and the sclera are prominent. A high-pitched, shrill cry; abnormal muscle tone of the legs; irritability; anorexia; and vomiting often occur. In adults and older children, indicators of hydrocephalus include decreased level of consciousness, ataxia, incontinence, and impaired intellect.

Diagnosis

In infants, abnormally large head size for the patient's age strongly suggests this diagnosis. Skull X-rays show thinning of the skull with separation of sutures and widening of fontanelles; ventriculography shows enlargement of the brain's ventricles. Angiography, pneumoencephalography, and a CAT scan can differentiate between hydrocephalus and intracranial lesions and can also demonstrate the Arnold-Chiari deformity, which occurs with hydrocephalus.

Treatment

Surgical correction is the only treatment for hydrocephalus. Usually, such surgery consists of insertion of a ventriculoperitoneal shunt, which transports excess fluid from the lateral ventricle into the peritoneal cavity. A less common procedure is insertion of a ventriculoatrial shunt, which drains fluid from the brain's lateral ventricle into the right atrium of the heart, where the fluid makes its way into the venous circulation.

Complications of surgery include septicemia (after ventriculoatrial shunt), adhesions and paralytic ileus, peritonitis, and intestinal perforation (with peritoneal shunt).

Additional considerations

On initial assessment, the hospital staff member should obtain a complete history from the patient or his family. This includes: noting general behavior, especially irritability or apathy, or decreased level of consciousness; performing a neurologic assessment; examining the eyes (pupils should be equal and reactive to light); in adults and older children, evaluating motor strength in extremities, and movements, watching especially for ataxia; asking the patient if he has headaches and watching for projectile vomiting (both are signs of increased intracranial pressure); watching for convulsions; noting changes in vital signs.

Before surgery to insert a shunt, the staff member should:
• encourage maternal/infant bonding when possible; feed the infant in a way that allows contact; stroke and cuddle him, and speak soothingly.
• feed the infant slowly; lessen arm strain from the weight of the infant's head while holding him during feeding by placing his head, neck, and shoulders on a pillow.
• prevent postfeeding aspiration and hypostatic pneumonia by placing the infant on his side and by repositioning him every 2 hours.
• check fontanelles for tension or fullness, and measure and record head circumference; draw a picture on the patient's chart showing where to measure the head so that other staff members measure it in the same place, or mark the forehead with ink.
• prevent skin breakdown by making sure his earlobe is flat, and by placing a sheepskin or foam rubber under his head.
• when turning the infant, move his head, neck, and shoulders with his body to reduce strain on his neck.

After surgery, the staff member should:
• place the infant on the side opposite the operative site, with his head level with his body unless the doctor's orders specify otherwise.
• check temperature, pulse rate, blood pressure, and level of consciousness; watch for increased intracranial pressure, a sign of possible shunt malfunction.
• watch for signs and symptoms of infection, especially meningitis: increased temperature, stiff neck, irritability, or tense fontanelles; watch for redness, swelling, or other signs of local infection over the shunt tract; check dressing often for drainage.
• listen for bowel sounds after ventriculoperitoneal shunt.
• check the infant's growth and development periodically; help the parents set goals consistent with ability and potential and focus on their child's strengths, not his weaknesses; discuss special education programs, and emphasize the infant's need for sensory stimulation appropriate for his age; teach parents to watch for signs of shunt malfunction, infection, and paralytic ileus; tell them that shunt insertion requires periodic surgery to lengthen the shunt as the child grows older, to correct malfunctioning shunts, or to treat infection.

ARNOLD-CHIARI SYNDROME

The Arnold-Chiari syndrome frequently accompanies hydrocephalus, especially when a myelomeningocele is also present. In this condition, an elongation or tonguelike downward projection of the cerebellum and medulla extends through the foramen magnum into the cervical portion of the spinal canal, impairing CSF drainage from the fourth ventricle.

In addition to signs and symptoms of hydrocephalus, infants with this syndrome have nuchal rigidity, noisy respirations, irritability, vomiting, weak sucking reflex, and a preference for hyperextension of neck.

Treatment requires surgery to insert a shunt like that used in hydrocephalus. Surgical decompression of the cerebellar tonsils at the foramen magnum is sometimes indicated.

Mental Retardation

Mental retardation is a syndrome of subnormal intellectual development associated with impaired learning and social adjustment. Related to a variety of causes, mental retardation is a major health problem throughout the world, with incidence highest in urban areas.

Causes

Many possible causes exist; however, in more than half of all cases of mental retardation, no specific cause can be identified.

Signs and symptoms

Mental retardation is immediately apparent in most adults and older children. Its obvious signs include poor motor development, faulty concepts of space and time, dismal performance in school (a retarded student may have an IQ as low as 60 and may fail to go beyond sixth grade), an inability to find or keep a job or to perform anything more than menial tasks, and difficulty with even the simplest social interactions. In a clinical situation, retarded adults often fail to give reliable personal histories; they may display inappropriate behavior.

The severely retarded infant displays a poor sucking reflex, an unhealthy physical appearance (sallow complexion and cachexia), and delayed sitting, walking, and standing. The retarded toddler speaks poorly and fails to develop self-help skills; the preschooler's development of skills is delayed; the school-age child has difficulty in comprehending abstract concepts.

Diagnosis

The dominant clues to mental retardation are overt anomalies or developmental lags. For example, Down's syndrome (trisomy 21) is easily recognized at birth, as are other forms of mental retardation accompanied by multiple anomalies. Down's syndrome represents only 1% of all mentally impaired persons but accounts for about one third of admissions to institutional care. It produces mild to severe mental impairment and is associated with dwarfed stature and facial anomalies (small head, sloping forehead, large protruding tongue, low-set ears, slanted eyes), as well as other physical abnormalities.

When mental retardation is not accompanied by obvious physical defects, it may be more difficult to detect and consequently may go unrecognized until later in life. Severe retardation becomes obvious in the first year of life by a clear lag in motor and adaptive development. (Lagging motor development alone may have some physical cause and doesn't necessarily point to mental retardation.) Moderate retardation also delays motor and adaptive development but may not be obvious unless it markedly delays speech. Mild retardation may go unrecognized until school age, when the child's deficient mental capacity causes great difficulty with reasoning and abstract thought. However, certain developmental tests (Denver Developmental Screening Examination, Bayley Developmental Scales) can help screen infants and toddlers for mental impairment. Used sequentially and for a prolonged period, they can accurately evaluate developmental progress.

Diagnosis requires a team approach, including a doctor, nurse, psychologist, and social worker, who assess the child's mental, physical, and social development in the context of both the family and school. Diagnosis also rules out vision, hearing, and speech defects, and other disorders that similarly impair development. The younger the child, the more difficult it is to make the diagnosis. For example, there is no test for range of intelligence for infants. In older persons, intelligence testing and other tests help confirm this diagnosis but should not be the only bases for it. When a patient is diagnosed as being mentally retarded, his retardation level is classified according to severity. However, these categories have little impact on treatment.

Treatment

When retardation is secondary to other curable conditions, accurate identification is essential to allow for early treatment and to limit the extent of retardation. For example, a change in diet can almost completely reverse rare metabolic disorders such as phenylketonuria; neurosurgery can correct hydrocephalus. With complex multifactorial mental retardation, all contributing factors (organic, psychologic, genetic, environmental) must be considered in treatment.

However, for most mentally retarded persons, no specific treatment exists. Their management is primarily nonmedical and emphasizes education, training in self-care and socialization, recreational and social services, vocational training, and custodial arrangements. Ideally, such management requires the cooperation of a team of specialists to develop a personalized and realistic plan of care. Whenever possible, care plans emphasize home care, early maximum stimulation, and an education program that includes modeling (having children imitate parents and teachers), behavior modification, and direct stimulation and teaching.

Additional considerations

Caring for the mentally retarded patient can often be frustrating, since there is little immediate help that can be given the patient. In addition, improvement is not always visible, and when it occurs, it's usually gradual. Still, such care is essential to the patient's treatment.

• Mentally retarded patients, like all patients, should be treated with respect. Their feelings of self-worth can be enhanced with positive reinforcement.

• Mentally retarded children need the same love, security, and help as normal children. Therefore, they should be cared for at home, if possible, through the preschool years.

• A daily routine should be developed for the patient.

• Behavior modification techniques, such as immediately giving patients rewards, will encourage positive behavior. Consistency is important. Such techniques increase the chances that the desired behavior will be repeated, and help patients learn complex behavior in small steps. Discipline and limit-setting should also be consistent and immediate.

• The patient must know about body functions. If the patient is a child, nor-

---

CAUSES OF MENTAL RETARDATION

Prenatal causes
• metabolic disorders (phenylketonuria, cretinism)
• hereditary disorders (Hunter's syndrome)
• chromosomal abnormalities (cri-du-chat, Down's syndrome)
• cranial malformation (microencephaly, hydroencephaly)
• maternal infections (rubella, syphilis, cytomegalic inclusion disease)
• maternal factors (multiple pregnancy, anoxia, malnutrition, isoimmunization, toxemia)

Natal causes
• intracranial hemorrhage
• anoxia (birth trauma)
• prematurity

Postnatal causes
• intracranial injury (falls, accidents, child abuse)
• CNS infections (meningitis, encephalitis)
• lead or drug poisoning
• anoxia (near-drowning, plastic bag asphyxiation)
• neoplasms
• recurrent convulsions
• degenerative diseases (Tay-Sachs, Huntington's chorea)
• cerebral hemorrhage, thrombosis, embolism
• social, cultural, and environmental factors (deprivation, emotional disturbance, nutritional deficiency).

MENTAL RETARDATION CLASSIFIED BY SEVERITY

Mildly retarded (75% of retarded)
- IQ: 51 to 70 (educable)
- Mental age: 8 to 12 years
- Abilities: can learn reading and arithmetic
- Outlook: capable of employment in simple job; functions well at home

Moderately retarded (20% of retarded)
- IQ: 21 to 50 (trainable)
- Mental age: 3 to 7 years
- Abilities: can understand and use language fairly well; ability to concentrate varies
- Outlook: needs adult supervision throughout life; may function in a sheltered workshop

Severely retarded (5% of retarded)
- IQ: 0 to 20
- Mental age: 0 to 2 years
- Abilities: completely dependent on others
- Outlook: needs lifelong custodial care.

mal growth and development will be delayed. Skills that are appropriate for the child's mental age should be taught.
- Teaching should be done by example, not verbal instruction. For instance, to teach a patient how to wash his face, the teacher should wash his own face so the patient can see how it is done. The patient's family should also follow this method of teaching.
- The child needs to be stimulated with toys, simple games, and recreational activities appropriate for his mental age.
- Family members must understand the retarded patient's potential so they can accept diagnosis and make realistic long-range plans; for example, whether or not the patient should be institutionalized. Also, they'll need to evaluate the physical and emotional capabilities necessary to care for a retarded family member on a day-to-day basis. Parents should involve their entire family in this difficult decision, because ultimately it will affect all of them. After they make their decision, the health care professional should respect it, whatever it is. Parents may feel that caring for a retarded child will take too much time away from their other children.
- The family will have to deal with initial feelings of shame or guilt so they can develop a healthy love for the retarded patient. The health care professional must not confuse his feelings with theirs. He should explore his own feelings and make sure they don't interfere with patient care.
- The family should know about community resources, public education benefits, and legislation designed to improve conditions for the retarded.
- To prevent retardation, families should know about controllable factors that may cause it, such as malnutrition, environmental deprivation, and poisoning. They should also know about the importance of good prenatal care, and genetic counseling.

For more information, families should contact the Association for Children with Retarded Mental Development, the Association for Retarded Citizens, and the President's Committee on Mental Retardation.

Cerebral Aneurysm

Cerebral aneurysm is a localized dilation of a cerebral artery that results from a weakness in the arterial wall. Its most common form is the berry aneurysm, a saclike outpouching in a cerebral artery. Cerebral aneurysms usually arise at an arterial junction in the circle of Willis, the circular anastomosis forming the major cerebral arteries at the base of the brain. Cerebral aneurysms often rupture and cause subarachnoid hemorrhage.

Prognosis is guarded. Probably half the patients suffering subarachnoid hemorrhages die immediately; of those persons who survive untreated, 40% die from the effects of hemorrhage; another 20% die later from recurring hemorrhage. With new and better treatment, prognosis is improving.

Causes and incidence

Cerebral aneurysm may result from a congenital defect, a degenerative process, or a combination of both. For example, hypertension and atherosclerosis may disrupt blood flow and exert pressure against a congenitally weak arterial wall, stretching it like an overblown balloon and making it likely to rupture. After such rupture, blood spills into the space normally occupied by CSF (subarachnoid hemorrhage). Sometimes, it also spills into brain tissue and subsequently forms a clot. This may result in potentially fatal increased intracranial pressure (ICP) and brain tissue damage.

Incidence is slightly higher in women than in men, especially those in their late 40s or early to mid-50s, but cerebral aneurysm may occur at any age, in both women and men.

Signs and symptoms

Occasionally, rupture of a cerebral aneurysm causes premonitory symptoms that last several days, such as headache, nuchal rigidity, stiff back and legs, and intermittent nausea. Normally, however, onset is abrupt and without warning, causing a sudden severe headache, nausea, vomiting, and depending on the severity and location of bleeding, altered consciousness (including deep coma).

Bleeding causes meningeal irritation, causing nuchal rigidity, back and leg pain, fever, restlessness, irritability, occasional seizures, and blurred vision. Bleeding into the brain tissues causes hemiparesis, hemisensory defects, dysphagia, and visual defects. If the aneurysm is near the internal carotid artery, it compresses the oculomotor nerve and causes diplopia, ptosis, dilated pupil, and inability to rotate the eye.

The severity of symptoms varies considerably from patient to patient, depending on the site and amount of bleeding. To better describe their con-

ditions, patients with ruptured cerebral aneurysms are grouped as follows:

• *Grade I: Minimal bleed.* Patient is alert with no neurologic deficit; he may have a slight headache and nuchal rigidity.
• *Grade II: Mild bleed.* Patient is alert, with a mild to severe headache, nuchal rigidity, and possibly, third-nerve palsy.
• *Grade III: Moderate bleed.* Patient is confused or drowsy, has nuchal rigidity, and possibly, a mild focal deficit.
• *Grade IV: Moderate to severe bleed.* Patient is stuporous, has nuchal rigidity, and possibly, mild to severe hemiparesis.
• *Grade V: Severe bleed (often fatal).* If nonfatal, patient is in deep coma or decerebrate.

Generally, cerebral aneurysm poses three major threats:

• *Death from increased ICP:* Increased ICP may push the brain downward, impair brain stem function, and cut off blood supply to the part of the brain that supports vital functions.
• *Rebleed:* Generally, after initial bleeding episode, a clot forms and seals the rupture, reinforcing the wall of the aneurysm for 7 to 10 days. However, after the seventh day, fibrinolysis begins to dissolve the clot and increases the risk of rebleeding. This rebleeding produces symptoms similar to those accompanying the initial hemorrhage. Rebleeds during the first 48 to 72 hours following initial hemorrhage are not uncommon and contribute to the high mortality.
• *Vasospasm:* Why this occurs isn't clearly understood. Usually, vasospasm occurs in blood vessels adjacent to the aneurysm, but it may extend to major vessels of the brain, causing ischemia and altered brain function.

Other complications include acute hydrocephalus (a result of abnormal accumulation of CSF within the cranial cavity because of CSF blockage by blood or adhesions) and pulmonary embolism (a possible side effect of aneurysm treat-

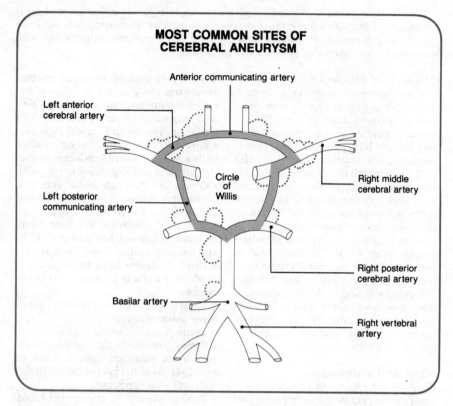

MOST COMMON SITES OF CEREBRAL ANEURYSM

Anterior communicating artery

Left anterior cerebral artery

Right middle cerebral artery

Circle of Willis

Left posterior communicating artery

Right posterior cerebral artery

Basilar artery

Right vertebral artery

ment with aminocaproic acid or deep vein thrombosis).

Diagnosis

Angiography can pinpoint an unruptured cerebral aneurysm. Unfortunately, diagnosis of cerebral aneurysm usually follows its rupture. Then, diagnostic evaluation includes patient history, physical examination, and certain laboratory tests.

• *Lumbar puncture* can detect blood in CSF and increased ICP.

• *Skull X-ray* may show calcification in the walls of a large aneurysm.

• *EKG* often shows flattened or depressed T waves.

• *CAT scan* locates the clot and identifies hydrocephalus, areas of infarction, and extent of blood spillage within the cisterns around the brain.

Other baseline laboratory studies in-clude CBC, urinalysis, measurement of arterial blood gases, coagulation studies, serum osmolality, and electrolyte and glucose levels.

Treatment

Treatment aims to reduce the risk of rebleeding by repairing the aneurysm. Usually, surgical repair (by clipping, ligation, or wrapping the aneurysm neck with muscle) takes place 7 to 10 days after the initial bleed. When surgical correction is risky (in very elderly patients or those with heart, lung, or other serious diseases), or when the aneurysm is in a particularly dangerous location or surgery is delayed because of vasospasm, conservative treatment includes:

• bed rest in a quiet, darkened room; if immediate surgery isn't possible, such bed rest may continue for 4 to 6 weeks.

• avoidance of coffee, other stimulants, and aspirin.

- codeine or another analgesic, as needed.
- hydralazine or another hypotensive agent if the patient is hypertensive.
- corticosteroids to reduce edema.
- phenobarbital or another sedative to reduce stress.
- aminocaproic acid, a fibrinolytic inhibitor, to minimize the risk of rebleed by delaying blood clot lysis.

After surgical repair, the patient's condition depends on the extent of damage from the initial bleed and the degree of success of the treatment of the resulting complications. Surgery cannot improve the patient's neurologic condition unless it removes a hematoma or reduces the compression effect.

Additional considerations
An accurate neurologic assessment, good patient care, patient and family teaching, and psychological support can speed recovery and reduce complications.

During initial treatment after hemorrhage, the hospital staff member should: establish and maintain a patent airway, since the patient may need supplementary oxygen; position the patient to promote pulmonary drainage and prevent upper airway obstruction; perform preoxygenation with 100% oxygen before suctioning the intubated patient to prevent hypoxia and vasodilation from CO_2 accumulation; give frequent nose and mouth care.

The staff member must impose aneurysm precautions to minimize the risk of rebleed and to avoid increased ICP. Such precautions include bed rest in a quiet, darkened room (keeping the head of the bed flat or under 30°, as ordered);

limited visitors; avoidance of coffee, other stimulants, and strenuous physical activity; and restricted fluid intake. The patient must know why these restrictive measures are necessary.

Along with these preventive measures, good patient care, to minimize other complications includes:
- turning the patient often; encouraging deep breathing and leg movement; warning the patient to avoid all unnecessary physical activity; assisting with active range-of-motion exercises (unless the doctor has forbidden them); performing regular passive range-of-motion exercises if the patient is paralyzed.
- monitoring arterial blood gases, level of consciousness, and vital signs often, and accurately measuring intake and output; not taking temperature rectally, since vagus nerve stimulation may cause cardiac arrest.
- watching for danger signals—decreased level of consciousness, unilateral enlarged pupil, onset or worsening of hemiparesis or motor deficit, increased blood pressure, slowed pulse, worsening of headache or sudden onset of a new headache, renewed or worsened nuchal rigidity, renewed or persistent vomiting—all of which may indicate an enlargement of the aneurysm, rebleeding, intracranial clot, vasospasm, or another complication.
- restricting fluids, as ordered, and monitoring I.V. infusions to avoid increased ICP; giving meticulous catheter care, if appropriate, to prevent infection; noting the color, consistency, and odor of urine.
- assisting the patient with facial weak-

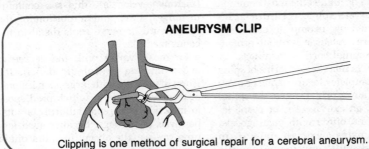

ANEURYSM CLIP

Clipping is one method of surgical repair for a cerebral aneurysm.

ness during meals by placing food in the unaffected side of his mouth; inserting a nasogastric tube if he can't swallow, and giving all tube feedings slowly; preventing skin breakdown by taping the tube so it doesn't press against the nostril.

• providing a high-bulk diet (bran, salads, and fruit) to the patient who can eat to prevent straining at stool, which can increase ICP; getting an order for a stool softener such as dioctyl sodium sulfosuccinate, or a mild laxative, and administering, as ordered; not forcing fluids; implementing a bowel program based on the patient's previous habits; checking the stool for blood if the patient is receiving steroids.

• administering artificial tears to the affected eye, and taping the eye shut at night to prevent corneal damage.

• minimizing stress by giving a sedative, as ordered; watching for signs of oversedation, and reporting them immediately; raising the side rails if the patient is confused—but not using restraints, if possible, since these can cause agitation and raise ICP.

• administering hydralazine or another hypotensive agent, as ordered; monitoring blood pressure and reporting *any* significant change, especially a rise in systolic pressure, immediately.

• administering aminocaproic acid I.V. in 5% dextrose in water, P.O., or as ordered; giving it at least every 2 hours to maintain therapeutic blood levels (renal insufficiency may require dosage adjustment); watching for adverse reactions, such as nausea and diarrhea (most common with oral administration), and phlebitis (most common with I.V. administration); minimizing deep vein thrombosis by applying elastic stockings.

• establishing a simple means of communication with the patient who can't speak; limiting conversation to topics that won't further frustrate the patient; encouraging his family to speak to him in a normal tone, even if he doesn't seem to respond.

• providing emotional support, and including the patient's family in his care as much as possible; encouraging family members to adopt a positive attitude, but discouraging unrealistic goals.

• before discharge, making a referral to a visiting nurse or a rehabilitation center when necessary.

Spinal Cord Defects

(Spina bifida, meningocele, myelomeningocele)

Defective embryonic neural tube closure during the first trimester of pregnancy results in various malformations of the spine. Generally, these defects occur in the lumbosacral area but are occasionally found in the sacral, thoracic, and cervical areas.

Spina bifida occulta is the most common and least severe spinal cord defect. It's characterized by incomplete closure of one or more vertebrae without protrusion of the spinal cord or meninges.

However, in more severe forms of spina bifida, incomplete closure of one or more vertebrae causes protrusion of the spinal contents in an external sac or cystic lesion. In spina bifida with meningocele, this sac contains meninges and CSF. In spina bifida with myelomeningocele (meningomyelocele), this sac contains meninges, CSF, and a portion of the spinal cord or nerve roots distal to the conus medullaris.

Prognosis varies with the degree of accompanying neurologic deficit. It's worst in patients with large open lesions, neurogenic bladders (which predispose to infection and renal failure), or total paralysis of the legs. Because such features are usually absent in spina bifida occulta and meningocele, prognosis is

TYPES OF SPINAL CORD DEFECTS

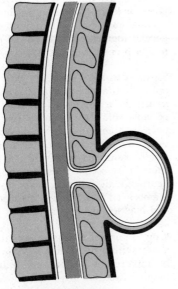

Meningocele

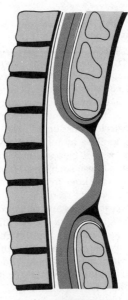

Myelocele

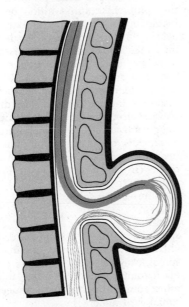

Myelomeningocele

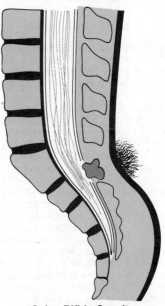

Spina Bifida Occulta

much better than in myelomeningocele, and many patients with this condition can lead normal lives.

Causes and incidence

Normally, about 20 days after conception, the embryo develops a neural groove in the dorsal ectoderm. This groove rapidly deepens, and the two edges fuse to form the neural tube. By about day 23, this tube is completely closed except for an opening at each end. Theoretically, if the posterior portion of this neural tube fails to close by the fourth week of gestation, or if it closes but then splits open from a cause such as an abnormal increase in CSF later in the first trimester, a spinal defect results.

Viruses, radiation, and other environmental factors may be responsible for such defects. However, spinal cord defects occur more often in offspring of women who have previously had children with similar defects, so genetic factors may also be responsible.

Spina bifida is relatively common and

occurs in about 5% of live births. In the United States, each year, about 12,000 infants are born with some form of spina bifida; spina bifida with myelomeningocele is less common than spina bifida occulta and spina bifida with meningocele. Incidence is highest in persons of Welsh or Irish ancestry.

Signs and symptoms

Spina bifida occulta is often accompanied by a depression or dimple, tuft of hair, soft fatty deposits, port wine nevi, or a combination of these abnormalities on the skin over the spinal defect; however, such signs may be absent. Spina bifida occulta doesn't usually cause neurologic dysfunction but occasionally is associated with foot weakness or bowel and bladder disturbances. Such disturbances are especially likely during rapid growth phases, when the spinal cord's ascent within the vertebral column may be impaired by its abnormal adherence to other tissues.

In both meningocele and myelomeningocele, a saclike structure protrudes over the spine. Like spina bifida occulta, meningocele rarely causes neurologic deficit. But myelomeningocele, depending on the level of the defect, causes permanent neurologic dysfunction, such as flaccid or spastic paralysis, and bowel and bladder incontinence. Associated disorders include trophic skin disturbances (ulcerations, cyanosis), clubfoot, knee contractures, hydrocephalus (in about 90% of patients), and possibly, mental retardation, Arnold-Chiari syndrome (in which part of the brain protrudes into the spinal canal), and curvature of the spine.

Diagnosis

Spina bifida occulta is often overlooked, although it's occasionally palpable and spinal X-ray can show the bone defect. Myelography can differentiate it from other spinal abnormalities, especially spinal cord tumors.

Usually, meningocele and myelomeningocele are obvious on examination; transillumination of the protruding sac

---

ENCEPHALOCELE

An encephalocele is a congenital saclike protrusion of the meninges and brain through a defective opening in the skull. Usually, it's in the occipital area, but it may also occur in the parietal, nasopharyngeal, or frontal area.

Clinical effects of encephalocele vary with the degree of tissue involvement and location of the defect. Paralysis and hydrocephalus are common.

Treatment includes surgery during infancy to place protruding tissues back in the skull, excise the sac, and correct associated craniofacial abnormalities. The infant with encephalocele must be handled carefully to avoid pressure on the sac. Both before and after surgery, the infant may show signs of increased intracranial pressure (bulging fontanelles). As the child grows older, his parents should watch for developmental deficiencies that may signal mental retardation.

can sometimes distinguish between them. (In meningocele, it typically transilluminates; in myelomeningocele, it doesn't.) In myelomeningocele, a pinprick examination of the legs and trunk shows the level of sensory and motor involvement; skull X-rays, cephalic measurements, and CAT scan demonstrate associated hydrocephalus. Other appropriate laboratory tests in patients with myelomeningocele include urinalysis, urine cultures, and tests for renal function in older children and adults with urinary incontinence.

Although amniocentesis can detect only open defects, such as myelomeningocele and meningocele, this procedure is recommended for all pregnant women who have previously had children with spinal cord defects, since these women are at an increased risk of having children with similar defects. If these defects are present, amniocentesis shows increased alpha-fetoprotein levels by 14 weeks of gestation.

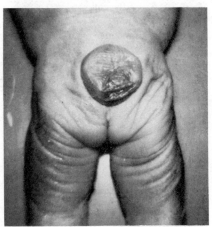

In myelomeningocele, a saclike structure protrudes over the spinal column. This structure contains meninges, cerebrospinal fluid, and a portion of the spinal cord.

Treatment

Spina bifida occulta usually requires no treatment. However, if neuromuscular problems occur during growth, surgery may be indicated.

Treatment for meningocele consists solely of surgical closure of the protruding sac and continual assessment of growth and development. Treatment of myelomeningocele requires surgical repair of the sac and supportive measures to promote independence and prevent further complications. Unfortunately, surgery can't reverse neurologic deficit. Usually, a shunt is necessary to relieve associated hydrocephalus.

In older children or adults, rehabilitation measures include:
• waist supports, long leg braces, walkers, crutches, and other orthopedic appliances.
• management of fecal incontinence with diet and bowel training or, possibly, colostomy.
• neurogenic bladder management with a urinary antiseptic, regular application of Credé's method (manual compression of bladder) to reduce urinary stasis, possible intermittent catheterization, antispasmodics such as bethanechol or propantheline, and in severe cases, possibly, urinary diversion.

Additional considerations

Effective care of the patient with severe spinal defect requires a team approach, which involves the neurosurgeon, orthopedist, urologist, nurse, social worker, both occupational and physical therapists, and parents. Obviously, care is most complex when the neurologic deficit is severe. Immediate goals include psychologic support to help parents accept the diagnosis, and pre- and postoperative care. Long-term goals include patient and family teaching, and measures to prevent contractures, decubitus ulcers, urinary tract infection, and other complications.

Before surgery for meningocele or myelomeningocele, the hospital staff member should:
• prevent local infection by cleansing the defect gently with sterile saline solution or other solutions, as ordered; inspect the defect often for signs of infection, and cover it with sterile dressings moist-

ened with sterile saline solution (ointments should not be used on the defect, since they may cause skin maceration); prevent skin breakdown by placing sheepskin or a foam pad under the infant; keep skin clean, and apply lotion to knees, elbows, chin, and other pressure areas; give antibiotics, as ordered.

• handle the infant carefully, without applying pressure to the defect; keep him warm in an infant incubator (Isolette)—he usually can't wear a diaper or a shirt until after surgical correction because it will irritate the sac; position him on his abdomen to prevent contamination of the sac with urine or feces; hold and cuddle the infant, but avoid pressure on the sac; position the infant's abdomen down when he is on someone's lap.

• measure head circumference daily, and watch for signs of hydrocephalus and meningeal irritation, such as fever or nuchal rigidity.

• minimize contractures through passive range-of-motion exercises and casting; prevent hip dislocation by moderately abducting hips with a pad between the knees, or sandbags and ankle rolls.

• monitor intake and output; watch for decreased skin turgor, dryness, or other signs of dehydration; prevent urinary tract infection by Credéing the bladder every 2 hours during the day and once during the night; provide meticulous skin care to genitals and buttocks to prevent infection.

• make sure the infant receives adequate nutrition.

After surgical repair of the defect, the staff member should:

• watch for hydrocephalus, which often follows such surgery; measure the child's head circumference every other day or as ordered.

• monitor vital signs often; watch for signs of shock, infection, and increased intracranial pressure (projectile vomiting). (Before age 2, infants don't show typical signs of increased intracranial pressure, since suture lines aren't fully closed. In infants, the most telling sign is bulging fontanelles.)

• change the dressing regularly, as ordered, and check for drainage, wound rupture, and infection.

• if a leg cast has been applied to prevent deformities, watch for signs that the child is outgrowing the cast; use a blow-dryer to dry skin under the cast; check for foul odor, and be alert for indications of skin breakdown.

Parents must be taught how to cope with the infant's physical problems and successfully meet long-range treatment goals. For example, they should be taught how to:

• recognize early signs of complications, such as hydrocephalus, decubitus ulcers, and urinary tract infection.

• provide psychological support for each other and maintain a positive attitude.

• Credé the bladder regularly. Parents must begin training their child in a bladder routine by age 3, and understand the need for increased fluid intake to prevent urinary tract infection. Intermittent catheterization and conduit hygiene may also be ordered.

• prevent bowel obstruction. The child needs increased fluid intake, a high-bulk diet, exercise, and use of a stool softener, as ordered. Parents should empty their child's bowel by exerting slight pressure on his abdomen, telling him to bear down, and giving a glycerin suppository, as needed.

• recognize developmental lags early (a possible result of hydrocephalus). Parents must know the importance of follow-up IQ assessment to help plan realistic educational goals. The child may need to attend a school with special facilities. Also, the child needs adequate stimulation to ensure maximum mental development. Parents should plan activities appropriate to their child's age and abilities.

Parents should be referred for genetic counseling and should have amniocentesis performed in future pregnancies. For more information on these disorders, parents can contact the Spina Bifida Association of America. This organization can also supply the names of community support groups for parents of children with similar problems.

PAROXYSMAL DISORDERS

Headache

The most common patient complaint, headache usually occurs as a symptom of an underlying disorder. Headaches are commonly classified as vascular, muscle contraction (tension), and traction-inflammatory. Migraine headaches, probably the most intensively studied, are throbbing, vascular headaches that usually begin to appear in childhood or adolescence and recur throughout adulthood. Affecting up to 10% of Americans, they're more common in females and have a strong familial incidence.

Causes

The cause of migraine headaches is unknown, but most chronic headaches result from tension, which may be caused by emotional stress, fatigue, menstruation, or environmental stimuli (noise, crowds, bright lights). Other causes include glaucoma; inflammation of the eyes or mucosa of the nasal or paranasal sinuses; diseases of the scalp, teeth, extracranial arteries, or external or middle ear; and muscle spasms of the face, neck, or shoulders. Headaches may also be caused by vasodilators (nitrates, alcohol, histamine); systemic disease, hypoxia, hypertension, head trauma and tumor, intracranial bleeding, abscess, or aneurysm.

Headache pain may emanate from structures above the tentorium cerebelli and pass through the trigeminal nerves to the parietal, temporal, or frontal area. Pain may also emanate from below the tentorium cerebelli and pass through upper cervical spinal roots, and glossopharyngeal and vagal nerves to the back of the head and neck.

Signs and symptoms

Both muscle contraction and traction-inflammatory headaches produce a dull, persistent ache, tender spots on the head and neck, and a feeling of tightness around the head, with a characteristic "hatband" distribution. The pain is often severe and unrelenting, occasionally bilateral. If caused by intracranial bleed-

ing, these headaches may result in neurologic deficits, such as paresthesias and muscle weakness; narcotics fail to relieve pain in these cases. If caused by a tumor, pain is most severe when the patient awakens.

Cluster headaches (paroxysmal nocturnal cephalalgia, migrainous neuralgia, histamine headache, or Horton's syndrome) are vascular headaches that usually occur in men at night, after an hour or two of sleep. These headaches recur over a period of days or weeks, causing closely spaced attacks of intense pain, followed by remissions that may last months or even years. Such headaches may be associated with lacrimation, nasal congestion, rhinorrhea, flushing, ptosis, and edema of the cheek. Prodromal symptoms are uncommon.

Diagnosis

Diagnosis requires a history of recurrent headaches and physical examination of the head and neck. Such examination includes percussion, auscultation for bruits, inspection for signs of infection, and palpation for defects, crepitus, or tender spots (especially after trauma). Firm diagnosis also requires a complete neurologic examination, assessment for other systemic diseases—such as hypertension—and a psychosocial evaluation, when such factors are suspected. Diagnostic tests include skull X-rays (including cervical spine and sinus), EEG, CAT scan, brain scan, and lumbar puncture.

CLINICAL FEATURES OF MIGRAINE HEADACHES

TYPE	SIGNS AND SYMPTOMS
Common migraine (*most prevalent*) Usually occurs on weekends and holidays	• Prodromal symptoms (fatigue, nausea and vomiting, and fluid imbalance) precede headache by about a day. • Sensitivity to light and noise (most prominent feature) • Headache pain (unilateral or bilateral, aching or throbbing)
Classic migraine Usually occurs in compulsive personalities and within families	• Prodromal symptoms include visual disturbances, such as zigzag lines and bright lights (most common), sensory disturbances (tingling of face, lips, and hands), or motor disturbances (staggering gait). • Recurrent and periodic headaches
Hemiplegic and ophthalmoplegic migraine (*rare*) Usually occurs in young adults	• Severe, unilateral pain • Extraocular muscle palsies (involving third cranial nerve) and ptosis • With repeated headaches, possible permanent third cranial nerve injury • In hemiplegic migraine, neurologic deficits (hemiparesis, hemiplegia) may persist after headache subsides.
Basilar artery migraine Occurs in young women before their menstrual periods	• Prodromal symptoms usually include partial vision loss followed by vertigo; ataxia; dysarthria; tinnitus; and sometimes, tingling of fingers and toes, lasting from several minutes to almost an hour. • Headache pain, severe occipital throbbing, vomiting

Treatment

Depending on the type of headache, analgesics ranging from aspirin to codeine or meperidine may provide symptomatic relief. A tranquilizer, such as diazepam, may be beneficial during acute attacks. Other measures include identification and elimination of causative factors, and if necessary, supportive psychotherapy for headaches caused by emotional stress. Chronic tension headaches may also require muscle relaxants.

For migraine headache, ergotamine alone or in combination with caffeine is the most effective treatment. These drugs and other analgesics work best when taken early in the course of an attack. If nausea and vomiting make oral administration impossible, these drugs may be given as rectal suppositories. Although migraine attacks can't be pre-vented, methysergide can help reduce frequency and intensity.

Additional considerations

Headaches rarely necessitate hospitalization unless they're caused by a serious underlying disorder. If this is the case, patient care must be directed to the primary problem.
• A complete patient history should include: duration and location of the headache; time of day it usually begins; nature of the pain (intermittent or throbbing); concurrence with other symptoms, such as blurred vision; precipitating factors, such as tension, menstruation, loud noises, menopause, alcohol; medications being taken, such as oral contraceptives; or prolonged fasting.
• Using the history as a guide, the patient can come to understand the reason

for his headaches. Knowing this, he can avoid exacerbating factors. During an attack, he should lie down in a dark, quiet room and place ice packs on his forehead or a cold cloth over his eyes.
• The patient must take the prescribed medication at the onset of migraine symptoms, prevent dehydration by drinking plenty of fluids after nausea and vomiting subside, and use other headache relief measures.
• The patient with migraine headaches usually needs to be hospitalized only if nausea and vomiting are severe enough to result in dehydration and possible shock.

Epilepsy
(Seizure disorder)

Epilepsy is a condition of the brain characterized by a susceptibility to recurrent seizures (paroxysmal events associated with abnormal electrical discharges of neurons in the brain). Epilepsy probably affects 1% to 2% of the population; incidence is higher among people with a family history of this disorder. Prognosis is good if the patient adheres strictly to prescribed treatment.

Causes
About half the cases of epilepsy probably result from some undiscovered abnormality in brain chemistry, which causes electrical instability and a low seizure threshold (idiopathic epilepsy). Other possible causes of epilepsy include:
• birth trauma (inadequate oxygen supply to the brain, blood incompatibility, hemorrhage)
• perinatal infection
• anoxia
• infectious diseases (meningitis, encephalitis, or brain abscess)
• ingestion of toxins (mercury, lead, or carbon monoxide)
• tumors of the brain
• inherited disorders or degenerative disease, such as phenylketonuria or tuberous sclerosis
• head injury or trauma
• metabolic disorders, such as hypoglycemia or hypoparathyroidism
• cerebrovascular accident (hemorrhage, thrombosis, embolism).

Signs and symptoms
The hallmarks of epilepsy are recurring seizures, which can be classified as partial or generalized (some patients may be affected by more than one type).
Partial seizures arise from a localized area of the brain, causing specific symptoms. In some patients, partial seizure activity may spread to the entire brain, causing a generalized seizure. Partial seizures include jacksonian and complex partial seizures (psychomotor or temporal lobe).
A jacksonian seizure begins as a localized motor seizure, characterized by a spread of abnormal activity to adjacent areas of the brain. It typically produces a stiffening or jerking in one extremity, accompanied by a tingling sensation in the same area. For example, it may start in the thumb and spread to the entire hand and arm. The patient seldom loses consciousness. Jacksonian seizure may progress to a generalized tonic-clonic seizure.
The symptoms of a complex partial seizure are variable but usually include purposeless behavior. This seizure may begin with an aura, a sensation the patient feels immediately before a seizure. An aura represents the beginning of abnormal electrical discharges within a focal area of the brain and may include a pungent smell, gastrointestinal distress (nausea or indigestion), a rising or sinking feeling in the stomach, a dreamy feeling, an unusual taste, or a visual disturbance. Overt signs of a complex

partial seizure include a glassy stare, picking at one's clothes, aimless wandering, lip-smacking or chewing motions, and unintelligible speech. Mental confusion may last several minutes after the seizure; as a result, an observer may mistakenly suspect intoxication with alcohol or drugs, or psychosis.

Generalized seizures, as the term suggests, cause a generalized electrical abnormality within the brain and include several distinct types:

Absence (petit mal) seizures occur most often in children, although they may affect adults as well. They usually begin with a brief change in level of consciousness, indicated by blinking or rolling of the eyes, a blank stare, and slight mouth movements. The patient retains his posture and continues preseizure activity without difficulty. (Absence seizures rarely occur during vigorous exercise.) Each seizure lasts from 1 to 10 seconds; if not properly treated, seizures can recur as often as 100 times a day. An absence seizure may progress to generalized tonic-clonic seizures.

The *myoclonic (bilateral massive epileptic myoclonus)* seizure is characterized by brief involuntary muscular jerks of the body or extremities, which may occur in a rhythmic fashion.

A *generalized tonic-clonic (grand mal)* seizure typically begins with a loud cry, precipitated by air rushing from the lungs through the vocal cords. The patient then falls to the ground, losing consciousness. The body stiffens (tonic phase), then alternates between episodes of muscular spasm and relaxation (clonic phase). Tongue-biting, incontinence, labored breathing, apnea, and subsequent cyanosis may also occur. The seizure stops in 2 to 5 minutes, when abnormal electrical conduction of the neurons is completed. The patient then regains consciousness but is somewhat confused and may have difficulty talking. If he can talk, he may complain of drowsiness, fatigue, headache, muscle soreness, and arm or leg weakness. He may fall into deep sleep following the seizure.

An *atonic* seizure produces falling and unconsciousness for only a few seconds; consequently, it's sometimes called a "drop attack." However, this sudden fall and unconsciousness may cause the patient to injure himself seriously.

Status epilepticus is a continuous seizure state, which can occur in all seizure types. The most life-threatening example is generalized tonic-clonic status epilepticus, a continuous generalized tonic-clonic seizure without intervening return of consciousness. Status epilepticus is accompanied by respiratory distress. It can result from abrupt withdrawal of antiepileptic medications, hypoxic encephalopathy, acute head trauma, metabolic encephalopathy, or septicemia secondary to encephalitis or meningitis.

Diagnosis

Clinically, the diagnosis of epilepsy is based on the occurrence of one or more seizures and proof or the assumption that the condition which led to them is still present.

Important diagnostic information is obtained from the patient's history and description of seizure activity, family history, thorough physical and neurologic examinations, and CAT scan. This scan offers density readings of the brain and may indicate abnormalities in internal structures. Paroxysmal abnormalities on the EEG confirm the diagnosis of epilepsy by providing evidence of the continuing tendency to have seizures. A negative EEG does not rule out epilepsy, since the paroxysmal abnormalities occur intermittently. Other helpful tests may include serum glucose and calcium studies, skull X-rays, lumbar puncture, brain scan, cerebral angiography, and pneumoencephalography.

Treatment

Generally, treatment for epilepsy consists of drug therapy specific to the type of seizure. The most commonly prescribed drugs include phenytoin, carbamazepine, phenobarbital, or primidone administered individually for generalized tonic-clonic seizures and in combinations of two for complex partial seizures. Valproic acid, clonazepam, and ethosuximide are commonly prescribed for absence seizures.

A patient taking antiepileptic medications requires constant monitoring for toxic signs, such as nystagmus, ataxia, lethargy, dizziness, drowsiness, slurred speech, irritability, nausea, and vomiting. If drug therapy fails, treatment may include surgical removal of a demonstrated focal lesion to attempt to bring an end to seizures. Emergency treatment for status epilepticus usually consists of diazepam, phenytoin, or phenobarbital; 50% dextrose I.V. (when seizures are secondary to hypoglycemia); and thiamine I.V. (in the presence of chronic alcoholism or withdrawal).

Additional considerations

A key to support is a true understanding of the nature of epilepsy and of the myths and misconceptions that surround this disorder. This includes:

• encouraging the patient and family to express their feelings about the patient's condition, and answering their questions. This will help dispel some of the myths about epilepsy. An example is the myth that epilepsy is contagious. They need to be assured that epilepsy is controllable for most patients who follow a prescribed regimen of medication, and that most patients can maintain a normal lifestyle.

• stressing the need for compliance with the prescribed drug schedule and assuring the patient that antiepileptic drugs are safe *when taken as ordered*. Dosage instructions should be reinforced and methods found to help the patient remember to take medications. He must be advised to monitor the amount of medication that he has left so he doesn't run out.

• warning against possible side effects—drowsiness, lethargy, hyperactivity, confusion, visual and sleep disturbances—all of which indicate the need for dosage adjustment. Phenytoin therapy may lead to hyperplasia of the gums, which may be relieved by conscientious oral hygiene. The patient should be told to report side effects immediately.

• using a large vein when administering phenytoin intravenously, and monitoring vital signs frequently. I.M. administration and mixing with dextrose solutions should be avoided.

• emphasizing the importance of having antiepileptic drug blood levels checked at regular intervals, even if the seizures are under control.

• warning the patient against drinking alcoholic beverages.

• knowing which social agencies in the community can help epileptic patients. The patient can contact the Epilepsy Foundation of America for general information and the state motor vehicle department for information about a driver's license.

Generalized tonic-clonic seizures may necessitate first aid. The patient's family should be taught how to give such aid correctly. This includes: not restraining the patient during a seizure; helping him to a lying position; loosening any tight clothing, and placing something flat and soft, such as a pillow, jacket, or hand, under his head. The area should be cleared of hard objects. Nothing should be forced into the patient's mouth if his teeth are clenched—a tongue blade or spoon could lacerate mouth and lips or displace teeth, precipitating respiratory distress. However, if the patient's mouth is open, his tongue can be protected by placing a soft object (such as folded cloth) between his teeth. His head should be turned to provide an open airway. After the seizure subsides, the patient will need assurance that he's all right. He should be oriented to time and place, and informed that he's had a seizure.

If the patient has a complex partial seizure, he should not be restrained during it. The area must be cleared of any hard objects. He can be protected from injury by gently calling his name and directing him away from any source of danger. After the seizure subsides, he'll need assurance that he's all right, and should be told that he's just had a seizure.

BRAIN & SPINAL CORD DISORDERS

Cerebrovascular Accident
(Stroke)

A cerebrovascular accident (CVA) is a sudden impairment of cerebral circulation in one or more of the blood vessels supplying the brain. CVA interrupts or diminishes oxygen supply and often causes serious damage or necrosis in brain tissues. The sooner circulation returns to normal after CVA, the better chances are for complete recovery. However, about half of those who survive a CVA remain permanently disabled and experience a recurrence within weeks, months, or years.

Causes and incidence

CVA is the third most common cause of death in the United States today and the most common cause of neurologic disability. It strikes 500,000 people each year; half of them die as a result.

Factors that increase the risk of CVA include history of transient ischemic attacks, atherosclerosis, hypertension, arrhythmias, EKG changes, rheumatic heart disease, diabetes mellitus, gout, postural hypotension, cardiac or myocardial enlargement, high serum triglyceride levels, lack of exercise, use of oral contraceptives, cigarette smoking, and family history of CVA.

The major causes of CVA are thrombosis, embolism, and hemorrhage. *Thrombosis* is the most common cause of CVA in middle-aged and elderly persons, among whom there is a higher incidence of atherosclerosis, diabetes, and hypertension. CVA results from obstruction of a blood vessel. Typically, the main site of the obstruction is in extracerebral vessels, but sometimes it is intracerebral. Thrombosis causes ischemia in brain tissue supplied by the affected vessel, as well as congestion and edema; the latter may produce more clinical effects than thrombosis itself, but these symptoms subside with the edema. Thrombosis tends to develop while the patient is asleep or shortly after he awakens; however, it can also occur during surgery or following a myocardial infarction. The risk of thrombosis increases with obe-

sity, smoking, or the use of oral contraceptives.

Embolism, the second most common cause of CVA, is an occlusion of a blood vessel, caused by a fragmented clot, a tumor, fat, bacteria, or air. It can occur at any age, especially among patients with a history of rheumatic heart disease, endocarditis, post-traumatic valvular disease, myocardial fibrillation and other cardiac arrhythmias, or following open-heart surgery. It usually develops rapidly—in 10 to 20 seconds—and without warning. When an embolus reaches the cerebral vasculature, it cuts off circulation by lodging in a narrow portion of an artery, most often the middle cerebral artery, causing necrosis and edema. If the embolus is septic and infection extends beyond the vessel wall, an abscess or encephalitis may develop. If the infection is within the vessel wall, an aneurysm may form, which could lead to cerebral hemorrhage.

Hemorrhage, the third most common cause of CVA, like embolism, may occur suddenly, at any age. Such hemorrhage results from chronic hypertension or aneurysms, which cause sudden rupture of a cerebral artery. The rupture diminishes blood supply to the area served by this artery. In addition, blood accumulates deep within the brain, further compressing neural tissue and causing even greater damage.

CVAs are classified according to their course of progression. The least severe is the transient ischemic attack (TIA), or "little stroke," which results from a temporary interruption of blood flow, most often in the carotid and vertebrobasilar arteries. A progressive stroke, or stroke-in-evolution (thrombus-in-evolution), begins with slight neurologic deficit, and the condition worsens in a day or two. In a completed stroke, deficits are maximal at onset.

Signs and symptoms
Clinical features of CVA vary with the artery affected (and, consequently, the portion of the brain it supplies), the severity of damage, and extent of collateral circulation that develops to help the brain compensate for decreased blood supply. If the CVA occurs in the left hemisphere, it produces symptoms on the right side; if in the right hemisphere, symptoms are on the left side. However, a CVA that causes cranial nerve damage produces signs of cranial nerve dysfunction on the same side as the hemorrhage. Symptoms are usually classified according to the artery affected:

• *middle cerebral artery:* aphasia, dysphasia, and visual-field cuts and hemiparesis on affected side (more severe in the face and arm than in the leg)
• *carotid artery:* weakness, paralysis, numbness, sensory changes, and visual disturbances on affected side; altered level of consciousness, bruits, headaches, aphasia, ptosis
• *vertebrobasilar artery:* weakness on affected side, numbness around lips and mouth, visual-field cuts, diplopia, poor coordination, dysphagia, slurred speech, dizziness, amnesia, ataxia
• *anterior cerebral artery:* confusion, weakness and numbness (especially in the leg) on affected side, incontinence, loss of coordination, personality changes, impaired motor and sensory functions
• *posterior cerebral arteries:* visual-field cuts, sensory impairment, dyslexia, coma, cortical blindness. Usually, paralysis is absent.

Symptoms can also be classified as premonitory, generalized, and focal. Premonitory symptoms, such as drowsi-

---

TRANSIENT ISCHEMIC ATTACK (TIA)

A TIA is a recurrent episode of neurologic deficit, lasting from seconds to hours, that clears within 12 to 24 hours. It's usually considered a warning sign of an impending thrombotic CVA. In fact, TIAs have been reported in 50% to 80% of patients who have had a cerebral infarction from such thrombosis. The age of onset varies. Incidence rises dramatically after age 50 and is highest among Blacks and men.

In TIA, microemboli released from a thrombus probably temporarily interrupt blood flow, especially in the small distal branches of the arterial tree in the brain. Small spasms in those arterioles may impair blood flow and also precede TIA. Predisposing factors are the same as for thrombotic CVAs. The most distinctive characteristics of TIAs are the transient duration of neurologic deficits and complete return of normal function. The symptoms of TIA easily correlate with the location of the affected artery. These symptoms include double vision, speech deficits (slurring or thickness), unilateral blindness, staggering or uncoordinated gait, unilateral weakness or numbness, falling because of weakness in the legs, and dizziness.

During an active TIA, the aim of treatment is to prevent a completed stroke and consists of aspirin or anticoagulants to minimize the risk of thrombosis. After or between attacks, preventive treatment includes carotid endartectomy or cerebral microvascular bypass.

---

ness, dizziness, headache, and mental confusion, are rare. Generalized symptoms, such as headache, vomiting, mental impairment, convulsions, coma, nuchal rigidity, fever, and disorientation, are typical. Focal symptoms, sensory and reflex changes, reflect the site of hemorrhage or infarct and may worsen.

Diagnosis
Diagnosis of CVA is based on observation of clinical features, a history of risk fac-

tors, and the results of diagnostic tests. Definitive tests for CVA victims are:

• *CAT scan*—shows evidence of thrombotic or hemorrhagic stroke, tumor, or hydrocephalus

• *brain scan*—shows ischemic areas but may not be positive for up to 2 weeks after the CVA.

Other supportive tests include:

• *lumbar puncture*—in hemorrhagic stroke, CSF may be bloody

• *ophthalmoscopy*—may show signs of hypertension and atherosclerotic changes in retinal arteries

• *angiography*—outlines blood vessels and pinpoints the site of occlusion or rupture

• *EEG*—may help to localize the area of damage.

Other baseline laboratory studies include urinalysis, coagulation studies, CBC, serum osmolality, and electrolyte, glucose, triglyceride, creatinine, and BUN levels.

Treatment

Surgery to improve cerebral circulation for patients with thrombotic or embolic CVA includes endarterectomy (removal of atherosclerotic plaques from inner arterial wall) or microvascular bypass (extracranial vessel is surgically anastomosed to an intracranial vessel).

Medications useful in CVA include:

• anticonvulsants, such as phenytoin or phenobarbital, to treat or prevent seizures

• stool softeners, such as dioctyl sodium sulfosuccinate, to avoid straining, which increases intracranial pressure (ICP)

• corticosteroids, such as dexamethasone, to minimize associated cerebral edema

• analgesics, such as codeine, to relieve headache that may follow hemorrhagic CVA. Usually, aspirin is contraindicated in hemorrhagic CVA, since it increases bleeding tendencies, but it may be useful in preventing TIAs.

Additional considerations

Health care of patients with CVA is complex and demands careful application of health care skills, keen observation, precise assessment, and supportive care. During the acute phase, such care emphasizes continuing neurologic assessment, support of respiration, continuous monitoring of vital signs, careful positioning to prevent aspiration and contractures, management of gastrointestinal problems, and careful monitoring of fluid, electrolyte, and nutritional intake. Also, care must prevent complications, such as infection. During care, the hospital staff member should:

• maintain patent airway and oxygenation; loosen constricting clothes; watch for ballooning of the cheek with respiration—the side that balloons is the side affected by the stroke; keep the patient in a lateral position to allow secretions to drain naturally, or suction secretions, as needed, since the patient could aspirate saliva if he is unconscious; insert an artificial airway, and start mechanical ventilation or supplemental oxygen, if necessary.

• check vital signs and neurologic status, record observations, and report any significant changes to the doctor; monitor blood pressure, level of consciousness, pupillary changes, motor function (voluntary and involuntary movements), sensory function, speech, skin color, temperature, signs of increased ICP, and nuchal rigidity or flaccidity; watch for signs of impending CVA, such as blood pressure rising suddenly, pulse rapid and bounding, and patient complaints of headache; watch for signs of pulmonary emboli, such as chest pains, shortness of breath, dusky color, tachycardia, fever, and changed sensorium; monitor the patient's blood gases often if the patient is unresponsive, and alert the doctor to increased PCO_2 or decreased PO_2.

• maintain fluid and electrolyte balance; if the patient can take liquids P.O., offer them as often as fluid limitations permit; administer I.V. fluids, as ordered, without giving too much too fast, since this can increase ICP; offer the urinal or bedpan every 2 hours (an incontinent patient may need a Foley catheter, but this should be avoided, if possible, because of the risk of infection).

• ensure adequate nutrition; check for gag reflex before offering small oral feedings of semisolid foods; place the food tray within the patient's visual field; if oral feedings aren't possible, insert a nasogastric tube.

• manage gastrointestinal problems; be alert for signs that the patient is straining at stool, since this increases ICP; modify diet, administer stool softeners, as ordered, and give laxatives, if necessary; keep the patient positioned on his side to prevent aspiration if he vomits (usually during the first few days).

• give careful mouth care; clean and irrigate the patient's mouth to remove food particles; care for his dentures, as needed.

• provide meticulous eye care; remove secretions with a cotton ball and sterile normal saline solution; instill eyedrops, as ordered; patch the patient's affected eye if he can't close the lid.

• position the patient, and align his extremities correctly; use high-topped sneakers to prevent footdrop and contracture; use egg crate, flotation, pulsating mattresses, or sheepskin to prevent decubitus ulcers; turn the patient at least every 2 hours to prevent pneumonia; elevate the affected hand to control dependent edema, and place it in a functional position.

• assist the patient with exercise; perform range-of-motion exercises for both the affected and unaffected sides; teach and encourage the patient to use his unaffected side to exercise his affected side.

• give medications, as ordered, and watch for and report side effects.

• establish and maintain communication with the patient. If he is aphasic, a simple method of communicating basic needs will be needed. Then questions should be phrased so he'll be able to answer using this system. The patient should be spoken to quietly and calmly (he isn't deaf!) and gestures used if necessary to help him understand. Even the unresponsive patient can hear, so nothing should be said in his presence that he shouldn't hear.

The patient will need psychological support and help setting realistic short-term goals. The patient's family should be involved in his care when possible.

Rehabilitation of the CVA patient must begin on admission. The amount of teaching needed will depend on the extent of neurologic deficit. This will include:

• establishing rapport with the patient; spending time with him, and providing a means of communication; simplifying language, asking yes-or-no questions whenever possible; not correcting his speech or treating him like a child; keeping in mind that building rapport may be difficult because of the mood changes that may result from brain damage or as a reaction to being dependent.

• teaching the patient, if necessary, to comb his hair, dress, and wash; obtaining appliances, such as walking frames, hand bars by the toilet, and ramps, with the aid of a physical and an occupational therapist; if speech therapy is indicated, encouraging the patient to begin as soon as possible and follow through with the speech pathologist's suggestions; involving the patient's family in all aspects of rehabilitation; devising a realistic discharge plan, with the patient's cooperation and support and letting the family help decide when the patient can return home.

• warning the patient or his family, before discharge, to report premonitory signs of CVA (severe headache, drowsiness, confusion, and dizziness); stressing the importance of follow-up visits.

• telling the patient, if aspirin has been prescribed to minimize the risk of embolic stroke, to watch for possible gastrointestinal bleeding related to ulcer formation; making sure the patient realizes that he cannot substitute acetaminophen for aspirin.

CVAs can be prevented by:

• stressing the need to control diseases such as diabetes or hypertension; teaching all patients (especially those at high risk) the importance of following a low-cholesterol, low-salt diet; watching body weight; increasing activity; avoiding smoking and prolonged bed rest; and minimizing stress.

Meningitis

In meningitis, the brain and the spinal cord meninges become inflamed, usually as a result of bacterial infection. Such inflammation may involve all three meningeal membranes—the dura mater, the arachnoid, and the pia mater. Prognosis is good and complications are rare, especially if the disease is recognized early and the infecting organism responds to antibiotics. However, mortality in untreated meningitis is 70% to 100%. Prognosis is poorer for infants and the elderly.

Causes

Meningitis is almost always a complication of another bacterial infection—bacteremia (especially from pneumonia, empyema, osteomyelitis, and endocarditis), sinusitis, otitis media, encephalitis, myelitis, or brain abscess—usually caused by *Neisseria meningitidis*, *Hemophilus influenzae*, *Streptococcus (Diplococcus) pneumoniae*, and *Escherichia coli*. Meningitis may also follow skull fracture, a penetrating head wound, lumbar puncture, or ventricular shunting procedures.

Aseptic meningitis may result from a virus or other organism. Sometimes, no causative organism can be found.

Meningitis often begins as an inflammation of the pia-arachnoid, which may progress to congestion of adjacent tissues, with some resultant nerve cell destruction.

Signs and symptoms

The cardinal signs of meningitis are those of infection (fever, chills, malaise) and of increased intracranial pressure (headache, vomiting, and rarely, papilledema). Signs of meningeal irritation include nuchal rigidity, positive Brudzinski's and Kernig's signs, exaggerated and symmetric deep tendon reflexes, and opisthotonos (a spasm in which the back and extremities arch backward so that the body rests on the head and heels). Other manifestations of meningitis are sinus arrhythmias; irritability; photophobia, diplopia, and other visual problems; and delirium, deep stupor, and coma. An infant may show signs of infection but often is simply fretful and refuses to eat. Such an infant may vomit a great deal, leading to dehydration; this prevents a bulging fontanelle and thus masks this important sign of increased intracranial pressure (ICP). As this illness progresses, twitching, seizures (in 30% of infants), or coma may develop. Most older children have the same symptoms as adults. In subacute meningitis, onset maybe insidious.

Diagnosis

A lumbar puncture showing typical CSF findings and positive Brudzinski's and Kernig's signs usually establish this diagnosis. The following tests can uncover the primary sites of infection: cultures of blood, urine, and nose and throat secretions; a chest X-ray; an EKG; and a complete physical examination, with special attention to skin, ears, and sinuses. CSF pressure is elevated, resulting from obstruction of CSF outflow at the arachnoid villi. The fluid may appear cloudy or milky white, depending on the number of WBCs present. CSF protein levels tend to be high; glucose levels may be low. (However, in subacute meningitis, CSF findings may vary.) CSF culture and sensitivity usually identify the infecting organism, unless it is a virus. Leukocytosis and serum electrolyte abnormalities are also common. CAT scan can rule out cerebral hematoma, hemorrhage, or tumors.

Treatment

Treatment of meningitis includes appropriate antibiotic therapy and vigorous supportive care. Usually, I.V. antibiotics are given for at least 2 weeks and are

TWO TELLTALE SIGNS OF MENINGITIS

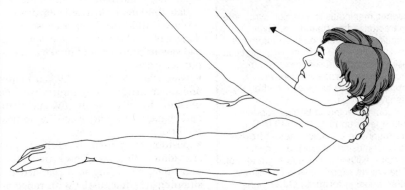

To test for *Brudzinski's sign,* the patient is placed in a dorsal recumbent position, and his hands are positioned behind his neck to bend it forward. Pain and resistance may indicate meningeal inflammation, neck injury, or arthritis. But if the patient also flexes the hips and knees in response to this manipulation, chances are he has meningitis.

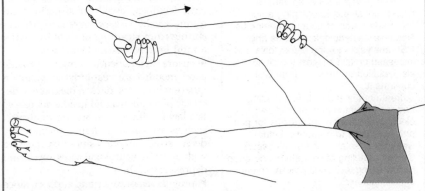

To test for *Kernig's sign,* the patient is placed in a supine position. His leg is flexed at the hip and knee, and then straightened. Pain or resistance points to meningitis.

followed by oral antibiotics. Such antibiotics include penicillin G, ampicillin, or nafcillin. However, if the patient is allergic to penicillin, anti-infective therapy includes tetracycline, chloramphenicol, or kanamycin. Other drugs include a cardiac glycoside, such as digoxin, to control arrhythmias, mannitol to decrease cerebral edema, an anticonvulsant (usually given I.V.) or a sedative to reduce restlessness, and aspirin or acetaminophen to relieve headache and fever. Supportive measures include bed rest, hypothermia, and measures to prevent dehydration. Isolation is necessary if nasal cultures are positive. Of course, treatment includes appropriate therapy for any coexisting conditions, such as endocarditis or pneumonia.

To prevent meningitis, prophylactic antibiotics are sometimes used after ventricular shunting procedures, skull fracture, or penetrating head wounds, but this use is controversial.

ASEPTIC MENINGITIS

Aseptic meningitis is a benign syndrome characterized by headache, fever, vomiting, and meningeal symptoms. It results from some form of virus infection including enteroviruses (most common), arboviruses, herpes simplex virus, mumps virus, or lymphocytic chorio-meningitis virus.

Aseptic meningitis begins suddenly with a fever up to 104° F. (40.0° C.), alterations in consciousness (drowsiness, confusion, stupor), and neck or spine stiffness, which is slight at first. (The patient experiences such stiffness when bending forward.) Other signs and symptoms include headaches, nausea, vomiting, abdominal pain, poorly defined chest pain, and sore throat.

Patient history of recent illness and knowledge of seasonal epidemics are essential in differentiating among the many forms of aseptic meningitis. Negative bacteriologic cultures and CSF analysis showing pleocytosis and increased protein suggest the diagnosis. Isolation of the virus from CSF confirms it.

Treatment is supportive, including bed rest, maintenance of fluid and electrolyte balance, analgesics for pain, and exercises to combat residual weakness. Isolation is not necessary. Careful handling of excretions and good handwashing technique prevent spreading the disease.

Additional considerations

The hospital staff member caring for the patient with meningitis should:

• assess neurologic function often; observe level of consciousness and signs of increased ICP (plucking at the bedcovers, vomiting, convulsions, a change in motor function and vital signs); watch for signs of cranial nerve involvement.

• watch for deterioration; be especially alert for a temperature increase up to 102° F. (38.9° C.), deteriorating level of consciousness, onset of seizures, and altered respirations, all of which may signal an impending crisis.

• monitor fluid balance; maintain adequate fluid intake to avoid dehydration, but avoid fluid overload because of the danger of cerebral edema; measure central venous pressure and intake and output accurately.

• watch for side effects of I.V. antibiotics and other drugs; avoid infiltration and phlebitis by checking the I.V. site often, and changing the site according to hospital policy.

• position the patient carefully to prevent joint stiffness and neck pain; turn him often, according to a planned positioning schedule; assist with range-of-motion exercises.

• maintain adequate nutrition and elimination; provide small, frequent meals, as necessary, or supplement these meals with nasogastric tube or parenteral feedings; avoid constipation and minimize the risk of increased ICP resulting from straining at stool by giving a mild laxative or stool softener.

• ensure the patient's comfort; provide good mouth care regularly; maintain a quiet environment; darken the room to decrease photophobia and headache; relieve headache with a nonnarcotic analgesic, such as aspirin or acetaminophen, as ordered; avoid narcotics, since they interfere with accurate neurologic assessment, and depress respiration.

• provide reassurance and support, since the patient may be frightened by his illness and frequent lumbar punctures; attempt to reassure the patient and his family that the delirium and behavior changes caused by meningitis usually disappear; refer the patient whose severe neurologic deficit appears permanent to a rehabilitation program as soon as the acute phase of this illness has passed.

• help prevent meningitis by teaching patients with chronic sinusitis or other chronic infections the importance of proper medical treatment, and by following strict aseptic technique when treating patients with head wounds or skull fractures.

Encephalitis

Encephalitis is a severe inflammation of the brain, usually caused by a mosquito-borne or, in some areas, a tick-borne virus. However, transmission by means other than arthropod bites may occur through ingestion of infected goat's milk and accidental injection or inhalation of the virus. Eastern equine encephalitis may produce permanent neurologic damage and is often fatal.

In encephalitis, intense lymphocytic infiltration of brain tissues and the leptomeninges causes cerebral edema, degeneration of the brain's ganglion cells, and diffuse nerve cell destruction.

Causes

Encephalitis generally results from infection with arboviruses specific to rural areas. However, in urban areas, encephalitis is most frequently caused by enteroviruses (coxsackievirus, poliovirus, and echovirus). Other causes include herpesvirus, mumps virus, adenoviruses, and demyelinating diseases following measles, varicella, rubella, or vaccination.

Between World War I and the Depression, a type of encephalitis known as lethargic encephalitis, von Economo's disease, or sleeping sickness occurred with some regularity. The virus that caused this disease was never clearly identified, and the disease is rarely seen today. Even so, the term sleeping sickness persists and is often mistakenly used to describe other types of encephalitis as well.

Signs and symptoms

All viral forms of encephalitis have similar clinical features, although certain differences do occur. Usually, the acute illness begins with sudden onset of fever, headache, and vomiting, and progresses to include signs of meningeal irritation (stiff neck and back) and neuronal damage (drowsiness, coma, paralysis, convulsions, ataxia, organic psychoses). After the acute phase, coma may persist for days or weeks. Severity of arbovirus encephalitis may range from subclinical to rapidly fatal necrotizing disease. Herpes encephalitis also produces symptoms that vary from subclinical to acute

and often fatal fulminating disease. Associated signs include disturbances of taste or smell.

Diagnosis

During an encephalitis epidemic, diagnosis is readily made on clinical findings and patient history. However, sporadic cases are difficult to distinguish from other febrile illnesses, such as gastroenteritis or meningitis. When possible, identification of the virus in CSF or blood confirms this diagnosis. The common viruses that also cause herpes, measles, and mumps are easier to identify than arboviruses. Arboviruses and herpesviruses can be isolated by inoculating young mice with a specimen taken from the patient. In herpes encephalitis, serologic studies may show rising titers of complement-fixing antibodies.

In all forms of encephalitis, CSF pressure is elevated, and despite inflammation, the fluid is often clear. WBC and protein levels in CSF are slightly elevated, but the glucose level remains normal. An EEG reveals abnormalities. Occasionally, a CAT scan may be ordered to rule out cerebral hematoma.

Treatment

The antiviral agent vidarabine is effective only against herpes encephalitis. Treatment of all other forms of encephalitis is entirely supportive. Drug therapy includes phenytoin or another anticonvulsant, usually given I.V.; glucocorticoids to reduce cerebral inflammation and resulting edema; sedatives for restlessness; and aspirin or acetaminophen to relieve headache and reduce fever. Other supportive measures include adequate fluid and electrolyte intake to prevent dehydration, and appropriate antibiotics for associated infections, such as pneumonia or sinusitis. Isolation is unnecessary.

Additional considerations

During the acute phase of the illness, the hospital staff member should:
• assess neurologic function often; observe level of consciousness and watch for signs of increased intracranial pressure (increasing restlessness, plucking at the bedcovers, vomiting, convulsions, and changes in pupil size, motor function, and vital signs); watch for cranial nerve involvement (signs include ptosis, strabismus, diplopia), abnormal sleep patterns, and behavior changes.
• maintain adequate fluid intake to prevent dehydration, but avoid fluid overload, which may increase cerebral edema; measure and record intake and output accurately.
• give vidarabine by slow I.V. infusion only; watch for side effects, such as tremor, dizziness, hallucinations, anorexia, nausea, vomiting, diarrhea, pruritus, rash, and anemia; also watch for side effects of other drugs; check the infusion site often to avoid infiltration and phlebitis.
• carefully position the patient to prevent joint stiffness and neck pain, and turn him often; assist with range-of-motion exercises.
• maintain adequate nutrition; if necessary, provide small, frequent meals or supplement these meals with nasogastric tube or parenteral feedings.
• give a mild laxative or stool softener, to prevent constipation and minimize the risk of increased intracranial pressure resulting from straining at stool.
• maintain a quiet environment; darken the room to decrease photophobia and headache; if the patient naps during the day and is restless at night, plan daytime activities to minimize napping and promote sleep at night.
• provide emotional support and reassurance, since the patient is apt to be frightened by the illness and frequent diagnostic tests.
• attempt to reorient the delirious or confused patient often; provide the patient with a calendar or a clock, to help in the reorientation.
• reassure the family that personality and behavior changes caused by encephalitis usually disappear; if a neurologic deficit is severe and appears permanent, refer the patient to a rehabilitation program as soon as the acute phase has passed.

Brain Abscess

(Intracranial abscess)

Brain abscess is a free or encapsulated collection of pus usually found in the temporal lobe, cerebellum, or frontal lobes. It can vary in size and may occur singly or multilocularly. Brain abscess has a relatively low incidence. Although it can occur at any age, it is most common in persons between ages 10 and 35, and is rare in the elderly.

Untreated brain abscess is usually fatal; with treatment, prognosis is only fair, and about 30% of patients develop focal seizures. Multiple metastatic abscesses secondary to systemic or other infections have the poorest prognosis.

Causes

Brain abscess is usually secondary to some other infection, especially otitis media, sinusitis, dental abscess, and mastoiditis. Other causes include subdural empyema; bacterial endocarditis;

bacteremia; pulmonary or pleural infection; pelvic, abdominal, and skin infections; and cranial trauma, such as a penetrating head wound or compound skull fracture. Brain abscess also occurs in about 2% of children with congenital heart disease, possibly because the hypoxic brain is a good culture medium for bacteria. The most common infecting organisms are pyogenic bacteria, such as *Staphylococcus aureus, Streptococcus viridans,* and *Streptococcus hemolyticus.* Penetrating head trauma or bacteremia usually leads to staphylococcal infection; pulmonary disease, to streptococcal infection.

Brain abscess usually begins with localized inflammatory necrosis and edema, septic thrombosis of vessels, and suppurative encephalitis. This is followed by thick encapsulation of accumulated pus, and adjacent meningeal infiltration by neutrophils, lymphocytes, and plasma cells.

Signs and symptoms
Onset varies according to cause, but generally, brain abscess produces clinical effects similar to those of a brain tumor. Early symptoms result from increased intracranial pressure (ICP) and include constant intractable headache, worsened by straining; nausea; vomiting; and focal or generalized seizures. Typical later symptoms include ocular disturbances, such as nystagmus, decreased vision, and inequality of pupils. Other features differ with the site of the abscess:
• *temporal lobe abscess:* auditory-receptive dysphasia, central facial weakness, hemiparesis
• *cerebellar abscess:* dizziness, coarse nystagmus, gaze weakness on lesion side, tremor, ataxia
• *frontal lobe abscess:* expressive dysphasia, hemiparesis with unilateral motor seizure, drowsiness, inattention, mental function impairment.

Signs of infection, such as fever, pallor, and bradycardia, are absent until late stages unless they result from the predisposing condition. If the abscess is encapsulated, they may never appear.

Depending on abscess size and location, level of consciousness varies from drowsiness to deep stupor.

Diagnosis
A history of infection—especially of the middle ear, mastoid, nasal sinuses, heart, or lungs—or a history of congenital heart disease, along with a physical examination showing characteristic clinical features such as increased ICP, point to brain abscess. An EEG, CAT scan, and occasionally, arteriography (highlights abscess by a halo) help locate the site.

Examination of CSF can help confirm infection, but most doctors agree that lumbar puncture is usually too risky, because it can release the increased ICP and provoke cerebral herniation. Other tests include culture and sensitivity of drainage from underlying infection to identify the causative organism, skull X-rays (for views of sinuses and mastoids), radioisotope scan (also helps locate abscess), and rarely, ventriculography.

Treatment
Therapy consists of antibiotics to combat the underlying infection, and surgical aspiration or drainage of the abscess. However, surgery is delayed until the abscess becomes encapsulated (CAT scan helps determine this) and is contraindicated in patients with congenital heart disease or another debilitating cardiac condition. Administration of a penicillinase-resistant antibiotic, such as nafcillin or methicillin, for at least 2 to 3 weeks before surgery can reduce the risk of spreading infection. Other treatment during the acute phase is palliative and supportive, and includes mechanical ventilation, administration of I.V. fluids with diuretics (urea, mannitol), and glucocorticoids (dexamethasone) to combat increased ICP and cerebral edema. Anticonvulsants, such as phenytoin and phenobarbital, help prevent seizures.

Additional considerations
During the acute stage, brain abscess requires intensive care monitoring, in-

cluding:
• frequently assessing neurologic status, paying particular attention to level of consciousness, speech, and motor, sensory, and cranial nerve functions; watching for signs of increased ICP (decreased level of consciousness, unexpected vomiting, abnormal pupil response, and depressed respirations), which may lead to cerebral herniation (fixed and dilated pupils, widened pulse pressure, tachycardia, absent or depressed respirations).
• recording vital signs at least every 1 to 2 hours.
• monitoring fluid intake and output carefully, since fluid overload could contribute to cerebral edema.

If surgery is necessary, the procedure should be explained to the patient and family, and any questions answered.

After surgery, the hospital staff member should:
• continue frequent neurologic assessment; monitor vital signs, and intake and output.

• watch for signs of meningitis (nuchal rigidity, headaches, chills, sweats).
• change any damp dressings often, using aseptic technique and noting amount of drainage; never allow bandages to remain damp; position the patient on the operative side, to promote drainage and prevent reaccumulation of the abscess.
• give meticulous skin care to the stuporous or comatose patient to prevent decubitus ulcers, and position him to preserve function and prevent contractures.
• make sure the patient who requires isolation because of postoperative drainage and his family understand the reason for it.
• ambulate the patient as soon as possible to prevent immobility and encourage independence.
• to prevent brain abscess, stress the need for adequate treatment of otitis media, mastoiditis, dental abscess, and other predisposing infections; administer prophylactic antibiotics, as ordered, after compound skull fracture or penetrating head wound.

Huntington's Disease

(Huntington's chorea, hereditary chorea, chronic progressive chorea, adult chorea)

Huntington's disease is a hereditary disease in which degeneration in the cerebral cortex and basal ganglia causes chronic progressive chorea and mental deterioration, ending in dementia. Huntington's disease usually strikes persons between ages 25 and 55 (the average age is 35); however, 2% of cases occur in children, and 5%, as late as age 60. Death usually results 10 to 15 years after onset, from suicide, congestive heart failure, or pneumonia.

Causes and incidence
The cause of Huntington's disease is unknown. Because this disease is transmitted as an autosomal dominant trait, either sex can transmit and inherit it. Each child of a parent with this disease has a 50% chance of inheriting it; however, the child who doesn't inherit it can't pass it on to his own children. Because of hereditary transmission, Huntington's disease is prevalent in areas where affected families have lived for

several generations. A study is being made of children in families with Huntington's disease in order to develop ways of identifying this disease before onset of symptoms.

Signs and symptoms
Onset is insidious. The patient eventually becomes totally dependent—emotionally and physically—through loss of musculoskeletal control. Gradually, the patient develops progressively severe choreic

movements. Such movements are rapid, often violent, and purposeless. Initially, they are unilateral and more prominent in the face and arms than in the legs, progressing from mild fidgeting to grimacing, tongue smacking, dysarthria (indistinct speech), athetoid movements (especially of the hands) related to emotional state, and torticollis.

Ultimately, the patient with Huntington's disease develops dementia, although the dementia doesn't always progress at the same rate as the chorea. Dementia can be mild at first but eventually severely disrupts the personality. Such personality changes include obstinacy, carelessness, untidiness, moodiness, apathy, inappropriate behavior, loss of memory and concentration, and sometimes, paranoia.

Diagnosis

There is no reliable confirming test for Huntington's disease. Diagnosis is based on a characteristic clinical history: progressive chorea and dementia, onset in early middle age (35 to 40), and confirmation of a genetic link. Helpful tests include pneumoencephalography, which shows characteristic butterfly dilation of the brain's lateral ventricles, and CAT scan, which shows brain atrophy.

Treatment and additional considerations

Since Huntington's disease has no known cure, treatment is supportive, protective, and symptomatic. Tranquilizers, as well as chlorpromazine, haloperidol, or imipramine, can't stop mental deterioration, but they do help control choreic movements. They also alleviate discomfort and depression, making the patient easier to manage. However, tranquilizers increase patient rigidity, so choline has recently been prescribed to control choreic movements without rigidity. Institutionalization is often necessary because of mental deterioration.

Physical support can be provided by attending to the patient's basic needs, such as general hygiene, skin care, bowel and bladder care, and adequate nutrition. This support should be increased as mental and physical deterioration makes the patient more immobile.

Emotional support should be offered to the patient and family. They must be taught about the disease, and given a chance to voice their concerns and special problems. Because of his dysarthria, the patient will need time to express himself. The family should participate in his care.

Staff members must watch for possible suicide attempts, and control the patient's environment to protect him from suicide or other self-inflicted injury. This includes padding the side rails of the bed, but avoiding restraints, which may cause the patient to injure himself with violent, uncontrolled movements.

Families affected by the disease need genetic counseling, and family members affected should realize that each of their offspring has a 50% chance of inheriting this disease.

The patient and family should be referred to appropriate community organizations: visiting nurse service, social services, psychiatric counseling, and long-term care facility. For more information about this disease, the patient and family can contact the Committee to Combat Huntington's Disease or the National Huntington's Disease Association.

Parkinson's Disease

(Parkinsonism, paralysis agitans, shaking palsy)

Named for James Parkinson, the English doctor who wrote the first accurate description of the disease, in 1817, Parkinson's disease characteristically produces progressive muscle rigidity, akinesia, and involuntary tremor. Deterioration pro-

gresses for an average of 10 years, at which time death usually results from aspiration pneumonia or some other infection. Parkinson's disease, one of the most common crippling diseases in the United States, affects men more often than women. According to current statistics, Parkinson's strikes 1 in every 100 people over age 60. Because of increased longevity, this amounts to roughly 60,000 new cases diagnosed annually in the United States alone.

Causes

Although the cause of Parkinson's disease is unknown, study of the extrapyramidal brain nuclei (corpus striatum, globus pallidus, substantia nigra) has established that a dopamine deficiency prevents affected brain cells from performing their normal inhibitory function within the central nervous system.

Signs and symptoms

The cardinal symptoms of Parkinson's disease are muscle rigidity and akinesia, and an insidious tremor that begins in the fingers (unilateral pill-roll tremor), increases during stress or anxiety, and decreases with purposeful movement and sleep. Muscle rigidity results in resistance to passive muscle stretching, which may be uniform (lead-pipe rigidity) or jerky (cogwheel rigidity). Akinesia causes the patient to walk with difficulty (gait lacks normal parallel motion and may be retropulsive or propulsive). It also produces a high-pitched, monotone voice, drooling, a masklike facial expression, loss of posture control (the patient walks with body bent forward), and dysarthria, dysphagia, or both. Occasionally, akinesia may also cause oculogyric crises (eyes are fixed upward, with involuntary tonic movements) or blepharospasm (eyelids are completely closed). Parkinson's disease itself doesn't impair the intellect, but a coexisting disorder, such as arteriosclerosis, may.

Diagnosis

Generally, laboratory data are of little value in identifying Parkinson's disease; consequently, diagnosis is based on the patient's age and history, and the characteristic clinical picture. However, urinalysis may support the diagnosis by revealing decreased dopamine levels. Conclusive diagnosis is possible only after ruling out other causes of tremor, involutional depression, cerebral arteriosclerosis, and in patients under age 30, intracranial tumors, Wilson's disease, or phenothiazine or other drug toxicity.

Treatment

Since there's no cure for Parkinson's disease, the primary aim of treatment is to relieve symptoms and keep the patient functional as long as possible. Treatment consists of drugs, physical therapy, and in severe disease states unresponsive to drugs, stereotactic neurosurgery.

Drug therapy usually includes levodopa, a dopamine replacement that is most effective during early stages. This drug is given in increasing doses until symptoms are relieved or side effects appear. Because these side effects can be serious, levodopa is now frequently given in combination with carbidopa to halt peripheral dopamine synthesis. When levodopa proves ineffective or too toxic, alternative drug therapy includes anticholinergics, such as trihexyphenidyl; antihistamines, such as diphenhydramine; and amantadine, an antiviral agent.

When drug therapy fails, stereotactic neurosurgery is sometimes an effective alternative. In this procedure, electrical coagulation, freezing, radioactivity, or ultrasound destroys the ventrolateral nucleus of the thalamus to prevent involuntary movement. Such neurosurgery is most effective in comparatively young, otherwise healthy persons with unilateral tremor or muscle rigidity. Like drug therapy, neurosurgery is a palliative measure that can only *relieve* symptoms.

Individually planned physical therapy complements drug treatment and neurosurgery to maintain normal muscle tone and function. Appropriate physical therapy includes both active and passive range-of-motion exercises, routine daily activities, walking, and baths and massage to help relax muscles.

Additional considerations
Effective care for the patient with Parkinson's disease requires careful monitoring of drug treatment, emphasis on teaching self-reliance, and generous psychological support.
• Drug treatment must be monitored so dosage can be adjusted to minimize side effects.
• If the patient has surgery he should be watched for signs of hemorrhage and increased intracranial pressure.
• Independence should be encouraged, but fatigue may make this impossible. The patient with excessive tremor may achieve partial control of his body by sitting on a chair and using its arms to steady himself.
• The patient will need help overcoming problems related to eating and elimination. For example, if he has difficulty eating, supplementary or small, frequent meals will increase caloric intake. A regular bowel routine can be established by having him drink at least 2,000 ml of liquids daily and eat high-bulk foods. He may need an elevated toilet seat to assist him from a standing to a sitting position.
• The patient and family will need emotional support, and teaching about the disease, its progressive stages, and drug side effects. The family should be shown how to prevent decubitus ulcers and contractures by proper positioning. They should understand the dietary restrictions levodopa imposes, and the necessity of household safety measures to prevent accidents. The patient and family must express their feelings and frustrations about the progressively debilitating effects of the disease and establish long- and short-term treatment goals. The patient must get intellectual stimulation and diversion.

The patient and family can get more information from the National Parkinson Foundation or the United Parkinson Foundation.

Myelitis and Acute Transverse Myelitis

Myelitis, or inflammation of the spinal cord, can result from several diseases. Poliomyelitis affects the cord's gray matter and produces motor dysfunction; leukomyelitis affects only the white matter and produces sensory dysfunction. These types of myelitis can attack any level of the spinal cord, causing partial destruction or scattered lesions. Acute transverse myelitis, which affects the entire thickness of the spinal cord, produces both motor and sensory dysfunctions. This latter form of myelitis, which has a rapid onset, is the most devastating.

The prognosis depends on the severity of cord damage and prevention of complications. If spinal cord necrosis occurs, prognosis for complete recovery is poor. Even without necrosis, residual neurologic deficits usually persist after recovery. Patients who develop spastic reflexes early in the course of the illness are more likely to recover than those who don't.

Causes
Acute transverse myelitis has a variety of causes. It often follows acute infectious diseases, such as measles or pneumonia (the inflammation occurs after the infection has subsided), and primary infections of the spinal cord itself, such as syphilis or acute disseminated encephalomyelitis. Acute transverse myelitis can accompany demyelinating diseases, such as acute multiple sclerosis, and inflammatory and necrotizing disorders of the spinal cord, such as hematomyelia.

Certain toxic agents (carbon monoxide, lead, and arsenic) can cause a type of myelitis in which acute inflammation (followed by hemorrhage and possible necrosis) destroys the entire circumference (myelin, axis cylinders, and neurons) of the spinal cord. Other forms of myelitis may result from poliovirus, herpes zoster, herpesvirus B, rabies virus; disorders that cause meningeal inflammation, such as syphilis, abscesses and other suppurative conditions, and tuberculosis; smallpox or polio vaccination; parasitic and fungal infections; and chronic adhesive arachnoiditis.

Signs and symptoms

In acute transverse myelitis, onset is rapid, with motor and sensory dysfunctions below the level of spinal cord damage appearing in 1 to 2 days.

Patients with acute transverse myelitis develop flaccid paralysis of the legs (sometimes beginning in just one leg) with loss of sensory and sphincter functions. Such sensory loss may follow pain in the legs or trunk. Reflexes disappear in the early stages but may reappear later. The extent of damage depends on the level of the spinal cord affected; transverse myelitis rarely involves the arms. If spinal cord damage is severe, it may cause shock (hypotension, hypothermia).

Diagnosis

Paraplegia of rapid onset usually points to acute transverse myelitis. In such patients, neurologic examination confirms paraplegia or neurologic deficit below the level of the spinal cord lesion, and absent or, later, hyperactive reflexes. CSF may be normal or show increased lymphocytes or elevated protein levels.

Diagnostic evaluation must rule out spinal cord tumor and identify the cause of any underlying infection.

Treatment

No effective treatment exists for acute transverse myelitis. However, this condition requires appropriate treatment of any underlying infection. Some patients with postinfectious or multiple sclerosis-induced myelitis have received steroid therapy, but its benefits aren't clear.

Additional considerations

Hospital care includes:
• frequently assessing vital signs; watching carefully for signs of spinal shock (hypotension, excessive sweating).
• preventing contractures with range-of-motion exercises and proper alignment.
• watching for signs of urinary tract infections from Foley catheters.
• preventing skin infections and decubitus ulcers with meticulous skin care; checking pressure points often and keeping skin clean and dry; using a water bed or other pressure-relieving device.
• initiating rehabilitation immediately; assisting the patient with physical therapy, bowel and bladder training, and life-style changes his condition requires.

Reye's Syndrome

Reye's syndrome is an acute childhood illness that causes fatty infiltration of the liver with concurrent hyperammonemia, encephalopathy, and increased intracranial pressure (ICP). In addition, fatty infiltration of the kidneys leads to azotemia, and possible infiltration of the myocardium may cause myocardial damage. Reye's syndrome affects children from infancy to adolescence and occurs equally in boys and girls. It affects Caucasians over age 1 more often than Blacks.

Prognosis depends on the severity of CNS depression. Previously, mortality was as high as 90%. Today, though, ICP monitoring and, consequently, early treatment of increased ICP, along with other treatment measures, have cut mortality to about 20%. Death is usually a result of cerebral edema, respiratory arrest, or coma. Comatose patients who survive may have residual brain damage.

STAGES OF TREATMENT FOR REYE'S SYNDROME

SIGNS AND SYMPTOMS	BASELINE TREATMENT	BASELINE CLINICAL INTERVENTION
Stage I: vomiting, lethargy, hepatic dysfunction	• To decrease intracranial pressure and brain edema, I.V. fluids are given at ⅓ maintenance with additional fluids, as needed. Also, an osmotic diuretic or furosemide is given. • To treat hypoprothrombinemia, vitamin K is given; if vitamin K is unsuccessful, fresh frozen plasma is given. • Serum ammonia, blood glucose, and plasma osmolality monitored every 4 to 8 hours.	• Vital signs require monitoring. Level of consciousness must be checked for increasing lethargy. • Fluid intake and output need monitoring to prevent fluid overload. Urine output should be maintained at 1.0 ml/kg/hr; plasma osmolality at 290 mOsm; and blood glucose at 150 mg/ml. (*Goal:* glucose should be high, osmolality, normal, and ammonia, low.)
Stage II: hyperventilation, delirium, hepatic dysfunction, hyperactive reflexes	• Baseline treatment continues. • Phenytoin P.O. or I.V. is given to prevent seizures (routine depends on severity).	• Seizures are watched for and seizure precautions maintained. • Signs of coma that require invasive, supportive therapy, such as intubation, must be reported. • Head of bed positioned at 30° angle.
Stage III: coma, hyperventilation, decorticate rigidity, hepatic dysfunction	• Baseline and seizure treatment continues. • ICP is monitored with a subarachnoid screw or other invasive device. • Endotracheal intubation and mechanical ventilation are provided to control Pco_2 levels. A paralyzing agent, such as pancuronium I.V., may be used to help maintain ventilation. • Mannitol I.V. or glycerol is given, by nasogastric tube, if necessary, to treat rising serum osmolality.	• ICP is monitored (should be <20 before suctioning) or thiopental given I.V., as ordered; the patient may need hyperventilation. • If patient lapses into coma, 50% dextrose in water I.V. is given immediately, as ordered. • During ventilation the patient's Pco_2 is maintained between 23 and 30 mmHg, and his Po_2 is maintained between 80 and 100 mmHg. • Cardiovascular status is closely monitored with a pulmonary artery catheter or central venous pressure line. • Skin and mouth care is given, and range-of-motion exercises performed.
Stage IV: deepening coma; decerebrate rigidity; large, fixed pupils; minimal hepatic dysfunction	• Baseline and supportive care continues. • If all previous measures fail, some pediatric centers use barbiturate coma, decompressive craniotomy, hypothermia, exchange transfusion, or hemodialysis.	• Patient is checked for loss of reflexes and signs of flaccidity. • The family needs extra support, considering their child's poor prognosis.
Stage V: seizures, loss of deep tendon reflexes, flaccidity, respiratory arrest, ammonia above 300 mg/100 ml	• Baseline and supportive care continued.	• The family must be helped to face the patient's impending death.

Causes and incidence

Reye's syndrome almost always follows within 1 to 3 days of an acute viral infection, such as an upper respiratory infection, type B influenza, or varicella (chickenpox). Incidence often rises during influenza outbreaks.

In Reye's syndrome, damaged hepatic mitochondria disrupt the urea cycle, which normally changes ammonia to urea for its excretion from the body. This results in hyperammonemia, hypoglycemia, and an increase in serum short-chain fatty acids, leading to encephalopathy. Simultaneously, renal tubular cells undergo fatty infiltration, and neuronal tissue degenerates.

Signs and symptoms

The severity of symptoms varies with the degree of encephalopathy and cerebral edema. In any case, Reye's syndrome develops in five stages: After the initial viral infection, a brief recovery period follows when the child doesn't seem seriously ill. A few days later, he develops intractable vomiting; lethargy; rapidly changing mental status (mild to severe agitation, confusion, irritability, delirium); rising blood pressure, respiratory rate, and pulse rate; and hyperactive reflexes.

Reye's syndrome often progresses to coma, shown by fixed dilated pupils. As coma deepens, seizures develop, followed by decreased tendon reflexes and, frequently, respiratory failure.

Increased ICP, a serious complication, results from cerebral edema. Such edema develops because brain endothelial cells fail to pump out sodium; therefore, an excess of water accumulates within the cells, and they become swollen, blocking the capillary lumen.

Diagnosis

A patient history of a preceding viral disorder with characteristic clinical features strongly suggests Reye's syndrome. An increased serum ammonia level confirms it. Testing serum salicylate level rules out aspirin overdose. Absence of jaundice despite increased liver transaminases rules out acute hepatic failure and hepatic encephalopathy.

Typical abnormal laboratory results include:
- *liver function studies:* SGOT and SGPT elevated to twice normal levels; bilirubin usually normal
- *liver biopsy:* typical pattern of fatty droplets uniformly distributed throughout cells, revealed by cutaneous needle biopsy
- *CSF analysis:* WBC less than 10/mm^3; with coma, increased CSF pressure
- *coagulation studies:* PT and PTT prolonged
- *blood values:* serum ammonia elevated; serum glucose normal or, in 15%, low; serum fatty acid and lactate levels increased; HCO$_3$ decreased
- *arterial blood gases:* decreased PCO$_2$.

For more information, parents should be referred to the National Reye's Syndrome Foundation. This organization can help them contact local chapters in both the United States and Canada.

Guillain-Barré Syndrome

(Infectious polyneuritis, Landry-Guillain-Barré syndrome, acute idiopathic polyneuritis)

Guillain-Barré syndrome is an acute, rapidly progressive and potentially fatal form of polyneuritis that causes muscle weakness and mild distal sensory loss. This syndrome can occur at any age but is most common between ages 30 and 50; it affects both sexes equally. Recovery is spontaneous and complete in about 95% of patients, although mild motor or reflex deficits in the feet and legs may persist. Prognosis is best when symptoms clear between 15 and 20 days after onset.

Causes and incidence

Precisely what causes Guillain-Barré syndrome is unknown, but it may be a cell-mediated immunologic attack on peripheral nerves in response to a virus. Since this syndrome causes inflammation and degenerative changes in both the posterior (sensory) and anterior (motor) nerve roots, signs of sensory and motor losses occur simultaneously.

Signs and symptoms

About 50% of patients with Guillain-Barré syndrome have a history of minor febrile illness, usually an upper respiratory tract infection or, less often, gastroenteritis. When infection precedes onset of Guillain-Barré syndrome, signs of infection subside before neurologic features appear. Other possible precipitating factors include surgery, rabies or swine influenza vaccination, viral illness, Hodgkin's or some other malignant disease, and lupus erythematosus.

Muscle weakness, the dominant neurologic sign, usually appears in the legs first, then extends to the arms and facial nerves within 24 to 72 hours. Occasionally, muscle weakness develops in the arms first, or in the arms and legs simultaneously. In milder forms of this disease, muscle weakness may not occur at all.

Another common neurologic sign is paresthesia, which sometimes precedes muscle weakness but tends to vanish quickly. However, some patients with this disorder never develop this symptom. Other clinical features may include facial diplegia (possibly with ophthalmoplegia [ocular paralysis]), dysphagia or dysarthria, and less often, weakness of the muscles supplied by the 11th cranial (spinal accessory) nerve. Muscle weakness develops so quickly that muscle atrophy doesn't occur, but hypotonia and areflexia do. Pain is uncommon.

In 25% of patients, muscle weakness progresses to total motor paralysis and life-threatening respiratory failure, peaking in severity after only 10 to 14 days. Flaccid quadriplegia may occur. Some patients display progressive paralysis over a period of weeks or months. Affected areas may recover, only to relapse; in other areas, paralysis may progress unremittingly.

Occasionally, increased intracranial pressure (due to respiratory distress or failure, or impaired CSF absorption) causes choked disk (papilledema)—a swelling of the optic nerve head, with engorged retinal veins and hemorrhage into the nerve and adjacent retina. Unexplained autonomic nervous system involvement may cause sinus tachycardia or bradycardia, hypertension, postural hypotension, or loss of bladder and bowel sphincter control.

Diagnosis

A history of preceding febrile illness (usually a respiratory tract infection) and typical clinical features (especially leg weakness that progresses upward) suggest Guillain-Barré syndrome. Several days after onset of symptoms, CSF protein level begins to rise, peaking in 4 to 6 weeks, probably as a result of widespread inflammatory disease of the nerve roots. CSF white blood count remains normal, but in severe disease, CSF pressure may rise above normal. Probably because of predisposing infection, CBC shows leukocytosis and a shift to immature forms early in the illness, but blood studies soon return to normal. Electromyography may show repeated firing of the same motor unit, instead of widespread sectional stimulation. Nerve conduction velocities are slowed soon after paralysis develops. Diagnosis must rule out similar diseases, such as acute poliomyelitis.

Treatment

Treatment is basically supportive, consisting of endotracheal intubation or tracheotomy if the patient has difficulty clearing secretions, and a trial dose of prednisone if the course of the disease is relentlessly progressive. If prednisone produces no noticeable improvement after 7 days, it's discontinued; if it does produce improvement, the dosage is gradually reduced.

TESTING FOR THORACIC SENSATION

When Guillain-Barré syndrome progresses rapidly, ascending sensory loss can be tested for by touching the patient or pressing his skin lightly with a pin every hour. This should be done systematically from the iliac crest (T-12) to the scapula, occasionally substituting the blunt end of the pin to test the patient's ability to discriminate between sharp and dull. The level of diminished sensation must be marked to measure any change. If diminished sensation ascends to T-8 or higher, the patient's intercostal muscle function (and consequently respiratory function) will probably be impaired. As Guillain-Barré syndrome subsides, sensory and motor weakness descends to the lower thoracic segments, heralding a return of intercostal and extremity muscle function.

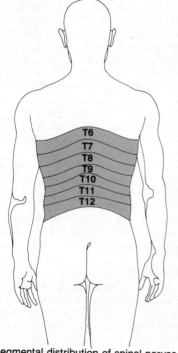

Segmental distribution of spinal nerves to back of the body

KEY
T = thoracic segments

Additional considerations

When caring for a patient with Guillain-Barré syndrome the hospital staff member should:

• watch for ascending sensory loss, which precedes motor loss.

• assess and treat respiratory dysfunction; take serial vital capacity recordings if respiratory muscles are weak; use a respirometer with a mouthpiece or a face mask for bedside testing; seal the mouthpiece tightly, if the patient has facial weakness.

• obtain arterial blood gas measurements; watch for PO_2 below 70 mmHg (this disease can cause primary hypoventilation with hypoxemia and hypercarbia, resulting in respiratory failure); be alert for signs of rising PCO_2 (confusion, tachypnea).

• auscultate breath sounds, turn and position the patient, and encourage coughing and deep breathing; begin respiratory support at the first sign of dyspnea (in adults, vital capacity less than 800 ml; in children, less than 12 ml/kg body weight) or decreasing PO_2.

• if respiratory failure becomes imminent, establish an emergency airway with an endotracheal tube; do pharyngeal suctioning before tracheal to remove secretions accumulated above the endotracheal tube cuff.

• give meticulous skin care to prevent skin breakdown and contractures; establish a strict turning schedule; inspect the skin (especially sacrum, heels, and ankles) for breakdown, and reposition the patient every 2 hours; stimulate circulation after each position change by carefully massaging pressure points; use foam, gel, or alternating pressure pads at points of contact.

• perform passive range-of-motion exercises within the patient's pain limits, perhaps using a Hubbard tank (although this disease doesn't produce pain, exercising little-used muscles will). The proximal muscle group of the thighs, shoulders, and trunk will be the most tender, and will cause the most pain on passive movement and turning. Gentle stretching and active assistance exercises should be used when the patient's condition stabilizes.

• prevent aspiration by testing the gag reflex, and elevating the head of the bed before giving the patient anything to eat; give nasogastric feedings, if the gag reflex is absent, until this reflex returns.

• be alert for postural hypotension as the patient regains strength and can tolerate a vertical position; monitor blood pressure and pulse during tilting periods, and if necessary, apply toe-to-groin elastic bandages or an abdominal binder to prevent postural hypotension.

• inspect the patient's legs regularly for signs of thrombophlebitis (localized pain, tenderness, erythema, edema, positive Homans' sign), a common complication of Guillain-Barré syndrome; to prevent thrombophlebitis, apply antiembolism stockings and give prophylactic anticoagulants, as ordered.

• give eye and mouth care every 4 hours if the patient has facial paralysis; protect the corneas with isotonic eyedrops and conical eye shields.

• watch for urinary retention; measure and record intake and output every 8 hours, and offer the bedpan every 3 to 4 hours; encourage adequate fluid intake (2,000 ml/day), unless contraindicated; if urinary retention develops, begin intermittent catheterization, as ordered; since the abdominal muscles may be weak, use manual pressure on the bladder (Credé's method), as needed.

• prevent and relieve constipation, by offering prune juice and a high-bulk diet; give daily or alternate-day suppositories (glycerin or bisacodyl), or Fleet enemas, as necessary.

• before discharge, prepare a home care plan; teach the patient how to transfer from bed to wheelchair, from wheelchair to toilet, from wheelchair to tub (using a tub seat), and how to walk short distances with the aid of a walker or a cane; teach the family how to help the patient eat, compensating for facial weakness, and how to help him avoid skin breakdown; stress the need for a regular bowel and bladder routine; refer the patient for follow-up physical therapy, as needed.

Paraplegia

Paraplegia is motor or sensory loss in the lower extremities, with or without involvement of the abdominal and back muscles. Paralysis may be complete or incomplete, spastic or flaccid, symmetric or asymmetric, and permanent or temporary. Almost half of the 10,000 to 12,000 spinal cord injuries reported each year result in paraplegia. This condition occurs twice as often in men as in women; incidence is highest between ages 16 and 35.

Causes
Most spinal cord injuries result from trauma, especially automobile, motorcycle, and sporting accidents; gunshot wounds; and falls. Less common causes are nontraumatic lesions, such as spina bifida, scoliosis, and chordoma.

Signs and symptoms
In many patients, onset of total or partial paralysis is immediate, resulting in loss of motion, sensation, and reflexes below the level of the lesion, with urinary retention and absence of perspiration in the paralyzed parts. In some patients, careful questioning and gentle examination are necessary to determine the extent of motor or sensory loss. Spinal cord injuries with motor and sensory loss may result in bowel, bladder, and sexual dysfunctions, depending on the level of the lesion and whether damage to the cord is complete or incomplete. In an incomplete spinal cord injury, perianal sensation, voluntary toe flexion, or sphincter control is still present; in a

complete spinal cord injury, lack of sensation or voluntary muscle control is apparent and persists for 24 hours. Any return of functional muscle power distal to the injury is unlikely.

Diagnosis

Diagnosis requires clinical history, neurologic examination, and X-rays. A lumbar puncture may rule out blocked CSF circulation. Laboratory studies include CBC, prothrombin time, electrolytes, 24-hour urine for creatinine clearance, serum creatinine, and urinalysis. After stabilization, hip, knee, and chest X-rays, and intravenous pyelography provide a baseline to detect any pathologic changes. Weekly urine samples for culture and sensitivity are advisable during the entire rehabilitation period.

Treatment

The four goals of treatment for any spinal cord injury include:
• restoration of normal alignment of the spine
• early insurance of complete stability of the injured spinal area
• decompression of compressed neurologic structures
• early rehabilitation to an active and productive life.

Treatment starts at the scene of the accident by *not* moving the patient until his spine and head have been stabilized by strapping him to a board. Even after reaching the hospital, the patient *is not* removed from the board but placed on a stretcher while still strapped to it. Such stabilization helps prevent reversible damage from becoming permanent through additional injury to the neuraxis. Supportive treatment corrects systemic shock and controls local hemorrhage. Insertion of a Foley catheter insures uninterrupted urine drainage.

Whenever possible, the care of spinal cord injuries emphasizes conservative treatment, such as closed reduction of fractures. However, unstable fractures and fracture dislocations require fusion following reduction, combined with recumbent immobilization until healing occurs. Bone fragments pressing on the spinal cord may require laminectomy. Drug therapy may include nitrofurantoin to prevent bladder infection; large doses of vitamin C to enhance utilization of protein and help minimize infection by acidifying the urine; diazepam, baclofen, or dantrolene sodium to relieve skeletal muscle spasms from upper motor neuron disorders; and, sparingly, analgesics and narcotics to relieve pain. The extent of paralysis can't be accurately assessed until a year after the spinal cord injury.

Additional considerations

The most effective care of the patient with spinal cord injury combines excellent health care skills with the ability to become an interested and knowledgeable friend, confidant, and teacher. Specific care includes:
• teaching assigned staff how to use a special bed (Stryker Frame, Circoelectric, Roto-Rest), if applicable.
• providing proper wound care after a laminectomy.
• providing meticulous catheter care; using intermittent catherization to reestablish bladder control, maintain adequate bladder capacity, and prevent infection.
• keeping skin clean and dry, giving back rubs, inspecting pressure areas daily, and massaging reddened skin areas; teaching the patient and family to inspect pressure areas for skin breakdown (the patient can do this himself with a handheld mirror) and reporting it immediately; instructing the patient to shift position at least every 15 minutes while sitting in a wheelchair.
• maintaining proper body alignment and position to prevent contractures in the immobilized patient.
• monitoring intake and output; restricting fluids to 2,000 to 2,500 ml/day if the patient is on an intermittent catheterization program (fluids can be increased to 4,000 ml/day in a patient with a Foley catheter).
• watching for orthostatic hypotension as the patient progresses from bed rest

to a wheelchair; providing an abdominal binder and thigh-length antiembolism hose (later replaced by knee-length) to help the body compensate for a sitting position after prolonged restriction to recumbent position.
• providing an appropriate high-bulk diet to prevent constipation; giving protein supplements to compensate for energy expenditure during therapy and to build up body tissues; initiating a bowel retraining program; establishing a time for daily defecation (the gastro-colic reflex is strongest 20 to 30 minutes after eating); providing laxatives, stool softeners, and suppositories, as needed; administering suppositories at the same time each day (if suppositories are ineffective, digital stimulation may be helpful).
• encouraging family and friends to become involved in his rehabilitation, since

the patient's paraplegia affects them as well; setting aside time to talk with them, teach and comfort them.
• being ready for psychological problems such as an altered body image, loss of self-esteem, denial, and anger; providing emotional support, and understanding the patient's castastrophic life change; reinforcing skills learned in therapy; emphasizing the strengths and abilities of patients with spinal cord injuries; encouraging the patient to assume the responsibility for a new purpose and direction to his life.

To prevent spinal cord injuries, everyone should wear seat belts, even while driving short distances; check the depth of the water before diving into a pond, creek, or swimming pool; wear appropriate protective equipment and stress safety when playing in strenuous sports.

Quadriplegia

A devastating, permanent injury that affects all body systems, quadriplegia is paralysis of the arms, legs, and body below the level of the injury to the spinal cord. Usually the result of trauma, this condition affects 150,000 Americans, most of whom are men between ages 20 and 40.

Causes
Quadriplegia may result from spinal cord injury, especially in the area of the fifth to seventh cervical vertebrae (C5 to C7). Such injury usually follows trauma or vertebral pressure on the soft tissue of the cord (see also PARAPLEGIA).

Signs and symptoms
Quadriplegia causes flaccidity in the arms and legs, and loss of power and sensation below the level of injury. Spinal cord injuries above C5 dramatically affect other body systems as well; for example, cardiovascular complications result from a block in the sympathetic nervous system that allows the parasympathetic system to dominate. Possible complications include:
• hypotension with blood pressure below 90/60, resulting from vasodilation,

which allows blood to pool in the veins of the extremities, thereby slowing the venous blood return to the heart
• low body temperature (96° F. [35.5° C.] or lower) from inability of blood vessels to constrict efficiently, allowing constant close blood vessel contact with the body surface and consequent heat loss
• bradycardia from stimulation of the heart by the vagus nerve and absence of the inhibiting effects of the sympathetic system
• decreased peristalsis from various types of shock
• respiratory complications, a major cause of death, from damage to the upper cervical cord
• autonomic dysreflexia (in injuries above T4), in which severed connection between the brain and the spinal cord produces an exaggerated autonomic response

to such stimuli as distended bladder, fecal impaction, infection, decubitus ulcers, or surgical manipulation; the key symptom of autonomic dysreflexia is hypertension.

Diagnosis

A complete physical and neurologic examination must assess remaining motor function and determine if the cord injury is complete or partial. Detailed information about the trauma may help anticipate other related injuries. Spinal X-rays and myelography identify fractures, dislocations, subluxation, and blockage in the spinal cord. Other tests include X-rays of the head, chest, and abdomen to rule out underlying injuries. Since this type of injury has such far-reaching physiologic effects, significant laboratory data assessing respiratory, hepatic, and pancreatic functions are necessary to provide a baseline.

Treatment

Treatment begins at the scene of the accident, with immobilization of the neck and spine. At the hospital, methods of immobilization include insertion of Gardner Wells tongs or halo traction. A turning frame, such as the Roto Rest bed, helps prevent pulmonary (atelectasis, pneumonia, pulmonary embolus) and cardiovascular (thrombus formation, orthostatic hypotension) complications, renal calculi, muscle atrophy, decubitus ulcers, and infections.

After stabilization, therapy consists of steroids, glycopyrrolate I.V. to maintain the integrity of the gastrointestinal tract, insertion of a Foley catheter, and administration of a potent diuretic (20% mannitol). This protocol is followed for 10 days to decrease spinal cord edema; unchecked edema further compromises the blood supply to sensitive cord tissue, producing irreversible cord damage. Prevention of ascending cord edema preserves higher cord segments and maximum function in the upper extremities. Each cord segment preserved means greater potential for rehabilitation.

After 10 days of this therapy, surgical fusion stabilizes the unstable spine. Surgery must also remove bone fragments that can irritate the spinal cord and, in later stages, aggravate spasticity.

Another necessary part of treatment is aggressive respiratory therapy that, in the intubated patient, includes instilling normal saline solution, and hyperventilating the patient, using a hand-held resuscitator, before thorough suctioning to remove secretions and prevent mucous plugs. In cervical cord injuries above C5, intubation and ventilator assistance are required.

Additional considerations

• The first priority in caring for a patient with quadriplegia is maintaining adequate respiration. The patient should be asked to cough and blow through his nose (a patient with poor diaphragmatic excursion and intercostal weakness can't effectively clear the airway). The hospital staff member needs to watch closely for signs of respiratory insufficiency (rising PCO_2, decreasing oxygen and pH).

• During I.V. therapy, the staffer must be careful not to overhydrate the patient because of vasodilation and venous pooling below the level of injury.

• The staffer must watch for gastrointestinal complications, especially paralytic ileus, bleeding, and pancreatic dysfunction. He should listen for bowel sounds every 8 hours, record amount and type of nasogastric drainage, and test coffee-ground secretions for blood.

• If bradycardia occurs, the patient must be connected to a cardiac monitor, and given 0.1 mg atropine I.V. If signs of hypotension develop, the patient should be placed in slight Trendelenburg position, and his respiratory function constantly checked. When placing the patient in an upright position, an abdominal binder and antiembolism stockings can be used to aid venous return and prevent orthostatic hypotension.

• If hypothermia occurs (temperature below 90° F. [32° C.]), the patient may be warmed with blankets. Hot-water bottles or mechanical heat devices *should not* be used because they may burn the patient.

• The staff member must watch for severe hypertension, which may lead to heart failure, retinal hemorrhage, or intracranial bleeding, and is usually a sign of autonomic dysreflexia in the patient with an injury above T4. If hypertension occurs, the head of the patient's bed should be elevated to decrease blood pressure. The staff member should make sure that bladder distention isn't due to an obstructed catheter. If hypertension is due to fecal impaction, the rectum *must not* be manipulated; this worsens the symptoms. Before removing the impaction, a topical anesthetic ointment, such as tetracaine, can be applied to lessen risk of further rise in blood pressure. If blood pressure doesn't return to normal levels, the doctor should be notified. He may order smooth-muscle relaxant or an antihypertensive. Persistent rise in blood pressure may require treatment with an alpha-adrenergic blocking agent.

• The patient will need help establishing nonverbal communication if he is intubated or has a tracheostomy.

Hemiplegia

Hemiplegia is unilateral paralysis that follows severe cortical or pyramidal tract damage. Usually, such damage results from a cerebrovascular accident, but it can also result from tumor, CNS infection, degenerative neurologic disease, or trauma. Less severe damage results in paresis (weakness) rather than in paralysis.

Because nerves cross in the pyramidal tract before descending to the spinal cord, damage to the right side of the brain causes left-sided hemiplegia; damage to the left side causes right-sided hemiplegia. Thoracic, abdominal, or other muscles innervated by both sides of the brain generally are not affected by this paralysis. Prognosis varies with neurologic complications, patient age, and cause, site, and extent of brain damage.

Causes
Any injury to the cerebral cortex, subcortical and corticospinal regions, brain stem, pons, or one side of the spinal cord can cause hemiplegia:
• *cerebrovascular accident (CVA)* or other vascular diseases that affect the brain
• *trauma,* including subdural, epidural, or intracerebral hemorrhage or hematoma, and cerebral contusion and laceration
• *tumors*
• *degenerative neurologic disease,* such as multiple sclerosis
• *CNS infection,* including encephalitis, syphilis, and abscesses.

Signs and symptoms
Depending on the site of injury, hemiplegia produces unilateral weakness or paralysis of the arm, leg, face, and tongue, although midline brain lesions may cause bilateral leg weakness. Such paralysis may be sudden (resulting from CVA) or gradual (from a tumor). Initially, this paralysis is flaccid but often progresses to spasticity within days or weeks.

Most patients with hemiplegia recover some function as initial edema and swelling at the site of injury subside, but additional improvement after a year is

---

FIVE A's OF HEMIPLEGIA

Hemiplegics often have related neurologic complications:
• *aphasia:* defect in comprehending speech or written language
• *agnosia:* inability to recognize the meaning of sensory stimuli
• *apraxia:* inability to use an object for its intended purpose
• *agraphia:* inability to express oneself in writing
• *alexia:* word blindness, or inability to read

unlikely. In many patients, paralysis causes complications, such as contractures, muscle shortening, impaired circulation, decubitus ulcers, and footdrop. Although bladder dysfunction is uncommon, many patients become incontinent because concurrent problems, such as decreased level of consciousness or aphasia, make it difficult for them to communicate their needs.

Also, depending on the site of injury, hemiplegia is associated with neurologic deficits, such as aphasia, agnosia, apraxia, agraphia, and alexia. Cranial nerve damage decreases corneal reflex and causes hemianopia (half-field blindness); weakness of the palate, tongue, and lower part of the face; and disturbed position sense.

Diagnosis

Usually, patient history and physical examination make this diagnosis obvious, but a neurologic workup is necessary to determine the cause, locate the site of the lesion, and provide baseline data:
• *brain studies* (CAT scan, brain scan, cerebral angiography, ventriculography, skull films, and an EEG to locate brain lesions and vascular damage)
• *blood workup*, including a CBC, electrolytes, glucose, PT, and PTT
• *chest X-ray*
• *EKG*.

If baseline tests confirm a cerebral lesion, further tests aren't necessary. Otherwise, additional testing depends on the suspected underlying cause and may include:
• *spinal X-rays* and *myelography* in suspected spinal cord damage
• *lumbar puncture* in suspected neurologic infection or degenerative disease. In multiple sclerosis, lumbar puncture shows increased cells in the CSF and increased gamma globulin levels. In intracerebral hemorrhage, it shows blood in CSF. In meningitis, it shows high protein levels, low glucose levels, and WBCs; and a culture can often determine the causative organisms. In encephalitis, it shows elevated CSF pressure, slightly elevated protein levels, and WBCs.

• *serologic tests* for suspected syphilis.

Treatment

During the acute phase, the primary goal of treatment is to control the precipitating disorder (CVA, tumor). Later goals include prevention of complications (for instance, splints to prevent contractures), correction of deformities, and rehabilitation to foster independence and promote recovery. Rehabilitation should begin early, and usually includes antispasmodics, orthopedic and assistive devices (hand bars in the shower, low toilet seat), and occupational, recreational, physical, and speech therapy.

Additional considerations

Because hemiplegia is often a permanent impairment, rehabilitation is an arduous process that demands much from the patient and his family. It also demands much from the health care professional, who's responsible for direct health care, measures to prevent complications, and patient and family teaching.

In the acute stage, direct care of the patient with hemiplegia focuses on observation and assessment for signs of deterioration until the patient is physiologically stable. This includes:
• monitoring vital signs hourly, or more often if the level of consciousness is altered; watching for complications, such as increased intracranial pressure (deteriorating level of consciousness, vomiting, altered respirations, progressive motor deficit, and sluggish pupillary reaction to light, which may progress to unilateral dilation); being alert for respiratory failure (tachypnea, tachycardia, abnormal blood gas values), and accurately monitoring intake and output; giving medications, as ordered, and watching for side effects.

During the acute phase and throughout rehabilitation care includes:
• preventing decubitus ulcers by giving good skin care; by using a pulsating or egg crate mattress, sheepskin, or heel pads; by repositioning often; by checking pressure areas for signs of decubitus ulcer formation.

• preventing contractures and frozen joints by assisting in range-of-motion exercises and by placing arms, legs, and hands in a functional position; preventing footdrop by using a footboard or by applying high-topped sneakers.

• encouraging early out-of-bed activities, and helping the patient move about as soon as possible; offering assistance when he first tries to sit up, stand, and walk, since hemiplegia alters position sense and he may have hemianopia; teaching him to use the unaffected side, and discouraging total neglect of the weakened or paralyzed side; making arrangements early with the physical therapist for assistive devices, and then encouraging and helping the patient learn to use them.

Nutrition and personal hygiene must be maintained. The patient will need psychological support and training:

• Food should be placed in the unaffected side of the patient's mouth.

• To prevent incontinence, the patient will need to be trained in a bowel and bladder routine.

• Communication must be established and maintained. Aphasics will need a simple method of communicating basic needs. They should be talked to quietly and calmly (such a patient isn't deaf), with gestures to help comprehension. If he can write, he should be given a Magic Slate or a pad and pencil. If the patient has hemianopia, anyone speaking to him should stand directly in front of him when speaking.

• A positive attitude and realistic goals are necessary. The family should be encouraged to participate in the patient's care. Their expectations about recovery and rehabilitation must be realistic.

• Before discharge, the patient must be taught what he needs to know about maintenance drugs, such as antihypertensives and anticoagulants. His family might want a visiting nurse. The patient should be referred for speech, physical, and occupational therapy, and vocational counseling as soon as possible.

NEUROMUSCULAR DISORDERS

Myasthenia Gravis

Myasthenia gravis produces sporadic but progressive weakness and abnormal fatigability of striated (skeletal) muscles, which are exacerbated by exercise and repeated movement but improved by anticholinesterase drugs. Usually, this disorder affects muscles innervated by the cranial nerves (face, lips, tongue, neck, and throat), but it can affect any muscle group. Myasthenia gravis follows an unpredictable course of recurring exacerbations and periodic remissions. There's no known cure. Drug treatment has improved prognosis and allows patients to lead relatively normal lives except during exacerbations. When the disease involves the respiratory system, it may be life-threatening.

Causes and incidence

Myasthenia gravis causes a failure in transmission of nerve impulses at the neuromuscular junction. Theoretically, such impairment may result from an autoimmune response, ineffective acetylcholine release, or inadequate muscle fiber response to acetylcholine.

Myasthenia gravis affects 1 in 25,000 persons. It occurs at any age, but incidence is highest between ages 20 and 40. It is three times more common in women than in men. About 20% of infants born to myasthenic mothers have transient (or occasionally persistent) myasthenia. Frequently, myasthenia gravis coexists with immunologic and thyroid disorders. In fact, 15% of myasthenic patients have thymomas. Unexplained, spontaneous remissions occur in about 25% of myasthenic patients.

Signs and symptoms

The dominant symptoms of myasthenia gravis are skeletal muscle weakness and fatigability, which may be severe enough to cause paralysis. Typically, myasthenic muscles are strongest in the morning but weaken throughout the day, especially after exercise. Short rest periods temporarily restore muscle function. Muscle weakness is progressive; more and more muscles become weak, and eventually some muscles may lose function entirely. Resulting symptoms depend on the muscle group affected; they become more intense during menses, and after emotional stress, prolonged exposure to sunlight or cold, or infections.

Onset may be sudden or insidious. In many patients, weak eye closure, ptosis, and diplopia are the first signs that something is wrong. Myasthenic patients usually have blank and expressionless faces and nasal vocal tones. They experience frequent nasal regurgitation of fluids and have difficulty chewing and swallowing. Because of this, they often worry about choking. Their eyelids droop, and they may have to tilt their heads back to see. Their neck muscles may become too weak to support their heads, without bobbing.

In patients with weakened respiratory muscles, decreased tidal volume and vital capacity make breathing difficult, and predispose to pneumonia and other respiratory tract infections. Respiratory muscle weakness (myasthenic crisis) may be severe enough to require an emergency airway and mechanical ventilation.

Diagnosis

Muscle fatigability that improves with rest strongly suggests this diagnosis. Tests for this condition record the effect of exercise and subsequent rest on muscle weakness. Electromyography, with repeated neural stimulation, may help confirm this diagnosis.

 But the classic proof of myasthenia gravis is improved muscle function after an I.V. injection of edrophonium or neostigmine. In myasthenic patients, muscle function improves within 30 to 60 seconds and lasts up to 30 minutes. However, long-standing ocular muscle dysfunction often fails to respond to such testing. This same test can differentiate a myasthenic crisis from a cholinergic crisis (caused by acetylcholine overactivity at the neuromuscular junction, possibly due to anticholinergic overdose).

Diagnostic evaluation should rule out thyroid disease and, in all adults, thymoma (by X-ray of the mediastinum).

Treatment

Treatment is symptomatic. Anticholinesterase drugs, such as neostigmine and pyridostigmine, counteract fatigue and muscle weakness, and allow about 80% of normal muscle function. However, these drugs become less effective as the disease worsens. Corticosteroids may be beneficial in relieving symptoms.

Patients with thymomas require thymectomy, which may cause remission in some cases of adult-onset myasthenia. Acute exacerbations that cause severe respiratory distress necessitate emergency treatment. Tracheotomy, ventilation with a positive-pressure ventilator, and vigorous suctioning to remove secretions usually bring improvement in a few days. Because anticholinesterase drugs aren't effective in myasthenic crisis, they're discontinued until respiratory function begins to improve. Such crisis requires immediate hospitalization and vigorous respiratory support.

Additional considerations

Careful baseline assessment, early recognition and treatment of potential crises, supportive measures, and thorough patient teaching can minimize exacerbations and complications. Continuity of care is essential. A hospital staff member caring for the patient with myasthenia gravis should:

• establish an accurate neurologic and respiratory baseline, and monitor tidal volume and vital capacity regularly. The patient may need a ventilator and frequent suctioning to remove accumulating secretions.

• be alert for signs of an impending crisis (increased muscle weakness, respiratory distress, difficulty in talking or chewing).

• evenly space administration of drugs, and give them on time, as ordered, to prevent relapses; keep atropine on hand and be prepared to give it in case of anticholinesterase overdose or toxicity.

• plan exercise, meals, patient care, and activities to make the most of energy peaks. For example, medication should be given 20 to 30 minutes before meals to facilitate chewing or swallowing during meals. The patient should be encouraged to participate in his care as much as possible.

• give soft, solid foods instead of liquids, when swallowing is difficult, to lessen the risk of choking.

• try to increase social activity as soon as possible after a severe exacerbation.

Patient teaching is essential, since myasthenia gravis is usually a lifelong condition. The patient should:

• plan daily activities to coincide with energy peaks and rest frequently throughout the day.

• understand that periodic remissions, exacerbations, and day-to-day fluctuations are common.

• know how to recognize side effects and signs of toxicity of anticholinesterase drugs (these include headaches, weakness, sweating, abdominal cramps, nausea, vomiting, diarrhea, excessive salivation, and bronchospasm).

• avoid strenuous exercise, stress, infection, and needless exposure to the sun or cold weather. All these may worsen symptoms. Wearing an eye patch, or glasses with one frosted lens may be useful for the patient with diplopia.

For more information and an opportunity to meet myasthenics who lead full, productive lives, the patient should be referred to the Myasthenia Gravis Foundation.

Amyotrophic Lateral Sclerosis
(Lou Gehrig's disease)

Amyotrophic lateral sclerosis (ALS) is the most common motor neuron disease of muscular atrophy. Other motor neuron diseases include progressive muscular atrophy and progressive bulbar palsy. Generally, onset occurs between ages 40 and 70. ALS is fatal within 3 to 10 years after onset, usually a result of aspiration pneumonia or respiratory failure.

Causes and incidence

ALS occurs in 2 to 7 of every 100,000 persons. Generally, it affects men four times more often than women, and is more common in Caucasians than in Blacks. In about 10% of cases, ALS is inherited as an autosomal dominant trait. This form of the disease affects men and women equally. In noninherited ALS, incidence is highest among persons whose occupations require strenuous physical labor.

ALS and other motor neuron diseases possibly result from several causes:

• nutritional deficiency of motor neurons related to a disturbance in enzyme metabolism

• deficiency of vitamin E, which damages the cell membranes

• metabolic interference in nucleic acid production by the nerve fibers

• autoimmune disorders that affect immune complexes in the renal glomerulus and basement membrane.

Precipitating factors include trauma, acute viral infections, and physical ex-

---

MOTOR NEURON DISEASE

In its final stages, motor neuron disease affects both upper and lower motor neuron cells. However, the site of initial cell damage varies:
- *progressive bulbar palsy:* degeneration of upper motor neurons in the medulla oblongata
- *progressive muscular atrophy:* degeneration of lower motor neurons in the spinal cord
- *amyotrophic lateral sclerosis:* degeneration of upper motor neurons in the medulla oblongata and lower motor neurons in the spinal cord

---

haustion. Associated disorders include spinal cord syphilis, multiple sclerosis, spinal cord tumors, and syringomyelia.

Signs and symptoms
Patients with ALS develop fasciculations, accompanied by atrophy and weakness, especially in the muscles of the forearms and the hands. Other signs include impaired speech; difficulty chewing, swallowing, and breathing, particularly if the brain stem is affected; and occasionally, choking and excessive drooling. Mental deterioration doesn't usually occur, but patients may become depressed as a reaction to the disease. Progressive bulbar palsy may cause crying spells or inappropriate laughter.

Diagnosis
Characteristic clinical features indicate a combination of upper and lower motor neuron involvement without sensory impairment. Electromyography and muscle biopsy help show nerve, rather than muscle, disease. Protein content of CSF is increased in one third of patients, but this finding alone doesn't confirm ALS. Diagnosis must rule out multiple sclerosis, spinal cord neoplasm, polyarteritis, syringomyelia, myasthenia gravis, and progressive muscular dystrophy.

Treatment
No effective treatment exists for ALS. Management aims to control symptoms and provide emotional, psychologic, and physical support.

Additional considerations
This neurologic disease challenges the patient's and health care professional's ability to cope. Since mental status remains intact while progressive physical degeneration takes place, the patient acutely perceives every change.

Health care begins with a complete neurologic assessment, a baseline for future evaluations of progressing disease.

During the course of the disease, health care includes:
- implementing a rehabilitation program designed to maintain independence as long as possible.
- helping the patient obtain equipment such as a walker and a wheelchair; arranging for a visiting nurse to oversee the patient's status, to provide support, and to teach the family about the illness.
- assisting with bathing, personal hygiene, and transfers from wheelchair to bed, depending on the patient's muscular capacity; helping establish a regular bowel and bladder routine.
- helping the patient handle increased accumulation of secretions and dysphagia by teaching him to suction himself (the patient should have a suction machine readily accessible in his home to reduce fear of choking).
- preventing skin breakdown by providing good skin care when the patient is bedridden, including turning the patient often, keeping his skin clean and dry, and using sheepskins or a pressure-relieving device.
- giving soft, solid foods to the patient who has trouble swallowing, and positioning him upright during meals; teaching the patient, if he's still able to feed himself, or family how to administer gastrostomy feedings (gastrostomy and nasogastric tube feedings may be necessary if he can no longer swallow).
- providing emotional support; preparing the patient and family for his eventual death, and encouraging the start of the grieving process. Patients with ALS may benefit from a hospice program.

Multiple Sclerosis

Multiple sclerosis (MS) is characterized by exacerbations and remissions caused by progressive demyelination of the white matter of the brain and the spinal cord. It's a major cause of chronic disability in young adults. Sporadic patches of demyelination in various parts of the central nervous system induce widely disseminated and varied neurologic dysfunction.

Prognosis is variable. MS may progress rapidly, disabling the patient by early adulthood or causing death within months of onset. However, 70% of patients lead active, productive lives with prolonged remissions.

Incidence

Onset occurs between ages 20 and 40 (average age is 27). The disease affects women to men in a ratio of 3:2; Caucasians to Blacks, 5:1. Incidence is low in Japan; it is generally higher among urban populations and upper socioeconomic groups. Family history of MS and living in a cold, damp climate increase the risk.

Causes

The exact cause of MS is unknown, but current theories suggest a slow-acting viral infection, an autoimmune response of the nervous system, or an allergic response to an infectious agent. Other theoretical causes include trauma, anoxia, toxins, nutritional deficiencies, vascular lesions, and anorexia, all of which may contribute to destruction of axons and the myelin sheath. Emotional stress, overwork, fatigue, pregnancy, and acute respiratory infections all have been known to precede onset of this illness. Endogenous, constitutional, and genetic factors may also contribute.

Signs and symptoms

Clinical findings in MS correspond to the extent and site of myelin destruction, the extent of remyelination, and the adequacy of subsequent restored synaptic transmission. Symptoms may be transient or may last for hours or weeks; they may wax and wane with no predictable pattern, vary from day to day, and be bizarre and difficult for the patient to describe.

DEMYELINATION IN MULTIPLE SCLEROSIS

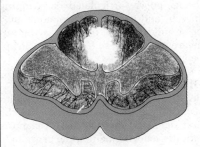

Transverse section of cervical vertebra shows partial loss of myelin, characteristic of multiple sclerosis. This degenerative process is called demyelination.

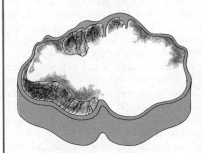

In this illustration, the loss of myelin is nearly complete. Clinical features of multiple sclerosis depend on the extent of demyelination.

In most patients, visual problems and sensory impairment, such as numbness and tingling sensations (paresthesia), are the first signs that anything is wrong. Other characteristic changes include:
• *ocular disturbances:* optic neuritis, diplopia, ophthalmoplegia, blurred vision, and nystagmus
• *muscle dysfunction:* weakness, paralysis ranging from monoplegia to quadriplegia, spasticity, hyperreflexia, intention tremor, gait ataxia
• *urinary disturbances:* incontinence, frequency, urgency, and frequent infections
• *emotional lability:* mood swings, irritability, euphoria, or depression.

Other clinical effects include paresthesia, poorly articulated or scanning speech, and dysphagia. Symptoms may be so mild that the patient may be unaware of them, or so bizarre that he appears hysterical.

Diagnosis

Because early symptoms may be mild, years may elapse between onset of the first signs and the diagnosis. Diagnosis requires evidence of multiple neurologic attacks, and characteristic remissions and exacerbations. Since diagnosis is so difficult, periodic testing and close observation are necessary, perhaps for years, depending on the course of the disease.

Abnormal EEG occurs in one third of patients. Lumbar puncture shows elevated gamma globulin fraction of IgG but normal total CSF protein levels. Such elevated CSF gamma globulin is significant only when serum gamma globulin levels are normal, and it reflects hyperactivity of the immune system because of chronic demyelinization. In addition, CSF white blood count is slightly increased. Diagnosis also may include a psychologic evaluation.

Differential diagnosis must rule out spinal cord compression, foramen magnum tumor (often, such a tumor exactly mimics the exacerbations and remissions of MS), multiple small strokes, syphilis or other infection, and psychologic disturbances.

Treatment

The aim of treatment is to shorten exacerbations and, if possible, relieve neurologic deficits, so the patient can resume a normal life-style. Because MS is thought to have allergic and inflammatory causes, ACTH, prednisone, or dexamethasone is used to reduce the associated edema of the myelin sheath during exacerbations. ACTH and corticosteroids seem to relieve symptoms and hasten remission but don't prevent future exacerbations.

Other drugs used with ACTH and corticosteroids include chlordiazepoxide to mitigate mood swings, baclofen or dantrolene to relieve spasticity, and bethanechol or oxybutynin to relieve urinary retention, and minimize frequency and urgency. During acute exacerbation, supportive measures include bed rest, comfort measures such as baths and massages, prevention of excessive fatigue, prevention of decubitus ulcers, bowel and bladder training (if necessary), treatment of bladder infections with antibiotics, physical therapy, and counseling.

Additional considerations

Appropriate health care depends on the severity of the disease and the symptoms.
• Physical therapy will probably be necessary. Massages and relaxing baths may make the patient more comfortable. The bathwater must not be too hot, since it may temporarily intensify otherwise subtle symptoms. Active, resistive, and stretching exercises will help maintain muscle tone and joint mobility, decrease spasticity, improve coordination, and boost morale.
• The patient and family will have to be educated about the disease's chronic course. They must understand the need to avoid stress, infections, and fatigue, and to maintain independence by developing new ways of performing daily activities.
• The patient should avoid exposure to infections.
• The patient must get a nutritious, well-balanced diet that contains sufficient roughage to prevent constipation.
• Bowel and bladder training, if needed,

should be given during hospitalization. The patient should take adequate fluids and urinate regularly. Eventually, the patient may require urinary drainage by self-catheterization or, in men, condom drainage. The patient will need to be taught correct use of suppositories to help establish a regular bowel schedule.

• The patient must be observed for drug side effects. For instance, dantrolene may cause muscle weakness and decreased muscle tone.

• The patient will need help in estab-lishing a daily routine to maintain an optimal level of functioning; his activity level will be regulated by his tolerance level. The patient will need regular rest periods to prevent fatigue, and daily physical exercise.

• Since the exacerbations are unpre-dictable, the patient has to make some physical and emotional adjustments in life-style.

• The patient should be referred to the National Multiple Sclerosis Society for additional information.

PERIPHERAL NERVE DISORDERS

Trigeminal Neuralgia
(Tic douloureux)

Trigeminal neuralgia is a painful disorder of one or more branches of the fifth cranial (trigeminal) nerve that produces paroxysmal attacks of excruciating facial pain precipitated by stimulation of a trigger zone. It occurs mostly in people over 40, in women more often than men, and on the right side of the face more often than the left. Trigeminal neuralgia can subside spontaneously, with remissions lasting from several months to years.

Causes
Although the cause remains undeter-mined, trigeminal neuralgia may reflect an afferent reflex phenomenon located centrally in the brain stem or more pe-ripherally in the sensory root of the tri-geminal nerve. Such neuralgia may also be related to compression of the nerve root by posterior fossa tumors, middle fossa tumors, or vascular lesions (sub-clinical aneurysm), although such le-sions usually produce simultaneous loss of sensation. Occasionally, trigeminal neuralgia is a manifestation of multiple sclerosis or herpes zoster. Whatever the cause, the pain is probably produced by an interaction or short-circuiting of touch and pain fibers.

Signs and symptoms
Typically, the patient reports a searing or burning pain that occurs in light-ninglike jabs and lasts from 1 to 15 min-utes (usually 1 to 2 minutes) in an area innervated by one of the divisions of the trigeminal nerve, primarily the superior mandibular or maxillary division. The pain rarely affects more than one divi-sion, and seldom the first division (ophthalmic) or both sides of the face. It affects the second (maxillary) and third (mandibular) divisions of the tri-geminal nerve equally.

These attacks characteristically follow stimulation of a trigger zone, usually by a light touch to a hypersensitive area, such as the tip of the nose, the cheeks, or the gums. Although attacks can occur at any time, they may follow a draft of air, exposure to heat or cold, eating, smiling, talking, or drinking hot or cold beverages. The frequency of attacks var-ies greatly, from many times a day to several times a month or year.

Between attacks, most patients are free of pain, although some have a constant, dull ache. No patient is ever free of the fear of the next attack.

Diagnosis

The patient's pain history is the basis for diagnosis, since trigeminal neuralgia produces no objective clinical or pathologic changes. Physical examination shows no impairment of sensory or motor function; indeed, sensory impairment implies a space-occupying lesion as the cause of pain.

Observation during the examination shows the patient favoring (splinting) the affected area. To ward off a painful attack, the patient often holds his face immobile when talking. He may also leave the affected side of his face unwashed and unshaven, or protect it with a coat or shawl. When asked where the pain occurs, he points to—but never touches—the affected area. Witnessing a typical attack helps to confirm diagnosis. Rarely, a tumor in the posterior fossa can produce pain that is clinically indistinguishable from trigeminal neuralgia. Skull X-rays, tomography, and CAT scan rule out sinus or tooth infections, and tumors.

Treatment

Oral administration of carbamazepine or phenytoin, or alcohol or phenol injections into the terminal branch of the nerve may temporarily relieve or prevent pain. Narcotics may be helpful during the pain episode. When these medical measures fail or attacks become increasingly frequent or severe, neurosurgical procedures may provide permanent relief. The preferred procedure is percutaneous electrocoagulation of nerve rootlets, under local anesthetic. New techniques using microsurgery allow more precise dissection of nerve rootlets.

Additional considerations

• The characteristics of each attack, in-

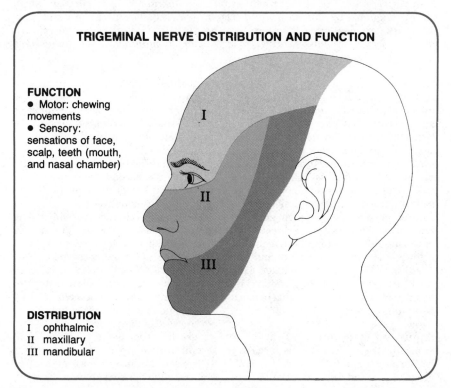

TRIGEMINAL NERVE DISTRIBUTION AND FUNCTION

FUNCTION
• Motor: chewing movements
• Sensory: sensations of face, scalp, teeth (mouth, and nasal chamber)

DISTRIBUTION
I   ophthalmic
II maxillary
III mandibular

cluding the patient's protective mechanisms, must be noted before treatment begins.
• The patient should eat small, frequent meals served at room temperature.
• If the patient is receiving carbamazepine, side effects may include cutaneous and hematologic reactions (pruritic and erythematous rashes, urticaria, photosensitivity, exfoliative dermatitis, leukopenia, agranulocytosis, eosinophilia, aplastic anemia, thrombocytopenia), and possibly, urinary retention and transient drowsiness. For the first 3 months of carbamazepine therapy, CBC and liver function should be monitored weekly, then monthly thereafter. The patient taking carbamazepine should immediately report fever, sore throat, mouth ulcers, easy bruising, or petechial or purpuric hemorrhage, since these may signal thrombocytopenia or aplastic anemia. Such complications may require discontinuation of drug therapy.
• Side effects associated with phenytoin include ataxia, skin eruptions, gingival hyperplasia, and nystagmus.

• After resection of the first branch of the trigeminal nerve, the patient must avoid rubbing his eyes and using aerosol spray. He should wear glasses or goggles outdoors and blink often.
• After surgery to sever the second or third branch, the patient must avoid hot foods and drinks, which could burn his mouth, and chew carefully to avoid biting his mouth. He should place food in the unaffected side of his mouth, brush his teeth and rinse his mouth often, and see the dentist twice a year to detect cavities. (Cavities in the area of the severed nerve won't cause pain.)
• After surgical decompression of the root or partial nerve dissection, neurologic and vital signs must be checked often.
• The patient will need emotional support, and encouragment to express his fear and anxiety. Independence can be promoted through self-care and maximum physical activity. Natural avoidance of stimulation (air, heat, cold) of trigger zones (lips, cheeks, gums) should be reinforced.

Glossopharyngeal Neuralgia

Glossopharyngeal neuralgia is a rare disease of the ninth cranial (glossopharyngeal) nerve, which extends from the medulla in the brain stem. It produces paroxysms of sharp, darting pain that vary in intensity and usually affect the ear, the posterior pharynx, or the base of the tongue or the jaws. Prognosis after surgery is good.

Causes
The cause of this disorder is unknown. Rarely, it may result from pressure on the ninth cranial nerve from intracranial tumors in the cerebellum or pons, or nasopharyngeal tumors. Other possible causes include penetrating wounds of the neck, vascular lesions, or ossification of the ligament attached to the hyoid bone. Glossopharyngeal neuralgia affects men more often than women. Incidence is highest after age 40.

Signs and symptoms
Glossopharyngeal neuralgia affects the

area within the sensory distribution of the glossopharyngeal nerve and, in some cases, branches of the adjacent vagus nerve. The dominant symptom is sharp paroxysms of pain lasting from seconds to minutes. The pain may vary in intensity—in some cases it may be so mild that it is not incapacitating—and may be associated with loss of gag reflex and taste on the posterior third of the tongue.
Swallowing, talking, chewing, coughing, or external pressure on the ear may precipitate an attack. This painful attack may be accompanied by salivation and excess coughing. Rarely, glossopharyn-

geal neuralgia also affects the vagus nerve, in which case syncope or cardiac arrest may accompany the attack.

Diagnosis

The pain of glossopharyngeal neuralgia, except for its distribution, is often identical to that of trigeminal neuralgia. To differentiate between these two neuralgias, the tonsillar area in the throat is stimulated with a cotton-tipped applicator. If this procedure produces pain, or if a local anesthetic eliminates the pain, the patient may have glossopharyngeal neuralgia. Diagnosis must rule out tonsillar, pharyngeal, and cerebellopontile angle tumors, which can induce similar symptoms.

Treatment

In most patients, the treatment of choice is intracranial sectioning of the glossopharyngeal nerve. However, carbamazepine, alone or in combination with phenytoin, may induce remission in a high percentage of patients.

Additional considerations

Supportive care and careful monitoring minimize complications. Carbamazepine therapy may cause cutaneous and hematologic reactions: pruritic and erythematous rashes, urticaria, photosensitivity, or exfoliative dermatitis; leukopenia, agranulocytosis, eosinophilia, aplastic anemia, or thrombocytopenia. Other side effects include urinary retention and transient drowsiness. A patient receiving carbamazepine requires weekly monitoring of CBC and liver function for the 3 months after drug therapy begins, then monthly checks thereafter. Since aplastic anemia and thrombocytopenia can be fatal, the patient must report any of these side effects: fever, sore throat, mouth ulcers, easy bruising, or the development of petechiae or purpura. The doctor will probably then discontinue carbamazepine. If the patient also receives phenytoin, side effects may also include ataxia, gingival hyperplasia, and nystagmus.

If treatment involves surgical nerve resection, before surgery the hospital staff member should:

• reinforce what the neurosurgeon has told the patient about the effects and possible complications of this surgery; make sure the patient understands this information, clarify anything he doesn't understand, and offer support.

• because the patient will most likely go to ICU after surgery, describe the ICU environment to him and his family to minimize anxiety; explain probable postoperative procedures, such as nasogastric intubation, I.V. fluid replacement, bladder catheterization, and the need for frequent neurologic checks.

After nerve resection the staff member should:

• assess respiratory status every 15 to 30 minutes until the patient is stable; since damage to the ninth and tenth cranial nerves during surgery may cause partial to complete paralysis of the vocal cords or muscles used in swallowing or coughing, watch carefully for signs of dysphagia or inability to swallow; check the gag and swallow reflexes before administering feeding to prevent aspiration; ensure adequate oxygenation and prevent CO_2 retention, which contributes to cerebral edema; suction as needed, making sure the airway is clear; provide good mouth care.

• evaluate neurologic status frequently; check level of consciousness, pupillary response, cranial nerve function, reflexes, motion, and coordination every 30 to 60 minutes for at least 2 days after surgery; watch for signs of vasospasm of the small vessels of the brain stem (for example, changes in pupillary response, or depressed respirations), which may indicate brain stem infarction; stay alert for signs of cerebral edema, such as restlessness and decreased level of consciousness.

• assess gastrointestinal status; watch for evidence of blood in the patient's nasogastric drainage and stool, since gastrointestinal hemorrhage may occur after surgery; monitor for normal bowel sounds, since impairment of the autonomic fibers of the vagus nerve may

cause paralytic ileus.
• warn the patient to be careful when eating, since surgery causes permanent unilateral loss of taste and sensation of the posterior third of the tongue and anesthesia of the gag reflex; instruct him to place food in the anterior portion of his mouth, to chew his food slowly and always chew carefully, and to swallow gently; stress the importance of and teach good oral hygiene.
• assess psychosocial status; encourage the patient to regain independence and mobility as soon as possible.

Bell's Palsy

Bell's palsy is a disease of the seventh cranial nerve (facial) that produces unilateral facial weakness or paralysis. Onset is rapid. While it affects all age-groups, it occurs most often in persons under age 60. In 80% to 90% of patients, it subsides spontaneously, with complete recovery in 1 to 8 weeks; however, recovery may be delayed in the elderly. If recovery is partial, contractures may develop on the paralyzed side of the face. Bell's palsy may recur on the same or opposite side of the face.

Causes
Bell's palsy blocks the seventh cranial nerve, which is responsible for motor innervation of the muscles of the face. The conduction block is due to an inflammatory reaction around the nerve, usually at the internal auditory meatus, which is often associated with infections and can result from hemorrhage, tumor, meningitis, or local trauma.

Signs and symptoms
Bell's palsy usually produces unilateral facial weakness, occasionally with aching pain around the angle of the jaw or behind the ear. On the weak side, the mouth droops (causing the patient to drool saliva from the corner of his mouth), and taste perception is distorted over the affected anterior portion of the tongue. In addition, the forehead appears smooth, and the patient's ability to close his eye on the weak side is markedly impaired. When he tries to close this eye, it rolls upward (Bell's phenomenon) and shows excessive tearing. Although Bell's phenomenon occurs in normal persons, it's not apparent, since the eye closes completely and covers this motion of the eye. In Bell's palsy, however, incomplete eye closure makes this upward movement obvious.

Diagnosis
Diagnosis is based on clinical presentation: distorted facial appearance, and inability to raise the eyebrow, close the eyelid, smile, show the teeth, or puff out the cheek. After 10 days, electromyography helps predict the level of expected recovery by distinguishing temporary conduction defects from a pathologic interruption of nerve fibers.

Treatment and additional considerations
Treatment consists of prednisone, an oral corticosteroid that reduces facial nerve edema and improves nerve conduction and blood flow. After the 14th day of prednisone therapy, electrotherapy may help prevent atrophy of facial muscles.
• During treatment with prednisone, the patient should be watched for steroid side effects, especially gastrointestinal distress and fluid retention. If gastrointestinal distress is troublesome, a concomitant antacid usually provides relief. If the patient has diabetes, prednisone must be used with caution and necessitates frequent monitoring of serum glucose levels.
• To reduce pain, moist heat can be applied to the affected side of the face, with care taken not to burn the skin.

• To help maintain muscle tone, the patient's face should be massaged, with a gentle upward motion two to three times daily for 5 to 10 minutes, or he can massage his face himself. When he's ready for active exercises, he should exercise his facial muscles by grimacing in front of a mirror.

• The patient must protect his eye by covering it with an eyepatch, especially when outdoors. He should keep warm and avoid exposure to dust and wind. When exposure is unavoidable, he should cover his face.

• The patient must be taught to cope with difficulty in eating and drinking, to prevent excessive weight loss. He should chew on the unaffected side of his mouth, eating a soft, nutritionally balanced diet, with no hot foods and fluids. He may want privacy at mealtimes to reduce embarrassment. A facial sling will improve lip alignment. Also, frequent and complete mouth care is necessary, with particular care taken to remove food that collects between the cheeks and gums.

• The patient will need psychological support. He should be reassured that complete recovery from Bell's palsy is likely within 1 to 8 weeks.

Peripheral Neuritis

(Multiple neuritis, peripheral neuropathy, polyneuritis)

Peripheral neuritis is the degeneration of peripheral nerves supplying mainly the distal muscles of the extremities. It results in muscle weakness with sensory loss and atrophy, and decreased or absent tendon reflexes. This syndrome is associated with a noninflammatory degeneration of the axon and myelin sheaths, chiefly affecting the distal muscles of the extremities. Although peripheral neuritis can occur at any age, incidence is highest in men between ages 30 and 50. Because onset is usually insidious, patients may compensate by overusing unaffected muscles; however, onset is rapid with severe infection and chronic alcohol intoxication. If the cause can be identified and eliminated, prognosis is good.

Causes
Causes of peripheral neuritis include:
• chronic intoxication (ethyl alcohol, arsenic, lead, carbon disulfide, benzene, phosphorus, and sulfonamides)
• infectious diseases (meningitis, diphtheria, syphilis, tuberculosis, pneumonia, mumps, and Guillain-Barré syndrome)
• metabolic and inflammatory disorders (gout, diabetes mellitus, rheumatoid arthritis, polyarteritis nodosa, systemic lupus erythematosus)
• nutritive diseases (beriberi and other vitamin deficiencies, and cachectic states).

Signs and symptoms
The clinical effects of peripheral neuritis develop slowly, and the disease usually affects the motor and sensory nerve fibers. Neuritis typically produces flaccid paralysis, wasting, loss of reflexes, pain of varying intensity, loss of ability to perceive vibratory sensations, and paresthesia, hyperesthesia, or anesthesia in the hands and feet. Deep tendon reflexes are diminished or absent, and atrophied muscles are tender or hypersensitive to pressure or palpation. Footdrop may also be present. Cutaneous manifestations include glossy red skin and decreased sweating. Patients often have a history of clumsiness and may complain of frequent vague sensations.

Diagnosis
Patient history and physical examination delineate characteristic distribution of motor and sensory deficits. Electromyography may show a delayed action potential if this condition impairs motor nerve function.

Treatment

Effective treatment of peripheral neuritis consists of supportive measures to relieve pain, adequate bed rest, and physical therapy, as needed. Most important, however, the underlying cause must be identified and corrected. For instance, it's essential to identify and remove the toxic agent, correct nutritional and vitamin deficiencies (the patient needs a high-calorie diet rich in vitamins, especially B complex), or counsel the patient to avoid alcohol.

Additional considerations

• Pain can be relieved with correct positioning, analgesics, or possibly, phenytoin, which has been used experimentally for neuritic pain, especially if associated with diabetic neuropathy.

• The patient should rest and refrain from using the affected extremity. A foot cradle can prevent pressure sores. To prevent contractures, the patient may need splints, boards, braces, or other orthopedic appliances.

• After the pain subsides, passive range-of-motion exercises or massage may be beneficial. Electrotherapy is advocated for nerve and muscle stimulation to help prevent atrophy.

Selected References

Alpers, Bernard J. and Elliott L. Mancall. CLINICAL NEUROLOGY, 6th ed. Philadelphia: F.A. Davis Co., 1971.

Baker, A., et al. CORE CURRICULUM FOR NEUROSURGICAL NURSING. Baltimore: American Association of Neurosurgical Nurses, 1977.

Baxter, R., and A. Linn. *Sex Counseling and the SCI Patient,* NURSING78. 8:46-52, September 1978.

Blount, M. *Symposium on Care of the Patient with Neuromuscular Disease, Management of the Patient with Amyotrophic Lateral Sclerosis,* NURSING CLINICS OF NORTH AMERICA. 14:157-171, March 1979.

Clark, Ronald G. MANTER & GATZ'S ESSENTIALS OF CLINICAL NEUROANATOMY AND NEUROPHYSIOLOGY, 5th ed. Philadelphia: F.A. Davis Co., 1975.

Conway, B. CARINI AND OWENS' NEUROLOGICAL AND NEUROSURGICAL NURSING, 7th ed. St. Louis: C.V. Mosby Co., 1978.

Donohoe, K. *Symposium on Care of the Patient with Neuromuscular Disease, An Overview of Neuromuscular Disease,* NURSING CLINICS OF NORTH AMERICA. 14:95-106, March 1979.

Flynn, I., et al. *Symposium on Care of the Patient with Neuromuscular Disease, Muscular Dystrophy: Comprehensive Nursing Care,* NURSING CLINICS OF NORTH AMERICA. 14:123-132, March 1979.

Heilman, K., et al. HANDBOOK FOR DIFFERENTIAL DIAGNOSIS OF NEUROLOGIC SIGNS AND SYMPTOMS. New York: Appleton-Century-Crofts, 1977.

Merritt, H. Houston. A TEXTBOOK OF NEUROLOGY, 6th ed. Philadelphia: Lea & Febiger, 1978.

Mutchie, K., and G. Burckart. *Drug Therapy of Reye's Syndrome,* AMERICAN JOURNAL OF HOSPITAL PHARMACY. 36:767-773, June 1979.

O'Brien, M., and P. Pallett. TOTAL CARE OF THE STROKE PATIENT. Boston: Little, Brown & Co., 1978.

Pierce, Donald S., and Vernon H. Nickel, eds. THE TOTAL CARE OF SPINAL CORD INJURIES. Boston: Little, Brown & Co., 1977.

Reeves, Alexander. NEUROLOGICAL DISORDERS. Chicago: Year Book Medical Publishers, 1981.

Suchenwirth, R. POCKETBOOK OF CLINICAL NEUROLOGY, 2nd ed. Chicago: Year Book Medical Publishers, 1979.

Swift, N., and R. Mabel. MANUAL OF NEUROLOGICAL NURSING. Boston: Little, Brown & Co., 1978.

Van Allen, M. PICTORIAL MANUAL OF NEUROLOGIC TESTS. Chicago: Year Book Medical Publishers, 1969.

Wehrmaker, S., and J. Wintermute. CASE STUDIES IN NEUROLOGICAL NURSING. Boston: Little, Brown & Co., 1978.

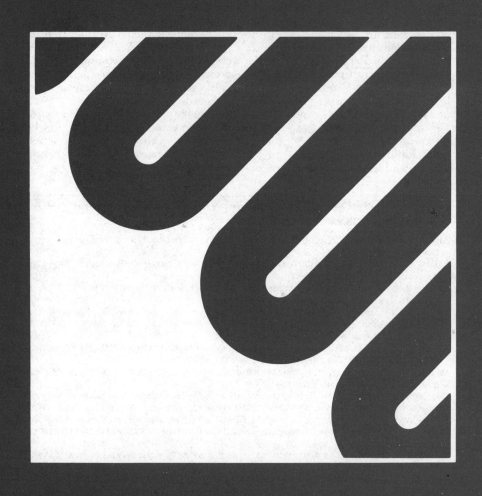

10 Gastrointestinal Disorders

Gastrointestinal Disorders

Introduction

The gastrointestinal (GI) tract, also known as the alimentary canal, is a long hollow tube with glands and accessory organs (salivary glands, liver, gallbladder, and pancreas). The GI tract breaks down food—carbohydrates, fats, and proteins—into molecules small enough to permeate cell membranes, thus providing cells with the necessary energy to function properly; it prepares food for cellular absorption by altering its physical and chemical composition. Consequently, a malfunction along the GI tract can produce far-reaching metabolic effects, eventually threatening life itself. The GI tract is an unsterile system filled with bacteria and other flora; these organisms can cause superinfection during or after antibiotic therapy, or they can infect other systems when a GI organ (such as the esophagus) ruptures. A common indication of GI problems is often referred pain, which makes diagnosis especially difficult.

Accurate assessment is vital

Assessment of the patient with suspected GI disease must begin with a careful history that includes race, marital status, occupation, and family history. Medical history should include previous hospital admissions, any surgery (including recent tooth extraction), family history of ulcers, colitis, or cancer, and any medications being taken currently, such as aspirin, steroids, or anticoagulants.

Next, a history of the chief complaint offers valuable diagnostic information. The patient should describe his complaint in his own words. How long has he had it? Does he have abdominal pain, indigestion, heartburn, or rectal bleeding? What relieves these symptoms or makes them worse? Has he experienced nosebleeds or difficulty in swallowing recently? Has any weight loss or gain occurred lately? Is he on a special diet? Does he drink alcoholic beverages? How much and how often? Have his bowel habits changed recently? How frequent are his bowel movements? What color are the stools? Does he regularly use laxatives or enemas? If he experiences nausea and vomiting, what does the vomitus look like? Does changing his position relieve nausea?

The next step is to try to define and locate any pain. This is essential for both diagnosis and treatment. The patient should describe the pain and point to it. How long does the pain last? Is it dull, sharp, burning, aching, spasmodic, intermittent? When does it occur (after meals, at night)? Does it radiate? What relieves it (use of antacids, a bowel movement)?

Visual assessment

How the patient looks and acts should be noted while monitoring vital signs or talking with the patient and family. Is he well nourished, thin, or obese? Is his behavior appropriate? Changes in fluid and electrolyte balance, severe infection, drug toxicity, and hepatic disease may cause abnormal behavior. Visual examination includes checking:

• *skin*—loss of turgor, jaundice, cyanosis, pallor, diaphoresis, petechiae, bruises, edema, texture (dry or oily)
• *head*—color of sclerae, sunken eyes, dentures, caries, lesions, tongue (color, swelling, dryness), breath odor
• *chest*—shape
• *lungs*—rate, rhythm, and quality of respirations
• *abdomen*—size and shape (distention, contour, visible masses, protrusions), abdominal scars or fistulae, excessive skin folds (may indicate wasting), abnormal respiratory movements (inflammation of diaphragm).

Auscultation and palpation

Auscultation provides helpful clues to GI abnormalities. For example, absence of bowel sounds over the area to the lower right of the umbilicus may indicate peritonitis. High-pitched sounds that coincide with colicky pain may indicate small bowel obstruction. Less intense, low-pitched rumbling noises may accompany minor irritation.

Palpating the abdomen helps detect tenderness, muscle guarding, and abdominal masses. Boardlike rigidity in muscle tone points to peritonitis. Transient rigidity in muscle tone suggests severe pain. Rebound tenderness may indicate peritoneal inflammation.

HISTOLOGY OF THE GI TRACT

The GI tract consists of four tissue layers whose structure varies in different organs:
• *mucous membrane:* innermost layer; secretes gastric juice and protects the tract
• *submucosa:* connective tissue that contains the major blood vessels
• *external muscle coat (muscularis externa):* double layer of smooth-muscle fibers; inner circular and outer longitudinal layers propel gastric contents downward by peristalsis
• *fibroserous coat (serosa):* outermost protective layer of connective tissue; forms the largest serous membrane of the body—the peritoneum. The peritoneum's parietal layer covers the walls of the abdominal cavity; the visceral layer drapes most of the abdominal organs, covering the upper surface of the pelvic organs.

PRIMARY SOURCE OF DIGESTIVE HORMONES

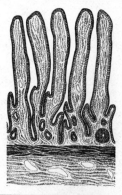

PYLORIC MUCOSA

Gastrin, which originates in the G cells of the pyloric antral mucosa (also from the duodenal and jejunal mucosa), stimulates secretion of HCl by parietal cells, and pepsinogen by chief cells.

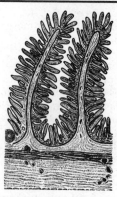

JEJUNAL MUCOSA

Gastric inhibitory peptide (GIP), which originates in the jejunal mucosa (also from duodenal mucosa), stimulates secretion of intestinal juice and insulin, and inhibits gastric acid secretion and motility.

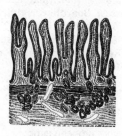

DUODENAL MUCOSA

Secretin, which originates in the duodenal mucosa, stimulates the pancreas to secrete alkaline fluid (water and HCO_3^-) into the duodenum, which neutralizes acid from the stomach.

Cholecystokinin-pancreozymin (CCK-PZ), which originates in the duodenal mucosa, stimulates pancreatic enzyme secretion, and contraction and evacuation of the gallbladder.

Motilin, which originates in the duodenal mucosa, slows gastric emptying and stimulates gastric acid and pepsin secretion.

Other digestive hormones

Three other digestive hormone-like substances are thought to originate in the hypothalamus, gastrointestinal tract, and neurons of the brain. These substances include substance P, which increases small bowel motility; bombesin, which increases gastrin secretion and small bowel motility; and somatosin, which inhibits secretion of gastrin, vasoactive intestinal polypeptide, GIP, secretin, and motilin. Other possible digestive hormones include enterogastrone, enteroglucagon, and somatostatin. More research is needed to confirm and clarify the existence and function of these hormones.

REVIEW OF ANATOMY AND PHYSIOLOGY

The GI tract includes the mouth, pharynx, esophagus, stomach (fundus, body, antrum), small intestine (duodenum, jejunum, ileum), and large intestine (cecum, colon, rectum, anal canal).

Digestion begins in the mouth through chewing and through the action of an enzyme, ptyalin (amylase), secreted in saliva, which breaks down starch. Digestion continues in the stomach, where the lining secretes gastric juice that contains hydrochloric acid and the enzymes pepsin (begins protein digestion), lipase (speeds hydrolysis of emulsified fats), and in infants, rennin (curdles milk). Through a churning motion, the stomach breaks food into tiny particles, mixes them with gastric juice, and pushes the mass toward the pylorus. The liquid portion (chyme) enters the duodenum in small amounts; any solid material remains in the stomach until it liquefies (usually from 1 to 6 hours). The stomach also produces an intrinsic factor necessary for the absorption of vitamin B_{12}. Although limited amounts of water, alcohol, and some drugs are absorbed in the stomach, chyme passes unabsorbed into the duodenum. Most digestion and absorption occur in the small intestine, where the surface area is increased by millions of villi in the mucous membrane lining. For digestion, the small intestine relies on a vast array of enzymes produced by the pancreas or by the intestinal lining itself. Pancreatic enzymes include tryspin, which digests protein to amino acids; lipase, which digests fat to fatty acids and glycerol; and amylase, which digests starches to sugars. Intestinal enzymes include erepsin, which digests protein to amino acids; lactase, maltase, and sucrase, which digest complex sugars like glucose, fructose, and galactose; and enterokinase, which activates trypsin.

In addition, bile, secreted by the liver, helps neutralize stomach acid and aids the small intestine to emulsify and absorb fats and fat-soluble vitamins.

By the time ingested material reaches the ileocecal valve (where the small intestine joins the large intestine), all its nutritional value has been absorbed.

The large intestine, so named because it's larger in diameter than the small intestine, absorbs water from the digestive material before passing it on for elimination. Rectal distention by feces stimulates the defecation reflex, which, when assisted by voluntary sphincter relaxation, permits defecation.

Throughout the GI tract, peristalsis propels ingested material along; sphincters prevent its reflux.

Diagnostic tests

After physical assessment, several tests can identify GI malfunction.

• *Barium swallow* primarily examines the esophagus.

• In an *upper GI series (UGI)*, swallowed barium sulfate proceeds into the esophagus, stomach, and small intestine, to reveal abnormalities. The barium outlines stomach walls and delineates ulcer craters and filling defects.

• A *small bowel series*—an extension of UGI—visualizes barium flowing through the entire small intestine to the ileocecal valve.

• A *barium enema (lower GI)* allows X-ray visualization of the colon.

• A *stool specimen* is useful with suspected GI bleeding, infection, or malabsorption. Guaiac test for occult blood, microscopic stool examination for ova and parasites, and tests for fat require several specimens.

• In *upper gastrointestinal endoscopy*, insertion of a fiberoptic scope allows direct visual inspection of the esophagus, stomach, and sometimes, duodenum; *proctosigmoidoscopy* permits inspection of the rectum and distal sigmoid colon; *colonoscopy*, inspection of descending, transverse, and ascending colon.

Intubation

Certain GI disorders require intubation to empty the stomach and intestine, to aid diagnosis and treatment, to decompress obstructed areas, to detect and treat GI bleeding, and to administer medications or feedings. Tubes generally inserted through the nose are the short nasogastric tubes (the Levin, the Salem Sump, and the specialized Sengstaken-Blakemore) and the long intestinal tubes (Cantor, and Miller-Abbott). The larger Ewald tube is usually inserted orally.

When caring for patients with tubes, the hospital staff member should:

• explain the procedure before intubation.

• maintain accurate intake and output records; measure gastric drainage every 8 hours; record amount, color, odor, and consistency; note the amount of saline solution instilled and aspirated when irrigating the tube; check for fluid and electrolyte imbalances.

• provide good oral and nasal care; brush the patient's teeth frequently; provide lemon and glycerine swabs, and mouthwash; make sure the tube is secure but isn't causing too much pressure on the nostrils; gently wash the area around the tube, and apply a water-soluble lubricant to soften crusts. These measures will help prevent sore throat and nose, dry lips, nasal excoriation, and parotitis.

• ensure maximum patient comfort; instruct the patient to turn from side to side after insertion of a long intestinal tube to facilitate its passage through the GI tract; note the tube's progress.

• anchor a short tube to the patient's clothing to support its weight.

• tell the patient to expect a feeling of dryness or a lump in the throat with both types of tubes; suggest he chew gum or eat hard candy if allowed, to relieve these discomforts.

• always keep a pair of scissors taped to the wall near the bed when the patient has a Sengstaken-Blakemore tube in place; cut the lumen to the balloon immediately if the tube should dislodge and obstruct the bronchus (sometimes the tube is taped to the face piece of a football-helmet–type headgear worn by the patient to prevent the tube from dislodging).

• after removing the tube from a patient with GI bleeding, watch for signs of recurrent bleeding, such as hematemesis, decreased hemoglobin, pallor, chills, and clamminess.

• provide emotional support. Many people panic at the sight of a tube. A calm, reassuring manner can help minimize their fear.

MOUTH & ESOPHAGUS

Stomatitis and Other Oral Infections

Stomatitis, inflammation of the oral mucosa, which may also extend to the buccal mucosa, lips, and palate, is a common infection. It may occur alone or as part of a systemic disease. There are two main types: acute herpetic stomatitis (herpetic gingivostomatitis) and aphthous stomatitis (recurrent aphthous stomatitis, canker sore). Acute herpetic stomatitis is usually self-limiting; however, it may be severe and, in newborns, may be generalized and potentially fatal. Aphthous stomatitis usually heals spontaneously, without a scar, in 10 to 14 days. Other oral infections include gingivitis, periodontitis, and Vincent's angina.

Causes and incidence

Acute herpetic stomatitis results from herpes simplex virus. It's a common cause of stomatitis in children between ages 1 and 3. Aphthous stomatitis is common in girls and female adolescents. Its predisposing factors include stress, fatigue, anxiety, and menstruation.

ORAL INFECTIONS

DISEASE AND CAUSES	SIGNS AND SYMPTOMS	TREATMENT
Gingivitis (inflammation of the gingiva) • Early sign of hypovitaminosis, diabetes, blood dyscrasias • Occasionally related to use of oral contraceptives	• Inflammation with painless swelling, redness, change of normal contours, bleeding, and periodontal pocket (gum detachment from teeth)	• Removal of irritating factors (calculus, faulty dentures) • Good oral hygiene; regular dental check-ups; vigorous chewing
Periodontitis (progression of gingivitis; inflammation of the oral mucosa) • Early sign of hypovitaminosis, diabetes, blood dyscrasias • Occasionally related to use of oral contraceptives • Dental factors: calculus, poor oral hygiene, malocclusion. Major cause of tooth loss after middle-age	• Acute onset of bright red gum inflammation, painless swelling of interdental papillae, easy bleeding • Loosening of teeth, typically without inflammatory symptoms, progressing to loss of teeth and alveolar bone • Acute systemic infection (fever, chills)	• Scaling, root planing, and curettage for infection control • Periodontal surgery to prevent recurrence • Good oral hygiene, regular dental checkups, vigorous chewing
Vincent's angina (trench mouth, necrotizing ulcerative gingivitis) • Fusiform bacillus or spirochete infection • Predisposing factors: stress, poor oral hygiene, insufficient rest, nutritional deficiency, smoking	• Sudden onset: painful, superficial bleeding gingival ulcers (rarely, on buccal mucosa) covered with a gray-white membrane • Ulcers become punched out lesions after slight pressure or irritation. • Malaise, mild fever, excessive salivation, bad breath, pain on swallowing or talking, enlarged submaxillary lymph nodes	• Removal of devitalized tissue with ultrasonic cavitron • Antibiotics (penicillin or erythromycin P.O.) for infection • Analgesics, as needed • Hourly mouth rinses (with equal amounts of hydrogen peroxide and warm water) • Soft, nonirritating diet; rest; no smoking • With treatment, improvement common within 24 hours
Glossitis (inflammation of the tongue) • Streptococcal infection • Irritation or injury; jagged teeth; ill-fitting dentures; biting during convulsions; alcohol; spicy foods; smoking; sensitivity to toothpaste or mouthwash • Vitamin B deficiency; anemia • Skin conditions: lichen planus, erythema multiforme, pemphigus vulgaris	• Reddened ulcerated or swollen tongue (may obstruct airway) • Painful chewing and swallowing • Speech difficulty • Painful tongue without inflammation	• Treatment of underlying cause • Topical anesthetic mouthwash or systemic analgesics (aspirin and acetaminophen) for painful lesions • Good oral hygiene; regular dental checkups; vigorous chewing • Avoidance of hot, cold, or spicy foods, and alcohol.

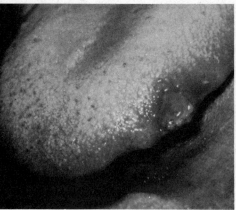

In aphthous stomatitis, numerous small round vesicles appear, soon breaking and leaving shallow ulcers with red areolae.

Signs and symptoms

Acute herpetic stomatitis begins suddenly with sore throat, malaise, lethargy, mouth pain, anorexia, irritability, and fever, with temperature as high as 104° F. (40° C.), which may persist for 1 to 2 weeks. Gums are swollen and bleed easily, and the mucous membrane is extremely tender. Papulovesicular ulcers appear in the mouth and throat, and eventually become punched-out lesions with reddened areolae. Submaxillary lymphadenitis is common. Pain usually disappears from 2 to 4 days before healing of ulcers is complete. If the child with stomatitis sucks his thumb, these lesions spread to the hand.

Aphthous stomatitis causes burning, tingling, and slight swelling of the mucous membrane. Single or multiple shallow ulcers with whitish centers and red borders appear and heal at one site but then appear at another.

Diagnosis

Diagnosis depends on physical examination and, in Vincent's angina, a smear of ulcer exudate allows identification of the causative organism.

Treatment and additional considerations

For acute herpetic stomatitis, treatment is conservative. For local symptoms, management includes warm-water mouth rinses (antiseptic mouthwashes are contraindicated because they are irritating) and a topical anesthetic to relieve mouth ulcer pain. Supplementary treatment includes bland or liquid diet and, in severe cases, I.V. fluids and bed rest.

For aphthous stomatitis, primary treatment involves application of a topical anesthetic. If anxiety is an obvious predisposing factor, tranquilizers may be appropriate. The patient should be warned to avoid foods that cause irritation.

Gastroesophageal Reflux

Gastroesophageal reflux is the backflow of gastric and/or duodenal contents into the esophagus, past the lower esophageal sphincter (LES), without associated belching or vomiting. Reflux may or may not cause symptoms or pathologic changes. Persistent reflux may cause reflux esophagitis (inflammation of the esophageal mucosa). Prognosis varies with the underlying cause.

Causes

The function of the LES—a high-pressure area in the lower esophagus, just above the stomach—is to prevent gastric contents from backing up into the esophagus. Normally, the LES creates pressure, closing the lower end of the esophagus, but relaxes after each swallow to allow food into the stomach. Reflux occurs when LES pressure is deficient or when pressure within the stomach exceeds LES pressure.

Studies have shown that a person with symptomatic reflux can't swallow often

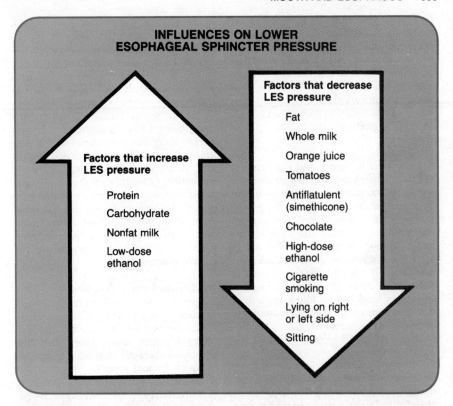

INFLUENCES ON LOWER ESOPHAGEAL SPHINCTER PRESSURE

Factors that increase LES pressure

Protein

Carbohydrate

Nonfat milk

Low-dose ethanol

Factors that decrease LES pressure

Fat

Whole milk

Orange juice

Tomatoes

Antiflatulent (simethicone)

Chocolate

High-dose ethanol

Cigarette smoking

Lying on right or left side

Sitting

enough to create sufficient peristaltic amplitude to clear gastric acid from the lower esophagus. This results in prolonged periods of acidity in the esophagus when reflux occurs.

Predisposing factors include:
• pyloric surgery (alteration or removal of the pylorus), which allows reflux of bile or pancreatic juice
• long-term nasogastric intubation (more than 4 or 5 days)
• any agent that lowers LES pressure, such as food, alcohol, cigarettes, anticholinergics (atropine, belladonna, propantheline), other drugs (morphine, diazepam, and meperidine)
• hiatal hernia (especially in children).
• any condition or position that increases intra-abdominal pressure.

Signs and symptoms
Gastroesophageal reflux doesn't always cause symptoms, and in patients showing clinical effects, physiologic reflux is not always confirmable. The most common feature of gastroesophageal reflux is heartburn, which may become more severe with vigorous exercise, bending, or lying down, and may be relieved by antacids or sitting upright. The pain of esophageal spasm resulting from reflux esophagitis tends to be chronic and may mimic angina pectoris, radiating to the neck, jaws, and arms. Other symptoms include: odynophagia, which may be followed by a dull substernal ache from severe, long-term reflux; dysphagia from esophageal spasm, stricture, or esophagitis; and bleeding (bright red or dark brown). Rarely, nocturnal regurgitation wakens the patient with coughing, choking, and a mouthful of saliva. Reflux may be associated with hiatal hernia. Direct hiatal hernia becomes clinically significant *only* when reflux is confirmed.

Pulmonary symptoms result from reflux of gastric contents into the throat and subsequent aspiration, and include nocturnal wheezing, bronchitis, asthma, morning hoarseness and cough, or chronic pulmonary disease. In children, other signs consist of failure to thrive and forceful vomiting from esophageal irritation. Such vomiting sometimes causes aspiration pneumonia.

Diagnosis

After a careful history and physical examination, tests to confirm gastroesophageal reflux include barium swallow fluoroscopy, esophageal pH probe, and manometric studies. In children, barium esophagography under fluoroscopic control can show reflux. Recurrent reflux after age 6 weeks is abnormal. An acid perfusion (Bernstein) test can show that reflux is the cause of symptoms. Finally, endoscopy and biopsy allow visualization and confirmation of any pathologic changes in the mucosa.

Treatment

Effective management relieves symptoms by reducing reflux through gravity, strengthening the LES with drug therapy, neutralizing gastric contents, and reducing intra-abdominal pressure. To reduce intra-abdominal pressure, the patient should sleep in a reverse Trendelenburg position (with the head of the bed elevated) and should avoid lying down after meals and late-night snacks. In uncomplicated cases, positional therapy is especially useful in infants and children. Antacids given 1 hour and 3 hours after meals, and at bedtime are effective for intermittent reflux. Hourly administration is necessary for intensive therapy. A nondiarrheal, nonmagnesium antacid (aluminum carbonate, aluminum hydroxide) may be preferred, depending on the patient's bowel status. A drug to increase LES pressure, bethanechol, stimulates smooth-muscle contraction and decreases esophageal acidity after meals (proven with pH probe). Metoclopramide and cimetidine have also been used with benefit. If possible, nasogastric intubation should not be continued for more than 4 or 5 days, because the tube interferes with sphincter integrity and itself allows reflux, especially when the patient lies flat.

Surgery may be necessary to control severe and refractory symptoms, such as pulmonary aspiration, hemorrhage, obstruction, severe pain, perforation, incompetent LES, or associated hiatal hernia. Surgical procedures that create an artificial closure at the gastroesophageal junction include Belsey Mark IV operation (invaginates the esophagus into the stomach) or Hill or Nissen procedure (creates a gastric wraparound with or without fixation). Also, vagotomy or pyloroplasty may be combined with an antireflux regimen to modify gastric contents.

Additional considerations

Supportive measures include:
• teaching the patient what causes reflux, how to avoid reflux with an antireflux regimen (medication, diet, and positional therapy), and what symptoms to watch for and report.
• instructing the patient to avoid any circumstance that increases intra-abdominal pressure (bending, coughing, vigorous exercise, tight clothing, constipation, and obesity) or any substance that reduces sphincter control (cigarettes, alcohol, fatty foods, and certain drugs).
• advising the patient to sit upright, particularly after meals, and to eat small, frequent meals. He must avoid highly seasoned food, acidic juices, alcoholic beverages, bedtime snacks, and foods high in fat or carbohydrates, which reduce LES pressure. He should eat meals at least 2 to 3 hours before lying down.
• telling the patient to take antacids, as ordered (usually 1 hour and 3 hours after meals and at bedtime).
• teaching correct preparation for diagnostic testing—for example, the patient should not eat for 6 to 8 hours before barium X-ray or endoscopy.
• carefully watching and recording chest tube drainage and respiratory status after surgery using a thoracic approach.

If needed, the patient should be given chest physiotherapy and oxygen. The patient with a nasogastric tube must be placed in semi-Fowler's position to help prevent reflux. He may need reassurance and emotional support.

Tracheoesophageal Fistula and Esophageal Atresia

Tracheoesophageal fistula is a developmental anomaly characterized by an abnormal connection between the trachea and the esophagus. It usually accompanies esophageal atresia, in which the esophagus is closed off at some point. Although these malformations have numerous anatomic variations, the most common, by far, is esophageal atresia with fistula to the distal segment.

These disorders, two of the most serious surgical emergencies in newborns, require immediate diagnosis and correction. They may coexist with other serious anomalies, such as congenital heart disease, imperforate anus, genitourinary abnormalities, and intestinal atresia. Esophageal atresia occurs in about 1 of every 4,000 live births; about one third of these infants are born prematurely.

Causes

Tracheoesophageal fistula and esophageal atresia result from failure of the embryonic esophagus and trachea to develop and separate correctly. The most common abnormality is type C tracheoesophageal fistula with esophageal atresia. In this type, the upper section of the esophagus terminates in a blind pouch, and the lower section ascends from the stomach and connects with the trachea by a short fistulous tract.

In type A atresia, both esophageal segments are blind pouches, and neither is connected to the airway. In type E (or H-type)—tracheoesophageal fistula without atresia—the fistula may occur anywhere between the level of the cricoid cartilage and the midesophagus but is usually higher in the trachea than in the esophagus. Such a fistula may be as small as a pinpoint. In types B and D, the upper portion of the esophagus opens into the trachea; infants with this anomaly may experience life-threatening aspiration of saliva or food.

Signs and symptoms

A newborn with type C tracheoesophageal fistula with esophageal atresia appears to swallow normally, but soon after swallowing coughs, struggles, becomes cyanotic, and stops breathing, as he aspirates fluids returning from the blind pouch of the esophagus through his nose and mouth. In such an infant, stomach distention may cause respiratory distress; air and gastric contents (bile and gastric secretions) may reflux through the fistula into the trachea, resulting in chemical pneumonitis.

An infant with type A esophageal atresia appears normal at birth. The infant swallows normally, but as secretions fill the esophageal sac and overflow into the oropharynx, he develops mucus in the oropharynx and drools excessively. When the infant is fed, regurgitation and respiratory distress follow aspiration. Suctioning the mucus and secretions temporarily relieves these symptoms. Excessive secretions and drooling in the newborn strongly suggest esophageal atresia.

Repeated episodes of pneumonitis, pulmonary infection, and abdominal distention may signal type E (or H-type) tracheoesophageal fistula. When a child with this disorder drinks, he coughs, chokes, and becomes cyanotic. Excessive mucus builds up in the oropharynx. Crying forces air from the trachea into

TYPES OF TRACHEOESOPHAGEAL ANOMALIES

Congenital malformations of the esophagus occur in about 1 in 4,000 live births. The American Academy of Pediatrics classification of the anatomic variations of tracheoesophageal anomalies is:

• **Type A** (7.7%): esophageal atresia without fistula

• **Type B** (0.8%): esophageal atresia with tracheoesophageal fistula to the proximal segment

• **Type C** (86.5%): esophageal atresia with fistula to the distal segment

• **Type D** (0.7%): esophageal atresia with fistula to both segments

• **Type E (or H-Type)** (4.2%): tracheoesophageal fistula without atresia

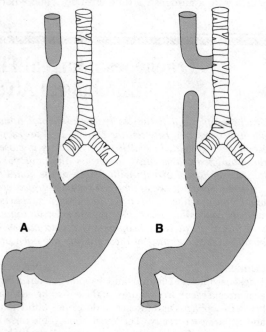

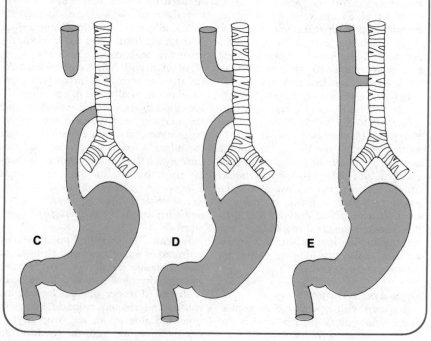

the esophagus, producing abdominal distention. Since such a child may appear normal at birth, this type of tracheoesophageal fistula may be overlooked, and diagnosis may be delayed as long as a year.

Both type B (proximal fistula) and type D (fistula to both segments) cause immediate aspiration of saliva into the airway, and bacterial pneumonitis.

Diagnosis

Respiratory distress and drooling in a newborn suggest tracheoesophageal fistula and esophageal atresia. The following procedures confirm it:

• *A size 10 or 12 French catheter passed through the nose* meets an obstruction (esophageal atresia) approximately 4" to 5" (10 to 13 cm) distal from the nostrils. Aspirate of gastric contents is less acidic than normal.

• *Chest X-ray* demonstrates the position of the catheter and can also show a dilated, air-filled upper esophageal pouch; pneumonia in the right upper lobe; or bilateral pneumonitis. Both pneumonia and pneumonitis suggest aspiration.

• *Abdominal X-ray* shows gas in the bowel in a distal fistula (type C) but none in a proximal fistula (type B) or in atresia without fistula (type A).

• *Cinefluorography* allows visualization on a fluoroscopic screen. After a size 10 or 12 French catheter is passed through the patient's nostril into the esophagus, a small amount of contrast medium is instilled to define the tip of the upper pouch and to differentiate between overflow aspiration from a blind end (atresia) and aspiration due to passage of liquids through a tracheoesophageal fistula.

Treatment

Tracheoesophageal fistula and esophageal atresia require surgical correction and are usually surgical emergencies. The type of surgical procedure and when it's performed depend on the nature of the anomaly, the patient's general condition, and the presence of coexisting congenital defects. For example, in a premature infant, a poor surgical risk, correction of combined tracheoesophageal fistula and esophageal atresia is done in two stages: first, gastrostomy (for gastric decompression, prevention of reflux, and feeding) and closure of the fistula; then 1 to 2 months later, anastomosis of the esophagus.

Both before and after surgery, positioning varies with the doctor's philosophy and the child's anatomy; the child may be placed supine, with his head low to facilitate drainage, or with his head elevated to prevent aspiration.

The child should receive I.V. fluids, as necessary, and appropriate antibiotics for superimposed infection.

Postoperative complications after correction of tracheoesophageal fistula include recurrent fistulas, esophageal motility dysfunction, esophageal stricture, recurrent bronchitis, pneumothorax, and failure to thrive. Esophageal motility dysfunction or hiatal hernia may develop after surgical correction of esophageal atresia.

Correction of esophageal atresia alone requires anastomosis of the proximal and distal esophageal segments in one or two stages. End-to-end anastomosis often produces postoperative stricture; end-to-side anastomosis is less likely to do so. If the esophageal ends are widely separated, treatment may include a colonic interposition (grafting a piece of the colon) or elongation of the proximal segment of the esophagus by bougienage. About 10 days after surgery, and again 1 month and 3 months later, X-rays are required to evaluate the effectiveness of surgical repair.

Postoperative treatment includes placement of a suction catheter in the upper esophageal pouch to control secretions and prevent aspiration; maintaining the infant in an upright position to avoid reflux of gastric juices into the trachea; I.V. fluids and nothing by mouth; gastrostomy to prevent reflux and allow feeding; and appropriate antibiotics for pneumonia.

Postoperative complications may include impaired esophageal motility (in one third of patients), hiatal hernia, and reflux esophagitis.

Additional considerations
Bedside care includes:
* monitoring respiratory status; administering oxygen, performing pulmonary physiotherapy and suctioning, as needed, and providing a humid environment.
* administering antibiotics and parenteral fluids, as ordered, and keeping accurate intake and output records.
* checking chest tubes, if appropriate, for patency; maintaining proper suction, measuring and marking drainage periodically, and milking tubing, as necessary.
* observing carefully for signs of complications, such as abnormal esophageal motility, recurrent fistulas, pneumothorax, and esophageal stricture.
* maintaining gastrostomy tube feed-

ings, as ordered. Such feedings initially consist of dextrose and water (not more than 5% solution); later, a proprietary formula (first diluted and then full strength) is added. If the infant develops gastric atony, an iso-osmolar formula is used. Oral feedings can usually resume 8 to 10 days postoperatively. If gastrostomy feedings and oral feedings are impossible due to decreased intestinal motility or intolerance to them, the infant requires total parenteral nutrition.
* giving the infant a pacifier to satisfy his sucking needs but *only* when he can safely handle secretions, since sucking stimulates secretion of saliva.
* offering the parents support and guidance in dealing with their infant's acute illness; encouraging them to participate in the infant's care, and to hold and touch him as much as possible to facilitate bonding.

Corrosive Esophagitis and Stricture

Corrosive esophagitis is inflammation and damage to the esophagus after ingestion of a harmful chemical. Similar to a burn, this injury may be temporary or may lead to permanent stricture (narrowing or stenosis) of the esophagus that is correctable only through surgery. Severe burns can quickly lead to esophageal perforation, mediastinitis, and death from infection, shock, and massive hemorrhage (due to aortic perforation).

Causes
The most common chemical injury to the esophagus follows the ingestion of lye or other strong alkalies; less often, the ingestion of strong acids. The type and amount of chemical ingested determine the severity and location of the damage. In children, household chemical ingestion is accidental; in adults, it's usually a suicide attempt or gesture. The chemical may damage only the mucosa or submucosa, or may damage all layers of the esophagus.

Esophageal tissue damage occurs in three phases: the acute phase, edema and hyperemia; latent phase, ulceration, exudation, and tissue sloughing; and chronic phase, diffuse scarring.

Signs and symptoms
Shortly after ingestion, the victim develops intense pain in the mouth and anterior chest, marked salivation, inability to swallow, and tachypnea. Bloody vomitus containing pieces of esophageal tissue signals severe damage. Signs of esophageal perforation and mediastinitis, especially crepitation, indicate destruction of the entire esophagus. Inability to speak implies laryngeal damage.

The acute phase subsides in 3 to 4 days, enabling the patient to eat again. Fever suggests secondary infection. Symptoms of dysphagia return if stricture develops, usually within weeks; rarely, stricture is delayed and develops several years after the injury.

Diagnosis

A history of chemical ingestion and physical examination revealing oropharyngeal burns (including white membranes and edema of the soft palate and uvula) usually confirm the diagnosis. The type and amount of the chemical ingested must be identified; this may sometimes be done by examining empty containers of the ingested material.

The following two procedures are helpful in evaluating the severity of the injury.

• *Endoscopy* (in the first 24 hours after ingestion) delineates the extent of the esophageal injury and assesses depth of the burn. This procedure may also be performed a week after ingestion to assess stricture development.

• *Barium swallow* (1 week after ingestion and every 3 weeks thereafter) may identify segmental spasm but doesn't always show mucosal injury.

Treatment

Conservative treatment for corrosive esophagitis and stricture includes monitoring the victim's condition; administering corticosteroids, such as prednisone and hydrocortisone, to control inflammation and inhibit fibrosis; and administering a broad-spectrum antibiotic, such as ampicillin, to protect the corticosteroid-immunosuppressed patient against infection by his own mouth flora.

Aggressive treatment includes administering corticosteroids and antibiotics, and performing endoscopy early. It may also include bougienage. This procedure involves passing a slender, flexible, cylindrical instrument called a bougie into the esophagus to dilate it and minimize stricture. Some doctors begin bougienage immediately and continue it regularly to maintain a patent lumen and prevent stricture; others delay it for a week to avoid the risk of esophageal perforation.

Surgery is necessary immediately for esophageal perforation, or later to correct stricture untreatable with bougienage. Corrective surgery may involve transplanting a piece of the colon to the damaged esophagus. However, even after surgery, stricture may recur at the site of the anastomosis.

Supportive treatment includes I.V. therapy to replace fluids or total parenteral nutrition while the patient can't swallow, gradually progressing to clear liquids and a soft diet.

Additional considerations

The quality of emergency care given by the first health care professional to see the patient who has ingested a corrosive chemical is critical.

At this time, the health care professional *should not*:

• *induce vomiting,* as this will burn the esophagus and oropharynx a second time.

• *perform gastric lavage,* as the corrosive chemical may cause further damage to the mucous membrane of the gastrointestinal lining.

Health care support for the patient will include:

• providing vigorous support of vital functions, as needed, such as oxygen, mechanical ventilation, I.V. fluids, and treatment for shock depending on severity of injury.

• carefully observing and recording intake and output.

• explaining the procedures before X-rays and endoscopy to the patient to lessen anxiety during the tests and to obtain cooperation.

• encouraging and assisting an adult patient and his family to seek psychologic counseling, since the adult who has ingested a corrosive agent has usually done so with suicidal intent.

• providing emotional support for parents whose child has ingested a chemical. They'll be distraught and may feel guilty about the accident. After the emergency and without emphasizing blame, they should be taught appropriate preventive measures, such as locking accessible cabinets and keeping all corrosive agents out of a child's reach.

Mallory-Weiss Syndrome

The Mallory-Weiss syndrome is mild to massive and usually painless bleeding due to a tear in the mucosa or submucosa of the cardia or lower esophagus. Such a tear, usually singular and longitudinal, results from prolonged or forceful vomiting. Sixty percent of these tears involve the cardia; 15%, the terminal esophagus; and 25%, the region across the esophagogastric junction. Mallory-Weiss syndrome is most common in men over age 40, especially alcoholics.

Causes

The direct cause of a tear in Mallory-Weiss syndrome is forceful or prolonged vomiting, probably when the upper esophageal sphincter fails to relax during vomiting; this lack of sphincter coordination seems more common after excessive intake of alcohol. Other factors and conditions that may also increase intra-abdominal pressure and predispose to esophageal tearing include coughing, straining during bowel movements, trauma, convulsions, childbirth, hiatal hernia, esophagitis, gastritis, and atrophic gastric mucosa.

Signs and symptoms

Typically, Mallory-Weiss syndrome begins with vomiting of blood or passing large amounts of blood rectally a few hours to several days after normal vomiting. This bleeding, which may be accompanied by epigastric or back pain, may range from mild to massive but is generally more profuse than in esophageal rupture. In Mallory-Weiss syndrome, the blood vessels are only partially severed, preventing retraction and closure of the lumen. Massive bleeding—most likely when the tear is on the gastric side, near the cardia—may quickly lead to fatal shock.

Diagnosis

 Identifying esophageal tears by fiberoptic endoscopy confirms Mallory-Weiss syndrome. These lesions, which usually occur near the gastroesophageal junction, appear as erythematous longitudinal cracks in the mucosa when recently produced and as raised, white streaks surrounded by erythema in older tears. Other helpful diagnostic measures include the following:

• *Angiography* (selective celiac arteriography) can determine the bleeding site but not the cause; this is used when endoscopy is not available
• *Gastrotomy* may be performed at the time of surgery.
• *Hematocrit* helps quantify blood loss.

Treatment

Treatment varies with the severity of bleeding. Usually, gastrointestinal bleeding stops spontaneously, and requires supportive measures and careful observation but no definitive treatment. However, if bleeding continues, treatment may include:

• angiography, with infusion of a vasoconstrictor (vasopressin) into the superior mesenteric artery or direct infusion into a vessel that leads to the bleeding artery.
• transcatheter embolization or thrombus formation with an autologous blood clot or other hemostatic material (insertion of artificial material, such as shredded absorbable gelatin sponge, or, less often, the patient's own clotted blood through a catheter into the bleeding vessel to aid thrombus formation).
• surgery to suture each laceration (for massive recurrent or uncontrollable bleeding).

Additional considerations

When treating a patient with Mallory-Weiss syndrome, the hospital staff member should:

• evaluate respiratory status, monitor arterial blood gas measurements, and administer oxygen, as necessary.

• assess the amount of blood loss, and record related symptoms, such as hematemesis and melena (including color, amount, consistency, and frequency); monitor hematologic status (hemoglobin, hematocrit, RBC); draw blood for coagulation studies (prothrombin time, partial thromboplastin time, and platelet count), and type and crossmatch (3 units of matched whole blood should be kept on hand at all times); insert a large-bore (14 to 18 gauge) I.V. line and start a temporary infusion of normal saline solution until blood is available.

• monitor vital signs, central venous pressure, urinary output, and overall clinical status.

• insert a large-bore nasogastric tube to detect fresh bleeding.

• explain diagnostic procedures carefully to facilitate cooperation and promote psychologic well-being.

• obtain a history of recent medications taken, dietary habits, and use of alcohol; avoid giving medications that may cause nausea or vomiting; administer antiemetics to prevent postoperative retching and vomiting.

• reassure the patient.

• advise the patient to avoid alcohol, aspirin, and other irritating substances.

Esophageal Diverticula

Esophageal diverticula are hollow outpouchings of one or more layers of the esophageal wall. They occur in three main areas: just above the upper esophageal sphincter (Zenker's, or pulsion, diverticulum, the most common type), near the midpoint of the esophagus (traction), and just above the lower esophageal sphincter (epiphrenic). Generally, esophageal diverticula occur later in life—although they can affect infants and children—and are three times more common in men than in women. Epiphrenic diverticula usually occur in middle-aged men; Zenker's, in men over age 60.

Causes

Esophageal diverticula are due either to primary muscular abnormalities that may be congenital or to inflammatory processes adjacent to the esophagus. Zenker's diverticulum occurs when the pouch results from increased intraesophageal pressure; traction diverticulum, when the pouch is pulled out by adjacent inflamed tissue. However, many authorities classify all diverticula as traction diverticula.

Zenker's diverticulum results from developmental muscular weakness of the posterior pharynx above the border of the cricopharyngeal muscle. The pressure of swallowing aggravates this weakness, as does contraction of the pharynx before relaxation of the sphincter. A midesophageal (traction) diverticulum is a response to scarring and pulling on esophageal walls by an ex-

ternal inflammatory process, such as tuberculosis. An epiphrenic diverticulum (rare) is generally right-sided and usually accompanies an esophageal motor disturbance, such as esophageal spasm or achalasia. It's thought to be caused by traction and pulsation.

Signs and symptoms

Both midesophageal and epiphrenic diverticula with an associated motor disturbance (achalasia or spasm) seldom produce symptoms but may cause dysphagia and heartburn. However, Zenker's diverticulum produces distinctly staged symptoms: initially, throat irritation and, later, dysphagia and near-complete obstruction. In early stages, regurgitation occurs soon after eating; in later stages (as the diverticulum enlarges), regurgitation after eating is delayed and may even occur during sleep, leading to food aspiration and pulmonary infection. Other symptoms include noise when liquids are swallowed, chronic cough, hoarseness, a bad taste in the mouth or foul breath, and rarely, bleeding.

Diagnosis

 X-rays taken following a barium swallow usually confirm diagnosis by showing characteristic outpouching. Esophagoscopy can rule out another lesion; however, the procedure risks rupturing the diverticulum by passing the scope into it rather than into the lumen of the esophagus, a special danger with Zenker's diverticulum.

Treatment

Treatment of Zenker's diverticulum is usually palliative, and includes a bland diet, thorough chewing, and drinking water after eating to flush out the sac. However, severe symptoms or a large diverticulum necessitates surgical removal of the sac. An esophagomyotomy may be necessary to prevent recurrence.

A midesophageal diverticulum seldom requires therapy except when coexistent esophagitis aggravates the risk of rupture. Then, treatment includes antacids and an antireflux regimen: keeping the head elevated, maintaining an upright position for 2 hours after eating, eating small meals, controlling chronic coughing, and avoiding tight clothing.

Epiphrenic diverticulum requires treatment of accompanying motor disorders, such as achalasia, by repeated dilations of the esophagus; of acute spasm by anticholinergic administration and diverticulum excision; of dysphagia or severe pain by surgical excision or suspending the diverticulum to promote drainage. Depending on the patient's nutritional status, treatment may also include insertion of a nasogastric tube (passed carefully to prevent perforation) and tube feedings to prepare for the stress of surgery.

Additional considerations

The patient should understand the causes and treatment of this disorder, and also any diagnostic procedures which will be used.

The patient should be carefully observed and his symptoms documented. Also, his nutritional status (weight, caloric intake, appearance) must be regularly and carefully assessed.

If the patient regurgitates food and mucus, he can protect against aspiration by careful positioning (head elevated or turned to one side). To prevent aspiration, he should empty any visible outpouching in the neck by massage or postural drainage before retiring.

If the patient has dysphagia, he must be given only the foods he can tolerate. The circumstances that ease swallowing should also be determined. He should eat a blenderized diet, with vitamin or protein supplements, chewing thoroughly.

Hiatal Hernia
(Hiatus hernia)

Hiatal hernia is a defect in the diaphragm that permits a portion of the stomach to pass through the diaphragmatic opening into the chest. Three types of hiatal hernia can occur: direct (or "sliding") hernia, paraesophageal (or "rolling") hernia, or mixed hernias, which include features of both. In direct hernia, both the stomach and the gastroesophageal junction slip up into the chest, so the gastroesophageal junction is above the diaphragmatic hiatus. In paraesophageal hernia, a part of the greater curvature of the stomach rolls through the diaphragmatic defect. Treatment can prevent complications, such as strangulation of the herniated intrathoracic portion of the stomach.

Causes and incidence

Direct hernia is three to ten times more common than paraesophageal and mixed hernias combined. The incidence of hiatal hernia increases with age, and prevalence is higher in women than in men (especially the paraesophageal type).

Usually, hiatal hernia results from muscle weakening that's common with aging and may be secondary to esophageal carcinoma, kyphoscoliosis, trauma, or certain surgical procedures. It may also result from certain diaphragmatic malformations that may cause congenital weakness.

In hiatal hernia, the muscular collar around the esophageal and diaphragmatic junction loosens, permitting the lower portion of the esophagus and the stomach to rise into the chest when intra-abdominal pressure increases (possibly causing gastroesophageal reflux). Such increased intra-abdominal pressure may result from ascites, pregnancy, obesity, constrictive clothing, bending, straining, coughing, Valsalva's maneuver, or extreme physical exertion.

Signs and symptoms

Typically, a paraesophageal hernia produces no symptoms; it's usually an incidental finding on barium swallow. Since this type of hernia leaves the closing mechanism of the cardiac sphincter unchanged, it rarely causes acid reflux and reflux esophagitis. Symptoms result from displacement or stretching of the stomach and may include a feeling of fullness in the chest or pain resembling angina pectoris. Even if it produces no symptoms, this type of hernia needs surgical treatment because of the high risk of strangulation.

A direct hernia without an incompetent sphincter produces no reflux or symptoms and, consequently, doesn't require treatment. When direct hernia causes symptoms, they are typical of gastric reflux, resulting from the incompetent lower esophageal sphincter, and may include the following:

• *Pyrosis* (heartburn) occurs from 1 to 4 hours after eating and is aggravated

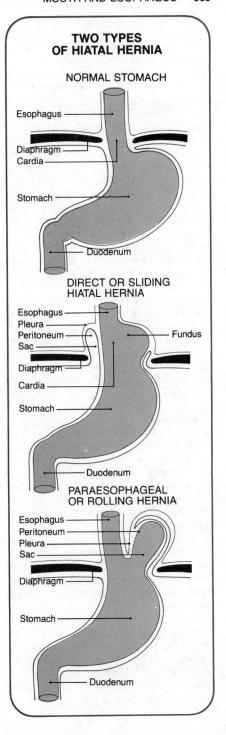

TWO TYPES OF HIATAL HERNIA

NORMAL STOMACH

Esophagus
Diaphragm
Cardia
Stomach
Duodenum

DIRECT OR SLIDING HIATAL HERNIA

Esophagus
Pleura
Peritoneum
Sac
Diaphragm
Cardia
Stomach
Fundus
Duodenum

PARAESOPHAGEAL OR ROLLING HERNIA

Esophagus
Peritoneum
Pleura
Sac
Diaphragm
Stomach
Duodenum

by reclining, belching, and increased intra-abdominal pressure. It may be accompanied by regurgitation or vomiting.

• *Retrosternal or substernal chest pain* results from reflux of gastric contents, distention of the stomach, and spasm or altered motor activity. Chest pain occurs most often after meals or at bedtime and is aggravated by reclining, belching, and increased intra-abdominal pressure.

Other common symptoms reflect possible complications:

• *Dysphagia* occurs when the hernia produces esophagitis, esophageal ulceration, or stricture, especially with ingestion of very hot or cold foods, alcoholic beverages, or a large amount of food.

• *Bleeding* may be mild or massive, frank or occult; the source may be esophagitis or erosions of the gastric pouch.

• *Severe pain and shock result from incarceration,* in which a large portion of the stomach is caught above the diaphragm (usually occurs with paraesophageal hernia). Incarceration may lead to perforation of gastric ulcer, and strangulation and gangrene of the herniated portion of the stomach. It requires immediate surgery.

Diagnosis

Diagnosis of hiatal hernia is based on typical clinical features and on the results of the following laboratory studies and procedures:

• *Chest X-ray* occasionally shows air shadow behind the heart with large hernia; infiltrates in lower lobes if patient has aspirated.

• In *barium study,* hernia may appear as an outpouching containing barium at the lower end of the esophagus. (Small hernias are difficult to recognize.) This study also shows diaphragmatic abnormalities.

• *Endoscopy and biopsy* differentiate between hiatal hernia, varices, and other small gastroesophageal lesions; identify the mucosal junction and the edge of the diaphragm indenting the esophagus; and can rule out malignancy that otherwise may be difficult to detect.

• *Esophageal motility studies* assess the presence of esophageal motor abnormalities before surgical repair of the hernia.

• *pH studies* assess for reflux of gastric contents.

• *Acid perfusion (Bernstein) test* indicates that heartburn results from esophageal reflux when perfusion of HCl through the nasogastric tube provokes this symptom.

Laboratory tests may indicate gastrointestinal bleeding as a complication of hiatal hernia:

• *CBC* may show hypochromic microcytic anemia when bleeding from esophageal ulceration occurs.

• *Stool guaiac test* may be positive.

• *Analysis of gastric contents* may reveal blood.

Treatment

The primary goals of treatment are to relieve symptoms by minimizing or correcting the incompetent cardia and to manage and prevent complications. Medical therapy is used first, because symptoms usually respond to it and because hiatal hernia tends to recur after surgery. Such therapy attempts to modify or reduce reflux by changing the quantity or quality of refluxed gastric contents; by strengthening the lower esophageal sphincter muscle pharmacologically; or by decreasing the amount of reflux through gravity. Such measures include restricting any activity that increases intra-abdominal pressure (coughing, straining, bending), giving antiemetics and cough suppressants, avoiding constrictive clothing, modifying diet, giving stool softeners or laxatives to prevent straining at stool, and discouraging smoking, because it stimulates gastric acid production. Modifying the diet means eating small, frequent, bland meals at least 2 hours before lying down (no bedtime snack); eating slowly; and avoiding spicy foods, fruit juices, alcoholic beverages, and coffee. Antacids also modify the fluid refluxed into the esophagus and are probably the best treatment for intermittent reflux. Intensive antacid therapy may call for hourly administration; however, the choice of antacid should take into consideration the patient's bowel function.

To reduce the amount of reflux, the overweight patient should lose weight to decrease intra-abdominal pressure. Elevating the head of the bed approximately 6″ (15 cm) reduces gastric reflux by using gravity.

Drug therapy to strengthen cardiac sphincter tone may include a cholinergic agent, such as bethanechol. Metoclopramide has also been used to stimulate smooth-muscle contraction, increase cardiac sphincter tone, and decrease reflux after eating.

Failure to control symptoms by medical means, or onset of complications, such as stricture, significant bleeding, pulmonary aspiration, strangulation or incarceration, necessitates surgical repair. Techniques for such repair vary greatly, but most create an artificial closing mechanism at the gastroesophageal junction to strengthen the lower esophageal sphincter's barrier function. The surgeon may use an abdominal or a thoracic approach.

Additional considerations
The health care professional caring for the patient with hiatal hernia should:
• teach the patient about the disorder, treatment, and diagnostic measures to enhance compliance.
• prepare the patient for diagnostic tests, as needed. After endoscopy, the professional must watch for signs of perforation (falling blood pressure, rapid pulse, shock, sudden pain).
• if surgery is scheduled, reinforce the explanation of the surgical technique and what the patient can expect. The patient probably won't be allowed to eat or drink and will have a nasogastric tube in place, with low suction, for 2 to 3 days postoperatively.
• carefully record intake and output after surgery, including nasogastric or wound drainage.
• provide meticulous mouth and nose care while the nasogastric tube is in place. Ice chips can be given to the patient to moisten oral mucous membranes; this ice must be included in his intake and output record.
• carefully observe chest tube drainage and respiratory status, if appropriate, and perform diligent pulmonary physiotherapy.
• before discharge, tell the patient what foods he can eat (he may require a bland diet), and recommend small, frequent meals. He should not perform activities that cause increased intra-abdominal pressure. A slow return to normal functions is urged. He'll probably be able to resume regular activity in 6 to 8 weeks.

STOMACH, INTESTINE & PANCREAS

Gastritis

Gastritis, an inflammation of the gastric mucosa, may be acute or chronic. Acute gastritis, the most common stomach disorder, produces mucosal reddening, edema, hemorrhage, and erosion. Gastritis is common in persons with pernicious anemia (as chronic atrophic gastritis). Although gastritis can occur at any age, it is more prevalent in the elderly.

Causes
Acute gastritis usually results from chronic ingestion of irritating foods, such as hot peppers (or an allergic reaction to them); alcoholic beverages; drugs, such as aspirin; or poisons, especially DDT, ammonia, mercury, and carbon tetrachloride. It can be part of hepatic

disorders, such as portal hypertension; GI disorders, such as sprue; or infectious diseases, such as viruses, influenza, and typhoid fever. Other causes include Curling's ulcer (after a burn), Cushing's ulcer (from a CNS disorder), and gastrointestinal injury that may be thermal (ingestion of hot fluids) or mechanical (swallowing a foreign object).

Corrosive gastritis results from the ingestion of strong acids or alkalies. Acute phlegmonous gastritis results from a rare bacterial (usually streptococcal) infection of the stomach wall.

Signs and symptoms

Typical clinical features of acute gastritis are GI bleeding (most common) and mild epigastric discomfort, such as post-prandial distress. Sometimes epigastric discomfort is the only symptom. Other possible signs of gastritis include upper abdominal pain, belching, fever, malaise, nausea, and vomiting (frank hematemesis may occur). Abdominal tenderness is rare.

Diagnosis

Patient history suggesting exposure to a GI irritant in a person with epigastric discomfort, or other GI symptoms (particularly bleeding) suggest gastritis. A gastroscopy (often with biopsy) confirms it, when done before lesions heal (usually within 24 hours). However, gastroscopy is contraindicated after ingestion of a corrosive agent. X-rays rule out other diseases.

Treatment

Symptoms are usually relieved by eliminating the gastric irritant or other cause. For instance, the treatment for corrosive gastritis is neutralization with the appropriate antidote (emetics are contraindicated). Treatment for gastritis caused by other poisons includes emetics. Anticholinergics, such as methantheline bromide, and antacids relieve GI distress. When gastritis causes massive bleeding, treatment includes blood replacement; iced saline lavage, possibly with norepinephrine; angiography, with catheter in left gastric artery through which vasopressin is infused in normal saline solution; and surgery. Treatment for bacterial gastritis includes antibiotics, bland diet, and an antiemetic. Treatment for acute phlegmonous gastritis is vigorous antibiotic therapy, followed by surgical repair.

Additional considerations

When caring for the patient with gastritis, the health care professional should:
- give antacids, anticholinergics, and antibiotics, as ordered.
- explain all diagnostic procedures.
- give antiemetics if the patient is vomiting and, as ordered, replace I.V. fluids; monitor fluid intake and output, and

---

CHRONIC GASTRITIS

Chronic gastritis results from recurring ingestion of an irritating substance or from pernicious anemia. The main types of chronic gastritis are fundal gland gastritis and chronic antral gastritis (pyloric gland gastritis). Fundal gland gastritis includes:
- superficial gastritis—reddened edematous mucosa, with hemorrhages and small erosions
- atrophic gastritis—inflammation in all stomach layers, with decreased number of parietal and chief cells
- gastric atrophy—dull and nodular mucosa, with irregular, thickened, or nodular rugae.

Many patients with chronic gastritis, particularly those with chronic antral gastritis, have no symptoms. When symptoms develop, they are typically indistinct and may include loss of appetite, feeling of fullness, belching, vague epigastric pain, nausea, and vomiting. Diagnosis requires biopsy.

Usually no treatment is necessary, except for avoiding aspirin and spicy or irritating foods, and taking antacids if symptoms persist. If pernicious anemia is the underlying cause, then vitamin B_{12} should be administered. Chronic gastritis often progresses to acute gastritis.

watch electrolyte balance.
• watch for signs of GI bleeding (hematemesis, drop in hematocrit, bloody nasogastric drainage, melena) or hemorrhagic shock (hypotension, tachycardia, or restlessness); in corrosive gastritis, watch for signs of obstruction, perforation, or peritonitis, such as nausea, diarrhea, abdominal pain, or fever.
• urge the patient to seek immediate attention for recurring symptoms (hematemesis, nausea, or vomiting).
• stress the importance of taking prescribed prophylactic medication as ordered to prevent recurrence of gastritis.
• advise patients to prevent gastric irritation by taking steroids with milk, food, or antacids; by taking antacids between meals and at bedtime; by avoiding aspirin-containing compounds, spicy foods, hot fluids, alcohol, caffeine, and tobacco.

Gastroenteritis
(Intestinal flu, traveler's diarrhea, viral enteritis, food poisoning)

A self-limiting disorder, gastroenteritis is characterized by diarrhea, nausea, vomiting, and abdominal cramping. It occurs in persons of all ages and is a major cause of morbidity and mortality in underdeveloped nations. In the United States, gastroenteritis ranks second to the common cold as a cause of lost work time, and fifth as the cause of death among young children. It also can be life-threatening in the elderly and the debilitated.

Causes
Gastroenteritis has many possible causes:
• bacteria (responsible for acute food poisoning): *Staphylococcus aureus, Salmonella, Shigella, Clostridium botulinum, Escherichia coli, Clostridium perfringens*
• amebae: especially *Entamoeba histolytica*
• parasites: *Ascaris, Enterobius,* and *Trichinella spiralis*
• viruses (may be responsible for traveler's diarrhea): adeno-, echo-, or coxsackieviruses
• ingestion of toxins: plants or toadstools
• drug reactions: antibiotics
• enzyme deficiencies
• food allergens.
The bowel reacts to any of these enterotoxins with hypermotility, producing severe diarrhea and secondary depletion of intracellular fluid.

Signs and symptoms
Clinical manifestations vary depending on the pathologic organism and on the level of GI tract involved. However, gastroenteritis in adults is usually a self-limiting, nonfatal disease producing diarrhea, abdominal discomfort (ranging from cramping to pain), nausea, and vomiting. Other possible symptoms include fever, malaise, and borborygmi. In children, the elderly, and the debilitated, gastroenteritis produces the same symptoms, but these patients' intolerance to electrolyte and fluid losses leads to a higher mortality.

Diagnosis
Patient history can aid diagnosis of gastroenteritis. Stool culture (by direct rectal swab) or blood culture identifies causative bacteria or parasites.

Treatment
Treatment is usually supportive and consists of bed rest, nutritional support, and increased fluid intake. When gastroenteritis is severe or affects a young child or an elderly or debilitated person, treatment may necessitate hospitalization; specific antimicrobials; I.V. fluid and

electrolyte replacement; antidiarrheals, such as a diphenoxylate compound; and antiemetics (P.O., I.M., or rectal suppository), such as prochlorperazine or trimethobenzamide.

Additional considerations

When caring for patients with gastroenteritis, the health care professional should:
• administer medications, as ordered; correlate dosages, routes, and times appropriately with the patient's meals and activities (for example, give antiemetics 30 to 60 minutes before meals).
• replace lost fluids and electrolytes, if the patient can eat, with broth, ginger ale, and lemonade, as tolerated; vary the diet to make it more enjoyable, and allow some choice of foods; warn the patient to avoid milk and milk products, which may provoke recurrence.
• record intake and output carefully; watch for signs of dehydration, such as dry skin and mucous membranes, fever, and sunken eyes.
• wash hands thoroughly after giving care to avoid spreading infection.
• provide warm sitz baths or apply witch hazel compresses, to ease anal irritation.
• contact public health authorities, if food poisoning is probable, so they can interview patients and food handlers, and take samples of the suspected contaminated food.

Gastroenteritis patients must learn to thoroughly cook foods, especially pork; to refrigerate perishable foods, such as milk, mayonnaise, potato salad, and cream-filled pastry; to always wash hands with warm water and soap before handling food, especially after using the bathroom; to clean utensils thoroughly; to avoid drinking water or eating raw fruit or vegetables when visiting a foreign country; to eliminate flies and roaches in the home.

Peptic Ulcers

Peptic ulcers—circumscribed lesions in the gastric mucosal membrane—can develop in the lower esophagus, stomach, pylorus, duodenum, or jejunum from contact with gastric juice (especially hydrochloric acid and pepsin). About 80% of all peptic ulcers are duodenal ulcers, which affect the proximal part of the small intestine and occur most often in men between ages 20 and 50. Gastric ulcers, which affect the stomach mucosa, are most common in both middle-aged and elderly men, especially among the poor and undernourished, and chronic users of aspirin or alcohol. Benign gastric ulcers tend to recur. Duodenal ulcers often follow a chronic course, with remissions and exacerbations; 5% to 10% of patients develop complications that necessitate surgery.

Causes

Decreased mucosal resistance, inadequate mucosal blood flow, and defective mucus have all been associated with the development of peptic ulcers, but a precise cause has not been determined. Psychogenic factors may stimulate long-term overproduction of gastric secretions that can erode the stomach, duodenum, or esophagus. Normally, tightly packed epithelial cells protect the stomach against irritation. Back diffusion of acid through mucosa damaged by chronic gastritis or irritants, such as aspirin or alcohol, is a likely cause of gastric ulcers. In the elderly, the pylorus begins to wear down, permitting the reflux of bile into the stomach, a common cause of gastric ulcers in this age-group. For unknown reasons, these ulcers often strike people with type A blood and may become malignant more often than duodenal ulcers.

Acid hypersecretion, possibly caused by an overactive vagus nerve, contributes to the formation of duodenal ulcers.

These ulcers tend to afflict people with type O blood, perhaps because such people don't secrete blood group antigens (mucopolysaccharides, which may serve to protect the mucosa) in their saliva and other body fluids. Duodenal ulcers may persist for life; when they do heal, they usually leave scars that can later break down and ulcerate again under hyperacidic conditions.

Signs and symptoms

Heartburn and indigestion usually signal the start of a gastric ulcer attack. Eating a large meal stretches the gastric wall, causing pain in the left epigastrium and a feeling of fullness and distention. Other typical effects include weight loss and repeated episodes of massive GI bleeding.

Duodenal ulcers produce heartburn, well-localized midepigastric pain (relieved by food), weight gain (since the patient eats to relieve discomfort), and a peculiar sensation of hot water bubbling in the back of the throat. Attacks usually occur about 2 hours after meals, whenever the stomach is empty, or after consumption of orange juice, coffee, aspirin, or alcohol. Exacerbations tend to recur several times a year, then fade into remission. Vomiting and other digestive disturbances are rare.

Both kinds of ulcers may be asymptomatic or may penetrate the pancreas and cause severe back pain. Other complications of peptic ulcers include perforation, hemorrhage, and pyloric obstruction.

Diagnosis

Upper GI tract X-rays show abnormalities in mucosa; gastric secretory studies show hyperchlorhydria.

 The presence of an ulcer is confirmed by upper GI endoscopy or esophagogastroduodenoscopy. Biopsy rules out malignancy. Stools may test positive for occult blood.

Treatment

Treatment is essentially symptomatic and emphasizes drug therapy and rest:

• antacids to reduce gastric acidity.

• cimetidine, a histamine receptor antagonist, to reduce gastric secretion; for short-term therapy (up to 8 weeks).

• anticholinergics, such as propantheline, to inhibit the vagus nerve effect on the parietal cells, and reduce gastrin production and excessive gastric activity in *duodenal ulcers;* these drugs are usually contraindicated in gastric ulcers, since they prolong gastric emptying and can aggravate the ulcer.

• physical rest and, for gastric ulcers only, sedatives and tranquilizers, such as chlordiazepoxide and phenobarbital.

If GI bleeding occurs, emergency treatment begins with passage of a nasogastric tube to allow for iced saline lavage, possibly containing norepinephrine. Angiography facilitates placement of an intra-arterial catheter, followed by infusion of vasopressin to constrict blood vessels and control bleeding. This allows postponement of surgery until the patient's condition stabilizes. Surgery is indicated for perforation, unresponsiveness to conservative treatment, and suspected malignancy. Surgical procedures for peptic ulcers include:

• *vagotomy and pyloroplasty:* severing one or more branches of the vagus nerve to reduce hydrochloric acid secretion, and refashioning the pylorus to create a larger lumen and facilitate gastric emptying

• *distal subtotal gastrectomy* (with or without vagotomy): excising the antrum of the stomach, thereby removing the hormonal stimulus of the parietal cells, followed by anastomosis of the rest of the stomach to the duodenum or the jejunum.

Additional considerations

Management of peptic ulcers requires careful administration of medications, thorough patient teaching, and skillful postoperative care. The hospital staff member should:

• administer medications, as ordered, and watch for cimetidine and anticholinergic side effects—dizziness, rash,

mild diarrhea, muscle pain, leukopenia, and gynecomastia for cimetidine, and dry mouth, blurred vision, headache, constipation, and urinary retention for anticholinergics (which are usually most effective when given 30 minutes prior to meals).
• instruct the patient to take antacids 1 hour after meals; advise the patient with a history of cardiac disease or on a sodium-restricted diet to take only low-sodium antacids; warn that antacids may cause changes in bowel habits (diarrhea with magnesium-containing antacids, constipation with aluminum-containing antacids).
• warn the patient about taking aspirin-containing drugs, reserpine, indomethacin, and phenylbutazone, because they irritate the gastric mucosa; tell the patient to avoid excessive use of coffee, stressful situations, and alcoholic beverages during exacerbations (although alcohol may be consumed in moderation during remission); advise the patient to stop smoking, because smoking of any sort stimulates gastric secretion.

After gastric surgery, the staffer should:
• keep nasogastric tube patent; notify the surgeon promptly if the tube isn't functioning, without repositioning it, since this may damage the suture line or anastomosis.
• monitor intake and output, including nasogastric tube drainage; check bowel sounds, and allow nothing by mouth until peristalsis resumes and the nasogastric tube is removed or clamped.
• replace fluids and electrolytes; assess for signs of dehydration, sodium deficiency, and metabolic alkalosis, which may occur secondary to gastric suction.
• control postoperative pain with narcotics and analgesics, as ordered.
• watch for complications such as hemorrhage; shock; iron, folate, or vitamin B_{12} deficiency anemia (from malabsorption or continued blood loss); and dumping syndrome (weakness, nausea, flatulence, diarrhea, distention, and palpitations within 30 minutes after a meal).
• prevent dumping syndrome by advising the patient to lie down after meals, to drink fluids *between* meals rather than with meals, to avoid eating large amounts of carbohydrates, and to eat four to six small, high-protein, low-carbohydrate meals during the day.

Ulcerative Colitis

Ulcerative colitis is an inflammatory, often chronic disease that affects the mucosa and submucosa of the colon. It usually begins in the rectum and sigmoid colon, and often extends upward into the entire colon; it rarely affects the small intestine, except for the terminal ileum. Ulcerative colitis produces congestion, edema (leading to mucosal friability), and ulcerations that eventually develop into abscesses. Severity ranges from a mild, localized disorder to a fulminant disease that may cause a perforated colon, progressing to potentially fatal peritonitis and toxemia.

Causes and incidence
Ulcerative colitis occurs primarily in young adults, especially women; it is also more prevalent among Jews and in higher socioeconomic groups. Overall, incidence is rising.

Although the etiology of ulcerative colitis is unknown, possible predisposing factors include:
• family history of the disease
• bacterial infection
• allergic reaction to food, milk, or other substances that release inflammatory histamine in the bowel
• overproduction of enzymes that break down the mucous membranes
• emotional stress
• autoimmune reactions, such as arthritis, hemolytic anemia, erythema nodosum, and uveitis.

Signs and symptoms

The hallmark of ulcerative colitis is recurrent bloody diarrhea, often containing pus and mucus, interspersed with asymptomatic remissions. The intensity of these attacks varies with the extent of inflammation. Other symptoms include spastic rectum and anus, abdominal pain, irritability, weight loss, weakness, anorexia, nausea, and vomiting.

Ulcerative colitis may lead to complications affecting many body systems.

• *Blood:* anemia from iron deficiency, coagulation defects due to vitamin K deficiency

• *Skin:* erythema nodosum on the face and arms; pyoderma gangrenosum on the legs and ankles

• *Eye:* uveitis

• *Liver:* pericholangitis, sclerosing cholangitis, cirrhosis, possible cholangiocarcinoma

• *Musculoskeletal:* arthritis, ankylosing spondylitis, loss of muscle mass

• *Gastrointestinal:* hemorrhoids, strictures, pseudopolyps, anal fissures, abscesses, stenosis, and perforated colon, leading to peritonitis and toxemia.

Patients with ulcerative colitis run a greater-than-normal risk of developing colorectal cancer, especially if onset of the disease occurs before age 15 or if it has persisted for longer than 10 years.

Diagnosis

Sigmoidoscopy showing increased mucosal friability, decreased mucosal detail, and thick inflammatory exudate suggests this diagnosis. Biopsy can help confirm it. Colonoscopy may be required to determine the extent of the disease and also to evaluate strictured areas and pseudopolyps. (Biopsy would then be done during colonoscopy.) Barium enema can assess the extent of the disease and detect complications, such as strictures, pseudopolyposis, and carcinoma.

Supportive laboratory values include decreased serum levels of potassium, magnesium, hemoglobin, and albumin, as well as leukocytosis and increased prothrombin time. Elevated ESR correlates with the severity of the attack.

Treatment

The goals of treatment are to control inflammation, replace nutritional losses and blood volume, and prevent complications. Supportive treatment includes bed rest, I.V. fluid replacement, and a clear-liquid diet. For patients awaiting surgery or those showing signs of severe dehydration and debilitation from excessive diarrhea, I.V. hyperalimentation rests the intestinal tract, decreases stool volume, and restores positive nitrogen balance. Blood transfusions or iron supplements may be necessary to correct anemia.

Drug therapy to control inflammation includes ACTH and adrenal corticosteroids, such as prednisone, prednisolone, and hydrocortisone; sulfasalazine, which has anti-inflammatory and antimicrobial properties, may also be used. Antispasmodics, such as tincture of belladonna, and antidiarrheals, such as diphenoxylate compound, are used only for patients with frequent, troublesome diarrheal stools whose ulcerative colitis is under control. These drugs may precipitate massive dilation of the colon (toxic megacolon) and are generally contraindicated.

Surgery is the treatment of last resort if the patient has toxic megacolon, fails to respond to drugs and supportive measures, or finds symptoms unbearable. The most common surgical technique is proctocolectomy with ileostomy. Total colectomy and ileorectal anastomosis is done less often because of its mortality (2% to 5%). This procedure removes the entire colon and anastomoses the rectum and the terminal ileum; it requires observation of the remaining rectal stump for any signs of malignancy or colitis.

Pouch ileostomy, in which a pouch is created from a small loop of the terminal ileum and a nipple valve formed from the distal ileum, is gaining popularity in some areas. The resulting stoma opens just above the pubic hairline; the pouch empties through a catheter inserted in the stoma several times a day. In ulcerative colitis, colectomy to prevent colon cancer is controversial.

Additional considerations

The hospital staff member caring for a patient with ulcerative colitis should:

• accurately record intake and output, particularly the frequency and volume of stools; watch for signs of dehydration (poor skin turgor, furrowed tongue) and electrolyte imbalances, especially signs of hypokalemia (muscle weakness, paresthesia) and hypernatremia (tachycardia, flushed skin, fever, dry tongue); monitor hemoglobin and hematocrit, and give blood transfusions, as ordered; provide good mouth care for the patient who is allowed nothing by mouth.

• thoroughly clean the skin around the rectum after each bowel movement; provide an air mattress or sheepskin to help prevent skin breakdown.

• administer medication, as ordered, and watch for side effects of prolonged corticosteroid therapy (moonface, hirsutism, edema, gastric irritation). Such therapy may mask infection.

• change dressings of the patient receiving hyperalimentation, assess for inflammation at the insertion site, and check urine every 6 hours for sugar and acetone.

• take precautionary measures if the patient is prone to bleeding, and watch closely for signs of complications, such as a perforated colon and peritonitis (fever, severe abdominal pain, abdominal rigidity and tenderness, cool clammy skin), and toxic megacolon (abdominal distention, decreased bowel sounds).

If surgery is required, the hospital staff member should:

• explain what a stoma is, what it looks like, and how it differs from normal anatomy; provide information (available from the United Ostomy Association),

and arrange for the patient to be visited by an enterostomal therapist and a recovered ileostomate, if possible.

• encourage the patient to verbalize his feelings and provide emotional support and a quiet environment.

• do a bowel prep, as ordered. This usually involves keeping the patient on a clear-liquid diet, using cleansing enemas, and administering antimicrobials, such as neomycin.

After surgery, the hospital staff member should:

• keep the nasogastric tube patent and, after removal of the tube, provide a clear-liquid diet, gradually advancing to a low-residue diet, as tolerated.

• teach good stoma care after a proctocolectomy and ileostomy; wash the skin around the stoma with soapy water and dry thoroughly; apply karaya gum around the base of the stoma to avoid irritation and provide a watertight seal; attach the pouch over the karaya ring, cut an opening in the ring to fit over the stoma, and secure the pouch to the skin; empty the pouch when it's one-third full. The patient should be encouraged to take over this care.

• after a pouch ileostomy, uncork the catheter every hour to allow contents to drain; after 10 to 14 days, gradually increase the length of time the catheter is left corked until it can be opened every 3 hours and then, remove the catheter and reinsert it every 3 to 4 hours for drainage. The patient must be taught how to insert the catheter and how to take care of the stoma.

• encourage the patient with ulcerative colitis to have regular physical examinations, since he risks developing colorectal cancer.

Necrotizing Enterocolitis

Necrotizing enterocolitis (NEC) is characterized by diffuse or patchy intestinal necrosis, accompanied by sepsis. Sepsis involves normal bowel flora: Escherichia coli, Salmonella, *or* Klebsiella. *Initially, necrosis is localized, occurring anywhere along the intestine, but most often it is right-sided (in the ileum, ascending colon, or rectosigmoid). With early detection, the survival rate is 60% to 80%; however, if surgical resection is necessary, mortality climbs to 50%. If diffuse bleeding occurs, NEC usually results in disseminated intravascular coagulation (DIC).*

Causes and incidence

NEC occurs most often among premature infants (less than 34 weeks gestation) and those of similar birth weight (less than 5 lb [2.25 kg]). NEC is becoming more prevalent; perhaps this increase is due to the higher incidence and survival of premature infants, and newborns who have low birth weights. One in five infants who develops NEC is full-term. Among premature infants in intensive care nurseries, incidence is about 3% to 8%. NEC is related to 2% of all infant deaths.

The exact cause of NEC is unknown; however, it may be a dynamic alteration in the integrity of the mucosal cells. Suggested predisposing factors include birth asphyxia, postnatal hypotension or respiratory distress, umbilical vessel catheterization, or patent ductus arteriosus. NEC may also be a response to significant perinatal stress, such as premature rupture of membranes, placenta previa, maternal sepsis, toxemia of pregnancy, or breech or cesarean birth.

According to current theory, NEC develops when the infant suffers perinatal hypoxia, which causes shunting of blood from the gut to more vital organs. Subsequent mucosal ischemia provides an ideal medium for bacterial growth. Hypertonic formula may increase bacterial activity because—unlike maternal breast milk—it doesn't provide protective immunologic activity, and because it contributes to the production of hydrogen gas. As the bowel swells and breaks down, gas-forming bacteria invade damaged areas, producing free air in the intestinal wall. This is often followed by fatal perforation and peritonitis.

Signs and symptoms

Any infant who has suffered from hypoxia or who consistently doesn't absorb glucose or formula feeding has the potential for developing NEC. A distended (especially tense or rigid) abdomen, with gastric retention, is the earliest and most common sign of oncoming NEC, usually appearing from 1 to 10 days after birth. Other clinical features are increasing residual gastric contents (which may contain bile), bile-stained vomitus, and occult blood in the stool. One fourth of patients have bloody diarrhea. A red or shiny, taut abdomen may indicate peritonitis. Nonspecific symptoms include thermal instability, lethargy, metabolic acidosis, jaundice, and DIC. The major complication is perforation, which requires surgery. Recurrence of NEC and postoperative mechanical and functional abnormalities of the intestine, especially stricture and short-gut syndrome, are the usual cause of intestinal malfunction in any infant who survives acute NEC, and may develop as late as 3 months postoperatively.

Diagnosis

Successful treatment of NEC relies on early recognition.

Anteroposterior and lateral abdominal X-rays confirm the diagnosis. X-rays show nonspecific intestinal dilation and, in later stages, pneumatosis cystoides intestinalis (gas or air in the intestinal wall).

Blood studies show several abnormalities. Platelet count may fall below $50,000/\text{mm}^3$. Serum sodium levels are decreased, and arterial blood gases show metabolic acidosis (a result of sepsis). Infection-induced RBC breakdown elevates bilirubin levels. Blood and stool cultures identify the infecting organism; clotting studies and hemoglobin levels, associated DIC; guaiac test detects occult blood in the stool.

Treatment

The first signs of NEC necessitate removal of the umbilical catheter (arterial or venous) and discontinuation of oral intake for 7 to 10 days to rest the injured bowel. I.V. fluids, including hyperalimentation (possibly intralipid solutions), maintain nutrition during this time; passage of a nasogastric tube aids bowel decompression. If coagulation studies indicate a need for transfusion, the infant usually receives dextran to promote hemodilution, increase mesenteric blood flow, and reduce platelet aggregation. Antibiotic therapy consists of parenteral administration of gentamicin, kanamycin, or ampicillin to suppress bacterial flora and prevent bowel perforation. Anteroposterior and lateral X-rays every 4 to 6 hours monitor disease progression.

Surgery is indicated if the patient shows any of the following symptoms: signs of perforation (free intraperitoneal air on X-ray or symptoms of peritonitis), respiratory insufficiency (caused by severe abdominal distention), progressive and intractable acidosis, or DIC. Surgery removes all necrotic and acutely inflamed bowel, and creates a temporary colostomy or ileostomy. Such surgery must leave at least 12" (30.5 cm) of bowel, or the infant may suffer from malabsorption or chronic vitamin B_{12} deficiency.

Additional considerations

 • The hospital staff member caring for patients with NEC should be alert for signs of perforation, such as apnea, cardiovascular shock, sudden drop in temperature, bradycardia, sudden listlessness, rag-doll limpness, increasing abdominal tenderness, edema, erythema, or involuntary rigidity of the abdomen. Axillary temperatures should be taken to avoid perforating the bowel.
• Cross-contamination can be prevented by disposing of soiled diapers properly and washing hands with povidone-iodine after diaper changes.
• A staff member should prepare parents for potential deterioration in their infant's condition by being honest with them, and explaining all treatments, including why feedings are being withheld.
• After surgery, the infant needs mechanical ventilation. Secretions must be gently suctioned, and respiration assessed.
• Fluids lost through nasogastric tube and stoma drainage must be replaced and those drainage losses included in output records. The infant should be weighed daily. Daily weight gain of 0.35 to 0.7 oz (9.9 to 19.8 g) indicates a good response to therapy.
• An infant with a temporary colostomy or ileostomy needs special care. The parents need to know what a colostomy or ileostomy is and why it's necessary. They should participate in their infant's physical care after his condition is no longer critical.
• Because of the infant's small abdomen, the suture line is near the stoma; therefore, keeping the suture line clean is a problem. Good skin care is essential, since the immature infant's skin is fragile and vulnerable to excoriation, and the active enzymes in bowel secretions are corrosive. Premature-sized colostomy bags can be made from urine collection bags, medicine cups, or condoms. Karaya is helpful in making a seal. The patient must be watched for wound disruption, infection, and excoriation—potential dangers because of severe catabolism.
• The patient should be watched for intestinal malfunction from stricture or short-gut syndrome. Such complications usually develop 1 month after the infant resumes normal feedings.

To help prevent NEC, mothers should be encouraged to breast-feed, since breast milk contains live macrophages that fight infection and has a low pH that inhibits the growth of many organisms. Also, colostrum—fluid secreted before the milk—contains high concentrations of IgA, which directly protects the gut from infection and which the newborn lacks for several days postpartum. If needed mothers may refrigerate their milk for 48 hours but shouldn't freeze it, since this destroys antibodies.

Crohn's Disease

(Regional enteritis, granulomatous colitis)

Crohn's disease is an inflammation of any part of the GI tract (usually the terminal ileum), which extends through all layers of the intestinal wall. It may also involve regional lymph nodes and the mesentery. Crohn's disease is most prevalent in adults aged 20 to 40. It is two to three times more common in Jews and least common in Blacks.

Causes

Although the exact cause of Crohn's disease is unknown, possible causes include allergies and other immune disorders, lymphatic obstruction, and infection. However, no infecting organism has been isolated. Several factors also implicate a genetic cause: Crohn's disease sometimes occurs in monozygotic twins, and up to 5% of patients with Crohn's disease have one or more affected relatives. However, no simple pattern of Mendelian inheritance is clear. Whatever the cause of Crohn's disease, lacteal blockage in the intestinal wall leads to edema and, eventually, to inflammation, ulceration, stenosis, and abscess and fistula formation.

Signs and symptoms

Symptoms vary according to the location and extent of the lesion, and at first may be mild and nonspecific. However, acute inflammatory symptoms mimic appendicitis and include lower right quadrant pain, cramping, tenderness, flatulence, nausea, fever, and diarrhea. Bleeding may occur, and although usually mild, it may be massive. Bloody stools also occur.

Chronic symptoms, which are more typical of the disease, are more persistent and less severe; they include diarrhea (four to six stools a day) with lower right quadrant pain, steatorrhea, marked weight loss, and rarely, clubbing of fingers. The patient may complain of weakness, lack of ambition, and inability to cope with everyday stress. Complications include intestinal obstruction, fistula formation between the small bowel

and the bladder, perianal and perirectal abscesses and fistulas, intra-abdominal abscesses, and perforation.

Diagnosis

Laboratory findings often indicate increased WBC and ESR, hypokalemia, hypocalcemia, hypomagnesemia, and decreased hemoglobin. Barium enema showing the string sign (segments of stricture separated by normal bowel) supports this diagnosis. Sigmoidoscopy and colonoscopy may show patchy areas of inflammation, thus helping to rule out ulcerative colitis. However, definitive diagnosis is possible only after biopsy.

Treatment

Treatment is symptomatic. In debilitated patients, therapy includes parenteral hyperalimentation to maintain nutrition while resting the bowel. During acute stages and in severely ill patients, corticosteroids, such as prednisone, are administered to decrease inflammation. If the patient's condition allows oral intake, sulfasalazine may be given for its anti-inflammatory and antibacterial effects, but it isn't always effective. Opium tincture and diphenoxylate may help combat diarrhea but are contraindicated in patients with significant intestinal obstruction. Effective treatment requires important changes in life-style: physical rest and restricted fiber diet (no fruit or vegetables) for intestinal stenosis; low-fat diet for steatorrhea; and elimination of dairy products for lactose deficiency.

Surgery may be necessary to correct bowel perforation, massive hemorrhage, fistulas, or acute intestinal obstruction.

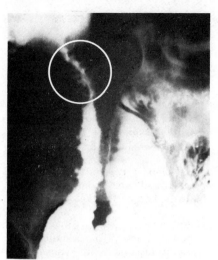

In Crohn's disease, the characteristic "string sign" (marked narrowing of the bowel), from inflammatory disease and scarring, strengthens the diagnosis.

Colectomy with ileostomy is often necessary in patients with extensive disease of the large intestine and rectum.

Additional considerations

The hospital staff member caring for the patient with Crohn's disease should:
- record fluid intake and output (including the amount of stool), and weigh the patient daily; watch for dehydration (decreased urinary output, poor skin turgor), and maintain fluid and electrolyte balance; be alert for signs of intestinal bleeding (bloody stools); check stools daily for occult blood.
- watch the patient receiving steroids for side effects, such as GI bleeding; keep in mind that steroids can mask signs of infection.
- check hemoglobin and hematocrit regularly; give iron supplements, blood transfusions and analgesics, as ordered.
- provide meticulous mouth care if the patient is restricted to nothing by mouth; give good skin care after each bowel movement; keep a clean, covered bedpan within the patient's reach; ventilate the room to eliminate odors.
- watch for fever and pain on urination, which may signal bladder fistula; watch for abdominal pain, fever, and hard, distended abdomen, which may indicate intestinal obstruction.
- arrange for an enterostomal therapist if the patient's to have an ileostomy.
- after surgery, frequently check the patient's I.V. and nasogastric tube for proper functioning; monitor vital signs, and fluid intake and output; watch for wound infection; provide meticulous stoma care, and teach it to the patient and family; realize that ileostomy changes the patient's body image, so offer reassurance and emotional support.
- emphasize the importance of severely restricted diet and bed rest, which may be trying, particularly for the young patient; encourage the patient to try to reduce the tension in his life; refer the patient for counseling, if stress is clearly an important aggravating factor in the patient's condition.

Pseudomembranous Enterocolitis

Pseudomembranous enterocolitis is an acute inflammation and necrosis of the small and large intestines, which usually affects the mucosa but may extend into submucosa and, rarely, other layers. Marked by severe diarrhea, this rare condition is generally fatal in 1 to 7 days from severe dehydration and toxicity, peritonitis, or perforation.

Causes

The exact cause of pseudomembranous enterocolitis is unknown. *Staphylococcus aureus* has been isolated in some but not all patients. Pseudomembranous enterocolitis has occurred postoperatively in debilitated patients who undergo abdominal surgery or patients who have been treated with broad-spectrum antibiotics. Whatever the cause, necrosed mucosa is replaced by a pseudomembrane filled with staphylococci, leukocytes, mucus, fibrin, and inflammatory cells.

Signs and symptoms

Pseudomembranous enterocolitis begins suddenly with copious watery or bloody diarrhea, which rapidly progresses to shock. Other symptoms include nausea, vomiting, fever, tachycardia, oliguria, colicky pain, and disorientation. Potentially fatal complications include peritonitis or bowel perforation.

Diagnosis

Diagnosis is often difficult because of the abrupt onset of enterocolitis and the emergency situation it creates, so consideration of patient history is essential. A rectal biopsy through sigmoidoscopy confirms pseudomembranous enterocolitis. Stool cultures can identify staphylococci, but the results usually arrive too late to determine treatment.

Treatment

Diarrhea and hypotension in a postoperative patient who is receiving broad-spectrum antibiotics signal rapidly progressive deterioration and require immediate discontinuation of the antibiotics. During attempts to isolate *S. aureus*, aggressive treatment with oxacillin and steroids may be lifesaving. Concomitant supportive treatment must maintain fluid and electrolyte balance and combat hypotension and shock with pressors, such as dopamine and levarterenol.

Additional considerations

The patient's vital signs, skin color, and level of consciousness require monitoring. Signs of shock must be reported.

Fluid intake and output, including fluid lost in stools, should be recorded. The patient must be watched for dehydration (poor skin turgor, sunken eyes, and decreased urine output).

Serum electrolytes must be checked daily, and the patient watched for signs of hypokalemia, especially malaise, and weak, rapid, irregular pulse.

Irritable Bowel Syndrome

(Spastic colon, spastic colitis)

Irritable bowel syndrome is a common condition marked by chronic or periodic diarrhea, alternating with constipation, and accompanied by straining and abdominal cramps. Prognosis is good. Supportive treatment or avoidance of a known irritant often relieves symptoms.

Causes

This functional disorder is generally associated with psychologic stress; however, it may result from physical factors, such as diverticular disease, ingestion of irritants (coffee, raw fruits or vegetables), lactose intolerance, abuse of laxatives, food poisoning, or colon cancer.

Signs and symptoms

Irritable bowel syndrome characteristically produces lower abdominal pain

(usually relieved by defecation or passage of gas), and diarrhea that typically occurs during the day. These symptoms alternate with constipation or normal bowel function. Stools are often small and contain visible mucus. Dyspepsia and abdominal distention may occur.

Diagnosis

Diagnosis of irritable bowel syndrome requires a careful history to determine contributing psychologic factors, such as a recent stressful life change. Diagnosis must also rule out other disorders, such as amebiasis, diverticulitis, colon cancer, and lactose intolerance. Appropriate diagnostic procedures include sigmoidoscopy, colonoscopy, barium enema, rectal biopsy, and stool examination for blood, parasites, and bacteria.

Treatment
Therapy aims to relieve symptoms, and includes counseling to help the patient understand the relationship between stress and his illness. Strict dietary restrictions aren't beneficial, but food irritants should be investigated and the patient instructed to avoid them. Rest and heat applied to the abdomen are helpful, as is judicious use of sedatives (phenobarbital) and antispasmodics (propantheline, or diphenoxylate with atropine sulfate). However, with chronic use, the patient may become dependent on these drugs. If the cause of irritable bowel syndrome is chronic laxative abuse, bowel training may help correct the condition.

Additional considerations
Since the patient with irritable bowel syndrome isn't hospitalized, care focuses on patient teaching.
• The patient must avoid irritating foods, not use laxatives, and try to develop regular bowel habits.
• The patient must learn how to deal with stress in ways other than using drugs. He must avoid becoming dependent on sedatives or antispasmodics.
• The patient should get regular checkups, since irritable bowel syndrome is associated with a higher-than-normal incidence of diverticulitis and colon cancer. Patients over age 40 should get an annual sigmoidoscopy and rectal examination, as well.

Tropical Sprue

Tropical sprue causes the mucosa of the small intestine to atrophy, and produces malabsorption, secondary malnutrition, and folic acid deficiency. Incidence is high among those who visit or live in the Tropics. The disease affects adults more often than children. Its distribution is sporadic: in the Western hemisphere, it occurs primarily in Puerto Rico, Cuba, and Haiti but rarely in Jamaica; in Asia, primarily in Hong Kong and India but not in Singapore.

Causes
The cause of tropical sprue is unknown. No single organism, parasite, or virus has been implicated, but because sprue often occurs in epidemics, a bacterial cause is considered possible.

Signs and symptoms
The first sign of sprue is usually severe diarrhea with mucus- and blood-tinged stools. Other clinical effects include abdominal distention, borborygmi, nausea, vomiting, anorexia, severe weight loss, fatigability, and steatorrhea. In advanced stages, macrocytic anemia is present.

Approximately 10% of patients with tropical sprue have anemia or edema without GI symptoms. Some may develop intolerance to alcohol and milk products. If patients live in or return to tropical climates, they may suffer relapses. Malnourished patients manifest sprue symptoms more quickly than those with adequate levels of vitamin B_{12} and folate.

Diagnosis
In general, diagnosis of tropical sprue may be difficult. Jejunal biopsy and a blood test showing evidence of malabsorption of two unrelated substances (such as vitamin B_{12} and xylose) suggest tropical sprue. Analyzing stool specimens for fat (after a 72-hour collection)

is the most reliable index of malabsorption. In tropical sprue, X-rays of the small bowel show a pattern that's also typical of celiac disease—widened mucosal folds, barium flocculation, delayed movement of barium through the small bowel—although this pattern is more dramatic in patients with celiac disease.

In early stages of tropical sprue, an oral postprandial glucose tolerance test doesn't show normal rise in blood sugar. In addition, the urine level of xylose and serum levels of sodium, potassium, chloride, and calcium may be low. In later stages, bone marrow biopsy shows macrocytosis; blood studies show anemia, and low serum iron, vitamin B_{12}, and folate levels. Diagnosis must rule out parasitic and other GI disorders.

Treatment
Treatment necessitates prolonged antimicrobial therapy and control of accompanying diarrhea. Antimicrobial therapy, which must continue for 6 months, includes tetracycline or oxytetracycline and poorly absorbed sulfonamides, such as phthalylsulfathiazole. Antidiarrheals, such as diphenoxylate with atropine sulfate, can minimize diarrhea; iron, folic acid, or vitamin B_{12} supplements combat anemia.

Additional considerations
The hospital staff member caring for the patient with tropical sprue should:
• assess fluid status, and administer fluid replacement, as ordered; look for signs of dehydration, and check electrolyte balance; watch for signs of hypokalemia (weakness, faint pulse, fall in blood pressure, malaise, anorexia, vomiting).
• record intake and output accurately (including frequency and characteristics of stools).
• monitor hematocrit and hemoglobin levels; administer iron, folate, and vitamin B_{12} supplements, as ordered.
• give antibiotics and antidiarrheals, as ordered; tell the patient that antibiotic therapy will continue for 6 months.

Celiac Disease
(Idiopathic steatorrhea, nontropical sprue, gluten-induced enteropathy, celiac sprue)

Celiac disease is characterized by poor food absorption and intolerance of gluten, a protein in wheat and wheat products. Such malabsorption in the small bowel results from atrophy of the villi, and a decrease in the activity and amount of enzymes in the surface epithelium. With treatment (eliminating gluten from the patient's diet), prognosis is good, but residual bowel changes may persist in adults.

Causes and incidence
This relatively uncommon disorder probably results from environmental factors and a genetic predisposition, but the exact mechanism is unknown. Two theories prevail. The first suggests that ingesting gluten may trigger a preexisting immunologic response in a genetically susceptible patient. (The presence of HLA-B8 antigen in such a person may be the primary determinant of celiac disease, according to recent studies.)

The second theory proposes that a patient with celiac disease may have an intramucosal enzyme defect that causes an inability to digest gluten. Resulting tissue toxicity produces rapid cell turnover, increases epithelial lymphocytes, and damages surface epithelium of the small bowel.

Celiac disease affects twice as many females as males and occurs more often among relatives, especially siblings. Incidence in the general population is approximately 1 in 3,000. This disease primarily affects Caucasians of northwestern European ancestry; it's rare among Blacks, Jews, Orientals, and people of Mediterranean ancestry. It usually affects children but may occur in adults.

Signs and symptoms
This disorder produces clinical effects in many body systems.

• *Gastrointestinal:* recurrent attacks of diarrhea, steatorrhea, abdominal distention due to flatulence, stomach cramps, weakness, anorexia, and occasionally, increased appetite without weight gain. Atrophy of intestinal villi leads to malabsorption of fat, carbohydrates, and protein. It also causes loss of calories, fat-soluble vitamins (A, D, and K), calcium, and essential minerals and electrolytes (including magnesium and potassium). In adults, celiac disease produces multiple, nonspecific ulcers in the small bowel, which may perforate or bleed.

• *Hematologic:* normochromic, hypochromic, or macrocytic anemia due to poor absorption of folate, iron, and vitamin B_{12}, and to hypoprothrombinemia from jejunal loss of vitamin K

• *Musculoskeletal:* osteomalacia, osteoporosis, tetany, and bone pain (especially in the lower back, rib cage, and pelvis). These symptoms are due to calcium loss and vitamin D deficiency, which weakens the skeleton, causing rickets in children and compression fractures in adults.

• *Neurologic:* peripheral neuropathy, convulsions, or paresthesia

• *Dermatologic:* dry skin, eczema, psoriasis, dermatitis herpetiformis, and acne rosacea. Deficiency of sulfur-containing amino acids may cause generalized fine, sparse, prematurely gray hair; brittle nails; and localized hyperpigmentation on the face, lips, or mucosa.

• *Endocrine:* amenorrhea, hypometabolism, and possibly, with severe malabsorption, adrenocortical insufficiency

• *Psychosocial:* mood changes and irritability.

Symptoms may develop during the first year of life, when gluten is introduced into the child's diet as cereal. Clinical effects may disappear during adolescence and reappear in adulthood. One theory proposes that the age at which symptoms first appear depends on the strength of the genetic factor: a strong factor produces symptoms during the child's first 4 years; a weak factor, in late childhood, or adulthood.

Diagnosis

 Histologic changes seen on small bowel biopsy specimens confirm the diagnosis: a mosaic pattern of alternating flat and bumpy areas on the bowel surface due to an almost total absence of villi and an irregular, blunt, and disorganized network of blood vessels. These changes appear most prominently in the jejunum.

Malabsorption and tolerance studies support the diagnosis. A glucose tolerance test shows poor absorption of glucose. A D-xylose tolerance test shows low urine and blood levels of xylose (less than 3 g over a 5-hour period); however, the presence of renal disease may cause a false positive result. Serum carotene levels measure absorption. (The patient ingests carotene for several days before the test; since the body neither stores nor manufactures carotene, low serum levels indicate malabsorption.) Analyses of stool specimens (after a 72-hour stool collection) show excess fat.

Barium X-rays of the small bowel show protracted barium passage. The barium shows up in a segmented, coarse, scattered, and clumped pattern; the jejunum shows generalized dilation.

The following lab findings also support the diagnosis:

• low hemoglobin, hematocrit, leukocyte, and platelet counts

• reduced albumin, sodium, potassium, cholesterol, and phospholipid levels

• reduced prothrombin time.

Treatment
Effective treatment necessitates elimination of gluten from the patient's diet for life. Even with this exclusion, full return to normal absorption and bowel

histology may not occur for months, or may never occur.

Supportive treatment may include supplemental iron, vitamin B_{12}, and folic acid, reversal of electrolyte imbalance (by I.V. infusion, if necessary), I.V. fluid replacement for dehydration, corticosteroids (prednisone, hydrocortisone) to treat accompanying adrenal insufficiency, and vitamin K for hypoprothrombinemia.

Additional considerations

The hospital staff member caring for the patient with celiac disease should:

• explain the necessity of a gluten-free diet to the patient (and to his parents, if the patient is a child); advise elimination of wheat, barley, rye, and oats, and foods made from them, such as breads and baked goods; suggest substitution of corn or rice; advise the patient to consult a dietitian for a gluten-free diet, which is high in protein but low in carbohydrates and fats (depending on individual tolerance, the diet initially consists of proteins and gradually expands to include other foods); assess the patient's acceptance and understanding of the disease.

• observe nutritional status and progress by daily calorie counts and weight checks; also, evaluate tolerance to new foods; in the early stages, offer small, frequent meals to counteract anorexia.

• record fluid intake, urine output, and number of stools (may exceed 10 per day); watch for dehydration (dry skin and mucous membranes).

• check serum electrolyte levels; watch for signs of hypokalemia (weakness, lethargy, rapid pulse, nausea, and diarrhea) and low calcium levels (impaired blood clotting, muscle twitching, and tetany).

• monitor prothrombin time, hemoglobin, and hematocrit; protect the patient from bleeding and bruising; administer vitamin K, iron, folic acid, and vitamin B_{12}, as ordered; early in treatment, give hematinic supplements I.M., using a separate syringe for each; use the Z-track method to give iron I.M.; give oral iron between meals, when absorption is best; dilute oral iron preparations, and give them through a straw to prevent teeth stains.

• protect patients with osteomalacia from injury by keeping the side rails up and assisting with ambulation, as necessary.

• give steroids, as ordered, and assess regularly for cushingoid side effects.

Whipple's Disease

(Intestinal lipodystrophy, lipophagia granulomatosis)

Whipple's disease, a rare disorder, is characterized by chronic diarrhea and progressive wasting. With treatment, prognosis is good; however, untreated persons die of malnutrition due to malabsorption.

Causes and incidence

Approximately 200 cases of Whipple's disease have been reported, primarily in the United States, England, continental Europe, and occasionally, South America. Whipple's disease generally affects Caucasian men aged 20 to 67.

Although the cause is unknown, this disorder may be due to an infection, since electron microscopy shows bacilliform bodies in affected patients. However, the exact role of these organisms is unclear.

Signs and symptoms

Patients typically have arthralgia, vague abdominal pain, diarrhea, steatorrhea, impaired intestinal absorption, progressive weight loss, slight fever, hyperpigmentation, and peripheral, mesenteric, periaortic, and celiac lymphadenopathy, as well as occasional splenomegaly.

Diagnosis

Biopsy of the small intestine by endoscopy is the most reliable diagnostic procedure.

 A biopsy specimen showing macrophages, and large cytoplasmic granules that stain a brilliant magenta color with periodic acid–Schiff (PAS) stain confirms this diagnosis. Diagnosis may also include a biopsy of the peripheral lymph nodes, but this method is less reliable than a biopsy of the small intestine. X-rays, although not in themselves diagnostic, reveal marked, coarse, edematous folds in the upper small bowel. Other laboratory findings that support this diagnosis include iron deficiency anemia, elevated urine xylose levels, hypoalbuminemia, hypocalcemia, low serum cholesterol levels, and in 93% of patients, excessive fat in the stool.

Treatment

Treatment consists of hospitalization and a 14-day course of therapy with penicillin G procaine and streptomycin, followed by daily administration of tetracycline for 10 to 12 months. In addition to antibiotics, treatment during the acute phase includes corticosteroids (prednisone or ACTH). Patients with iron deficiency anemia need iron supplements. Treatment also necessitates follow-up of intestinal biopsy specimen, because relapses can occur.

Additional considerations

Supportive care includes:
• maintaining fluid and electrolyte balance; administering I.V. fluids, as needed.
• measuring intake and output and watching for signs of dehydration.
• checking serum calcium levels, and watching for signs of hypocalcemia (tingling of fingers, tetany, abdominal cramps).
• monitoring hemoglobin and hematocrit; administering iron supplements, antibiotics, and steroids, as ordered; telling the patient to continue antibiotic therapy even after he feels better.

Diverticular Disease

In diverticular disease, bulging pouches (diverticula) in the gastrointestinal wall push the mucosal lining through the surrounding muscle. The most common site for diverticula is in the sigmoid colon, but they may develop anywhere, from the proximal end of the pharynx to the anus. Other typical sites are the duodenum, near the pancreatic border or the ampulla of Vater, and the jejunum. Diverticular disease of the stomach is rare and is often a precursor of peptic or neoplastic disease. Diverticular disease of the ileum (Meckel's diverticulum) is the most common congenital anomaly of the GI tract.

Diverticular disease has two clinical forms. In diverticulosis, diverticula are present but do not cause symptoms. In diverticulitis, diverticula are inflamed and may cause potentially fatal obstruction, infection, or hemorrhage.

Causes

Diverticular disease is most prevalent in men over age 40. Diverticula probably result from high intraluminal pressure on areas of weakness in the gastrointestinal wall, where blood vessels enter.

Diet may also be a contributing factor, since lack of roughage reduces fecal residue, narrows the bowel lumen, and leads to higher intra-abdominal pressure during defecation. The fact that diverticulosis is most prevalent in Western industrialized nations, where processing removes much of the roughage from foods, supports this theory. Diverticulosis is less common in nations where the diet contains more natural bulk and fiber.

In diverticulitis, retained undigested food mixed with bacteria (fecalith) accumulates in the diverticular sac, forming a hard mass. This substance cuts off the blood supply to the thin walls of the sac, making them more susceptible to attack by colonic bacteria. Inflammation follows, possibly leading to perforation, abscess, peritonitis, obstruction, or hemorrhage. Occasionally, the inflamed colon segment may produce a fistula by adhering to the bladder or other organs.

Signs and symptoms

Diverticulosis usually produces no symptoms but may cause recurrent lower left quadrant pain without clinical evidence of acute diverticulitis. Such pain, often accompanied by alternating constipation and diarrhea, is relieved by defecation or the passage of flatus. These symptoms resemble irritable bowel syndrome and suggest that both disorders may coexist.

In elderly patients, a rare complication of diverticulosis (without diverticulitis) is hemorrhage from colonic diverticula, usually in the right colon. Such hemorrhage is usually mild to moderate and easily controlled but may occasionally be massive and life-threatening.

Mild diverticulitis produces moderate lower left abdominal pain, mild nausea, gas, irregular bowel habits, low-grade fever, and leukocytosis. In severe diverticulitis, the diverticula can rupture and produce abscesses or peritonitis. Such rupture occurs in up to 20% of such patients; its symptoms include abdominal rigidity and lower left quadrant pain. Peritonitis follows release of fecal material from the rupture site and causes signs of sepsis and shock (high fever, chills, hypotension). Rupture of diverticulum near a blood vessel may cause either microscopic or massive hemorrhage, depending on the size of the ruptured vessel.

Chronic diverticulitis may cause fibrosis and adhesions that narrow the bowel's lumen and lead to bowel obstruction. Symptoms of incomplete obstruction are constipation, ribbonlike

MECKEL'S DIVERTICULUM

In Meckel's diverticulum, a congenital abnormality, a blind tube, like the appendix, opens into the distal ileum near the ileocecal valve. This disorder results from failure of the intra-abdominal portion of the yolk sac to close completely during fetal development. It occurs in 2% of the population, mostly in males.

Uncomplicated Meckel's diverticulum produces no symptoms, but complications cause abdominal pain, especially around the umbilicus, and dark red melena. The lining of the diverticulum may be either gastric mucosa or pancreatic tissue. This disorder may lead to peptic ulceration, perforation, and peritonitis, and may resemble acute appendicitis.

Meckel's diverticulum may also cause bowel obstruction when a fibrous band that connects the diverticulum to the abdominal wall, the mesentery, or other structures snares a loop of the intestine. This may cause intussusception into the diverticulum, or volvulus near the diverticular attachment to the back of the umbilicus or another intra-abdominal structure. Meckel's diverticulum should be considered in cases of gastrointestinal obstruction or hemorrhage, especially when routine gastrointestinal X-rays are negative.

Treatment is surgical resection of the inflamed bowel, and antibiotic therapy if infection is present.

stools, intermittent diarrhea, and abdominal distention. As obstruction increases, abdominal distention causes abdominal rigidity, diminishing or absent bowel sounds, nausea, vomiting, and abdominal pain.

Diagnosis

Diverticular disease frequently produces no symptoms, and is often found incidental to an upper GI barium X-ray series. Upper GI series confirms or rules out diverticulosis of the esophagus and upper bowel; a barium enema confirms or rules out diverticulosis of the lower bowel. Barium-filled diverticula can be single, multiple, or clustered like grapes, and may have a wide or narrow mouth. Barium outlines but does not fill diverticula blocked by impacted feces. In patients with acute diverticulitis, a barium enema may rupture the bowel, so this procedure requires caution. If irritable bowel syndrome accompanies diverticular disease, X-rays may reveal colonic spasm.

Biopsy rules out cancer; however, a colonoscopic biopsy is not recommended during acute diverticular disease because of the strenuous bowel preparation it requires. Blood studies may show elevated ESR in diverticulitis, especially if the diverticula are infected.

Treatment

Asymptomatic diverticulosis generally doesn't necessitate treatment. Intestinal diverticulosis with pain, mild GI distress, constipation, or difficult defecation may respond to a liquid or bland diet, stool softeners, and occasional doses of mineral oil. These measures relieve symptoms, minimize irritation, and lessen the risk of progression to diverticulitis. After pain subsides, patients also benefit from a high-residue diet and bulk medication, such as psyllium.

Treatment of mild diverticulitis without signs of perforation must prevent constipation and combat infection. It may include bed rest, a liquid diet, stool softeners, a broad-spectrum antibiotic, meperidine to control pain and relax smooth muscle, and an antispasmodic, such as propantheline, to control muscle spasms.

Diverticulitis that is refractory to medical treatment requires a colon resection to remove the involved segment. Perforation, peritonitis, obstruction, or fistula that accompanies diverticulitis may require a temporary colostomy to drain abscesses and rest the colon, followed by later anastomosis.

Patients who hemorrhage need blood replacement and careful monitoring of fluid and electrolyte balance. Such bleeding usually stops spontaneously. If it continues, angiography for catheter placement and infusion of vasopressin into the bleeding vessel is effective. Rarely, surgery may be required.

Additional considerations

Management of uncomplicated diverticulosis chiefly involves thorough patient teaching about bowel and dietary habits.
• The patient should understand what diverticula are and how they form.
• The patient must understand the importance of dietary roughage and the harmful effects of constipation and straining at stool. He should increase his intake of foods high in undigestible fiber, including fresh fruits and vegetables, whole grain bread, and wheat or bran cereals. This diet may temporarily cause flatulence and discomfort. The patient can relieve constipation with stool softeners or bulk-forming cathartics. But he shouldn't take bulk-forming cathartics without plenty of water; if swallowed dry, they may absorb enough moisture in the mouth and throat to swell and obstruct the esophagus or trachea.
• If the patient with diverticulosis is hospitalized, a staff member should administer medication, as ordered; observe his stools carefully for frequency, color, and consistency; and keep accurate pulse and temperature charts to check for developing inflammation or complications.

Management of diverticulitis depends on severity of symptoms:
• In mild disease, a staff member should administer medications, as ordered; explain diagnostic tests and preparations; observe stools carefully; and accurately record temperature, pulse, respirations, and intake and output.
• If the patient requires angiography and catheter placement for vasopressin infusion, he'll need careful monitoring. This includes inspecting the insertion site for bleeding, checking pedal pulses often, and keeping the patient from flexing his legs at the groin.
• The patient may exhibit signs of vasopressin-induced fluid retention (apprehension, abdominal cramps, convulsions, oliguria, or anuria) and severe

hyponatremia (hypotension; rapid, thready pulse; cold, clammy skin; and cyanosis.)

After surgery to resect diverticula, a staff member should:

• watch for signs of infection; provide meticulous wound care, since perforation may have already infected the area; check drain sites frequently for signs of infection (pus on dressing, foul odor) or fecal drainage; change dressings, as necessary.

• encourage coughing and deep breathing to prevent atelectasis.

• watch for signs of postoperative bleeding (hypotension, and decreased hemoglobin and hematocrit).

• record intake and output accurately.

• keep the nasogastric tube patent; notify the surgeon if it becomes dislodged and avoid moving it.

• teach colostomy care, if applicable, and arrange for a visit by an enterostomal therapist.

Appendicitis

The most common major surgical disease, appendicitis is inflammation of the vermiform appendix due to an obstruction. Appendicitis may occur at any age and affects both sexes equally; however, between puberty and age 25, it's more prevalent in men. Since the advent of antibiotics, the incidence and the death rate of appendicitis have declined; if untreated, this disease is invariably fatal.

Causes

Appendicitis probably results from an obstruction of the intestinal lumen caused by a fecal mass, stricture, barium ingestion, or viral infection. This obstruction sets off an inflammatory process that can lead to infection, thrombosis, necrosis, and perforation. If the appendix ruptures or perforates, the infected contents spill into the abdominal cavity, causing peritonitis, the most common and most perilous complication of appendicitis.

Signs and symptoms

Typically, appendicitis begins with generalized or localized abdominal pain in the upper right abdomen, followed by anorexia, nausea, and vomiting (rarely profuse). Pain eventually localizes in the lower right abdomen (McBurney's point) with abdominal "boardlike" rigidity, retractive respirations, increasing tenderness, increasingly severe abdominal spasms, and almost invariably, rebound tenderness. (Rebound tenderness on the opposite side of the abdomen suggests peritoneal inflammation.)

Later symptoms include constipation (although diarrhea is also possible), slight

fever, and tachycardia. Sudden cessation of abdominal pain indicates perforation or infarction of the appendix.

Diagnosis

Diagnosis of appendicitis is based on physical findings and characteristic clinical symptoms. Findings that support this diagnosis include a temperature of 99° to 102° F. (37.2° to 38.9° C.) and a moderately elevated WBC (12,000 to 15,000/mm³), with increased immature cells. Diagnosis must rule out illnesses with similar symptoms: gastritis, gastroenteritis, ileitis, colitis, diverticulitis, pancreatitis, renal colic, bladder infection, ovarian cyst, and uterine disease.

Treatment

Appendectomy is the only effective treatment. If peritonitis develops, treatment involves gastrointestinal intubation, parenteral replacement of fluids and electrolytes, and administration of antibiotics.

Additional considerations

If appendicitis is suspected, or the patient's being prepared for appendectomy,

a hospital staff member should:
• administer I.V. fluids to prevent dehydration; *never* administer cathartics or enemas, as they may rupture the appendix; give the patient nothing by mouth, and administer analgesics judiciously, since they may mask symptoms.
• place the patient in Fowler's position to lessen pain (this is also helpful postoperatively); *never* apply heat to the lower right abdomen—this may cause the appendix to rupture.
• never give the patient an enema.

After appendectomy, a staffer should:
• monitor vital signs, and intake and output; give analgesics, as ordered.
• encourage the patient to cough, deep breathe, and turn frequently to prevent pulmonary complications.
• document bowel sounds, passing of flatus, or bowel movements—signs of the return of peristalsis. (These signs in a patient whose nausea and abdominal rigidity have subsided indicate readiness to resume oral fluids.)
• watch closely for possible surgical complications—continuing pain and fever may signal an abscess; suspect wound dehiscence if the patient complains that "something gave way"; prepare the patient for an incision and drainage if an abscess or peritonitis develops; assess the dressing for wound drainage.
• assist the patient to ambulate as soon as possible—usually within 12 hours.
• insert a nasogastric tube, as ordered, to decompress the stomach and reduce nausea and vomiting if peritonitis complicated appendicitis; record drainage, and give good mouth and nose care.

Peritonitis

Peritonitis is an acute or chronic inflammation of the peritoneum, the membrane that lines the abdominal cavity and covers the visceral organs. Such inflammation may extend throughout the peritoneum or may be localized as an abscess. Peritonitis commonly decreases intestinal motility and causes intestinal distention with gas. Mortality is 10%, with death usually a result of bowel obstruction; this mortality rate was much higher before the introduction of antibiotics.

Causes and incidence
Although the GI tract normally contains bacteria, the peritoneum is sterile. In peritonitis, however, bacteria invade the peritoneum. Generally, such infection results from inflammation and perforation of the GI tract, allowing bacterial invasion. Usually, this is a result of appendicitis, diverticulitis, peptic ulcer, ulcerative colitis, volvulus, strangulated obstruction, abdominal neoplasm, or a stab wound. Peritonitis may also result from chemical inflammation, as in rupture of the fallopian or an ovarian tube, or the bladder; perforation of a gastric ulcer; or released pancreatic enzymes.

In both chemical and bacterial inflammation, accumulated fluids containing protein and electrolytes make the transparent peritoneum opaque, red, inflamed, and edematous. Because the peritoneal cavity is so resistant to contamination, such infection is often localized as an abscess instead of disseminated as a generalized infection.

Signs and symptoms
The key symptom of peritonitis is sudden, severe, and diffuse abdominal pain that tends to intensify and localize in the area of the underlying disorder. For instance, if appendicitis causes the rupture, pain eventually localizes in the lower right quadrant. The patient often displays weakness, pallor, excessive sweating, and cold skin as a result of excessive loss of fluid, electrolytes, and protein into the abdominal cavity. Decreased intestinal motility and paralytic ileus result from the effect of bacterial

toxins on the intestinal muscles. Intestinal obstruction causes nausea, vomiting, and abdominal rigidity.

Other clinical characteristics include hypotension, tachycardia, signs of dehydration (oliguria, thirst, dry swollen tongue, pinched skin), acutely tender abdomen associated with rebound tenderness, temperature of 103° F. (39.4° C.) or higher, and hypokalemia. Inflammation of the diaphragmatic peritoneum may cause shoulder pain and hiccups. Abdominal distention and resulting upward displacement of the diaphragm may decrease respiratory capacity. Typically, the patient with peritonitis tends to breathe shallowly and move as little as possible to minimize pain.

Diagnosis

Severe abdominal pain in a person with direct or rebound tenderness suggests peritonitis. Abdominal X-rays showing edematous and gaseous distention of the small and large bowel support the diagnosis. In the case of perforation of a visceral organ, the X-ray shows air in the abdominal cavity. Other appropriate tests include:
• *chest X-ray:* may show elevation of the diaphragm
• *blood studies:* leukocytosis (more than 20,000/mm³)
• *paracentesis:* reveals bacteria, exudate, blood, pus, or urine
• *laparotomy:* may be necessary to identify the underlying cause.

Treatment

Early treatment of GI inflammatory conditions, and pre- and postoperative antibiotic therapy help prevent peritonitis. After peritonitis develops, emergency treatment must combat infection, restore intestinal motility, and replace fluids and electrolytes.

Massive antibiotic therapy usually includes administration of penicillin G, streptomycin, clindamycin, or chloramphenicol, depending on the infecting organisms. To decrease peristalsis and prevent perforation, the patient should receive nothing by mouth; he should receive supportive fluids and electrolytes parenterally.

Other supplementary treatment measures include pre- and postoperative administration of an analgesic, such as meperidine; nasogastric intubation to decompress the bowel; and possible use of a rectal tube to facilitate passage of flatus.

When peritonitis results from perforation, surgery is necessary as soon as the patient's condition is stable enough to tolerate it. The aim of surgery is to eliminate the source of infection by evacuating the spilled contents and inserting drains. Occasionally, abdominocentesis may be necessary to remove accumulated fluid. Irrigation of the abdominal cavity with antibiotic solutions during surgery may be appropriate.

Additional considerations

Health care of the patient with peritonitis includes:
• regularly monitoring vital signs, fluid intake and output, and amount of nasogastric drainage or vomitus.
• placing the patient in semi-Fowler's position to help him deep breathe with less pain and thus prevent pulmonary complications.
• counteracting mouth and nose dryness due to fever and nasogastric intubation with regular cleansing and lubrication.

After surgery, to evacuate the peritoneum, health care includes:
• maintaining parenteral fluid and electrolyte administration; accurately recording fluid intake and output, including nasogastric and incisional drainage.
• placing the patient in Fowler's position to promote drainage (through drainage tube) by gravity; moving him carefully, since the slightest movement will intensify the pain.
• implementing safety procedures, such as keeping the bed rails up, because the patient may be disoriented.
• encouraging and assisting ambulation, usually on the first postoperative day.
• watching for signs of dehiscence (the patient may complain that "something

gave way") and abscess formation (continued abdominal tenderness and fever).
• frequently assessing for peristaltic activity by listening for bowel sounds and checking for gas, bowel movements, and soft abdomen.

When peristalsis returns, and temperature and pulse rate are normal, parenteral fluids should be gradually decreased and oral fluids increased. If the patient has a nasogastric tube in place, it should be clamped for short intervals. If nausea or vomiting does not result, oral fluids can be started.

Intestinal Obstruction

Intestinal obstruction is the partial or complete blockage of the lumen of the small or large bowel. Small bowel obstruction is far more common (90% of patients) and usually more serious. Complete obstruction in any part of the bowel, if untreated, can cause death within hours from shock and vascular collapse. Intestinal obstruction is most likely to occur after abdominal surgery or in persons with congenital bowel deformities.

Causes

Adhesions and strangulated hernias usually cause small bowel obstruction; carcinomas, large bowel obstruction. Mechanical intestinal obstruction results from foreign bodies (fruit pits, gallstones, worms) or compression of the bowel wall due to stenosis, intussusception, volvulus of the sigmoid or cecum, tumors, or atresia. Nonmechanical obstruction results from physiologic disturbances, such as paralytic ileus, electrolyte imbalances, toxicity (uremia, generalized infection), neurogenic abnormalities (spinal cord lesions), and thrombosis or embolism of mesenteric vessels.

Intestinal obstruction develops in three forms:
• *Simple:* Blockage prevents intestinal contents from passing, with no other complications.
• *Strangulated:* Blood supply to part or all of the obstructed section is cut off, in addition to blockage of the lumen.
• *Close-looped:* Both ends of a bowel section are occluded, isolating it from the rest of the intestine.

In all three forms, the physiologic effects are similar: When intestinal obstruction occurs, fluid, air, and gas collect near the site. Peristalsis increases temporarily, as the bowel tries to force its contents through the obstruction, injuring intestinal mucosa and causing distention at and above the site of the obstruction. This distention blocks the flow of venous blood and halts normal absorptive processes. As a result, the bowel begins to secrete water, sodium, and potassium into the fluid pooled in the lumen. Obstruction in the upper intestine results in metabolic alkalosis from dehydration and loss of gastric hydrochloric acid; lower obstruction causes slower dehydration and loss of intestinal alkaline fluids, resulting in metabolic acidosis. Ultimately, intestinal obstruction may lead to ischemia, necrosis, and death.

Signs and symptoms

Colicky pain, nausea, vomiting, constipation, and abdominal distention characterize small bowel obstruction. It may also cause drowsiness, intense thirst, malaise, and aching, and may dry up oral mucous membranes and the tongue. Auscultation reveals bowel sounds, borborygmi, and rushes; occasionally, these are loud enough to be heard without a stethoscope. Palpation elicits abdominal tenderness, with moderate distention; rebound tenderness occurs when obstruction has caused strangulation with ischemia. In late stages, signs of hypovolemic shock result from progressive dehydration and plasma loss.

In complete upper intestinal (small bowel) obstruction, vigorous peristaltic waves propel bowel contents toward the mouth instead of the rectum. Spasms may occur every 3 to 5 minutes and last about 1 minute each, with persistent epigastric or periumbilical pain. Passage of small amounts of mucus and blood may occur. The higher the obstruction, the earlier and more severe the vomiting. Vomitus initially contains gastric juice, then bile, and finally fecal contents of the ileum.

Symptoms of large bowel obstruction develop more slowly, because the colon can absorb fluid from its contents and distend well beyond its normal size. Constipation may be the only clinical effect for days. Colicky abdominal pain may then appear suddenly, producing spasms that last less than 1 minute each and recur every few minutes. Continuous hypogastric pain and nausea may develop, but vomiting is usually absent at first. Large bowel obstruction can cause dramatic abdominal distention: loops of large bowel may become visible on the abdomen. Eventually, complete large bowel obstruction may cause fecal vomiting, continuous pain, or localized peritonitis.

Patients with partial obstruction may display any of the above symptoms in a milder form. However, leakage of liquid stool around the obstruction is common in partial obstruction.

Diagnosis

Progressive, colicky, abdominal pain and distention, with or without nausea and vomiting, suggest bowel obstruction; X-rays confirm it. Abdominal films show the presence and location of intestinal gas or fluid. In small bowel obstruction, a typical "stepladder" pattern emerges, with alternating fluid and gas levels apparent in 3 to 4 hours. In large bowel obstruction, barium enema reveals a distended, air-filled colon or a closed loop of sigmoid with extreme distention (in sigmoid volvulus).

PARALYTIC (ADYNAMIC) ILEUS

Paralytic ileus is a physiologic form of intestinal obstruction that usually develops in the small bowel after abdominal surgery. It causes decreased or absent intestinal motility that usually disappears spontaneously after 2 to 3 days. This condition can develop as a response to trauma, toxemia, or peritonitis, or as a result of electrolyte deficiencies (especially hypokalemia) and the use of certain drugs, such as ganglionic blocking agents and anticholinergics. It can also result from vascular causes, such as thrombosis or embolism. Excessive air swallowing may contribute to it, but paralytic ileus brought on by this factor alone seldom lasts more than 24 hours.

Clinical effects of paralytic ileus include severe abdominal distention, extreme distress, and possibly, vomiting. The patient may be severely constipated or may pass flatus and small, liquid stools. Paralytic ileus lasting longer than 48 hours necessitates intubation for decompression and nasogastric suctioning. Because of the absence of peristaltic activity, a weighted Cantor tube may be necessary in the patient with extraordinary abdominal distention. However, such procedures must be used with extreme caution, because any additional trauma to the bowel can aggravate ileus. When paralytic ileus results from surgical manipulation of the bowel, treatment may also include cholinergic agents, such as neostigmine or bethanechol.

When caring for patients with paralytic ileus, a hospital staff member should warn those receiving cholinergic agents to expect side effects, such as intestinal cramps and diarrhea, and remember that neostigmine produces cardiovascular side effects, usually bradycardia and hypotension. The staffer must check for returning bowel sounds.

Laboratory results supporting this diagnosis include:
- decreased sodium, chloride, and potassium levels (due to vomiting)
- slightly elevated WBC (with necrosis, peritonitis, or strangulation)

• increased serum amylase level (possibly from irritation of pancreas by bowel loop).

Treatment

Preoperative therapy consists of correction of fluid and electrolyte imbalances, decompression of the bowel to relieve vomiting and distention, and treatment of shock and peritonitis. Strangulated obstruction usually necessitates blood replacement as well as I.V. fluid administration. Passage of a Levin tube, followed by use of the longer and weighted Miller-Abbott tube, usually accomplishes decompression, especially in small bowel obstruction. Close monitoring of the patient's condition determines duration of treatment; if the patient fails to improve or his condition deteriorates, surgery is necessary. In large bowel obstruction, surgical resection with anastomosis, colostomy, or ileostomy commonly follows decompression with a Levin tube.

Hyperalimentation may be appropriate if the patient suffers a protein deficit from chronic obstruction, postoperative or paralytic ileus, or infection. Drug therapy includes analgesics or sedatives, such as meperidine or phenobarbital (but not opiates, since they inhibit GI motility), and antibiotics for peritonitis caused by strangulation or infarction of the bowel.

Additional considerations

Effective management of intestinal obstruction, a life-threatening condition that often causes overwhelming pain and distress, requires skillful supportive care and keen observation.

• Vital signs must be monitored and the patient observed for signs of shock (pallor, rapid pulse, and hypotension). A drop in blood pressure may indicate reduced circulating blood volume due to blood loss from a strangulated hernia. Also, as much as 10 liters of fluid can collect in the small bowel, drastically reducing plasma volume.

• The patient may slow signs of metabolic alkalosis (changes in sensorium, slow, shallow respirations, hypertonic muscles, tetany) or acidosis (shortness of breath on exertion, disorientation, and later, deep, rapid breathing, weakness, and malaise), or possibly, secondary infection (fever, chills).

• Urinary output must be monitored carefully to assess renal function, circulating blood volume, and possible urinary retention due to bladder compression by the distended intestine. If bladder compression is suspected the patient should be catheterized for residual urine immediately after he has voided. Progressive distention can be detected by frequently measuring abdominal girth.

• Fastidious mouth and nose care is necessary if the patient has undergone decompression by intubation or vomited. He should be watched for signs of dehydration (thick, swollen tongue, dry, cracked lips and dry oral mucous membranes). Amount and color of drainage from the decompression tube should be recorded. If necessary, the tube should be irrigated with normal saline solution to maintain patency. If a weighted tube has been inserted, it must be checked periodically to make sure it's advancing. Turning the patient from side to side (or walking around, if he can) will facilitate passage of the tube.

• The patient should stay in Fowler's position as much as possible to promote pulmonary ventilation and ease respiratory distress from abdominal distention. He should be periodically checked for bowel sounds and signs of returning peristalsis (passage of flatus and mucus through the rectum).

• The patient must understand all diagnostic and therapeutic procedures, and that they are necessary to relieve the obstruction and reduce pain. The patient should lie on his left side for about a half hour before X-rays are taken. He and his family should be prepared for the possibility of surgery, and given emotional support and positive reinforcement afterward. The patient with a colostomy should see an enterostomal therapist.

Inguinal Hernia
(Rupture)

A hernia occurs when part of an internal organ protrudes through an abnormal opening in the containing wall of its cavity. Most hernias occur in the abdominal cavity. Although many kinds of abdominal hernias are possible, inguinal hernias are most common. In an inguinal hernia, the large or small intestine, omentum, or bladder protrudes into the inguinal canal. Hernias can be reducible (if the hernia can be manipulated back into place with relative ease), incarcerated (if the hernia can't be reduced because adhesions have formed in the hernial sac), or strangulated (part of the herniated intestine becomes twisted or edematous, seriously interfering with normal blood flow and peristalsis, and possibly leading to intestinal obstruction and necrosis).

Causes and incidence

An inguinal hernia may be indirect or direct. An indirect inguinal hernia, the more common form, results from weakness in the fascial margin of the internal inguinal ring. In an indirect hernia, abdominal viscera leave the abdomen through the inguinal ring and follow the spermatic cord (in males) or round ligament (in females); they emerge at the external ring and extend down the inguinal canal, often into the scrotum or labia. An indirect inguinal hernia may develop at any age, is three times more common in males, and is especially prevalent in infants under age 1.

Direct inguinal hernia results from a weakness in the fascial floor of the inguinal canal. Instead of entering the canal through the internal ring, the hernia passes through the posterior inguinal wall, protrudes directly through the transverse fascia of the canal (in an area known as Hesselbach's triangle), and comes out at the external ring.

In males, during the seventh month of gestation, the testicle normally descends into the scrotum, preceded by the peritoneal sac. If the sac closes improperly, it leaves an opening through which the intestine can slip. In either sex, a hernia can result from weak abdominal muscles (caused by congenital malformation, trauma, or aging) or increased intra-abdominal pressure (due to heavy lifting, pregnancy, obesity, or straining).

Signs and symptoms

Inguinal hernia usually causes a lump to appear over the herniated area when the patient stands or strains. The lump disappears when the patient is supine. Tension on the herniated contents may cause a sharp, steady pain in the groin, which fades when the hernia is reduced. Strangulation produces severe pain, and may lead to partial or complete bowel obstruction and even intestinal necrosis. Partial bowel obstruction may cause anorexia, vomiting, pain and tenderness in the groin, an irreducible mass, and diminished bowel sounds. Complete obstruction may cause shock, high fever, absent bowel sounds, and bloody stools. In an infant, an inguinal hernia often coexists with an undescended testicle or a hydrocele.

Diagnosis

In a patient with a large hernia, physical examination reveals an obvious swelling or lump in the inguinal area. In the patient with a small hernia, the affected area may simply appear full. Palpation of the inguinal area while the patient is performing Valsalva's maneuver confirms the diagnosis. To detect a hernia in a male patient, the patient is asked to stand with his ipsilateral leg slightly flexed and his weight resting on the other leg. The examiner inserts an index finger into the lower part of the scrotum and invaginates the scrotal skin so the finger

COMMON SITES OF HERNIA

• *Umbilical hernia* results from abnormal muscular structures around the umbilical cord. This hernia is quite common in newborns but also occurs in women who are obese or who have had several pregnancies. Since most umbilical hernias in infants close spontaneously, surgery is warranted only if the hernia persists for more than 4 or 5 years. Taping or binding the affected area or supporting it with a truss may relieve symptoms until the hernia closes. Severe congenital umbilical hernia allows the abdominal viscera to protrude outside the body. This condition necessitates immediate repair.

• *Incisional (ventral) hernia* develops at the site of previous surgery, usually along vertical incisions. This hernia may result from a weakness in the abdominal wall, perhaps as a result of an infection or impaired wound healing. Inadequate nutrition, extreme abdominal distention, or obesity also predispose to incisional hernia. Palpation of an incisional hernia may reveal several defects in the surgical scar. Effective repair requires pulling the layers of the abdominal wall together without creating tension. If this isn't possible, surgical reconstruction uses Teflon, Marlex mesh, or tantalum mesh to close the opening.

• *Inguinal hernia* can be direct or indirect. Indirect inguinal hernia causes the abdominal viscera to protrude through the inguinal ring and follow the spermatic cord (in males); or round ligament (in females). Direct inguinal hernia results from a weakness in the fascial floor of the inguinal canal.

• *Femoral hernia* occurs where the femoral artery passes into the femoral canal. Typically, a fatty deposit within the femoral canal enlarges and eventually creates a hole big enough to accommodate part of the peritoneum and bladder. A femoral hernia appears as a swelling or bulge at the pulse point of the large femoral artery. It's usually a soft, pliable, reducible, nontender mass, but often becomes incarcerated or strangulated.

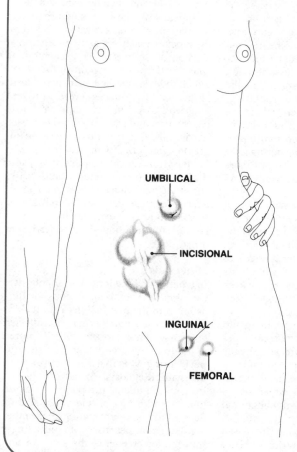

UMBILICAL

INCISIONAL

INGUINAL

FEMORAL

advances through the external inguinal ring to the internal ring (about 1½" to 2" [4 to 5 cm] through the inguinal canal). The patient is then told to cough. If the examiner feels pressure against the fingertip, an indirect hernia exists; if pressure is felt against the side of the finger, a direct hernia exists.

Patient history of sharp or "catching" pain when lifting or straining may help confirm the diagnosis. Suspected bowel obstruction requires X-rays and a WBC count (may be elevated).

Treatment

If the hernia is reducible, the pain may be temporarily relieved by pushing the hernia back into place. A truss may keep the abdominal contents from protruding into the hernial sac, although it won't cure the hernia. This device is especially beneficial for an elderly or debilitated patient, since any surgery is potentially hazardous to him.

For infants, adults, and otherwise healthy elderly patients, herniorrhaphy is the treatment of choice. Herniorrhaphy replaces the contents of the hernial sac into the abdominal cavity and closes the opening. This procedure is often performed under local anesthestic in a short-term unit, or as a single-day admission. Another effective surgical procedure for repairing hernia is hernioplasty, which reinforces the weakened area with steel mesh, fascia, or wire.

A strangulated or necrotic hernia necessitates bowel resection. Rarely, an extensive resection may require temporary colostomy. In either case, bowel resection lengthens postoperative recovery and requires massive doses of antibiotics, parenteral fluids, and electrolyte replacements.

Additional considerations

A truss is applied only after a hernia has been reduced. For best results, it should be applied in the morning, before the patient gets out of bed.

To prevent skin irritation, the patient should bathe daily and apply liberal amounts of cornstarch or baby powder.

He should not apply the truss over clothing, since this reduces the effectiveness of the truss and may make it slip.

Any signs of incarceration and strangulation should be reported immediately. Trying to reduce an incarcerated hernia may result in bowel perforation. The doctor should be informed immediately if severe intestinal obstruction arises because of hernial strangulation. A nasogastric tube may be inserted promptly to empty the stomach and relieve pressure on the hernial sac.

Health care before surgery includes:
• closely monitoring vital signs; administering I.V. fluids, and analgesics for pain; controlling fever with acetaminophen or tepid sponge baths; placing the patient in Trendelenburg position to reduce pressure on the hernia site.
• giving special reassurance and support to a child scheduled for hernia repair; encouraging him to ask questions, and answering them as simply as possible; offering appropriate diversions to distract him from the impending surgery.

Health care after surgery includes:
• making sure the patient voids within 8 to 12 hours; checking the incision and dressing at least three times a day for drainage, inflammation, or swelling; checking for normal bowel sounds and watching for fever.
• observing the patient carefully for postoperative scrotal swelling; supporting the scrotum with a rolled towel and applying an ice bag to reduce such swelling.
• encouraging fluid intake to maintain hydration and prevent constipation; teaching deep-breathing exercises, and showing the patient how to splint the incision before coughing.
• warning the patient before discharge against lifting or straining; telling him to watch for signs of infection (oozing, tenderness, warmth, redness) at the incision site, and to keep the incision clean and covered until the sutures are removed.
• advising the patient not to resume normal activity or return to work without the surgeon's permission.

Intussusception

Intussusception is a telescoping (invagination) of a portion of the bowel into an adjacent distal portion. Intussusception may be fatal, especially if treatment is delayed more than 24 hours.

Causes and incidence

Intussusception is most common in infants and occurs three times more often in males than in females; 87% of children with intussusception are under age 2; 70% of these children are between ages 4 and 11 months.

Studies suggest that intussusception may be linked to viral infections, since seasonal peaks are noted—in the spring-summer, coinciding with peak incidence of enteritis, and in the midwinter, coinciding with peak incidence of respiratory tract infections.

The cause of most cases of intussusception in infants is unknown. In older children, polyps, alterations in intestinal motility, hemangioma, lymphosarcoma, lymphoid hyperplasia, or Meckel's diverticulum may trigger the process. In

This barium study confirms retrograde intussusception following gastrojejunostomy by showing the characteristic "coiled spring" appearance caused by barium coating on the outer layers of the jejunum. Barium also outlines the stomach pouch.

adults, intussusception usually results from benign or malignant tumors (65% of patients). It may also result from polyps, Meckel's diverticulum, gastroenterostomy with herniation, or an appendiceal stump.

When a bowel segment (the intussusceptum) invaginates, peristalsis propels it along the bowel, pulling more bowel along with it; the receiving segment is the intussuscipiens. This invagination produces edema, hemorrhage from venous engorgement, incarceration, and obstruction. If treatment is delayed for longer than 24 hours, strangulation of the intestine usually occurs, with gangrene, shock, and perforation.

Signs and symptoms

In an infant or child, intussusception produces four cardinal clinical effects:
• *intermittent attacks of colicky pain,* which cause the child to scream, draw his legs up to his abdomen, turn pale and diaphoretic, and possibly, display grunting respirations
• initially, *vomiting of stomach contents;* later, of bile-stained or fecal material
• *"currant jelly" stools,* which contain a mixture of blood and mucus
• *tender, distended abdomen, with a palpable, sausage-shaped abdominal mass;* often, the viscera are absent from the lower right quadrant.

In adults, intussusception produces nonspecific, chronic, and intermittent symptoms, including colicky abdominal pain and tenderness, vomiting, diarrhea (occasionally constipation), bloody stools, and weight loss. Abdominal pain usually localizes in the lower right quadrant, radiates to the back, and increases with eating. Adults with severe intussusception may develop strangulation with excruciating pain, abdominal distention, and tachycardia.

Diagnosis

 Barium enema confirms colonic intussusception when it shows the characteristic coiled spring sign; it also delineates the extent of intussusception. Upright abdominal X-rays may show a soft-tissue mass and signs of complete or partial obstruction, with dilated loops of bowel. WBC up to 15,000/mm³ indicates obstruction; greater than 15,000/mm³, strangulation; more than 20,000/mm³, bowel infarction should be considered.

Treatment

In children, therapy may include hydrostatic reduction or surgery. Surgery is indicated for children with recurrent intussusception, for those who show signs of shock or peritonitis, and for those in whom symptoms have been present longer than 24 hours. In adults, surgery is always the treatment of choice.

During hydrostatic reduction, the radiologist drips a barium solution into the rectum from a height of not more than 3' (0.9 m); fluoroscopy traces the progress of the barium. If the procedure is successful, the barium backwashes into the ileum, and the mass disappears. If not, the procedure is stopped, and the patient is prepared for surgery.

During surgery, manual reduction is attempted first. After compressing the bowel above the intussusception, the doctor attempts to milk the intussusception back through the bowel. However, if manual reduction fails, or if the bowel is gangrenous or strangulated, the doctor will perform a resection of the affected bowel segment. In addition, he'll probably perform a prophylactic appendectomy at this time.

Additional considerations

• Vital signs must be monitored before and after surgery. A change in temperature may indicate sepsis; infants may become hypothermic at onset of infection. Rising pulse rate and falling blood pressure may be signs of peritonitis.

• The patient should be watched for signs of dehydration and bleeding, and intake and output checked. If he is in shock, blood or plasma may be ordered.

• A nasogastric tube is inserted to decompress the intestine and minimize vomiting. Tube drainage should be monitored, and any lost fluids replaced.

• After surgery, broad-spectrum antibiotics may be ordered. Meticulous wound care must be given, even though most incisions heal without complications. The incision should be closely checked for inflammation, drainage, or suture separation.

• Turning the patient from side to side will encourage productive coughing. The incision should be splinted when he coughs, or he should be taught to do so himself. In addition, he should take 10 deep breaths an hour.

• Oral fluids may be resumed when bowel sounds and peristalsis return, nasogastric tube drainage is minimal, the abdomen remains soft, and vomiting does not occur when the nasogastric tube is clamped briefly for a trial period. When the patient tolerates oral fluids well, the tube can be removed and the patient's diet gradually returned to normal.

• After the patient resumes a normal diet he should be checked for abdominal distention, and his general condition monitored.

• The child and parents will need special reassurance and emotional support. This condition is considered a pediatric emergency, and parents are often unprepared for their child's hospitalization and possible surgery; they may feel guilty for not seeking medical aid when their child first began exhibiting symptoms. Similarly, the child is unprepared for an abrupt separation from his parents and familiar environment.

To minimize the stress of hospitalization, parents should be encouraged to participate in their child's care as much as possible. Flexible visiting hours will promote this participation.

Anomalies of Rotation and Fixation

In anomalies of rotation and fixation, the bowel fails to rotate and fixate within the abdominal cavity because of an arrest in embryonic development.

Causes and incidence

Anomalies of rotation result from faulty development in one of three embryonic stages. In the first stage, about the eighth week of gestation, the fetal midgut from the yolk sac should migrate through the umbilical ring into the peritoneal cavity and rotate 180° counterclockwise. If this process is impaired, the midgut and other organs (liver, stomach, spleen, and colon) remain in an umbilical sac as an omphalocele.

In the second stage, about the tenth to twelfth week of gestation, the midgut should return to the peritoneal cavity, rotating an additional 90° counterclockwise and coming to rest in the lower right quadrant. An arrest in the second stage of development may result in nonrotation, malrotation, or reverse rotation. In nonrotation, the midgut returns to the abdomen but doesn't rotate. In malrotation (most common in children), the midgut rotates incompletely, and the small bowel is supported on a slender mesentery and is very vulnerable to volvulus. In reverse rotation (rare), the midgut rotates 90° clockwise instead of counterclockwise; this can lead to volvulus of the right colon.

In the third stage, between the twelfth week and the fifth month, the duodenum, descending colon, and mesentery of the small bowel should attach to the posterior abdominal wall, and the cecum descend to its normal position in the lower right quadrant. Failure to do so may produce retroperitoneal bands that stretch across the duodenum.

Signs and symptoms

The clinical effects of anomalies of rotation and fixation usually result from obstruction or vascular compression. Symptoms vary according to the patient's age and may not appear until later in life. When symptoms appear in infancy, they usually begin in the first week of life, with bile-stained vomiting, upper abdominal distention, and visible peristaltic waves. In midgut volvulus, complete obstruction (no stools) and vascular compression may result in strangulation and shock. In older children, obstruction can be partial, with intermittent, bile-stained vomiting. In reverse rotation, signs include colon obstruction and bowel incarceration. Adults may have no symptoms, intermittent chronic symptoms (dyspepsia and distention), or acute abdominal distention and vomiting. In all age-groups, such anomalies predispose the patient to intestinal herniation.

Diagnosis

Signs of abdominal obstruction, distention, and incarceration may suggest volvulus. X-rays are required to confirm it. Abdominal X-rays show abnormal air-fluid levels. Contrast studies (barium enema or swallow, upper GI series) locate the level of obstruction, identify abnormal portions of the intestinal tract, and reveal any enlargement and dilation.

Treatment and additional considerations

Surgery is the primary treatment, and includes lysis of peritoneal bands, and the proper placement and stabilization of the cecum, ileum, and small bowel. Hyperalimentation may be necessary following resection, particularly in infants, to rest the intestinal tract and allow for nutritional adaption.

After surgery to correct the anomaly, the health care professional should:
• monitor vital signs, watching especially for changes in temperature (a sign of sepsis), and rising pulse rate and fall-

ing blood pressure (signs of shock); check fluid intake and output, electrolytes, and CBC; record amount of drainage from the nasogastric tube and drains; replace lost volume with saline solution, as ordered.

• promote coughing and deep breathing; position the infant to prevent aspiration, and suction, as needed.

• keep dressings clean and dry; record any excessive or unusual drainage; check for incisional inflammation and separation of sutures.

• begin oral feedings with clear liquids, as ordered, usually when bowel sounds and peristalsis return; clamp the nasogastric tube, before removing it, for a trial period and watch for abdominal distention; when appropriate, slowly add solid foods to the patient's diet.

• offer reassurance and support to the patient and family, and explain all diagnostic tests and procedures; if the patient is a child, encourage parents to participate in his care to help minimize the stress of hospitalization.

Volvulus

Volvulus is a twisting of the intestine at least 180° on its mesentery, which results in blood vessel compression.

Causes and incidence
In volvulus, twisting may result from an anomaly of rotation, an ingested foreign body, or an adhesion; in some cases, however, the cause is unknown. Volvulus usually occurs in a bowel segment with a mesentery long enough to twist. The most common area, particularly in adults, is the sigmoid; the small bowel is a common site in children. Other common sites include the stomach and cecum. Volvulus can occur in patients with cystic fibrosis.

Signs and symptoms
Vomiting and rapid, marked abdominal distention follow sudden onset of severe abdominal pain. Without immediate treatment, volvulus can lead to strangulation of the twisted bowel loop, ischemia, infarction, perforation, and fatal peritonitis.

Diagnosis
Sudden onset of severe abdominal pain, and physical examination that may reveal a palpable mass suggest volvulus. Appropriate special tests include:

• *X-rays:* Abdominal X-rays may show obstruction and abnormal air-fluid levels in the sigmoid and cecum; in midgut

volvulus, abdominal X-rays may be normal.

• *Barium enema:* In cecal volvulus, barium fills the colon distal to the section of cecum; in sigmoid volvulus in children, barium may twist to a point, and in adults, barium may take on an "ace of spades" configuration.

• *Upper GI series:* In midgut volvulus, obstruction and possibly a twisted contour show in a narrow area near the duodenojejunal junction, where barium will not pass.

• *WBC:* In strangulation, the count is greater than $15,000/mm^3$; in bowel infarction, greater than $20,000/mm^3$.

Treatment and additional considerations
Treatment varies according to the severity and location of the volvulus. For children with midgut volvulus, treatment is surgical. For adults with sigmoid volvulus, nonsurgical treatment includes proctoscopy to check for infarction, and reduction by careful insertion of a sigmoidoscope or a long rectal tube to deflate the bowel. Success of nonsurgical reduction is indicated by expulsion of gas and immediate relief of abdominal pain. For all types of volvulus, if the

bowel is distended but viable, surgery consists of detorsion (untwisting); if the bowel is necrotic, surgery includes resection and anastomosis. Prolonged hyperalimentation and I.V. antibiotics are usually necessary. Occasionally, sedatives are needed.

After surgical correction of volvulus, the hospital staff member should:
• monitor vital signs, watching for temperature changes (a sign of sepsis), and a rapid pulse rate and falling blood pressure (signs of shock and peritonitis); monitor fluid intake and output (including stool), electrolytes, and CBC; measure and record drainage from nasogastric tube and drains.
• encourage frequent coughing and deep breathing; turn and reposition the patient often, and suction him, as needed.
• keep dressings clean and dry; record any excessive or unusual drainage; later, check for incisional inflammation and separation of sutures.
• begin oral feedings with clear liquids, as ordered, when bowel sounds and peristalsis return; clamp the nasogastric tube for a trial period before removing it and watch for abdominal distention; gradually expand the diet when solid food can be tolerated; reassure the patient and family, and explain all diagnostic procedures. If the patient is a child, parents should be encouraged to participate in their child's care to minimize the stress of hospitalization.

Hirschsprung's Disease
(Congenital megacolon, congenital aganglionic megacolon)

Hirschsprung's disease is a congenital disorder of the large intestine, characterized by absence or marked reduction of parasympathetic ganglion cells in the colorectal wall. This disorder impairs intestinal motility and causes severe, intractable constipation. Without prompt treatment, an infant with colonic obstruction may die within 24 hours from enterocolitis that leads to severe diarrhea and hypovolemic shock. With prompt treatment, prognosis is good.

Causes and incidence
In Hirschsprung's disease, the aganglionic bowel segment contracts without the reciprocal relaxation needed to propel feces forward. In 90% of patients, this aganglionic segment is in the rectosigmoid area, but it occasionally extends to the entire colon and parts of the small intestine.

Hirschsprung's disease is believed to be a familial, congenital defect, and occurs in 1 in 2,000 to 1 in 5,000 live births. It's up to seven times more common in males than in females (although the aganglionic segment is usually shorter in males than in females) and is more prevalent in Caucasians. Total aganglionosis affects both sexes equally. Females with Hirschsprung's disease are at higher risk of having affected children. This disease often coexists with other congenital anomalies, particularly trisomy 21 and anomalies of the urinary tract, such as megaloureter.

Signs and symptoms
Clinical effects usually appear shortly after birth, but mild symptoms may not be recognized until later in childhood, or during adolescence (usually) or adulthood (rarely). The newborn with Hirschsprung's disease commonly fails to pass meconium within 24 to 48 hours, shows signs of obstruction (bile-stained or fecal vomiting, abdominal distention), irritability, feeding difficulties (poor sucking, refusal to take feedings), failure to thrive, dehydration (pallor, loss of skin turgor, sunken eyes), and overflow diarrhea. The infant may also exhibit abdominal distention that causes rapid breathing, and grunting. Rectal exami-

nation reveals a rectum empty of stool and, when the examining finger is withdrawn, an explosive gush of malodorous gas and liquid stool. Such examination may temporarily relieve GI symptoms. In infants, the main cause of death is enterocolitis, caused by fecal stagnation that leads to bacterial overgrowth, intestinal irritation, profuse diarrhea, hypovolemic shock, and perforation.

The older child has intractable constipation (usually requiring laxatives and enemas), abdominal distention, and easily palpated fecal masses. In severe cases, failure to grow is characterized by wasted extremities and loss of subcutaneous tissue, with a large protuberant abdomen.

Adult megacolon (rare) usually affects men. The patient has abdominal distention, rectal bleeding (rare), and a history of chronic intermittent constipation. He is generally in poor physical condition.

Diagnosis

 Rectal biopsy provides definitive diagnosis by showing absence of ganglion cells. Suction aspiration using a small tube inserted into the rectum may be performed initially. If findings of suction aspiration are inconclusive, diagnosis requires full-thickness surgical biopsy under general anesthetic. In older infants, barium enema showing a narrowed segment of distal colon with a sawtooth appearance and a funnel-shaped segment above it confirms the diagnosis and assesses the extent of intestinal involvement. Significantly, infants with Hirschsprung's disease retain barium longer than the usual 12 to 24 hours, so delayed films are often helpful when other characteristic signs are absent. Other tests include rectal manometry, which detects failure of the internal anal sphincter to relax and contract, and upright plain films of the abdomen, which show marked colonic distention.

Treatment

Surgical treatment involves pulling the normal ganglionic segment through to the anus. However, such corrective surgery is usually delayed until the infant is at least 10 months old and better able to withstand it. Management of an infant until the time of surgery consists of daily colonic lavage to empty the bowel. If total obstruction is present in the newborn, a temporary colostomy or ileostomy is necessary to decompress the colon. A preliminary bowel prep with an antibiotic, such as neomycin or nystatin, is necessary before surgery. The surgical technique used is based on the three main corrective procedures: the Duhamel, Soave, or Swenson pull-through procedure.

Additional considerations

Before emergency decompression surgery, the hospital staff member should:
• maintain fluid and electrolyte balance, and prevent shock; provide adequate nutrition (by hyperalimentation, if necessary), and hydrate with I.V. fluids, as needed. Transfusions may be necessary to correct shock or dehydration. Respiratory distress can be relieved by keeping the patient upright.

After colostomy or ileostomy, the staff member should:
• place the infant in a heated incubator, with the temperature set at 98° to 99° F. (36.7° to 37.2° C.), or in a radiant warmer; monitor vital signs, watching for sepsis and enterocolitis (increased respiratory rate with abdominal distention).
• carefully monitor and record fluid intake and output (including drainage from ileostomy or colostomy), and electrolytes (ileostomy is especially likely to cause excessive electrolyte loss); also, measure and record nasogastric drainage, and replace fluids and electrolytes, as ordered; check stools carefully for excess water—a sign of fluid loss.
• check urine for specific gravity, glucose (hyperalimentation may lead to osmotic diuresis), and blood.
• turn and reposition the patient often to prevent aspiration pneumonia and skin breakdown; suction the nasopharynx frequently.

• keep the area around the stoma clean and dry, and cover it with dressings, or a colostomy or ileostomy appliance to absorb drainage; use aseptic technique until the wound heals; watch for prolapse, discoloration, or excessive bleeding (slight bleeding is common); to prevent excoriation, use a powder such as karaya gum or a protective stoma disk.

• begin oral feeding when bowel sounds return (an infant may tolerate predigested formulas best).

• teach parents to recognize the signs of fluid loss and dehydration (decreased urinary output, sunken eyes, poor skin turgor), and enterocolitis (sudden marked abdominal distention, vomiting, diarrhea, fever, lethargy).

• before discharge, make sure the parents consult with an enterostomal therapist, for valuable tips for colostomy and ileostomy care.

Before corrective surgery, the staffer should:

• at least once a day, perform colonic lavage with normal saline solution to evacuate the colon, since ordinary enemas and laxatives won't clean it adequately; keep accurate records of how much lavage solution is instilled; repeat lavage until the return solution is completely free of fecal particles.

• administer antibiotics for bowel prep, as ordered.

After corrective surgery, the staffer should:

• keep the wound clean and dry, and check for significant inflammation (some inflammation is normal); avoid using a rectal thermometer or suppository until the wound has healed. After 3 to 4 days, the infant will have a first bowel movement, a liquid stool, which will probably create discomfort. The number of stools must be recorded.

• check urine for blood, especially in a boy—extensive surgical manipulation may cause bladder trauma.

• watch for signs of anastomic leaks (sudden development of abdominal distention unrelieved by gastric aspiration, temperature spike, and extreme irritability), which may lead to pelvic abscess.

• begin oral feedings with clear fluids, increasing bulk as tolerated, when active bowel sounds begin and nasogastric drainage decreases. As an additional check, the nasogastric tube can be clamped for brief, intermittent periods. If abdominal distention develops, the patient isn't ready to begin oral feedings.

• instruct parents to watch for foods that increase the number of stools and to avoid offering these foods; reassure them that their child will probably gain sphincter control and be able to eat a normal diet but warn that complete continence may take several years to develop and constipation may recur at times.

Because an infant with Hirschsprung's disease needs surgery and hospitalization so early in life, parents have difficulty establishing an emotional bond with their child. To promote bonding, they should be encouraged to participate in their child's care as much as possible.

Inactive Colon

(Lazy colon, colonic stasis, atonic constipation)

Inactive colon is a state of chronic constipation that, if untreated, may lead to fecal impaction. It's common in elderly persons and invalids because of their inactivity.

Causes

Inactive colon usually results from some deficiency in the three elements necessary for normal bowel activity: dietary bulk, fluid intake, and exercise. Other causes include habitual disregard of the impulse to defecate, emotional conflicts, chronic use of laxatives, or prolonged dependence on enemas, which dull rectal sensitivity to the presence of feces.

Inactive colon may also occur secondary to hypothyroidism, stricture, or neoplastic obstruction.

Signs and symptoms
The primary symptom of inactive colon is chronic constipation. The patient often strains to produce hard, dry, stools; such effort is accompanied by mild abdominal discomfort. Straining can aggravate preexisting rectal conditions, such as hemorrhoids.

Diagnosis
A patient history of dry, hard, infrequent stools suggests inactive colon. A digital rectal examination reveals stool in the lower portion of the rectum and a palpable colon. Proctoscopy may show an unusually small colon lumen, prominent veins, and an abnormal amount of mucus. Tests to rule out other causes include upper GI series, barium enema, and examination of stool for occult blood from neoplasms.

Treatment
Treatment varies according to the patient's age and condition. A higher bulk diet, sufficient exercise, and increased fluid intake often relieve constipation. Treatment for severe constipation may include bulk-forming laxatives, such as psyllium, or well-lubricated glycerin suppositories; for fecal impaction, manual removal of feces is necessary. Administration of an oil-retention enema usually precedes feces removal; an enema is also necessary afterward. For lasting relief of constipation, the patient with inactive colon must modify bowel habits.

Additional considerations
Patient education can help break the constipation habit. The patient should:
• drink at least eight to ten glasses of liquid every day (particularly important in the older patient), since fluids help keep the intestinal contents in a semisolid state for easier passage. The patient should stimulate the bowel with a drink of hot or cold water—plain or with lemon—or prune juice before breakfast

or in the evening.
• add fiber to the diet with foods such as whole grain cereals (rolled oats, bran, oatmeal) to contribute bulk and induce peristalsis. However, too much bran can create an irritable bowel, so the patient should check labels on foods for fiber content (low fiber—0.3 to 1 g; moderate fiber—1.1 to 2 g; high fiber—2.1 to 4.2 g). Bulk content of the diet should be increased slowly to prevent flatulence, which is sometimes a transient effect of a high-bulk diet.
• use fat-containing foods, such as bacon, butter, cream, and oil, in moderation, since they will help to soften intestinal contents but sometimes cause diarrhea.
• avoid highly refined foods, such as white rice, cream of wheat, farina, white pastries, pie or cake, macaroni, spaghetti, noodles, and ice cream.
• rest at least 6 hours every night.
• incorporate moderate exercise, such as walking, into the daily routine.
• avoid overuse of laxatives, and maintain a regular time for bowel movements (usually after breakfast). Autosuggestion, relaxation, and use of a small footstool to promote thigh flexion while sitting on the toilet may be helpful. The patient should respond promptly to the urge to defecate. If he worries about constipation, he can be reassured that a 2- to 3-day interval between bowel movements can be normal.
• take bulk-forming laxatives, such as psyllium, with at least 8 oz (240 ml) of liquid. Juices, soft drinks, or other pleasant-tasting liquids help mask this drug's grittiness.
  If the patient with inactive colon is hospitalized, some special supportive measures are needed.
  The elderly patient should be assisted to a bedside commode for a bowel movement, since using a bedpan causes additional strain. However, if the patient must use a bedpan, he should sit in Fowler's position, or on the pan at the side of his bed, to facilitate elimination. Occasional digital rectal stimulation or abdominal massage near the sigmoid area

may help stimulate a bowel movement. *Caution:* If the patient has a history of arteriosclerosis, congestive heart failure, or hypertension, constipation and straining may induce a "bathroom coronary" or a cerebrovascular accident.

Enemas should not be overused, since they may cause dependence. If the patient requires enemas, sodium biphosphate enema must not be used too often. Its hypertonic solution can absorb as much as 10% of the colon's sodium content or draw intestinal fluids into the colon, causing dehydration.

Pancreatitis

Pancreatitis, inflammation of the pancreas, occurs in acute and chronic forms and may be due to edema, necrosis, or hemorrhage. In men, this disease is commonly associated with alcoholism, trauma, or peptic ulcer; in women, with biliary tract disease. Prognosis is good when pancreatitis follows biliary tract disease but poor when it follows alcoholism. Mortality rises as high as 60% when pancreatitis is associated with necrosis and hemorrhage.

Causes

The most common causes of pancreatitis are biliary tract disease and alcoholism, but it can also result from pancreatic carcinoma, trauma (blunt, penetrating, or surgical), or use of certain drugs, such as glucocorticoids, sulfonamides, chlorothiazide, and azathioprine. This disease also may develop as a complication of peptic ulcer (especially duodenal), mumps, or hypothermia. Rarer causes include stenosis or obstruction of the sphincter of Oddi, hyperlipemia, metabolic endocrine disorders (hyperparathyroidism, hemochromatosis), vasculitis or vascular disease, viral infections (such as coxsackievirus B), mycoplasmal pneumonia, and pregnancy.

Afro-Asian syndrome (diabetes, pancreatic insufficiency, and pancreatic calcification) occurs in young persons, probably from the combined effects of malnutrition and alcoholism, and leads to pancreatic atrophy. Regardless of the cause, the pathogenesis of pancreatitis involves autodigestion: the enzymes normally excreted by the pancreas (especially trypsin) digest pancreatic tissue.

Signs and symptoms

In many patients, the first and only symptom of mild pancreatitis is steady epigastric pain centered close to the umbilicus, radiating between the tenth thoracic and sixth lumbar vertebrae, and unrelieved by vomiting. However, a severe attack causes extreme pain, persistent vomiting, abdominal rigidity, diminished bowel activity (suggesting peritonitis), rales at lung bases, and left pleural effusion. Severe pancreatitis may produce extreme malaise and restlessness, with mottled skin, tachycardia, low-grade fever (100° to 102° F. [37.8° to 38.9° C.]), and cold, sweaty extremities. Proximity of the inflamed pancreas to the bowel may cause ileus.

If pancreatitis damages the islets of Langerhans, complications may include diabetes mellitus. Fulminant pancreatitis causes massive hemorrhage and total destruction of the pancreas, resulting in diabetic acidosis, shock, or coma.

Diagnosis

A careful patient history (especially for alcoholism) and physical examination are the first steps in diagnosis, but the retroperitoneal position of the pancreas makes physical assessment difficult.

 Dramatically elevated serum amylase levels—frequently over 500 units—confirm pancreatitis and rule out perforated peptic ulcer, acute cholecystitis, appendicitis, and bowel

infarction or obstruction. Similarly dramatic elevations of amylase also occur in urine, ascites, or pleural fluid. Characteristically, amylase levels return to normal 48 hours after onset of pancreatitis, despite continuing clinical manifestations. Supportive laboratory values include:
• increased serum lipase levels, which rise more slowly than serum amylase
• low serum calcium (hypocalcemia) from fat necrosis and formation of calcium soaps
• WBC counts range from 8,000 to 20,000/ mm³, with increased polymorphonuclear leukocytes
• elevated glucose levels—as high as 500 to 900 mg/100 ml, indicating hyperglycemia
• hematocrit occasionally exceeding 50% concentrations.

In addition, EKG changes (prolonged QT segment but normal T wave) help diagnose hypocalcemia. Abdominal X-rays show dilation of the small or large bowel, or calcification of the pancreas; GI series, extrinsic pressure on the duodenum or stomach due to edema of the pancreas head; chest X-rays show left-sided pleural effusion. I.V. cholangiography helps distinguish acute cholecystitis from acute pancreatitis. Analysis of abdominal fluid obtained by paracentesis may detect amylase levels as high as 7,000 units; in the patient with a perforated bowel, it may also detect bacteria or bile.

Treatment

Effective treatment must maintain circulation and fluid volume, relieve pain, and decrease pancreatic secretions. Emergency treatment for shock (the most common cause of death in early-stage pancreatitis) consists of vigorous I.V. replacement of electrolytes and proteins. Metabolic acidosis secondary to hypovolemia and impaired cellular perfusion requires vigorous fluid volume replacement.

Parenteral anticholinergics, such as atropine or propantheline, may reduce pancreatic activity but may also aggravate an associated ileus, and thus accelerate pancreatic deterioration.

Treatment may also include meperidine for pain (although it may cause spasm of the sphincter of Oddi); diazepam for restlessness and agitation; and antibiotics, such as gentamicin, clindamycin, or chloramphenicol, for bacterial infections. Hypocalcemia requires infusion of 10% calcium gluconate; serum glucose levels greater than 300 to 350 mg/100 ml require insulin therapy.

After the emergency phase, continuing I.V. therapy should provide adequate electrolytes and protein solutions that don't stimulate the pancreas (glucose or free amino acids), for 5 to 7 days. If the patient is not ready to resume oral feedings by then, hyperalimentation may be necessary. Nonstimulating elemental

---

CHRONIC PANCREATITIS

Chronic pancreatitis is usually associated with alcoholism (in over half of all patients), but can also follow hyperparathyroidism, hyperlipemia, or infrequently, gallstones, trauma, or peptic ulcer. Inflammation and fibrosis cause progressive pancreatic insufficiency and eventually destroy the pancreas. Symptoms of chronic pancreatitis include constant dull pain with occasional exacerbations, malabsorption, severe weight loss, and hyperglycemia (leading to diabetic symptoms). Relevant diagnostic measures include patient history, X-rays showing pancreatic calcification, elevated ESR, and examination of stool for steatorrhea.

The severe pain of chronic pancreatitis often requires large doses of analgesics or narcotics, making addiction a serious problem. Treatment also includes a low-fat diet and oral administration of pancreatic enzymes, such as pancreatin or pancrelipase to control steatorrhea, insulin or oral hypoglycemics to curb hyperglycemia, and occasionally, surgical repair of biliary or pancreatic ducts, or the sphincter of Oddi to reduce pressure and promote the flow of pancreatic juice. Prognosis is good if the patient can avoid alcohol; poor if he can't.

ANATOMY OF THE PANCREAS

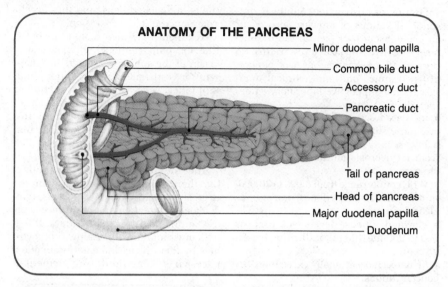

- Minor duodenal papilla
- Common bile duct
- Accessory duct
- Pancreatic duct
- Tail of pancreas
- Head of pancreas
- Major duodenal papilla
- Duodenum

gavage feedings may be safer because of the decreased risk of infection and overinfusion. In extreme cases, laparotomy to drain the pancreatic bed, 95% pancreatectomy, or a combination of cholecystostomy-gastrostomy, feeding jejunostomy, and drainage may be necessary.

Additional considerations

Acute pancreatitis is a life-threatening emergency. A care plan should emphasize meticulous supportive care and continuous monitoring of the patient's vital systems, such as:
- monitoring vital signs and pulmonary artery pressure closely; if the patient has a central venous pressure line instead of a pulmonary artery catheter, monitoring it closely for volume expansion (it shouldn't rise above 10 cmH$_2$O); giving plasma or albumin, if ordered, to maintain blood pressure; carefully recording fluid intake and output; checking urine output hourly, and monitoring electrolyte levels; assessing for rales, rhonchi, or decreased breath sounds.
- for bowel decompression, maintaining constant nasogastric suctioning, and giving nothing by mouth; performing good mouth and nose care.
- staying alert for signs of calcium deficiency—tetany, muscle cramps, carpopedal spasm, and convulsions; keeping airway and suction apparatus handy, and keeping side rails padded in suspected cases of hypocalcemia.
- administering analgesics, as needed, to relieve pain and anxiety; remembering that anticholinergics reduce salivary and sweat gland secretions; warning the patient that he may experience dry mouth and facial flushing (*caution:* Narrow-angle glaucoma contraindicates the use of atropine or its derivatives).
- watching for adverse reactions to antibiotics, such as nephrotoxicity with gentamicin, pseudomembranous enterocolitis with clindamycin, and blood dyscrasias with chloramphenicol.
- not confusing thirst due to hyperglycemia (indicated by serum glucose levels as high as 350 mg/100 ml, and sugar and acetone in urine) with dry mouth due to nasogastric intubation and effects of anticholinergics.
- watching for complications due to hyperalimentation, such as sepsis, hypokalemia, overhydration, and metabolic acidosis; watching for fever, cardiac irregularities, changes in arterial blood gas measurements, and deep respirations; using strict aseptic technique when caring for the catheter insertion site.

Intestinal Lymphangiectasia

Intestinal lymphangiectasia is dilation and possible rupture of the intestinal lymphatic vessels, resulting in hypoproteinemia and steatorrhea due to loss of fat and albumin into the intestinal lumen. This uncommon, chronic, and usually mild disease develops most often before age 30.

Causes

Lymphangiectasia may be a congenital anomaly, or it may be acquired as a result of increased pressure in the lymphatics from obstruction, valvular heart disease, or constrictive pericarditis.

Signs and symptoms

Patients with intestinal lymphangiectasia have massive edema due to excessive enteric protein loss; such a loss probably occurs when plasma proteins cross the tissue barrier due to damaged intestinal mucosa, or when enlarged lymph vessels rupture and discharge protein into the intestinal lumen. The resulting edema is intermittent at first but later becomes chronic. Typically, such edema is present in both hands; it may lead to ascites and hydrothorax, perhaps related to effusion into serous cavities. Gradually, recurrent diarrhea and steatorrhea develop. Lymphocytopenia is common, and is associated with delayed hypersensitivity reactions, such as impaired cutaneous response to antigens like mumps virus. Other clinical effects include hypocalcemia and impaired vitamin B_{12} absorption.

Diagnosis

Dilated and telangiectatic lymphatic vessels on jejunal biopsy confirm intestinal lymphangiectasia. Other tests and procedures that support this diagnosis include:

• *lymphangiography:* dilation of the peripheral and visceral lymphatics and absent groups of retroperitoneal lymph nodes
• *X-rays of the small bowel:* thickened jejunal folds, mucosal edema, and a malabsorption pattern
• *blood studies:* lymphocytopenia (400 to 1,000/mm³); hypoproteinemia (extremely low serum albumin and gamma globulin levels; IgA and IgG components severely depressed; IgM reduced); hypocholesterolemia (less than 150 mg); and hypocalcemia (less than 9 mg)
• *stool studies:* increased stool fat; increased degradation rate of I.V. radioactive serum albumin on radioactive excretion tests (decreased half life of I-labeled albumin).

In young children, diagnosis should also include echocardiography to rule out constrictive pericarditis, a curable cause of secondary intestinal lymphangiectasia.

Treatment

Elimination of fat from the diet decreases lymph flow and consequent loss of protein, calcium, and albumin. Treatment may also include replacement of dietary sources of long-chain triglycerides with medium-chain triglycerides. These are transported as medium-chain fatty acids through the portal vein rather than the lymphatic system. Consequently, they prevent fat overload in the lymphatic channels and dramatically improve ascites and edema.

Patients with impaired vitamin B_{12} absorption may need supplementary B_{12} injections.

Additional considerations

• Medium-chain triglycerides should be administered in frequent, small doses to minimize GI side effects, such as nausea, vomiting, and diarrhea. Mixing with fruit juice or in salad dressing will make them more palatable. Medium-chain triglycerides are easier to absorb than long-chain fatty acids, so they're a source of quick energy.

• The patient should fully understand the nature of this disorder, especially if he has steatorrhea. In this case stool may be bulky, foamy, greasy, gray, and foul-smelling (depending on the degree of steatorrhea) until treatment fully corrects the disorder.

• The patient should watch for signs of continued malnutrition (weakness, weight loss, and general lack of well-being), which may develop after discharge, and report these to the doctor immediately, because they may require reevaluation of treatment.

• Because edematous skin is fragile, meticulous skin care is necessary for the patient with flare-ups of edema to prevent skin breakdown. Edematous extremities should be elevated.

• The patient must understand that the condition is chronic and that dietary fat must be permanently excluded. He should get regular medical follow-ups.

ANORECTUM

Hemorrhoids

Hemorrhoids are varicosities in the superior or inferior hemorrhoidal venous plexus. Dilation and enlargement of the superior plexus produce internal hemorrhoids; dilation and enlargement of the inferior plexus produce external hemorrhoids that may protrude from the rectum. Generally, incidence is highest between ages 20 and 50, and includes both sexes.

Causes
Hemorrhoids probably result from increased intravenous pressure in the hemorrhoidal plexus. Predisposing factors include occupations that require prolonged standing or sitting; straining due to constipation, diarrhea, coughing, sneezing, or vomiting; heart failure; hepatic disease, such as cirrhosis, amebic abscesses, or hepatitis; alcoholism; anorectal infections; loss of muscle tone due to old age, rectal surgery, or episiotomy; anal intercourse; and pregnancy.

Signs and symptoms
Although hemorrhoids may be asymptomatic, they characteristically cause painless, intermittent bleeding, which occurs on defecation. Bright-red blood appears on stool or on toilet paper due to injury of the fragile mucosa covering the hemorrhoid. These first-degree hemorrhoids may itch due to poor anal hygiene. When second-degree hemorrhoids prolapse, they're usually painless, and spontaneously return to the anal canal following defecation. Third-degree hemorrhoids cause constant discomfort and prolapse in response to any increase in intra-abdominal pressure. They must be manually reduced. Thrombosis of external hemorrhoids produces sudden rectal pain and a subcutaneous, large, firm lump that the patient can feel. If hemorrhoids cause severe or recurrent bleeding, they may lead to secondary anemia with significant pallor, fatigue, and weakness. However, such systemic complications are rare.

Diagnosis
Physical examination confirms external hemorrhoids. Proctoscopy confirms internal hemorrhoids and rules out rectal polyps.

Treatment
Treatment depends on the type and severity of the hemorrhoid, and the patient's overall condition. Generally,

TYPES OF HEMORRHOIDS

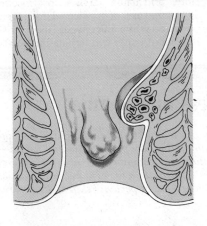

Frontal and cross section view of internal hemorrhoids.
Covered by mucosa, internal hemorrhoids bulge into the rectal lumen and may prolapse during defecation.

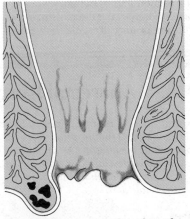

Frontal and cross section view of external hemorrhoids.
Covered by skin, external hemorrhoids protrude from the rectum and are more likely to thrombose than internal hemorroids.

treatment includes measures to ease pain, combat swelling and congestion, and regulate bowel habits. Patients can relieve constipation by increasing the amount of raw vegetables, fruit, and whole grain cereal in the diet, or by using stool softeners. Venous congestion can be prevented by avoiding prolonged sitting on the toilet, and local swelling and pain decreased with local anesthetic agents (lotions, creams, or suppositories), astringents, or cold compresses, followed by warm sitz baths or thermal packs. Rarely, the patient with chronic, profuse bleeding may require blood transfusion.

Other nonsurgical treatments include the injection of a sclerosing solution to produce scar tissue that decreases the prolapse, manual reduction of hemorrhoids, and ligation or freezing of the hemorrhoids.

Hemorrhoidectomy, the most effective treatment, is necessary for patients with severe bleeding, intolerable pain and pruritus, and large prolapse. This procedure is contraindicated in patients with blood dyscrasias (acute leukemia, aplastic anemia, hemophilia) or gastrointestinal carcinoma, and during the first trimester of pregnancy.

Additional considerations

Supportive care includes:
• preoperatively, administering an enema, as ordered (usually 2 to 4 hours before surgery), and recording the results; shaving the perianal area, and cleaning the anus and surrounding skin.
• postoperatively, checking for signs of prolonged rectal bleeding, and providing adequate analgesics (usually morphine or meperidine) and sitz baths.
• administering a bulk medication, such as psyllium, as soon as the patient can resume oral feedings; giving the medication about 1 hour after the evening meal to ensure a daily stool; warning against using stool-softening medications soon after hemorrhoidectomy, since a firm stool acts as a natural dilator to prevent anal stricture from the scar tissue (some patients may

need repeated digital dilation to prevent such narrowing).

• keeping the wound site clean to prevent infection and irritation.

• before discharging the patient, stressing the importance of regular bowel habits and good anal hygiene; warning against too vigorous wiping with washcloths and using harsh soaps; encouraging the use of medicated astringent pads and white toilet paper (the fixative in colored paper can irritate the skin).

Anorectal Abscess and Fistula

Anorectal abscess is a localized collection of pus due to inflammation of the soft tissue near the rectum or anus. Such inflammation may produce an anal fistula— an abnormal opening in the anal skin—that may communicate with the rectum. Such disorders develop four times as often in men as in women, possibly because men wear rougher clothing that produces friction on the perianal skin and interferes with air circulation.

Causes

The inflammatory process that leads to abscess may begin with an abrasion or tear in the lining of the anal canal, rectum, or perianal skin, and subsequent infection by *Escherichia coli*, staphylococci, or streptococci. Such trauma may result from injections for treatment of internal hemorrhoids, enema-tip abrasions, puncture wounds from ingested eggshells or fishbones, or insertion of foreign objects. Other preexisting lesions include infected anal fissure, infections from the anal crypt through the anal gland, ruptured anal hematoma, prolapsed thrombosed internal hemorrhoids, and septic lesions in the pelvis, such as acute appendicitis, acute salpin-

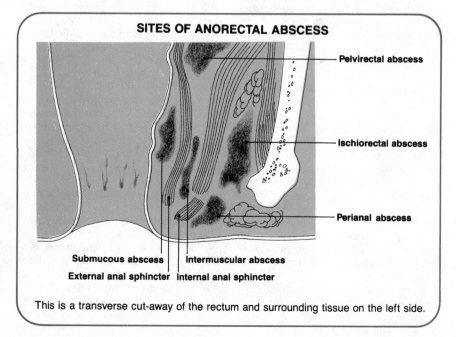

SITES OF ANORECTAL ABSCESS

Pelvirectal abscess

Ischiorectal abscess

Perianal abscess

Submucous abscess   Intermuscular abscess

External anal sphincter   Internal anal sphincter

This is a transverse cut-away of the rectum and surrounding tissue on the left side.

gitis, and diverticulitis. Systemic illnesses that may cause abscesses include ulcerative colitis and Crohn's disease. However, many abscesses develop without preexisting lesions.

As the abscess produces more pus, a fistula may form in the soft tissue beneath the muscle fibers of the sphincters (especially the external sphincter). The internal (primary) opening of the abscess/fistula is usually near the anal glands and crypts; the external (secondary) opening, in the perianal skin.

Signs and symptoms

Characteristic symptoms are throbbing pain and tenderness at the site of the abscess. A hard, painful lump develops on one side, preventing the patient from sitting comfortably.

Diagnosis

Anorectal abscess is detectable on physical examination:

• *Perianal abscess* (80% of patients) is a red, tender, localized, oval swelling close to the anus. Sitting or coughing increases pain, and pus may drain from the abscess. Digital examination reveals no abnormalities.

• *Ischiorectal abscess* (15% of patients) involves the entire perianal region on the affected side of the anus. It's tender but may not produce drainage. Digital examination reveals a tender induration bulging into the anal canal.

• *Submucous or high intermuscular abscess* (5% of patients) may produce a dull, aching pain in the rectum, tenderness, and occasionally, induration. Digital examination reveals a smooth swelling of the upper part of the anal canal or lower rectum.

• *Pelvirectal abscess* (rare) produces fever, malaise, and myalgia but no local anal or external rectal signs or pain. Digital examination reveals a tender mass high in the pelvis, perhaps extending into one of the ischiorectal fossae.

If the abscess drains by forming a fistula, the pain usually subsides and the predominant signs become pruritic drainage and subsequent perianal irritation. The external opening of a fistula generally appears as a pink or red, elevated, discharging sinus or ulcer on the skin near the anus. Depending on the severity of the infection, the patient may have chills, fever, nausea, vomiting, and malaise. Digital examination may reveal a palpable indurated tract and a drop or two of pus on palpation. The internal opening may be palpated as a depression or ulcer in the midline anteriorly or at the dentate line posteriorly. A complete examination with a probe may require an anesthetic.

Sigmoidoscopy rules out associated conditions, such as Crohn's disease, carcinoma, or retrorectal tumors.

Treatment

Anorectal abscesses require surgical incision under caudal anesthesia to promote drainage. Fistulas require a fistulotomy—removal of the fistula and associated granulation tissue—under caudal anesthesia. If the fistula tract is epithelialized, treatment requires fistulectomy—removal of the fistulous tract—followed by insertion of drains, which remain in place for 48 hours.

Additional considerations

After the patient's had an incision to drain anorectal abscess, the hospital staff member should:

• provide adequate medication for pain relief, as ordered.

• examine the wound frequently to assess proper healing, which should progress from the inside out. Healing should be complete in 4 to 5 weeks for perianal fistulas and in 12 to 16 weeks, for deeper wounds.

• tell the patient that recovery takes time and offer encouragement.

• stress the importance of perianal cleanliness.

• dispose of soiled dressings properly.

• be alert for the first postoperative bowel movement. The patient may suppress the urge to defecate because of anticipated pain. The resulting constipation increases pressure at the wound site. He should get a stool-softening laxative.

Rectal Polyps

Rectal polyps are masses of tissue that rise above the mucosal membrane and protrude into the gastrointestinal tract. Types of polyps include common polypoid adenomas, villous adenomas, hereditary polyposis, focal polypoid hyperplasia, and juvenile polyps (hamartomas). Most rectal polyps are benign. However, villous and hereditary polyps show a marked inclination to become malignant. Indeed, a striking feature of familial polyposis is its frequent association with rectosigmoid adenocarcinoma.

Causes and incidence

Villous adenomas are most prevalent in men over age 55; common polypoid adenomas, in Caucasian women between ages 45 and 60. Incidence in both sexes rises after age 70. Juvenile polyps occur most frequently among children under age 10 and are characterized by rectal bleeding. Predisposing factors include heredity, age, infection, and diet. Formation of polyps results from unrestrained cell growth in the upper epithelium.

Signs and symptoms

Because rectal polyps don't generally cause symptoms, they are usually discovered incidentally during a digital examination or rectosigmoidoscopy. Their most common sign is rectal bleeding: high rectal polyps leave a streak of blood on the stool; low rectal polyps bleed freely.

Rectal polyps vary in appearance:
• *Common polypoid adenomas* are small (usually less than 1 cm), multiple lesions (typically two to five) that are redder than normal mucosa. These lesions are frequently pedunculated—attached to rectal mucosa by a long, thin stalk—and granular, with a red, lobular, or eroded surface.
• *Villous adenomas* are sessile—attached to the mucosa by a wide base—and vary in size from 0.5 to 12 cm. They are soft, friable, and finely lobulated. They may grow large and cause painful defecation; however, because adenomas are soft, they rarely cause bowel obstruction. Sometimes adenomas prolapse out-

side the anus, expelling parts of the adenoma with the feces. These polyps may cause diarrhea, bloody stools, and subsequent fluid and electrolyte depletion, with hypotension and oliguria.
• In *hereditary polyposis,* rectal polyps resemble benign adenomas but occur in hundreds of small (0.5 cm) lesions, filling the entire mucosal surface. Accompanying signs include diarrhea, bloody stools, and secondary anemia. In a patient with hereditary polyposis, a change in bowel habits with abdominal pain usually signals rectosigmoid cancer.
• *Juvenile polyps* are large, inflammatory lesions, often without an epithelial covering. Mucus-filled cysts cover their usually smooth surface.
• *Focal polypoid hyperplasia* produces small (less than 3 mm), granular, sessile lesions, similar to the colon in color, or gray or translucent. They usually occur at the rectosigmoid junction.

Diagnosis

 Firm diagnosis of rectal polyps requires identification of the polyps through proctosigmoidoscopy or colonoscopy, and rectal biopsy. Barium enema can help identify polyps that are located high in the colon. Supportive laboratory findings include occult blood in the stool, low hemoglobin and hematocrit (with anemia), and possibly, serum electrolyte imbalances.

Treatment

Treatment varies according to the type and size of polyps, and their location within the colon. Common polypoid adenomas less than 1 cm in size require polypectomy, frequently by fulguration (destruction by high-frequency electricity) during endoscopy. For common polypoid adenomas over 4 cm and all invasive villous adenomas, treatment usually consists of abdominoperineal resection. Focal polypoid hyperplasia requires local fulguration. Depending on gastrointestinal involvement, hereditary polyps necessitate total abdominoperineal resection with a permanent ileostomy, subtotal colectomy with ileoproctostomy, or ileal anal anastomosis. Juvenile polyps are prone to autoamputation; if this doesn't occur, snare removal during colonoscopy is the treatment of choice.

Additional considerations

During diagnostic evaluation, a hospital staff member should:
• check sodium, potassium, and chloride levels daily in the patient with fluid imbalance; adjust fluid and electrolytes, as necessary; administer normal saline solution with potassium I.V., as ordered; weigh the patient daily, and record the amount of diarrhea; watch for signs of dehydration (decreased urine, increased BUN levels).
• tell the patient to watch for and report evidence of rectal bleeding.

After biopsy and fulguration, the staff member should:
• check for signs of perforation and hemorrhage, such as sudden hypotension, decrease in hemoglobin or hematocrit, shock, abdominal pain, and passage of red blood through the rectum.
• record the first bowel movement, which may not occur for 2 to 3 days.
• ambulate the patient within 24 hours of the procedure.
• provide sitz baths for 3 days.
• stress the need for routine follow-up studies for the patient with benign polyps to check the polypoid growth rate.
• prepare the patient with precancerous or familial lesions for abdominoperineal resection; provide emotional support and preoperative instruction.
• properly care for abdominal dressings, I.V. lines, and Foley catheter in the patient with an ileostomy or subtotal colectomy with ileoproctostomy; record intake and output, and check vital signs for hypotension and surgical complications; administer pain medication, as ordered; ambulate the patient as soon as possible to prevent embolism, and apply antiembolism stockings; encourage range-of-motion exercises; provide enterostomal therapy and teach stoma care.

Anorectal Stricture, Stenosis, or Contracture

In anorectal stricture, anorectal lumen size decreases; stenosis prevents dilation of the sphincter.

Causes
Anorectal stricture results from scarring after anorectal surgery or inflammation, inadequate postoperative care, or laxative abuse.

Signs and symptoms
The patient with anorectal stricture strains excessively when defecating and is unable to completely evacuate his bowel. Other clinical effects include pain, bleeding, and pruritus ani.

Diagnosis
Visual inspection reveals narrowing of the anal canal. Digital examination reveals tenderness and tightness.

Treatment and additional considerations
Surgical removal of scar tissue is the most effective treatment. Digital or instrumental dilation may be beneficial but may cause additional tears and splits. If the cause of stricture is inflammation,

correction of the underlying inflammatory process is necessary.

The hospital staff member should:
• prepare the patient for the digital examination and testing by explaining procedures thoroughly.
• after surgery, check vital signs often until the patient is stable and watch for signs of hemorrhage (excessive bleeding on rectal dressing).

• record first leg motion if surgery was performed under spinal anesthetic, and keep the patient lying flat for 6 to 8 hours after surgery.
• resume normal diet when the patient's condition is stable, and record time of first bowel movement; administer stool softeners, as ordered; give analgesics, provide sitz baths, and change perianal dressing, as ordered.

Pilonidal Disease

In pilonidal disease, a coccygeal cyst—which usually contains hair—becomes infected and produces an abscess, a draining sinus, or a fistula. Incidence is highest among hirsute, Caucasian men aged 18 to 30.

Causes
Pilonidal disease may develop congenitally from a tendency to hirsutism, or it may be acquired from stretching or irritation of the sacrococcygeal area (intergluteal fold) from prolonged rough exercise (such as horseback riding), heat, excessive perspiration, or constricting clothing.

Signs and symptoms
Generally, a pilonidal cyst produces no symptoms until it becomes infected, causing local pain, tenderness, swelling, or heat. Other clinical features include continuous or intermittent purulent drainage, chills, fever, headache, and malaise.

Diagnosis
Physical examination confirms the diagnosis and may reveal a series of openings along the midline, with thin, brown, foul-smelling drainage or a protruding tuft of hair. Pressure on the sinus tract may produce a purulent drainage. Passing a probe back through the sinus tract toward the sacrum should not reveal a perforation between the anterior sinus and anal canal. Cultures of discharge from the infected sinus may show staphylococci or skin bacteria but do not usually contain bowel bacteria.

Treatment
Conservative treatment of pilonidal disease consists of incision and drainage of abscesses, regular extraction of protruding hairs, and sitz baths (four to six times daily). However, persistent infections may necessitate surgical excision of the entire affected area. After excision of a pilonidal abscess, the patient requires regular follow-up care to monitor wound healing. The surgeon may periodically palpate the wound during healing with a cotton-tipped applicator, curette excess granulation tissue, and extract loose hairs to promote wound healing from the inside out and to prevent dead cells from collecting in the wound. Complete healing may take several months.

Additional considerations
Before incision and drainage of pilonidal abscess, the patient will need to be assured that he will receive adequate relief from pain.

After surgery, the compression dressing must be checked for signs of excessive bleeding and changed as directed.

The patient should walk within 24 hours. He must wear a gauze sponge over the wound site after the dressing is removed to allow ventilation and prevent friction from clothing. He should take sitz baths frequently, followed by air-drying instead of rubbing or patting dry with a towel.

After healing, the patient should briskly wash the area daily with a washcloth to remove loose hairs. Obese patients should be encouraged to change their diet to lose weight.

Rectal Prolapse

Rectal prolapse is the circumferential protrusion of one or more layers of the mucous membrane through the anus. Prolapse may be complete (with displacement of the anal sphincter or bowel herniation) or partial (mucosal layer).

Causes and incidence

Rectal prolapse usually occurs in men under age 40, in women around age 45 (three times more often than men), and in children aged 1 to 3 (especially those with cystic fibrosis). Predisposing factors include increased intra-abdominal pressure, especially from straining at stool; conditions that affect the pelvic floor or rectum, such as weak sphincters; or weak longitudinal, rectal, or levator ani muscles due to neurologic disorders, injury, tumors, aging, and chronic wasting diseases, such as tuberculosis, cystic fibrosis, or whooping cough; and nutritional disorders.

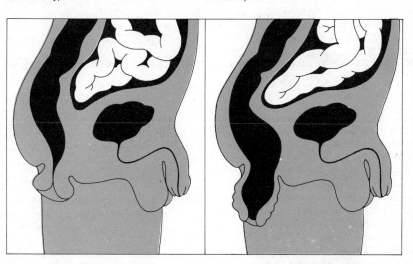

RECTAL PROLAPSE

Partial rectal prolapse (involves rectal mucosa only)

Complete prolapse (involves all layers of rectum)

Partial rectal prolapse involves only the mucosa and a small mass of radial mucosal folds. However, in complete rectal prolapse (also known as procidentia), the full rectal wall, sphincter muscle, and a large mass of concentric mucosal folds protrude. Ulceration is possible after complete prolapse.

Signs and symptoms
In rectal prolapse, protrusion of tissue from the rectum may occur during defecation or walking. Other symptoms include a persistent sensation of rectal fullness, bloody diarrhea, and pain in the lower abdomen due to ulceration. Hemorrhoids or rectal polyps may coexist with a prolapse.

Diagnosis
Typical clinical features and visual examination confirm diagnosis. In complete prolapse, examination reveals the full thickness of the bowel wall and, possibly, the sphincter muscle protruding, and mucosa falling into bulky, concentric folds. In partial prolapse, examination reveals only partially protruding mucosa and a smaller mass of radial mucosal folds. Straining during examination may disclose the full extent of prolapse.

Treatment and additional considerations
Treatment varies according to the underlying cause. Sometimes eliminating this cause (straining, coughing, nutritional disorders) is the only treatment necessary. In a child, prolapsed tissue usually diminishes as the child grows. In an older patient, injection of a sclerosing agent to cause a fibrotic reaction fixes the rectum in place. Severe or chronic prolapse requires surgical repair by strengthening or tightening the sphincters with wire or by anterior or rectal resection of prolapsed tissue.

The hospital staff member should:
• help the patient prevent constipation by teaching correct diet and stool-softening regimen; advise the patient with severe prolapse and incontinence to wear a perineal pad.
• before surgery, explain possible complications, including permanent rectal incontinence.
• after surgery, watch for immediate complications (hemorrhage) and later ones (pelvic abscess, fever, pus drainage, pain, rectal stenosis, constipation, or pain on defecation). The patient should learn perineal strengthening exercises, which include: lying down, with his back flat on the mattress, then pulling in his abdomen and squeezing while taking a deep breath; or repeatedly squeezing and relaxing his buttocks while sitting on a chair.

Anal Fissure

Anal fissure is a laceration or crack in the lining of the anus that extends to the circular muscle. Posterior fissure, the most common, is equally prevalent in males and females. Anterior fissure, the rarer type, is 10 times more common in females. Prognosis is very good, especially with fissurectomy and good anal hygiene.

Causes and incidence
Posterior fissure results from passage of large, hard stools that stretch the lining beyond its limits. Anterior fissure usually results from strain on the perineum during childbirth and, rarely, from scar stenosis. Occasionally, anal fissure is secondary to proctitis, anal tuberculosis, or carcinoma.

Signs and symptoms
Onset of an acute anal fissure is characterized by tearing, cutting, or burning pain during or immediately after bowel movement. A few drops of blood may streak toilet paper or underclothes. Painful anal sphincter spasms result from ulceration of a "sentinel pile" (swelling at the lower end of the fissure). A fissure may heal spontaneously and completely, or it may partially heal and break open again. Chronic fissure produces scar tissue that hampers normal bowel evacuation.

Diagnosis

Anoscopy showing longitudinal tear and typical clinical features help establish diagnosis. Digital examination that elicits pain and bleeding supports this diagnosis. Also, gentle traction on perianal skin can create sufficient eversion to visualize the fistula directly.

Treatment and additional considerations

Treatment varies according to severity of the tear. For superficial fissures without hemorrhoids, forcible digital dilation of anal sphincters under local anesthetic stretches the lower portion of the anal sphincter. For complicated fissures, treatment includes surgical excision of tissue, adjacent skin, and mucosal tags, and division of internal sphincter muscle from external. Other treatment includes:

• preparing the patient for rectal examination, and explaining the necessity for the procedure.
• providing hot sitz baths, warm soaks, and local anesthetic ointment to relieve pain, and low–residue diet, adequate fluid intake, and stool softeners to prevent straining during defecation.
• controlling diarrhea with diphenoxylate or other antidiarrheals.

Pruritus Ani

Pruritus ani is perianal itching, irritation, or superficial burning. This disorder is more common in men than in women and is rare in children.

Causes and incidence

Factors that contribute to pruritus ani include overcleaning of perianal area (harsh soap, vigorous rubbing with washcloth or toilet paper); minor trauma caused by straining to defecate; poor hygiene; sensitivity to spicy foods, coffee, alcohol, food preservatives, perfumed or colored toilet paper, detergents, or certain fabrics; specific medications (antibiotics, antihypertensives, or antacids that cause diarrhea); excessive sweating (in occupations associated with physical labor or high stress levels); anal skin tags; systemic disease, especially diabetes; certain skin lesions, such as squamous cell carcinoma, basal cell carcinoma, Bowen's disease, Paget's disease, melanoma, syphilis, and tuberculosis; fungus or parasite infection; and local anorectal disease (fissure, hemorrhoids, fistula).

Signs and symptoms

The key symptom of pruritus ani is perianal itching or burning after a bowel movement, during stress, or at night. In acute pruritus ani, scratching produces reddened skin, with weeping excoriations; in chronic pruritus ani, skin becomes thick and leathery, with excessive pigmentation.

Diagnosis

Detailed patient history is essential. Rectal examination rules out fissures and fistulas; biopsy rules out carcinoma. Allergy testing may also be helpful.

Treatment and additional considerations

After elimination of the underlying cause, treatment is symptomatic.

The patient should understand his condition and the causes. He should not scratch the area, since this may cause secondary infection. He should also avoid self-prescribed creams or powders, perfumed soaps, and colored toilet paper, because they may be irritating. Also, he should keep the perianal area clean and dry. Witch hazel pads can be used for wiping, and cotton balls can be tucked between buttocks to absorb moisture.

Proctitis

Proctitis is acute or chronic inflammation of the rectal mucosa. Prognosis is good unless massive bleeding occurs.

Causes and incidence
Contributing factors include chronic constipation, habitual laxative use, emotional upset, radiation (especially for cancer of the cervix and of the uterus), endocrine dysfunction, rectal injury, rectal medications, bacterial infections, allergies (especially to milk), vasomotor disturbance that interferes with normal muscle control, and food poisoning.

Signs and symptoms
Key symptoms include tenesmus, constipation, a feeling of rectal fullness, and left abdominal cramps. The patient feels an intense urge to defecate, which produces a small amount of stool that may contain blood and mucus.

Diagnosis
In acute proctitis, sigmoidoscopy shows edematous, bright red or pink rectal mucosa that's thick, shiny, friable, and possibly, ulcerated. In chronic proctitis, sigmoidoscopy shows thickened mucosa, loss of vascular pattern, and stricture of the rectal lumen. Other supportive tests include biopsy to rule out carcinoma and a bacteriologic examination. Detailed patient history is essential.

Treatment and additional considerations
Primary treatment eliminates the underlying cause (fecal impaction, laxatives, other medications). Soothing enemas, or steroid (hydrocortisone) suppositories or enemas may be helpful if proctitis is due to radiation. Tranquilizers may be appropriate for the patient with emotional stress.

The patient must be told to watch for and report bleeding and other persistent symptoms. Proctitis and its treatment should be fully explained to help him understand the disorder and prevent its recurrence. As appropriate, emotional support and reassurance can be offered during rectal examinations and treatment.

Selected References

Almy, T. *Wrestling with the Irritable Colon,* MEDICAL CLINICS OF NORTH AMERICA. 62:203-210, January 1978.

Bockus, Henry, ed. GASTROENTEROLOGY, 3rd ed. Philadelphia: W.B. Saunders Co., 1976.

Bouchier, I.A. GASTROENTEROLOGY, 2nd ed. New York: Macmillan Publishing Co., 1978.

Brooks, Frank P., et al. GASTROINTESTINAL PATHOPHYSIOLOGY, 2nd ed. New York: Oxford University Press, 1978.

Crane, R. GASTROINTESTINAL PHYSIOLOGY, Vol. 3. Baltimore: University Park Press, 1979.

Flores, R. *Necrotizing Enterocolitis: Symposium on Neonatal Care... Children's Hospital of Los Angeles,* NURSING CLINICS OF NORTH AMERICA. 13:39-45, March 1978.

Fradd, E.H. *Containment of Salmonellosis in a Baby Ward,* NURSING TIMES. 75:630-632, April 12, 1979.

Gaeke, R.F., et al. *When I Say "Colitis" I Mean...,* JOURNAL OF NURSING CARE. 11:14-15, March 1978.

Gitnick, G. PRACTICAL DIAGNOSIS OF GASTRO-INTESTINAL DISEASE. Boston: Houghton Mifflin Co., 1979.

Given, Barbara A., and Sandra J. Simmons. GASTROENTEROLOGY IN CLINICAL NURSING, 3rd ed. St. Louis: C.V. Mosby Co., 1979.

Greenberger, Norton J., and Daniel H. Winship. GASTROINTESTINAL DISORDERS: A PATHOLOGIC APPROACH. Chicago: Year Book Medical Publishers, 1976.

Grossman, M.B. *Gastrointestinal Endoscopy*, CLINICAL SYMPOSIA. 32:2-36, 1980.

Jones, K. *Love and Lavage: The Urgent Needs of Children with Hirschsprung's Disease*, NURSING78. 8:32-39, July 1978.

Kumar, P. *Sprue*, NURSING MIRROR. 146:25-26, January 12, 1978.

Long, G. *GI Bleeding: What to Do and When*, NURSING78. 8:44-50, March 1978.

Lynch, M., ed. BURKET'S ORAL MEDICINE, 7th ed. Philadelphia: J.B. Lippincott Co., 1977.

McCraw, V. *The Role of Dietary Fiber in Gastrointestinal Disorders*, ENTEROSTOMAL JOURNAL. 6:21-23, September-October 1979.

McLeod, James H. A METHOD OF PROCTOLOGY. New York: Harper & Row, 1976.

Palmer, E.D. *Gastrointestinal Problems in the Elderly*, HOSPITAL MEDICINE. 14:32, December 1978.

Ravitch, M. M., et al. PEDIATRIC SURGERY, 3rd ed. Chicago: Year Book Medical Publishers, 1978.

Rice, H. GASTROINTESTINAL NURSING. Flushing, N.Y.: Medical Examination Publishing Co., Inc., 1978.

Sleisenger, Marvin H., and John S. Fordtran. GASTROINTESTINAL DISEASE: PATHOPHYSIOLOGY, DIAGNOSIS, MANAGEMENT, 2nd ed. Philadelphia: W.B. Saunders Co., 1978.

Spiro, H.M. CLINICAL GASTROENTEROLOGY, 2nd ed. New York: Macmillan Publishing Co., 1977.

Trier, J., et al. *Celiac Sprue and Refractory Sprue*, GASTROENTEROLOGY. 75:307-316, August 1978.

Whitley, N.O., et al. *Angiography in the Diagnosis and Management of Gastrointestinal Bleeding*, APPLIED RADIOLOGY AND NUCLEAR MEDICINE. 8:63-66, November-December 1979.

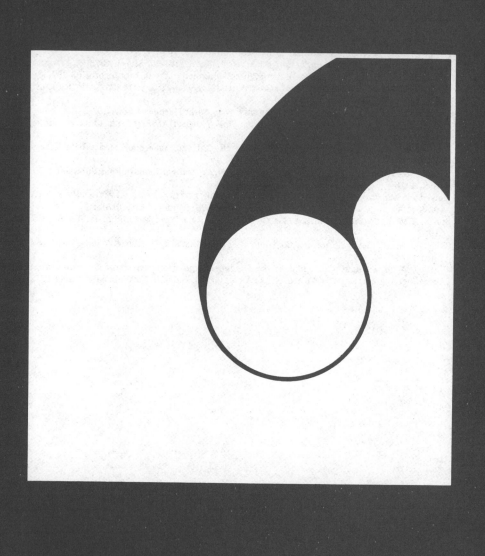

11 Hepatobiliary Disorders

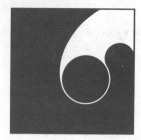

Hepatobiliary Disorders

Introduction

The liver is the largest internal organ in the human body, weighing slightly more than 3 lb (1,200 to 1,600 g) in the average adult. It's also one of the busiest, performing well over 100 separate functions. The most important of these are the formation and secretion of bile, detoxification of harmful substances, storage of vitamins, and metabolism of carbohydrates, fats, and proteins. This remarkably resilient organ serves as the body's warehouse and is absolutely essential to life.

Lobular structure

Located above the right kidney, stomach, pancreas, and intestines, and immediately below the diaphragm, the liver divides into a left and a right lobe (the right lobe is six times larger than the left), which are separated by the falciform ligament. Glisson's capsule, a network of connective tissue, covers the entire organ and extends into the parenchyma along blood vessels and bile ducts. Within the parenchyma, cylindrical lobules comprise the basic functional units of the liver, consisting of cellular plates that radiate from a central vein—like spokes in a wheel. Small bile canaliculi fit between the cells in the plates and empty into terminal bile ducts. These ducts join two larger ones, which merge into a single hepatic duct upon leaving the liver. The hepatic duct then joins the

cystic duct to form the common bile duct.

The liver receives blood from two major sources: the hepatic artery and the portal vein. These two vessels carry approximately 1,500 ml of blood per minute to the liver, nearly 75% of which is supplied by the portal vein. Sinusoids—offshoots of both the hepatic artery and portal vein—run between each row of hepatic cells. Phagocytic Kupffer's cells, part of the reticuloendothelial system, line the sinusoids, destroying old or defective red blood cells and detoxifying harmful substances. The liver has a large lymphatic supply, and consequently, cancer frequently metastasizes there.

One of the liver's most important functions is the conversion of bilirubin, a breakdown product of hemoglobin, into bile. Liberated by the spleen into plasma and bound loosely to albumin, bilirubin reaches the liver in an unconjugated (water-insoluble) state. The liver then conjugates or dissociates it, converting it to a water-soluble derivative before excreting it as bile. All hepatic cells continually form bile.

The liver also detoxifies many substances through inactivation as well as through conjugation. Inactivation involves reduction, oxidation, and hydroxylation. To inactivate gonadal and adrenocortical hormones, for example, the liver reduces them to their derivatives, making them more soluble so they can be excreted in bile and urine. Another important liver function is the inactivation of many drugs. All the barbiturates (except phenobarbital and barbital), for example, are metabolized primarily in the liver. Such drugs must be used with caution in hepatic disease, since their effects may be markedly prolonged. As still another example of its amazing versatility, the liver forms vitamin A from certain vegetables and stores vitamins K, D, and B_{12}. It also stores iron in the form of ferritin.

Metabolic functions
Finally, the liver figures indispensably in the metabolism of the three major food groups: carbohydrates, fats, and proteins. In carbohydrate metabolism, the liver plays one of its most vital roles by extracting excess glucose from the blood and reserving it for times when blood glucose levels fall below normal; at such times, the liver releases glucose into the circulation, and then replenishes the supply by a process called glyconeogenesis (gluconeogenesis). To prevent dangerously low blood glucose levels, the liver can also convert galactose or amino acids into glucose. The liver also forms many critical chemical compounds from the intermediate products of carbohydrate metabolism.

Liver cells metabolize fats more quickly and efficiently than do any other body cells, breaking them down into glycerol and fatty acids, then converting the fatty acids into small molecules that can be oxidized. The liver performs more than half the body's preliminary breakdown of fats. This remarkable organ also produces great quantities of cholesterol and phospholipids, manufactures lipoproteins, and synthesizes fat from carbohydrates and proteins, to be transported in lipoproteins for eventual storage in adipose tissue.

Like so many of its functions, the liver's role in protein metabolism is essential to life. The liver deaminates amino acids so they can be used for energy or converted into fats or carbohydrates. It forms urea to remove ammonia from body fluids and all plasma proteins (as much as 50 to 100 g/day) except gamma globulin. The liver is such an effective synthesizer of protein that it can replenish as much as half its plasma proteins in 4 to 7 days. The liver also synthesizes nonessential amino acids and forms other important chemical compounds from amino acids.

Assessing for liver disease
A careful physical examination and patient history can often detect telltale signs of hepatic disease. Cardinal signs of the disease are: The jaundice (a result of increased serum bilirubin levels), ascites (often accompanied by hemodilu-

tion, edema, and oliguria), and hepatomegaly. Its symptoms may include right upper quadrant abdominal pain, lassitude, anorexia, nausea, and vomiting. To detect hepatomegaly, the liver's left lobe is palpated, in the epigastrium between the xiphoid process and the umbilicus. Another primary sign is portal hypertension, or portal vein pressure greater than 6 to 12 cmH_2O. Auscultating a venous hum over the patient's abdomen suggests portal hypertension. Another test for portal hypertension is surgical insertion of a catheter into the portal vein to measure hepatic vein pressure.

The patient's neurologic status must be carefully assessed, since neurologic symptoms such as those associated with hepatic encephalopathy (confusion, muscle tremors, and asterixis) may signal onset of life-threatening hepatic failure.

Other common manifestations of hepatic disease include pallor (often linked to cirrhosis or carcinoma), parotid gland enlargement (in alcoholism-induced liver damage), Dupuytren's contracture, gynecomastia, testicular atrophy, decreased axillary or pubic hair, bleeding disorders (ecchymosis, purpura), spider angiomas, and palmar erythema. Careful abdominal palpation and auscultation can also detect hepatoma or metastasis (either turns the liver rock-hard and causes abdominal bruits) and postnecrotic cirrhosis. In hepatitis, palpation may elicit tenderness at the liver's edge. In neoplastic disease or hepatic abscess, auscultation may detect a pleural friction rub.

Comprehensive history essential

This includes: asking if the patient has ever had jaundice, anemia, or a splenectomy; asking about occupation and possible contact with rodents or exposure to toxins (carbon tetrachloride, beryllium, or vinyl chloride may all predispose to hepatic disease); asking about recent trips to other countries, especially to areas where hepatic disease is endemic.

Also important is alcohol consumption, which holds paramount significance in suspected hepatic disease. Since the alcoholic often deliberately underestimates how much he drinks, friends and relatives should be interviewed as well. Other important parts of patient history are: recent contact with a jaundiced person and any recent blood or plasma transfusions, blood tests, tattoos, or dental work; if the patient takes any drugs (especially parenteral narcotics, hallucinogens, or stimulants); if onset of symptoms was abrupt or insidious, or followed a recent abdominal injury that could have damaged the liver; if the patient bruises or bleeds easily; the color of stools and urine, and any change in bowel habits; if the patient's weight has fluctuated recently.

Liver function studies

The numerous tests that are available to detect hepatic disease reflect the liver's multiple functions. Perhaps the most useful tests are the so-called liver function studies, which measure serum enzymes and other substances. The following results are typical in hepatic disease:

• increased serum and urine bilirubin
• increased alkaline phosphatase and 5'-nucleotidase
• elevated transaminase levels (aminotransferases)—serum glutamic-pyruvic transaminase (SGPT) and serum glutamic oxaloacetic transaminase (SGOT); these enzymes are particularly useful in detecting hepatocellular damage, viral hepatitis, and acute hepatic necrosis.
• elevated gamma glutamyl transpeptidase (GGT)—this test is especially helpful, because this enzyme level rises even while hepatic damage is still minimal.
• hypoalbuminemia—suggests subacute or massive hepatic necrosis, cirrhosis
• hyperglobulinemia—suggests chronic inflammatory disorders
• prolonged prothrombin (PT) or partial thromboplastin time (PTT)—suggests hepatitis or cirrhosis
• elevated serum ammonia
• decreased serum total cholesterol
• positive lupus erythematosus (LE) cell

test in chronic active hepatitis and presence of hepatitis B antigen.

After liver trauma, liver function studies are less reliable. For instance, tests done long after the injury might miss an initial rise in serum transaminase levels. Less specific, and therefore less useful, tests include elevated urine urobilinogen, lactic dehydrogenase (LDH), and ornithine carbamyl transferase (OCT).

Other useful diagnostic tests include:

• *abdominal X-rays*—may indicate gross hepatomegaly and hepatic masses by elevation or distortion of the diaphragm, and may show calcification in the gallbladder, biliary tree, pancreas, and liver
• *barium studies*—may indicate an elevated left hepatic lobe by displacing the barium-filled stomach laterally and posteriorly
• *oral cholecystography*—useful because parenchymal dysfunction and impaired bile excretion decrease excretion of contrast material and prevent visualization of the gallbladder
• *I.V. cholangiography*—visualizes the intrahepatic and extrahepatic bile ducts and localizes obstructing lesions in the major ducts
• *percutaneous transhepatic cholangiography*—distinguishes between mechanical biliary obstruction and intrahepatic cholestasis
• *angiography*—demonstrates hepatic arterial circulation (deranged in cirrhosis) and helps diagnose primary or secondary hepatic tumor masses
• *radioisotope liver scans (scintiscans)*—may show an area of decreased uptake (a "hole") using colloidal or bengal scan, or an area of increased uptake (a "hot spot") using gallium scan in hepatoma or hepatic abscess
• *portal and hepatic vein manometry*—localizes obstructions in the extrahepatic portion of the portal vein, portal inflow system, or pressure in the presinusoidal vessels
• *percutaneous liver biopsy*—can determine the cause of unexplained hepatomegaly, hepatosplenomegaly, cholestasis, or persistent abnormal liver function tests; also useful in suspected systemic infiltrative disease (sarcoidosis, for example) and suspected primary or metastatic hepatic tumors
• *peritoneoscopy*—visualizes the serosal lining, liver, gallbladder, spleen, and other organs; useful in unexplained hepatomegaly, ascites, or abdominal mass
• *laparotomy*—used only when thorough clinical, laboratory, and biopsy studies fail to identify hepatic disease.

Gallbladder anatomy

The gallbladder is a pear-shaped organ that lies in the fossa on the underside of the liver, and is capable of holding 50 ml of bile. Attached to the large organ above by connective tissue, the peritoneum, and blood vessels, the gallbladder is divided into four parts: the fundus, or broad inferior end; the body, which is funnel-shaped and bound to the duodenum; the neck, which empties into the cystic duct; and the infundibulum, which lies between the body and the neck, and sags to form Hartmann's pouch.

The hepatic artery supplies both the cystic and hepatic ducts with blood, which drains out of the gallbladder through the cystic vein. Rich lymph vessels in the submucosal layer also drain the gallbladder, as well as the head of the pancreas.

The biliary duct system provides a passage for bile from the liver to the intestine and regulates bile flow. The gallbladder itself collects, concentrates, and stores bile. The normally functioning gallbladder also removes water and electrolytes from hepatic bile, increases the concentration of the larger solutes, and lowers its pH below 7. In gallbladder disease, bile becomes more alkaline, altering bile salts and cholesterol, and predisposing the organ to stone formation.

Mechanisms of contraction

The gallbladder responds to both sympathetic and parasympathetic innervation. Sympathetic stimulation inhibits muscle contraction; mild vagal stimulation causes the gallbladder to contract and the sphincter of Oddi to relax; stronger stimulation causes the sphincter to contract. The gallbladder also responds to substances released by the intestine. For instance, after chyme (semiliquid, partially digested food) enters the duodenum from the stomach, the duodenum releases cholecystokinin (CCK) and pancreozymin (PCZ) into the bloodstream, and stimulates the gallbladder to contract. The gallbladder also produces secretin, which stimulates the liver to secrete bile and CCK-PCZ. The gallbladder may also respond to some type of hormonal control, a theory based in part on the fact that the gallbladder empties more slowly during pregnancy.

Assessing for gallbladder disease

During physical examination of a patient with suspected gallbladder disease, there are telltale signs: pain, jaundice (a result of blockage of the common bile duct), fever, chills, indigestion, nausea, and intolerance of fatty foods. Pain may range from vague discomfort (as when pressure within the common bile duct gradually increases) to deep visceral pain (as when the gallbladder suddenly distends). Abrupt onset of pain with epigastric distress indicates gallbladder inflammation or obstruction of bile outflow by a stone or spasm.

Onset of jaundice also varies. If the gallbladder is healthy, jaundice may be delayed several days after bile duct blockage; if the gallbladder is absent or diseased, jaundice may appear within 24 hours after the blockage. Other effects of obstruction—pruritus, steatorrhea, and bleeding tendencies—may accompany jaundice. Gallbladder disorders rarely cause internal bleeding, but when they do—as in cholecystitis or obstructive clots in the biliary tree from gastrointestinal bleeding—they can be fatal.

Diagnostic tests

After a thorough patient history and careful assessment of clinical features, accurate diagnosis of gallbladder disease begins with oral *cholecystography*, which visualizes the gallbladder after the patient has ingested radiopaque dye. However, visualization depends on absorption of the dye from the small intestine, the liver's capacity to remove the dye from the blood and excrete it in bile, the patency of the ductal system, and the ability of the gallbladder to concentrate and store the dye. (This test may be repeated to rule out inadequate preparation.) Normally, the gallbladder fills about 13 hours after ingestion of the dye. Presence of stones or failure to visualize the gallbladder is significant.

Other diagnostic tests for gallbladder disease include:

• *percutaneous transhepatic cholangiography*—differentiates obstructive from intrahepatic types of jaundice, and detects hepatic dysfunction and calculi. Needle insertion in a bile duct permits withdrawal of bile and injection of dye. Fluoroscopic tests evaluate the filling of the hepatic and biliary trees.

• *duodenal drainage*—diagnoses cholelithiasis, choledocholithiasis, biliary obstruction, hepatic cirrhosis, and pancreatic disease, and differentiates types of jaundice. This test is especially useful when gallbladder function is poor or absent; when cholecystography fails to visualize the gallbladder or yields negative results despite continuing symptoms; or when cholecystography is contraindicated because of the patient's condition. In this test, a tube is passed through the gastrointestinal tract into the duodenum and CCK-PCZ is given to stimulate the gallbladder. This permits measurement of bile flow and also specimen collection, which is examined for mucus, blood, cholesterol crystals, pancreatic enzymes, cancer cells, bacteria, or calcium bilirubinate.

• *endoscopic retrograde cholangiopancreatography*—duodenal endoscopy dye injection and fluoroscopy are used to visualize and cannulate Vater's papilla. This test is particularly useful in locating obstruction, stones, carcinoma, or stricture.

Other appropriate tests for biliary disease are the same as those for hepatic disease, since their symptoms are similar and diagnosis often must distinguish between them.

LIVER DISEASES

Viral Hepatitis

A fairly common systemic disease, viral hepatitis is marked by liver cell destruction, necrosis, and autolysis, leading to anorexia, jaundice, and hepatomegaly. More than 70,000 cases are reported annually in the United States. This disease has three forms: type A (infectious or short-incubation hepatitis), type B (serum or long-incubation hepatitis), and type non-A, non-B hepatitis. All three types are found worldwide. Type B hepatitis rarely occurs in epidemics but has a higher mortality than type A hepatitis, which tends to be benign and self-limiting. Type non-A, non-B hepatitis has the mildest course.

Causes and incidence

Type A hepatitis is highly contagious and is usually transmitted by the fecal-oral route, although occasionally it's transmitted parenterally. The most common cause is ingestion of contaminated food, water, or milk. Outbreaks of type A hepatitis often occur after people have eaten seafood that came from polluted water. Type B hepatitis, which is generally transmitted parenterally, can also be spread through contact with human secretions and feces. Nurses, doctors, laboratory technicians, blood bank workers, and dentists are frequent victims of type B hepatitis, often as a result of wearing defective gloves while working. In addition, the incidence of both type A and type B hepatitides appears to be rising among homosexuals, presumably because of oral and anal sexual contact. Type non-A, non-B hepatitis accounts for 60% to 90% of post-transfusion hepatitis in the United States, and transmission usually results from commercial blood donations.

In most patients with hepatitis, liver cells eventually regenerate with little or no residual damage. Patients usually recover readily, with a lifelong immunity to type A hepatitis (but not to type B). Old age and serious underlying disor-

DIFFERENCES BETWEEN HEPATITIS A AND B		
	TYPE A (infectious)	**TYPE B (serum)**
Age incidence	Children, young adults	Any age
Seasonal incidence	Fall, winter	Any time
Transmission	Food, water, semen, tears, stools, and possibly urine	Serum, blood and blood products, and semen
Incubation	15 to 45 days	40 to 180 days
Onset	Sudden	Insidious
Serum markers	Anti-HAV	HB_sAg + anti HB_s
Prognosis	Good	Worsens with age
Carrier state	No	Yes

ders (congestive heart failure, severe anemia, diabetes, malignancy) make complications more likely. Prognosis is poor if edema and hepatic encephalopathy develop.

Signs and symptoms

The preicteric phase of viral hepatitis begins with a wide range of clinical features: fatigue, malaise, arthralgia, myalgia, headache, anorexia, photophobia, pharyngitis, cough, and coryza. This disease also causes nausea and vomiting, often with alterations in the senses of taste and smell; the patient may lose all desire to drink alcohol or smoke. Fever, with temperature of 100° to 101° F. (37.8° to 38.3° C.), may be associated with liver and lymph node enlargement. Symptoms begin suddenly in type A hepatitis and insidiously in type B; they disappear with the onset of jaundice. Type non-A, non-B hepatitis has a clinical course similar to type B hepatitis but is milder.

Mild weight loss, dark urine, clay-colored stools, and yellow scleras and skin signal the start of the icteric phase of hepatitis. In this second phase, anorexia may continue, the liver remains enlarged and tender, and the patient complains of discomfort and pain in the right upper abdominal quadrant. During this phase, splenomegaly, cervical adenopathy, and bile obstruction (cholestatic hepatitis) may develop; the patient may also be irritable and experience severe pruritus.

Jaundice, which may last from 1 to 2 weeks, results from the damaged liver cells' inability to remove bilirubin from the blood but doesn't indicate the severity of the disease. Occasionally, hepatitis occurs without jaundice (anicteric hepatitis). After jaundice disappears, the patient continues to experience fatigue, flatulence, abdominal pain or tenderness, and indigestion, although appetite usually returns and liver enlargement subsides. The posticteric, or convalescent phase generally lasts from 2 to 6 weeks, with full recovery in 6 months.

Complications include chronic hepatitis, which may be benign (chronic persistent hepatitis) or active (chronic aggressive hepatitis). About 25% of patients with chronic aggressive hepatitis die from hepatic failure. Fulminant hepatitis, a life-threatening complication, develops in about 1% of patients, causing unremitting hepatic failure, with encephalopathy. Progression is commonly to coma and death within 2 weeks.

Diagnosis

Patient history revealing recent exposure to drugs, chemicals, or jaundiced persons, or recent blood transfusions or injections, in the presence of typical clinical features, strongly suggests viral hepatitis. Recent piercing of the patient's ears may also be significant, since contaminated instruments can cause hepatitis.

 The presence of hepatitis B surface antigens (HBsAg) and hepatitis B antibodies (anti-HBs) confirms a diagnosis of type B hepatitis. HBsAg— sometimes called Australia antigen because it was originally discovered in the serum of an Australian aborigine—appears early in the disease, but blood levels may be negative later, giving a false negative reading if drawn too late. Detection of an antibody to type A hepatitis (anti-HAV) confirms diagnosis.

In the presence of HBsAg, anti-HBs, and anti-HAV, other laboratory results support a diagnosis of viral hepatitis, type A or type B; in their absence, these tests confirm type non-A, non-B hepatitis:

• prolonged prothrombin time (more than 3 seconds longer than the normal 12 to 15 seconds indicates severe liver damage)

• elevated SGOT and SGPT levels and slightly elevated serum alkaline phosphatase, reflecting the presence of enzymes in the blood

• elevated serum and urine bilirubin (with jaundice)

• low serum albumin and high serum globulin

• increased cephalin flocculation and thymol turbidity levels

- liver biopsy and scan showing patchy necrosis.

Hepatitis may be mistaken for infectious mononucleosis, although patients with mononucleosis have more prominent lymphadenopathy. During the preicteric phase of acute type B hepatitis, a serum sickness-like syndrome sometimes occurs, causing arthralgia, arthritis, rash, angioedema, and sometimes, hematuria and proteinuria, which may be misdiagnosed as rheumatoid arthritis or lupus erythematosus.

Treatment

No specific treatment exists for hepatitis. The patient should rest—at least in the early stages of the illness—and combat anorexia by eating small meals high in calories and protein. (Protein intake should be reduced if signs of precoma—lethargy, confusion, mental changes—develop.) Large meals are usually better tolerated in the morning. Antiemetics (trimethobenzamide or benzquinamide) may be given ½ hour before meals to relieve nausea and prevent vomiting; phenothiazines have a cholestatic effect and should be avoided. If vomiting persists, the patient will require I.V. infusions.

In severe clinical hepatitis, administration of corticosteroids may give the patient a sense of well-being and stimulate appetite, while decreasing itching and inflammation. Corticosteroids should be given sparingly, however, since their use in hepatitis is controversial.

All cases of hepatitis should be reported to public health officials. The patient should name anyone he had contact with recently who might have contracted the disease.

Additional considerations

The hospital staff member should design a plan around supportive care, close observation, and emotional support. This includes:

- isolating the patient in a single room with a private bath; wearing gloves when handling fluids and feces, and when drawing blood from a patient with type B

PREVENTION OF VIRAL HEPATITIS

Immune serum globulin (ISG)—commonly known as gamma globulin—has been studied extensively and found to be 80% to 90% effective in preventing type A hepatitis when promptly and properly administered. In confirmed type A cases, ISG should be given as soon as possible after exposure but within 2 weeks after onset of jaundice. ISG should also be administered prophylactically to contacts of the infected person who may have been exposed. Transmission of the disease is usually through the fecal-oral route, and persons at high risk include household, sexual, and institutional contacts. Natural disease is believed to produce permanent immunity.

Most gamma globulin manufactured in the United States contains low titers of antibody against type B hepatitis (anti-HBs), which probably transmits some passive protection against type B hepatitis. A high-titer hepatitis B immune globulin (HBIG) is also available and is approximately 70% effective in preventing type B hepatitis. A recently developed vaccine for type B hepatitis shows great promise. It's made from fragments of the virus' surface coat, which stimulate the body's immune system to produce antibodies against the virus.

High-risk factors include oral or percutaneous contact with an HBsAg-positive fluid or sexual contact within the 4 weeks before onset of jaundice.

hepatitis; lining wastebaskets with disposable plastic bags; seeing that the patient wears pajama bottoms, to minimize contamination of bedsheets.

- limiting visitors and imposing isolation precautions.
- encouraging the patient to eat as much as possible; not overloading his meal tray because too much food on the tray will only diminish his appetite; not overmedicating since this too will diminish his appetite; forcing fluids (at least 4,000 ml/day) and encouraging the anorectic patient to drink fruit juices; offering chipped

ice and soft drinks to maintain hydration without inducing vomiting.

• recording weight daily, and keeping accurate intake and output records; observing feces for color, consistency, frequency, and amount.

• watching for signs of hepatic coma, dehydration, pneumonia, vascular problems, and decubitus ulcers.

• maintaining electrolyte balance and a patent airway, and controlling bleeding in the fulminant hepatitis patient; correcting hypoglycemia and other complications in the fulminant hepatitis patient awaiting liver regeneration and repair.

• explaining the nature of hepatitis so the patient understands the need for isolation; explaining all diagnostic tests.

• urging the patient, before discharge, to have regular medical checkups for at least 1 year; warning him not to drink any alcohol during this time, and telling him how to recognize recurrence; refering him for follow-up, as needed.

Nonviral Hepatitis

Nonviral inflammation of the liver (toxic or drug-induced hepatitis) is a form of hepatitis that usually results from exposure to certain chemicals or drugs. Most patients recover from this illness, although a few develop fulminating hepatitis or cirrhosis.

Causes
Various hepatotoxins—carbon tetrachloride, trichloroethylene, poisonous mushrooms, vinyl chloride—can cause the toxic form of this disease. Following exposure to these agents, liver damage (diffuse fatty infiltration of liver cells and necrosis) usually occurs within 24 to 48 hours, depending on the size of the dose. Alcohol, anoxia, and preexisting liver disease exacerbate the toxic effects of some of these agents.

Drug-induced (idiosyncratic) hepatitis may stem from a hypersensitivity reaction unique to the affected individual, unlike toxic hepatitis, which appears to affect all persons indiscriminately. Among the drugs that may cause this type of hepatitis are halothane, sulfonamides, isoniazid, alphamethyldopa, and chlorpromazine (cholestasis-induced hepatitis). In hypersensitive persons, symptoms of hepatic dysfunction may appear at any time during or after exposure to these drugs but usually emerge after 2 to 5 weeks of therapy. Not all adverse drug reactions are toxic. Oral contraceptives, for example, may impair liver function and produce jaundice without causing necrosis, fatty infiltration of liver cells, or a hypersensitive reaction.

Signs and symptoms
Clinical features of toxic and drug-induced hepatitis vary with the severity of liver damage and the causative agent. In most patients, symptoms resemble those of viral hepatitis: anorexia, nausea, vomiting, jaundice, dark urine, hepatomegaly, possible abdominal pain (with acute onset and massive necrosis), and clay-colored stools or pruritus with the cholestatic form of hepatitis. In addition, carbon tetrachloride poisoning produces headache, dizziness, drowsiness, and vasomotor collapse; in halothane-related hepatitis, fever, moderate leukocytosis, and eosinophilia; with chlorpromazine, abrupt fever, rash, arthralgias, lymphadenopathy, and epigastric or upper right quadrant pain.

Diagnosis
Diagnostic findings include elevations in serum transaminase (SGOT, SGPT), both total and direct bilirubin (with cholestasis), alkaline phosphatase (unusually high), WBC, and eosinophils (possible in drug-induced type). Liver biopsy may help identify the underlying pathology,

especially infiltration with WBCs and eosinophils. Liver function tests have limited value in distinguishing between nonviral and viral hepatitis.

Treatment and additional considerations
Effective treatment must remove the causative agent by lavage, catharsis, or hyperventilation, depending on the route of exposure. Dimercaprol may serve as an antidote for toxic hepatitis caused by gold or arsenic poisoning but doesn't prevent drug-induced hepatitis caused by other substances. Corticosteroids may be ordered for patients with the drug-induced type. Thioctic acid, an investigational drug, has been tried successfully for mushroom poisoning.

Measures that can be taken to prevent poisoning include knowing about the proper use of prescription drugs, and about the proper handling of cleaning agents and solvents.

Cirrhosis and Fibrosis

Cirrhosis is a chronic hepatic disease characterized by diffuse destruction and fibrotic regeneration of hepatic cells. As necrotic tissue yields to fibrosis, this disease alters liver structure and normal vasculature, impairs blood and lymph flow, and ultimately causes hepatic insufficiency. It's twice as common in men as in women and is especially prevalent among malnourished chronic alcoholics over age 50. Mortality is high; many patients die within 5 years of onset. Prognosis is better in noncirrhotic forms of hepatic fibrosis, which cause minimal hepatic dysfunction and don't destroy liver cells.

Causes
The following clinical types of cirrhosis reflect its diverse etiology:
• *Portal, nutritional, or alcoholic cirrhosis* (Laennec's type), the most common, accounts for 30% to 50% of patients, up to 90% of whom have a history of alcoholism. Liver damage results primarily from malnutrition, especially of dietary protein, which causes scar tissue to form around the portal area.
• *Biliary cirrhosis* (15% to 20% of patients) results from bile duct diseases, which suppress bile flow.
• *Postnecrotic (posthepatitic) cirrhosis* (10% to 30% of patients) stems from various types of hepatitis.
• *Pigment cirrhosis* (5% to 10% of patients) may stem from disorders such as hemochromatosis.
• *Cardiac cirrhosis* (rare) refers to liver damage caused by right heart failure.
• *Idiopathic cirrhosis* (about 10% of patients) has no known cause.

Noncirrhotic fibrosis may result from schistosomiasis or congenital hepatic fibrosis, or may be idiopathic.

Signs and symptoms
Clinical manifestations of cirrhosis and fibrosis are similar for all types, regardless of cause. Early indications are vague but usually include gastrointestinal symptoms (anorexia, indigestion, nausea, vomiting, constipation, or diarrhea) and dull abdominal ache. Major and late symptoms develop as a result of hepatic insufficiency and portal hypertension, and involve the entire body. These clinical features include:
• *respiratory*—limited thoracic expansion due to abdominal ascites, interfering with efficient gas exchange and leading to hypoxia
• *CNS*—various symptoms of hepatic encephalopathy, including lethargy, mental changes, slurred speech, asterixis, peripheral neuritis, paranoia, and hallucinations, progressing to extreme obtundation and coma
• *hematologic*—bleeding tendencies (nosebleeds, easy bruising, bleeding

PORTAL HYPERTENSION AND ESOPHAGEAL VARICES

Portal hypertension—elevated pressure in the portal vein—occurs when blood flow through the porta hepatis meets increased resistance. The disorder is a common result of cirrhosis but may also stem from mechanical obstruction of the portal veins by thrombosis, or tumor and occlusion of the hepatic veins (Budd-Chiari syndrome). As portal pressure rises, blood backs up into the spleen and flows through collateral channels to the venous system, bypassing the liver. Consequently, portal hypertension produces splenomegaly with thrombocytopenia, dilated collateral veins (esophogeal varices, hemorrhages, or prominent abdominal veins), and ascites. Nevertheless, in many patients the first sign of portal hypertension is bleeding from esophageal varices—dilated tortuous veins in the submucosa of the lower esophagus. Such varices often cause massive hematemesis, requiring emergency treatment to control hemorrhage and prevent hypovolemic shock.

• *Endoscopy* identifies the ruptured varix as the bleeding site and excludes other potential sources in the upper gastrointestinal tract.

• *Angiography* may aid diagnosis but is less precise than endoscopy.

• *Vasopressin* infused into the superior mesenteric artery may temporarily stop bleeding; when angiography is unavailable, vasopressin may be infused by I.V. drip, diluted with 5% dextrose in water (except in patients with coronary vascular disease), but this route is usually less effective.

• *A Sengstaken-Blakemore tube* may also help control hemorrhage by applying pressure on bleeding site. Iced saline lavage through the tube may help control bleeding.

The use of vasopressin or a Sengstaken-Blakemore tube is a temporary measure, especially in the patient with a severely deteriorated liver. Fresh blood and fresh frozen plasma, if available, are preferred for blood transfusions, to replace clotting factors. Treatment with lactulose promotes elimination of old blood from the gastrointestinal tract and combats excessive production and accumulation of ammonia.

Appropriate surgical bypass procedures include portosystemic anastomosis, splenorenal shunt, and mesocaval shunt. A portacaval or a mesocaval shunt decreases pressure within the liver, as well as reduces ascites, plasma loss, and risk of hemorrhage by directing blood from the liver into collateral vessels. Emergency shunts carry a mortality of 25% to 50%. Evidence suggests that the portosystemic bypass does not prolong survival time; it usually means the patient will eventually die of hepatic coma rather than of hemorrhage.

The patient with portal hypertension with esophageal varices must be carefully monitored for hemorrhage and subsequent hypotension, compromised oxygen supply, and altered level of consciousness. The hospital staff member should:

• monitor vital signs, urinary output, and central venous pressure to determine fluid volume status.

• assess mental status and level of consciousness often.

• provide emotional support and reassurance in the wake of massive gastrointestinal bleeding, which is always a frightening experience.

• keep the patient as quiet and comfortable as possible, but remember that tolerance for sedatives and tranquilizers may be decreased because of liver damage.

• clean the patient's mouth, which may be dry and flecked with dried blood, with a mixture of mouthwash and water on gauze dressing.

• monitor the patient with a Sengstaken-Blakemore tube carefully for persistent bleeding in gastric drainage, signs of asphyxiation from tube displacement, proper inflation of balloons, and correct traction to maintain tube placement.

CIRCULATION IN PORTAL HYPERTENSION

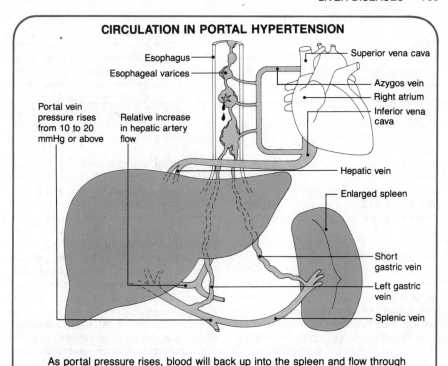

As portal pressure rises, blood will back up into the spleen and flow through collateral channels to the venous system, bypassing the liver and causing esophageal varices.

gums), anemia

- *endocrine*—testicular atrophy, menstrual irregularities, gynecomastia, and loss of chest and axillary hair
- *skin*—severe pruritus, extreme dryness, poor tissue turgor, abnormal pigmentation, spider angiomas, palmar erythema, and possibly, jaundice
- *hepatic*—jaundice, hepatomegaly, ascites, edema of the legs, hepatic encephalopathy, and hepatorenal syndrome comprise the other major effects of full-fledged cirrhosis
- *miscellaneous*—musty breath, enlarged superficial abdominal veins, muscle atrophy, pain in the upper right abdominal quadrant that worsens when the patient sits up or leans forward, palpable liver or spleen, and temperature of 101° to 103° F. (38.3° to 39.4° C.). Bleeding from esophageal varices results from portal hypertension.

Diagnosis

Liver biopsy, the definitive test for cirrhosis, detects destruction and fibrosis of hepatic tissue; liver scan shows abnormal thickening and a liver mass. Cholecystography and cholangiography visualize the gallbladder and the biliary duct system, respectively; splenoportal venography, the portal venous system. Percutaneous transhepatic cholangiography differentiates extrahepatic from intrahepatic obstructive jaundice and discloses hepatic pathology and presence of gallstones.

The following laboratory findings support this diagnosis:

- decreased WBC, hemoglobin and hematocrit, albumin, serum electrolytes (sodium, potassium, chlorides, and magnesium), and cholinesterase
- elevated globulin, serum ammonia, total bilirubin, alkaline phosphatase,

transaminase (SGOT and SGPT), lactic dehydrogenase (LDH), and thymol turbidity
- anemia, neutropenia, and thrombocytopenia, with prolonged prothrombin and partial thromboplastin times
- deficiencies of vitamins A, B_{12}, C, and K; folic acid; and iron
- abnormal Bromsulphalein (BSP) excretion and glucose tolerance test (possible)
- positive tests for galactose tolerance and urine bilirubin
- fecal urobilinogen greater than 40 to 280/mg in 24 hours, urine urobilinogen greater than 0 to 1.16/mg for the same period.

Treatment

Treatment is designed to remove or alleviate the underlying cause of cirrhosis or fibrosis, prevent further liver damage, and prevent or treat complications. The patient may benefit from a high-calorie and moderate- to high-protein diet, but developing hepatic encephalopathy mandates restricted protein intake. In addition, sodium is usually restricted to 200 to 500 mg/day, fluids to 1,000 to 1,500 ml/day.

If the patient's condition continues to deteriorate, he may need tube feedings or hyperalimentation. Other supportive measures include supplemental vitamins—A, B complex, D, and K—to compensate for the liver's inability to store them, and vitamin B_{12}, folic acid, and thiamine for deficiency anemia. Rest, moderate exercise, and avoidance of exposure to infections and toxic agents are essential.

Drug therapy requires special caution, since the cirrhotic liver can't detoxify harmful substances efficiently. Alcohol is prohibited; sedatives should be avoided or prescribed with great care. When absolutely necessary, antiemetics, such as trimethobenzamide or dimenhydrinate, may be given for nausea; vasopressin, for esophageal varices; and diuretics, such as furosemide or spironolactone, for edema. However, diuretics require careful monitoring, since fluid and electrolyte imbalance may precipitate hepatic encephalopathy.

Paracentesis and infusions of salt-poor albumin may alleviate ascites. Surgical procedures include ligation of varices, splenectomy, esophagogastric resection, and splenorenal or portacaval anastomosis to relieve portal hypertension. Programs for prevention of cirrhosis usually emphasize avoidance of alcohol.

Additional considerations

Cirrhotic patients need close observation, first-rate supportive care, and sound nutritional counseling.
- The patient's skin, gums, stools, and emesis must be checked regularly for bleeding. Pressure applied to injection sites will prevent bleeding. The patient must not take aspirin, strain at stool, and blow his nose or sneeze too vigorously. He should use an electric razor and a soft toothbrush.
- Signs of behavioral or personality changes, such as increasing stupor, lethargy, hallucinations, or neuromuscular dysfunction require monitoring and must be reported. The patient should be aroused periodically to determine level of consciousness. He must especially be watched for asterixis, a clear sign of developing hepatic encephalopathy.
- To assess fluid retention, the patient's weight should be checked, abdominal girth measured daily, ankles and sacrum inspected for dependent edema, and intake and output accurately recorded. The patient must be evaluated before, during, and after paracentesis; this drastic loss of fluid may induce shock.
- To prevent skin breakdown associated with edema and pruritus, soap should not be used when bathing the patient; instead, lubricating lotion or moisturizing agents can be applied. The patient must be handled gently, and repositioned often to keep skin intact.
- Rest and good nutrition will conserve the patient's energy and decrease metabolic demands on the liver. He should eat frequent, small meals, avoid infections and abstain from alcohol. He may need to be referred to Alcoholics Anonymous.

Budd-Chiari Syndrome

Budd-Chiari syndrome is a rare disorder in which hepatic vein obstruction impairs blood flow out of the liver. Incidence is rising in young women and is thought to be related to the increased risk of venous thrombosis associated with oral contraceptives. This disease usually progresses slowly, eventually becoming a chronic condition; however, acute Budd-Chiari syndrome may prove rapidly fatal.

Causes

Conditions that can obstruct blood flow from the hepatic veins include:
- fibrotic obliteration of the hepatic veins
- thrombosis of the hepatic veins due to myeloproliferative disease
- pregnancy and use of oral contraceptives
- generalized blood disorders, such as polycythemia, leukemia, or sickle cell disease
- trauma
- tumors of the liver, kidneys, pancreas, or adrenal glands
- formation of a fibrous web across the inferior vena cava just above the point where the hepatic veins empty into it— this may be a congenital disorder related to closure of the ductus venosus
- severe right heart failure or constrictive pericarditis
- sclerosis of the hepatic veins due to radiation therapy to the liver
- liver abscess or cyst (rare).

When hepatic outflow diminishes, the liver becomes congested with blood, and liver cells atrophy, causing thrombosclerosis in the liver, hepatic veins, and sometimes, the inferior vena cava. Death results from hepatic failure.

Signs and symptoms

Clinical features of Budd-Chiari syndrome vary with rapidity of onset and the extent of the disease, as well the nature of the underlying illness. Typically, this disorder begins with abdominal discomfort, followed by massive ascites and hepatomegaly several weeks or even months later. Nausea and vomiting occur intermittently; jaundice may develop but is usually mild. Portal hypertension eventually causes hematemesis and esophageal varices. If the inferior vena cava becomes blocked, collateral veins may be visible on the abdomen and back.

Diagnosis

Liver biopsy may detect tissue changes consistent with pathology (dilated liver sinusoids, thrombosclerotic changes, central lobular congestion and necrosis). Abnormal liver function tests, however, show only moderate impairment (elevated serum transaminase) and are not specific for Budd-Chiari syndrome.

Angiography detects abnormalities in hepatic circulation. As part of this test, splenoportography (injection of dye into the spleen) may show collateral portal circulation, but portal veins may not be visible because of retrograde blood flow— a compensatory mechanism for obstructed hepatic veins. Angiography of the inferior vena cava helps identify abnormalities of blood flow and obstruction of vena cava. These angiographic studies may be performed percutaneously or directly during exploratory laparotomy.

Hepatic vein catheterization may show a narrow or occluded segment of the vein, displaying a "spider web" pattern. Because of hepatomegaly, ascites, and pulmonary hypertension, Budd-Chiari syndrome is often misdiagnosed as cirrhosis.

Treatment

Treatment of Budd-Chiari syndrome is symptomatic and essentially the same as that for chronic hepatic disease. It includes diuretics and fluid restriction, and depending on the underlying cause,

SURGICAL SHUNTS FOR PORTAL HYPERTENSION

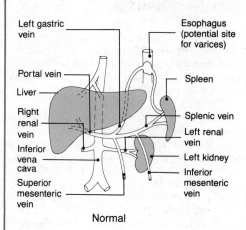

Left gastric vein

Esophagus (potential site for varices)

Portal vein

Liver

Spleen

Right renal vein

Splenic vein

Inferior vena cava

Left renal vein

Left kidney

Superior mesenteric vein

Inferior mesenteric vein

Normal

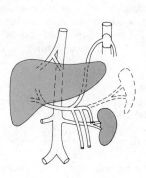

End-to-side splenorenal shunt

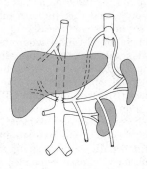

End-to-side portacaval shunt

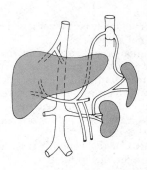

Distal end-to-side splenorenal shunt

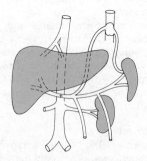

Side-to-side portacaval shunt

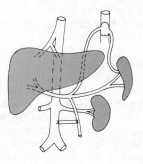

Side-to-side mesocaval shunt

sometimes includes surgery. Portacaval shunt procedures, for example, may improve liver function and decrease portal hypertension; they have shown some promise, especially in patients with fibrous web in the vena cava. However, mortality is high during the early postoperative period, and those patients who survive often suffer intractable ascites.

Additional considerations
The hospital staff member should:
• administer diuretics, as ordered; weigh the patient, and measure abdominal girth daily to assess ascites; test stools and emesis for blood.

• explain thoroughly all necessary diagnostic and surgical procedures, as well as all drugs and dietary restrictions; warn the patient to avoid foods and activities that may cause esophageal varices to bleed.
• guide and support critically ill patients who cannot be treated successfully through the various stages of dying; provide emotional support for the family, through the grieving process.
• help to detect Budd-Chiari syndrome early by warning patients taking oral contraceptives to report abdominal pain and to be examined regularly for hepatomegaly.

Liver Abscess

A liver abscess occurs when bacteria or protozoa destroy hepatic tissue, producing a cavity, which fills with infectious organisms, liquefied liver cells, and leukocytes. Necrotic tissue then walls off the cavity from the rest of the liver.

While liver abscess is relatively uncommon, it carries a mortality of 30% to 50%. This rate soars to more than 80% with multiple abscesses, and to more than 90% with complications, such as rupture into the peritoneum, pleura, or pericardium. About 70% of pyogenic liver abscesses occur among men, usually between ages 20 and 30.

Causes
In pyogenic liver abscesses, the common infecting organisms are *Escherichia coli, Klebsiella, Enterobacter, Salmonella, Staphylococcus,* and *Enterococcus.* Such organisms may invade the liver directly after a liver wound, or they may spread from the lungs, skin, or other organs by the hepatic artery, portal vein, or biliary tract. Pyogenic abscesses are generally multiple and often follow cholecystitis, peritonitis, pneumonia, and bacterial endocarditis.

An amebic abscess results from infection with the protozoa *Entamoeba histolytica,* the organism that causes amebic dysentery. Amebic liver abscesses usually occur singly, in the right lobe.

Signs and symptoms
The clinical manifestations of a liver abscess depend on the degree of involvement: some patients are acutely ill; in others, the abscess is recognized only at autopsy, after death from another illness. Onset of symptoms of a pyogenic abscess is usually sudden; in an amebic abscess, onset is more insidious. The most common signs include right abdominal and shoulder pain, weight loss, fever, chills, diaphoresis, nausea, vomiting, and anemia. Signs of right pleural effusion, such as dyspnea and pleural pain, develop if the abscess extends through the diaphragm. Extensive liver damage may cause jaundice.

Diagnosis
 A liver scan showing filling defects at the area of the abscess more than ¾″ (1.9 cm), together with characteristic clinical features, confirms this diagnosis. A liver ultrasound may indi-

cate defects caused by the abscess but is less definitive than a liver scan. In a chest X-ray, the diaphragm on the affected side appears raised and fixed. After discovery of the abscess, hepatic arteriography differentiates it from a malignancy. Relevant laboratory values include elevated serum transaminase (SGOT, SGPT), alkaline phosphatase, bilirubin, and WBC (usually more elevated in pyogenic abscess than in amebic), and decreased serum albumin. In pyogenic abscess, a blood culture can identify the bacterial agent; in amebic abscess, a stool culture and serologic and hemagglutination tests can isolate *E. histolytica.*

Treatment

If the organism causing the abscess is unknown, long-term antibiotic therapy begins immediately with gentamicin, cephalothin, clindamycin, or chloramphenicol. If cultures demonstrate that the infectious organism is *E. coli*, treatment includes ampicillin; if *E. histolytica*, it includes emetine, chloroquine, or metronidazole. Therapy continues for 2 to 4 months. Surgical drainage is indicated only for a single pyogenic abscess or for an amebic abscess that fails to respond to drug therapy.

Additional considerations

Care by a hospital staff member includes:
• providing supportive care, monitoring vital signs (especially temperature), and maintaining adequate fluid and nutritional intake.
• administering anti-infectives and antibiotics, as ordered, watching for possible side effects, and stressing the importance of compliance with therapy.
• explaining diagnostic and surgical procedures.
• watching carefully for complications of abdominal surgery, such as hemorrhage or infection.

Fatty Liver
(Steatosis)

A common clinical finding, fatty liver is the accumulation of triglycerides and other fats in liver cells. In severe fatty liver, fat comprises as much as 40% of the liver's weight (as opposed to 5% in a normal liver), and the weight of the liver may increase from 3.31 lb (1.5 kg) to as much as 11 lb (5 kg). Minimal fatty changes are temporary and asymptomatic; severe or persistent changes may cause liver dysfunction. Fatty liver is usually reversible by simply eliminating the cause; however, this disorder may result in recurrent infection or sudden death from fat emboli to the lungs.

Causes

The most common cause of fatty liver in the United States and in Europe is chronic alcoholism, with the severity of hepatic disease directly related to the amount of alcohol consumed. Other causes include malnutrition (especially protein deficiency), obesity, diabetes mellitus, jejunoileal bypass surgery, Cushing's syndrome, Reye's syndrome, pregnancy, large doses of hepatotoxins—such as I.V. tetracycline—carbon tetrachloride intoxication, prolonged I.V. hyperalimentation, and DDT poisoning. Whatever the cause, fatty infiltration of the liver probably results from mobilization of fatty acids from adipose tissues or altered fat metabolism.

Signs and symptoms

Clinical features of fatty liver vary with the degree of lipid infiltration, and many patients are asymptomatic. The most typical sign is a large, tender liver (hepatomegaly). Common symptoms include upper right quadrant pain (with massive or rapid infiltration), ascites, edema, jaundice, and fever (all with hepatic necrosis or biliary stasis). Nausea, vomiting, and anorexia are less common. Splenomegaly usually accompanies cirrhosis. Rarer changes are spider angiomas, varices, transient gynecomastia, and menstrual disorders.

Diagnosis

Typical clinical features—especially in patients with chronic alcoholism, malnutrition, poorly controlled diabetes mellitus, or obesity—suggest fatty liver.

A liver biopsy confirms excessive fat in the liver. Liver function tests support this diagnosis:

• *albumin*—somewhat low
• *globulin*—usually elevated
• *cholesterol*—usually elevated
• *total bilirubin*—elevated
• *alkaline phosphatase*—elevated
• *transaminase*—usually low (less than 300 units)
• *prothrombin time*—possibly prolonged.

Other possible findings include anemia, leukocytosis, occasionally elevated WBC, albuminuria, hyper- or hypoglycemia, and deficiencies of iron, folic acid, and vitamin B_{12}.

Treatment and additional considerations

Treatment for fatty liver is essentially supportive and consists of correcting the underlying condition or eliminating its cause. For instance, when fatty liver results from I.V. hyperalimentation, decreasing the rate of carbohydrate infusion may correct it. In alcoholic fatty liver, abstinence from alcohol and a proper diet can begin to correct liver changes within 4 to 8 weeks. Such correction requires comprehensive patient teaching:

• Alcoholics should seek counseling. They and their families will need emotional support.
• Diabetics and their families need to know about proper care, such as the purpose of insulin injections, diet, and exercise. Public health nurses or group classes will help promote compliance with treatment. Diabetics may need long-

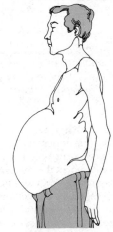

MASSIVE ASCITES IN FATTY LIVER

A possible effect of fatty liver is massive ascites. Emaciated extremities and upper thorax are also typical of ascites.

term medical supervision, and should report any changes in their health immediately.

• Obese patients and their families should learn about a proper diet. They must avoid fad diets, which may be nutritionally inadequate. Medical supervision will be needed for those patients more than 20% overweight. They should attend group diet and exercise programs and, if necessary, behavior modification programs to correct eating habits. Their progress should be checked and they should be given positive reinforcement for any weight loss.
• Patients with chronic illness must be checked for malnutrition, especially protein deficiency, and given an adequate diet.
• Patients receiving hepatotoxins and those who risk occupational exposure to DDT should watch for and immediately report signs of toxicity.
• All patients need to know that fatty liver is reversible *only* if they strictly follow the therapeutic program; otherwise, they risk permanent liver damage.

Wilson's Disease
(Hepatolenticular degeneration)

Wilson's disease is a rare, inherited metabolic disorder characterized by retention of excessive amounts of copper in the liver, brain, kidneys, and corneas. These deposits eventually lead to tissue necrosis and fibrosis, causing a variety of clinical effects, especially hepatic disease and neurologic changes. Wilson's disease is progressive and, if untreated, leads to fatal hepatic failure.

Causes and incidence

Wilson's disease is inherited as an autosomal recessive trait when *both* parents carry the abnormal gene. There is a 25% chance that parents will transmit Wilson's disease (and a 50% chance they will transmit the carrier state) to each of their offspring. The disease occurs most often among eastern European Jews, Sicilians, and southern Italians, probably as a result of consanguineous marriages.

This genetic disorder causes excessive intestinal absorption of copper and subsequent decreased excretion of copper in the stool. Copper accumulates first in the liver, and as liver cells necrose, they release copper into the bloodstream, which then carries it to other tissues. For example, in the kidneys, excretion of excessive amounts of unbound copper

in the urine (hypercupriuria) results from deficiency of ceruloplasmin, a serum enzyme normally bound to copper. The deposition of copper in the tissue decreases serum copper (hypocupremia).

Signs and symptoms

Clinical manifestations of Wilson's disease usually appear between ages 6 and 20, although they can occur as late as age 40. Symptoms result from the damage to the body tissues from progressive deposition of copper, and vary according to the individual and the progress of the disease.

The most characteristic symptom of Wilson's disease (by itself sufficient for diagnosis) is Kayser-Fleischer rings—rusty brown rings of pigment at the periphery of the corneas. Fever may also occur in acute disease or with intercurrent infection. Other clinical features depend on the area affected:
- *liver* (including spleen): hepatomegaly, splenomegaly, ascites, jaundice, hematemesis, spider angiomas, and thrombocytopenia, eventually leading to cirrhosis or subacute necrosis of the liver
- *blood*: anemia and leukopenia
- *CNS*: "wing-flapping" tremors in arms, "pill-rolling" tremors in hands, facial and muscular rigidity, dysarthria, unsteady gait, emotional and behavioral changes
- *genitourinary tract*: aminoaciduria, proteinuria, peptidiuria, uricosuria, glycosuria, and phosphaturia
- *musculoskeletal system:* (in severe disease): muscle-wasting, contractures, deformities, osteomalacia, and pathologic fractures.

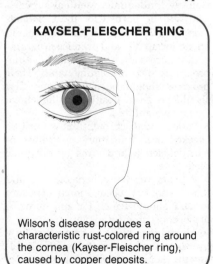

KAYSER-FLEISCHER RING

Wilson's disease produces a characteristic rust-colored ring around the cornea (Kayser-Fleischer ring), caused by copper deposits.

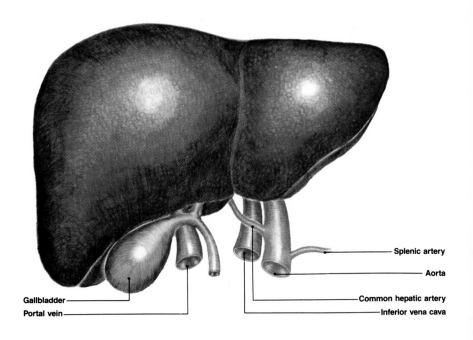

Splenic artery

Aorta

Gallbladder

Common hepatic artery

Portal vein

Inferior vena cava

Microscopic view of liver lobule

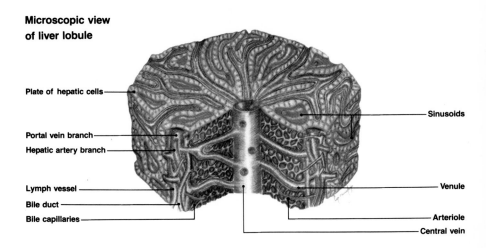

Plate of hepatic cells

Sinusoids

Portal vein branch

Hepatic artery branch

Lymph vessel

Venule

Bile duct

Bile capillaries

Arteriole

Central vein

Hypothalamus and pituitary

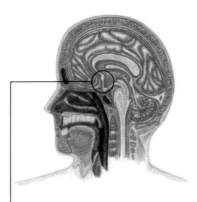

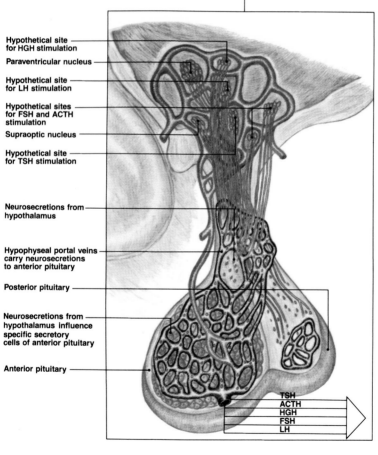

Hypothetical site for HGH stimulation

Paraventricular nucleus

Hypothetical site for LH stimulation

Hypothetical sites for FSH and ACTH stimulation

Supraoptic nucleus

Hypothetical site for TSH stimulation

Neurosecretions from hypothalamus

Hypophyseal portal veins carry neurosecretions to anterior pituitary

Posterior pituitary

Neurosecretions from hypothalamus influence specific secretory cells of anterior pituitary

Anterior pituitary

TSH
ACTH
HGH
FSH
LH

Endocrine target organs

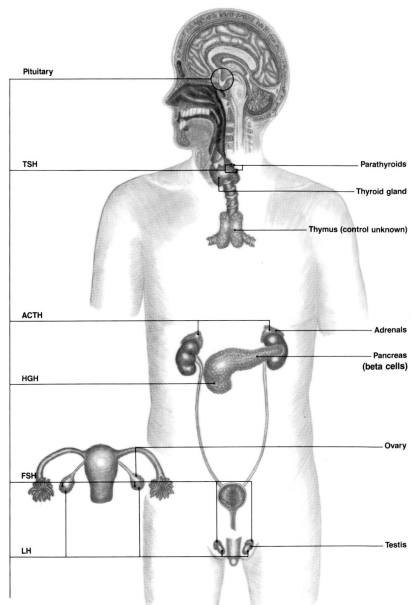

- Pituitary
- TSH
- ACTH
- HGH
- FSH
- LH

- Parathyroids
- Thyroid gland
- Thymus (control unknown)
- Adrenals
- Pancreas (beta cells)
- Ovary
- Testis

GASTROINTESTINAL TRACT

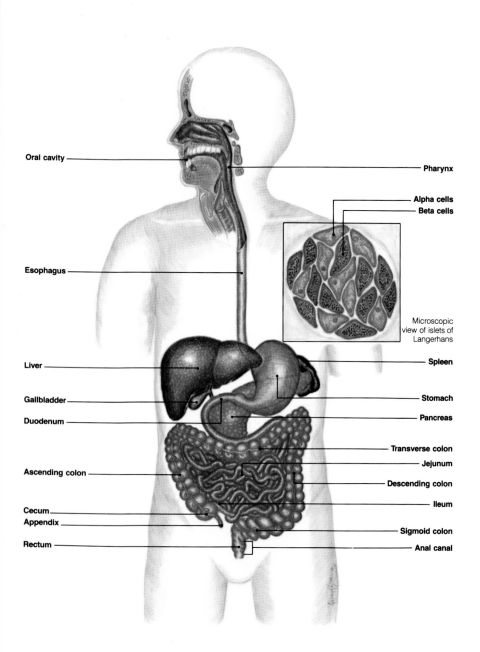

Oral cavity

Pharynx

Alpha cells

Beta cells

Esophagus

Microscopic view of islets of Langerhans

Liver

Spleen

Gallbladder

Stomach

Duodenum

Pancreas

Transverse colon

Jejunum

Ascending colon

Descending colon

Ileum

Cecum

Appendix

Sigmoid colon

Rectum

Anal canal

Diagnosis

Several tests suggest Wilson's disease:

- *serum ceruloplasmin:* less than 20 mg/100 ml
- *serum copper:* less than 80 mcg/100 ml
- *urine copper:* more than 100 mcg/24 hours (may be as high as 1,000 mcg)
- *liver biopsy:* excessive copper deposits (250 mcg/g dry weight), tissue changes indicative of chronic active hepatitis, fatty liver, or cirrhosis.

However, revelation of Kayser-Fleischer rings during slit-lamp ophthalmic examination confirms diagnosis.

Treatment

Treatment aims to reduce the amount of copper in the tissues, prevent additional accumulation, and manage hepatic disease. The most effective treatment for Wilson's disease consists of lifetime therapy with D-penicillamine, a copper-chelating agent that mobilizes copper from the tissues and promotes its excretion in the urine. However, about one third of patients are sensitive to this drug, necessitating dosage adjustment or discontinuation. If an adverse reaction recurs after the second dosage adjustment, the patient may require treatment with corticosteroids, such as prednisone. If the reaction is so severe that therapy can't continue, triethylenetetramine dihydrochloride is an effective substitute; however, it's not commercially available. Treatment also includes potassium and sodium supplements before meals, to prevent gastrointestinal absorption of copper.

Additional considerations

- Since penicillamine is chemically related to penicillin, whether or not the patient is allergic to penicillin should be determined before administering the first dose. He must be watched closely for allergic reactions, such as fever, skin rash, adenopathy, severe leukopenia, and thrombocytopenia. Penicillamine should always be given on an empty stomach. If gastrointestinal irritation develops, enteric-coated tablets may be provided.
- Patient and family must know which foods to avoid on a low-copper diet (mushrooms, nuts, chocolate, dried fruit, liver, and shellfish). The patient should use distilled water, since most tap water flows through copper pipes.
- The patient will need lifetime therapy, and he and his family should be helped with arrangements for continuing education, physical or vocational rehabilitation, and community nursing services.
- Because the neurologic changes that Wilson's disease produces often lead to its misdiagnosis as a psychiatric disorder, the patient should be reassured that his condition has a treatable physical basis.
- For a patient in an advanced stage of the disease, self-care is needed to prevent further mental and physical deterioration. He'll need an exercise schedule. Sensory deprivation or overload should be avoided and accidents and injuries that could occur as a result of neurologic deficits should be prevented.
- If the patient is in a terminal stage, the family will need emotional support.
- Couples who are blood relatives or who have a relative with Wilson's disease should get genetic counseling. The chance of their having a child with Wilson's disease is 25% with *each* pregnancy. Parents should know the early symptoms of this disease, so they can seek prompt treatment for their child; regular pediatric examinations are important for detection.

Hepatic Encephalopathy

(Hepatic coma)

Hepatic encephalopathy is a neurologic syndrome that develops as a complication of chronic liver disease. Most common in patients with cirrhosis, this syndrome is due primarily to ammonia intoxication of the brain. It may be acute and self-limiting, or chronic and progressive. Treatment requires correction of the precipitating cause and reduction of blood ammonia levels. In advanced stages, prognosis is extremely poor despite vigorous treatment.

Causes

Hepatic encephalopathy follows rising blood ammonia levels. Normally, the ammonia produced by protein breakdown in the bowel is metabolized to urea in the liver. When portal blood shunts past the liver, ammonia directly enters the systemic circulation and is carried to the brain. Such shunting may result from the collateral venous circulation that develops in portal hypertension or from surgically created portal-systemic shunts. Cirrhosis further compounds this problem, because impaired hepatocellular function prevents conversion of ammonia that reaches the liver.

Other factors that predispose to rising ammonia levels include excessive protein intake, sepsis, excessive accumulation of nitrogenous body wastes (from constipation or gastrointestinal hemorrhage), and bacterial action on protein and urea to form ammonia. Certain other factors heighten the brain's sensitivity to ammonia intoxication: fluid and electrolyte imbalance (especially metabolic alkalosis), hypoxia, azotemia, impaired glucose metabolism, infection, and administration of sedatives, narcotics, and general anesthetics.

Signs and symptoms

Clinical manifestations of hepatic encephalopathy vary, depending on the severity of neurologic involvement, and develop in four stages:
* *prodromal stage*—early symptoms are often overlooked because they're so subtle: slight personality changes (disorientation, forgetfulness, slurred speech) and a slight tremor
* *impending stage*—tremor progresses into asterixis (liver flap, flapping tremor)—the hallmark of hepatic encephalopathy—which is characterized by quick, irregular extensions and flexions of the wrists and fingers when the

wrists are held out straight and the hands flexed upward. Lethargy, aberrant behavior, and apraxia also occur.
* *stuporous stage*—hyperventilation; patient stuporous but noisy and abusive when aroused
* *comatose stage*—hyperactive reflexes, a positive Babinski's sign, fetor hepaticus (musty, sweet odor to the breath), and coma.

Diagnosis

Clinical features, a positive history of liver disease, and elevated serum ammonia levels in venous and arterial samples confirm hepatic encephalopathy. Other supportive lab values include EEG, which slows as the disease progresses, elevated bilirubin, and prolonged prothrombin time.

Treatment

Effective treatment stops progression of encephalopathy by reducing blood ammonia levels. Such treatment eliminates ammonigenic substances from the gastrointestinal tract by administration of neomycin to suppress bacterial flora (preventing them from converting amino acids into ammonia); by sorbitol-induced catharsis to produce osmotic diarrhea; by continuous aspiration of blood from the stomach; by administration of lactulose to suppress bacterial production of ammonia; and by decreasing dietary protein intake. Lactulose traps ammonia in the bowel and promotes its excretion. It's effective because bacterial enzymes change lactulose to lactic acid and thereby render the colon too acid for bacterial growth. At the same time, the resulting increase in free hydrogen ions prevents diffusion of ammonia through the mucosa; lactulose promotes conversion of systemically absorbable NH_3 to NH_4, which is poorly absorbed and can be excreted. Lactulose syrup may be given 30 to 45 ml P.O. three or four times daily. For acute hepatic coma, 300 ml diluted with 700 ml water may be administered by retention enema. Lactulose therapy requires careful monitoring of fluid and electrolyte balance. The usual dose of neomycin is 3 to 4 g/day P.O. or by retention enema. Although neomycin is nonabsorbable at recommended dosages, an amount that exceeds 4 g/day may produce irreversible hearing loss and nephrotoxicity.

Treatment may also include potassium supplements (80 to 120 mEq/day, P.O. or I.V.) to correct alkalosis (from increased ammonia levels), especially if the patient is taking diuretics. Sometimes, hemodialysis can temporarily clear toxic blood. Exchange transfusions may provide dramatic but temporary improvement; however, these require a particularly large amount of blood. Salt-poor albumin may be used to maintain fluid and electrolyte balance, replace depleted albumin levels, and restore plasma.

Additional considerations

Care for a patient with hepatic enceph-alopathy includes:

• frequently recording level of consciousness; continually orienting the patient to place and time; recording patient's handwriting daily to monitor progression of neurologic involvement.

• monitoring intake, output, and fluid and electrolyte balance; checking daily weight and measuring abdominal girth; watching for and immediately reporting signs of anemia (decreased hemoglobin), infection, alkalosis (increased serum bicarbonate), and gastrointestinal bleeding (melena, hematemesis).

• giving drugs, as ordered, and watching for side effects.

• asking the dietary department to provide the specified low-protein diet, with carbohydrates for calories; providing good mouth care.

• promoting rest, comfort, and quiet; discouraging stressful exercise.

• using restraints, if necessary, but avoiding sedatives; protecting the comatose patient's eyes from corneal injury by using artificial tears or eyepatches.

• providing emotional support for the patient's family in the terminal stage of encephalopathy.

GALLBLADDER & DUCT DISEASES

Cholelithiasis, Choledocholithiasis, Cholangitis, Cholecystitis, Cholesterolesis, Biliary Cirrhosis, and Gallstone Ileus

Diseases of the gallbladder and biliary tract are common and often painful conditions that usually require surgery and may be life-threatening. They are commonly associated with deposition of calculi and inflammation.

Causes and incidence

Cholelithiasis, stones or calculi (gallstones) in the gallbladder, results from changes in bile components. Gallstones are made of cholesterol, calcium bilirubinate, or a mixture of cholesterol and bilirubin pigment. They arise during periods of sluggishness in the gallbladder due to pregnancy, oral contraceptives, diabetes mellitus, celiac disease, cirrhosis of the liver, and pancreatitis. Cholelithiasis is the fifth leading cause of hospitalization among adults, and accounts for 90% of all gallbladder and

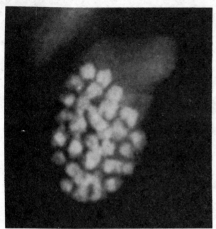

Oral cholecystography shows stones in the gallbladder.

duct diseases. Prognosis is usually good with treatment unless infection occurs, in which case prognosis depends on its severity and response to antibiotics.

One out of every ten patients with gallstones develops *choledocholithiasis* or gallstones in the common bile duct (sometimes called "common duct stones"). This occurs when stones passed out of the gallbladder lodge in the hepatic and common bile ducts and obstruct the flow of bile into the duodenum. Prognosis is also good unless infection occurs.

Cholangitis, infection of the bile duct, is often associated with choledocholithiasis and may follow percutaneous transhepatic cholangiography. Predisposing factors may include bacterial or metabolic alteration of bile acids. Widespread inflammation may cause fibrosis and stenosis of the common bile duct. Prognosis for this rare condition is poor— stenosing or primary sclerosing cholangitis is almost always fatal.

Cholecystitis, acute or chronic inflammation of the gallbladder, is usually associated with a gallstone impacted in the cystic duct, causing painful distention of the gallbladder. Cholecystitis accounts for 10% to 25% of all patients requiring gallbladder surgery. The acute form is most common during middle age; the

chronic form, among the elderly. Prognosis is good with treatment.

Cholesterolesis, cholesterol polyps or deposits of cholesterol crystals in the submucosa of the gallbladder, may result from bile secretions containing high concentrations of cholesterol and insufficient bile salts. These polyps may be localized or speckle the entire gallbladder with yellow spots. Cholesterolesis, the most common pseudotumor, is not related to widespread inflammation of the mucosa or lining of the gallbladder. Prognosis is good with surgery.

Biliary cirrhosis, ascending infection of the biliary system, sometimes follows viral destruction of liver and duct cells, but the primary cause is unknown. This condition usually leads to obstructive jaundice and involves the portal and periportal spaces of the liver. It strikes women aged 40 to 60 nine times more often than men. Prognosis is poor—about 75% of patients die within 1 to 5 years from hepatic coma, variceal hemorrhage, or superimposed hepatoma.

Gallstone ileus results from a gallstone lodging at the terminal ileum. This condition is more common in the elderly. Prognosis is good with surgery.

Generally, gallbladder and duct diseases occur during middle age. Between ages 20 and 50, they're six times more common in women, but incidence between men and women becomes equal after age 50. Incidence rises with each succeeding decade.

Signs and symptoms

Although gallbladder disease may be asymptomatic (even when X-rays reveal gallstones), acute cholelithiasis, acute cholecystitis, choledocholithiasis, and cholesterolesis produce the symptoms of a classic gallbladder attack. Such an attack often follows meals rich in fats (such as fried foods, creams, and chocolates) or may occur in the middle of the night, suddenly awakening the individual. It begins with acute abdominal pain in the upper right quadrant. This pain may radiate to the back, between the shoulders, or to the front of the chest; it may be so severe that the patient seeks emergency room care. Other clinical features may include recurring fat intolerance, biliary colic, belching that leaves a sour taste in the mouth, flatulence, indigestion, diaphoresis, nausea, vomiting, chills, and low-grade fever. Jaundice may occur if a stone obstructs the common bile duct (small stones are more likely to do this than larger ones). Clay-colored stools may also occur with choledocholithiasis.

Clinical features of cholangitis include a rise in eosinophils, jaundice, abdominal pain, high fever and chills; biliary cirrhosis may produce jaundice, related itching, weakness, fatigue, slight weight loss, and abdominal pain. Gallstone ileus produces signs of small bowel obstruction—nausea, vomiting, abdominal distention, and absence of bowel sounds if the bowel is completely obstructed. Its most telling sign is the intermittent recurrence of colicky pain.

Diagnosis

Echography and X-rays detect gallstones. Specific procedures include:

• *flat plate of the abdomen:* identifies calcified, but not cholesterol, stones

• *oral cholecystography:* shows stones in the gallbladder and biliary duct obstruction

• *percutaneous transhepatic cholangiography:* an imaging technique done under fluoroscopic control, distinguishes between gallbladder disease and cancer of the head of the pancreas in patients with jaundice

• *intravenous cholangiography:* visualizes the ductal system

• *hida scan:* of the gallbladder; detects obstruction of the cystic duct

• *CAT scan:* although not used routinely, helps to distinguish between obstructive and nonobstructive jaundice.

Elevated icteric index, total bilirubin, urine bilirubin, and alkaline phospha-

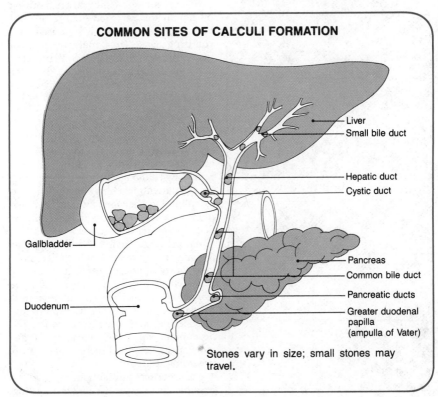

COMMON SITES OF CALCULI FORMATION

Liver
Small bile duct
Hepatic duct
Cystic duct
Pancreas
Common bile duct
Pancreatic ducts
Greater duodenal papilla (ampulla of Vater)
Gallbladder
Duodenum

Stones vary in size; small stones may travel.

tase support the diagnosis. WBC is slightly elevated during a cholecystitis attack. Differential diagnosis is essential, because gallbladder disease can mimic several other diseases (myocardial infarction, angina, pancreatitis, cancer of the head of the pancreas, pneumonia, peptic ulcer, hiatal hernia, esophagitis, gastritis). Serum amylase differentiates between gallbladder disease and pancreatitis. With suspected heart disease, serial enzyme tests and EKG should precede gallbladder and upper gastrointestinal diagnostic tests.

Treatment

Surgery, usually an elective procedure, is the treatment of choice for gallbladder and duct disease. Surgery may include cholecystectomy, cholecystectomy with choledochostomy, or cholecystojejunostomy (palliative anastomosis of gallblad-

der to jejunum to bypass an obstruction of bile flow). Other treatment includes a low-fat diet to prevent acute attacks, and vitamin K for itching, jaundice, and bleeding tendencies due to vitamin K deficiency. Initial treatment during an acute attack includes insertion of nasogastric tube and administration of anticholinergics and antispasmodics. Treatment for cholangitis should also include antibiotics.

Additional considerations

Health care for gallbladder and duct disease focuses on supportive care and close postoperative observation. This includes:

• before surgery, teaching the patient to deep-breathe, cough, expectorate, perform leg exercise, repositioning, and ambulation techniques that are necessary after surgery.

• after surgery, monitoring vital signs carefully; allowing the patient nothing by mouth for 24 to 48 hours, or until bowel sounds return and nausea and vomiting cease (postoperative nausea may indicate a full bladder); percussing over the symphysis pubis for bladder distention if the patient doesn't void within 8 hours, or if the amount voided is inadequate, based on the amount of I.V. fluids received per hour (especially important in patients receiving anticholinergics, since catheterization should be avoided); encouraging coughing and deep breathing, although this will be painful for the patient; teaching the patient how to splint the incision area to decrease pain; auscultating lungs to determine if deep breathing is effective.

• reporting any pain other than that at the site of the incision (which normally lasts 24 to 48 hours), especially sudden pain which the patient describes as a tearing of the incision (possible wound dehiscence) and chest or back pain; administering adequate medication to relieve pain, since the proximity of the incision to the diaphragm makes deep breathing difficult.

• encouraging ambulation as soon as possible, usually the evening or morning

SYMPTOMS OF VIRAL HEPATITIS	
PREICTERIC PHASE	**ICTERIC PHASE**
Headache	Yellow scleras
Photophobia	
Coryza	Cervical adenopathy
Altered sense of smell	Liver enlargement
Altered sense of taste	Splenomegaly
Fever	Anorexia
Pharyngitis	Bile obstruction
Cough	Pain in upper right abdominal quadrant
Lymph node enlargement	
Liver enlargement	Dark urine
Nausea, vomiting, and anorexia	Mild weight loss
Fatigue	Yellow skin
Myalgia	Severe pruritus
Arthralgia	

after surgery; providing elastic stockings to support leg muscles and promote venous blood flow, and discouraging sitting in a chair, thus preventing stasis and possible clot formation; checking daily for a positive Homans' sign (pain on dorsiflexion of the foot) or calf tenderness, both signs of phlebitis and thrombophlebitis; having the patient rest in slight Fowler's position as much as possible to direct any abdominal drainage into the pelvic cavity rather than allowing it to accumulate under the diaphragm; evaluating the incision site for bleeding (serosanguineous and bile drainage is common during the first 24 to 48 hours if the patient has a wound drain); making sure there is no kink in the drainage tube if, after a choledochostomy, a T tube drain is placed in the duct and attached to a drainage bag; checking for adequate connecting tubing from the T tube that's well secured to the patient to prevent dislodgement; measuring and recording drainage daily (200 to 300 ml is normal); teaching patients

who will be discharged with a T tube how to empty it, change the dressing, and perform proper skin care.

Abdominal distention is common the second and third postoperative days but should resolve spontaneously in most patients.

About 4 to 6 days after surgery, behavioral changes may occur due to fluid and electrolyte imbalances, especially potassium and sodium disturbances, with the discontinuation of I.V. fluids and inadequate oral intake. Before judging the patient as depressed, fluid intake and output and electrolyte status for the past 24 hours should be assessed. Dehydration may result from inadequate intake or fluid shift into extravascular spaces.

At discharge, the patient must avoid doing any heavy lifting or straining for 6 weeks. He should walk daily. Food restrictions are unnecessary unless he has an intolerance to a specific food or some underlying condition (diabetes, atherosclerosis, obesity) that requires such restriction.

Selected References

Bates, Robin. *The Illusive Illness*, NOVA. WGBH Educational Foundation, 1980.

Bell, Judy. *Just Another Patient with Gallstones*, NURSING79. 9:26, October 1979.

Bockus, Henry, ed. GASTROENTEROLOGY, 3rd ed. Philadelphia: W.B. Saunders Co., 1976.

Boyer, Carol A., and Susan M. Oehlberg, eds. *Symposium on Diseases of the Liver*, NURSING CLINICS OF NORTH AMERICA. 12:257-356, June 1977.

Corey, L., and K. Holmes. *Sexual Transmission of Hepatitis A in Homosexual Men: Incidence and Mechanism*, NEW ENGLAND JOURNAL OF MEDICINE. 302:435, February 21, 1980.

Cossart, Yvonne E. VIRUS HEPATITIS AND ITS CONTROL. New York: Macmillan Co., 1978.

Dolan, Patricia, and Harry Greene. *Conquering Cirrhosis of the Liver*, NURSING76. 6:44-53, December 1976.

Given, Barbara A., and Sandra J. Simmons. GASTROENTEROLOGY IN CLINICAL NURSING, 3rd ed. St. Louis: C.V. Mosby Co., 1979.

Greenberger, Norton J., and Daniel H. Winship. GASTROINTESTINAL DISORDERS: A PATHO-PHYSIOLOGIC APPROACH. Chicago: Year Book Medical Publishers, 1976.

Hoofnagle, J.H., et al. *Transmission of Non-A, Non-B Hepatitis*, ANNALS OF INTERNAL MEDICINE. 87:14-20, 1977.

Leevy, Carroll M., et al. DISEASES OF THE LIVER AND BILIARY TRACT. Chicago: Year Book Medical Publishers, 1977.

Riely, Caroline A. DISEASES OF THE LIVER AND BILIARY TRACT: STANDARDIZATION OF NOMENCLATURE, DIAGNOSTIC CRITERIA AND DIAGNOSTIC METHODOLOGY. Washington, D.C.: Dept. of Health, Education and Welfare, 1976.

Schiff, Leon, ed. DISEASES OF THE LIVER, 4th ed. Philadelphia: J.B. Lippincott Co., 1975.

Zimmerman, Hyman J. HEPATOTOXICITY: THE ADVERSE EFFECTS OF DRUGS AND OTHER CHEMICALS IN THE LIVER. New York: Appleton-Century-Crofts, 1978.

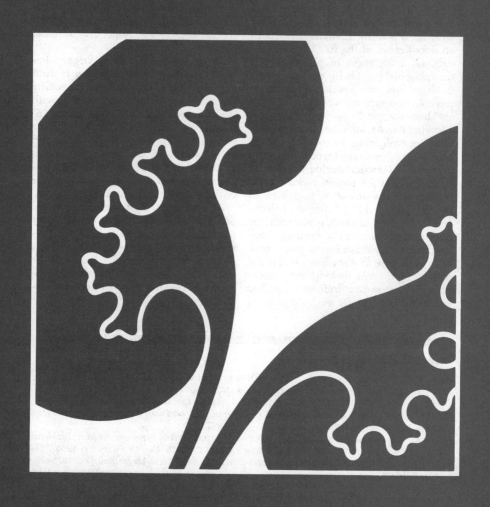

12 Renal and Urologic Disorders

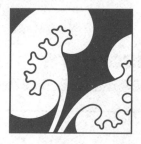

Renal and Urologic Disorders

Introduction

Renal and urologic diseases currently affect more than 8 million Americans. Symptoms can range from inconsequential to life-threatening. But because of technological advances in treatment and care, persons even with chronic renal disease can expect to live longer, more normal lives.

Kidneys and homeostasis
Through the production and elimination of urine, the kidneys maintain homeostasis. These vital organs regulate the volume, electrolyte concentration, and acid-base balance of body fluids; detoxify the blood and eliminate wastes; regulate blood pressure; and aid in erythropoiesis. The kidneys eliminate wastes from the body through urine formation (by glomerular filtration, tubular reabsorption, and tubular secretion) and excretion. Glomerular filtration, the process of filtering the blood flowing through the kidneys, depends on the permeability of the capillary walls, vascular pressure, and filtration pressure. The normal glomerular filtration rate (GFR) is about 120 ml/minute.

Clearance measures function
Clearance, the volume of plasma that can be cleared of a substance per unit of time, depends on how renal tubular cells handle the substance that has been filtered by the glomerulus:

- If the tubules don't reabsorb or secrete the substance, clearance equals the GFR.
- If the tubules reabsorb it, clearance is less than the GFR.
- If the tubules secrete it, clearance is greater than the GFR.
- If the tubules reabsorb and secrete it, clearance is less than, equal to, or greater than the GFR.

The most accurate measure of glomerular function is creatinine clearance, since this substance is filtered only by the glomerulus and is not reabsorbed by the tubules.

The transport of filtered substances in tubular reabsorption or secretion may be active—requiring the expenditure of energy—or passive—requiring none. For example, energy is required to move sodium across tubular cells (active transport), but none is required to move urea (passive transport). The amount of reabsorption or secretion of a substance depends on the maximum tubular transport capacity (Tm) for that substance—that is, the amount of a substance reabsorbed or secreted per minute.

Water regulation
Hormones partially control water regulation by the kidneys. Hormonal control depends on the response of osmoreceptors to changes in osmolality. The two hormones involved are antidiuretic hormone (ADH), produced by the pituitary

gland, and aldosterone, produced by the adrenal cortex. ADH alters the collecting tubules' permeability to water. When plasma concentration of ADH is high, the tubules are very permeable to water, so a greater amount of water is reabsorbed, creating a highly concentrated but small volume of urine. The reverse is true if ADH concentration is low.

Aldosterone, however, regulates sodium reabsorption from the distal tubules. High plasma aldosterone concentration promotes sodium reabsorption from the tubules and decreases sodium

ASSESSMENT OF SERUM AND URINE VALUES IN RENAL DISEASE

	NORMAL SERUM VALUE	DEVIATION	NORMAL URINE VALUE	DEVIATION
Sodium	136-146 mEq/L	↑ or N	50-130 mEq/L	V
Potassium	3.5-5.5 mEq/L	↑	20-70 mEq/L	↓
Chloride	96-106 mEq/L	↑	50-130 mEq/L	↓
Calcium	8.5-10.5 mg/ 100 ml	↓	5-12 mEq/L	↓
Phosphorus	2-4.5 mg/100 ml	↑	1 g/24 hr	V
Magnesium	1.6-2.2 mEq/L	↑ or N	2-18 mEq/L	↓
CO_2 combining power	24 mEq/L	↓		
Specific gravity			1.003-1.030	↓
pH			5.0-8.0	↑
BUN/Urea	9-18 mg/100 ml	↑	10-20 g/L	↓
Creatinine	0.7-1.5 mg/100 ml	↑	1.0-1.6 g/24 hr	↓
Osmolality	280-295 mOsm/kg	V	500-1,200 mOsm/ kg	↓
Uric acid	3-7 mg/100 ml	↑		
Glucose	70-100 mg/100 ml	↑ or N	0	V
Protein	6-8 g/100 ml	↓ or N	0	V
Hematocrit	40%-50%	↓		
Hemoglobin	12-16 g/100 ml	↓		
WBC	4,000-10,000/mm³	V	<2,000,000/24 hr	V
RBC			<1,000,000/24 hr	V
Casts			<100,000/24 hr	V
Bacteria			<100,000 organisms/ml	V
Alkaline phosphatase	5-13 K-A-U	↑		

KEYS: ↑ = increased, ↓ = decreased, N = normal, V = varies

STRUCTURE OF THE KIDNEYS

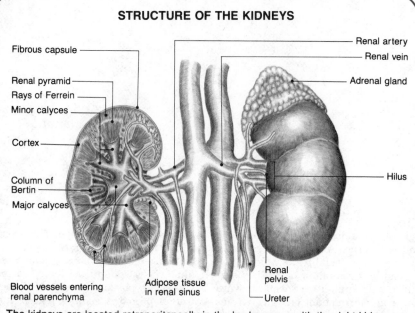

Fibrous capsule

Renal pyramid
Rays of Ferrein
Minor calyces

Cortex

Column of
Bertin
Major calyces

Renal artery
Renal vein
Adrenal gland

Hilus

Blood vessels entering
renal parenchyma

Adipose tissue
in renal sinus

Renal
pelvis
Ureter

The kidneys are located retroperitoneally in the lumbar area, with the right kidney a little lower than the left because of the liver mass above it. The left kidney is slightly longer than the right and closer to the midline. The kidneys assume different locations with changes in body position. The coverings of the kidneys consist of the true or fibrous capsule, perirenal fat, renal fascia, and pararenal fat.

Renal arteries branch into five segmental arteries that supply different areas of the kidneys. The segmental arteries then branch into several divisions from which the afferent arterioles and vasa recta arise. Renal veins follow a similar branching pattern, characterized by stellate vessels and locking segmental branches, and empty into the inferior vena cava. The tubular system receives its blood supply from a peritubular capillary network of vessels.

excretion in the urine; low plasma aldosterone concentration promotes sodium excretion.

Aldosterone also helps control the distal tubular secretion of potassium. Other factors that determine potassium secretion include the amount of potassium ingested, number of hydrogen ions secreted, level of intracellular potassium, amount of sodium in the distal tubule, and the GFR.

The countercurrent mechanism is the method by which the kidneys concentrate urine; this mechanism is composed of a multiplication system and an exchange system, which occur in the renal medulla via the limbs of the loops of Henle and the vasa recta. This mechanism achieves active transport of sodium and chloride between the loops of Henle and the medullary interstitial fluid. Failure of this mechanism produces polyuria and nocturia.

To regulate acid-base balance, the kidneys secrete hydrogen ions, reabsorb sodium and bicarbonate ions, acidify phosphate salts, and synthesize ammonia—all of which keep the blood at its normal pH of 7.38 to 7.42.

The kidneys assist in regulating blood pressure by synthesizing and secreting renin in response to an actual, or perceived, decreased extracellular fluid volume. Renin, in turn, clears a substrate

REVIEW OF RENAL AND
UROLOGIC ANATOMY

The gross structure of each kidney includes the lateral and medial margins, the hilus, the renal sinus, and renal parenchyma. The hilus, located at the medial margin, is the indentation where the blood and lymph vessels enter the kidney and the ureter emerges. The hilus leads to the renal sinus, which is a spacious cavity filled with adipose tissue, branches of the renal vessels, calyces, the renal pelvis, and the ureter. The renal sinus is surrounded by parenchyma, which consists of a cortex and a medulla. The cortex (outermost layer of the kidney) contains glomeruli (parts of the nephron), cortical arches (areas that separate the medullary pyramids from the renal surface), columns of Bertin (areas that separate the pyramids from one another), and medullary rays of Ferrein (long, delicate processes from the bases of the pyramids that mix with the cortex).

The medulla contains pyramids (cone-shaped structures of parenchymal tissue), papillae (apical ends of the pyramids through which urine oozes into the minor calyces), and papillary ducts of Bellini (collecting ducts in the pyramids that empty into the papillae).

The ureters are a pair of retroperitoneally located, mucosa-lined, fibromuscular tubes that transport urine from the renal pelvis to the urinary bladder. Although the ureters have no sphincters, their oblique entrance into the bladder creates a mucosal fold that may produce a sphincterlike action.

The adult urinary bladder is a spherical, hollow muscular sac, with a normal capacity of 300 to 500 ml. It is located anterior and inferior to the peritoneal cavity, and posterior to the pubic bones. The gross structure of the bladder includes the fundus (large central, posterosuperior portion of the bladder), the apex (anterosuperior region), the body (posteroinferior region containing the ureteral orifices), and the urethral orifice, or neck (most inferior portion of the bladder). The three orifices comprise a triangular area called the trigone.

Functional units
The functional units of each kidney are its 1 to 3 million nephrons. Each nephron is composed of the renal corpuscle and the tubular system. The renal corpuscle includes the glomerulus (a network of minute blood vessels) and Bowman's capsule (an epithelial sac surrounding the glomerulus that is part of the tubular system). The renal corpuscle has a vascular pole, where the afferent arteriole enters and the efferent arteriole emerges, and a urinary pole that narrows to form the beginning of the tubular system. The tubular system includes the proximal convoluted tubule, the loop of Henle, and the distal convoluted tubule. The last portion of the nephron consists of the collecting duct.

Innervation and vasculature
The kidneys are innervated by sympathetic branches from the celiac plexus, upper lumbar splanchnic and thoracic nerves, and the intermesenteric and superior hypogastric plexuses, which form a plexus around the kidneys. Similar numbers of sympathetic and parasympathetic nerves from the renal plexus, superior hypogastric plexus, and intermesenteric plexus innervate the ureters. Nerves that arise from the inferior hypogastric plexuses innervate the bladder. The parasympathetic nerve supply to the bladder controls micturition.

The ureters receive their blood supply from the renal, vesical, gonadal, and iliac arteries, and the abdominal aorta. The ureteral veins follow the arteries and drain into the renal vein. The bladder receives blood through vesical arteries. Vesical veins unite to form the pudendal plexus, which empties into the iliac veins. A rich lymphatic system drains the renal cortex, the kidneys, the ureters, and the bladder.

to form angiotensin I, which is cleared again to form angiotensin II. Angiotensin II increases arterial blood pressure by peripheral vasoconstriction and stimulates aldosterone secretion. The increased aldosterone level increases the reabsorption of sodium and water to correct the fluid deficit.

The kidneys secrete erythropoietin in response to decreased oxygen tension in the renal blood supply. Erythropoietin then acts on the bone marrow to increase the production of RBCs.

Renal tubular cells synthesize active vitamin D. Thus, the kidneys regulate calcium balance and bone metabolism.

Clinical assessment

Assessment of the renal and urologic systems begins with an accurate patient history; assessment also requires a thorough physical examination, and certain laboratory data and test results from invasive and noninvasive procedures. A patient history should include questions about symptoms that pertain specifically to the pathology of the renal and urologic systems, such as frequency and bedwetting; and about the presence of any systemic diseases that can produce renal or urologic dysfunction, such as hypertension, diabetes mellitus, or bladder infections. Family history may also suggest a genetic predisposition to certain renal diseases, such as glomerulonephritis or polycystic kidney disease. What medications the patient has been taking is also important; abuse of analgesics or antibiotics may cause nephrotoxicity.

Physical examination for renal disease

The first step in physical examination is careful observation of the patient's overall appearance, since renal disease affects all body systems. The patient's skin should be examined for color, turgor, intactness, texture; mucous membranes, color, secretions, odor, and intactness; eyes, for periorbital edema and vision; general activity, for motion, gait, and posture; muscle movement, for motor function and general strength;

and mental status, for level of consciousness, orientation, and response to stimuli.

Renal disease causes distinctive changes in vital signs: hypertension due to fluid and electrolyte imbalances and hyperactivity of the renin-angiotensin system; hyperventilation to compensate for metabolic acidosis; and an increased susceptibility to infection due to overall decreased resistance. Palpation and percussion reveal little, since the kidneys and bladder are difficult to palpate unless they are enlarged or distended.

Relevant laboratory data

Laboratory tests analyze serum levels of chemical substances, such as uric acid, creatinine, and BUN; tests also determine urine characteristics, including the presence of RBCs, WBCs, casts, or bacteria; specific gravity and pH; and physical properties, such as clarity, color, and characteristic ammonia odor.

Noninvasive monitoring of the renal and urologic systems includes the following:

• *Intake and output assessment:* Intake and output measurement helps assess the patient's hydration state but is not a valid evaluation of renal function, since urine output varies with different types of renal failure. However, to provide the most useful and accurate information, calibrated containers are used, baseline values for each patient established, measurement patterns compared, and intake and output measurements validated by weighing the patient daily. Also, monitoring all fluid losses—including blood, vomitus, diarrhea, and wound and stoma drainage—should be done.

• *Specimen collection:* Meticulous collection is vital for valid laboratory data. If the patient is collecting the specimen, he needs to know the importance of cleaning the meatal area thoroughly. The culture specimen should be caught midstream, in a sterile container; a specimen for urinalysis, in a clean container, preferably at the first voiding of the day. A 24-hour specimen collection should begin after discard-

INVASIVE DIAGNOSTIC TESTS FOR ASSESSING THE RENAL AND UROLOGIC SYSTEM

PROCEDURE AND PURPOSE	CLINICAL CONSIDERATIONS
Cystoscopy: Visualizes the inside of the bladder with a fiberoptic scope	*Before:* Sedatives given. *After:* Increased fluids offered; analgesics administered; the patient is watched for hematuria and signs of perforation, hemorrhage, and infection (chills, fever, increased pulse rate, shock).
Cystourethrography: Determines size and shape of bladder and urethra through X-rays and instilled contrast medium	*During:* The patient is catheterized. *After:* Increased fluids offered; the patient is observed for hypersensitivity reaction (chills, fever, increased pulse rate, itching, hives).
Cystometry: Evaluates micturition	*Before:* Voiding observed; the patient is catheterized for residual urine. *After:* Catheter removed; the patient is watched for stress incontinence when coughing; voiding is observed; the patient is catheterized for residual urine and given analgesics, as necessary, for discomfort.
Intravenous pyelography: Visualizes renal parenchyma, calyces, pelves, ureters, and bladder with X-rays and contrast medium	*After:* Patient is observed for hypersensitivity reaction (chills, fever, increased pulse rate, itching, hives) and watched for hematomas at injection site.
Nephrotomography: Visualizes parenchyma, calyces, and pelves in layers after I.V. injection of contrast medium, followed by tomography	*After:* Patient is observed for hypersensitivity reaction (chills, fever, increased pulse rate, itching, hives).
Renal angiography: Visualizes arterial tree, capillaries, and venous drainage of the kidney, using contrast medium injected into a catheter in the femoral artery or vein	*After:* Patient is observed for hypersensitivity reaction (chills, fever, increased pulse rate, itching, hives), hematomas and hemorrhage at injection site, and nephrotoxicity. Increased fluids are offered.
Renal scan: Determines renal function by visualizing the appearance and disappearance of radioisotopes within the kidney	*After:* Patient observed for hypersensitivity reaction (chills, fever, increased pulse rate, itching, hives).
Renal biopsy: Obtains specimen for developing histologic diagnosis and determines therapy and prognosis	*Before:* Patient's clotting times, prothrombin times, and platelet count are recorded on his chart as well as the fact that he has had an IVP. Patient is placed in prone position with his side slightly elevated on a towel or pillow, and the skin over the area to be biopsied is cleaned. *During:* Patient is helped to maintain proper position—lying still and holding his breath—if the biopsy is done at bedside. Often, however, it's done in the O.R. *After:* Patient breathes normally; gentle pressure is applied to the bandage site; the patient is watched for hemorrhage and hematoma at the biopsy site and for hematuria; bed rest is enforced for 24 hours postprocedure; increased fluids are offered.

COMMON RENAL SYMPTOMS

SYMPTOM	POSSIBLE CAUSE
Frequency	Infection, diabetes
Nocturia	Infection, prostatic disease
Urgency	Infection, prostatic disease
Hesitancy	Prostatic enlargement
Oliguria	Failure, insufficiency, neoplasms
Dysuria	Infection
Dribbling	Prostatic enlargement, strictures
Hematuria	Glomerular diseases, trauma, neoplasms
Pyuria	Infection
Edema	Nephrotic syndrome, failure
Incontinence	Infection, neoplasms, prolapsed uterus
Renal colic	Calculi

ing the first voiding; such specimens often necessitate special handling or preservatives. When obtaining a urine specimen from a catheterized patient, the specimen should not be taken from the collection bag; instead, a sample can be aspirated through the latex catheter, with a sterile needle and a syringe.

• *X-ray:* A plain film of the abdomen (kidney-ureter-bladder) assesses the size, shape, position, and possible areas of calcification of renal and urologic systems.

If the patient needs invasive diagnostic procedures such as cystoscopy, intravenous pyelography, and renal angiography, each procedure should be carefully explained to allay anxiety and encourage cooperation. He has to be prepared for the procedure, as appropriate, and afterward, observed for complications, such as hypersensitivity and hemorrhage. This is done by carefully monitoring vital signs, intake and output, and general status.

Treatment methods
Treatment of intractable renal or urinary system dysfunction may require urinary diversion, dialysis, or renal transplantation. Urinary diversion is the creation of an abnormal outlet for excreting urine. Several methods of urinary diversion are performed: ileal conduit, cutaneous ureterostomy, ureterosigmoidostomy, and the creation of a rectal bladder.

In dialysis, a machine or other artificial process imitates the kidneys' function by eliminating excess body fluids, maintaining or restoring plasma electrolyte and acid-base balances, and removing waste products and dialyzable poisons from the blood. Dialysis is most commonly used for patients with acute or chronic renal failure. The two most frequently used types of dialysis are peritoneal dialysis and hemodialysis.

In peritoneal dialysis, a dialysate solution is infused into the peritoneal cavity. Substances then diffuse through the peritoneal membrane into the solution. Waste products remain in the solution and are removed.

Hemodialysis separates solutes by differential diffusion through a cellophane membrane placed between the blood and the dialysate solution, in an external receptacle. Since the blood must actually pass out of the body into a dialysis machine, hemodialysis requires an access route to the blood supply by an arteriovenous fistula or cannula, or a bovine or synthetic graft. When caring for a patient with such vascular access routes, the health care professional should: monitor the patency of the shunt; prevent infection, and promote safety and adequate function; watch for complications after dialysis, which may include headache, vomiting, agitation, and twitching.

Patients with end-stage renal disease may benefit from renal transplantation, despite its great limitations: a shortage of donor kidneys, the chance of transplant rejection, and the necessity to take medications and receive lifelong follow-up care. After renal transplantation, the hospital staff member should maintain fluid and electrolyte balance, prevent infection, monitor for rejection, and promote psychologic well-being.

CONGENITAL ANOMALIES

Medullary Sponge Kidney

In medullary sponge kidney, the collecting ducts in the renal pyramids dilate, and cavities, clefts, and cysts form in the medulla. This disease may affect only a single pyramid in one kidney or all pyramids in both kidneys. The kidneys are usually somewhat enlarged but may be of normal size; they appear spongy.

Since this disorder is usually asymptomatic and benign, it's often overlooked until the patient reaches adulthood. Although medullary sponge kidney may be found in both sexes and in all age-groups, it primarily affects men aged 40 to 70. It occurs in about 1 in every 5,000 to 20,000 persons. Prognosis is generally very good. Medullary sponge kidney is unrelated to medullary cystic disease; these conditions are similar only in the presence and location of the cysts.

Causes
Medullary sponge kidney may be transmitted as an autosomal dominant trait, but this remains unproven. Most nephrologists still consider it a congenital abnormality.

Signs and symptoms
Symptoms usually appear only as a result of complications and are seldom present before adulthood. Such complications include formation of calcium phosphate stones, which lodge in the dilated cystic collecting ducts or pass through a ureter, and infection secondary to dilation of the ducts. These complications, which occur in about 30% of patients, are likely to produce severe colic, hematuria, lower urinary tract infection (burning on urination, urgency, frequency), and pyelonephritis.

Secondary impairment of renal function from obstruction and infection occurs in only about 10% of patients.

Diagnosis
Intravenous pyelography is usually the key to diagnosis, often showing a characteristic flowerlike appearance of the pyramidal cavities when they fill with contrast material. Retrograde pyelography or excretory urography may show renal calculi, but these tests are usually avoided because of the risk of infection.

Urinalysis is generally normal unless complications develop; however, it may show a slight reduction in concentrating ability or hypercalciuria.

Diagnosis must distinguish medullary sponge kidney from renal tuberculosis, renal tubular acidosis, and papillary necrosis.

Treatment
Treatment focuses on preventing or treating complications caused by stones and infection. Specific measures include increasing fluid intake and routine, periodic checks of renal function and urine. New symptoms necessitate immediate evaluation.

Since medullary sponge kidney is a benign condition, surgery is seldom necessary, except to remove stones during acute obstruction. Only serious, uncontrollable infection or hemorrhage requires nephrectomy.

Additional considerations
When caring for a patient with medullary sponge kidney, the hospital staff member should:
• explain the disease to the patient and family; stress that the condition is benign and the prognosis good.
• instruct the patient to bathe often and use proper toilet hygiene to prevent infection. (Such hygiene is especially im-

portant for a female patient, since the proximity of the urinary meatus and the anus increases the risk of infection.)
• stress the importance of completing the prescribed course of antibiotic therapy if infection occurs.
• explain all diagnostic procedures, and provide emotional support; demonstrate how to collect a clean-catch urine specimen for culture.
• when the patient is hospitalized for a stone, strain all urine, administer analgesics freely, and force fluids; tell the patient before discharge to watch for and report any signs of stone passage and urinary tract infection.

Medullary Cystic Disease
(Juvenile nephronophthisis)

Medullary cystic disease is a rare congenital renal disorder marked by cyst formation, primarily in the medulla and the corticomedullary junction. This disease occurs predominantly in young people of both sexes. Medullary cystic disease usually progresses to end-stage renal disease in late childhood or adolescence. Treatment doesn't halt progression of this disease, and most patients don't survive beyond their 30s without dialysis or kidney transplantation.

Causes
Medullary cystic disease appears to be transmitted as an autosomal recessive or dominant trait. The autosomal dominant pattern of inheritance seems to apply to adult onset.

Signs and symptoms
Anemia, which characteristically produces fatigue, lassitude, and pallor, is usually the presenting sign and often leads to the discovery of uremia as the underlying cause. Other signs are polyuria, nocturia, hyponatremia, and possibly, severe vascular volume depletion and hypotension due to renal salt-wasting. Parathyroid hyperplasia, which results in bone demineralization, may lead to renal rickets and retarded growth in children.

Proteinuria (possibly preceded by azotemia) and hypertension are usually absent until late stages, when medullary cystic disease progresses to end-stage renal failure. In fact, blood pressure is usually normal or even slightly below normal unless an underlying disorder causes hypertension.

For reasons still unknown, approximately half the patients with medullary cystic disease suffer a high-frequency hearing loss; the degree of loss increases with the severity of renal impairment. Also, 10% to 12% of patients with medullary cystic disease have ocular abnormalities.

Diagnosis
A typical pattern of symptoms or a positive family history of medullary cystic disease suggests this diagnosis.

 Arteriography and intravenous pyelography demonstrate small kidneys, and a biopsy confirms structural abnormalities.

Abnormal laboratory results include profound anemia, and high alkaline phosphatase (in young patients), low serum bicarbonate, and high BUN and serum creatinine. Urinalysis shows low specific gravity.

Treatment
Symptomatic treatment includes adequate intake of sodium, needed electrolytes, and fluids. Transplantation or dialysis may prolong survival.

Additional considerations
The patient's age, life-style, and degree of renal insufficiency should be considered

in health care planning. The patient must understand that although treatment relieves symptoms, this disease will permanently alter his life-style and can never be cured. He will need psychologic support, and must be taught ways to prevent complications of salt and water imbalances.

Health care includes: supervising daily care; monitoring vital signs, intake and output, and daily weight; watching for signs of dehydration (sunken eyes, poor skin turgor) and severe vascular volume depletion (rapid pulse rate, cold skin, and possibly, dyspnea); providing appropriate recreational activities, and enlisting the aid of hospital departments (social services, dietary, psychiatric), as needed.

The patient's family should be involved in his care as much as possible. They will need help understanding and adjusting to the prognosis, and preparing for changes as the patient approaches the uremic stage. Community support groups can help them cope with these problems.

Polycystic Kidney Disease

An inherited disorder, polycystic kidney disease is characterized by multiple, bilateral, grapelike clusters of fluid-filled cysts that grossly enlarge the kidneys, compressing and eventually replacing functioning renal tissue. This disease appears in two distinct forms. The infantile form causes stillbirth or early neonatal death. A few infants with this disease survive for 2 years and then develop fatal renal, congestive heart, or respiratory failure. Onset of the adult form is insidious but usually becomes obvious between ages 30 and 50; rarely, it may not cause symptoms until the patient is in his 70s. In the adult form, renal deterioration is more gradual but, like the infantile form, progresses relentlessly to fatal uremia.

Prognosis in adults is extremely variable. Progression may be slow, even after symptoms of renal insufficiency appear. However, after uremic symptoms develop, polycystic disease is usually fatal within 4 years, unless the patient receives treatment with dialysis.

Causes and incidence

While both types of polycystic kidney disease are genetically transmitted, the incidence in two distinct age-groups and different inheritance patterns suggest two unrelated disorders. The infantile type appears to be inherited as an autosomal recessive trait; the adult type, as an autosomal dominant trait. Both types affect males and females equally.

Signs and symptoms

The newborn with infantile polycystic disease often has pronounced epicanthal folds, a pointed nose, a small chin (Potter facies), and floppy, low-set ears. At birth, he has huge bilateral masses on the flanks that are symmetric, tense, and cannot be transilluminated. He characteristically shows signs of respiratory distress and congestive heart failure.

Eventually, he develops uremia and renal failure. Accompanying hepatic fibrosis may cause portal hypertension and bleeding varices to develop also.

Adult polycystic kidney disease is often asymptomatic while the patient's in his 30s and 40s, but may induce nonspecific symptoms, such as hypertension, polyuria, and urinary tract infection. Later, the patient develops overt symptoms related to the enlarging kidney mass, such as lumbar pain, widening girth, and swollen or tender abdomen. Such abdominal pain is usually worsened by exertion and relieved by lying down. In advanced stages, this disease may cause recurrent hematuria; life-threatening retroperitoneal bleeding resulting from cyst rupture; proteinuria; and colicky, abdominal pain from the ureteral passage of clots or calculi. Gen-

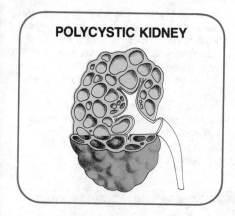

POLYCYSTIC KIDNEY

erally, about 10 years after symptoms appear, progressive compression of kidney structures by the enlarging mass causes renal insufficiency and failure, and uremia.

Diagnosis

A positive family history and a physical examination revealing large bilateral, irregular masses in the flanks strongly suggest polycystic kidney disease. In advanced stages, grossly enlarged and palpable kidneys make the diagnosis obvious. In patients with these findings, the following laboratory results are typical:

• *Intravenous or retrograde pyelography* reveals enlarged kidneys, with elongation of pelvis, flattening of the calyces, and indentations caused by cysts. Excretory urography of the newborn shows poor excretion of contrast medium.

• *X-ray and tomography* show kidney enlargement; tomography demonstrates multiple areas of cystic damage.

• *Urinalysis and creatinine clearance tests*—nonspecific tests that evaluate renal function—indicate abnormalities.

Diagnosis must rule out renal tumors.

Treatment

Polycystic kidney disease can't be cured, but careful management of urinary tract infections and secondary hypertension may prolong life. Progressive renal failure requires treatment similar to that for other types of renal disease, including dialysis or, rarely, kidney transplant.

When adult polycystic kidney disease is discovered in the asymptomatic stage, careful monitoring is required, including urine cultures and creatinine clearance tests repeated at 6-month intervals. When urine culture detects infection, prompt and vigorous antibiotic treatment is necessary even for asymptomatic infection. As renal impairment progresses, selected patients may undergo dialysis, transplantation, or both. Cystic abscess or retroperitoneal bleeding may require surgical drainage; intractable pain (rare) may also require surgery. However, since this disease is bilateral, nephrectomy usually isn't recommended, because it aggravates the risk of infection in the remaining kidney.

Additional considerations

Since polycystic kidney disease is usually relentlessly progressive, comprehensive patient teaching and emotional support are essential. The health care professional should:

• refer the young adult patient or parents of infants with this disease for genetic counseling. Such parents will probably have many questions about the risk to other offspring.

• provide supportive care to minimize symptoms; assess the patient's physical and mental state, and lifestyle; determine how rapidly the disease is progressing; use this information to plan individualized care.

• be familiar with all aspects of end-stage renal disease, including dialysis and transplantation; provide appropriate care and teaching as the disease progresses.

• explain all diagnostic procedures; ask the patient, before intravenous pyelography and other procedures using an iodine-based contrast medium, if he has ever had an allergic reaction to iodine or shellfish; watch for a possible allergic reaction after the test even if the patient has no history of allergy.

• administer antibiotics, as ordered, for urinary tract infection; stress the need to take medication exactly as prescribed, even if symptoms are minimal or absent.

ACUTE RENAL DISORDERS

Acute Renal Failure

Acute renal failure is the sudden interruption of kidney function due to obstruction, reduced circulation, or renal parenchymal disease. It's usually reversible with medical treatment; otherwise, it may progress to end-stage renal disease, uremic syndrome, and death.

Causes

The causes of acute renal failure are classified as prerenal, intrinsic (or parenchymal), and postrenal. Prerenal failure is associated with diminished blood flow to the kidneys. Such decreased flow may result from hypovolemia, shock, embolism, blood loss, sepsis, pooling of fluid in ascites or burns, and cardiovascular disorders, such as congestive heart failure, arrhythmias, and tamponade.

Intrinsic or parenchymal renal failure results from damage to the kidneys themselves, usually due to acute tubular necrosis. Such damage may also result from acute poststreptococcal glomerulonephritis, systemic lupus erythematosus, polyarteritis nodosa, vasculitis, sickle cell disease, bilateral renal vein thrombosis, nephrotoxins, ischemia, renal myeloma, and acute pyelonephritis.

Postrenal failure results from bilateral obstruction of urinary outflow. Its multiple causes include kidney stones, blood clots, papillae from papillary necrosis, tumors, benign prostatic hypertrophy, strictures, and urethral edema from catheterization.

Signs and symptoms

Acute renal failure is a critical illness. Its early signs are oliguria, azotemia, and rarely, anuria. Electrolyte imbalance, metabolic acidosis, and other severe effects follow, as the patient becomes increasingly uremic and renal dysfunction disrupts other body systems.

• *Gastrointestinal:* anorexia, nausea, vomiting, diarrhea or constipation, stomatitis, bleeding, hematemesis, dry mucous membranes, uremic breath

• *Central nervous system:* headache, drowsiness, irritability, confusion, personality changes, decreased concentration, convulsions, coma, minimal peripheral neuropathy

• *Cutaneous:* dryness, pruritus, pallor, purpura, and rarely, uremic frost

• *Cardiovascular:* early in the disease, hypotension; later, hypertension, dysrhythmias, fluid overload, congestive failure, systemic edema, anemia, altered clotting mechanisms

• *Respiratory:* pulmonary edema, Kussmaul's respirations.

Fever and chills indicate infection, a common complication.

Diagnosis

Patient history of renal disease suggests possible causes.

Blood tests indicating acute renal failure include elevated BUN, serum creatinine, and potassium; and low blood pH, bicarbonate, hematocrit, and hemoglobin. Urine samples show casts, cellular debris, decreased specific gravity, and in glomerular diseases, proteinuria and urine osmolality close to serum osmolality. Urine sodium level is less than 20 mEq/liter if oliguria results from decreased perfusion; urine sodium is greater than 300 mEq/liter if it results from an intrinsic problem.

Other appropriate diagnostic studies include ultrasound of the kidneys, plain films of the abdomen and the kidney-ureter-bladder, intravenous pyelography, renal scan, retrograde pyelography, and nephrotomography.

Treatment

Supportive measures include a diet high in calories and low in protein, sodium, and potassium, with supplemental vitamins and restricted fluids. Meticulous electrolyte monitoring is essential to detect hyperkalemia. If hyperkalemia occurs, acute therapy may include dialysis, hypertonic glucose and insulin infusions, and sodium bicarbonate—all administered I.V.—and sodium polystyrene sulfonate, P.O. or by enema, to permanently remove potassium from the body.

If measures fail to control uremic symptoms (hyperkalemia, congestive heart failure, and acidosis), hemo- or peritoneal dialysis may be necessary.

Additional considerations

When caring for an acute renal failure patient, the hospital staff member should:
• measure and record intake and output, including all body fluids, such as wound drainage, nasogastric output, and diarrhea; weigh the patient daily.
• assess hematocrit and hemoglobin levels, and replace blood components, as ordered; *not* use whole blood if the patient is prone to congestive heart failure and can't tolerate extra fluid volume.
• monitor vital signs; watch for and report any signs of pericarditis (pleuritic chest pain, tachycardia, pericardial friction rub), inadequate renal perfusion (hypotension), and acidosis.
• maintain proper electrolyte balance; strictly monitor potassium levels; watch for and report symptoms of hyperkalemia (malaise, anorexia, paresthesia, muscle weakness) and EKG changes (tall peaked T waves, widening QRS segment, disappearing P waves); avoid administering medications containing potassium.
• assess the patient frequently, especially during emergency treatment to lower potassium levels; monitor blood glucose levels and watch for signs of hyper- and hypoglycemia if the patient receives hypertonic glucose and insulin infusions: make sure the patient doesn't retain any sodium polystyrene sulfonate given rectally, to avoid constipation.
• maintain nutritional status; provide a high-calorie, low-protein, low-sodium, and low-potassium diet, with vitamin supplements; give the anorectic patient small, frequent meals.
• use aseptic technique, since the patient with acute renal failure is highly susceptible to infection; not allow personnel with upper respiratory tract infections to care for the patient.
• prevent complications of immobility by encouraging frequent coughing and deep breathing and by performing passive range-of-motion exercises; help the patient walk as soon as possible; add lubricating lotion to the patient's bathwater to combat skin dryness.
• provide good mouth care frequently, since mucous membranes are dry; provide an antibiotic solution, as ordered, if stomatitis occurs; have the patient swish the solution around in his mouth before swallowing.
• watch for gastrointestinal bleeding by guaiac-testing all stools for blood; administer medications appropriately, especially antacids and stool softeners.
• use appropriate safety measures, such as side rails and restraints, since the patient with CNS involvement may be dizzy or confused.
• provide reassurance and emotional support; fully explain all procedures to the patient and family.
• position the patient carefully during peritoneal dialysis; elevate the head of the bed to reduce pressure on the diaphragm and aid respiration; be alert for signs of infection (cloudy drainage, elevated temperature) and, rarely, bleeding; reduce the amount of dialysate if pain occurs; monitor blood sugars periodically, and administer insulin, as ordered; watch for complications, such as peritonitis, atelectasis, hypokalemia, pneumonia, and shock.
• check the site of the arteriovenous shunt or fistula every 2 hours for patency and signs of clotting if the patient requires hemodialysis; avoid using the arm with the shunt or fistula for taking blood pressures or drawing blood; keep two bulldog clips attached to the dressing over the shunt—use them to clamp off

the shunt if it becomes disconnected; monitor vital signs, clotting times, blood flow, the function of the vascular access site, and arterial and venous pressures during dialysis; watch for complications, such as septicemia, embolism, hepatitis, and rapid fluid and electrolyte loss; monitor vital signs and the vascular access site after dialysis; watch for signs of fluid and electrolyte imbalances.

Acute Pyelonephritis
(Acute infective tubulointerstitial nephritis)

One of the most common renal diseases, acute pyelonephritis is a sudden inflammation caused by bacteria that primarily affects the interstitial area and the renal pelvis; or less often, the renal tubules. With treatment and continued follow-up, prognosis is good and extensive permanent damage is rare.

Causes and incidence

Acute pyelonephritis results from bacterial infection of the kidneys. Infecting bacteria usually are normal intestinal and fecal flora that grow readily in urine. The most common causative organism is *Escherichia coli*, but *Proteus, Pseudomonas, Staphylococcus aureus*, and *Streptococcus faecalis* (enterococcus) may also cause such infections.

Typically, the infection spreads from the bladder to the ureters, then to the kidneys, as in vesicoureteral reflux. Vesicoureteral reflux may result from congenital weakness at the junction of the ureter and the bladder. Bacteria refluxed to intrarenal tissues may create colonies of infection within 24 to 48 hours. Infection may also result from instrumentation (catheterization, cystoscopy, urologic surgery), hematogenic infection (as in septicemia or endocarditis), or possibly, lymphatic infection.

Pyelonephritis may also result from an inability to empty the bladder (neurogenic bladder), urinary stasis, or urinary obstruction due to tumors, strictures, or benign prostatic hypertrophy.

Pyelonephritis occurs more often in females, probably because of a shorter urethra and the proximity of the urinary meatus to the vagina and the rectum—both conditions allow bacteria to reach the bladder more easily—and a lack of the antibacterial prostatic secretions produced in the male.

Incidence increases with age and is higher in the following groups:

• *Sexually active women:* Intercourse in-

CHRONIC PYELONEPHRITIS

Chronic pyelonephritis is a persistent kidney inflammation that can scar the kidneys and may lead to chronic renal failure. Its etiology may be bacterial, metastatic, or urogenous. This disease is most common in patients who are predisposed to recurrent acute pyelonephritis, such as those with urinary obstructions or vesicoureteral reflux.

Patients with chronic pyelonephritis may have a childhood history of unexplained fevers or bed-wetting. The clinical effects of chronic pyelonephritis may include flank pain, anemia, low urine specific gravity, proteinuria, leukocytes in urine, and especially in late stages, hypertension. Uremia rarely develops from chronic pyelonephritis unless structural abnormalities exist in the excretory system. Bacteriuria may be intermittent. When no bacteria are found in the urine, diagnosis depends on intravenous pyelography (renal pelvis may appear small and flattened) and renal biopsy.

Effective treatment of chronic pyelonephritis requires control of hypertension, elimination of the existing obstruction (when possible), and long-term antimicrobial therapy.

creases the risk of bacterial contamination.

• *Pregnant women:* About 5% develop asymptomatic bacteriuria; if untreated, about 40% develop pyelonephritis.

• *Diabetics:* Neurogenic bladder causes incomplete emptying and urinary stasis; glycosuria may support bacterial growth in the urine.

• *Persons with other renal diseases:* Compromised renal function aggravates susceptibility.

Signs and symptoms

Typical clinical features include urgency, frequent burning during urination, dysuria, nocturia, and hematuria (usually microscopic but may be gross). Urine may appear cloudy and have an ammoniacal or fishy odor. Other common symptoms include a temperature of 102° F. (38.9° C.) or higher, shaking chills, flank pain, anorexia, and general fatigue.

These symptoms characteristically develop rapidly over a few hours or a few days. Although these symptoms may disappear within days, even without treatment, residual bacterial infection is likely and may cause later recurrence of symptoms.

Diagnosis

Diagnosis requires urinalysis and culture. Typical findings include:

• *Pyuria* (pus in urine): Urine sediment reveals the presence of leukocytes singly, in clumps, and in casts; and possibly, a few RBCs.

• *Significant bacteriuria:* Urine culture reveals more than 100,000 organisms/mm^3 of urine.

• *Low specific gravity and osmolality:* These findings result from a temporarily decreased ability to concentrate urine.

• *Slightly alkaline urine pH.*

• *Proteinuria, glycosuria, and ketonuria:* These conditions are less common.

X-rays also help in the evaluation of acute pyelonephritis. A plain film of the kidneys-ureters-bladder may reveal calculi, tumors, or cysts in the kidneys and the urinary tract. Intravenous pyelography may show asymmetric kidneys.

Treatment

Treatment centers on antibiotic therapy appropriate to the specific infecting organism after identification by urine culture and sensitivity studies. For example, enterococcus requires treatment with ampicillin, penicillin G, or vancomycin. *Staphylococcus* requires penicillin G or, if resistance develops, a semisynthetic penicillin, such as nafcillin, or a cephalosporin. *Escherichia coli* may be treated with sulfisoxazole, nalidixic acid, and nitrofurantoin; *Proteus,* with ampicillin, sulfisoxazole, nalidixic acid, and a cephalosporin; and *Pseudomonas,* with gentamicin, tobramycin, and carbenicillin. When the infecting organism cannot be identified, therapy usually consists of a broad-spectrum antibiotic, such as ampicillin or cephalexin. If the patient is pregnant, antibiotics must be prescribed cautiously. Urinary analgesics, such as phenazopyridine, are also appropriate.

Symptoms may disappear after several days of antibiotic therapy. Although urine usually becomes sterile within 48 to 72 hours, the course of such therapy is 10 to 14 days. Follow-up treatment includes reculturing urine 1 week after drug therapy stops, then periodically for the next year to detect residual or recurring infection. Most patients with uncomplicated infections respond well to therapy and don't suffer reinfection.

In infection from obstruction or vesicoureteral reflux, antibiotics may be less effective; treatment may then necessitate surgery to relieve the obstruction or correct the anomaly. Patients at high risk of recurring urinary tract and kidney infections—such as those with prolonged use of an indwelling catheter, or maintenance antibiotic therapy—require long-term follow-up.

Additional considerations

• Fluids should be forced to achieve urinary output of more than 2,000 ml/day. This helps to empty the bladder of contaminated urine. However, intake of

more than 2 to 3 liters should be discouraged, because this may decrease the effectiveness of the antibiotics.
• An acid-ash diet will help prevent stone formation.
• The patient should learn proper technique for collecting a clean-catch urine specimen. Urine specimens should be refrigerated or cultured within 30 minutes of collection to prevent bacterial overgrowth.
• The patient must complete prescribed antibiotic therapy, even after symptoms subside. High-risk patients may need long term follow-up care.

Acute pyelonephritis can be prevented by:
• observing strict sterile technique during catheter insertion and care.
• instructing females to prevent bacterial contamination by wiping the perineum from front to back after defecation.
• advising routine checkups for patients with a history of urinary tract infections; teaching them to recognize signs of infection (cloudy urine, burning on urination, urgency, frequency), especially when accompanied by a low-grade fever.

Acute Poststreptococcal Glomerulonephritis
(Acute glomerulonephritis)

Acute poststreptococcal glomerulonephritis (APSGN) is a relatively common bilateral inflammation of the glomeruli. It follows a streptococcal infection of the respiratory tract or, less often, a skin infection, such as impetigo. APSGN is most common in boys aged 3 to 7, but can occur at any age. Up to 95% of children and up to 70% of adults with APSGN recover fully; the rest may progress to chronic renal failure within months.

Causes
APSGN results from the entrapment and collection of antigen-antibody complexes (produced as an immunologic mechanism in response to streptococcus) in the glomerular capillary membranes, inducing inflammatory damage and impeding glomerular function. Sometimes, the immune complement further damages the glomerular membrane. The damaged and inflamed glomerulus loses the ability to be selectively permeable, and allows RBCs and proteins to filter through as the glomerular filtration rate falls. Uremic poisoning may result.

Signs and symptoms
Generally, APSGN begins within 1 to 3 weeks after untreated pharyngitis. The most common symptoms are mild to moderate edema, proteinuria, azotemia, hematuria (smoky or coffee-colored urine), oliguria (400 to 600 ml/24 hours), and fatigue. Mild to severe hypertension may result from either sodium or water retention (caused by decreased glomerular filtration rate), or inappropriate renin release. Congestive heart failure from hypervolemia leads to symptoms of pulmonary edema: shortness of breath, dyspnea, and orthopnea.

Diagnosis
Diagnosis requires a detailed patient history, and assessment of clinical symptoms and laboratory tests. Blood values (elevated electrolytes, BUN, and creatinine) and urine values (RBCs, WBCs, mixed cell casts, and protein) indicate renal failure. In addition, elevated antistreptolysin-O titers (in 80% of patients), elevated streptozyme and anti-DNase B titers, and low-serum complement levels verify recent streptococcal infection. A throat culture may also show group A beta-hemolytic streptococcus. Kidney-ureter-bladder X-rays show bilateral kidney enlargement. A renal biopsy may be necessary to confirm diagnosis or assess renal tissue status.

Treatment

The goals of treatment are relief of symptoms and prevention of complications. Vigorous supportive care includes bed rest, fluid and dietary sodium restrictions, and correction of electrolyte imbalances (possibly with dialysis, although this is rarely necessary). Therapy may include diuretics, such as metolazone or furosemide, to reduce extracellular fluid overload, and an antihypertensive, such as hydralazine. The use of antibiotics to prevent secondary infection or transmission to others is controversial.

Additional considerations

APSGN usually resolves within 2 weeks, so health care is primarily supportive. When caring for an APSGN patient, the hospital staff member should:
• check vital signs and electrolyte values; monitor intake and output, and daily weight; assess renal function daily through serum creatinine, BUN, and urine creatinine clearance; watch for and immediately report signs of acute renal failure (oliguria, azotemia, and acidosis).
• consult the dietitian to provide a diet high in calories and low in protein, sodium, potassium, and fluids.

• protect the debilitated patient against secondary infection by providing good nutrition, using good hygienic technique, and preventing contact with infected persons.
• allow the patient to *gradually* resume normal activities as symptoms subside.
• provide emotional support for the patient and family; explain dialysis procedure fully, if appropriate.

Appropriate follow-up care of an APSGN patient includes:
• advising the patient with a history of chronic upper respiratory tract infections to immediately report signs of infection (fever, sore throat).
• telling the patient that follow-up examinations are necessary to detect chronic renal failure; stressing the need for regular blood pressure, urinary protein, and renal function assessments during the convalescent months to detect recurrence. (After APSGN, gross hematuria may recur during nonspecific viral infections; abnormal urinary findings may persist for years.)
• encouraging pregnant women with histories of APSGN to have frequent medical evaluations, since pregnancy further stresses the kidneys and increases the risk of chronic renal failure.

Acute Tubular Necrosis
(Acute tubulointerstitial nephritis)

Acute tubular necrosis (ATN) accounts for about 75% of all cases of acute renal failure, and is the most common cause of acute renal failure in critically ill patients. ATN injures the tubular segment of the nephron, causing renal failure and uremic syndrome. Mortality ranges from 40% to 70%, depending on complications from other underlying diseases. Nonoliguric forms of ATN have a better prognosis.

Causes

ATN results from ischemic or nephrotoxic injury, most commonly in debilitated patients, such as the critically ill or those who have undergone extensive surgery. In ischemic injury, disruption of blood flow to the kidneys may result from circulatory collapse, severe hypotension, trauma, hemorrhage, dehydration, cardiogenic or septic shock, surgery, anesthetics, or reactions to transfusions. Nephrotoxic injury may follow ingestion of certain chemical agents or result from a hypersensitive reaction of the kidneys. Since nephrotoxic ATN doesn't damage the basement membrane of the nephron, it's potentially reversible. However, ischemic ATN can damage the epithelial and basement membranes, and can cause lesions that extend into the renal interstitium.

ATN may progress to oliguria or anuria and may result from:

• diseased tubular epithelium that allows leakage of glomerular filtrate across the membranes and reabsorption of filtrate into the blood.

• obstruction of urine flow by the collection of damaged cells, casts, RBCs, and other cellular debris within the tubular walls.

• ischemic injury to glomerular epithelial cells, resulting in cellular collapse and decreased glomerular capillary permeability.

• ischemic injury to vascular endothelium, resulting in damage to ion pumps that causes cellular swelling and obstruction.

Signs and symptoms

ATN is difficult to recognize in its early stages, because effects of the critically ill patient's primary disease may mask its symptoms. The first recognizable effect may be decreased urine output. Generally, hyperkalemia and the characteristic uremic syndrome soon follow, with oliguria or, rarely, anuria and confusion, which may progress to uremic coma. Other possible complications may include congestive heart failure, uremic pericarditis, pulmonary edema, uremic lung, anemia, anorexia, intractable vomiting, and poor wound healing due to debilitation. Fever and chills signify onset of infection, the leading cause of death in ATN.

Diagnosis

Diagnosis is usually delayed until the condition has progressed to an advanced stage. The most significant laboratory clues are urinary sediment containing RBCs and casts, and dilute urine of a low specific gravity (1.010), low osmolality (less than 400 mOsm/kg), and high sodium level (40 to 60 mEq/liter). Blood studies reveal elevated BUN and serum creatinine, anemia, defects in platelet

---

NEPHROTOXIC INJURY INCREASING

Incidence of acute tubular necrosis (ATN) from ingestion or inhalation of toxic substances is rising. This exposure may occur in the hospital, while the patient is already debilitated, from such toxic agents as antibiotics (kanamycin, gentamicin, cephaloridine, and tobramycin, for example) and contrast media. Other nephrotoxic agents include pesticides, fungicides, heavy metals (mercury, arsenic, lead, bismuth, uranium), and organic solvents containing carbon tetrachloride or ethyl glycol, such as cleaning fluids or industrial solvents. Ingestion of these substances may be accidental or intentional.

Nephrotoxic injury causes multiple symptoms similar to those of renal failure, particularly azotemia, anemia, acidosis, overhydration, and hypertension; and less often, fever, skin rash, and eosinophilia. Treatment consists of identifying the nephrotoxic substance, eliminating its use, and removing it from the body by any means available, such as hemodialysis in extreme cases. Treatment is supportive during the course of acute renal failure.

---

adherence, metabolic acidosis, and hyperkalemia. EKG may show arrhythmias (from electrolyte imbalances) and, with hyperkalemia, widening QRS segment, disappearing P waves, and tall, peaked T waves.

Treatment

Treatment for ATN consists of vigorous supportive measures during the acute phase until kidney function resumes.

Initial treatment may include administration of diuretics and infusion of a large volume of fluids to flush tubules of cellular casts and debris, and to replace fluid loss. However, this treatment carries a risk of fluid overload. Long-term fluid management requires daily replacement of projected and calculated losses (including insensible loss).

Other appropriate measures to control complications include transfusion of packed RBCs for anemia and administration of antibiotics for infection. Hyperkalemia may require emergency I.V. administration of 50% glucose, regular insulin, and sodium bicarbonate. Sodium polystyrene sulfonate with sorbitol may be given P.O. or by enema to reduce extracellular potassium levels. Peritoneal dialysis or hemodialysis may be needed if the patient is catabolic.

Additional considerations

The hospital staff member caring for the patient with acute tubular necrosis should:

• maintain fluid balance; watch for fluid overload, a common complication of therapy; record intake and output, including wound drainage, nasogastric output, and peritoneal dialysis and hemodialysis balances; weigh the patient daily.

• monitor hemoglobin and hematocrit, and administer blood products, as needed; use fresh packed cells instead of whole blood to prevent fluid overload and congestive heart failure.

• maintain electrolyte balance; monitor laboratory results, and report imbalances; enforce dietary restriction of foods containing sodium and potassium, such as bananas, orange juice, and baked potatoes; check for potassium content in prescribed medications; provide adequate calories and essential amino acids, while restricting protein intake to maintain an anabolic state; provide total parenteral nutrition, as ordered, in the severely debilitated or catabolic patient.

• use aseptic technique, particularly when handling catheters, since the debilitated patient is vulnerable to infection; report fever, chills, delayed wound healing, or flank pain immediately if the patient has a Foley catheter in place.

• watch for complications; administer RBCs, as ordered, if anemia worsens (pallor, weakness, lethargy with decreased hemoglobin); give sodium bicarbonate for acidosis, or, in severe cases, assist with dialysis; watch for signs of diminishing renal perfusion (hypotension and decreased urinary output); encourage coughing and deep breathing to prevent pulmonary complications.

• perform passive range-of-motion exercises; provide good skin care by applying lotion or bath oil for dry skin; help the patient to walk as soon as possible, but guard against exhaustion.

• provide reassurance and emotional support; encourage the patient and family to express their fears; help the patient and family set realistic goals according to individual prognosis.

To prevent ATN, all patients should be well hydrated before surgery, or after X-rays that use a contrast medium. Mannitol may be administered to high-risk patients before and during these procedures. Patients receiving blood transfusions must be carefully monitored to detect early signs of transfusion reaction (fever, rash, chills). In such cases, the transfusion must be discontinued immediately.

Renal Infarction

Renal infarction is the formation of a coagulated, necrotic area in one or both kidneys that results from renal blood vessel occlusion. The location and size of the infarction depend on the site of vascular occlusion. Most often, infarction affects the renal cortex, but can extend into the medulla. Residual renal function after infarction depends on the extent of the damage from the infarction.

Causes

In 75% of patients, renal infarction results from renal artery embolism secondary to mitral stenosis, infective endocarditis, atrial fibrillation, microthrombi in the left ventricle, rheumatic valvular disease, or recent myocardial infarction. The embolism reduces the rate of blood flow to renal tissue and leads to ischemia. The rate and degree of blood flow reduction determine whether or not the insult will be acute or chronic as arterial narrowing progresses.

Less common causes of renal infarction are atherosclerosis, with or without thrombus formation; and thrombus from flank trauma, sickle cell anemia, scleroderma, and arterionephrosclerosis.

Signs and symptoms

Although renal infarction may be asymptomatic, typical symptoms include severe upper abdominal pain or gnawing flank pain and tenderness, costovertebral tenderness, fever, anorexia, nausea, and vomiting. When arterial occlusion causes infarction, the affected kidney is small and not palpable. Renovascular hypertension, a frequent complication that may occur several days after infarction, results from reduced blood flow, which stimulates the renin-angiotensin mechanism.

Diagnosis

A history of predisposing cardiovascular disease or other factors in a patient with typical clinical features strongly suggests renal infarction. Firm diagnosis requires appropriate laboratory tests:
• *Urinalysis* reveals proteinuria and microscopic hematuria.
• *Urine enzyme levels,* especially lactic dehydrogenase (LDH) and alkaline phosphatase, are often elevated as a result of tissue destruction.
• *Serum enzyme levels,* especially SGOT, alkaline phosphatase, and LDH, are elevated. Blood studies may also reveal leukocytosis and increased ESR.
• *Intravenous pyelography* shows diminished or absent excretion of contrast dye, indicating vascular occlusion or urethral obstruction; retrograde pyelography differentiates renal infarction from urinary tract obstruction when it shows normal excretion.
• *Isotopic renal scan,* a benign, nonin-

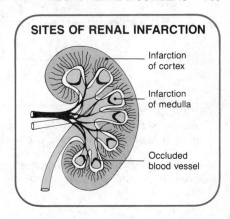

SITES OF RENAL INFARCTION

Infarction of cortex

Infarction of medulla

Occluded blood vessel

vasive technique, demonstrates absence of or reduced blood flow to the kidneys.

• *Renal arteriography* provides absolute proof of existing infarction but is used as a last resort, since it is a high-risk procedure.

Treatment

Infection in the infarcted area or significant hypertension may require surgical repair of the occlusion, or nephrectomy. Surgery to establish collateral circulation to the area can relieve renovascular hypertension. Persistent hypertension may respond to antihypertensives and a low-sodium diet.

Additional considerations

The first step in the health care of a patient with renal infarction is assessing the degree of renal function and offering supportive care to maintain homeostasis. Further care includes:
• monitoring intake and output, vital signs (particularly blood pressure), electrolytes, and daily weight; watching for signs of fluid overload, such as dyspnea, tachycardia, pulmonary edema, and electrolyte imbalances.
• providing reassurance and emotional support for the patient and family.
• encouraging the patient to return for follow-up examination. Such examination usually includes intravenous pyelography or a renal scan to assess regained renal function.

Renal Calculi
(Kidney stones)

Renal calculi may form anywhere in the urinary tract but usually develop in the renal pelvis or the calyces of the kidneys. Such formation follows precipitation of substances normally dissolved in the urine (calcium oxalate, calcium phosphate, magnesium ammonium phosphate, or occasionally, urate or cystine). Renal calculi vary in size and may be solitary or multiple. They may remain in the renal pelvis or enter the ureter and may damage renal parenchyma; large calculi cause pressure necrosis. In certain locations, calculi cause obstruction, with resultant hydronephrosis, and tend to recur.

Causes

Among Americans, renal calculi develop in 1 in 1,000 persons, are more common in men (especially those aged 30 to 50) than in women, and are rare in Blacks and children. They're particularly prevalent in certain geographic areas, such as southeastern United States (stone belt), possibly because a hot climate promotes dehydration or because of regional dietary habits. Although the exact cause of renal calculi is unknown, predisposing factors include the following:

• *Dehydration:* Decreased urine production concentrates calculus-forming substances.

• *Infection:* Infected, damaged tissue serves as a site for calculus development; pH changes provide a favorable medium for calculus formation (especially for magnesium ammonium phosphate or calcium phosphate calculi); or infected calculi (usually magnesium ammonium phosphate or staghorn calculi) may develop if bacteria serve as the nucleus in calculus formation. Such infections may promote destruction of renal parenchyma.

• *Obstruction:* Urinary stasis (as in immobility from spinal cord injury) allows calculus constituents to collect and adhere, forming calculi. Obstruction also promotes infection, which, in turn, compounds the obstruction.

• *Metabolic factors:* These factors may predispose to renal calculi: hyperparathyroidism, renal tubular acidosis, elevated uric acid (usually with gout), defective metabolism of oxalate, genetic defect in metabolism of cystine, and excessive intake of vitamin D or dietary calcium.

Signs and symptoms

Clinical effects vary with size, location, and etiology of the calculi. Pain, the key symptom, usually results from obstruction; large, rough calculi occlude the opening to the ureter and increase the frequency and force of peristaltic contractions. The pain of classic renal colic travels from the costovertebral angle to the flank, to the suprapubic region and external genitalia. The intensity of this pain fluctuates and may be excruciating at its peak. If calculi are in the renal pelvis and calyces, pain may be more constant and dull. Back pain (from calculi that produce an obstruction within a kidney) and severe abdominal pain (from calculi traveling down a ureter) may also occur. Nausea and vomiting usually accompany severe pain.

Other associated signs include fever, chills, hematuria (when calculi abrade a ureter), abdominal distention, pyuria, and rarely, anuria (from bilateral obstruction, or unilateral obstruction in the patient with one kidney).

Diagnosis

Diagnosis is based on the clinical picture and the following tests:

• *Kidney-ureter-bladder X-rays* reveal most renal calculi.

• *Stone analysis* shows mineral content.

TYPES OF RENAL CALCULI

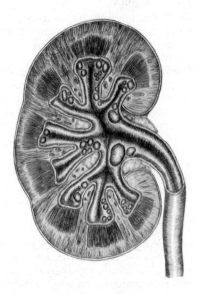

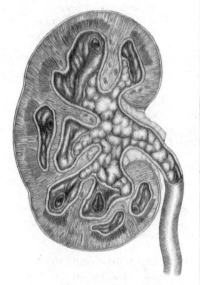

Multiple small calculi may vary in size; they may remain in the renal pelvis or pass down the ureter.

A staghorn calculus (a cast of the calyceal and pelvic collecting system) may form from a stone that stays in the kidney.

- *Intravenous pyelography* confirms the diagnosis and determines size and location of calculi.
- *Kidney ultrasonography* is an easily performed noninvasive, nontoxic test to detect obstructive changes, such as hydronephrosis.
- *Urine culture* of midstream sample may indicate urinary tract infection.
- *Urinalysis* may be normal, or may show increased specific gravity and acid or alkaline pH suitable for different types of stone formation. Other urinalysis findings include hematuria (gross or microscopic), crystals (urate, calcium, or cystine), casts, and pyuria with or without bacteria and WBCs.
- A *24-hour urine collection* is evaluated for calcium oxalate, phosphorus, and uric acid excretion levels.

Other laboratory results support this diagnosis:

- *Serial blood calcium and phosphorus levels* detect hyperparathyroidism and show increased calcium level in proportion to normal serum protein.
- *Blood protein level* determines level of free calcium unbound to protein.
- *Blood chloride and bicarbonate levels* may show renal tubular acidosis.
- *Increased blood uric acid levels* may indicate gout as the cause.

Diagnosis must rule out appendicitis, cholecystitis, peptic ulcer, and pancreatitis as potential sources of pain.

Treatment

Since 90% of renal calculi are smaller than 5 mm in diameter, treatment usually consists of measures to promote their natural passage. Along with vigorous hydration, such treatment includes antimicrobial therapy (varying with the cultured organism) for infection; analgesics, such as meperidine, for pain; and diuretics to prevent urinary stasis and further calculus formation (thiazides decrease calcium excretion into the urine). Prophylaxis to prevent calculus formation includes a low-calcium diet for absorptive hypercalciuria, parathyroidectomy for hyperparathyroidism, allopurinol for uric acid calculi, and daily administration of ascorbic acid P.O. to acidify the urine.

Calculi too large for natural passage require surgical removal to relieve pain and prevent infection or deterioration of renal function. When a calculus is in the ureter, a cystoscope may be inserted through the urethra, and the calculus manipulated with catheters or retrieval instruments. Extraction of calculi from other areas (kidney calyx, renal pelvis) may necessitate a flank or lower abdominal approach.

Additional considerations

• To aid diagnosis, a 24- to 48-hour record of urine pH, with nitrazine pH paper, should be maintained. All urine must be strained through gauze or a tea strainer, and all recovered solid material saved for analysis.

• To facilitate spontaneous passage, the patient should walk, if possible. Fluid intake should be sufficient to maintain a urinary output of 3 to 4 liters/day (urine should be very dilute and colorless). Fruit juices, particularly cranberry juice, will help acidify urine. If the patient can't drink the required amount of fluid, supplemental I.V. fluids may be ordered. Intake and output, and daily weight must be accurately recorded to assess fluid status and renal function.

• Proper diet and compliance with drug therapy are very important. For example, if the patient's stone is caused by a hyperuricemic condition, the patient or whoever prepares his meals should know which foods are high in purine. Hypercalciuria requires limiting the intake of dietary calcium. The patient might discuss his needs with a dietitian.

• If surgery is necessary, the patient can be reassured by supplementing and reinforcing what the surgeon has told him. He is apt to be fearful, especially if a kidney will be removed, so the fact that the body can adapt well to one kidney should be emphasized. If he is to have an abdominal or flank incision, he should be taught deep breathing and coughing exercises.

• After surgery, the patient will probably have a Foley catheter. Unless a kidney was removed, there will be bloody

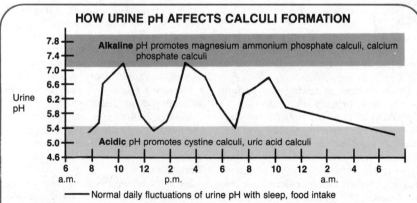

HOW URINE pH AFFECTS CALCULI FORMATION

Urine pH

Alkaline pH promotes magnesium ammonium phosphate calculi, calcium phosphate calculi

Acidic pH promotes cystine calculi, uric acid calculi

————— Normal daily fluctuations of urine pH with sleep, food intake

Normally, the pH of urine fluctuates from slightly acidic to slightly alkaline over a 24-hour period. This fluctuation has the periodicity shown above. If urine pH is consistently acidic or alkaline, the urine provides a medium suitable for calculi formation: acidic urine promotes formation of cystine and uric acid calculi; alkaline urine promotes formation of calcium phosphate and magnesium ammonium phosphate calculi. Calcium oxalate calculi can form in urine of varying pH.

drainage from the catheter. The catheter must never be irrigated without a doctor's order. Dressings should be checked regularly for bloody drainage. Suspected hemorrhage (excessive drainage, rising pulse rate) must be reported immediately. Sterile technique should be used when changing dressings or providing catheter care.

• Signs of infection (rising fever, chills) may indicate the need for antibiotics. To prevent pneumonia, the patient should be encouraged to make frequent position changes, and to ambulate as soon as possible. He can hold a small pillow over the operative site to splint the incision and thereby facilitate deep breathing and coughing exercises.

• Before discharge, the patient and family must understand the importance of following the prescribed dietary and medication regimens to prevent recurrence of calculi. If appropriate, the patient should be shown how to check his urine pH, and instructed to keep a daily record. He should immediately report symptoms of acute obstruction (pain, inability to void).

Renal Vein Thrombosis

Renal vein thrombosis, clotting in the renal vein, results in renal congestion, engorgement, and possibly, infarction. Such thrombosis may affect both kidneys and may occur in an acute or a chronic form. Chronic thrombosis usually impairs renal function, causing nephrotic syndrome. Abrupt onset of thrombosis that causes extensive damage may precipitate rapidly fatal renal infarction. If thrombosis affects both kidneys, prognosis is poor. However, less severe thrombosis that affects only one kidney, or gradual progression that allows development of collateral circulation may preserve partial renal function.

Causes
Renal vein thrombosis often results from a tumor that obstructs the renal vein (usually hypernephroma). Other causes include thrombophlebitis of the inferior vena cava (may result from abdominal trauma) or blood vessels of the legs, congestive heart failure, and periarteritis. In infants, renal vein thrombosis usually follows diarrhea that causes severe dehydration. Chronic renal vein thrombosis is often a complication of other glomerulopathic diseases, such as amyloidosis, diabetic nephropathy, and membranoproliferative glomerulonephritis.

Signs and symptoms
Clinical features of renal vein thrombosis vary with speed of onset. Rapid onset of venous obstruction produces severe lumbar pain, and tenderness in the epigastric region and the costovertebral angle. Other characteristic features include fever, leukocytosis, pallor, hematuria, proteinuria, peripheral edema, and when the obstruction is bilateral, oliguria and other uremic signs. The kidneys enlarge and become easily palpable. Hypertension is unusual, but may develop.

Gradual onset causes symptoms of nephrotic syndrome. Peripheral edema is possible, but pain is generally absent. Other clinical signs include proteinuria, hypoalbuminemia, and hyperlipemia.

Infants with this disease have enlarged kidneys, oliguria, and renal insufficiency that may progress to acute or chronic renal failure.

Diagnosis
• *Intravenous pyelography* provides reliable diagnostic evidence. In acute renal vein thrombosis, the kidneys appear enlarged and excretory function diminishes. Contrast medium seems to "smudge" necrotic renal tissue. In chronic

thrombosis, it may show ureteral indentations that result from collateral venous channels. Renal arteriography and biopsy may also confirm the diagnosis.

• *Urinalysis* reveals gross or microscopic hematuria, proteinuria (more than 2 g/day in chronic disease), casts, and oliguria.

• *Blood studies* show leukocytosis, hypoalbuminemia, and hyperlipemia.

Treatment

Treatment is most effective for gradual thrombosis that affects only one kidney. Anticoagulant therapy (heparin or warfarin) may prove helpful, particularly if long-term. Effective surgery must be performed within 24 hours of thrombosis but even then has limited success, since thrombi often extend into the small veins. Extensive intrarenal bleeding may necessitate nephrectomy.

Patients who survive abrupt thrombosis with extensive renal damage develop nephrotic syndrome and require treatment for renal failure, such as dialysis and, possibly, transplantation. Some infants with renal vein thrombosis recover completely following heparin therapy or surgical removal of the thrombus; others suffer irreversible kidney damage.

Additional considerations

• Renal function should be assessed and appropriate emotional support provided, particularly for an infant's parents.

• Vital signs, intake and output, daily weight, and electrolytes must be monitored. Diuretics may be ordered for edema, as well as dietary restrictions, such as limited sodium and potassium intake.

• The patient must be watched closely for signs of pulmonary emboli.

• If heparin is given by constant I.V. infusion, prothrombin time must be monitored frequently to determine the response to it. The drug should be diluted and administered by infusion pump or controller, so the patient receives the least amount necessary.

• During anticoagulant therapy, signs of bleeding must be watched for and reported (tachycardia, hypotension, hematuria, bleeding from nose or gums, ecchymoses, petechiae, and tarry stools). The patient on maintenance warfarin therapy should use an electric razor and a soft toothbrush, and avoid trauma. Also, he must avoid taking aspirin, which aggravates bleeding tendencies. He may want to wear a medical identification bracelet. He needs to understand the need for close medical follow-up.

CHRONIC RENAL DISORDERS

Nephrotic Syndrome

Nephrotic syndrome (NS) is a condition characterized by marked proteinuria, hypoalbuminemia, hyperlipemia, and edema. Although NS is not a disease itself, it results from a specific glomerular defect and indicates renal damage. Prognosis is highly variable, depending on the underlying cause. Some forms may progress to end-stage renal failure.

Causes and incidence

About 75% of NS results from primary (idiopathic) glomerulonephritis. Classifications include the following:

• In *lipid nephrosis (nil lesions)*—main cause of NS in children—glomerulus appears normal by light microscopy.

Some tubules may contain increased lipid deposits.

• *Membranous glomerulonephritis*—most common lesion in adult idiopathic NS—is characterized by uniform thickening of the glomerular basement membrane containing dense deposits and eventually progresses to renal failure.

• *Focal glomerulosclerosis* can develop spontaneously at any age, follow renal transplantation, or result from heroin abuse. Reported incidence is 10% in children with NS, and up to 20% in adults. Lesions initially affect the deeper glomeruli, causing hyaline sclerosis, with later involvement of the superficial glomeruli. These lesions generally cause slowly progressive deterioration in renal function. Remissions occur occasionally.

• In *membranoproliferative glomerulonephritis,* slowly progressive lesions develop in the subendothelial region of the basement membrane. These lesions may follow infection, particularly streptococcal infection. This disease occurs primarily in children and young adults.

Other causes of NS include metabolic diseases, such as diabetes mellitus; collagen-vascular disorders, such as systemic lupus erythematosus and periarteritis nodosa; circulatory diseases, such as congestive heart failure, sickle cell anemia, and renal vein thrombosis; nephrotoxins, such as mercury, gold, and bismuth; allergic reactions; and infections, such as tuberculosis and enteritis. Other possible causes are pregnancy, hereditary nephritis, multiple myeloma, and other neoplastic diseases.

These diseases increase glomerular protein permeability, leading to increased urinary excretion of protein, especially albumin, and subsequent hypoalbuminemia.

Signs and symptoms

The dominant clinical feature of nephrotic syndrome is mild to severe dependent edema of the ankles or sacrum, or periorbital edema, especially in children. Such edema may lead to ascites, pleural effusion, and swollen external genitalia (labia, vulva, scrotum). Accompanying symptoms may include orthostatic hypotension, lethargy, fatigue, anorexia, depression, and pallor. Major complications are malnutrition, infection, coagulation disorders, thromboembolic vascular occlusion, and accelerated atherosclerosis.

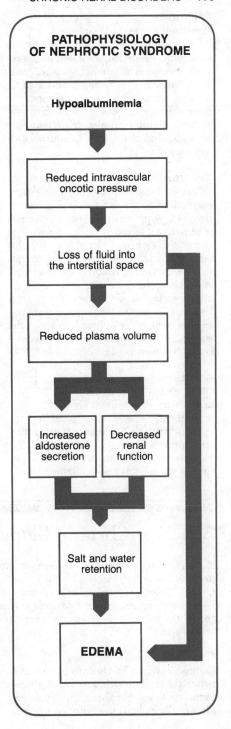

PATHOPHYSIOLOGY OF NEPHROTIC SYNDROME

Hypoalbuminemia

Reduced intravascular oncotic pressure

Loss of fluid into the interstitial space

Reduced plasma volume

Increased aldosterone secretion

Decreased renal function

Salt and water retention

EDEMA

Diagnosis

Consistent proteinuria in excess of 3.5 g/24 hours strongly suggests nephrotic syndrome; examination of urine also reveals increased number of hyaline, granular, and waxy, fatty casts, and oval fat bodies. Serum values that support the diagnosis are increased cholesterol and decreased albumin levels. Histologic identification of the lesion requires kidney biopsy.

Treatment

Effective treatment of NS necessitates correction of the underlying cause, if possible. Supportive treatment consists of protein replacement with a nutritional diet of 3 to 4 g protein/kg of body weight, with restricted sodium intake; diuretics for edema; and antibiotics for infection.

Corticosteroid therapy produces variable results, depending on the type of lesion. Treatment may include cytotoxic agents, such as cyclophosphamide, if the patient is unresponsive to corticosteroids, but therapeutic results vary.

Additional considerations

When caring for a patient with NS, the health care professional should:
• frequently check urine protein with appropriate tests. (Urine containing protein appears frothy.)
• measure blood pressure while the patient is supine and also while he's standing; immediately report a drop in blood pressure that exceeds 20 mmHg.
• watch for bleeding and shock after kidney biopsy.
• monitor intake and output, and daily weight at about the same time each morning, after the patient voids, before he eats, and while he's wearing approximately the same clothing; ask the dietitian to plan a high-protein, low-sodium diet.
• give good skin care, since the patient with NS usually has edema.
• encourage activity and exercise to avoid thrombophlebitis; provide antiembolism stockings, as ordered.
• watch for and teach the patient and family how to recognize drug therapy side effects, such as bone marrow toxicity from cytotoxic immunosuppressives, and cushingoid symptoms (muscle weakness, mental changes, acne, moon face, hirsutism, girdle obesity, purple striae, amenorrhea) from steroids. Other steroid complications include masked infections, increased susceptibility to infections, ulcers, and gastrointestinal bleeding; a steroid crisis may occur if the drug is discontinued abruptly. To prevent gastrointestinal complications, steroids should be given with an antacid. The patient should know that steroid side effects will subside when therapy stops.
• offer the patient and family reassurance and support, especially during the acute phase, when edema is severe.

Chronic Glomerulonephritis

A slowly progressive disease, chronic glomerulonephritis is characterized by inflammation of the glomeruli, which results in sclerosis, scarring, and eventual renal failure. This condition usually remains subclinical until the progressive phase begins, with proteinuria, cylindruria (presence of granular tube casts), and hematuria. By the time it produces symptoms, chronic glomerulonephritis is usually irreversible.

Causes

Common causes of chronic glomerulonephritis include primary renal disorders, such as membranoproliferative glomerulonephritis, membranous glomerulopathy, focal glomerulosclerosis, rapidly progressive glomerulonephritis, and less often, poststreptococcal glomerulonephritis. Systemic disorders that may cause chronic glomerulonephritis include lupus erythematosus, Goodpasture's syndrome, and hemolytic-uremic syndrome.

Signs and symptoms

Chronic glomerulonephritis usually develops insidiously and asymptomatically, often over many years. At any time, however, it may suddenly become progressive, producing nephrotic syndrome, hypertension, proteinuria, and hematuria. In late stages of progressive chronic glomerulonephritis, it may accelerate to uremic symptoms, such as azotemia, nausea, vomiting, pruritus, dyspnea, malaise, and fatigability. Mild to severe edema and anemia may accompany these symptoms. Severe hypertension may cause cardiac hypertrophy, leading to congestive heart failure, and may accelerate the development of advanced renal failure, eventually necessitating dialysis or transplantation.

Diagnosis

Patient history and physical assessment seldom suggest glomerulonephritis. Suspicion develops from urinalysis revealing proteinuria, hematuria, cylindruria, and RBC casts. Rising BUN and serum creatinine indicate advanced renal insufficiency. Kidney biopsy is performed to identify underlying disease and provides data needed to determine therapy.

Treatment

Treatment is essentially nonspecific and symptomatic, with its goals to control hypertension with various antihypertensives and a sodium-restricted diet; to correct fluid and electrolyte imbalances through restrictions and replacement measures; to reduce edema with diuretics, such as metolazone and furosemide; and to prevent congestive heart failure. Treatment may also include antibiotics to treat symptomatic urinary tract infections. Immunosuppressive therapy remains controversial.

Additional considerations

Health care is primarily supportive, focusing on continual observation and sound patient teaching. This includes:

• accurately monitoring vital signs, intake and output, and daily weight to evaluate fluid retention; monitoring renal function daily, and observing for signs of fluid, electrolyte, and acid-base imbalances; asking the dietitian to plan low-sodium, high-calorie meals that contain adequate protein.

• administering medications, as ordered, and providing good skin care (because of pruritus and edema) and oral hygiene; instructing the patient to continue taking prescribed antihypertensives exactly as scheduled, even if he's feeling better, and to report any side effects; advising the patient to take diuretics in the morning, so he won't have to disrupt his sleep to void; teaching him how to assess ankle edema.

• warning the patient to report signs of infection, particularly urinary tract infection, and to avoid contact with persons who have infections; urging him to have follow-up examinations to assess renal function.

• facilitating the patient's adjustment to this illness by encouraging him to verbalize his feelings; explaining all necessary procedures beforehand, and answering his questions about them.

Cystinuria

An autosomal recessive disorder, cystinuria is an inborn error of amino acid transport in the kidneys and intestine that allows excessive urinary excretion of cystine and other dibasic amino acids, and results in recurrent cystine renal calculi. It is the most common defect of amino acid transport, but with proper treatment, prognosis is good.

Causes and incidence

Cystinuria is inherited as an autosomal recessive defect, and occurs in approximately 1 in 15,000 live births. It is more prevalent in persons of short stature; the reason for this is unknown. Although this disorder affects both sexes, it is more severe in males.

Impaired renal tubular reabsorption of dibasic amino acids (cystine, lysine, arginine, and ornithine) results in excessive amino acid concentration and excretion in the urine. When cystine concentration exceeds its solubility, it precipitates and forms crystals, precursors of cystine calculi. Excessive excretion of the other three amino acids produces no ill effects.

Signs and symptoms

The clinical effects of cystinuria result from cystine or mixed cystine calculi, which develop most frequently between ages 10 and 30. Typically, such calculi may cause dull flank pain from renal parenchymal and capsular distention, nausea, vomiting, abdominal distention from acute renal colic (due to smooth-muscle spasm and hyperperistalsis), hematuria, and tenderness in the costovertebral angle or over the kidneys.

Renal calculi may also cause urinary tract obstruction, with resultant secondary infection (chills; fever; burning, itching, or pain on urination; frequency; and foul-smelling urine) and, with prolonged ureteral obstruction, marked hydronephrosis and a visible or palpable flank mass.

Diagnosis

Typical clinical features and a positive family history of renal disease or kidney stones suggest cystinuria, but the following laboratory data confirm it:
• *Chemical analysis of calculi* shows cystine crystals, with a variable amount of calcium. Pure cystine stones are radiolucent on X-ray, but most contain some calcium. These stones are light yellow or brownish-yellow, and granular; they may be large.
• *Blood studies* may show elevated serum

WBC, especially with a urinary tract infection, and elevated clearance of cystine, lysine, arginine, and ornithine.
• *Urinalysis* with amino acid chromatography indicates aminoaciduria, consisting of cystine, lysine, arginine, and ornithine. Urine pH is usually less than 5.
• *Microscopic examination of urine* shows hexagonal, flat cystine crystals. When glacial acetic acid is added to chilled urine, cystine crystals resemble benzene rings.
• *Cyanide-nitroprusside test* is positive. In cystinuria, a urine specimen made alkaline by adding ammonia turns magenta when nitroprusside is added to it.

Confirming tests also include excretory urography to determine renal function, and kidney-ureter-bladder X-rays to determine size and location of calculi.

Treatment

No effective treatment exists to decrease cystine excretion. Increasing fluid intake to maintain a minimum 24-hour urine volume of 3,000 ml and reduce urine cystine concentration is the primary means of dissolving excess cystine and preventing cystine stones. Sodium bicarbonate and an alkaline-ash diet (high in vegetables and fruit, low in protein) alkalinize urine, increasing cystine solubility. However, this therapy may provide a favorable environment for formation of calcium phosphate stones. Penicillamine can also increase cystine solubility but should be used with caution because of its toxic side effects and high incidence of allergic reaction. Treatment may also include surgical removal of renal calculi, when necessary, and appropriate measures to prevent and treat urinary tract infection.

Additional considerations

In addition to general supportive care, management of cystinuria focuses on careful patient teaching to promote compliance with the treatment regimen. The health care professional should:
• emphasize the need to maintain increased, evenly spaced fluid intake, even through the night.

• teach the patient how to recognize signs of renal calculi and urinary tract infection, and tell him to report any symptoms immediately.
• teach the patient to check urine pH and record the results.
• carefully monitor sodium bicarbonate administration, since metabolic alkalosis may develop. Arterial bicarbonate level can be estimated by subtracting 2 from the serum CO_2 level.
• explain to the patient receiving penicillamine that it may cause an allergic or serum sickness–type reaction. Other side effects include severe proteinuria— a sign of evolving nephrotic syndrome— and neutropenia, tinnitus, and taste impairment.

Renovascular Hypertension

Renovascular hypertension is a rise in systemic blood pressure resulting from stenosis of the major renal arteries or their branches, or from intrarenal atherosclerosis. This narrowing or sclerosis may be partial or complete, and the resulting blood pressure elevation, benign or malignant. Approximately 5% to 10% of patients with high blood pressure display renovascular hypertension; it is most common in persons under age 30 or over age 50.

Causes
Atherosclerosis (especially in older men) and fibromuscular diseases of the renal artery wall layers—such as medial fibroplasia and, less commonly, intimal and subadventitial fibroplasia—are the primary causes in 95% of all patients with renovascular hypertension. Other causes include arteritis, anomalies of the renal arteries, embolism, trauma, tumor, and dissecting aneurysm.

Stenosis or occlusion of the renal artery stimulates the affected kidney to release the enzyme renin, which converts angiotensin—a plasma protein—to angiotensin I. As angiotensin I circulates through the lungs and liver, it converts to angiotensin II, which causes peripheral vasoconstriction, increased arterial pressure and aldosterone secretion, and eventually, hypertension.

Signs and symptoms
In addition to elevated systemic blood pressure, renovascular hypertension usually produces symptoms common to hypertensive states, such as headache, palpitations, tachycardia, anxiety, lightheadedness, decreased tolerance of temperature extremes, retinopathy, and mental sluggishness. Significant complications include congestive heart failure, myocardial infarction, cerebrovascular accident, and occasionally, renal failure.

Diagnosis
In addition to thorough patient and family histories, diagnosis requires isotopic renal blood flow scan and rapid-sequence intravenous pyelography to identify abnormalities of renal blood flow and discrepancies of kidney size and shape. Renal arteriography reveals the actual arterial stenosis or obstruction; samples from both the right and left renal veins are obtained for comparison of plasma renin levels with those in the inferior vena cava. Increased renin level implicates the affected kidney and determines whether surgical correction can reverse hypertension.

Treatment
Surgery, the treatment of choice, is performed to restore adequate circulation, and to control severe hypertension or severely impaired renal function by renal artery bypass, endarterectomy, arterioplasty, or as a last resort, nephrectomy. Balloon catheter renal artery dilation is a relatively new procedure, used in selected cases to correct renal artery ste-

nosis without the risks and morbidity of surgery. Symptomatic measures include antihypertensives, diuretics, and a sodium-restricted diet.

Additional considerations
An appropriate health care plan must emphasize helping the patient and family understand renovascular hypertension and the importance of following prescribed treatment. Also, the hospital staff member should:

• accurately monitor intake and output, and daily weight; check blood pressure regularly, with the patient lying down and standing (a drop of 20 mmHg or more on arising may necessitate an adjustment in antihypertensive medications); assess renal function daily.

• administer drugs, as ordered; maintain fluid and sodium restrictions; explain the purpose of a low-sodium diet (to reduce constriction of arterioles and reduce blood pressure).

• explain the diagnostic tests, and prepare the patient appropriately; make sure the patient is not allergic to the dye used in diagnostic tests; watch for complications after intravenous pyelography or arteriography.

• reassure the patient if a nephrectomy is necessary that the remaining kidney can handle renal function adequately.

• watch for bleeding and hypotension postoperatively (if the sutures around the renal vessels slip, the patient can quickly go into shock, since kidneys receive 25% of cardiac output).

• provide a quiet, stressfree environment, if possible; urge the patient and family members to have regular blood pressure screenings.

Hydronephrosis

Hydronephrosis is an abnormal dilation of the renal pelvis and the calyces of one or both kidneys, caused by an obstruction of urine flow in the genitourinary tract. Although partial obstruction and hydronephrosis may not produce symptoms initially, the pressure built up behind the area of obstruction eventually results in symptomatic renal dysfunction.

Causes
Almost any type of obstructive uropathy can result in hydronephrosis. The most common ones include benign prostatic hypertrophy, urethral strictures, and calculi; less common causes include strictures or stenosis of the ureter or bladder outlet, congenital abnormalities, abdominal tumors, blood clots, and neurogenic bladder. If the site of obstruction is the urethra or bladder, hydronephrosis usually affects both kidneys; if a ureter, it usually affects only one kidney. Obstructions distal to the bladder cause the bladder to dilate and act as a buffer zone, delaying hydronephrosis. Total obstruction with dilation of the collecting system ultimately causes complete cortical atrophy and cessation of glomerular filtration.

Signs and symptoms
Clinical features of hydronephrosis vary with the cause of the obstruction. In some patients, hydronephrosis produces no symptoms or only mild pain and slightly decreased urinary flow; in others, this disorder may produce severe, colicky renal pain or dull flank pain that may radiate to the groin, and gross urinary abnormalities, such as hematuria, pyuria, dysuria, alternating oliguria and polyuria, or complete anuria. Other symptoms of hydronephrosis include nausea, vomiting, abdominal fullness, pain on urination, dribbling, or hesitancy. Unilateral obstruction may cause pain on only one side, usually in the flank area.

The most common complication of an obstructed kidney is infection (pyelonephritis), due to stasis that exacerbates renal damage and may create a life-threatening crisis. Paralytic ileus frequently accompanies acute obstructive uropathy.

Diagnosis

 While clinical features may suggest hydronephrosis, intravenous pyelography, retrograde pyelography, renal ultrasound, and renal func-‍tion studies confirm it.

Treatment

The goals of treatment are to preserve renal function and prevent infection through surgical removal of the obstruction, such as dilation for stricture of the urethra, or prostatectomy for benign prostatic hypertrophy.

If renal function has already been affected, therapy may include a diet low in protein, sodium, and potassium. This diet is designed to stop the progression of renal failure before surgery. Inoperable obstructions may necessitate decompression and drainage of the kidney using a nephrostomy tube placed temporarily in the renal pelvis. Concurrent infection requires appropriate antibiotic therapy.

Additional considerations

When caring for a patient with hydronephrosis, the hospital staff member should:
• explain hydronephrosis, as well as the purpose of intravenous pyelography and other diagnostic procedures; check the patient for allergy to intravenous pyelography dye.
• administer medication for pain, as needed and prescribed.
• closely monitor intake and output, vital signs, and fluid and electrolyte status postoperatively; watch for a rising pulse rate and cold, clammy skin, which indicate possible impending hemorrhage and shock; monitor renal function studies.
• check the nephrostomy tube frequently, if present, for bleeding and patency; irrigate the tube only as ordered, without clamping it.
• teach the patient to be discharged with a nephrostomy tube in place how to care for it properly.
• urge older men (especially those with family histories of benign prostatic hypertrophy or prostatitis) to have routine medical checkups to prevent progression of hydronephrosis to irreversible renal disease; teach them to recognize and report symptoms of hydronephrosis (colicky pain, hematuria) or urinary tract infection.

Renal Tubular Acidosis

Renal tubular acidosis (RTA)—a syndrome of persistent dehydration, hyperchloremia, hypokalemia, metabolic acidosis, and nephrocalcinosis—results from the kidneys' inability to conserve bicarbonate. This disorder occurs as distal RTA (Type I, or classic RTA) or proximal RTA (Type II). Prognosis is usually good but depends on the severity of renal damage that precedes treatment.

Causes and incidence

Metabolic acidosis usually results from renal excretion of bicarbonate. However, metabolic acidosis associated with RTA results from a defect in the kidneys' normal tubular acidification of urine.

Distal RTA results from an inability of the distal tubule to secrete hydrogen ions against established gradients across the tubular membrane. This results in decreased excretion of titratable acids and ammonium, increased loss of potassium and bicarbonate in the urine, and systemic acidosis. Prolonged acidosis causes mobilization of calcium from bone and, eventually, hypercalciuria, predisposing to the formation of renal calculi.

There are two classifications of distal RTA:

• *Primary distal RTA* may occur sporadically or through a hereditary defect, and is most prevalent in females, older children, adolescents, and young adults.
• *Secondary distal RTA* has been linked to many renal or systemic conditions, such as starvation, malnutrition, hepatic cirrhosis, and several genetically transmitted disorders.

Proximal RTA results from defective reabsorption of bicarbonate in the proximal tubule. This causes bicarbonate to flood the distal tubule, which normally secretes hydrogen ions, and leads to impaired formation of titratable acids and ammonium for excretion. Ultimately, metabolic acidosis results.

Proximal RTA occurs in two forms:
• In *primary proximal RTA,* the reabsorptive defect is idiopathic and is the only disorder present.
• In *secondary proximal RTA,* the reabsorptive defect may be one of several defects, and is due to proximal tubular cell damage from a disease, as Fanconi's syndrome.

Signs and symptoms

In infants, RTA produces anorexia, vomiting, occasional fever, polyuria, dehydration, growth retardation, apathy, weakness, tissue wasting, constipation, nephrocalcinosis, and rickets.

In children and adults, RTA may lead to urinary tract infection, rickets, and growth problems. Possible complications of RTA include nephrocalcinosis and pyelonephritis.

Diagnosis

 Demonstration of impaired acidification of urine with systemic metabolic acidosis confirms distal RTA. Demonstration of bicarbonate wasting due to impaired reabsorption confirms proximal RTA.

Other relevant laboratory results show:
• decreased serum bicarbonate, pH, potassium, and phosphorus

• increased serum chloride and alkaline phosphatase
• alkaline pH, with low titratable acids and ammonium content in urine; increased urinary bicarbonate and potassium, low specific gravity.

In later stages, X-rays may show nephrocalcinosis.

Treatment

Supportive treatment requires replacement of those substances being abnormally excreted, especially bicarbonate, and may include sodium bicarbonate tablets or Shohl's solution to control acidosis, potassium P.O. for dangerously low potassium levels, and vitamin D for bone disease. If pyelonephritis occurs, treatment may include antibiotics.

Treatment for renal calculi secondary to nephrocalcinosis varies, and may include supportive therapy until the calculi pass or surgery for severe obstruction is performed.

Additional considerations

The health care professional caring for a patient with RTA should:
• urge compliance with all medication instructions and inform the patient and his family that the prognosis for RTA and bone lesion healing is directly related to adequate treatment.
• monitor laboratory values, especially potassium, for hypokalemia.
• test urine for pH, and strain it for calculi.
• explain the condition and treatment of rickets to the patient and his family if he develops it.
• teach the patient how to recognize signs of calculi (hematuria, low abdominal or flank pain) and advise him to immediately report any such signs.
• instruct the patient with low potassium levels to eat foods with a high potassium content, such as bananas and baked potatoes. Orange juice is also high in potassium.
• encourage family members to seek genetic counseling for RTA since it may be caused by a genetic defect.

Fanconi's Syndrome

(de Toni-Fanconi syndrome)

Fanconi's syndrome is a renal disorder that produces malfunctions of the proximal renal tubules, leading to hyperkalemia, hypernatremia, glycosuria, phosphaturia, aminoaciduria, uricosuria, bicarbonate wasting, and eventually, retarded growth and development, and rickets. Since treatment of Fanconi's syndrome is usually unsuccessful, it commonly leads to end-stage renal failure, and the patient may survive only a few years after its onset.

Causes and incidence

Idiopathic congenital Fanconi's syndrome is most prevalent in children and affects both sexes equally. Onset of the hereditary form usually occurs during the first 6 months of life, although another hereditary form also occurs in adults. The more serious adult form of this disease is acquired Fanconi's syndrome; it is secondary to Wilson's disease, cystinosis, galactosemia, or exposure to a toxic substance (heavy metal poisoning).

Fanconi's syndrome produces characteristic changes in the proximal renal tubules, such as shortening of the connection to glomeruli by an abnormally narrow segment (swan's neck)—a result of the atrophy of epithelial cells and loss of proximal tubular mass volume.

Signs and symptoms

Changes in the proximal renal tubules result in decreased tubular reabsorption of glucose, phosphate, amino acid, bicarbonate, potassium, and occasionally, water. An infant with Fanconi's syndrome appears normal at birth, although birth weight may be low. At about age 6 months, the infant shows failure to thrive, weakness, dehydration (associated with polyuria, vomiting, and anorexia), constipation, acidosis, cystine crystals in the corneas and conjunctivas, and peripheral retinal pigment degeneration. Typically, the skin is yellow and has little pigmentation, even in summer. Refractory rickets or osteomalacia may be severe, and linear growth is slow. Bicarbonate loss causes acidosis; potas-

sium loss, weakness; water loss, dehydration. Renal calculi rarely occur.

In adults, symptoms of Fanconi's syndrome are secondary to hypophosphatemia, hypokalemia, and glycosuria. Their clinical effects include osteomalacia, muscle weakness and paralysis, and metabolic acidosis.

Diagnosis

Diagnosis requires evidence of excessive 24-hour urinary excretion of glucose, phosphate, amino acids, bicarbonate, and potassium (generally, serum values correspond to the decrease in these components). Other results include elevated phosphorus and nitrogen levels with increased renal dysfunction, and increased alkaline phosphatase with rickets. Hyperchloremic acidosis and hypokalemia support the diagnosis. (*Caution:* Glucose tolerance test is contraindicated for these patients, because it may cause a fatal shocklike reaction.) In a child with refractory rickets, growth retardation is evident; serum sample shows increased alkaline phosphatase and, with renal dysfunction, decreased calcium.

Treatment

Treatment is symptomatic, with replacement therapy appropriate to the patient's specific deficiencies. For example, a patient with rickets receives large doses of vitamin D; with acidosis and hypokalemia, supplements containing a flavored mixture of sodium and potassium citrate; and with hypocalcemia, calcium supplements (close monitoring is necessary to prevent hypercalcemia). When diminishing renal function causes hyperphosphatemia, treatment includes aluminum hydroxide antacids to bind phosphate in the intestine and prevent its absorption. Acquired Fanconi's syndrome requires treatment of the underlying cause. End-stage Fanconi's syndrome occasionally requires dialysis. Other treatment is symptomatic.

Additional considerations
• The patient with acquired Fanconi's syndrome or the parents of an infant with inherited Fanconi's syndrome must understand the seriousness of this disease (including possible dialysis) and the need to comply with drug and dietary therapy. If the patient has rickets he may need help accepting changes in his body image.

• Because prognosis is poor, the patient with acquired Fanconi's syndrome may be apathetic about taking medication. He may need encouragement to comply with therapy.
• Renal function must be monitored closely and 24-hour urine specimens collected accurately. The patient must be watched for fluid and electrolyte imbalances, particularly hypokalemia and hyponatremia; disturbed regulatory function characterized by anemia and hypertension; and uremic symptoms characteristic of renal failure (oliguria, anorexia, vomiting, muscle twitching, and pruritus).
• The patient with acquired Fanconi's sydrome should follow a diet for chronic renal failure, as ordered.

Chronic Renal Failure

Chronic renal failure is usually the end result of a gradually progressive loss of renal function; occasionally, it's the result of a rapidly progressive disease of sudden onset. Few symptoms develop until after more than 75% of glomerular filtration is lost; then the remaining normal parenchyma deteriorates progressively, and symptoms worsen as renal function decreases.

If this condition continues unchecked, uremic toxins accumulate and produce potentially fatal physiologic changes in all major organ systems. Maintenance dialysis and transplantation can temporarily sustain life.

Causes
Chronic renal failure may be the end result of:
• *chronic glomerular disease,* such as glomerulonephritis
• *chronic infections,* such as complicated chronic pyelonephritis or tuberculosis
• *congenital anomalies,* such as polycystic kidneys
• *vascular diseases,* such as renal nephrosclerosis
• *obstructive processes,* such as calculi
• *collagen diseases,* such as systemic lupus erythematosus
• *nephrotoxic agents,* such as chronic phenacetin overdose
• *endocrine diseases,* such as diabetic neuropathy.

Such conditions gradually destroy the nephrons and eventually cause irreversible renal failure. Similarly, acute renal failure that fails to respond to treatment becomes chronic renal failure.

This syndrome may progress through the following stages:
• renal insufficiency (glomerular filtration rate [GFR] can range from 40 to 70 ml/minute)
• renal failure (GFR 6 to 40 ml/minute)
• end-stage renal disease (GFR less than 6 ml/minute).

Signs and symptoms
Chronic renal failure produces major changes in all body systems:
• *Renal:* Initially, salt-wasting and consequent hyponatremia produce hypoten-

sion, dry mouth, loss of skin turgor, listlessness, fatigue, and nausea; later, this progresses to mental clouding, somnolence, and confusion. As the number of functioning nephrons decreases, so does the kidneys' capacity to excrete sodium, resulting in salt overload. Accumulation of potassium causes muscle irritability as the potassium level approaches 6.5 mEq/liter, then muscle weakness as the potassium level continues to rise. Fluid overload and metabolic acidosis also occur.

• *Cardiovascular:* Renal failure leads to hypertension, dysrhythmias (including life-threatening ventricular tachycardia or fibrillation), cardiomyopathy, uremic pericarditis, pericardial effusion with possible cardiac tamponade, congestive heart failure, and peripheral edema.

• *Respiratory:* Pulmonary changes include reduced pulmonary macrophage activity with increased susceptibility to infection, pulmonary edema, pleuritic pain, pleural friction rub and effusions, uremic pleuritis and uremic lung (or uremic pneumonitis), dyspnea due to congestive heart failure, and Kussmaul's respirations as a result of acidosis.

• *Gastrointestinal:* Inflammation and ulceration of gastrointestinal mucosa cause stomatitis, gum ulceration and bleeding, parotitis, esophagitis, gastritis, duodenal ulcers, lesions on the small and large bowel, uremic colitis, pancreatitis, and proctitis. Other gastrointestinal symptoms include a metallic taste in the mouth, uremic fetor (ammonia smell to breath), anorexia, nausea, vomiting, and constipation.

• *Cutaneous:* Typically, the skin is pallid, yellowish-bronze, dry, and scaly. Other cutaneous symptoms include severe itching, purpura, ecchymoses, uremic frost (a white, powdery covering that occurs most often in critically ill or terminal patients), thin brittle fingernails, and dry, brittle hair that may change color and fall out easily.

• *Neurologic:* Restless legs syndrome, one of the first signs of peripheral neuropathy, causes pain, burning, and itching in the legs and feet, which may be relieved by voluntarily shaking, moving, or rocking them. Eventually, this condition progresses to paresthesia and motor nerve dysfunction (usually bilateral footdrop) unless dialysis is initiated. Other signs and symptoms include muscle cramping and twitching, shortened memory and attention span, apathetic attitude, drowsiness, irritability, confusion, coma, and convulsions. EEG changes indicate metabolic encephalopathy.

• *Endocrine:* Common endocrine abnormalities include stunted growth patterns in children (even though growth hormone levels are usually elevated), infertility and decreased libido in both sexes, amenorrhea and cessation of menses in women, impotence and decreased sperm production in men, increased aldosterone secretion (related to increased renin production), and impaired carbohydrate metabolism (increased blood glucose levels similar to diabetes mellitus).

• *Hematopoietic:* Anemia, decreased RBC survival time, blood loss from dialysis and gastrointestinal bleeding, mild thrombocytopenia, and platelet defects occur. Other problems include increased bleeding and clotting disorders, demonstrated by purpura, hemorrhage from body orifices, easy bruising, ecchymoses, and petechiae.

• *Skeletal:* Calcium-phosphorus imbalance and consequent parathyroid hormone imbalances cause muscle and bone pain, skeletal demineralization, pathologic fractures, and calcifications in the brain, eyes, gums, joints, myocardium, and blood vessels. Arterial calcification may produce coronary artery disease.

Diagnosis

Diagnosis of chronic renal failure is based on clinical assessment, a history of chronic progressive debilitation, and gradual deterioration of renal function as determined by creatinine clearance tests. The following laboratory findings also aid in diagnosis:

• *Blood studies* show elevated BUN, and serum creatinine and potassium levels; decreased arterial pH and bicarbonate;

CONTINUOUS AMBULATORY PERITONEAL DIALYSIS

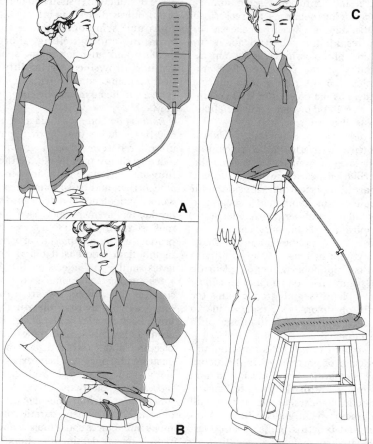

Continuous ambulatory peritoneal dialysis (CAPD) is a relatively new, increasingly useful alternative to hemodialysis in patients with renal failure. Using the peritoneum as a dialysis membrane, it allows almost uninterrupted exchange of dialysis solution. With this method, four to six exchanges of fresh dialysis solution are infused each day. The approximate dwell-time for the daytime exchanges is 5 hours; for the overnight exchange, the dwell-time is 8 to 10 hours. After each dwell-time, the patient removes the dialyzing solution by gravity drainage. This form of dialysis offers the unique advantages of a simple, easily taught procedure and patient independence from a special treatment center.

A. In this procedure, a Tenchkoff tube is surgically implanted in the abdomen, just below the umbilicus. A bag of dialysis solution is aseptically attached to the tube, and the fluid allowed to flow into the peritoneal cavity (this takes about 10 minutes).

B. The dialyzing fluid remains in the peritoneal cavity for about 4 to 6 hours. During this time, the bag may be rolled up and placed under a shirt or blouse, and the patient can go about normal activities while dialysis takes place.

C. The fluid is then drained out of the peritoneal cavity through gravity flow by unrolling the bag and suspending it below the pelvis (drainage takes about 20 minutes). After it drains, the patient aseptically connects a new bag of dialyzing solution and fills the peritoneal cavity again. He repeats this procedure four to six times a day.

COMPARISON OF PERITONEAL DIALYSIS AND HEMODIALYSIS

TYPE	ADVANTAGES	DISADVANTAGES	POSSIBLE COMPLICATIONS
Peritoneal dialysis	• Can be performed immediately • Requires less complex equipment and less specialized personnel than hemodialysis • Requires small amounts of heparin or none at all • No blood loss; minimal cardiovascular stress • Can be performed by patient anywhere (CAPD), without assistance and with minimal patient teaching • Allows patient independence without long interruptions in daily activities • Lower cost	• Contraindicated within 72 hours of abdominal surgery • Requires 48 to 72 hours for significant response to treatment • Severe protein loss necessitates high-protein diet (up to 100 g/day) • High risk of peritonitis; repeated bouts may cause scarring, preventing further treatments with peritoneal dialysis • Urea clearance less than with hemodialysis (60%)	• Bacterial or chemical peritonitis • Pain (abdominal, low back, shoulder) • Shortness of breath, or dyspnea • Atelectasis and pneumonia • Severe loss of protein into the dialysis solution in the abdominal cavity (10 to 20 g/day) • Fluid overload • Excessive fluid loss • Constipation • Catheter site inflammation, infection, or leakage
Hemodialysis	• Takes only 3 to 5 hours per treatment • Faster results in an acute situation • Total number of hours of maintenance treatment is only half that of peritoneal dialysis • In an acute situation, can use an I.V. route without a surgical access route	• Requires surgical creation of a vascular access between circulation and dialysis machine • Requires complex water treatment, dialysis equipment, and highly trained personnel • Requires administration of larger amounts of heparin • Confines patient to special treatment unit	• Septicemia • Air emboli • Rapid fluid and electrolyte imbalance (disequilibrium syndrome) • Hemolytic anemia • Metastatic calcification • Increased risk of hepatitis • Hypo- or hypertension • Itching • Pain (generalized or in chest) • Heparin overdose, possibly causing hemorrhage • Leg cramps • Nausea and vomiting • Headache

and low hemoglobin and hematocrit.
• *Urine specific gravity* becomes fixed at 1.010; urinalysis may show proteinuria, glycosuria, erythrocytes, leukocytes, and casts, depending on the etiology.
• *X-ray studies* include kidney-ureter-bladder films, intravenous pyelography, nephrotomography, renal scan, and renal arteriography to determine if any reversible components exist.
• *Kidney biopsy* allows a histologic identification of the underlying pathology.

Treatment

Dialysis therapy (hemo- or peritoneal) can eliminate or markedly decrease most manifestations of end-stage renal disease; altering dialyzing bath fluids can correct fluid and electrolyte disturbances. However, anemia, peripheral neuropathy, cardiopulmonary complications, sexual dysfunction, and skeletal defects may persist. In addition, maintenance dialysis may itself be associated with complications, including serum hepatitis (hepatitis B) due to numerous blood transfusions, protein-wasting, refractory ascites, and dialysis dementia.

The aim of conservative treatment is correction of specific symptoms. A low-protein diet reduces the production of end-products of protein metabolism that the kidneys can't excrete. (If the patient is receiving dialysis, no protein restriction is necessary, since dialysis removes such end-products.) A high-calorie diet prevents ketoacidosis and the negative nitrogen balance that results in catabolism and tissue atrophy. Such a diet also restricts sodium and potassium.

Maintaining fluid balance requires careful monitoring of vital signs, weight changes, and urine volume (if present). Diuretics (if some renal function remains) and fluid restriction can reduce fluid retention. Digitalis may be used to mobilize edema fluids; antihypertensives, to control blood pressure and associated edema. Antiemetics taken before meals may relieve nausea and vomiting; cimetidine may decrease gastric irritation. Methylcellulose or dioctyl sodium succinate prevents constipation.

Treatment may also include regular stool analysis (guaiac test) to detect occult blood, and, as needed, cleansing enemas to remove blood from the gastrointestinal tract. Anemia necessitates iron and folate supplements; severe anemia requires infusion of fresh frozen (leukocyte-poor) packed cells or washed packed cells. However, transfusions relieve anemia only temporarily. Androgen therapy (testosterone or nandrolone) may increase RBC production.

Drug therapy often relieves associated symptoms: an antipruritic, such as trimeprazine, diphenhydramine, or lidocaine (while on dialysis), to relieve itching; and aluminum hydroxide gel to lower serum phosphate levels. The patient may also benefit from supplementary vitamins and essential amino acids.

Careful monitoring of serum potassium levels is necessary to detect hyperkalemia. Emergency treatment for severe hyperkalemia includes dialysis therapy, and administration of 50% hypertonic glucose I.V., regular insulin, calcium gluconate I.V., sodium bicarbonate I.V., and cation exchange resins, such as sodium polystyrene sulfonate. Cardiac tamponade induced by uremia may require emergency pericardial tap or surgery.

Blood gas measurements may indicate acidosis; intensive dialysis and thoracentesis can relieve pulmonary edema and pleural effusions.

Additional considerations

Since chronic renal failure has such widespread clinical effects, it requires meticulous and carefully coordinated supportive care. The health care professional should:
• bathe the patient daily, using superfatted soaps, oatmeal baths, and skin lotion to ease pruritus; give good perineal care, using mild soap and water; pad the side rails to guard against ecchymoses; turn the patient often, and use an egg crate mattress to prevent skin breakdown.

• provide good oral hygiene by brushing the patient's teeth often with a soft brush or sponge tip to reduce breath odor; provide hard candy and mouthwash to minimize bad taste in the mouth and alleviate thirst.

• offer small, palatable meals that are also nutritious; try to provide favorite foods within dietary restrictions; encourage intake of high-calorie foods; instruct the outpatient to avoid high-sodium foods, such as cold cuts, diet beverages, processed cheeses, canned soups, bacon, and snack foods; tell him to avoid high-potassium foods also (citrus fruits and juices, bananas, dried fruits, and some green, leafy vegetables); encourage adherence to fluid and protein restrictions; prevent constipation, by stressing the need for exercise and sufficient dietary bulk.

• watch for hyperkalemia; observe for cramping of the legs and abdomen, and diarrhea; watch for muscle irritability and a weak pulse rate as potassium levels rise; monitor EKG for tall, peaked T waves, widening QRS segment, and disappearance of P waves, indicating hyperkalemia; report such changes immediately.

• assess hydration status carefully; check for jugular vein distention, and auscultate the lungs for rales; measure daily intake and output carefully, including all drainage, emesis, diarrhea, and blood loss; record daily weight, presence or absence of thirst, axillary sweat, dryness of tongue, hypertension, and peripheral edema.

• monitor for bone or joint complications; prevent pathologic fractures by turning the patient carefully; provide passive range-of-motion exercises for the bedridden patient.

• encourage deep breathing and coughing to prevent pulmonary congestion; listen often for rales, rhonchi, and decreased lung sounds; be alert for clinical effects of pulmonary edema (dyspnea, restlessness, rales); administer diuretics and other medications, as ordered.

• maintain strict aseptic technique; use a micropore filter during I.V. therapy; watch for signs of infection (listlessness, high fever, leukocytosis); urge the outpatient to avoid contact with infected persons during the cold and flu season.

• carefully observe and document seizure activity; infuse sodium bicarbonate for acidosis, and sedatives or anticonvulsants for seizures, as ordered; pad the side rails, and keep a padded tongue blade and suction setup at bedside; assess neurologic status periodically, and check for Chvostek's and Trousseau's signs, indicators of low serum calcium levels.

• observe for signs of bleeding (petechiae, ecchymoses); watch for prolonged bleeding at puncture sites and at the vascular access site used for hemodialysis; monitor hemoglobin and hematocrit, and check stool, urine, and vomitus for blood.

• report signs of pericarditis, such as a pericardial friction rub and chest pain.

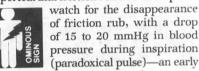 watch for the disappearance of friction rub, with a drop of 15 to 20 mmHg in blood pressure during inspiration (paradoxical pulse)—an early sign of pericardial tamponade.

• schedule medications carefully; give iron before meals, aluminum hydroxide gels after meals, and antiemetics, as necessary, a half hour before meals; administer antihypertensives at appropriate intervals; promote compliance by explaining the reason for medications; apply an emollient to soothe the perianal area if the patient requires a rectal infusion of sodium polystyrene sulfonate for dangerously high potassium levels; make sure the sodium polystyrene sulfonate enema is expelled or it will cause constipation; recommend antacid cookies as an alternative to aluminum hydroxide gels needed to bind gastrointestinal phosphate.

If the patient requires hemodialysis, the health care professional should:

• prepare the patient by fully explaining the procedure; make sure he understands how to protect and care for the arteriovenous shunt, fistula, or other vascular access; check the vascular access site every 2 hours for patency and the extremity for adequate blood supply and intact nervous function (temperature, pulse rate, capillary refill, and sensation); look for bright red blood pulsating in the tube, and listen for a bruit on auscultation if the patient has a shunt; feel for a thrill, and listen for a bruit on auscultation if a fistula is present; notify the doctor if clotting is suspected; avoid using the arm with the vascular access site to take blood pressure readings or draw blood; keep two bulldog clamps attached to the shunt dressing in case the shunt becomes disconnected.

• withhold the 6 a.m. (or morning dose) of antihypertensive on the morning of dialysis, and instruct the outpatient to do the same.

• check the patient's hepatitis antigen status. If it's positive, he is a carrier of hepatitis B and requires stool, needle, and blood precautions.

• monitor hemoglobin and hematocrit; instruct the anemic patient to conserve energy and to rest frequently.

• check for disequilibrium syndrome after dialysis, a result of sudden correction of blood chemistry abnormalities (symptoms range from a mild headache to convulsive seizures); check for excessive bleeding from the dialysis site; apply pressure dressing or absorbable gelatin sponge, as ordered and if indicated; monitor blood pressure carefully after dialysis.

A patient undergoing dialysis is under a great deal of stress, as is his family. They should be referred to appropriate counseling agencies for assistance in coping with chronic renal failure.

LOWER URINARY TRACT

Lower Urinary Tract Infection

Cystitis and urethritis, the two forms of lower urinary tract infection (UTI), are nearly 10 times more common in women than in men, and affect approximately 10% to 20% of all women at least once. Lower UTI is also a prevalent bacterial disease in children, with girls also most commonly affected. In men and children, lower UTIs are frequently related to anatomic or physiologic abnormalities and therefore require extremely close evaluation. UTIs often respond readily to treatment, but resistant bacterial flare-up during therapy, and recurrence are possible.

Causes

Most lower UTIs result from ascending infection by a single gram-negative enteric bacteria, such as *Escherichia coli, Klebsiella, Proteus, Enterobacter, Pseudomonas,* and *Serratia.* However, in a patient with neurogenic bladder, a Foley catheter, or a fistula between the intestine and bladder, lower UTI may result from simultaneous infection with multiple pathogens. Recent studies suggest that infection results from a breakdown in local defense mechanisms in the bladder that allow bacteria to invade the bladder mucosa and multiply. These bacteria cannot be readily eliminated by normal micturition.

Bacterial flare-up during treatment is generally caused by the pathogenic organism's resistance to antimicrobial therapy. The presence of even a small number (less than 10,000/ml) of bacteria in a midstream urine sample obtained during treatment casts doubt on the treatment's effectiveness.

In 99% of patients, recurrent lower UTI results from reinfection by the same organism or from some new pathogen; in the remaining 1%, recurrence reflects persistent infection, usually from renal calculi, chronic bacterial prostatitis, or a structural anomaly that may become a source of infection.

The high incidence of lower UTI among women may result from the shortness of the female urethra (1¼" to 2" [3 to

5 cm]), which allows infection from bacteria from the vagina, perineum, rectum, or a sexual partner. Men are less likely to become infected, because their urethras are longer (7¾″ [20 cm]), and prostatic fluid serves as an antibacterial shield. In both men and women, infection usually ascends from the urethra to the bladder.

Signs and symptoms
Lower UTI usually produces urgency, frequency, dysuria, cramps or spasms of the bladder, itching, a feeling of warmth during urination, nocturia, and possibly, discharge in males. Inflammation of the bladder wall also causes hematuria and fever. Other features include low back pain, malaise, nausea, vomiting, abdominal pain or tenderness over the bladder area, chills, and flank pain.

Diagnosis
Characteristic clinical features, and a microscopic urinalysis showing RBCs and WBCs greater than 10/high-power field suggest lower UTI.

 A clean, midstream urine specimen revealing a bacterial count of more than 100,000/ml confirms the diagnosis. Lower counts do not necessarily rule out infection, especially if the patient is voiding frequently, since bacteria require 30 to 45 minutes to reproduce in urine. Careful midstream, clean-catch collection is preferred to catheterization, which can reinfect the bladder with urethral bacteria. Sensitivity testing determines the appropriate antimicrobial agent. If patient history and physical examination warrant, a blood test or a stained smear of the discharge rules out venereal disease. Voiding cystourethrography or intravenous pyelography may detect congenital anomalies that predispose the patient to recurrent UTIs.

Treatment
Appropriate antimicrobials are the treatment of choice for most initial lower UTIs. In the past, a 7- to 10-day course of therapy was standard, but recent studies suggest that a single dose of an antibiotic or a 3- to 5-day course may be sufficient to render the urine sterile. After 3 days of therapy, urine culture should show no organisms. If the urine is not sterile, bacterial resistance has probably occurred, making the use of a different antimicrobial necessary.

Recurrent infections due to infected renal calculi, chronic prostatitis, or structural abnormality may necessitate surgery; prostatitis also requires long-term antibiotic therapy. In patients without these predisposing conditions, long-term, low-dosage antibiotic therapy is the treatment of choice.

Additional considerations
The care plan should include careful patient teaching, supportive measures, and proper specimen collection. The health care professional should:
• explain the nature and purpose of antimicrobial therapy; emphasize the importance of completing the prescribed course of therapy or, with long-term prophylaxis, of adhering strictly to ordered dosage; urge the patient to drink plenty of water (at least eight glasses a day) to prevent antimicrobial side effects, to help combat the infection, and to promote good hydration; stress the need to maintain a consistent fluid intake of about 2,000 ml/day. More or less than this amount may alter the effect of the prescribed antimicrobial. Fruit juices, especially cranberry juice, acidify the urine, which may decrease the rate of bacterial multiplication, although evidence to this effect is inconclusive.
• watch for gastrointestinal disturbances with antimicrobial therapy. Nitrofurantoin macrocrystals taken with milk or a meal prevents such distress. If therapy includes phenazopyridine as an analgesic for urgency, frequency, and spasms, pain, and burning in the urinary tract, the patient should be warned that this medication may turn urine red-orange.
• suggest warm sitz baths for relief of perineal discomfort; apply heat sparingly to the perineum if baths are not

effective, being careful not to burn the patient; apply topical antiseptics, such as povidone-iodine ointment, on the urethral meatus, as necessary.

• collect all urine samples for culture and sensitivity testing carefully and promptly; teach the female patient how to clean the perineum properly and keep the labia separated during voiding. A noncontaminated midstream specimen is essential for accurate diagnosis.

• prevent recurrent lower UTIs by teaching the female patient to carefully wipe the perineum from front to back and to clean it thoroughly with soap and water after defecation; advising an infection-prone woman to void immediately after sexual intercourse; stressing the need to drink plenty of fluids routinely and to avoid postponing urination; recommending frequent comfort stops during long car trips; stressing the need to completely empty the bladder.

• prevent recurrent infections in men by urging prompt treatment of predisposing conditions such as chronic prostatitis.

Vesicoureteral Reflux

In vesicoureteral reflux, urine flows from the bladder back into the ureters and eventually into the renal pelvis or the parenchyma. Because the bladder empties poorly, urinary tract infection may result, possibly leading to acute or chronic pyelonephritis with renal damage. Vesicoureteral reflux is most common during infancy in boys and during early childhood (ages 3 to 7) in girls. Primary vesicoureteral reflux that results from congenital anomalies is most prevalent in females and is rare in Blacks. Up to 25% of asymptomatic siblings of children with diagnosed primary vesicoureteral reflux also show reflux.

Causes and incidence

In patients with vesicoureteral reflux, incompetence of the ureterovesical junction allows backflow of urine into the ureter when the bladder contracts during voiding. Such incompetence may result from congenital anomalies, including short or absent intravesical ureter, ureteral ectopia lateralis (greater-than-normal lateral placement of ureters), and gaping or golf hole orifice. It also may be caused by inadequate detrusor muscle buttress in the bladder, stemming from congenital paraureteral bladder diverticulum, acquired diverticulum (from outlet obstruction), flaccid neurogenic bladder, and high intravesical pressure from outlet obstruction or an unknown cause. Reflux may also result from cystitis, with inflammation of the intravesical ureter, which causes edema and fixation of the intramural ureter and usually leads to vesicoureteral reflux in persons with congenital anomalies or other predisposing conditions.

Signs and symptoms

Vesicoureteral reflux usually manifests itself as a urinary tract infection: frequent, urgent, burning urination; hematuria; foul-smelling urine; and in infants, dark urine. With upper urinary tract involvement, symptoms usually include high fever, chills, flank pain, vomiting, and malaise. In children, fever, vague abdominal pain, and diarrhea may be the only clinical effects. Rarely, children with minimal symptoms remain undiagnosed until puberty or adulthood, when they develop clear signs of renal impairment—anemia, hypertension, and lethargy.

Diagnosis

Symptoms of urinary tract infection provide the first clues to diagnosis. In infants, hematuria or strong-smelling urine may be the first indication; palpation may reveal a hard, thickened bladder (hard mass deep in the pelvis) if posterior urethral valves are causing an ob-

struction in male infants. Cytoscopy, with instillation of a solution containing methylene blue or indigo carmine dye, may confirm the diagnosis. After the bladder is emptied and refilled with clear sterile water, color-tinged efflux from either ureter positively confirms reflux. Other pertinent studies include:
• *Clean-catch urinalysis* shows bacterial count greater than 100,000/mm³. Microscopic examination may reveal WBCs, RBCs, and an increased urine pH in the presence of infection. Specific gravity less than 1.010 demonstrates inability to concentrate urine.
• *Elevated creatinine* (greater than 1.2 mg/dl) and *BUN* (greater than 18 mg/dl) show advanced renal dysfunction.
• *Intravenous pyelography* may show dilated lower ureter, ureter visible for its entire length, hydronephrosis, calyceal distortion, and renal scarring.
• *Voiding cystourethrography* identifies and determines degree of reflux and shows when reflux occurs. It may also pinpoint the anomaly. In this procedure, contrast material is instilled in the bladder, and X-rays are taken before, during, and after voiding. Radioisotope scanning and renal ultrasound may also be used to detect reflux.
• *Catheterization of the bladder* after the patient voids determines the amount of residual urine.

Treatment

The goal of treatment is to prevent pyelonephritis and renal dysfunction with antibiotic therapy and, when necessary, vesicoureteral reimplantation. Appropriate surgical procedures create a normal valve effect at the junction by reimplanting the ureter into the bladder wall at a more oblique angle.

Antimicrobial therapy is effective for reflux that is secondary to infection, reflux related to neurogenic bladder, and in children, reflux related to a short intravesical ureter (which abates spontaneously with growth). Reflux related to infection generally subsides after the infection is cured. However, 80% of girls with vesicoureteral reflux will have recurrent urinary tract infections within a year. Recurrent infection requires long-term prophylactic chemotherapy and close patient follow-up (cystoscopy and intravenous pyelography every 4 to 6 months) to track the degree of reflux.

Urinary tract infection that recurs despite adequate prophylactic antibiotic therapy necessitates vesicoureteral reimplantation. Bladder outlet obstruction in neurogenic bladder requires surgery only if renal dysfunction is present. After surgery, as after antibiotic therapy, close medical follow-up is necessary (pyelography every 2 to 3 years and urinalysis once a month for a year), even if symptoms have not recurred.

Additional considerations

• To ensure complete emptying of the bladder, the patient with reflux should double void (void once and try to void again in a few minutes). Also, since his natural urge to urinate may be impaired, he must void every 2 to 3 hours, whether or not he feels the urge.
• Since the diagnostic tests may frighten the child, one of his parents may stay with him during all procedures. The procedures should be explained to the parents and the child, if he's old enough. If surgery is necessary, postoperative care includes: suprapubic catheter in the male, Foley catheter in the female; and in both, one or two ureteral catheters or splints brought out of the bladder through a small abdominal incision. The suprapubic or Foley catheter keeps the bladder empty and prevents pressure from stressing the surgical wound; ureteral catheters drain urine directly from the renal pelvis. After complicated reimplantations, all catheters remain in place for 7 to 10 days. The child will be able to move and walk with the catheters but must be very careful not to dislodge them.
• Postoperative supportive care includes: closely monitoring fluid intake and output; giving analgesics and antibiotics, as ordered; making sure the catheters are patent and draining well; maintaining sterile

technique during catheter care; watching for fever, chills, and flank pain, which suggest a blocked catheter.

• Before discharge, the importance of follow-up care and adequate fluid intake throughout childhood should be stressed. Parents should watch for and report recurring signs of urinary tract infection (painful, frequent, burning urination; foul-smelling urine). If the child is taking antimicrobials, the parents must understand the importance of completing the prescribed therapy or maintaining low-dose prophylaxis.

Neurogenic Bladder

(Neuromuscular dysfunction of the lower urinary tract, neurologic bladder dysfunction, neuropathic bladder)

Neurogenic bladder refers to all types of bladder dysfunction caused by an interruption of normal bladder innervation. Subsequent complications include incontinence, residual urine retention, urinary infection, stone formation, and renal failure. A neurogenic bladder can be spastic (hypertonic, reflex, or automatic) or flaccid (hypotonic, atonic, nonreflex, or autonomous).

Causes

At one time, neurogenic bladder was thought to result primarily from spinal cord injury; now, it appears to stem from a host of underlying conditions:

• *cerebral disorders,* such as cerebrovascular accident, brain tumor meningioma and glioma), Parkinson's disease, multiple sclerosis, dementia, and incontinence caused by aging

• *spinal cord disease or trauma,* spinal stenosis (causing cord compression) or arachnoiditis (causing adhesions between the membranes covering the cord), cervical spondylosis, myelopathies from hereditary or nutritional deficiencies, and rarely, tabes dorsalis

• *disorders of peripheral innervation,* including autonomic neuropathies resulting from endocrine disturbances, such as diabetes mellitus (most common)

• *metabolic disturbances,* such as hypothyroidism, porphyria, or uremia (infrequent)

• *acute infectious diseases,* such as Guillain-Barré syndrome

• *heavy metal toxicity*

• *chronic alcoholism*

• *collagen diseases,* such as systemic lupus erythematosus

• *vascular diseases,* such as atherosclerosis

• *distant effects of cancer,* such as primary oat cell carcinoma of the lung

• *herpes zoster*

• *sacral agenesis.*

An upper motor neuron lesion (above S_2 to S_4) causes spastic neurogenic bladder, with spontaneous contractions of detrusor muscles, elevated intravesical voiding pressure, bladder wall hypertrophy with trabeculation, and urinary sphincter spasms. A lower motor neuron lesion (below S_2 to S_4) causes flaccid neurogenic bladder, with decreased intravesical pressure, increased bladder capacity and large residual urine retention, and poor detrusor contraction.

Signs and symptoms

Neurogenic bladder produces a wide range of clinical effects, depending on the underlying cause and its effect on the structural integrity of the bladder. Usually, this disorder causes some degree of incontinence, changes in initiation or interruption of micturition, and inability to empty the bladder completely. Other effects of neurogenic bladder include vesicoureteral reflux, deterioration or infection in the upper urinary tract, and hydroureteral nephrosis.

Depending on the site and extent of the spinal cord lesion, *spastic neuro-*

genic bladder may produce involuntary or frequent scanty urination, without a feeling of bladder fullness, and possibly spontaneous spasms of the arms and legs. Anal sphincter tone may be increased. Tactile stimulation of the abdomen, thighs, or genitalia may precipitate voiding and spontaneous contractions of the arms and legs. With cord lesions in the upper thoracic (cervical) level, bladder distention can trigger hyperactive autonomic reflexes, resulting in severe hypertension, bradycardia, and headaches.

Flaccid neurogenic bladder may be associated with overflow incontinence, diminished anal sphincter tone, and a greatly distended bladder (evident on percussion or palpation), but without the accompanying feeling of bladder fullness due to sensory impairment.

Diagnosis
Since the causes of neurogenic bladder are so varied, diagnosis must begin with a meticulous patient history, including a thorough neurologic history (especially for injury to the spinal cord) and a history of bowel, urologic, and sexual function. Physical examination includes a complete assessment for overt neurologic disease and the following tests:
• *Spinal fluid analysis* showing increased protein level may indicate cord tumor; increased gamma globulin may indicate multiple sclerosis.
• *Skull and vertebral column X-rays* show fracture, dislocation, congenital anomalies, or metastasis.
• *Myelography* shows spinal cord compression (from tumor, spondylosis, or arachnoiditis).
• *EEG* may be abnormal in the presence of a brain tumor.
• *Electromyelography* confirms presence of peripheral neuropathy.
• *Brain and CAT scans* localize and identify brain masses.
Other tests assess bladder function:
• *Cystometry* evaluates bladder nerve supply and detrusor muscle tone.
• *Urethral pressure profile* determines urethral function.

• *Urinary flow study (uroflow)* shows diminished or impaired urinary flow.
• *Retrograde urethrography* reveals presence of strictures and diverticula.
• *Voiding cystography* evaluates bladder neck function and continence.

Treatment
The goals of treatment are to maintain the integrity of the upper urinary tract, control infection, and prevent urinary incontinence through evacuation of the bladder, drug therapy, surgery, or less often, neural blocks and electrical stimulation. Techniques of bladder evacuation include Credé's method, Valsalva's maneuver, and intermittent self-catheterization. Credé's method and Valsalva's maneuver are especially effective in patients with sacral cord lesions; those with thoracic lesions require Credé's method, since their abdominal muscles are weak. Patients with suprasacral lesions also require stimulation of bladder function to induce bladder contraction reflex through stimulation of sacral-lumbar dermatomes or by tactile stimulation of the rectum.

Intermittent self-catheterization has proven a major advance in the treatment of neurogenic bladder, since it allows complete emptying of the bladder without the risks of a Foley catheter. Generally, a male can perform this procedure more easily, but a female can learn self-catheterization with the help of a mirror. Intermittent self-catheterization, in conjunction with a bladder-retraining program, is especially useful in patients with flaccid neurogenic bladder.

Drug therapy for neurogenic bladder may include bethanechol and phenoxybenzamine to facilitate bladder emptying, and propantheline, belladonna, levodopa, propranolol, and imipramine to facilitate urine storage. When conservative treatment fails, surgery may correct the structural impairment through transurethral resection of the bladder neck, a Y-V plasty, urethral dilation, external sphincterotomy, or urinary diversion procedures. Implantation of an artificial urinary sphincter may be necessary if permanent incontinence follows surgery.

Additional considerations

Care for patients with neurogenic bladder varies according to the underlying cause and the method of treatment. When caring for such patients, the health care professional should:

• explain all diagnostic tests clearly so the patient understands the procedure, the time involved, and the possible results; assure the patient that the lengthy diagnostic process is necessary to identify the most effective treatment plan; explain the treatment plan to the patient in detail.

• use strict aseptic technique during insertion of a Foley catheter (a temporary measure to drain the incontinent patient's bladder); not interrupt the closed drainage system for any reason; obtain urine specimens with a syringe and small-bore needle inserted through the aspirating port of the catheter itself (below the junction of the balloon instillation site); irrigate in the same manner, if ordered.

• clean the catheter insertion site with soap and water at least twice a day; not allow the catheter to become encrusted; use a sterile applicator to apply antibiotic ointment around the meatus after catheter care; keep the drainage bag below the tubing, and avoid raising the bag above the level of the bladder; clamp the tubing, or empty the bag before transferring the patient to a wheelchair or stretcher to prevent accidental urine reflux; empty the bag more frequently than once every 8 hours if urinary output is considerable, since bacteria can multiply in standing urine and migrate up the catheter and into the bladder.

• watch for signs of infection (fever, cloudy or foul-smelling urine); encourage the patient to drink plenty of fluids to prevent calculus formation and infection from urinary stasis; try to keep the patient as mobile as possible; perform passive range-of-motion exercises, if necessary.

• arrange for consultation with an enterostomal therapist if urinary diversion procedure is to be performed, and coordinate the care plans.

• before discharge, teach the patient and his family evacuation techniques, (Credé's method, intermittent catheterization) and counsel him regarding sexual activities. The incontinent patient may feel embarrassed and distressed and may need emotional support.

Congenital Anomalies of the Ureter, Bladder, and Urethra

Congenital anomalies of the ureter, bladder, and urethra are among the most common birth defects, occurring in about 5% of all births. Some of these abnormalities are obvious at birth; others are not apparent and are recognized only after they produce symptoms.

Causes

The most common malformations include duplicated ureter, retrocaval ureter, ectopic orifice of the ureter, stricture or stenosis of the ureter, ureterocele, exstrophy of the bladder, congenital bladder diverticulum, hypospadias, and epispadias. Their causes are unknown; diagnosis and treatment vary.

Additional considerations

• Since these anomalies aren't always obvious at birth, the newborn's urogenital function must be evaluated. The amount and color of urine, voiding pattern, strength of stream, and any indications of infection, such as fever and urine odor, should be documented. Parents should watch for these signs at home.

CONGENITAL ANOMALIES OF THE URETER AND BLADDER

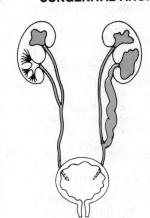

DUPLICATED URETER
PATHOPHYSIOLOGY
- Most common ureteral anomaly
- *Complete,* a double collecting system with two separate pelves, each with its own ureter and orifice
- *Incomplete* (y type), two separate ureters join before entering bladder

CLINICAL FEATURES
- Persistent or recurrent infection
- Frequency, urgency, or burning on urination
- Diminished urinary output
- Flank pain, fever, and chills

DIAGNOSIS AND TREATMENT
- Intravenous pyelography
- Voiding cystoscopy
- Cystoureterography
- Retrograde pyelography
- Surgery for obstruction, reflux, or severe renal damage

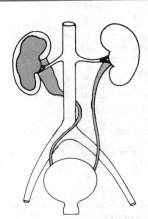

RETROCAVAL URETER (PREURETERAL VENA CAVA)
PATHOPHYSIOLOGY
- Right ureter passes behind the inferior vena cava before entering the bladder. Compression of the ureter between the vena cava and the spine causes dilation and elongation of the pelvis; hydroureter, hydronephrosis; fibrosis and stenosis of ureter in the compressed area.
- Relatively uncommon; higher incidence in males

CLINICAL FEATURES
- Right flank pain
- Recurrent urinary tract infection
- Renal calculi
- Hematuria

DIAGNOSIS AND TREATMENT
- Intravenous or retrograde pyelography demonstrates superior ureteral enlargement with spiral appearance.
- Surgical resection and anastomosis of ureter with renal pelvis, or reimplantation into bladder

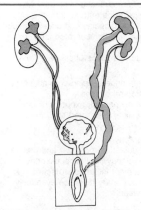

ECTOPIC ORIFICE OF URETER
PATHOPHYSIOLOGY
- Ureters single or duplicated. In females, ureteral orifice usually inserts in urethra or vaginal vestibule, beyond external urethral sphincter; in males, in prostatic urethra, or in seminal vesicles or vas deferens

CLINICAL FEATURES
- Symptoms rare when ureteral orifice opens between trigone and bladder neck
- Obstruction, reflux, and incontinence (dribbling) in 50% of females
- In males, flank pain, frequency, urgency

DIAGNOSIS AND TREATMENT
- Intravenous pyelography
- Urethroscopy, vaginoscopy
- Voiding cystourethrography
- Resection and ureteral reimplantation into bladder for incontinence

CONGENITAL ANOMALIES OF THE URETER AND BLADDER (continued)

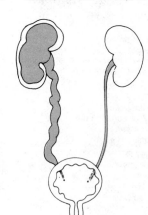

STRICTURE OR STENOSIS OF URETER

PATHOPHYSIOLOGY
- Most common site, the distal ureter above uretero-vesical junction; less common, ureteropelvic junction; rare, the midureter
- Discovered during infancy in 25% of patients; before puberty in most
- More common in males

CLINICAL FEATURES
- Megaloureter or hydroureter (enlarged ureter), with hydronephrosis when stenosis occurs in distal ureter
- Hydronephrosis alone when stenosis occurs at ureteropelvic junction

DIAGNOSIS AND TREATMENT
- Ultrasound
- Intravenous and retrograde pyelography
- Voiding cystography
- Surgical repair of stricture. Nephrectomy for severe renal damage

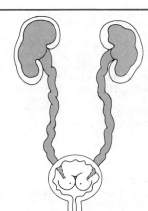

URETEROCELE

PATHOPHYSIOLOGY
- Bulging of submucosal ureter into bladder can be 1 or 2 cm, or can almost fill entire bladder
- Unilateral, bilateral, ectopic with resulting hydroureter, and hydronephrosis

CLINICAL FEATURES
- Obstruction
- Persistent or recurrent infection

DIAGNOSIS AND TREATMENT
- Voiding cystourethrography
- Intravenous pyelography and cystoscopy show thin, translucent mass.
- Surgical excision or resection of ureterocele, with reimplantation of ureter

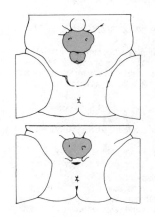

EXSTROPHY OF BLADDER

PATHOPHYSIOLOGY
- Absence of anterior abdominal and bladder wall allows the bladder to protrude onto abdomen.
- In males, associated epispadias and undescended testes; in females, cleft clitoris, separated labia, or absent vagina
- Skeletal or intestinal anomalies possible

CLINICAL FEATURES
- Obvious at birth, with urine seeping onto abdominal wall from abnormal ureteral orifices
- Surrounding skin is excoriated; exposed bladder mucosa ulcerated; infection; associated abnormalities

DIAGNOSIS AND TREATMENT
- Intravenous pyelography
- Surgical closure of defect, and bladder and urethra reconstruction during infancy to allow pubic bone fusion; alternative treatment includes protective dressing and diapering; urinary diversion eventually necessary for most patients

CONGENITAL ANOMALIES OF THE URETER AND BLADDER (continued)

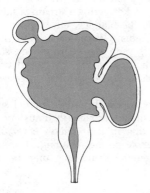

CONGENITAL BLADDER DIVERTICULUM
PATHOPHYSIOLOGY
- Circumscribed pouch or sac (diverticulum) of bladder wall
- Can occur anywhere in bladder, usually lateral to ureteral orifice. Large diverticulum at orifice can cause reflux.

CLINICAL FEATURES
- Fever, frequency, and painful urination
- Urinary tract infection
- Cystitis, particularly in males

DIAGNOSIS AND TREATMENT
- Intravenous pyelography shows diverticulum.
- Retrograde cystography shows vesicoureteral reflux in ureter.
- Surgical correction for reflux

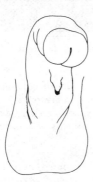

HYPOSPADIAS
PATHOPHYSIOLOGY
- Urethral opening is on ventral surface of penis or, in females, in the vagina.
- Occurs in 1 of 300 live male births. Genetic factor suspected in less severe cases

CLINICAL FEATURES
- Usually associated with chordee, making normal urination with penis elevated impossible
- Absence of ventral prepuce
- Vaginal discharge

DIAGNOSIS AND TREATMENT
- Mild disorder requires no treatment.
- Surgical repair of severe anomaly usually necessary before child reaches school age

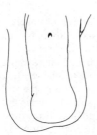

EPISPADIAS
PATHOPHYSIOLOGY
- Urethral opening on dorsal surface of penis; in females, a fissure of the upper wall of urethra
- A rare anomaly; usually develops in males; often accompanies bladder exstrophy.

CLINICAL FEATURES
- In mild cases, orifice appears along dorsum of glans; in severe cases, along dorsum of penis.
- In females, bifid clitoris and short, wide urethra

DIAGNOSIS AND TREATMENT
- Surgical repair, in several stages, almost always necessary

- All children should be watched for signs of obstruction, such as dribbling, oliguria or anuria, abdominal mass, hypertension, fever, bacteriuria, or pyuria.
- Renal function should be monitored daily and intake and output recorded.
- Strict aseptic technique should be followed in handling cystostomy tubes or Foley catheters.
- Ureteral, suprapubic, or urethral catheters must remain in place and stay uncontaminated. Type, color, and amount of drainage should be documented.
- Sterile saline pads will protect the exposed mucosa of the newborn with bladder exstrophy. Heavy clamps must not

be used on the umbilical cord, and dressing or diapering the infant should be avoided. By placing the infant in an incubator, and directing a stream of saline mist onto the bladder, the bladder can be kept moist. Warm water and mild soap will keep the surrounding skin clean. The area should be rinsed well, and kept as dry as possible to prevent excoriation.
- The parents will need emotional support and should verbalize their anxiety. By participating in their child's care, they will promote normal bonding. If appropriate, genetic counseling may be arranged.

PROSTATE DISORDERS

Prostatitis

Prostatitis, inflammation of the prostate gland, may be acute or chronic. Acute prostatitis most often results from gram-negative bacteria, and is easy to recognize and treat. However, chronic prostatitis, the most common cause of recurrent urinary tract infection (UTI) in men, is less easy to recognize. As many as 35% of men over age 50 have chronic prostatitis.

Causes
About 80% of bacterial prostatitis results from infection by *Escherichia coli*; the rest, from *Klebsiella, Enterobacter, Proteus, Pseudomonas, Streptococcus,* and *Staphylococcus.* Such infection probably spreads to the prostate gland by the hematogenous route or from ascending urethral infection, invasion of rectal bacteria by way of lymphatics, reflux of infected bladder urine into prostate ducts, or less commonly, infrequent or excessive sexual intercourse or urethral instrumentation, such as cystoscopy or catheterization. Chronic prostatitis usually develops as a result of bacterial invasion from the urethra.

Signs and symptoms
Acute prostatitis begins with sudden fever, chills, low back pain, a feeling of myalgia, perineal fullness, and arthral-

gia. Urination becomes more frequent and more urgent. Dysuria, nocturia, and some degree of urinary obstruction may also occur. The urine may appear cloudy. When palpated rectally, the prostate is markedly tender, indurated, swollen, firm, and warm.

Clinical features of chronic bacterial prostatitis vary. Although some patients are asymptomatic, this condition usually elicits the same urinary symptoms as the acute phase but to a lesser degree. Other possible signs include painful ejaculation, hemospermia, persistent urethral discharge, and sexual dysfunction. UTI is a common complication.

Diagnosis
Although a urine culture can often identify the infectious organism, and a rectal examination suggests prostatitis (especially in the acute phase), diagnosis de-

pends on the comparison of urine cultures of samples obtained by the Meares and Stamey technique. This test requires four specimens: one collected when the patient starts voiding (voided bladder one—VB1); another midstream (VB2); another after the patient stops urinating and the doctor massages the prostate gland to produce secretions (expressed prostate secretions—EPS); and finally, one more voided specimen (VB3). A significant increase in colony count of the prostatic specimens (EPS and VB3) confirms prostatitis.

Treatment
A 10-day course of therapy with carbenicillin indanyl sodium, tetracycline, or co-trimoxazole is the treatment of choice for both acute and chronic bacterial prostatitis. If the patient is allergic to penicillins, tetracyclines, or sulfonamides, gentamicin I.M. is an effective alternative. Supportive therapy includes bed rest, adequate hydration, analgesics, antipyretics, and stool softeners. If drug therapy is unsuccessful in chronic prostatitis, treatment may include transurethral resection of the prostate. To be effective, this procedure requires removal of all infected tissue, but it should not be performed on young adults, because it usually leads to retrograde ejaculation and sterility. Total prostatectomy is curative but may cause impotence and incontinence.

Additional symptomatic measures for chronic prostatitis include daily sitz baths and intercourse, as prescribed by the urologist, to promote drainage.

Additional considerations
The health care professional caring for a patient with prostatitis should:
• provide a calm atmosphere to ensure bed rest; promote adequate hydration; provide stool softeners to prevent pain and straining at stool; administer sitz baths to relieve pain and spasm.
• assist with suprapubic needle aspiration of the bladder to relieve acute urinary retention, or a suprapubic cystostomy for prolonged bladder drainage, since urethral instrumentation should be avoided.
• administer medications, as ordered; stress the need for strict adherence to the prescribed regimen; instruct the patient to drink at least eight glasses of water a day; tell him to immediately report signs of possible drug side effects, such as rash, nausea, vomiting, fever, chills, and gastrointestinal irritation.

Epididymitis

This infection of the epididymis, the testicle's cordlike excretory duct, is one of the most common infections of the male reproductive tract. It usually affects adults and is rare before puberty. Epididymitis may spread to the testicle itself, causing orchitis; bilateral epididymitis may cause sterility.

Causes
Epididymitis usually results from pyogenic organisms, such as staphylococci, *Escherichia coli*, and streptococci. Generally, such organisms result from established urinary tract infection or prostatitis, and reach the epididymis through the lumen of the vas deferens. Rarely, epididymitis is secondary to a distant infection, such as pharyngitis or tuberculosis, that spreads through the lymphatics or, less commonly, the bloodstream. Other causes include trauma, gonorrhea, syphilis, or a chlamydial infection. Trauma may reactivate a dormant infection or initiate a new one. Epididymitis is a complication of prostatectomy, and may also result from chemical irritation by extravasation of urine through the vas deferens.

ORCHITIS

Orchitis, infection of the testicles, is a serious complication of epididymitis. This infection may also result from mumps, which may lead to sterility, and, less often, from another systemic infection, testicular torsion, or severe trauma. Its typical effects include unilateral or bilateral tenderness, gradual onset of pain, and swelling of the scrotum and testicles. The affected testicle may be red and hot. Nausea and vomiting also occur. Sudden cessation of pain indicates testicular ischemia, which may result in permanent damage to one or both testicles.

Treatment consists of immediate antibiotic therapy or, in mumps orchitis, diethylstilbestrol (DES), which may relieve pain, swelling, and fever. Corticosteroids are still experimental. Severe orchitis may require surgery to incise and drain the hydrocele and to improve testicular circulation. Other treatment is similar to that for epididymitis. To prevent mumps orchitis, prepubertal males should receive mumps vaccine (or gamma globulin injection after contracting mumps).

Signs and symptoms

The key symptoms are pain, extreme tenderness, and swelling in the groin and scrotum from enlarged lymph nodes in the spermatic cord. Also, the scrotum may feel hot. Other clinical effects: high fever, malaise, and a characteristic waddle, an attempt to protect the groin and scrotum during walking. An acute hydrocele may also occur as a reaction to the inflammatory process.

Diagnosis

While typical clinical features strongly suggest epididymitis, firm diagnosis requires laboratory testing:
• *Urinalysis:* Increased WBC indicates infection.
• *Urine culture and sensitivity:* Findings may identify causative organism.
• *Serum WBC:* > 10,000/mm³ in infection.

However, in epididymitis accompanied by orchitis, diagnosis must be made cautiously, since symptoms mimic those of testicular torsion, a condition requiring urgent surgical intervention.

Treatment

The goal of treatment is to reduce pain and swelling, and combat infection. Therapy must begin immediately, particularly in the patient with bilateral epididymitis, since sterility is always a threat. During the acute phase, treatment consists of bed rest, scrotal elevation with towel rolls or adhesive strapping, broad-spectrum antibiotics, and analgesics. An ice bag applied to the area may reduce swelling and relieve pain (heat is contraindicated, since it may damage germinal cells, which are viable only at or below normal body temperature). When pain and swelling subside and allow walking, an athletic supporter may prevent pain. Occasionally, corticosteroids may be prescribed to help counteract inflammation, but their use is controversial.

In the older patient undergoing open prostatectomy, bilateral vasectomy may be necessary to prevent epididymitis as a postoperative complication; however, antibiotic therapy alone may prevent it. When epididymitis is refractory to antibiotic therapy, epididymectomy under local anesthetic is necessary.

Additional considerations

The hospital staff member should:
• watch closely for abscess formation (localized, hot, red, tender area) or extension of infection into the testes; monitor temperature closely, and ensure adequate fluid intake.
• administer analgesics, as necessary, since the patient is usually very uncomfortable; check often for proper scrotum elevation during bed rest.
• before discharge, emphasize the importance of completing prescribed antibiotic therapy, even after symptoms subside; suggest supportive counseling, as necessary, if sterility seems likely.

Benign Prostatic Hypertrophy

Although most men over age 50 have some prostatic enlargement, in benign prostatic hypertrophy or hyperplasia (BPH), the prostate gland enlarges sufficiently to compress the urethra and cause some overt urinary obstruction. Depending on the size of the enlarged prostate, the age and health of the patient, and the extent of obstruction, BPH is treated symptomatically or surgically.

Causes

Recent evidence suggests a link between BPH and hormonal activity. As men age, production of androgenic hormones decreases, causing an imbalance in androgen and estrogen levels, and high levels of dihydrotestosterone, the main prostatic intracellular androgen. Other theoretical causes include neoplasm, arteriosclerosis, inflammation, and metabolic or nutritional disturbances.

Whatever the cause, BPH begins with changes in periurethral glandular tissue. As the prostate enlarges, it may extend into the bladder and obstruct urinary outflow by compressing or distorting the prostatic urethra. BPH may also cause a pouch to form in the bladder, which retains urine when the rest of the bladder empties. This retained urine may lead to calculus formation or cystitis.

Signs and symptoms

Clinical features of BPH depend on the extent of prostatic enlargement and the lobes affected. Characteristically, the condition starts with a group of symptoms known as "prostatism": reduced urinary stream caliber and force, difficulty starting micturition (straining), feeling of incomplete voiding, and occasionally, urinary retention. As obstruction increases, urination becomes more frequent, with nocturia, incontinence, and possibly, hematuria. Physical examination indicates a visible midline mass (distended bladder) that represents an incompletely emptied bladder; rectal palpation discloses an enlarged prostate. Examination may detect secondary anemia and, possibly, renal insufficiency secondary to obstruction.

As BPH worsens, complete urinary obstruction may follow infection, or ingestion of decongestants, tranquilizers, alcohol, antidepressants, or anticholinergics. Possible complications include infection, renal insufficiency, hemorrhage, and shock.

Diagnosis

Clinical features and a rectal examination are usually sufficient for diagnosis. Other findings help to confirm this diagnosis.

• *Intravenous pyelography* may indicate urinary tract obstruction, calculi or tumors, and filling and emptying defects in the bladder.

• *Elevated BUN and creatinine levels* suggest impaired renal function.

• *Urinalysis and urine culture* show hematuria, pyuria, and when bacterial count is more than $100,000/mm^3$, urinary tract infection.

When symptoms are severe, a cystourethroscopy is the definitive diagnostic measure, but this examination is performed only immediately before surgery, to help determine the best operative procedure. It can show prostate enlargement, bladder wall changes, and a raised bladder.

Treatment

Conservative therapy includes prostatic massages, sitz baths, short-term fluid restriction (to prevent bladder distention), and if infection develops, antimicrobials. Regular sexual intercourse may help relieve prostatic congestion.

However, surgery is the only effective therapy for relief of acute urinary retention, hydronephrosis, severe hematuria, and recurrent urinary tract infection, or for palliative relief of intolerable symptoms. A transurethral resection may be performed if the prostate weighs less than 2 oz (60 g). (Weight is approximated by digital examination.) In this procedure, a resectoscope removes tissue with a wire loop and electric current. For patients who are at high risk, continuous drainage with a Foley catheter alleviates urinary retention.

Other appropriate procedures involve open surgical removal:
• *suprapubic* (transvesical): most common and especially useful when prostatic enlargement remains within the bladder
• *perineal:* for a large gland in an older patient; usually results in impotence and incontinence
• *retropubic* (extravesical): allows direct visualization; potency and continence are usually maintained.

Additional considerations
Care by a hospital staff member includes preparing the patient for diagnostic tests and surgery, as appropriate. The staff member should:
• monitor and record vital signs, intake and output, and daily weight; watch closely for signs of postobstructive diuresis (increased output, hypotension), which may lead to serious dehydration, lowered blood volume, shock, electrolyte loss, and anuria.
• administer antibiotics, as ordered, for urinary tract infection, urethral instrumentation, and cystoscopy.
• insert a Foley catheter if urinary retention is present, although this is usually difficult in a patient with BPH; assist with suprapubic cystostomy (under local anesthetic) if the catheter can't be passed transurethrally; watch for rapid bladder decompression.

After prostatic surgery, the staffer should:
• maintain patient comfort, and watch for and prevent complications; observe for immediate dangers—shock and hemorrhage—of prostate bleeding; check the catheter frequently (every 15 minutes for the first 2 to 3 hours) for patency and color, and the dressings for bleeding.
• keep a three-way catheter, if applicable, open at a rate sufficient to maintain returns that are clear and light pink (postoperatively, many urologists insert a three-way catheter and establish continuous bladder irrigation); watch for fluid overload from absorption of the irrigating fluid into systemic circulation; observe a regular catheter closely. If drainage stops because of clots, the catheter should be irrigated, as ordered, usually with 80 to 100 ml normal saline solution, while maintaining *strict* aseptic technique.
• watch for septic shock, the most serious complication of prostatic surgery; report immediately severe chills, sudden fever, tachycardia, hypotension, or other signs of shock; start rapid infusion of antibiotics I.V., as ordered; watch for pulmonary embolus, heart failure, and

---

BENIGN PROSTATIC HYPERPLASIA

NORMAL PROSTATE

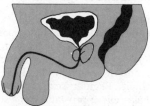

ENLARGED PROSTATE

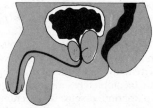

As the prostate gland expands, it compresses the urethra and bladder, obstructing urinary flow.

renal shutdown; monitor vital signs, central venous pressure, and arterial pressure continuously. The patient may need intensive supportive care in the ICU.
• give belladonna and opium suppositories or other anticholinergics, as ordered, to relieve painful bladder spasms after transurethral resection. Comfort measures after an open procedure include suppositories (except with perineal prostatectomy), analgesics to control incisional pain, and frequent dressing changes.
• continue I.V. fluids until the patient can drink enough (2,000 to 3,000 ml/day) to maintain an adequate intake.
• give stool softeners and laxatives, as ordered, to prevent straining; *not* check for impaction, since rectal examination

may precipitate bleeding.
• reassure the patient that, although he may experience frequency and dribbling after the catheter is removed, he will gradually regain urinary control; explain this to the patient's family so they can reinforce this reassurance.
• reinforce prescribed limits on activity; warn against lifting, strenuous exercise, and long automobile rides, since these increase bleeding tendency; caution the patient to restrict sexual activity for several weeks after discharge; instruct him to take antibiotics P.O., as prescribed, and tell him the indications for using gentle laxatives; urge him to seek medical care immediately if he can't void or has bloody urine, or if a fever develops.

Selected References

Brundage, Dorothy. NURSING MANAGEMENT OF RENAL PROBLEMS, 2nd ed. St. Louis: C.V. Mosby Co., 1980.
Early, Lawrence E., and Carl W. Gottschalk. STRAUSS AND WELT'S DISEASES OF THE KIDNEYS, 3rd ed. Boston: Little, Brown & Co., 1979.
Ellis, P.D. *Renal Failure*, CRITICAL CARE QUARTERLY. September 1978.
Friedman, Eli A. STRATEGY IN RENAL FAILURE (Nephrology and hypertension series). New York: John Wiley & Sons, 1978.
Harrington, Joan, and Etta R. Brener. PATIENT CARE IN RENAL FAILURE (Monographs in Clinical Nursing: No. 5). Philadelphia: W.B. Saunders Co., 1973.
Harrison, J., et al., eds. CAMPBELL'S UROLOGY, 4th ed. Philadelphia: W.B. Saunders Co., 1978.
Hekelman, Francine, and Carol Ostendarp. NEPHROLOGY NURSING: PERSPECTIVES OF CARE. New York: McGraw-Hill Book Co., 1979.
Kagan, Lynn. RENAL DISEASE: A MANUAL OF PATIENT CARE. New York: McGraw-Hill Book Co., 1979.
Lancaster, Larry E. THE PATIENT WITH END STAGE RENAL DISEASE. New York: John Wiley & Sons, 1979.
Leaf, Alexander, and Ramzi Cotran, eds. RENAL PATHOPHYSIOLOGY—RECENT ADVANCES. New York: Raven Press, 1980.
Marshall, Fray. *Embryology of the Lower Genitourinary Tract*, UROLOGIC CLINICS OF NORTH AMERICA. 5:1:3-15, February 1978.
Netter, Frank H. THE CIBA COLLECTION OF MEDICAL ILLUSTRATIONS, Volume VI: Kidneys, Ureters, and Urinary Bladder. Summit, N.J.: Ciba Pharmaceutical Co., 1973.
Papper, Solomon. CLINICAL NEPHROLOGY, 2nd ed. Boston: Little, Brown & Co., 1978.
Pitts, Robert. PHYSIOLOGY OF THE KIDNEY AND BODY FLUIDS, 3rd ed. Chicago: Year Book Medical Publishers, 1974.
Schrier, Robert W., ed. RENAL AND ELECTROLYTE DISORDERS, 2nd ed. Boston: Little, Brown & Co., 1980.
Thompson, Ian. *Transurethral Surgery*, UROLOGIC SURGERY, 2nd ed. New York: Harper & Row, 1975.
Valtin, Heinz. RENAL DYSFUNCTION: MECHANISMS INVOLVED IN FLUID SOLUTE IMBALANCE. Boston: Little, Brown & Co., 1979.
Vander, Arthur. RENAL PHYSIOLOGY. New York: McGraw-Hill Book Co., 1975.
Winter, Chester, and Alice Morel. NURSING CARE OF PATIENTS WITH UROLOGIC DISEASES, 4th ed. St. Louis: C.V. Mosby Co., 1977.

13 Endocrine Disorders

Endocrine Disorders

Introduction

Together with the nervous system, the endocrine system regulates and integrates the body's metabolic activities. The endocrine system meets the nervous system at the hypothalamus. The hypothalamus, the highest integrative center for the endocrine and autonomic nervous systems, controls endocrine organs by neural and hormonal pathways. A hormone is a chemical transmitter released from specialized cells into the bloodstream, which carries it to specialized organ-receptor cells that respond to it.

Neural pathways connect the hypothalamus to the posterior pituitary, or neurohypophysis. Neural stimulation to the posterior pituitary provokes the secretion of two effector hormones: antidiuretic hormone (ADH) and oxytocin.

Hypothalamic control

The hypothalamus also exerts hormonal control at the anterior pituitary through releasing and inhibiting factors, which arrive by a portal system. Hypothalamic hormones stimulate the pituitary to release trophic hormones (adrenocorticotropic hormone [ACTH], thyroid-stimulating hormone [TSH], luteinizing hormone [LH], and follicle-stimulating hormone [FSH]); and to release or inhibit effector hormones (human growth hormone [HGH], prolactin, and melanocyte-stimulating hormone [MSH]). In turn, secretion of trophic hormones stimulates the adrenal cortex, thyroid, and gonads. In a patient whose clinical condition suggests endocrine pathology, this complex hormonal sequence requires careful evaluation at each level to identify the dysfunction; dysfunction may result from defects of releasing, trophic, or effector hormones, or of the target tissue. Hyperthyroidism, for example, may result from an excess of thyrotropin-releasing hormone (TRH), of TSH, or of thyroid hormone.

In addition to hormonal and neural controls, a negative feedback system regulates the endocrine system. The mechanism of feedback may be simple or complex. Simple feedback occurs when the level of one substance regulates secretion of a hormone. For example, low serum calcium stimulates parathyroid hormone (PTH) secretion; high serum calcium inhibits it. Complex feedback occurs through the hypothalamic-pituitary-target organ axis. For example, secretion of the hypothalamic corticotropin-releasing hormone (CRH) releases pituitary ACTH, which, in turn, stimulates adrenal cortisol secretion. Subsequently, a rise in serum cortisol inhibits ACTH by decreasing CRH secretion. Steroid therapy disrupts the hypothalamic-pituitary-adrenal (HPA) axis by suppressing hypothalamic-pituitary secretion. Because abrupt withdrawal of steroids doesn't allow time for recovery of the HPA axis to stimulate cortisol secretion, it can induce life-threatening adrenal crisis.

Endocrine pathology

Common dysfunctions of the endocrine system are classified as hypo- and hyperfunction, inflammation, and tumor. The source of hypo- and hyperfunction may originate in the hypothalamus, or in the pituitary or effector glands. Inflammation may be acute or subacute, as in thyroiditis, but is usually chronic, often resulting in glandular hypofunction. Tumors can occur within a gland—as in thyroid carcinoma or pheochromocytoma—or outside a gland, resulting in ectopic hormone production. Certain lung tumors, for example, secrete ADH or PTH.

The study of endocrine function focuses on measuring the level or the effect of a hormone. Radioimmunoassay, for example, measures insulin levels; a fasting blood sugar test measures insulin's effects. Sophisticated techniques of hormone measurement have improved diagnosis of endocrine disorders. While diagnostic tests are needed to confirm endocrine disorders, clinical data usually provide the first clues to these disorders. Clinical assessment can reveal common signs and symptoms of endocrine dysfunction, such as excessive or delayed growth, wasting, weakness,

polydipsia, polyuria, and mental changes. The quality and distribution of hair, skin pigmentation, and distribution of body fat are also significant. Preparation of the patient for testing includes instruction and support by the health care professional. Patient specimens must be collected properly, particularly the 12- or 24-hour urine specimens.

Hormonal effects

In response to the hypothalamus, the *posterior pituitary* secretes oxytocin and ADH. Oxytocin stimulates contraction of the uterus and is responsible for the milk let-down reflex in lactating women. ADH controls the concentration of body fluids by altering the permeability of the distal convoluted tubules and collecting ducts of the kidneys, to conserve water. The secretion of ADH depends on the plasma osmolality as monitored by hypothalamic neurons. Circulatory shock and severe hemorrhage are the most powerful stimulators of ADH; other stimulators include pain, emotional stress, trauma, morphine, tranquilizers, certain anesthetics, and positive-pressure breathing. Paradoxically, in some patients, *low* plasma osmolality triggers excessive secretion of ADH; this is called the syndrome of inappropriate ADH (SIADH). Generally, however, overhydration suppresses ADH secretion (so,

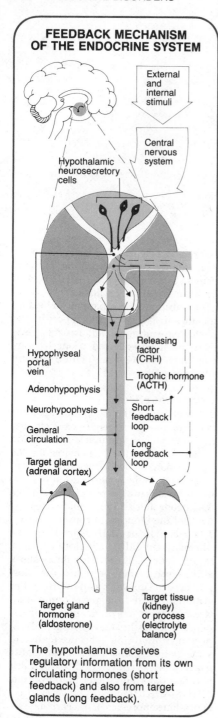

FEEDBACK MECHANISM OF THE ENDOCRINE SYSTEM

External and internal stimuli

Central nervous system

Hypothalamic neurosecretory cells

Hypophyseal portal vein

Adenohypophysis

Neurohypophysis

General circulation

Target gland (adrenal cortex)

Releasing factor (CRH)

Trophic hormone (ACTH)

Short feedback loop

Long feedback loop

Target gland hormone (aldosterone)

Target tissue (kidney) or process (electrolyte balance)

The hypothalamus receives regulatory information from its own circulating hormones (short feedback) and also from target glands (long feedback).

incidentally, does alcohol). Deficiency of ADH causes a condition of high urinary output known as diabetes insipidus.

The *anterior pituitary* secretes three effector hormones: MSH, which affects skin pigmentation; prolactin (formerly called luteotropic hormone), which stimulates milk secretion; and HGH, which affects most body tissues. HGH stimulates growth by increasing protein synthesis and fat mobilization, and decreasing carbohydrate utilization. Hyposecretion of HGH results in dwarfism; hypersecretion causes gigantism in children and acromegaly in adults.

The *thyroid gland* secretes the iodinated hormones thyroxine (T_4) and triiodothyronine (T_3). The overall function of thyroid hormone is to increase the metabolic rate of tissues by increasing essential metabolic activities—the rate of nutrient use for energy production, the rate of growth, and the activities of other endocrine glands. Deficiency of thyroid hormone causes varying degrees of hypothyroidism, from a mild, clinically insignificant form to the life-threatening extreme, myxedema coma. Congenital hypothyroidism causes cretinism. Hypersecretion causes hyperthyroidism and, in extreme cases, thyrotoxic crisis. Excessive secretion of TSH causes hyperplasia of the thyroid gland and results in goiter.

The *parathyroid glands* secrete PTH, which regulates calcium and phosphate metabolism. PTH elevates serum calcium levels by stimulating resorption of calcium and phosphate from bone, reabsorption of calcium and excretion of phosphate by the kidneys, and by combined action with vitamin D, absorption of calcium and phosphate from the gastrointestinal tract. Thyrocalcitonin, a secretion from the thyroid, opposes the effect of PTH and therefore decreases serum calcium. Hyperparathyroidism causes hypercalcemia; hypoparathyroidism causes hypocalcemia. Altered calcium levels may also result from nonendocrine causes, such as metastatic bone disease.

The *endocrine pancreas* produces glucagon from the alpha cells and insulin from the beta cells. Glucagon, the hormone of the fasting state, releases stored glucose to raise blood sugar level. Insulin, the hormone of the nourished state, facilitates glucose transport, promotes glucose storage, stimulates protein synthesis, and enhances free fatty acid uptake and storage. Insulin deficiency causes diabetes mellitus. Insulin excess can result from an insulinoma.

The *adrenal cortex* secretes mineralocorticoids, glucocorticoids, and sex steroids. Aldosterone, a mineralocorticoid, regulates the reabsorption of sodium and the excretion of potassium by the kidneys. Although affected by ACTH, aldosterone is also regulated by angiotensin II, which, in turn, is regulated by renin. Together, aldosterone, angiotensin, and renin may be implicated in the pathogenesis of hypertension. An excess of aldosterone (aldosteronism) can result primarily from hyperplasia or from cancer of the adrenal gland; or secondarily from many conditions, including congestive heart failure and cirrhosis.

Cortisol, a glucocorticoid, stimulates gluconeogenesis, increases protein breakdown and free fatty acid mobilization, suppresses the immune response, and provides for an appropriate response to stress. Hyperactivity of the adrenal cortex results in Cushing's syndrome; hypoactivity causes Addison's disease and, in extreme cases, adrenal crisis. Adrenogenital syndromes may result from overproduction of sex steroids.

The *adrenal medulla* is an aggregate of nervous tissue that produces the catecholamines epinephrine and norepinephrine, both of which cause vasoconstriction. Epinephrine also causes the "fight or flight" response—dilation of bronchioles and increased blood pressure, blood sugar, and heart rate. Pheochromocytoma, a tumor of the adrenal medulla, causes hypersecretion of catecholamines and results in characteristic sustained or paroxysmal hypertension.

The *testes* synthesize and secrete testosterone in response to gonadotropic hormones, especially LH, from the anterior pituitary gland; spermatogenesis occurs in response to FSH. The *ovaries* produce sex steroid hormones (primarily estrogen and progesterone) in response to anterior pituitary trophic hormones.

Chronic endocrine abnormalities are common health problems. For example, deficiencies of cortisol, thyroid hormone, or insulin require lifelong replacement of these hormones for survival. That fact places special demands on the health care professional. They include continually assessing the patient's condition, handling situations of acute illness, and teaching the patient.

PITUITARY DISORDERS

Hypopituitarism
(Panhypopituitarism and dwarfism)

Hypopituitarism is a complex syndrome marked by metabolic dysfunction, sexual immaturity, and growth retardation (when it occurs in childhood), resulting from a deficiency of the hormones secreted by the anterior pituitary gland. Panhypopituitarism refers to a generalized condition caused by partial or total failure of all six of this gland's vital hormones—ACTH, TSH, LH, FSH, HGH, and prolactin. However, deficiency of a single or all anterior pituitary hormones is quite rare. Hypopituitarism and panhypopituitarism occur in adults and children; in children, these diseases may cause dwarfism and pubertal delay. Prognosis may be good with adequate replacement therapy and correction of the underlying causes.

Causes

The most common cause of primary hypopituitarism is a lesion of the anterior pituitary gland, usually due an to intra- or extrasellar tumor. Other causes include congenital defects (hypoplasia or aplasia of the pituitary gland); pituitary infarction (most often from postpartum hemorrhage); or partial or total hypophysectomy by surgery, irradiation, or chemical agents; and rarely, granulomatous disease (tuberculosis, for example). Occasionally, hypopituitarism may have no identifiable cause. Secondary hypopituitarism stems from a deficiency of releasing hormones produced by the hypothalamus, a possible result of infection, trauma, or tumor.

Primary hypopituitarism usually develops in a predictable pattern of hormonal failures. It generally starts with hypogonadism or gonadotropin failure (decreased FSH and LH). In adults, it causes cessation of menses in women and impotence in men. Growth hormone deficiency follows; in children, this causes short stature, delayed growth, and failure to mature sexually at puberty. Subsequent failure of thyrotropin (decreased TSH) causes hypothyroidism; finally, adrenocorticotropic failure (decreased ACTH) results in adrenal insufficiency. However, when hypopituitarism follows surgical ablation or trauma, the pattern of hormonal events may not necessarily follow this sequence.

Occasionally, damage to the neurohypophysis from one of the above causes is extensive enough to cause diabetes insipidus.

Signs and symptoms

Clinical features of hypopituitarism usually develop slowly and vary greatly with the severity of the disorder and the number of deficient hormones. Symptoms of hypopituitarism in adults may include gonadal failure (secondary amenorrhea, impotence, infertility, decreased libido), diabetes insipidus, hypothyroidism (tiredness, lethargy, sensitivity to cold, menstrual disturbances), and adrenocortical insufficiency (hypoglycemia, anorexia, nausea, abdominal pain, hypotension). Postpartum necrosis of the pituitary (Sheehan's syndrome) characteristically causes failure of lactation, menstruation, and growth of pubic and axillary hair; symptoms of thyroid and adrenocortical failure; and diabetes insipidus.

In children, hypopituitarism causes retarded growth or delayed puberty. Dwarfism usually isn't apparent at birth, but early signs begin to appear during the first few months of life; by age 6 months, growth retardation is obvious. Although these children generally enjoy good health, pituitary dwarfism may cause chubbiness due to fat deposits in the lower trunk, delayed secondary tooth eruption, and possibly, hypoglycemia. Growth continues at less than half the normal rate—sometimes into the 20s or 30s—to an average height of 4′ (122 cm), with normal proportions.

When hypopituitarism strikes before puberty, it totally prevents development of secondary sexual characteristics (including facial and body hair). In males, it produces undersized testes, penis, and prostate gland; absent or minimal libido; and inability to initiate and maintain an erection. In females, it usually causes immature development of the breasts, sparse or absent pubic and axillary hair, and primary amenorrhea.

Panhypopituitarism may induce a host of mental and physiologic abnormalities, including lethargy, psychosis, orthostatic hypotension, bradycardia, anemia, and anorexia. However, clinical manifestations of hormonal deficiencies resulting from pituitary destruction don't become apparent until 75% of the gland is destroyed. Total loss of all hormones released by the anterior pituitary invariably proves fatal.

Neurologic signs associated with hypopituitarism and produced by pituitary tumors include headache, bilateral temporal hemianopia, loss of visual acuity, and possibly, blindness. Acute hypopituitarism resulting from surgery or infection is often associated with fever, hypotension, vomiting, and hypoglycemia—all characteristic of adrenal insufficiency.

Diagnosis

In persons with suspected hypopituitarism, diagnostic evaluation must confirm hormonal deficiency due to impairment or destruction of the anterior pituitary gland, and rule out disease of the target organs (adrenals, gonads, and thyroid) or the hypothalamus. Low serum levels of thyroxine (T_4), for example, indicate diminished thyroid gland function, but further tests are necessary to identify the source of this dysfunction as the thyroid, pituitary, or hypothalamus. Radioimmunoassay showing decreased plasma levels of some or all pituitary hormones (except ACTH, which requires more sophisticated testing), accompanied by end-organ hypofunction, suggests pituitary failure and eliminates target gland disease. Failure of TRH administration to increase TSH or prolactin concentrations rules out hypothalamic dysfunction as the cause of hormonal deficiency.

Provocative tests are helpful. To pinpoint the source of low hydroxycorticosteroid levels, P.O. administration of metyrapone blocks cortisol synthesis, which should stimulate pituitary secretion of ACTH. Insulin-induced hypoglycemia also stimulates ACTH secretion. Persistently low levels of ACTH, despite provocative testing, indicate pituitary or hypothalamic failure. These tests require careful medical supervision, because they may precipitate an adrenal crisis.

Diagnosis of dwarfism requires measurement of growth hormone levels in the blood after administration of regular insulin (inducing hypoglycemia) or levodopa (causing hypotension). These drugs should provoke increased secretion of growth hormone. Persistently low growth hormone levels, despite provocative testing, confirm growth hormone deficiency. CAT scan, pneumoencephalography, or cerebral angiography confirms the presence of intra- or extrasellar tumors.

Treatment

Replacement of hormones secreted by the target glands is the most effective treatment for hypopituitarism and panhypopituitarism. Hormonal replacement includes cortisol, thyroxine, and androgen or cyclic estrogen. Prolactin need not be replaced. The patient of reproductive age may benefit from administration of FSH and human chorionic gonadotropin (HCG) to boost fertility.

HGH, obtained from cadaver pituitaries, is effective for treating dwarfism and stimulates growth increases as great 4" to 6" (10 to 15 cm) in the first year of treatment. Growth rate tapers off in later years. After pubertal changes have occurred, the effects of HGH therapy are limited. (The National Pituitary Agency, which supplies HGH, currently withdraws treatment after the patient attains a height of 5' [152 cm].) Occasionally, a child becomes unresponsive to HGH therapy, even with larger doses, perhaps because of antibody formation against the hormone. In such refractory patients, small doses of androgen may again stimulate growth, but extreme caution is necessary to prevent premature closure of the epiphyses. Children with hypopituitarism may also need replacement of adrenal and thyroid hormones, and as they approach puberty, sex hormones.

Additional considerations

Caring for patients with hypopituitarism and panhypopituitarism requires an understanding of hormonal effects, and strong skills in offering physical and psychologic support. The health care professional should:
• keep track of the results of all laboratory tests for hormonal deficiencies and know what they mean; until replacement therapy is complete, check for signs of thyroid deficiency (increasing lethargy), adrenal deficiency (weakness, orthostatic hypotension, hypoglycemia, fatigue, and weight loss), and gonadotropin deficiency (decreased libido, lethargy, and apathy).
• watch for anorexia in the patient with panhypopituitarism; help plan a menu

containing favorite foods—ideally, high-calorie foods; monitor for weight loss or gain.

• encourage exercise during the day if the patient has trouble sleeping.

• record temperature, blood pressure, and heart rate every 4 to 8 hours; check eyelids, nailbeds, and skin for pallor, which indicates anemia.

• prevent infection by giving meticulous skin care; use oil or lotion instead of soap, since the patient's skin is probably dry; provide additional clothing and covers, as needed, to keep him warm, especially if body temperature is low.

• darken the room if the patient has a tumor that is causing headaches and visual disturbances; help with any activity that requires good vision, such as reading the menu; stand where he can be seen by the patient with bilateral hemianopia, and advise the family to do the same, since the patient may be able to see only out of the corners of his eyes.

• monitor closely during insulin testing for signs of hypoglycemia (initially, slow cerebration, tachycardia, and nervousness, progressing to convulsions); keep 50% dextrose in water available for I.V. administration to correct hypoglycemia rapidly.

• be sure to keep the patient supine during levodopa testing to prevent postural hypotension.

• instruct the patient to wear a medical identification bracelet; teach him to administer steroids parenterally in case of an emergency.

• refer the family of a child with dwarfism to appropriate community resources for psychologic counseling, since the emotional stress caused by this disorder increases as the child becomes more aware of his condition.

Hyperpituitarism
(Acromegaly and gigantism)

A chronic, progressive disease marked by hormonal dysfunction and startling skeletal overgrowth, hyperpituitarism appears in two forms: acromegaly occurs after epiphyseal closure, causing bone thickening, and transverse growth and visceromegaly; gigantism begins before epiphyseal closure and causes proportional overgrowth of all body tissues. Although prognosis depends on the causative factor, this disease usually reduces life expectancy.

Causes and incidence
In hyperpituitarism, oversecretion of HGH produces changes throughout the body, resulting in acromegaly and, when such oversecretion occurs before puberty, gigantism. Eosinophilic or mixed-cell adenomas of the anterior pituitary gland may cause this oversecretion, but the etiology of the tumors themselves remains unclear. Occasionally, hyperpituitarism occurs in more than one family member, suggesting a possible genetic cause.

In acromegaly, HGH oversecretion causes atrophy of skeletal muscle and formation of new bone and cartilage after epiphyseal closure. This form of hyperpituitarism is a rare disease of middle age and occurs equally among men and women, usually between ages 30 and 50.

In gigantism, proportional overgrowth of all body tissues starts before epiphyseal closure. This causes remarkable height increases of as much as 6″ (15 cm) a year. Gigantism affects infants and children, causing them to attain as much as three times the normal height for their age. As adults, they may ultimately reach a height of more than 80″ (203 cm).

Signs and symptoms
Acromegaly develops slowly, and typi-

cally produces diaphoresis, oily skin, hypermetabolism, and hypertrichosis. Severe headache, central and peripheral nervous system impairment, bitemporal hemianopia, loss of visual acuity, and blindness may result from the underlying intrasellar tumor.

Hypersecretion of HGH produces cartilaginous and connective tissue overgrowth, resulting in a characteristic hulking appearance, with an enlarged supraorbital ridge and thickened ears and nose. Prognathism becomes marked and may interfere with chewing. Laryngeal hypertrophy, paranasal sinus enlargement, and thickening of the tongue cause the voice to sound deep and hollow. Distal phalanges display an arrowhead appearance on X-rays, and the fingers are thickened. Irritability, hostility, and various psychologic disturbances may occur.

Prolonged effects of excessive HGH secretion include bowed legs, barrel chest, arthritis, osteoporosis, kyphosis, hypertension, and arteriosclerosis. Both gigantism and acromegaly may also cause signs of glucose intolerance and clinically apparent diabetes mellitus, due to the insulin-antagonistic character of HGH.

Gigantism develops abruptly, producing some of the same skeletal abnormalities seen in acromegaly. In infants, it may cause a highly arched palate, muscular hypotonia, slanting eyes, and exophthalmos. As the disease progresses, the pituitary tumor enlarges and invades normal tissue, resulting in the loss of other trophic hormones such as TSH, LH, FSH, and ACTH, which causes the target organ to stop functioning.

Diagnosis

Radioimmunoassay shows increased plasma HGH levels. However, since HGH is not secreted at a steady rate, a random sampling may be misleading. The glucose suppression test offers more reliable information. Glucose normally suppresses HGH secretion; therefore, a glucose infusion that fails to suppress the hormone level to below the accepted normal value of 5 ng, when combined with characteristic clinical features, strongly suggests hyperpituitarism.

In addition, skull X-rays, CAT scan, arteriography, and pneumoencephalography determine the presence and extent of the pituitary lesion. Bone X-rays showing a thickening of the cranium (especially of frontal, occipital, and parietal bones) and of the long bones, as well as osteoarthritis in the spine, support this diagnosis.

Treatment

The aim of treatment is to curb overproduction of HGH through removal of the underlying tumor by cranial or transsphenoidal hypophysectomy, or pituitary radiation therapy. In acromegaly, surgery is mandatory when a tumor causes blindness or other severe neurologic disturbances. Postoperative therapy often requires replacement of thyroid, cortisone, and gonadal hormones. Adjunctive treatment may include bromocriptine, which inhibits HGH synthesis.

Additional considerations

• Grotesque body changes characteristic of this disorder can cause severe psychologic stress. The patient will need emotional support to help him cope with an altered body image.

• Skeletal manifestations, such as arthritis of the hands and osteoarthritis of the spine, may require medications. Range-of-motion exercises will help promote maximum joint mobility.

• Patients, especially those with late-stage acromegaly, should be evaluated for muscular weakness. If the patient's handclasp is very weak, he may need help with such tasks as cutting food.

• Oily lotions should not be used, since the patient's skin is already oily.

• Urine should be tested for glucose, and the patient checked for signs of hyperglycemia (sweating, fatigue, polyuria, polydipsia).

• The tumor may cause visual problems. If the patient has hemianopia, visitors should stand where he can see them. This disease can also cause inexplicable mood changes. The family must understand that these changes result from the disease and can be modified with treatment.

• Before surgery, a health care professional should reinforce what the surgeon has told the patient, and try to allay the patient's fear with a clear and honest explanation of the scheduled operation. If the patient is a child, the parents should be told that such surgery prevents permanent soft-tissue deformities but won't correct bone changes that have already taken place. Counseling may be necessary to help the child and parents cope with these permanent defects.

• After surgery, the professional should diligently monitor vital signs and neurologic status and immediately report any alteration in level of consciousness, pupil equality, or visual acuity, as well as vomiting, falling pulse rate, or rising blood pressure. These changes may signal an increase in intracranial pressure due to intracranial bleeding.

• Blood sugar must be checked often, since HGH levels usually fall rapidly after surgery, removing an insulin-antagonist effect in many patients and possibly precipitating hypoglycemia. Intake and output should be measured hourly, and large increases reported. Transient diabetes insipidus, which sometimes occurs after surgery for hyperpituitarism, can cause such increases in urine output.

• If the transsphenoidal approach is used, a large nasal packing is kept in place for several days. Since the patient must breathe through his mouth, he will need good mouth care. Special attention should be paid to the mucous membranes—which usually become very dry—and the incision site under the upper lip, at the top of the gum line. The surgical site is packed with a piece of tissue generally taken from a midthigh donor site. The patient must be watched for increased external nasal drainage or drainage into the nasopharynx, which may be CSF leaking from the packed site. CSF leaks may necessitate additional surgery to repair the leak.

• The patient should walk around on the first or second day after surgery.

• Before discharge, the patient must understand the importance of continuing hormone replacement therapy, if ordered. He and his family should know which hormones are to be taken and why, as well as the correct times and dosages. The hormones must not be stopped suddenly.

• The patient should always wear a medical identification bracelet, and bring his hormone replacement schedule whenever he returns to the hospital.

• The patient should also have follow-up examinations at least once a year for the rest of his life, since a slight chance exists that the tumor which caused his hyperpituitarism may recur.

Diabetes Insipidus
(Pituitary diabetes insipidus)

Characterized by polyuria and excessive thirst, pituitary diabetes insipidus results from a deficiency of circulating vasopressin (also called ADH). This uncommon condition occurs equally among both sexes, usually between ages 10 and 20. Incidence is slightly higher today than in the past because of the increased use of hypophysectomy to treat breast cancer and other disorders. In uncomplicated diabetes insipidus, prognosis is good, even without treatment, and patients usually lead normal lives, with adequate water replacement. In cases complicated by an underlying disorder, such as breast cancer, prognosis varies. .

Causes
Primary diabetes insipidus (50% of patients) is familial or idiopathic in origin. Secondary diabetes insipidus results from

intracranial neoplastic or metastatic lesions, hypophysectomy or other neurosurgery, or head trauma—which damages the neurohypophyseal structures. It can also result from infection, granulomatous disease, and vascular lesions. (*Note:* Pituitary diabetes insipidus should not be confused with nephrogenic diabetes insipidus, a rare congenital disturbance of water metabolism that results from renal tubular resistance to vasopressin.)

Normally, the hypothalamus synthesizes vasopressin. The posterior pituitary gland (or neurohypophysis) stores vasopressin and releases it into general circulation, where it causes the kidneys to reabsorb water by making the distal and collecting tubule cells water-permeable. The absence of vasopressin in diabetes insipidus allows the filtered water to be excreted in the urine instead of being reabsorbed.

Signs and symptoms

Diabetes insipidus typically produces extreme polyuria (usually 4 to 16 liters/day of dilute urine, but sometimes as much as 30 liters/day). As a result, the patient is extremely thirsty and drinks great quantities of water to compensate for the body's water loss. This disorder may also result in slight to moderate nocturia and, in severe cases, extreme fatigue from inadequate rest caused by frequent voiding and excessive thirst. Other characteristic features of diabetes insipidus include signs of dehydration (poor tissue turgor, dry mucous membranes, constipation, muscle weakness, dizziness, and hypotension). These symptoms usually begin abruptly, commonly appearing within 1 to 2 days after basal skull fracture, cerebrovascular accident, or surgery. Relief of cerebral edema or intracranial pressure may cause all of these symptoms to subside just as rapidly as they began.

Diagnosis

Urinalysis reveals almost colorless urine of low osmolality (50 to 200 mOsm/kg, less than that of plasma) and low specific gravity (less than 1.005).

 However, diagnosis requires evidence of vasopressin deficiency, resulting in renal inability to concentrate urine during a water restriction test: After baseline vital signs, weight, and urine and plasma osmolalities are obtained, the patient is deprived of fluids and observed to make sure he doesn't drink anything surreptitiously. Hourly measurements record total volume of urine output, body weight, urine osmolality or specific gravity, and plasma osmolality. Blood pressure and pulse rate must be monitored for signs of postural hypotension. Fluid deprivation continues until the patient loses 3% of his body weight (indicating severe dehydration), or until severe postural hypotension occurs. This test may end sooner if no further rise in urine osmolality appears in three consecutive urine samples, and plasma osmolality is greater than normal (usually after 8 to 16 hours).

Hourly measurements of urine volume and specific gravity are continued after subcutaneous injection of 5 units of aqueous vasopressin. Patients with pituitary diabetes insipidus respond to vasopressin with decreased urine output and increased specific gravity. (Patients with nephrogenic diabetes insipidus show no response to vasopressin.)

Treatment

Until the cause of diabetes insipidus can be identified and eliminated, administration of various forms of vasopressin or of a vasopressin stimulant can control fluid balance and prevent dehydration:

• *vasopressin tannate:* an oil preparation administered I.M.; effective for 48 to 96 hours

• *vasopressin injection:* an aqueous preparation administered subcutaneously or I.M. several times a day, since effectiveness lasts only for 2 to 6 hours; often used in acute disease caused by trauma or surgery, for example

• *desmopressin:* nasal spray absorbed through the mucous membranes; effective up to 20 hours

• *lypressin:* short-acting nasal spray with significant disadvantages—variable dosage, nasal congestion and irritation, ulcerated nasal passages (with repeated use), substernal chest tightness, coughing, and dyspnea (after accidental inhalation of large doses)

• *chlorpropamide:* reduces the polyuria of diabetes insipidus by possibly releasing ADH or potentiating its effects.

Additional considerations

When caring for a patient with diabetes insipidus, the hospital staff member should:

• record fluid intake and output carefully; maintain fluid intake to prevent severe dehydration; watch for signs of hypovolemic shock, and monitor blood pressure, and heart and respiratory rates regularly, especially during the water deprivation test; check weight daily; keep the side rails up and assist the patient with walking if he is dizzy or has muscle weakness.

• monitor urine specific gravity between doses; watch for a decrease in specific gravity, with increasing urinary output, indicating the return of polyuria and necessitating administration of the next dose or a dosage increase.

• observe the patient receiving chlorpropamide for signs of hypoglycemia; tell the patient about possible drug side effects; make sure calorie intake is adequate; keep orange juice or another carbohydrate handy to treat hypoglycemic attacks; watch for decreasing urinary output and increasing specific gravity between doses; check laboratory values for hyponatremia and hypoglycemia.

• add more bulk foods and fruit juices to the diet if constipation develops; obtain an order for a mild laxative, such as milk of magnesia, if necessary; provide meticulous skin and mouth care; apply petrolatum, as needed, to cracked or sore lips.

• teach the patient before discharge how to monitor intake and output; instruct him to administer vasopressin I.M. or by nasal insufflation only after onset of polyuria—not before—to prevent excess fluid retention and water intoxication; tell him to report weight gain—it may mean dosage is too high (recurrence of polyuria, as reflected on the intake and output sheet, indicates dosage is too low); warn the patient never to administer vasopressin tannate while the suspension is cold, because of its viscosity; show him how to warm the vial in his hands and to rotate it gently to disperse the active particles throughout the oil.

• identify all patients with coronary artery disease—they need special periodic evaluations, since vasopressin constricts the arteries.

• advise the patient to wear a medical identification bracelet and to carry his medication with him at all times.

Hypothyroidism in Adults

Hypothyroidism, a state of low serum thyroid hormone, results from hypothalamic, pituitary, or thyroid insufficiency. Clinical effects range from mild fatigue and anorexia to life-threatening myxedema coma. Hypothyroidism is most prevalent in women; in the United States, incidence is rising significantly in persons aged 40 to 50.

Causes

Hypothyroidism results from inadequate production of thyroid hormone—usually because of dysfunction of the gland due to surgery (thyroidectomy), irradiation therapy (particularly ^{131}I), inflammation, chronic autoimmune thyroiditis (Hashimoto's disease), or inflammatory conditions, such as amyloidosis and sarcoidosis. It may also result from pituitary failure to produce TSH, hypothalamic failure to produce TRH, inborn errors of thyroid hormone synthesis, inability to synthesize the hormone because of iodine deficiency (usually dietary), or the use of antithyroid medications, such as propylthiouracil.

In patients with hypothyroidism, infection, exposure to cold, and sedatives may precipitate myxedema coma.

Signs and symptoms

Typically, the early clinical features of hypothyroidism are vague: fatigue, forgetfulness, sensitivity to cold, unexplained weight gain, and constipation. As the disorder progresses, characteristic myxedematous symptoms appear: decreasing mental stability; dry, flaky, inelastic skin; puffy face, hands, and feet; hoarseness; periorbital edema; upper eyelid droop; dry, sparse hair; and thick, brittle nails. Cardiovascular involvement leads to decreased cardiac output, slow pulse rate, signs of poor peripheral circulation, and occasionally, arteriosclerosis and cardiac enlargement. Other common clinical effects of hypothyroidism include anorexia, abdominal distention, menorrhagia, decreased libido, infertility, ataxia, intention tremor, and nystagmus. Reflexes show delayed relaxation time (especially in the Achilles tendon).

Progression to myxedema coma is usually gradual, but when stress aggravates severe or prolonged hypothyroidism, coma may develop abruptly. Signs of developing coma include progressive stupor, hypoventilation, hypoglycemia, hyponatremia, hypotension, and hypothermia.

Diagnosis

Radioimmunoassay confirms hypothyroidism with low T_3 and T_4 levels. Supportive laboratory findings include:
• increased TSH level with hypothyroidism due to thyroid insufficiency; decreased TSH level with hypothyroidism due to hypothalamic or pituitary insufficiency.
• elevated serum cholesterol, carotene, alkaline phosphatase, and triglycerides.

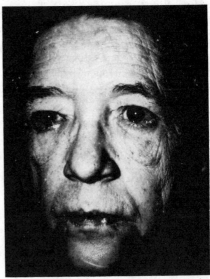

Characteristic myxedematous symptoms in adults include dry, flaky, inelastic skin; puffy face; and upper eyelid droop.

• normocytic normochromic anemia.

In myxedema coma, laboratory tests may also show low serum sodium, and decreased pH and increased PCO_2 in arterial blood gases, indicating respiratory acidosis.

Treatment

Therapy for hypothyroidism consists of gradual thyroid replacement with levothyroxine (T_4), liothyronine (T_3), liotrix, or thyroid USP (desiccated). During myxedema coma, effective treatment supports vital functions while restoring euthyroidism. To support blood pressure and pulse rate, treatment includes I.V. administration of levothyroxine and hydrocortisone to correct possible pituitary or adrenal insufficiency. Hypoventilation necessitates oxygenation and vigorous respiratory support (with ventilator, if necessary). Other supportive measures include careful fluid replacement, and antibiotics for infection.

Additional considerations

To manage the hypothyroid patient, the health care professional should:

- force fluids, provide a high-bulk, low-calorie diet, and encourage activity to combat constipation and promote weight loss; administer cathartics and stool softeners, as needed.
- watch for symptoms of hyperthyroidism (restlessness, nervousness, sweating, and excessive weight loss) after thyroid replacement therapy begins.
- tell the patient to report any signs of aggravated cardiovascular disease—chest pain, tachycardia.
- teach the patient on antithyroid medication to prevent myxedema coma by recognizing the clinical effects of hypothyroidism.
- warn the patient to report infection immediately and to make sure any doctor who prescribes drugs for him knows about the underlying hypothyroidism.

Treatment of myxedema coma requires meticulous and comprehensive supportive care. This includes:
- checking frequently for signs of decreasing cardiac output (such as falling urinary output).
- monitoring temperature frequently, until stable; providing extra blankets and clothing, and a warm room to compensate for hypothermia (rapid rewarming may cause vasodilation and vascular collapse).
- recording intake and output, and daily weight. As treatment begins, urinary output should increase and body weight decrease; if not, it must be reported.
- turning the edematous bedridden patient every 2 hours, and providing skin care, particularly around bony prominences, at least once a shift, to increase circulation and relieve dry, flaky skin.
- avoiding sedation when possible or reducing dosage, since hypothyroidism delays metabolism of many drugs.
- maintaining patent I.V. line; monitoring serum electrolytes carefully when administering I.V. fluids.
- monitoring vital signs carefully when administering levothyroxine, since rapid correction of hypothyroidism can cause adverse cardiac effects; reporting chest pain or tachycardia immediately; watching for hypertension and congestive heart failure in the elderly patient.
- checking arterial blood gases for indications of hypoxia and respiratory acidosis, and the need for ventilatory assistance.
- checking possible sources of infection, such as blood or urine, and obtaining sputum cultures. Myxedema coma can be precipitated by infection.

Hypothyroidism in Children
(Cretinism)

Deficiency of thyroid hormone secretion during fetal development or early infancy results in infantile cretinism (congenital hypothyroidism). Untreated hypothyroidism is characterized in infants by respiratory difficulties, persistent jaundice, and hoarse crying; in older children, by stunted growth (dwarfism), bone and muscle dystrophy, and mental deficiency. Cretinism occurs three times more often in girls than in boys. Early diagnosis and treatment allow the best prognosis; infants treated before age 3 months usually grow and develop normally. However, athyroid children who remain untreated beyond age 3 months, and children with acquired hypothyroidism who remain untreated beyond age 2 suffer irreversible mental retardation; their skeletal abnormalities are reversible with treatment.

Causes
In infants, cretinism usually results from defective embryonic development that causes congenital absence or underdevelopment of the thyroid gland, or from severe maternal iodine deficiency during pregnancy. Less frequently, it can be traced to an inherited enzymatic defect

in the synthesis of thyroxine (an iodine-containing hormone secreted by the thyroid gland), caused by an autosomal recessive gene. In children older than age 2, cretinism usually results from chronic autoimmune thyroiditis.

Signs and symptoms

At birth, the weight and length of an infant with infantile cretinism appear normal, but characteristic signs of hypothyroidism develop by the time he's 3 to 6 months old. An exception to this is the breast-fed infant, in whom onset of most symptoms may be delayed until weaning, because breast milk contains small amounts of thyroid hormone.

Typically, an infant with cretinism sleeps excessively, seldom cries (except for occasional hoarse crying), and is generally inactive. Because of this, his parents may describe him as a "good baby—no trouble at all." However, such behavior actually results from lowered metabolism and progressive mental impairment. The infant with cretinism also exhibits abnormal deep tendon reflexes, hypotonic abdominal muscles, a protruding abdomen, and slow, awkward movements. He has feeding difficulties, develops constipation, and because his immature liver can't conjugate bilirubin, becomes jaundiced.

His large, protruding tongue obstructs respiration, making breathing loud and noisy, and forcing him to open his mouth to breathe. He may have dyspnea on exertion, anemia, abnormal facial features—such as a short forehead; puffy, wide-set eyes (periorbital edema); wrinkled eyelids; a broad, short, upturned nose—and a dull expression, resulting from mental retardation. His skin is cold and mottled because of poor circulation, and his hair is dry, brittle, and dull. Teeth erupt late and tend to decay early; body temperature is below normal, and pulse rate is slow.

In the child who acquires hypothyroidism after age 2, appropriate treatment is likely to prevent mental retardation. However, growth retardation becomes apparent in short stature (due to delayed epiphyseal maturation, particularly in the legs), obesity, and a head that appears abnormally large because the arms and legs are stunted. An older child may show delayed or accelerated sexual development.

Diagnosis

A high serum level of TSH, associated with low T_3 and T_4 levels, points to cretinism. Since early detection and treatment can minimize the effects of cretinism, many states require measurement of infant thyroid hormone levels at birth.

Thyroid scan (^{131}I uptake test) shows decreased uptake levels and confirms the absence of thyroid tissue in athyroid children. Increased gonadotropin levels are compatible with sexual precocity in older children and may coexist with hypothyroidism. EKG shows bradycardia and flat or inverted T waves in untreated infants. Hip, knee, and thigh X-rays reveal absence of femoral or tibial epiphyseal line and delayed skeletal development markedly inappropriate for the child's chronologic age. A low T_4 level associated with a normal TSH level suggests hypothyroidism secondary to hypothalamic or pituitary disease, a rare condition.

Treatment

Early detection is mandatory to prevent irreversible mental retardation and permit normal physical development.

Treatment in infants younger than age 1 consists of replacement therapy with levothyroxine P.O., beginning with moderate doses. Dosage gradually increases to levels sufficient for lifelong maintenance. (Rapid increase in dosage may precipitate thyrotoxicity.) Doses are proportionately higher in children than in adults, because children metabolize thyroid hormone more quickly. Therapy in older children includes liothyronine and levothyroxine.

Additional considerations

Prevention, early detection, comprehensive parent teaching, and psychologic support are essential. The health care professional should know the early signs and be especially wary if parents emphasize how good their new baby is.

After cretinism is diagnosed, supportive care is necessary during hormonal replacement. The health care professional should:

• monitor blood pressure and pulse rate during early management of infantile cretinism; report hypertension and tachycardia immediately (normal infant heart rate is approximately 120 beats per minute); position the patient on his side if his tongue is unusually large and observe him frequently to prevent airway obstruction; check rectal temperature every 2 to 4 hours; keep the infant warm and his skin moist.

• inform parents that the child will require lifelong treatment with thyroid supplements; teach them to recognize signs of overdose—rapid pulse rate, irritability, insomnia, fever, sweating, and weight loss; stress the need to comply with treatment to prevent further mental impairment.

• provide the psychologic support parents need to deal with a child who may be mentally retarded; help them adopt a positive but realistic attitude and focus on their child's strengths rather than his weaknesses; encourage them to provide stimulating activities to help the child reach maximum potential; refer them to supportive community resources.

Infantile cretinism can be prevented during pregnancy with adequate nutrition, which includes iodine-rich foods and the use of iodized salt, or in case of sodium restriction, an iodine supplement.

Thyroiditis

Inflammation of the thyroid gland occurs as autoimmune thyroiditis (long-term inflammatory disease), subacute granulomatous thyroiditis (self-limiting inflammation), Riedel's thyroiditis (rare, invasive fibrotic process), and miscellaneous thyroiditis (acute suppurative, chronic infective, and chronic noninfective). Thyroiditis is more common in women than in men.

Causes
Although the causes of the four types of thyroiditis vary, all seem related to bacterial or viral infection, or the body's immune response to it.

Autoimmune thyroiditis is due to antibodies to thyroid antigens in the blood, as a result of a reaction within the thyroid gland. It may cause inflammation and lymphocytic infiltration (Hashimoto's thyroiditis). It can lead to Graves' disease, or glandular atrophy (myxedema), depending on the degree of lymphocytic infiltration and atrophy.

Subacute granulomatous thyroiditis usually follows mumps, influenza, or coxsackie- or adenoviral infection. *Riedel's thyroiditis* may be the result of an autoimmune or subacute process.

Miscellaneous thyroiditis results from bacterial invasion of the gland in suppurative thyroiditis; tuberculosis, syphilis, or actinomycosis in the chronic infective form; and sarcoidosis and amyloidosis in chronic noninfective thyroiditis.

Signs and symptoms
Autoimmune thyroiditis is usually asymptomatic and commonly occurs in women, with peak incidence in middle age. It's the most prevalent cause of spontaneous hypothyroidism.

In subacute granulomatous thyroiditis, moderate thyroid enlargement usually occurs 2 to 3 days after onset of fever, aching arms and legs, malaise, and other viral symptoms. The thyroid may be painful and tender, and dysphagia may occur.

In Riedel's thyroiditis, the gland enlarges suddenly, sometimes causing tracheal or esophageal compression. The thyroid feels firm.

Clinical effects of miscellaneous thyroiditis are characteristic of pyogenic infection: fever, pain, tenderness, and reddened skin over the gland.

Diagnosis
Precise diagnosis depends on the type of thyroiditis:
• *autoimmune:* positive precipitin test, high titers of thyroglobulin, microsomal antibodies present in serum
• *subacute granulomatous:* elevated ESR, increased thyroid hormone levels, decreased thyroidal radioiodine uptake
• *chronic infective and noninfective:* variance in findings, depending on underlying infection or other disease.

Treatment
Treatment varies with the type of thyroiditis. Drug therapy includes levothyroxine for accompanying hypothyroidism, analgesics and anti-inflammatory drugs for mild subacute granulomatous thyroiditis, propranolol for transient hyperthyroidism, and steroids for severe episodes of acute illness. Suppurative thyroiditis requires antibiotics. A partial thyroidectomy may be necessary to relieve compression in Riedel's thyroiditis.

Additional considerations
• Patient history will identify underlying diseases that may cause thyroiditis, such as tuberculosis or recent viral infection.

• Vital signs should be checked, and the patient's neck examined for unusual swelling, enlargement, or redness. A liquid diet should be used by the patient who has difficulty swallowing, especially when due to fibrosis. If the neck is swollen, the circumference must be measured and recorded daily to monitor progressive enlargement.
• Antibiotics may be given. Elevations in temperature, which may indicate developing resistance to the antibiotic, must be recorded and reported.
• The patient should watch for and report signs of hypothyroidism (lethargy, restlessness, sensitivity to cold, forgetfulness, or dry skin)—especially if he has Hashimoto's thyroiditis, which places him at risk. He should also watch for signs of hyperthyroidism (nervousness, tremor, weakness), which often occurs in subacute thyroiditis.
• After thyroidectomy, the hospital staff member should: check vital signs every 15 to 30 minutes until the patient's condition stabilizes; stay alert for signs of tetany secondary to accidental parathyroid injury during surgery; keep 10% calcium gluconate available for I.V. use; assess dressings frequently for excessive bleeding; watch for signs of airway obstruction, such as difficulty in talking or increased swallowing; keep tracheotomy equipment handy.
• The patient must know that lifelong thyroid hormone replacement therapy is necessary. He should watch for signs of overdosage, such as nervousness and palpitations.

Simple Goiter
(Nontoxic goiter)

Simple goiter, thyroid gland enlargement not caused by inflammation or a neoplasm, is commonly classified as endemic or sporadic. Endemic goiter usually results from geographically related nutritional factors, such as iodine-depleted soil or iodine deficiency that accompanies malnutrition. Areas in the United States where this deficiency is most common are called "goiter belts," and include the Midwest, the Northwest, and the Great Lakes region. Sporadic goiter follows ingestion of certain drugs or foods, and affects no particular segment of the population.

Simple goiter is found most frequently in females, especially during adolescence, pregnancy, and menopause. With treatment, prognosis is good.

Causes

Simple goiter occurs when the thyroid gland can't secrete enough thyroid hormone to meet metabolic requirements; as a result, the thyroid mass increases to compensate for inadequate hormone synthesis. Such compensation usually overcomes mild to moderate hormonal impairment. Since TSH levels are generally within normal limits in patients with simple goiter, goitrogenesis probably results from impaired intrathyroidal hormone synthesis and depletion of glandular iodine that increases the thyroid gland's sensitivity to TSH. However, increased levels of TSH may be transient and therefore missed. Endemic goiter is usually due to inadequate dietary intake of iodine, which leads to inadequate secretion of thyroid hormone. Iodized salt prevents this deficiency.

Sporadic goiter commonly results from ingestion of large amounts of goitrogenic foods or use of goitrogenic drugs. Goitrogenic foods contain agents that decrease thyroxine production, and include rutabagas, cabbage, soybeans, peanuts, peaches, peas, strawberries, spinach, and radishes. Goitrogenic drugs include propylthiouracil, iodides, phenylbutazone, para-aminosalicylic acid, cobalt, and lithium. In a pregnant woman, such substances may cross the placenta and affect the fetus.

Inherited defects may cause insufficient thyroxine synthesis or impaired iodine metabolism. Since families tend to congregate in one geographic area, this familial factor may contribute to endemic and sporadic goiters.

Signs and symptoms

Thyroid enlargement may range from a single, small nodule to massive, multinodular goiter. Because simple goiter doesn't alter the patient's metabolic state, clinical features arise solely from thyroid enlargement, and include respiratory distress and dysphagia from compression of the trachea and esophagus, and swelling and distention of the neck. In addition, large goiters may obstruct venous return, produce venous engorgement, and rarely, induce development of collateral venous circulation of the chest. Such obstruction may cause dizziness or syncope (Pemberton's sign) when the patient raises his arms above his head.

Diagnosis

Detailed patient history may reveal goitrogenic medications or foods, or endemic influence. Diagnostic laboratory tests include:
• *TSH or T_3 serum concentration:* high or normal
• *T_4 and PBI serum concentrations:* low-normal or normal
• *^{131}I uptake:* normal or increased (50% of the dose at 24 hours)
• *protein-bound iodine:* low or exceptionally high
• *urinary excretion of iodine:* low.

Diagnosis must rule out disorders with similar clinical effects: Graves' disease, Hashimoto's thyroiditis, and thyroid carcinoma.

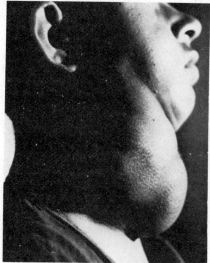

Massive multinodular goiter causes gross distention and swelling of the neck.

Treatment

The goal of treatment is to reduce thyroid hyperplasia. Exogenous thyroid hormone replacement with levothyroxine, desiccated thyroid, or liothyronine) is the treatment of choice; it inhibits TSH secretion and allows the gland to rest. Small doses of iodide (Lugol's or potassium iodide solution) are often effective in relieving goiter that results from iodine deficiency. Sporadic goiter requires avoidance of known goitrogenic drugs or food. A large goiter unresponsive to treatment may require subtotal thyroidectomy to relieve symptoms.

Additional considerations

• The patient must be watched for progressive thyroid gland enlargement and for hard nodules in the gland, which may indicate malignancy.

• To prevent insomnia, a side effect of thyroid hormone preparations, the patient should take the daily dose in the morning. Also, he should look for and report signs of thyrotoxicosis: increased pulse rate, palpitations, nausea, vomiting, diarrhea, sweating, tremors, agitation, and shortness of breath.

• The use of iodized salt is the most economic and effective way for the patient with endemic goiter to obtain the daily 150 to 300 mcg iodine necessary to prevent the disease.

• The patient taking goitrogenic drugs must be monitored for sporadic goiter.

Hyperthyroidism

(Graves' disease, Basedow's disease, Parry's disease, thyrotoxicosis)

Hyperthyroidism is a metabolic imbalance that results from thyroid hormone overproduction. The most common form of hyperthyroidism is Graves' disease, which increases thyroxine production, enlarges the thyroid gland (goiter), and causes multiple system changes. Incidence of Graves' disease is highest between ages 30 and 40, especially in persons with family histories of thyroid abnormalities; only 5% of hyperthyroid patients are younger than age 15. With treatment, most patients can lead normal lives. However, thyroid storm—an acute exacerbation of hyperthyroidism—is a medical emergency that may lead to life-threatening cardiac, hepatic, or renal failure.

Causes

Graves' disease may result from genetic and immunologic factors. Increased incidence in monozygotic twins, for example, points to an inherited factor, probably an autosomal recessive gene. This disease occasionally coexists with abnormal iodine metabolism and other endocrine abnormalities, such as diabetes mellitus, thyroiditis, and hyperparathyroidism. Graves' disease is also associated with production of autoantibodies (long-acting thyroid stimulator [LATS], LATS-protector, and human thyroid adenyl cyclase stimulator), possibly caused by a defect in suppressor T lymphocyte function that allows the formation of these autoantibodies.

In a person with latent hyperthyroidism, excessive dietary intake of iodine and, possibly, stress can precipitate clinical hyperthyroidism. Similarly, in a person with untreated or inadequately treated hyperthyroidism, stressful conditions—including surgery, infection, toxemia of pregnancy, and diabetic ketoacidosis—can precipitate thyroid storm.

Signs and symptoms

The classic symptoms of Graves' disease are an enlarged thyroid (goiter), nervousness, heat intolerance, weight loss despite increased appetite, sweating, diarrhea, tremor, and palpitations. Ex-

OTHER FORMS OF HYPERTHYROIDISM

• *Toxic adenoma*—a small, benign nodule in the thyroid gland that secretes thyroid hormone—is the second most common cause of hyperthyroidism. The cause of toxic adenoma is unknown; incidence is highest in the elderly. Clinical effects are essentially similar to those of Graves' disease, except that toxic adenoma doesn't induce ophthalmopathy, pretibial myxedema, or acropachy. Presence of adenoma is confirmed by radioactive iodine (131I) uptake and thyroid scan, which show a single hyperfunctioning nodule suppressing the rest of the gland. Treatment includes 131I therapy, or surgery to remove adenoma after antithyroid drugs achieve a euthyroid state.

• *Thyrotoxicosis factitia* results from chronic ingestion of thyroid hormone for thyrotropin suppression in patients with thyroid carcinoma, or from thyroid hormone abuse by persons who are trying to lose weight.

• *Functioning metastatic thyroid carcinoma* is a rare disease that causes excess production of thyroid hormone.

• *TSH-secreting pituitary tumor* causes overproduction of thyroid hormone.

• *Subacute thyroiditis* is a virus-induced granulomatous inflammation of the thyroid, producing transient hyperthyroidism associated with fever, pain, pharyngitis, and tenderness in the thyroid gland.

• *Silent thyroiditis* is a self-limiting, transient form of hyperthyroidism, with histologic thyroiditis but no inflammatory symptoms.

ophthalmos is considered most characteristic but is absent in many patients with hyperthyroidism. Many other symptoms are common, as hyperthyroidism profoundly affects virtually every body system:

• *CNS:* difficulty in concentrating because increased thyroxine secretion accelerates cerebral function; excitability or nervousness due to increased basal metabolic rate (BMR); fine tremor, shaky handwriting, and clumsiness from increased activity in the spinal cord area that controls muscle tone; emotional instability and mood swings, ranging from occasional outbursts to overt psychosis

• *Skin, hair, and nails:* smooth, warm, flushed skin (patient sleeps with minimal covers and little clothing); fine, soft hair; premature graying and increased hair loss in both sexes; friable nails and onycholysis (distal nail separated from the bed); pretibial myxedema (dermopathy), producing thickened skin, accentuated hair follicles, raised red patches of skin that are itchy and sometimes painful, with occasional nodule formation. Microscopic examination shows increased mucin deposits.

• *Cardiovascular system:* tachycardia; full, bounding pulse; wide pulse pressure; cardiomegaly; increased cardiac output and blood volume; visible point of maximal impulse (PMI); paroxysmal supraventricular tachycardia and atrial fibrillation (especially in the elderly); and occasionally, systolic murmur at the left sternal border

• *Respiratory system:* dyspnea on exertion and at rest, possibly from cardiac decompensation and increased cellular oxygen utilization

• *Gastrointestinal system:* possible anorexia; nausea and vomiting due to increased gastrointestinal mobility and peristalsis; increased defecation; soft stools or, with severe disease, diarrhea; and liver enlargement

• *Musculoskeletal system:* weakness, fatigue, and muscle atrophy; rare coexistence with myasthenia gravis; generalized or localized paralysis associated with hypokalemia may occur; and occasional acropachy—soft-tissue swelling, accompanied by underlying bone changes where new bone formation occurs.

• *Reproductive system:* in females, oligomenorrhea or amenorrhea, decreased fertility, higher incidence of spontaneous abortions; in males, gynecomastia due to increased estrogen levels; in both sexes, diminished libido

• *Eyes:* exophthalmos (produced by the combined effects of accumulation of mucopolysaccharides and fluids in the retroorbital tissues that force the eyeball outward, and of lid retraction that produces the characteristic staring gaze); occasional inflammation of conjunctivas, corneas, or eye muscles; diplopia; and increased tearing.

When hyperthyroidism escalates to thyroid storm, these symptoms can be accompanied by extreme irritability, hypertension, tachycardia, vomiting, temperature up to 106° F. (41.1° C.), delirium, and coma.

Diagnosis

Patient history and physical examination suggest hyperthyroidism. The following laboratory tests confirm it:

• *Radioimmunoassay* showing increased serum T_4 and T_3 concentrations confirms the diagnosis.

• *Thyroid scan* reveals increased uptake of ^{131}I.

• *Thyroid suppression test* determines whether the pituitary controls the thyroid gland. Following administration of thyroid hormone, uptake value must be less than 50% of pretest measurement to show suppression and rule out hyperthyroidism.

• *Thyroid-releasing hormone (TRH) stimulation test* indicates hyperthyroidism if thyroid-stimulating hormone (TSH) level fails to rise within 30 minutes after administration of TRH.

• *BMR* is elevated in hyperthyroidism, but this test has largely been superseded by the more reliable and efficient measurements of T_3 and T_4.

Other supportive test results show increased serum protein-bound iodine (PBI), and decreased serum cholesterol and total lipids. Ultrasonography confirms subclinical ophthalmopathy.

Treatment

The primary forms of treatment for hyperthyroidism are antithyroid drugs, ^{131}I, and surgery. Appropriate treatment depends on the size of the goiter, the patient's age and parity, and how long surgery will be delayed (if the patient is a candidate for it).

Antithyroid drug therapy is used for children, young adults, pregnant women, and patients who refuse surgery or ^{131}I treatment. Thyroid hormone antagonists include propylthiouracil (PTU) and methimazole, which block thyroid hormone synthesis. Although hypermetabolic symptoms subside from 4 to 8 weeks after such therapy begins, the patient must continue taking the medication for 6 months to 2 years. In many patients, particularly pregnant women, concomitant propranolol is used to manage tachycardia and other peripheral effects of excessive hypersympathetic activity.

During pregnancy, antithyroid medication should be kept at the minimum dosage required to keep maternal thyroid function normal until delivery and to minimize the risk of fetal hypothyroidism—even though most infants of hyperthyroid mothers are born with mild and transient hyperthyroidism. (Neonatal hyperthyroidism may even necessitate treatment with antithyroid drugs and propranolol for 2 to 3 months.) Because exacerbation of hyperthyroidism sometimes occurs in the puerperium, continuous control of maternal thyroid function is essential. Approximately 3 to 6 months postpartum, antithyroid drugs can be gradually tapered down and thyroid function reassessed (drugs may be discontinued at that time). Throughout antithyroid treatment, the mother should not breast-feed, as this may cause neonatal hypothyroidism.

Another major form of therapy for hyperthyroidism is a single P.O. dose of ^{131}I—the treatment of choice for patients not planning to have children. (Patients of reproductive age must give informed consent for this treatment, since small amounts of ^{131}I concentrate in the gonads.) During treatment with ^{131}I, the thyroid gland picks up the radioactive element as it would regular iodine. Subsequently, the radioactivity destroys some of the cells that normally concentrate iodine and produce thyroxine, thus decreasing thyroid hormone production and normalizing thyroid size and function. In most patients, hypermetabolic symptoms diminish from 6 to 8 weeks after such treatment. However, some patients, especially those with thyroid-stimulating antibodies, may require a second dose.

Subtotal (partial) thyroidectomy is indicated for the patient younger than age 40 who has a very large goiter, and whose hyperthyroidism has repeatedly relapsed after drug therapy. Thyroidectomy removes part of the thyroid gland, thus decreasing its size and capacity for hormone production. Preoperatively, the patient should receive iodides (Lugol's solution or saturated solution of potassium iodide) or an antithyroid drug for 10 days to 3 weeks, until thyroid function becomes normal. If euthyroidism is not achieved, surgery should be delayed and propranolol administered to decrease the systemic effects (cardiac arrhythmias) caused by hyperthyroidism.

After ablative treatment with ^{131}I or surgery, patients require regular, frequent medical supervision for the rest of their lives, because they usually develop hypothyroidism, sometimes as long as several years after treatment.

Therapy for hyperthyroid ophthalmopathy includes local applications of topical medications but may require high doses of corticosteroids, given systemically or, in severe cases, injected into the retrobulbar area. Severe exophthalmos that causes pressure on the optic nerve may require surgical decompression to lessen pressure on the orbital contents.

Treatment of thyroid storm includes administration of an antithyroid drug such as PTU, propranolol I.V. to block sympathetic effects, and an iodide to block release of thyroid hormone. Supportive measures include nutrients, vitamins, fluid administration, and sedation, as necessary.

Additional considerations

Patients with hyperthyroidism require vigilant care to prevent acute exacerbations and complications. This includes:
• recording vital signs and weight; monitoring serum electrolytes, and checking periodically for hyperglycemia and glycosuria; carefully monitoring cardiac function if the patient is elderly or has coronary artery disease; checking blood pressure and pulse rate often if the cardiac rate is more than 100 beats per minute; checking level of consciousness and urinary output; telling a patient who is pregnant to watch closely during the first trimester for signs of spontaneous abortion (spotting, occasional mild cramps) and to report such signs immediately.
• encouraging bed rest, and keeping the patient's room cool, quiet and dark. The patient with dyspnea will be most comfortable sitting upright or in high Fowler's position.
• remembering that extreme nervousness may produce bizarre behavior, and reassuring the patient and family that such behavior subsides with treatment; providing sedatives, as necessary.
• providing a balanced diet, with six meals a day, to promote weight gain; suggesting a low-sodium diet for the patient with edema.
• mixing iodide, if applicable, with milk to prevent gastrointestinal distress, and administering it through a straw to prevent tooth discoloration.
• watching for signs of thyroid storm (tachycardia, hyperkinesis, fever, vomiting, hypertension); checking intake and output carefully to ensure adequate hydration and fluid balance; closely monitoring blood pressure, cardiac rate and rhythm, and temperature; reducing high fever with appropriate hypothermic measures (sponging, hypothermia blankets, and acetaminophen; aspirin should be avoided because it raises thyroxine levels); maintaining an I.V. line and giving drugs, as ordered.
• suggesting sunglasses or eyepatches for the patient with exophthalmos or other ophthalmopathy to protect his eyes from light; moistening the conjunctivas often with isotonic eyedrops; warning the patient with severe lid retraction to avoid sudden physical movements that might cause the lid to slip behind the eyeball.

Thyroidectomy necessitates meticulous postoperative care to prevent com-

plications. The hospital staff member should:
- check often for respiratory distress, and keep a tracheotomy tray at bedside.
- watch for evidence of hemorrhage into the neck, such as a tight dressing with no blood on it; change dressings and perform wound care, as ordered; check the *back* of the dressing for drainage; keep the patient in semi-Fowler's position, and support his head and neck with sandbags to ease tension on the incision.
- check for dysphagia or hoarseness from possible laryngeal nerve injury.
- watch for signs of hypoparathyroidism (tetany, numbness), a complication that results from accidental removal of the parathyroid glands during surgery.
- stress the importance of regular medical follow-up after discharge, since hypothyroidism may develop from 2 to 4 weeks postoperatively.

Drug therapy and ^{131}I therapy require careful monitoring and comprehensive patient teaching.
- After ^{131}I therapy, the patient should not expectorate or cough freely, because his saliva is radioactive for 24 hours. The need for repeated measurement of serum thyroxine levels must be stressed. The patient must not resume antithyroid drug therapy.
- The patient taking PTU and methimazole must get CBC monitoring periodically to detect leukopenia, thrombocytopenia, and agranulocytosis. The patient should take these medications with meals to minimize gastrointestinal distress and must avoid over-the-counter cough preparations because many contain iodine. He should watch for and report fever, enlarged cervical lymph nodes, sore throat, mouth sores, and other signs of blood dyscrasia, and any rash or skin eruptions— signs of hypersensitivity.
- The patient taking propranolol must be watched for signs of hypotension (dizziness, decreased urinary output). Rising slowly after sitting or lying down will prevent orthostatic syncope.
- The patient taking antithyroid drugs or ^{131}I therapy should report any symptoms of hypothyroidism.

Hypoparathyroidism

Hypoparathyroidism is a deficiency of parathyroid hormone (PTH) from disease, injury, or congenital malfunction of the parathyroid glands. Since the parathyroid glands primarily regulate calcium balance, hypoparathyroidism causes hypocalcemia, producing neuromuscular symptoms ranging from paresthesia to tetany. The clinical effects of hypoparathyroidism are usually correctable with replacement therapy. However, some complications of this disorder, such as cataracts and basal ganglion calcifications, are irreversible.

Causes and incidence
Hypoparathyroidism may be acute or chronic and is classified as idiopathic, acquired, or reversible.

Idiopathic hypoparathyroidism may result from an autoimmune genetic disorder or the congenital absence of the parathyroid glands. *Acquired hypoparathyroidism* often results from accidental removal of or injury to one or more parathyroid glands during thyroidectomy or other neck surgery or, rarely, from massive thyroid irradiation. It may also result from ischemic infarction of the parathyroids during surgery, or from hemochromatosis, sarcoidosis, amyloidosis, tuberculosis, neoplasms, or trauma. An *acquired, reversible hypoparathyroidism* may result from hypomagnesemia-induced impairment of hormone synthesis, from suppression of normal gland function due to hypercalcemia, or from delayed maturation of parathyroid function.

PTH normally maintains blood calcium levels by increasing bone resorption and gastrointestinal absorption of calcium. It also maintains an inverse relationship between serum calcium and phosphate levels by inhibiting phosphate reabsorption in the renal tubules. Abnormal PTH production in hypoparathyroidism disrupts this delicate balance.

Incidence of the idiopathic and reversible forms is highest in children; that of the irreversible acquired form in older patients who have undergone surgery for hyperthyroidism.

Signs and symptoms

Although mild hypoparathyroidism may be asymptomatic, it usually produces hypocalcemia and high serum phosphate levels that affect the CNS and other body systems. Chronic hypoparathyroidism produces neuromuscular irritability, increased deep tendon reflexes, Chvostek's sign (hyperirritability of the facial nerve when tapped), dysphagia, organic brain syndrome, psychosis, mental deficiency in children, and tetany.

Acute (overt) tetany begins with a tingling in the fingertips, around the mouth, and occasionally, in the feet. This tingling spreads and becomes more severe, producing muscle tension and spasms, and consequent adduction of the thumbs, wrists, and elbows. Pain varies with the degree of muscle tension but rarely affects the face, legs, and feet. Chronic tetany is usually unilateral and less severe; it may cause difficulty in walking and a tendency to fall. Both forms of tetany can lead to laryngospasm, stridor, and eventually, cyanosis. They may also cause elementary partial, absence, or tonoclonic seizures. These CNS abnormalities tend to be exaggerated during hyperventilation, pregnancy, infection, withdrawal of thyroid hormone, and administration of diuretics; and before menstruation.

Other effects of hypoparathyroidism include abdominal pain; dry, lusterless hair; spontaneous hair loss; brittle fingernails that develop ridges or fall out; dry, scaly skin; cataracts; and weakened tooth enamel, which causes teeth to stain, crack, and decay easily. Hypocalcemia may induce cardiac arrhythmias and may eventually lead to congestive heart failure.

Diagnosis

The following test results confirm the presence of hypoparathyroidism:

• *radioimmunoassay for parathyroid hormone:* decreased

• *serum calcium levels:* decreased

• *serum phosphorus:* increased (more than 5.4 mg/100 ml)

• *qualitative urinary calcium (Sulkowitch) test:* decreased urine calcium levels (in 70% of patients)

• *X-rays:* increased bone density

• *EKG:* increased Q-T and S-T intervals due to hypocalcemia.

The following test may provoke clinical evidence of hypoparathyroidism: inflating a blood pressure cuff on the upper arm to above systolic blood pressure elicits Trousseau's sign (tetany and, finally, a typical attack of carpal spasm).

Treatment

Treatment initially includes vitamin D, with or without supplemental calcium. Such therapy is usually lifelong, except in patients with the reversible form of the disease. If the patient can't tolerate the pure form of vitamin D, alternatives include dihydrotachysterol if renal function is adequate, and calcitriol if renal function is severely compromised.

Acute life-threatening tetany calls for immediate I.V. administration of calcium gluconate to raise serum calcium levels. If the patient is awake and able to cooperate, he can help raise ionized serum calcium levels by breathing into a paper bag and then inhaling his own CO_2; this produces hypoventilation and mild respiratory acidosis. Sedatives and anticonvulsants may control spasms until calcium levels rise. Chronic tetany calls for maintenance of serum calcium levels with oral calcium supplements.

Additional considerations

• A patient with suspected hypoparathyroidism and a history of tetany will need a patent I.V. line maintained and calcium I.V. available. Because the patient is vulnerable to convulsions, seizure precautions should be taken. Also, a tracheotomy tray and endotracheal tube must be kept at bedside, since laryngospasm may result from hypocalcemia.

• For the patient with tetany, a 10% calcium gluconate slow I.V. (1 mg/minute) should be given and a patent airway maintained. Such a patient may also require intubation, and sedation with diazepam I.V. Vital signs must be monitored often after administration of diazepam I.V. to make certain blood pressure and heart rate return to normal.

• The patient should follow a high-calcium, low-phosphorus diet, and must know which foods are permitted.

• A patient with chronic disease, particularly a child, must be watched for minor muscle twitching (especially in the hands) and for signs of laryngospasm (respiratory stridor or dysphagia), since these effects may signal onset of tetany.

• The patient on drug therapy must understand the importance of having serum calcium levels checked at least three times a year. Also, he should watch for signs of hypercalcemia and keep his medications away from light.

• Because the patient with chronic disease has prolonged Q-T intervals on an EKG, he must be watched for heart block and signs of decreasing cardiac output. The patient receiving both digitalis and calcium must be watched closely, since calcium potentiates the effect of digitalis, and must be checked for signs of digitalis toxicity.

• The patient with scaly skin can use creams to soften his skin. He should keep his nails trimmed to prevent them from splitting.

Hyperparathyroidism

Hyperparathyroidism is characterized by overactivity of one or more of the four parathyroid glands, resulting in excessive secretion of parathyroid hormone (PTH). Such hypersecretion of PTH promotes bone resorption and leads to hypercalcemia and hypophosphatemia. In turn, increased renal and gastrointestinal absorption of calcium occurs.

Causes

Hyperparathyroidism may be primary or secondary. In primary hyperparathyroidism, one or more of the parathyroid glands enlarges, increasing PTH secretion and elevating serum calcium levels. The most common cause is a single adenoma. Other causes include a genetic disorder or other multiple endocrine disorders, such as Wermer's syndrome (tumors of the parathyroid, pituitary, and pancreatic islet cells) and Sipple's syndrome (pheochromocytoma, and parathyroid and medullary thyroid cancer). Primary hyperparathyroidism usually occurs between ages 30 and 50 but can also occur in children and the elderly. It affects women two to three times more frequently than men.

In secondary hyperparathyroidism, excessive compensatory production of PTH stems from a hypocalcemia-producing abnormality outside the parathyroid gland, which causes a resistance to the metabolic action of PTH. Some hypocalcemia-producing abnormalities are rickets, vitamin D deficiency, chronic renal failure, or osteomalacia due to phenytoin or laxative abuse.

Signs and symptoms

Clinical effects of primary hyperparathyroidism result from hypercalcemia and are present in several body systems:

• *Renal:* nephrocalcinosis due to elevated levels of calcium and phosphorus;

possibly, recurring nephrolithiasis, which may lead to renal insufficiency. Renal manifestations are the most common effects of hyperparathyroidism.

• *Skeletal and articular:* chronic low back pain and easy fracturing due to generalized osteoporosis; bone tenderness; chondrocalcinosis; occasional severe osteopenia, especially on the vertebrae; erosions of the juxta-articular surface; subchondral fractures; traumatic synovitis; and pseudogout

• *Gastrointestinal:* pancreatitis, causing constant, severe epigastric pain radiating to the back; peptic ulcers, causing abdominal pain, hematemesis, nausea, and vomiting

• *Neuromuscular:* marked muscle weakness and atrophy, particularly in the legs

• *CNS:* psychomotor and personality disturbances, depression, overt psychosis, stupor, coma

• *Other:* skin necrosis, cataracts, calcium microthrombi to lungs and pancreas, positive Trousseau's or Chvostek's sign, and subcutaneous calcification.

Similarly, in secondary hyperparathyroidism, decreased serum calcium levels may produce the same features of calcium imbalance, with skeletal deformities of the long bones (rickets, for example), as well as symptoms of the underlying disease.

Diagnosis

In primary disease, a high concentration of serum PTH on radioimmunoassay, with accompanying hypercalcemia, confirms the diagnosis. X-rays show diffuse demineralization of bones, bone cysts, outer cortical bone absorption, and subperiosteal erosion of the radial aspect of the middle fingers. Microscopic examination of the bone with tests such as X-ray spectrophotometry demonstrates increased bone turnover. Laboratory tests reveal elevated urine and serum calcium, chloride, and alkaline phosphatase levels, and decreased serum phosphorus.

Hyperparathyroidism may also raise uric acid and creatinine levels, and increase basal acid secretion and serum immunoreactive gastrin. Increased serum amylase levels may indicate acute pancreatitis.

Laboratory findings in secondary hyperparathyroidism show normal or slightly decreased serum calcium levels and variable serum phosphorus levels, especially when hyperparathyroidism is due to rickets, osteomalacia, or renal disease. Patient history may reveal familial renal disease, convulsive disorders, or drug ingestion. Other laboratory values and physical examination identify the cause of secondary hyperparathyroidism.

Treatment

Treatment varies, depending on the cause of the disease. Treatment for primary hyperparathyroidism may include surgery to remove the adenoma or, depending on the extent of hyperplasia, all but half of one gland (necessary to maintain normal PTH levels). Such surgery may relieve bone pain within 3 days. However, renal damage may be irreversible. Preoperatively—or if surgery isn't feasible or necessary—other treatments can decrease calcium levels: forcing fluids; limiting dietary intake of calcium; promoting sodium and calcium excretion through forced diuresis, using normal saline solution (up to 6 liters in life-threatening circumstances), furosemide, or ethacrynic acid; and administering sodium or potassium phosphate P.O., calcitonin, or mithramycin.

Therapy for potential postoperative magnesium and phosphate deficiencies includes I.V. administration of magnesium and phosphate, or sodium phosphate solution given P.O. or by retention enema. Also, during the first 4 or 5 days after surgery, when serum calcium falls to low normal levels, supplemental calcium may be necessary; vitamin D or calcitriol may also be beneficial.

Treatment of secondary hyperparathyroidism must correct the underlying cause of parathyroid hypertrophy, and includes vitamin D therapy or, in the patient with renal disease, aluminum hydroxide for hyperphosphatemia. In the patient with renal failure, peritoneal dialysis therapy is necessary to lower calcium levels and may have to continue for life. In the patient with chronic secondary hyperparathyroidism, the enlarged glands may not revert to normal size and function even after calcium levels have been controlled.

Additional considerations
Care emphasizes prevention of complications from the underlying disease and its treatment. The hospital staff member should:

• obtain pretreatment baseline serum potassium, calcium, phosphate, and magnesium levels, since these values may change abruptly during treatment.

• record intake and output accurately during hydration to reduce serum calcium level; strain urine to check for stones; provide at least 3 liters of fluid a day, including cranberry or prune juice; obtain blood and urine samples, as ordered, to measure sodium, potassium, and magnesium levels, especially for the patient taking furosemide.

• auscultate for lung sounds often; listen for signs of pulmonary edema in the patient receiving large amounts of saline solution I.V., especially if he has pulmonary or cardiac disease; monitor the patient on digitalis carefully, since elevated calcium levels can rapidly produce toxic effects.

• assist with walking, keep the bed at its lowest position, and raise the side rails since the patient is predisposed to pathologic fractures; lift the immobilized patient carefully to minimize bone stress, and check X-rays to determine which bones are weakest; schedule care to allow the patient with muscle weakness as much rest as possible.

• watch for signs of peptic ulcer, and administer antacids, as appropriate.

After parathyroidectomy, the staffer should:

• check frequently for respiratory distress, and keep a tracheotomy tray at

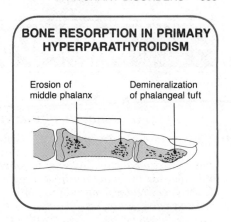

BONE RESORPTION IN PRIMARY HYPERPARATHYROIDISM

Erosion of middle phalanx

Demineralization of phalangeal tuft

bedside; watch for postoperative complications, such as renal colic, acute psychosis, laryngeal nerve damage, or rarely, hemorrhage; monitor intake and output carefully.

• check for swelling at the operative site, place the patient in semi-Fowler's position, and support his head and neck with sandbags to decrease edema, which may cause pressure on the trachea.

• watch for signs of mild tetany, such as complaints of tingling in the hands and around the mouth (these symptoms should subside quickly but may be prodromal signs of tetany, so calcium gluconate I.V. must be available for emergency administration); watch for increased neuromuscular irritability and other signs of severe tetany, and report them immediately; ambulate the patient as soon as possible postoperatively, even though he may find this uncomfortable, since pressure on bones speeds up bone recalcification.

• check laboratory results for low serum calcium and magnesium levels.

• monitor mental status, and watch for listlessness; check for muscle weakness and signs of psychosis in the patient with persistent hypercalcemia.

• advise the patient before discharge of the possible side effects of drug therapy; emphasize the need for periodic follow-up through laboratory blood tests; warn the patient to avoid calcium-containing antacids and thiazide diuretics if hyperparathyroidism was not corrected surgically.

ADRENAL DISORDERS

Adrenal Hypofunction
(Adrenal insufficiency, Addison's disease)

Primary adrenal hypofunction (Addison's disease) originates within the adrenal gland itself, and is characterized by decreased mineralocorticoid, glucocorticoid, and androgen secretion. Adrenal hypofunction can also occur secondary to a disorder outside the gland (such as pituitary tumor, with ACTH deficiency), but aldosterone secretion frequently continues intact. A relatively uncommon disorder, Addison's disease can occur at any age and in both sexes; incidence of secondary adrenal hypofunction is rising with the increasing use of steroid therapy. With early diagnosis and adequate replacement therapy, prognosis for adrenal hypofunction is good.

Adrenal crisis (Addisonian crisis), a critical deficiency of mineralocorticoids and glucocorticoids, generally follows acute stress in septic patients and in persons with chronic adrenal insufficiency. A medical emergency, adrenal crisis necessitates immediate, vigorous treatment.

Causes

Addison's disease occurs when more than 90% of the adrenal gland is destroyed. Such massive destruction usually results from an autoimmune process in which circulating antibodies react specifically against the adrenal tissue. Other causes include tuberculosis (once the chief cause but incidence is now less than 30%), bilateral adrenalectomy, hemorrhage into the adrenal gland, neoplasms, and fungal infections, such as histoplasmosis. Rarely, a familial tendency to autoimmune disease predisposes to Addison's disease as well as to other endocrinopathies.

Secondary adrenal hypofunction that results in glucocorticoid deficiency can stem from hypopituitarism (causing decreased ACTH secretion), abrupt withdrawal of long-term corticosteroid therapy, or removal of a nonendocrine, ACTH-secreting tumor (long-term exogenous corticosteroid stimulation suppresses pituitary ACTH secretion and results in adrenal gland atrophy). Adrenal crisis follows when trauma, surgery, or other physiologic stress (such as infection) exhausts the body's stores of glucocorticoids in a person with adrenal hypofunction.

Signs and symptoms

Addison's disease typically produces weakness, fatigue, weight loss, and various gastrointestinal disturbances, such as nausea, vomiting, anorexia, and chronic diarrhea. Addison's disease also causes a conspicuous bronze coloration of the skin. The patient appears to be deeply suntanned, especially on the creases of the hands and over the metacarpophalangeal joints, the elbows, and the knees. He shows a darkening of scars, areas of vitiligo (absence of pigmentation), and increased pigmentation on the mucous membranes, usually the buccal mucosa. Such abnormal skin and mucous membrane coloration results from decreased secretion of cortisol (one of the glucocorticoids), which causes the pituitary gland to simultaneously secrete excessive amounts of ACTH and melanocyte-stimulating hormone (MSH).

Associated cardiovascular abnormalities in Addison's disease include postural hypotension, decreased cardiac size and output, and a weak, irregular pulse. Other clinical effects include decreased tolerance for even minor stress, poor co-

SYMPTOMS OF CUSHINGOID SYNDROME

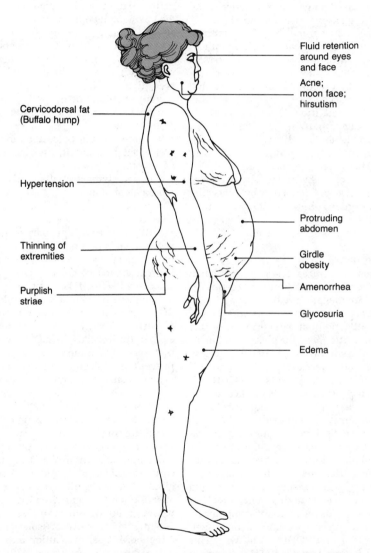

Cervicodorsal fat
(Buffalo hump)

Hypertension

Thinning of
extremities

Purplish
striae

Fluid retention
around eyes
and face

Acne;
moon face;
hirsutism

Protruding
abdomen

Girdle
obesity

Amenorrhea

Glycosuria

Edema

Long-term treatment with corticosteroids may produce a side effect called
cushingoid syndrome—a condition marked by obvious fat deposits between the
shoulders and around the waist, and widespread systemic abnormalities.

In addition to the symptoms shown in the illustration, other symptoms include
renal disorders, hyperglycemia, tissue wasting, muscular weakness, and labile
emotional state.

ordination, fasting hypoglycemia (due to decreased glyconeogenesis), and a craving for salty food. Addison's disease may also retard axillary and pubic hair growth in females, decrease libido (due to decreased androgen production), and in severe cases, cause amenorrhea.

Secondary adrenal hypofunction produces similar clinical effects but without hyperpigmentation, since ACTH and MSH levels are low. Because aldosterone secretion may continue at fairly normal levels in secondary adrenal hypofunction, this condition does not necessarily cause accompanying hypotension and electrolyte abnormalities.

Adrenal crisis produces profound weakness, fatigue, nausea, vomiting, hypotension, dehydration, and occasionally, high fever followed by hypothermia. If untreated, this condition can ultimately cause vascular collapse, renal shutdown, coma, and death.

Diagnosis

Diagnosis requires the demonstration of decreased concentrations of corticosteroids in the plasma or urine, and an accurate determination as to whether adrenal hypofunction is primary or secondary. After baseline plasma and urine steroid testing (24-hour urine collection for 17-ketosteroids [17-KS] and 17-hydroxycorticosteroids [17-OHCS]), special provocative tests are necessary.

The *metyrapone test* requires P.O. or I.V. administration of metyrapone, which blocks cortisol production and should stimulate the release of ACTH from the hypothalamic-pituitary system. In Addison's disease, the hypothalamic-pituitary system responds normally, and plasma reveals high levels of ACTH; however, plasma levels of compound S (cortisol precursor) and urinary concentration of 17-OHCS don't rise. This test is followed by the *ACTH stimulation test,* which involves I.V. administration of ACTH over 6 to 8 hours, after samples have been obtained to determine baseline plasma cortisol and 24-hour urine cortisol levels. In Addison's disease, plasma and urine cortisol levels fail to rise normally in response to ACTH; in secondary disease, repeated doses of ACTH over successive days produce a gradual increase in cortisol levels, until normal values are reached.

In a patient with typical symptoms, the following laboratory findings strongly suggest acute adrenal insufficiency:
• decreased cortisol levels in plasma (less than 10 mcg/dl in the morning, with lower levels in the evening). However, this test is time-consuming, and therapy shouldn't be delayed for results.
• decreased serum sodium and fasting blood sugar
• increased serum potassium and BUN
• elevated hematocrit, and lymphocyte and eosinophil counts
• X-rays showing a small heart, and adrenal calcification.

Treatment

For all patients with primary or secondary adrenal hypofunction, corticosteroid replacement, usually with cortisone or hydrocortisone (both also have mineralocorticoid effect), is the primary treatment and must continue for life. Addison's disease may also necessitate desoxycorticosterone I.M., a pure mineralocorticoid, or fludrocortisone P.O., a synthetic that acts as a mineralocorticoid; both prevent dangerous dehydration and hypotension. Women with Addison's disease who have muscle weakness and decreased libido may benefit from testosterone injections but risk unfortunate masculinizing effects.

Adrenal crisis requires prompt I.V. bolus administration of 100 mg hydrocortisone. Later, 50 to 100 mg doses are given I.M., or are diluted with dextrose in saline solution and given I.V. until the patient's condition stabilizes; up to 300 mg/day of hydrocortisone and 3 to 5 liters of I.V. saline solution may be required during the acute stage. With proper treatment, the crisis usually subsides quickly; blood pressure should stabilize, and water and sodium levels return to normal. After the crisis, maintenance doses of hydrocortisone preserve physiologic stability.

Additional considerations

• In adrenal crisis, vital signs must be monitored carefully, especially for hypotension, volume depletion, and other signs of shock (decreased level of consciousness and urinary output). The patient must be watched for hyperkalemia before treatment and for hypokalemia after treatment (from excessive mineralocorticoid effect).

• If the patient also has diabetes, blood sugar should be checked periodically, since steroid replacement may require adjusting of insulin dosage.

• Weight, and intake and output must be recorded carefully, since the patient may have volume depletion. Until onset of mineralocorticoid effect, fluids should be forced to replace excessive fluid loss.

To manage the patient receiving maintenance therapy, the health care professional should:

• arrange for a diet that maintains sodium and potassium balances.

• suggest six small meals a day to increase calorie intake if the patient is anorectic; provide a diet high in protein and carbohydrates; keep a late-morning snack available in case the patient becomes hypoglycemic.

• observe the patient receiving steroids for cushingoid signs, such as fluid retention around the eyes and face; watch for fluid and electrolyte imbalance, especially if the patient is receiving mineralocorticoids; monitor weight, and check blood pressure to assess body fluid status; remember that steroids administered in the late afternoon or evening may stimulate the CNS and cause insomnia in some patients; check for petechiae, since the patient bruises easily.

• watch for and report facial hair growth and other signs of masculinization in women receiving testosterone injections; adjust dosage, if necessary.

• observe for orthostatic hypotension or electrolyte abnormalities if the patient receives glucocorticoids alone since they may indicate a need for mineralocorticoid therapy.

• explain that lifelong steroid therapy is necessary; advise him of symptoms of over- and underdosage; tell him that dosage may need to be increased during times of stress (when he has a cold, for example); warn that infection, injury, or profuse sweating in hot weather may precipitate adrenal crisis.

• instruct the patient to always carry a medical identification card stating that he takes a steroid and giving the name of the drug and the dosage; teach the patient how to give himself an injection of hydrocortisone and tell him to keep an emergency kit available containing hydrocortisone in a prepared syringe for use in times of stress; warn that any stress may necessitate additional cortisone to prevent a crisis.

Cushing's Syndrome

Cushing's syndrome is a cluster of clinical abnormalities due to excessive levels of adrenocortical hormones (particularly cortisol) or related corticosteroids and, to a lesser extent, androgens and aldosterone. Its unmistakable signs include rapidly developing adiposity of the face (moon face), neck, and trunk, and purple striae on the skin. Cushing's syndrome is most common in females. Prognosis depends on the underlying cause; it is poor in untreated persons and in those with untreatable ectopic ACTH-producing carcinoma or metastatic adrenal carcinoma.

Causes

In approximately 70% of patients, Cushing's syndrome results from excess production of ACTH and consequent hyperplasia of the adrenal cortex. Overproduction of ACTH may stem from pituitary hypersecretion (Cushing's disease), an ACTH-producing tumor in another organ (particularly broncho-genic or pancreatic carcinoma), or administration of synthetic glucocorti-coids or ACTH. In the remaining 30% of patients, Cushing's syndrome results from a cortisol-secreting adrenal tumor, which is usually benign. In infants, the usual cause of Cushing's syndrome is adrenal carcinoma.

Signs and symptoms

Like other endocrine disorders, Cush-ing's syndrome induces changes in mul-tiple body systems, depending on the adrenocortical hormone involved:
• *Endocrine and metabolic systems:* "steroid diabetes," with decreased glu-cose tolerance, fasting hyperglycemia, and glucosuria
• *Musculoskeletal system:* muscle weak-ness due to hypokalemia or to loss of muscle mass from increased catabolism, pathologic fractures due to decreased bone mineral, skeletal growth retarda-tion in children
• *Skin:* striae (stretch marks); fat pads above the clavicles, over the upper back (buffalo hump), on the face (moon face), and throughout the trunk (truncal obe-sity, with slender arms and legs); little or no scar formation; poor wound heal-ing; acne and hirsutism in women
• *Gastrointestinal system:* peptic ulcer, resulting from increased gastric secre-tions and pepsin production, and de-creased gastric mucus
• *CNS:* irritability and emotional labil-ity, ranging from euphoric behavior to depression or psychosis; insomnia
• *Cardiovascular system:* hypertension due to sodium and water retention; left ventricular hypertrophy; capillary weakness due to protein loss, which leads to bleeding, petechiae, and ecchy-mosis
• *Immunologic system:* increased sus-ceptibility to infection due to decreased lymphocyte production and suppressed antibody formation; decreased resis-tance to stress. Suppressed inflammatory response may mask even a severe infec-tion.
• *Renal system:* sodium and secondary

fluid retention; increased potassium ex-cretion; inhibited ADH secretion; ure-teral calculi from increased bone demineralization, with hypercalciuria
• *Reproductive system:* increased an-drogen production, causing gynecomas-tia in males, and clitoral hypertrophy, mild virilism, and amenorrhea or oli-gomenorrhea in females.

Diagnosis

Initially, diagnosis of Cushing's syn-drome requires determination of plasma and urine steroid levels. In normal per-sons, plasma cortisol levels are elevated in the morning and decrease gradually through the day (diurnal variation). In patients with Cushing's syndrome, cor-tisol levels do not fluctuate, and remain consistently elevated; 24-hour urine sample demonstrates elevated free cor-tisol levels. Elevated 17-ketogenic steroid (17-KGS) or 17-hydroxycorticosteroid (17-OHCS)—both metabolites of adrenal hormones—suggests adrenal hyperac-tivity; elevated 17-KGS helps estimate the amount of urinary androgens present, and elevated 17-OHCS indicates primary or secondary hyperadrenalism.

 A low-dose dexamethasone suppression test confirms the diagnosis of Cushing's syn-drome. A high-dose dexa-methasone suppression test can determine if Cushing's syndrome results from pituitary dysfunction (Cushing's disease). In this test, dexa-methasone suppresses plasma cortisol levels, and urinary 17-OHCS and 17-KGS fall to 50% or less of basal levels. Failure to suppress these levels indicates that the syndrome results from an adrenal tumor or a nonendocrine, ACTH-secreting tu-mor. This test can produce false positive results.

In a stimulation test, administration of metyrapone, which blocks cortisol production by the adrenal glands, tests the ability of the pituitary gland and the hypothalamus to detect and correct low levels of plasma cortisol by increasing ACTH production. The patient with Cushing's disease reacts to this stimulus by secreting an excess of plasma ACTH as measured by levels of urinary compound S or 17-OHCS. If the patient has an adrenal or a nonendocrine, ACTH-secreting tumor, the pituitary gland—which is suppressed by the high cortisol levels—cannot respond normally, so steroid levels remain stable or fall.

Ultrasound, CAT scan, or angiography localizes adrenal tumors; CAT scan of the head identifies pituitary tumors.

Treatment

Management to restore hormone balance and reverse Cushing's syndrome may necessitate radiation or drug therapy, or surgery. For example, pituitary-dependent Cushing's syndrome with adrenal hyperplasia and severe cushingoid symptoms—such as psychosis, poorly controlled steroid diabetes, osteoporosis, and severe pathologic fractures—may require bilateral adrenalectomy, hypophysectomy, or pituitary irradiation. Nonendocrine, ACTH-producing tumors require excision of the tumor, followed by drug therapy (mitotane, metyrapone, or the experimental drug aminoglutethimide) to decrease cortisol levels if cushingoid symptoms persist.

Aminoglutethimide and cyproheptadine (another experimental drug used to treat Cushing's disease) decrease cortisol levels and have been beneficial for many cushingoid patients. Aminoglutethimide alone, or in combination with metyrapone, may also be useful in metastatic adrenal carcinoma.

Before surgery, the patient with cushingoid symptoms needs special management to control hypertension, edema, diabetes, and cardiovascular manifestations, and prevent infection. Glucocorticoid administration on the morning of surgery can help prevent acute adrenal insufficiency during surgery. Cortisol is essential during and after surgery, to help the patient tolerate the physiologic stress imposed by removal of the pituitary or adrenals. If normal cortisol production resumes, steroid therapy may be gradually tapered and eventually discontinued. However, bilateral adrenal-

ectomy or total hypophysectomy mandates lifelong steroid replacement therapy to correct hormonal deficiencies. Patients with pituitary-dependent Cushing's disease may develop Nelson's syndrome (pituitary chromophobe adenoma) after bilateral adrenalectomy.

Additional considerations

Patients with Cushing's syndrome require painstaking assessment and vigorous supportive care. This includes:

• frequently monitoring vital signs, especially blood pressure; carefully observing the hypertensive patient who also has cardiac disease.

• checking laboratory reports for hypernatremia, hypokalemia, hyperglycemia, and glycosuria.

• checking for edema, and monitoring daily weight, and intake and output carefully because the cushingoid patient is likely to retain sodium and water; providing a diet that is high in protein and potassium but low in calories, carbohydrates and sodium to minimize weight gain, edema, and hypertension.

• watching for infection—a particular problem in Cushing's syndrome.

• carefully performing passive range-of-motion exercises if the patient has osteoporosis and is bedridden.

• remembering that Cushing's syndrome produces emotional lability; recording incidents that upset the patient, and preventing such situations, if possible; helping him get the physical and mental rest he needs—by sedation, if necessary; offering support to the emotionally labile patient throughout the difficult testing period.

After bilateral adrenalectomy and pituitary surgery, the hospital staff member should:

• report wound drainage or temperature elevation immediately; use strict aseptic technique in changing dressings.

• administer analgesics and replacement steroids, as ordered.

• monitor urinary output, and check vital signs carefully, watching for signs of shock (decreased blood pressure, increased pulse rate, pallor, and cold, clammy skin); give vasopressors and increase the rate of I.V. fluids, as ordered, to counteract shock; assess neurologic and behavioral status, and warn the patient of CNS side effects because mitotane, aminoglutethimide, and metyrapone decrease mental alertness and produce physical weakness; watch for severe nausea, vomiting, and diarrhea.

• check laboratory reports for hypoglycemia due to removal of the source of cortisol, a hormone that maintains blood glucose levels.

• check for abdominal distention and return of bowel sounds following adrenalectomy.

• check regularly for signs of adrenal hypofunction—orthostatic hypotension, apathy, weakness, fatigue—indicators that steroid replacement is inadequate.

• check for and immediately report signs of increased intracranial pressure (confusion, agitation, changes in level of consciousness, nausea, and vomiting) in the patient undergoing pituitary surgery; watch for hypopituitarism.

The patient will need comprehensive teaching to cope with lifelong treatment. This includes:

• advising the patient to take replacement steroids with antacids or meals to minimize gastric irritation. (He should be encouraged to take two thirds of the dosage in the morning and the remaining third in the early afternoon to mimic diurnal adrenal secretion.)

• telling the patient to carry a medical identification card and to immediately report physiologically stressful situations, such as infections, which necessitate increased dosage.

• instructing the patient to watch closely for signs of inadequate steroid dosage (fatigue, weakness, dizziness) and of overdosage (severe edema, weight gain); emphatically warning against discontinuing steroid dosage, because this may produce a fatal adrenal crisis.

Hyperaldosteronism

In hyperaldosteronism, hypersecretion of the mineralocorticoid aldosterone by the adrenal cortex causes excessive reabsorption of sodium and water, and excessive renal excretion of potassium.

Causes and incidence

Hyperaldosteronism may be primary or secondary. Primary hyperaldosteronism (Conn's syndrome) is uncommon; in 70% of patients, it results from a benign aldosterone-producing adrenal adenoma. Incidence is three times higher in women than in men, and is highest between ages 30 and 50. In 15% to 30% of patients with primary hyperaldosteronism, the cause is unknown; rarely, the cause is adrenocortical hyperplasia (in children) or carcinoma.

In primary hyperaldosteronism, chronic aldosterone excess is independent of the renin-angiotensin system and, in fact, it suppresses plasma renin activity. This aldosterone excess enhances sodium reabsorption by the kidneys, which leads to hypernatremia and, simultaneously, hypokalemia and increased extracellular fluid volume. Expansion of intravascular fluid volume also occurs and results in volume-dependent hypertension and increased cardiac output.

Ingestion of an excessive amount of licorice or licoricelike substances can produce a syndrome similar to primary hyperaldosteronism, due to the mineralocorticoid activity of glycyrrhizic acid.

Secondary hyperaldosteronism results from extra-adrenal pathology, which stimulates the adrenal gland to increase production of aldosterone. For example, conditions that reduce renal blood flow (renal artery stenosis) and extracellular fluid volume or produce a sodium deficit activate the renin-angiotensin system and, subsequently, increase aldosterone secretion. Thus, secondary hyperaldosteronism may result from conditions that induce hypertension through increased renin production (such as Wilms' tumor), ingestion of oral contraceptives, and pregnancy.

However, secondary hyperaldosteronism may also result from disorders unrelated to hypertension. Such disorders may or may not cause edema. For example, nephrotic syndrome, hepatic cirrhosis with ascites, and congestive heart failure commonly induce edema; Bartter's syndrome and salt-losing nephritis do not.

Signs and symptoms

Most clinical effects of hyperaldosteronism result from hypokalemia, which increases neuromuscular irritability and produces muscular weakness; intermittent, flaccid paralysis; fatigue; headaches; paresthesia; and possibly, tetany, as a result of metabolic alkalosis, which can lead to hypocalcemia. Diabetes mellitus is common, perhaps because hypokalemia interferes with normal insulin secretion. Hypertension and its accompanying complications are also common. Other characteristic signs include visual disturbances and loss of renal concentrating ability, producing nocturnal polyuria and polydipsia. Azotemia and bacilluria indicate chronic potassium depletion nephropathy.

Diagnosis

Persistently low serum potassium levels in a nonedematous patient who isn't taking diuretics, doesn't have obvious gastrointestinal losses (from vomiting or diarrhea), and has a normal sodium intake suggest hyperaldosteronism. If hypokalemia develops in a hypertensive patient shortly after starting treatment with potassium-wasting diuretics (such as thiazides), and it persists after the diuretic has been discontinued and potassium replacement therapy has been instituted, evaluation for hyperaldosteronism is necessary.

 Low plasma renin level after volume depletion by diuretic administration and upright posture, and a high plasma aldosterone level after volume expansion by salt loading confirm primary (Conn's) hyperaldosteronism in a hypertensive patient without edema.

Serum bicarbonate level is often elevated, with ensuing alkalosis due to hydrogen and potassium ion loss in the distal renal tubules. Other tests show markedly increased urinary aldosterone levels, increased plasma aldosterone levels, and in secondary hyperaldosteronism, increased plasma renin levels.

A suppression test is useful to differentiate between primary and secondary hyperaldosteronism. During this test, the patient receives desoxycorticosterone P.O. for 3 days, while plasma aldosterone levels and urinary metabolites are continuously measured. These levels decrease in secondary hyperaldosteronism but remain the same in primary (Conn's). Simultaneously, renin levels are low in primary hyperaldosteronism and high in secondary hyperaldosteronism.

Other helpful diagnostic evidence includes an increase in plasma volume of 30% to 50% above normal, EKG signs of hypokalemia (ST segment depression and U waves), chest X-ray showing left ventricular hypertrophy from chronic hypertension, and localization of tumor by adrenal angiography or CAT scan.

Treatment

Although treatment for primary hyperaldosteronism may include unilateral adrenalectomy, administration of a potassium-sparing diuretic—spironolactone—and sodium restriction may control hyperaldosteronism without surgery. Bilateral adrenalectomy reduces blood pressure for most patients with idiopathic primary hyperaldosteronism. However, some degree of hypertension persists in most patients, even after surgery, necessitating treatment with spironolactone or other antihypertensive therapy. Such patients also require lifelong adrenal hormone replacement.

Treatment of secondary hyperaldosteronism must include correction of the underlying cause.

Additional considerations

• Urinary output, blood pressure, weight, and serum potassium levels of the patient must be monitored and recorded.

• The patient must be watched for signs of tetany (muscle twitching, Chvostek's sign) and for hypokalemia-induced cardiac arrhythmias, paresthesia, or weakness. Potassium replacement, as ordered, should be given and calcium gluconate

I.V. kept available.

• The patient should follow a low-sodium, high-potassium diet.

• After adrenalectomy, the patient must be watched for weakness, hyponatremia, rising serum potassium levels, and adrenal insufficiency, especially hypotension.

• If the patient is taking spironolactone, he should watch for signs of hyperkalemia. Impotence and gynecomastia may follow long-term use.

• The patient taking steroid hormone replacement should wear a medical alert bracelet.

Adrenogenital Syndrome

Adrenogenital syndrome results from disorders of adrenocortical steroid biosynthesis. This syndrome may be inherited (congenital adrenal hyperplasia [CAH]) or acquired, usually as a result of an adrenal tumor (adrenal virilism). Salt-losing CAH may cause fatal adrenal crisis in newborns.

Causes and incidence

CAH is the most prevalent adrenal disorder in infants and children; simple virilizing CAH and salt-losing CAH are the most common forms. Adrenal virilism is rare.

CAH is transmitted as an autosomal recessive trait that causes deficiencies in enzymes needed for adrenocortical secretion of cortisol and, possibly, aldosterone. Compensatory secretion of ACTH produces varying degrees of adrenal hyperplasia. In simple virilizing CAH, deficiency of the enzyme 21-hydroxylase results in underproduction of cortisol. In turn, this cortisol deficiency stimulates increased secretion of ACTH, producing large amounts of cortisol precursors and androgens that do not require 21-hydroxylase for synthesis. In salt-losing CAH, 21-hydroxylase is almost completely absent. ACTH secretion increases, causing excessive production of cortisol precursors, including salt-wasting compounds. However, plasma cortisol levels and aldosterone—both dependent on 21-hydroxylase—fall precipitously and, in combination with the

excessive production of salt-wasting compounds, precipitate acute adrenal crisis. ACTH hypersecretion stimulates adrenal androgens, possibly even more than in simple virilizing CAH, and produces masculinization.

Other rare CAH enzyme deficiencies (such as 17-hydroxylase deficiency) exist and lead to increased or decreased production of affected hormones.

Signs and symptoms

The newborn female with simple virilizing CAH has ambiguous genitalia (enlarged clitoris, with urethral opening at the base; some labioscrotal fusion) but normal genital tract and gonads. As she grows older, signs of progressive virilization develop: early appearance of pubic and axillary hair, deep voice, acne, and facial hair. The newborn male with this condition has no obvious abnormality; however, at prepuberty he shows accentuated masculine characteristics, such as deepened voice, and an enlarged phallus, with frequent erections. At puberty, females fail to begin menstruation, and males have small testes. Both males and females with this condition may be taller than other children their age due to rapid bone and muscle growth, but since excessive androgen levels hasten epiphyseal closure, abnormally short adult stature results.

Salt-losing CAH in females causes more complete virilization than the simple form and results in development of male external genitalia without testes. Since males with this condition have no external genital abnormalities, immediate neonatal diagnosis is difficult, and is commonly delayed until the infant develops severe systemic symptoms. Characteristically, such an infant is apathetic, fails to eat, and has diarrhea; he develops symptoms of adrenal crisis in the first week of life (vomiting, dehydration from hyponatremia, hyperkalemia). Unless this condition is treated promptly, dehydration and hyperkalemia may lead to cardiovascular collapse and cardiac arrest.

Diagnosis

Physical examination revealing pseudohermaphroditism in females, or precocious puberty in both sexes strongly suggests CAH.

 The following laboratory findings confirm the diagnosis: elevated urinary 17-ketosteroids (17-KS), which can be suppressed by administering dexamethasone P.O.; elevated urinary metabolites of hormones, particularly pregnanetriol; elevated plasma 17-hydroxyprogesterone; and normal or decreased urinary levels of 17-hydroxycorticosteroids.

Symptoms of adrenal hypofunction or adrenal crisis in the first week of life strongly suggest salt-losing CAH. Hyperkalemia, hyponatremia, and hypochloremia in the presence of excessive urinary 17-KS and pregnanetriol, and decreased urinary aldosterone confirm it.

Treatment

Simple virilizing CAH requires correction of the cortisol deficiency and inhibition of excessive pituitary ACTH production by daily administration of

ACQUIRED ADRENAL VIRILISM

Acquired adrenal virilism results from virilizing adrenal tumors, carcinomas, or adenomas. This rare disorder is twice as common in females as it is in males. Although acquired adrenal virilism can develop at any age, its clinical effects vary with the patient's age at onset:

- *prepubescent girls:* pubic hair, clitoral enlargement; at puberty, no breast development, menses delayed or absent
- *prepubescent boys:* hirsutism, macrogenitosomia precox (excessive body development, with marked enlargement of genitalia). Occasionally, the penis and prostate equal those of an adult male in size; however, testicular maturation fails to occur.
- *women (especially middle-aged):* dark hair on legs, arms, chest, back, and face; pubic hair extending toward navel; oily skin, sometimes with acne; menstrual irregularities; muscular hypertrophy (masculine resemblance); male pattern balding; and atrophy of breasts and uterus
- *men:* no overt signs; discovery of tumor usually accidental
- *all patients:* good muscular development; taller than average during childhood and adolescence; short stature as adults due to early closure of epiphyses.

Diagnostic tests:
- *urinary total 17-ketosteroids (17-KS):* greatly elevated, but levels vary daily; dexamethasone P.O. doesn't suppress 17-KS.
- *plasma levels of dehydroepiandrosterone (DHA):* greatly elevated
- *serum electrolytes:* normal
- *X-ray of kidneys:* may show downward displacement of kidneys by tumor.

Treatment requires surgical excision of tumor and metastases (if present), when possible, or radiation therapy and chemotherapy. Preoperative treatment may include glucocorticoids. With treatment, prognosis is very good in patients with slow-growing and nonrecurring tumors. Periodic follow-up urine testing (for increased 17-KS) to check for possible tumor recurrence is essential.

HERMAPHRODITISM

True hermaphroditism (hermaphrodism, intersexuality) is a rare condition characterized by both ovarian and testicular tissues. External genitalia are usually ambiguous but may be completely male or female, and thus can mask hermaphroditism until puberty. The hermaphrodite almost always has a uterus (fertility is rare) and ambiguous gonads distributed:
• *bilaterally:* testis and ovary on both sides, ovatestes
• *unilaterally:* ovary or testis on one side; an ovatestis opposite
• *asymmetrically or laterally:* an ovary and a testis on opposite sides.

Since the Y chromosome is needed to develop testicular tissue, hermaphroditism in infants with XX karyotypes is particularly perplexing but may possibly result from mosaicism (XX/XY, XX/XXY), hidden mosaicism, or hidden gene alterations. In patients with XX karyotype, ovaries are usually better developed than in those with XY karyotype. Fifty percent of hermaphrodites have 46,XX karyotype, 20% have XY, and 30% are mosaics.

Although ambiguous external genitalia suggest hermaphroditism, chromosomal studies (particularly a buccal smear for Barr bodies, indicating an XX karyotype), a 24-hour urine specimen for 17-ketosteroids to rule out congenital adrenal hyperplasia, and gonadal biopsy are necessary to confirm it.

Sexual assignment, based on the anatomy of the external genitalia, and prognosis for most successful plastic reconstruction should be made as early as possible to prevent physical and psychologic consequences of delayed reassignment. During such surgery, inappropriate reproductive organs are removed to prevent incongruous secondary sex characteristics at puberty. Hormonal replacement may be necessary.

Parents of the young hermaphrodite who is being treated surgically will need psychologic support and reinforcement of their choice of sexual assignment for their child.

cortisone or hydrocortisone. Such treatment returns androgen production to normal levels. Measurement of urinary 17-KS determines the initial dose of cortisone or hydrocortisone; this dose is usually large and is given I.M. Later dosage is modified according to decreasing urinary 17-KS levels. Infants must continue to receive cortisone or hydrocortisone I.M. until age 18 months; after that, they may take it P.O.

The infant with salt-losing CAH in adrenal crisis requires immediate I.V. sodium chloride and glucose infusion to maintain fluid and electrolyte balance and stabilize vital signs. If saline and glucose infusion doesn't control symptoms while diagnosis is being established, desoxycorticosterone I.M. and, occasionally, hydrocortisone I.V. are necessary. Later, maintenance includes mineralocorticoid (desoxycorticosterone) and glucocorticoid (cortisone or hydrocortisone) replacement.

Sex chromatin and karyotype studies determine the genetic sex of patients with ambiguous external genitalia. Females with masculine external genitalia require reconstructive surgery, such as correction of the labial fusion and of the urogenital sinus. Such surgery is usually scheduled between ages 1 and 3, after the effect of cortisone therapy has been assessed.

Additional considerations
• CAH should be suspected in infants hospitalized for failure to thrive, dehydration, or diarrhea, as well as in tall, sturdy-looking children with a record of numerous episodic illnesses.
• When caring for an infant with adrenal crisis, the hospital staff member should: keep the I.V. line patent, infuse fluids, and give steroids, as ordered; monitor body weight, blood pressure, and serum electrolytes carefully, especially sodium and potassium levels; watch for cyanosis, hypotension, tachycardia, tachypnea, and signs of shock; keep external stress to a minimum.
• If the child is receiving maintenance therapy with steroid injections, I.M. in-

jection sites should be rotated to prevent atrophy; parents should do the same. They should know the possible side effects (cushingoid symptoms) of long-term therapy. Maintenance therapy with hydrocortisone, cortisone, or implanted desoxycorticosterone pellets is essential for life. Parents must not withdraw these drugs suddenly, since potentially fatal adrenal insufficiency will result. Parents should report stress and infection, which require increased steroid dosages.

• The patient receiving desoxycorticosterone should be monitored for edema, weakness, and hypertension. He must be watched for significant weight gain and rapid changes in height, since normal growth is an important indicator of adequate therapy.

• The patient should wear a medical identification bracelet indicating that he's on prolonged steroid therapy and providing information about dosage.

• Parents of a female infant with male genitalia will need help understanding that she is physiologically a female and that this abnormality can be surgically corrected. Counseling may be necessary.

Pheochromocytoma

A pheochromocytoma is a chromaffin-cell tumor of the adrenal medulla that secretes an excess of the catecholamines epinephrine and norepinephrine, which results in severe hypertension, increased metabolism, and hyperglycemia. This disorder is potentially fatal, but prognosis is generally good with treatment. However, pheochromocytoma-induced kidney damage is irreversible.

Causes and incidence
A pheochromocytoma may result from an inherited autosomal dominant trait. According to some estimates, about 0.5% of newly diagnosed patients with hypertension have pheochromocytoma. While this tumor is usually benign, it may be malignant in as many as 10% of these patients. It affects all races and both sexes, occurring primarily between ages 30 and 40.

Signs and symptoms
The cardinal sign of pheochromocytoma is persistent or paroxysmal hypertension. Common clinical effects include palpitations, tachycardia, headache, diaphoresis, pallor, warmth or flushing, paresthesia, tremor, excitation, fright, nervousness, feelings of impending doom, abdominal pain, tachypnea, nausea, and vomiting. Postural hypotension and paradoxical response to antihypertensive drugs are common, as are associated glycosuria, hyperglycemia, and hypermetabolism. Patients with hypermetabolism may show marked weight loss, but some patients with pheochromocytomas are obese. Symptomatic episodes may recur as seldom as once every 2 months or as often as 25 times a day. They may occur spontaneously or may follow certain precipitating events, such as postural change, exercise, laughing, smoking, induction of anesthesia, urination, or a change in environmental or body temperature.

Often, pheochromocytoma is diagnosed during pregnancy, when uterine pressure on the tumor induces more frequent attacks; such attacks can prove fatal for both mother and fetus as a result of cerebrovascular accident, acute pulmonary edema, cardiac arrhythmias, or hypoxia. In such patients, the risk of spontaneous abortion is high, but most fetal deaths occur during labor or immediately after birth.

Diagnosis
A history of acute episodes of hypertension, headache, sweating, and tachycardia—particularly in a patient with hyperglycemia, glycosuria, and hyper-

metabolism—strongly suggests pheochromocytoma. In a patient with intermittent attacks, physical examination may show no abnormality during a latent phase. The tumor is rarely palpable; however, when it is, palpation of the surrounding area may induce a typical acute attack and help confirm the diagnosis. Generally, diagnosis depends on laboratory findings.

 Increased urinary excretion of total free catecholamine and its metabolites, vanillylmandelic acid (VMA) and metanephrine, as measured by an analysis of a 2- to 4-hour or a 24-hour urine collection, confirms pheochromocytoma. Labile blood pressure necessitates urine collection during a hypertensive episode and comparison of this specimen to a baseline specimen. Direct assay of total plasma catecholamines may show levels 10 to 50 times higher than normal.

Provocative tests with tyramine or glucagon, and depressor tests (phentolamine) suggest the diagnosis. However, because they may precipitate a hypertensive crisis or result in a false positive or negative, they're rarely used.

Angiography demonstrates an adrenal medullary tumor; intravenous pyelography with nephrotomography, adrenal venography, or CAT scan helps localize the tumor.

Treatment
Surgical removal of the tumor is the treatment of choice. To decrease blood pressure, alpha-adrenergic blocking agents (phentolamine or phenoxybenzamine) or, more recently, metyrosine (blocks catecholamine synthesis) is administered from 1 day to 2 weeks before surgery. A beta-adrenergic blocking agent (propranolol) may also be used after achieving alpha blockade. Postoperatively, I.V. fluids, plasma volume expanders, vasopressors, and possibly, transfusions may be required if marked hypotension occurs. However, persistent hypertension in the immediate postoperative period is more common.

If surgery isn't feasible, alpha- and beta-adrenergic blocking agents—such as phenoxybenzamine and propranolol, respectively—are beneficial in controlling catecholamine effects and preventing attacks.

Acute attack or hypertensive crisis requires I.V. administration of phentolamine (push or drip) or nitroprusside to normalize blood pressure.

Additional considerations
The hospital staff member should:
• make sure the patient avoids foods high in vanillin (such as coffee, nuts, chocolate, and bananas) for 2 days before urine collection of VMA to ensure the reliability of urine catecholamine measurements; be aware of possible drug therapy that may interfere with the accurate determination of VMA (such as guaifenesin and salicylates); collect the urine in a special container, with hydrochloric acid, prepared by the laboratory.
• obtain blood pressure readings often, since transient hypertensive attacks are possible; tell the patient to report headaches, palpitations, nervousness, or other symptoms of an acute attack; monitor blood pressure and heart rate every 2 to 5 minutes if hypertensive crisis develops, until blood pressure stabilizes at an acceptable level.
• check urine for glucose, and watch for weight loss from hypermetabolism.
• keep the patient quiet after surgery, and provide a private room, if possible, since blood pressure may rise or fall sharply and excitement may trigger a hypertensive episode. Postoperative hypertension is common, because the stress of surgery and manipulation of the adrenal gland stimulate secretion of catecholamines. Since this excess secretion causes profuse sweating, the room should be cool, and the patient's clothing and bedding should be changed often. If the patient receives phentolamine, blood pressure must be monitored closely. Possible side effects—dizziness, hypotension, tachycardia—should be recorded. The first 24 to 48 hours immediately after surgery are the most critical, since blood

pressure can drop drastically.
• check blood pressure every 3 to 5 minutes if the patient is receiving vasopressors I.V., and regulate the drip to maintain a safe pressure. Arterial pressure lines facilitate constant monitoring.
• watch for abdominal distention and return of bowel sounds.
• check dressings and vital signs for indications of hemorrhage (increased pulse rate, decreased blood pressure, cold and clammy skin, pallor, unresponsiveness).
• give analgesics for pain, as ordered, but monitor blood pressure carefully, since many analgesics, especially meperidine, can cause hypotension.

If autosomal dominant transmission of pheochromocytoma is suspected, the patient's family should also be evaluated for this condition.

PANCREATIC & MULTIPLE DISORDERS

Multiple Endocrine Neoplasia
(Wermer's syndrome, Sipple's syndrome)

Multiple endocrine neoplasia (MEN) is a hereditary disorder in which two or more endocrine glands develop hyperplasia, adenoma, or carcinoma, concurrently or consecutively. Two of the types that occur are well documented; a third may exist. MEN I (Wermer's syndrome) involves hyperplasia and adenomatosis of the parathyroids, islet cells of the pancreas, pituitary, and rarely, adrenals and thyroid gland; MEN II (Sipple's syndrome) involves medullary carcinoma of the thyroid, with hyperplasia and adenomatosis of the adrenal medulla (pheochromocytoma) and parathyroids. MEN I is the most common form.

Causes and incidence
MEN usually results from autosomal dominant inheritance, affects both males and females, and may occur at any time from adolescence to old age.

Signs and symptoms
Clinical effects of MEN may develop in various combinations and orders, depending on the glands involved. The most common symptom of MEN I is peptic ulceration, perhaps associated with hyperparathyroidism or Zollinger-Ellison syndrome (marked by increased gastrin production from non-beta islet cell tumors of the pancreas). Hypoglycemia may result from pancreatic beta islet cell tumors, with increased insulin production. When MEN I affects the parathyroids, it produces overt signs of hyperparathyroidism, including hypercalcemia (since the parathyroids are primarily responsible for the regulation of calcium and phosphorus levels). When MEN causes pituitary tumor, it usually triggers pituitary hypofunction but can also result in hyperfunction. MEN I rarely produces renal and skeletal complications.

Characteristic features of MEN II with medullary carcinoma of the thyroid include enlarged thyroid mass, with resultant increased calcitonin, and, occasionally, ectopic ACTH production, causing Cushing's syndrome. With tumors of the adrenal medulla, symptoms include headache, tachyarrhythmias, and hypertension; with adenomatosis or hyperplasia of the parathyroids, symptoms result from renal calculi.

Diagnosis
Investigating symptoms of pituitary tumor, hypoglycemia, hypercalcemia, or gastrointestinal hemorrhage may lead to a diagnosis of MEN. Diagnostic tests must be used to carefully evaluate each affected endocrine gland. For example,

radioimmunoassay showing increased levels of gastrin in patients with peptic ulceration and Zollinger-Ellison syndrome suggests the need for follow-up studies for MEN I, since 50% of patients with Zollinger-Ellison syndrome have MEN. After confirmation of MEN, family members must also be assessed for this inherited syndrome.

Treatment
Treatment must eradicate the tumors. Subsequent therapy controls residual symptoms. In MEN I, peptic ulceration is usually the most urgent clinical feature, so primary treatment emphasizes control of bleeding or resection of necrotic tissue. In hypoglycemia caused by insulinoma, P.O. administration of diazoxide or glucose can keep blood sugar within acceptable limits. In MEN II, treatment for adrenal medullary tumor includes antihypertensives and resection of the tumor.

Additional considerations
Supportive care depends on the body system involved.
• If MEN involves the pancreas, blood and urine glucose levels must be monitored frequently. If it affects the adrenal glands, blood pressure must be monitored closely, especially during drug therapy.
• Peptic ulceration, hypoglycemia, and other abnormalities or symptoms, should be treated, as appropriate.
• If pituitary tumor is suspected, the patient should be watched for signs of pituitary trophic hormone dysfunction, which may affect any of the endocrine glands. Also, pituitary apoplexy may cause sudden severe headache, altered level of consciousness, or visual disturbances.

Diabetes Mellitus

A chronic disease of insulin deficiency or resistance, diabetes mellitus is characterized by disturbances in carbohydrate, protein, and fat metabolism. A leading cause of death by disease in the United States, this syndrome contributes to about 50% of myocardial infarctions and about 75% of strokes, as well as to renal failure and peripheral vascular disease. It's also the leading cause of new blindness.

This condition occurs in two forms: insulin-dependent diabetes mellitus (IDDM, ketosis-prone, or juvenile diabetes) and noninsulin-dependent diabetes mellitus (NIDDM, ketosis-resistant, or maturity-onset diabetes). IDDM usually occurs before age 30 (although it may occur at any age); the patient is usually thin and requires exogenous insulin and dietary management to achieve control. Conversely, NIDDM is most prevalent among obese adults—however, it does occur occasionally in children—who respond to treatment with diet alone or in combination with hypoglycemic agents or insulin.

Causes and incidence
Diabetes mellitus affects an estimated 5% of the population of the United States (10 to 12 million persons), about half of whom are undiagnosed. Incidence is equal in males and females, and rises with age.

Although recent studies show that certain cases of IDDM are viral in origin, heredity strongly influences most diabetes. Precipitating factors include:

• obesity: causes resistance to endogenous insulin
• physiologic or emotional stress: causes prolonged elevation of stress hormones (cortisol, epinephrine, glucagon, and growth hormone), which raises blood glucose, placing increased demands on the pancreas
• pregnancy and oral contraceptives: increase levels of estrogen and placental hormones, which antagonize insulin

• other medications that are known insulin antagonists: thiazide diuretics, adrenal corticosteroids, phenytoin.

Insulin transports glucose into the cell for use as energy and storage as glycogen. It also stimulates protein synthesis and free fatty acid storage in the fat depots. Insulin deficiency compromises the body tissues' access to essential nutrients for fuel and storage.

Signs and symptoms
Diabetes may begin dramatically with ketoacidosis, or insidiously as in mild diabetes, which is often asymptomatic. Its most common symptom is fatigue, from energy deficiency and a catabolic state. Insulin deficiency causes hyperglycemia. The high blood glucose pulls fluid from body tissues, causing osmotic diuresis, polyuria, and ultimately, dehydration. Other symptoms include polydipsia, dry mucous membranes, and poor skin turgor. Edema and sugar deposits cause changes in the lens, which result in visual disturbances. When diabetes causes ketoacidosis or hyperglycemic hyperosmolar nonketotic coma, dehydration may cause hypovolemia and shock. Wasting of glucose in the urine usually produces weight loss and hunger in IDDM, even if the patient eats voraciously.

Long-term effects of diabetes include retinopathy, nephropathy, myocardial infarction and stroke, peripheral neuropathy, and autonomic neuropathy with nocturnal diarrhea. Because it impairs resistance to infection, uncontrolled diabetes may result in skin and urinary tract infections, vaginitis, and anal pruritus. Glucose content of the epidermis and urine encourages bacterial growth.

Diagnosis
Symptoms of uncontrolled diabetes, and random elevated blood sugars or glucosuria suggest diabetes. Confirmation requires a fasting plasma glucose above 140 mg/100 ml; or, with normal fasting glucose, a blood sugar level above 200 mg/100 ml during the first 2 hours of a glucose tolerance test (GTT). An ophthalmologic examination may show diabetic retinopathy. Other diagnostic and monitoring tests include the cortisone GTT to elicit stress-induced diabetes, blood insulin level determination, urine testing for sugar and acetone, and glycosylated hemoglobin (hemoglobin A_{1c}) determination, which reflects recent glucose control.

Treatment
The cornerstone of diabetic treatment is a strict diet carefully planned to meet nutritional needs, to control blood sugar levels, and to reach and maintain appropriate body weight. For the obese diabetic, weight reduction is a dietary goal. In IDDM, the calorie allotment may be high, depending on growth stage and activity level. However, to be successful, the diet must be followed consistently and meals eaten at regular times.

Although treatment with diet alone is effective in some patients, many require insulin injections or oral hypoglycemics. Multiple injections of regular insulin, or regular insulin mixed with NPH or with lente insulin generally control blood sugar better than a single daily injection of long-acting insulin. The effects of diet and insulin may also be modified by the patient's activity level, which affects blood sugar and lipid metabolism.

Treatment for long-term diabetic complications may include transplantation or dialysis for renal failure, photocoagulation for retinopathy, and vascular surgery for large vessel disease. Continued emphasis on meticulous blood sugar control is also essential.

Additional considerations
Clinical management of diabetes focuses on comprehensive teaching, recognition and care of the patient in crisis, and prevention of complications. Teaching the diabetic patient self-care begins during initial assessment.
• Compliance with the prescribed program is essential. The program should be tailored to the patient's needs, abilities, and developmental stage. It includes

PATIENT TEACHING AID

Mixing Regular and Long-acting Insulins

Your doctor has prescribed regular and long-acting insulins to control your diabetes. To avoid separate injections, you can mix these two types and administer them together. Here are the steps you must follow:

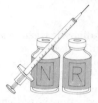 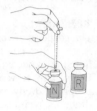 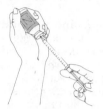

1. *Check your equipment.* Always wash your hands first, and prepare the mixture in a clean area. Make sure you have alcohol swabs, both types of insulin, and the proper syringe for the insulin concentration. Then, warm each vial by rolling it gently between your palms.

2. *Put air into the vial of long-acting insulin.* Clean the rubber stopper of the vial with an alcohol swab. To put air into the syringe, pull the plunger back to the appropriate number of units of long-acting insulin. Then, insert the needle into the top of the vial, making sure the point doesn't touch the insulin. Push in the plunger, and withdraw the syringe.

3. *Withdraw your dose of regular insulin.* Clean the rubber stopper of the regular insulin vial with an alcohol swab. Next, pull back the plunger to the necessary number of units of regular insulin, and inject air into the bottle. With the needle still in the bottle, turn the bottle upside down, and withdraw the proper dose of regular insulin.

4. *Withdraw your dose of long-acting insulin.* Clean the top of the long-acting insulin vial, and insert the needle into it, without pushing down the plunger. Then, invert the bottle, and withdraw the appropriate number of units. (Remember to pull the plunger back to the number of units needed for the *total* dose. For instance, if you have 10 units of regular insulin in the syringe and you need 20 units of long-acting insulin, pull the plunger back to 30 units.)

This patient teaching aid is intended for distribution to patients by doctors and nurses. It should not be used without a doctor's approval.

---

diet; administration of insulin or oral hypoglycemics, as applicable; exercise; urine testing; hygiene; and the prevention and recognition of hypo- and hyperglycemia. Meticulous control of blood sugar will have a significant effect on long-term health.

• The patient must be watched for acute complications of diabetes and diabetic therapy, especially hypoglycemia (vagueness, slow cerebration, dizziness, weakness, pallor, tachycardia, diaphoresis, seizures, and coma); if compli-

cations arise, carbohydrates can be given in the form of fruit juice, hard candy, honey, or if the patient is unconscious, glucagon or dextrose I.V. He must also be watched for signs of ketoacidosis (acetone breath, dehydration, weak and rapid pulse, Kussmaul's respirations) and hyperosmolar coma (polyuria, thirst, neurologic abnormalities, stupor)—both are hyperglycemic crises that require I.V. fluids, insulin, and possibly, potassium replacement.

• Diabetic control must be monitored

by testing urine for sugar and acetone, and obtaining blood glucose levels. (Urine sugar tests should be reported in mg% sugar instead of plus values.) Which urine test is most appropriate and how often it should be done depend on the patient's stability and on the accuracy of test results. For example, a patient with NIDDM may test once daily using glucose oxidase method (such as Testape); a patient with IDDM may test four times a day using the two-drop copper sulfate reduction method (such as Clinitest) and an acetone test; a patient with renal disease (in whom urine testing is unreliable) should monitor control of blood sugars using a home glucose-monitoring device.

• The patient must be watched for diabetic effects on the cardiovascular system, such as cerebral vascular, coronary artery, and peripheral vascular disease. All injuries, cuts, and blisters (particularly on the lower extremities) should be treated meticulously. He must also be watched for signs of urinary tract infection, renal failure, and Kimmelstiel-Wilson syndrome (protein and RBCs in urine, edema); the latter results from vascular deterioration in the kidneys and is a leading cause of death in young adult diabetics. Regular ophthalmologic examinations will aid early detection of diabetic retinopathy (microaneurysms, hemorrhages, and exudate on retina).

• The patient should be checked for signs of diabetic neuropathy (numbness, pain in the arms and legs, footdrop, and neurogenic bladder). He must try to avoid trauma, since he may have decreased sensation in his arms and legs, and can injure himself unknowingly. Maintaining strict blood glucose control will minimize complications.

To prevent diabetes, persons at high risk should avoid precipitive factors as much as possible; for example, females with family histories of diabetes should have thorough medical counseling about the use of contraceptives and the risks of pregnancy. Young adult diabetics who are planning families should obtain genetic counseling.

Further information about diabetes, and patient teaching aids may be obtained from the Juvenile Diabetes Foundation, the American Diabetes Association, the American Association of Diabetes Educators, and the manufacturers of products used by diabetics.

Selected References

Camuñas, C. *Transsphenoidal Hypophysectomy*, AMERICAN JOURNAL OF NURSING. 80:10:1820-1823, October 1980.

Cryer, Phillip. DIAGNOSTIC ENDOCRINOLOGY, 2nd ed. New York: Oxford University Press, 1979.

DeGroot, Leslie, et al. ENDOCRINOLOGY. New York: Grune & Stratton, 1979.

Eaton, R. Philip. *Lipids and Diabetes: The Case for Treatment of Macrovascular Disease*, DIABETES CARE. 2:46-49, January-February 1979.

Guthrie, Diana, and Richard Guthrie, eds. NURSING MANAGEMENT OF DIABETES MELLITUS. St. Louis: C.V. Mosby Co., 1977.

Hallal, Janice C. *Thyroid Disorders*, AMERICAN JOURNAL OF NURSING. 77:418-432 March 1977.

Hamburger, S.C. *Endocrine Metabolic Crisis*, CRITICAL CARE QUARTERLY. September 1980.

Krall, Leo P., ed. JOSLIN DIABETES MANUAL, 11th ed. Philadelphia: Lea & Febiger, 1978.

Kreuger J., and J. Ray. ENDOCRINE PROBLEMS IN NURSING: A PHYSIOLOGIC APPROACH. St. Louis: C.V. Mosby Co., 1976.

McCarthy, Joyce A. *Somogyi Effect*, NURSING79. 9:2:38-41, February 1979.

Montgomery, D.A. MEDICAL AND SURGICAL ENDOCRINOLOGY. Baltimore: Williams & Wilkins, 1975.

Pillitteri, Adele. NURSING CARE OF THE GROWING FAMILY: A CHILD HEALTH TEXT. Boston: Little, Brown & Co., 1977.

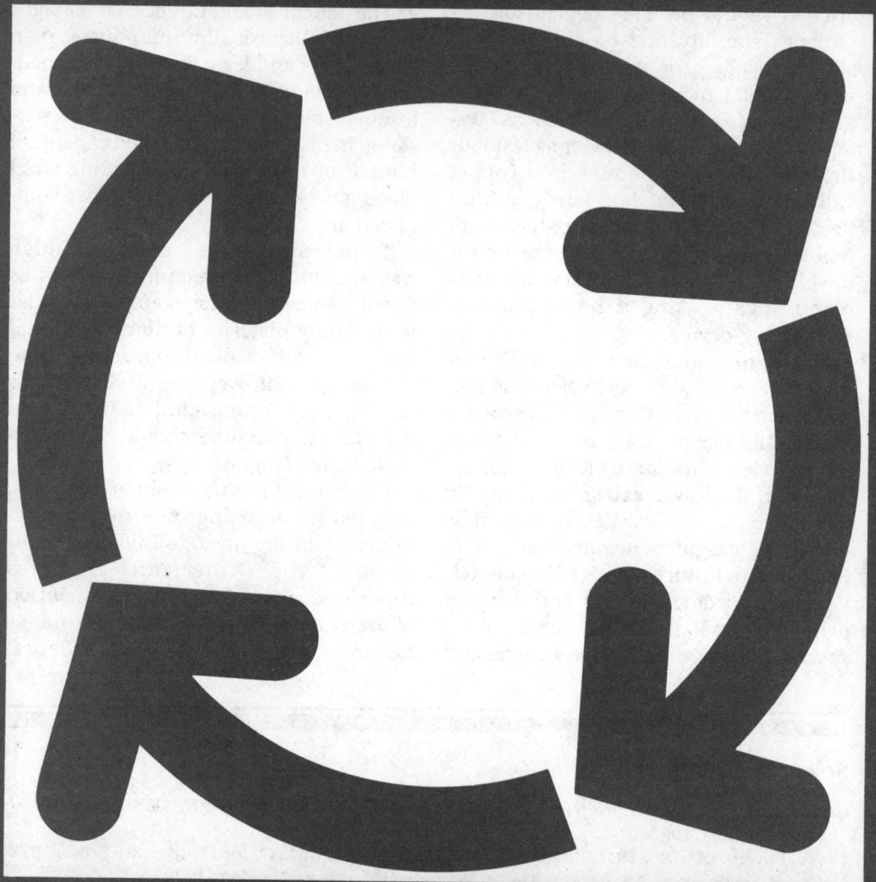

14 Metabolic and Nutritional Disorders

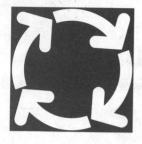

Metabolic and Nutritional Disorders

Introduction

Metabolism is the physiologic process that absorbs nutrients and converts them into forms that produce energy and continually rebuild body cells. Metabolism has two phases: catabolism and anabolism. In catabolism, the energy-producing phase of metabolism, the body breaks down large food molecules into smaller ones; in anabolism, the tissue-building phase, the body converts small molecules into larger ones (such as antibodies to keep the body capable of fighting infection). Both phases are accomplished by means of a chemical process using energy.

Carbohydrates: Primary energy source

The body gets most of its energy by metabolizing carbohydrate foods, especially glucose. Glucose catabolism proceeds in three phases:
• *Glycolysis,* a series of chemical reactions, converts glucose molecules into pyruvic acid.
• *The citric acid cycle* removes ionized hydrogen atoms from pyruvic acid and produces carbon dioxide.
• *Oxidative phosphorylation* traps energy from the hydrogen electrons and combines the hydrogen ions and electrons with oxygen to form water and the common form of biologic energy, adenosine triphosphate (ATP).

Other essential processes in carbohydrate metabolism include glycogenesis—the formation of glycogen, a storage form of glucose—which occurs when cells become saturated with glucose-6-phosphate (an intermediate product of glycolysis); glycogenolysis, the reverse process, which converts glycogen into glucose-6-phosphate in muscle cells and liberates free glucose in the liver; and glyconeogenesis, or "new" glucose formation from protein amino acids or fat glycerols.

A complex interplay of hormonal and neural controls regulates the homeostasis of glucose metabolism. Hormone secretions of five endocrine glands dominate this regulatory function:
• Beta cells of the islands of Langerhans secrete the glucose-regulating hormone *insulin,* which decreases blood sugar levels.
• Alpha cells of the islands of Langerhans secrete *glucagon,* which increases the blood glucose level by stimulating phosphorylase activity to accelerate liver glycogenolysis.
• The adrenal medulla, as a response to stress, secretes *epinephrine,* which stimulates liver and muscle glycogenolysis to increase the blood glucose level.
• *Adrenocorticotropic hormone (ACTH)* and *glucocorticoids* also increase blood glucose levels. Glucocorticoids accelerate glyconeogenesis by promoting the flow of amino acids to the liver, where

they are synthesized into glucose.

- *Growth hormone* (GH) limits the storage of fat and favors fat catabolism; consequently, it inhibits carbohydrate catabolism and thus raises blood glucose levels.
- *Thyroid-stimulating hormone (TSH)* and *thyroid hormone* have mixed effects on carbohydrate metabolism and may raise or lower blood glucose levels.

Fats: Catabolism and anabolism

The breaking up of triglycerides—lipolysis—yields fatty acids and glycerol. Beta-oxidation breaks down fatty acids into acetyl coenzyme A, which can then enter the citric acid cycle phase of glucose catabolism; glycerol can also undergo glyconeogenesis and enter the glycolytic pathways to produce energy. Conversely, lipogenesis is the chemical

---

ESSENTIAL NUTRIENTS AND THEIR FUNCTIONS

NUTRIENTS	FUNCTIONS
Carbohydrates	• Energy source
Fats and essential fatty acids	• Energy source; essential for growth, normal skin, and membranes
Proteins and amino acids	• Synthesis of all body proteins, growth, and tissue maintenance
Water-soluble vitamins:	
• Ascorbic acid (C)	• Collagen synthesis, wound healing, antioxidation
• Thiamine (B$_1$)	• Coenzyme in carbohydrate (CHO) metabolism
• Riboflavin (B$_2$)	• Coenzyme in energy metabolism
• Niacin	• Coenzyme in CHO, fat, energy metabolism, and tissue metabolism
• Vitamin B$_{12}$	• DNA and RNA synthesis; erythrocyte formation
• Folic acid	• Coenzyme in amino acid metabolism; heme and hemoglobin formation
Fat-soluble vitamins:	
• Vitamin A	• Vision in dim light, mucosal epithelium integrity, tooth development, endocrine function
• Vitamin D	• Regulation of calcium and phosphate absorption and metabolism; renal phosphate clearance
• Vitamin E	• Antioxidation; essential for muscle, liver, and RBC integrity
• Vitamin K	• Blood clotting (catalyzes synthesis of prothrombin by liver)

formation of fat from excess carbohydrates and proteins, or from the fatty acids and glycerol products of lipolysis. Adipose tissue is the primary storage site for excess fat, and thus is the greatest source of energy reserve. Certain unsaturated fatty acids are necessary for synthesis of vital body compounds. Because the body cannot produce these essential fatty acids, they must be provided through diet. Insulin, GH, catecholamines, ACTH, and glucocorticoids control fat metabolism in an inverse relationship with carbohydrate metabolism. In other words, large amounts of carbohydrates promote storage of fat; deficiency of available carbohydrates promotes the breakdown of fat for energy needs.

Proteins: Anabolism

The primary process in protein metabolism is anabolism; catabolism is relegated to a supporting role—a reversal of the roles played by these two processes in carbohydrate and fat metabolisms. By anabolizing proteins—the tissue-building foods—the body derives substances essential for life, such as plasma proteins, and can reproduce, control cell growth, and repair itself. However, when carbohydrates or fats are unavailable as energy sources, or energy demands are exceedingly high, protein catabolism converts protein into an available energy source. Protein metabolism consists of three processes:

• Deamination: a catabolic and energy producing process occurring in the liver with the splitting off of the amino acid to form ammonia and a keto acid
• Transamination: anabolic mechanism converts keto acids to amino acids
• Urea formation: a catabolic process occurring in the liver, producing urea, the end product of protein catabolism.

GH and the male hormone testosterone stimulate protein anabolism; ACTH prompts secretion of glucocorticoids, which, in turn, facilitate protein catabolism. Normally, the rate of protein anabolism equals the rate of protein catabolism, in a condition known as nitrogen balance (because ingested nitrogen equals nitrogen waste excreted in urine, feces, and sweat). When excessive catabolism causes the amount of nitrogen excreted to exceed the amount ingested, a state of *negative nitrogen balance* exists—usually the result of starvation and cachexia.

Fluid and electrolyte balance

A critical component of metabolism is fluid and electrolyte balance. Water is an essential body substance, and comprises almost 60% of an adult's body weight and more than 75% of a newborn's body weight. In both older and obese adults, the ratio of water to body weight drops; children and lean people have a higher proportion of water in their bodies.

Body fluids can be classified as intracellular (or cellular) and extracellular. Intracellular fluid comprises about 40% of total body weight and 60% of all body fluid, and contains large quantities of potassium and phosphates but very little sodium and chloride. Conversely, extracellular fluid contains mostly sodium and chloride but very little potassium and phosphates. Divided into interstitial, cerebrospinal, intraocular, and gastrointestinal fluids, and plasma, extracellular fluid supplies cells with nutrients and other substances needed for cellular function. The many components of body fluids have the important function of preserving osmotic pressure, and acid-base and anion-cation balance.

Homeostasis is a stable state—the equilibrium of chemical and physical properties of body fluid. Body fluids contain two kinds of dissolved substances: those that dissociate in solution (electrolytes) and those that do not. For example, glucose, when dissolved in water, does not break down into smaller particles; but sodium chloride dissociates in solution into sodium cations (+) and chloride anions (− 1). The composition of these electrolytes in body fluids is electrically balanced so the positively charged ions (cations: sodium, potassium, calcium, and magnesium) equal the negatively charged ions (anions:

FLUID HOMEOSTASIS

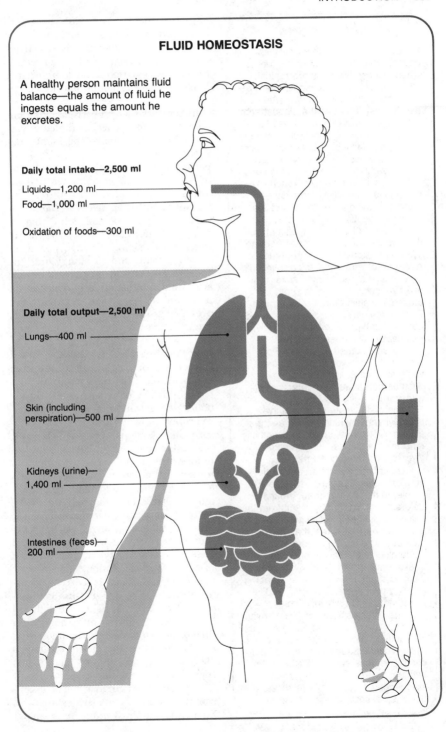

A healthy person maintains fluid balance—the amount of fluid he ingests equals the amount he excretes.

Daily total intake—2,500 ml

Liquids—1,200 ml

Food—1,000 ml

Oxidation of foods—300 ml

Daily total output—2,500 ml

Lungs—400 ml

Skin (including perspiration)—500 ml

Kidneys (urine)— 1,400 ml

Intestines (feces)— 200 ml

HYPOGLYCEMIA

Hypoglycemia is an abnormally low glucose level in the bloodstream. It occurs when glucose burns up too rapidly; when the glucose release rate falls behind tissue demands; and/or when excessive insulin enters the bloodstream.

Hypoglycemia may be classified in two ways: reactive (functional) hypoglycemia, and fasting (spontaneous) hypoglycemia. Reactive hypoglycemia may take several forms. In a diabetic patient, it may result from administration of too much insulin or—less commonly—too much oral hypoglycemia medication. In a mildly diabetic patient (or one in the early stages of diabetes mellitus), reactive hypoglycemia may result from delayed and excessive insulin production after carbohydrate ingestion. Similarly, a nondiabetic patient may suffer reactive hypoglycemia from a sharp increase in insulin output after a meal. Sometimes called postprandial hypoglycemia, this type of reactive hypoglycemia usually disappears when the patient eats something sweet. Postprandial hypoglycemia may also develop after gastrointestinal surgery, such as partial gastrectomy, gastroenterostomy, or pyloroplasty.

Signs and symptoms of reactive hypoglycemia include fatigue and malaise, nervousness, irritability, trembling, tension, headaches, hunger, cold sweats, and rapid heart rate.

Fasting hypoglycemia causes discomfort during fasting periods; for example, in the early morning hours before breakfast. It may result from the failure of glucose production caused by extensive hepatic disease. Other possible causes of fasting hypoglycemia include alcohol intake without food intake, panhypopituitarism, Addison's disease or steroid withdrawal, a fast-growing nonpancreatic tumor, and islet cell tumor (especially insulinoma).

Signs and symptoms of fasting hypoglycemia are usually the same as those of reactive hypoglycemia. But a fasting hypoglycemia attack may also cause central nervous system (CNS) disturbances; for example, blurry or double vision, confusion, motor weakness, hemiplegia, convulsions, or coma.

chloride, bicarbonate, sulfate, phosphate, proteinate, and carbonic and other organic acids). Although these particles are present in relatively low concentrations, any deviation from their normal levels can have profound physiologic effects.

In homeostasis—an ever-changing but balanced state—water, and electrolytes and other solutes move continually between cellular and extracellular compartments. Such motion is made possible by semipermeable membranes that allow diffusion, filtration, and active transport. Diffusion refers to the movement of particles or molecules from an area of greater concentration to one of lesser concentration. Normally, particles move randomly and constantly until the concentrations within given solutions are equal. Diffusion also depends on permeability, electrical gradient, and pressure gradient. Particles, however, cannot diffuse against any of these gradients without energy and a carrier substance (active transport). ATP is released from cells to aid particles needing energy to pass through the cell membrane.

The diffusion of water from a solution of low concentration to one of high concentration is called osmosis. The pressure that develops when a selectively permeable cell membrane separates solutions of different strengths or concentrations is known as osmotic pressure, expressed in terms of osmols or milliosmol (mOsm). Osmotic activity is described in terms of osmolality—the osmotic pull exerted by all particles per unit of water, expressed in mOsm/kg of water—or osmolarity, when expressed in mOsm/liter of solution.

The normal range of body fluid osmolality is 285 to 295 mOsm. Solutions of 50 mOsm above or below the high and low points of this normal range exert little or no osmotic effect (isosmolality). A solution below 240 mOsm contains a lower particle concentration than plasma (hypo-osmolar), while a solution over 340 mOsm has a higher particle concentration than plasma (hyperosmolar). Rapid I.V. administration of isosmolar solutions to patients who are debilitated, very old or very young, or who have cardiac or renal insufficiency could lead to extracellular fluid volume overload and induce pulmonary edema and congestive heart failure.

Continuous I.V. administration of hypo-osmolar solutions decreases serum osmolality and leads to excess intracellular fluid volume (water intoxication). Continuous I.V. administration of hyperosmolar solutions results in intracellular dehydration, increased serum osmolality, and eventually, extracellular fluid volume deficit due to excessive urinary excretion.

Regulation of pH
Primarily through the complex chemical regulation of carbonic acid by the lungs and of base bicarbonate by the kidneys, the body maintains the hydrogen ion concentration to keep the extracellular fluid pH between 7.35 and 7.45. Nutritional deficiency or excess, disease, injury, or metabolic disturbance can interfere with normal homeostatic mechanisms and cause a lowering of pH (acidosis) or a rise in pH (alkalosis).

Assessing homeostasis
The goal of metabolism and homeostasis is to maintain the complex environment of extracellular fluid—the plasma—which nourishes and supports every body cell. This special environment is subject to multiple interlocking influences and readily reflects any disturbance in nutrition, chemical or fluid content, and osmotic pressure. Such disturbances are detectable by various laboratory determinations. For example, measurements of albumin-transferrin and other blood proteins, electrolyte concentration, enzyme and immunologic levels, and urine and blood chemistry levels (lipoproteins, glucose, BUN, creatinine, and creatinine-height index) accurately reflect the state of metabolism, homeostasis, and nutrition throughout the body. Results of such laboratory tests supplement the information obtained from dietary history and physical examination—which offer gross clinical information about the quality, quantity, and efficiency of metabolic processes. To support such clinical information, anthropometry, height-weight ratio, and skin-fold thickness determinations offer specialized measures of tissue nutritional status.

• A complete dietary history is needed to determine if carbohydrate, fat, protein, vitamin, mineral, and water intake is adequate to meet the body's needs for energy production, and tissue repair and growth. During periods of rapid tissue synthesis (growth, pregnancy, healing), the need for protein increases.

• A dietitian should be consulted about any patient who may be malnourished (malabsorption syndromes, renal or hepatic disease, clear-liquid diets). Carefully planned meals that provide adequate amounts of carbohydrates, fats, and protein are necessary for convalescence. Supplementary carbohydrate snacks are often needed to spare protein and achieve a positive nitrogen balance.

• Intake and output, including intake of oral liquids or I.V. solutions, must be recorded as well as urine, gastric, and stool output.

• The patient must be weighed daily—at the same time, with the same type clothing, and on the same scale. A weight loss of 2.2 lb (1 kg) is equivalent to the loss of a liter of fluid.

• The patient should be observed for insensible water or unmeasured fluid losses (such as through diaphoresis). Fluid loss from the skin and lungs (normally 900 ml/day) can reach 2,000 ml/day from diaphoresis and hyperventilation.

• I.V. solutions that are hypo-osmolar, include 0.45% NaCl (half normal saline solution) and 5% dextrose in water. Isosmolar solutions include normal saline solution (0.9% NaCl), 5% dextrose in 0.2% NaCl, and Ringer's solutions. Examples of hyperosmolar solutions are 5% dextrose in normal saline solution, 10% dextrose in water, and 5% dextrose in lactated Ringer's solution.

• When continuously administering

hypo-osmolar solutions, the patient must be watched for signs of water intoxication: headaches, behavior changes (confusion or disorientation), nausea, vomiting, rising blood pressure, and falling pulse rate.

• When continuously administering hyperosmolar solutions, the patient must be checked for signs of hypovolemia: thirst, dry mucous membranes, slightly falling blood pressure, rising pulse rate and respirations, low-grade fever (99° F. [37.2° C.]), and elevated hematocrit, hemoglobin, and BUN.

• Fluid should be given cautiously, especially to the patient with cardiopulmonary disease. The patient must be watched for overhydration. Signs of overhydration include: constant and irritating cough, dyspnea, moist rales, rising central venous pressure, and pitting edema (late sign). When the patient is in an upright position, neck and hand vein engorgement is a common sign of fluid overload, possibly from administration of hyperosmolar solutions.

Elderly patients and others vulnerable to fluid imbalances should know what constitutes adequate fluid intake. Parents caring for newborns should know, too.

NUTRITIONAL IMBALANCE

Vitamin A Deficiency

A fat-soluble vitamin absorbed in the gastrointestinal tract, vitamin A maintains epithelial tissue and retinal function. Consequently, deficiency of this vitamin may result in night blindness, decreased color adjustment, keratinization of epithelial tissue, and poor bone growth. Healthy adults have adequate vitamin A reserves to last up to a year; children often do not. Each year, more than 80,000 persons worldwide—mostly children in underdeveloped countries—lose their sight from severe vitamin A deficiency. This condition is rare in the United States, although many disadvantaged children have substandard levels of vitamin A. With therapy, the chance of reversing symptoms of night blindness and milder conjunctival changes is excellent. When corneal damage is present, emergency treatment is necessary.

Causes

Vitamin A deficiency usually results from inadequate dietary intake of foods high in vitamin A (liver, kidney, butter, milk, cream, cheese, and fortified margarine) or carotene, a precursor of vitamin A found in dark green leafy vegetables, and yellow or orange fruits and vegetables.

Less common causes include:
• *malabsorption* due to celiac disease, sprue, obstructive jaundice, cystic fibrosis, giardiasis, or habitual use of mineral oil as a laxative.
• *massive urinary excretion* caused by cancer, tuberculosis, pneumonia, nephritis, or urinary tract infection.
• *decreased storage and transport* of vitamin A due to hepatic disease.

Signs and symptoms

Typically, the first symptom of vitamin A deficiency is night blindness (nyctalopia), which usually becomes apparent when the patient enters a dark place or is caught in the glare of oncoming headlights while driving at night. This condition can progress to xerophthalmia, or drying of the conjunctivas, with development of gray plaques (Bitot's spots); if unchecked, perforation, scarring, and blindness may result. Keratinization of epithelial tissue causes dry, scaly skin; follicular hyperkeratosis; and shrinking and hardening of the mucous membranes, possibly leading to infections of the eyes and the respiratory or genitourinary tract. An infant with severe vitamin A deficiency shows signs of failure to thrive, and apathy, along with dry skin and corneal changes, which can lead to ulceration and rapid destruction of the cornea.

Diagnosis
Dietary history and characteristic ocular lesions suggest vitamin A deficiency. Decreased carotene levels (less than 40 mcg/100 ml) also suggest vitamin A deficiency, but they fluctuate with seasonal ingestion of fruits and vegetables. Serum levels of vitamin A that fall below 20 mcg/100 ml confirm vitamin A deficiency.

Treatment
Mild conjunctival changes or night blindness requires vitamin A replacement in the form of cod liver or halibut liver oil. Acute deficiency requires aqueous vitamin A solution I.M., especially when corneal changes have occurred. Therapy for underlying biliary obstruction consists of administration of bile salts; for pancreatic insufficiency, pancreatin. Dry skin responds well to cream- or petrolatum-based products.

In patients with chronic malabsorption of fat-soluble vitamins, and in those with low dietary intake, prevention of vitamin A deficiency requires aqueous I.V. supplements or a water-miscible preparation P.O.

Additional considerations
• Oral vitamin A supplements should be administered with or after meals, or parenterally. Signs of overdosage include hypercarotenemia (orange coloration of the skin and eyes) and hypervitaminosis A (rash, hair loss, anorexia, transient hydrocephalus, and vomiting in children; bone pain, hepatosplenomegaly, diplopia, and irritability in adults). If these signs occur, supplements should be discontinued, and the doctor notified immediately. (Hypercarotenemia is relatively harmless; hypervitaminosis A may be toxic.)
• Since vitamin A deficiency usually results from dietary insufficiency, the patient and family will need nutritional counseling and, if necessary, should be referred to an appropriate community agency.

Vitamin B Deficiencies

Vitamin B complex is a group of water-soluble vitamins essential to normal metabolism, cell growth, and blood formation. The most common deficiencies involve thiamine (B_1), riboflavin (B_2), niacin, pyridoxine (B_6), and cobalamin (B_{12}).

Causes and incidence
Thiamine deficiency results from malabsorption or inadequate dietary intake of vitamin B_1. Beriberi, a serious thiamine-deficiency disease, is most prevalent in Orientals, who subsist mainly on diets of unenriched rice and wheat. Although this disease is uncommon in the United States, alcoholics may develop cardiac (wet) beriberi with high output congestive heart failure, neuropathy, and cerebral disturbances. In times of stress (pregnancy, for example), malnourished young adults may develop beriberi; infantile beriberi may appear in infants on low-protein diets or in those breast-fed by thiamine-deficient mothers.

Riboflavin deficiency (ariboflavinosis) results from a diet deficient in milk, meat, fish, green leafy vegetables, and legumes. Chronic alcoholism or prolonged diarrhea may also induce deficiency of riboflavin (or of any of the other water-soluble B complex vitamins). Exposure of milk to sunlight or treatment of legumes with baking soda can destroy riboflavin.

Niacin deficiency, in its advanced form,

produces pellagra, which affects the skin, central nervous system, and gastrointestinal tract. Although this deficiency is now rarely found in the United States, it was once common among Southerners who subsisted mainly on corn and consumed minimal animal protein. (Corn is low in niacin and in tryptophan, the amino acid from which the body synthesizes niacin.) Niacin deficiency is still common in parts of Egypt, Yugoslavia, Rumania, and Africa, where corn is the dominant staple food. Niacin deficiency can also occur secondary to carcinoid syndrome or Hartnup disease.

Pyridoxine deficiency usually results from destruction of pyridoxine by autoclaving infant formulas. A frank deficiency is uncommon in adults, except in patients taking pyridoxine antagonists, such as isoniazid and penicillamine.

Cobalamin deficiency most commonly results from an absence of intrinsic factor in gastric secretions, or an absence of receptor sites after ileal resection. Other causes include malabsorption syndromes associated with diverticulosis, sprue, intestinal infestation, regional ileitis, and gluten enteropathy, and a diet low in animal protein (due to strict vegetarianism or poverty).

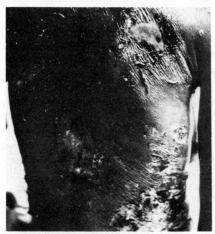

This patient with pellagra shows dark, scaly, advanced dermatitis. Such dermatitis usually occurs on areas exposed to the sun.

Signs and symptoms

Thiamine deficiency causes polyneuritis and, possibly, Wernecke's encephalopathy and Korsakoff's psychosis. In infants (infantile beriberi), this deficiency produces edema, irritability, abdominal pain, pallor, vomiting, loss of voice, and possibly, convulsions. In wet beriberi, severe edema starts in the legs and moves up through the body; dry beriberi causes multiple neurologic symptoms and an emaciated appearance. Thiamine deficiency may also cause cardiomegaly, palpitations, tachycardia, dyspnea, and circulatory collapse. Constipation and indigestion are common; ataxia, nystagmus, and ophthalmoplegia are also possible.

Riboflavin deficiency characteristically causes cheilosis (cracking of the lips and corners of the mouth), sore throat, and glossitis. It may also cause seborrheic dermatitis in the nasolabial folds, scrotum, and vulva, and possibly, generalized dermatitis involving the arms, legs, and trunk. This deficiency can also affect the eyes, producing burning, itching, light sensitivity, tearing, and vascularization of the corneas. Late-stage riboflavin deficiency causes neuropathy, mild anemia, and in children, growth retardation.

Niacin deficiency in its early stages produces fatigue, anorexia, muscle weakness, headache, indigestion, mild skin eruptions, weight loss, and backache. In advanced stages (pellagra), it produces dark, scaly dermatitis, especially on exposed parts of the body, that makes the patient appear to be severely sunburned. The mouth, tongue, and lips become red and sore, which may interfere with eating. Common gastrointestinal symptoms include nausea, vomiting, and diarrhea. Associated CNS aberrations—confusion, disorientation, and neuritis—may become severe enough to induce hallucinations and paranoia. Because of this triad of symptoms, pellagra is sometimes called a "3-D" syndrome—dementia, dermatitis, and diarrhea. If not reversed by therapeutic doses of niacin, pellagra can be fatal.

RECOMMENDED DAILY ALLOWANCE OF B-COMPLEX VITAMINS

VITAMIN	MEN (23-50)	WOMEN (23-50)	INFANTS	CHILDREN (1-10)
B$_1$*	1.4 mg	1.0 mg	0.4 mg	0.7 to 1.2 mg
B$_2$*	1.6 mg	1.2 mg	0.5 mg	0.8 to 1.2 mg
niacin*	18 mg	13 mg	5 to 8 mg	9 to 16 mg
B$_6$	2.0 mg	2.0 mg	0.4 mg	0.6 to 1.2 mg
B$_{12}$	3 mcg	3 mcg	0.3 mcg	1.0 to 2.0 mg

requirements per 1,000 kilocalories of dietary intake

Pyridoxine deficiency in infants causes a wide range of distressing symptoms: dermatitis, occasional cheilosis or glossitis that does not respond to riboflavin therapy, abdominal pain, vomiting, ataxia, and convulsions. This deficiency can also lead to CNS disturbances, particularly in infants.

Cobalamin deficiency causes pernicious anemia and may lead to demyelination of the large nerve fibers of the spinal cord—yellowing of skin, anorexia, weight loss, abdominal discomfort, dyspnea, megaloblastic anemia, peripheral neuropathy, ataxia, glossitis, and occasional depression.

Diagnosis

The following values confirm vitamin B deficiency:

• *Thiamine deficiency:* thiamine serum levels less than 5 mcg/100 ml; elevated levels of serum pyruvic and lactic acids, especially after exercise and glucose administration; low thiamine concentration in urine

• *Riboflavin deficiency:* riboflavin serum level less than 2 mcg/100 ml

• *Niacin deficiency:* serum niacin levels less than 30 mcg/100 ml; diminished or absent metabolites (N-methyl niacinamide and N-methylpyridone) in urine

• *Pyridoxine deficiency:* xanthurenic acid more than 50 mg/day in 24-hour urine collection after administration of 10 g L-tryptophan; decreased levels of serum and RBC transaminases; reduced excretion of pyridoxic acid in urine

• *Cobalamin deficiency:* cobalamin serum levels less than 150 pg/ml. Tests to discover the cause of the deficiency include gastric analysis and hemoglobin

studies. In addition, Schilling test measures absorption of radioactive cobalamin with and without intrinsic factor; X-rays must rule out gastric cancer, which is common among patients with pernicious anemia.

Prevention and treatment

Appropriate dietary adjustments and supplementary vitamins can prevent or correct vitamin B deficiencies:

• *Thiamine deficiency:* a high-protein diet, with adequate calorie intake, possibly supplemented by B complex vitamins for early symptoms. Thiamine-rich foods include pork, peas, wheat bran, oatmeal, and liver. Alcoholic beriberi may require thiamine supplements or administration of thiamine hydrochloride as part of a B complex concentrate.

• *Riboflavin deficiency:* supplemental riboflavin in patients with intractable diarrhea or increased demand for riboflavin as a result of growth, pregnancy, lactation, or wound healing. Good sources of riboflavin are meats, enriched flour, milk and dairy foods, green leafy vegetables, eggs, and cereal. Acute riboflavin deficiency requires daily oral doses of riboflavin alone or in combination with other B complex vitamins. Riboflavin supplements can also be administered I.V. or I.M. as the sodium salt of riboflavin phosphate.

• *Niacin deficiency:* supplemental B complex vitamins and dietary enrichment in patients at risk due to marginal diets or alcoholism. Meats, fish, peanuts, brewers' yeast, enriched breads, and cereals are rich in niacin; milk and eggs, in tryptophan. Confirmed niacin deficiency requires daily doses of niacin-

amide P.O. or I.V.
• *Pyridoxine deficiency*: prophylactic pyridoxine therapy in infants and epileptic children; supplemental B complex vitamins in patients with anorexia, malabsorption, or those taking isoniazid or penicillamine. Some women who take oral contraceptives may have to supplement their diets with pyridoxine. Confirmed pyridoxine deficiencies require oral or parenteral pyridoxine. Children with convulsive seizures stemming from metabolic dysfunction may require daily doses of 200 to 600 mg pyridoxine.
• *Cobalamin deficiency*: parenteral cyanocobalamin in patients with reduced gastric secretion of hydrochloric acid, lack of intrinsic factor, some malabsorption syndromes, or ileum resections. Strict vegetarians may have to supplement their diets with oral vitamin B_{12}. Depending on the severity of the deficiency, supplementary cyanocobalamin is usually given parenterally for 5 to 10 days, followed by monthly or daily vitamin B_{12} supplements.

Additional considerations
An accurate dietary history provides a baseline for effective dietary counseling. This includes:
• identifying and observing patients who risk vitamin B deficiencies—alcoholics, the elderly, pregnant women, and persons on limited diets.
• administering prescribed supplements; making sure patients understand how important it is that they adhere strictly to their prescribed treatment for the rest of their lives; watching for side effects from large doses of niacinamide, in patients with niacin deficiency (prolonged intake of niacin can cause hepatic dysfunction); cautioning patients with Parkinson's disease receiving pyridoxine that this drug can impair response to levodopa therapy.
• explaining all tests and procedures; reassuring patients that, with treatment, prognosis is good; referring patients to appropriate assistance agencies if their diets are inadequate due to socioeconomic conditions.

Vitamin C Deficiency
(Scurvy)

Vitamin C (ascorbic acid) deficiency leads to scurvy or inadequate production of collagen, an extracellular substance that binds the cells of the teeth, bones, and capillaries. Historically common among sailors and others deprived of fresh fruits and vegetables for long periods of time, vitamin C deficiency is uncommon today in the United States, except in alcoholics, persons on restricted-residue diets, and infants weaned from breast milk to cow's milk without a vitamin C supplement.

Causes
The primary cause of this deficiency is a diet lacking foods rich in vitamin C, such as citrus fruits, tomatoes, cabbage, broccoli, spinach, and berries. Since the body can't store this water-soluble vitamin in large amounts, the supply needs to be replenished daily. Other causes include:
• destruction of vitamin C in foods by overexposure to air or overcooking.
• excessive ingestion of vitamin C during pregnancy, which causes the new-

born to require large amounts of the vitamin after birth.
• marginal intake of vitamin C during periods of physiologic stress—caused by infectious disease, for example—which can deplete tissue saturation of vitamin C.

Signs and symptoms
Clinical features of vitamin C deficiency appear as capillaries become increasingly fragile. In an adult, it produces petechiae, ecchymoses, follicular hyper-

keratosis (especially on the buttocks and legs), anemia, anorexia, limb and joint pain (especially in the knees), pallor, weakness, swollen or bleeding gums, loose teeth, lethargy, insomnia, poor wound healing, and ocular hemorrhages in the bulbar conjunctivas. Vitamin C deficiency can also induce psychologic disturbances—irritability, depression, hysteria, and hypochondriasis.

In a child, vitamin C deficiency produces tender, painful swelling in the legs, causing the child to lie with his legs partially flexed. Other symptoms include fever, diarrhea, and vomiting.

Diagnosis

Dietary history revealing an inadequate intake of ascorbic acid suggests vitamin C deficiency; serum ascorbic acid levels less than 0.4 mg/100 ml and WBC ascorbic acid levels less than 25 mg/100 ml help confirm it.

Treatment

Since scurvy is potentially fatal, treatment begins immediately to restore adequate vitamin C intake by daily doses of 100 to 200 mg vitamin C in synthetic form or in orange juice in mild disease, and doses as high as 500 mg/day in severe disease. Symptoms usually subside in 2 to 3 days; hemorrhages and bone disorders, in 2 to 3 weeks.

To prevent vitamin C deficiency, patients unable or unwilling to consume foods rich in vitamin C, or those facing surgery should take daily supplements of ascorbic acid. Vitamin C supplements may also prevent this deficiency in recently weaned infants or those drinking formula not fortified with vitamin C.

Additional considerations

• Ascorbic acid is administered P.O. or by slow I.V. infusion. The patient should not be moved unnecessarily; it may cause irritation of painful joints and muscles.
• The patient must understand the importance of supplemental ascorbic acid. He should be encouraged to drink orange juice, if possible. He and his family may

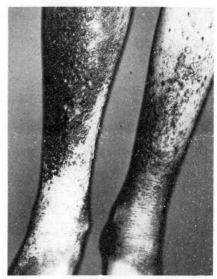

Follicular hyperkeratosis from scurvy usually occurs on the legs.

need counseling about other good dietary sources of vitamin C. Knowing that adequate amounts of vitamin C help wounds heal faster may encourage them to increase their intake.
• However, the patient should be discouraged from taking too much vitamin C, because large doses of ascorbic acid may cause nausea, diarrhea, and renal calculi, and may interfere with anticoagulant therapy.

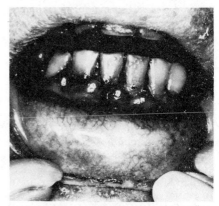

In adults, scurvy causes swollen or bleeding gums and loose teeth.

Vitamin D Deficiency

(Rickets)

Vitamin D deficiency causes failure of normal bone calcification, which results in rickets in infants and young children, and osteomalacia in adults. With treatment, prognosis is good. However, in rickets, bone deformities usually persist, while in osteomalacia, deformities may disappear.

Causes and incidence

Vitamin D deficiency results from inadequate dietary intake of preformed vitamin D, malabsorption of vitamin D, or too little exposure to sunlight.

Once a common childhood disease, rickets is now rare in the United States, but occasionally appears in breast-fed infants who do not receive a vitamin D supplement or in infants receiving a formula with a nonfortified milk base. This deficiency may also occur in overcrowded, urban areas where smog limits sunlight penetration; incidence is highest in Black children who, because of their pigmentation, absorb less sunlight. (Solar ultraviolet rays irradiate 7-dehydrocholesterol, a precursor of vitamin D, to form calciferol, a vitamin D complex.)

Osteomalacia, also uncommon in the United States, is most prevalent in the Orient, among young multiparas who eat a cereal diet and have minimal exposure to sunlight. Other causes include:

• *vitamin D–resistant rickets* (refractory rickets, familial hypophosphatemia) from an inherited impairment of renal tubular reabsorption of phosphate (from vitamin D insensitivity).

• *conditions that lower absorption of fat-soluble vitamin D,* such as chronic pancreatitis, celiac disease, Crohn's disease, cystic fibrosis, gastric or small bowel resections, fistulas, colitis, and biliary obstruction.

• *hepatic or renal disease,* which interferes with the formation of hydroxylated calciferol, necessary to initiate the formation of a calcium-binding protein in intestinal absorption sites.

• *malfunctioning parathyroid gland* (decreased secretion of parathyroid hormone), which contributes to calcium deficiency (normally, vitamin D controls absorption of calcium and phosphorus through the intestine) and interferes with activation of vitamin D in the kidneys.

Signs and symptoms

Early indications of vitamin D deficiency are profuse sweating, restlessness, and irritability. Chronic deficiency induces numerous bone malformations due to softening of the bones: bowlegs, knock-knees, rachitic rosary (beading of ends of ribs), enlargement of wrists and ankles, pigeon breast, delayed closing of the fontanelles, softening of the skull, and bulging of the forehead. Other rachitic features are poorly developed muscles (potbelly) and infantile tetany. These bone deformities may also produce difficulty in walking and in climbing stairs, spontaneous multiple fractures, and pain in the legs and lower back.

Diagnosis

Physical examination, dietary history, and laboratory tests establish diagnosis. Test results include plasma calcium serum levels <7.5 mg/100 ml, inorganic phosphorus serum levels <3 mg/100 ml, serum citrate levels <2.5 mg/100 ml, and alkaline phosphatase <4 Bodansky units/100 ml—all of which suggest vitamin D deficiency.

 X-rays confirm diagnosis by showing characteristic bone deformities and abnormalities, such as Looser's zones.

Treatment and additional considerations

For osteomalacia and rickets—except when

due to malabsorption—treatment consists of massive P.O. doses of vitamin D or cod liver oil. For rickets refractory to vitamin D or in rickets accompanied by hepatic or renal disease, treatment includes 25-hydroxycholecalciferol (active form of vitamin D).

• A dietary history should be obtained to assess the patient's current vitamin D intake. He should be encouraged to eat foods high in vitamin D—such as fortified milk, fish liver oils, herring, sardines, liver, and egg yolks—and get sufficient sun exposure. If the dietary deficiency is due to socioeconomic conditions, the patient or parents should be referred to an appropriate community agency for assistance.

• If the patient must take vitamin D for a prolonged period, he should watch for signs of vitamin D toxicity (headache, nausea, diarrhea, and after prolonged use, renal calculi).

• Measures that can be used to prevent rickets include administering supplementary aqueous preparations of vitamin D for chronic fat malabsorption, hydroxy-

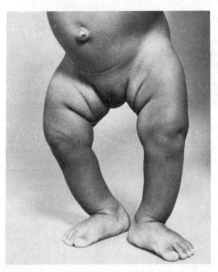

This infant with rickets shows characteristic bowing of the legs.

lated cholecalciferol for refractory rickets, and supplemental vitamin D for breast-fed infants.

Vitamin E Deficiency

Vitamin E (tocopherol) is necessary for reproductive function; development of smooth muscle, skeletal muscle, and vascular tissue; erythrocyte protection; and other biochemical functions. Deficiency of vitamin E usually manifests as hemolytic anemia in low–birth-weight or premature infants. With treatment, prognosis is good.

Causes and incidence
Vitamin E deficiency in infants usually results from formulas high in polyunsaturated fatty acids that are fortified with iron but not vitamin E. Such formulas increase the need for antioxidant vitamin E, because the iron supplement catalyzes the oxidation of RBC lipids. A newborn has low tissue concentrations of vitamin E to begin with, since only a small amount passes through the placenta; the mother retains most of it. Since vitamin E is a fat-soluble vitamin, deficiency develops in conditions associated with fat malabsorption, such as kwash-

iorkor, celiac disease, or cystic fibrosis. These conditions may induce megaloblastic or hemolytic anemia, and creatinuria, all of which are reversible with vitamin E administration.

Vitamin E deficiency is uncommon in adults but is possible in persons whose diets are high in polyunsaturated fatty acids, which increase consumption of vitamin E, and in persons with vitamin E malabsorption, which impairs red cell survival.

Signs and symptoms
Vitamin E deficiency is difficult to rec-

ognize, but its early symptoms include edema and skin lesions in infants, and muscle weakness or intermittent claudication in adults. In premature infants, vitamin E deficiency produces hemolytic anemia, thrombocytosis, and erythematous papular skin eruption, followed by desquamation.

Diagnosis

The patient's dietary and medical histories suggest vitamin E deficiency. Serum alpha-tocopherol levels below 0.5 mg/100 ml confirm it. Excessive creatinuria, increased creatine phosphokinase, hemolytic anemia, and elevated platelet count generally support the diagnosis.

Treatment and additional considerations

Replacement of vitamin E with a water-soluble vitamin E supplement, either P.O. or parenteral, is the only appropriate treatment.

• Vitamin E deficiency can be prevented by providing vitamin E supplements for low–birth-weight infants receiving formulas not fortified with vitamin E, and for adults with vitamin E malabsorption. Many commercial multivitamin supplements are easily absorbed by patients with vitamin E malabsorption.

• New mothers who plan to breastfeed should know that human milk provides adequate vitamin E.

• Adult patients should be encouraged to eat foods high in vitamin E: vegetable oils (corn, safflower, soybean, cottonseed), whole grains, dark green leafy vegetables, nuts, and legumes. Heavy consumption of polyunsaturated fatty acids increases their need for vitamin E.

• If vitamin E deficiency is related to socioeconomic conditions, the patient should be referred to appropriate community agencies.

Vitamin K Deficiency

Deficiency of vitamin K, an element necessary for formation of prothrombin and other clotting factors in the liver, produces abnormal bleeding. If the deficiency is corrected, prognosis is excellent.

Causes and incidence

Vitamin K deficiency is common among newborns in the first few days postpartum due to poor placental transfer of vitamin K and inadequate production of vitamin K-producing intestinal flora. Its other causes include prolonged use of drugs, such as the anticoagulant dicumarol and antibiotics that destroy normal intestinal bacteria; decreased flow of bile to the small intestine from obstruction of the bile duct or bile fistula; malabsorption of vitamin K due to sprue, pellagra, bowel resection, ileitis, or ulcerative colitis; chronic hepatic disease, with impaired response of hepatic ribosomes to vitamin K; and cystic fibrosis, with fat malabsorption. Vitamin K deficiency rarely results from insufficient dietary intake of this vitamin.

Signs and symptoms

The cardinal sign of vitamin K deficiency is an abnormal bleeding tendency, accompanied by prolonged prothrombin time; these signs disappear with administration of vitamin K. Without treatment, such bleeding may be severe and possibly fatal.

Diagnosis

A prothrombin time 25% longer than the normal range of 25 to 40 seconds when measured by the Quick method confirms the diagnosis after other causes of prolonged prothrombin time (such as anticoagulant therapy or hepatic disease) have been ruled out. Repetition of this test in 24 hours (and regularly during treatment) monitors success of therapy.

Treatment and additional considerations

Administration of vitamin K corrects abnormal bleeding tendencies. Measures that can be used to prevent vitamin K deficiency include:
• administering vitamin K to newborns and patients with fat malabsorption, or prolonged diarrhea due to colitis, ileitis,

or extended antibiotic therapy.
• warning against self-medication with or overuse of antibiotics, because these drugs destroy the intestinal bacteria necessary to generate significant amounts of vitamin K.
• if the deficiency has a dietary cause, helping the patient and family plan a diet that includes important sources of vitamin K, such as green leafy vegetables, cauliflower, tomatoes, cheese, egg yolks, and liver.

Hypervitaminoses A and D

Hypervitaminosis A is excessive accumulation of vitamin A; hypervitaminosis D, of vitamin D. Although these are toxic conditions, they usually respond well to treatment. They are most prevalent in infants and children, usually as a result of accidental or misguided overdosage by parents. A related, benign condition called hypercarotenemia results from excessive consumption of carotene, a chemical precursor of vitamin A.

Causes and incidence

Vitamins A and D are fat-soluble vitamins that accumulate in the body because they aren't dissolved and excreted in the urine. Generally, hypervitaminoses A and D result from ingestion of excessive amounts of supplemental vitamin preparations. A single dose of more than 1 million units of vitamin A can cause acute toxicity; daily doses of 15,000 to 25,000 units taken over weeks or months have proven toxic in infants

and children. For the same dose to produce toxicity in adults, ingestion over years is necessary. Ingestion of only 1,600 to 2,000 units of vitamin D is sufficient to cause toxicity.

Hypervitaminosis A may occur in patients receiving pharmacologic doses of vitamin A for dermatologic disorders. Hypervitaminosis D may occur in patients receiving high doses of the vitamin as treatment for hypoparathyroidism, rickets, and the osteodystrophy of chronic

IMPORTANT FACTS ABOUT VITAMINS A AND D

VITAMIN	SOURCES	RECOMMENDED DIETARY ALLOWANCE (RDA)	ACTION
Vitamin A	• Carrots, sweet potatoes, dark leafy green vegetables, butter, margarine, liver, egg yolk	• Children: 1,400 IU • Adults: 4,000 to 5,000 IU • Lactating women: 6,000 IU	• Produces retinal pigment and maintains epithelial tissue
Vitamin D	• Ultraviolet light, fortified foods (especially milk)	• 400 IU daily	• Promotes absorption and regulates metabolism of calcium and phosphorus

renal failure; and in infants who consume fortified milk and cereals, plus a vitamin supplement. Concentrations of vitamin A in common foods are generally low enough not to pose a danger of excessive intake. However, a benign condition called hypercarotenemia results from excessive consumption of vegetables high in carotene (a protovitamin that the body converts into vitamin A), such as carrots, sweet potatoes, and dark green leafy vegetables.

Signs and symptoms

Chronic hypervitaminosis A produces anorexia, irritability, headache, hair loss, malaise, itching, vertigo, bone pain, bone fragility, and dry, peeling skin. It may also cause hepatosplenomegaly and emotional lability. Acute toxicity may also produce transient hydrocephalus and vomiting. (Hypercarotenemia causes yellow or orange skin coloration.)

Hypervitaminosis D causes anorexia, headache, nausea, vomiting, weight loss, polyuria, and polydipsia. Since vitamin D promotes calcium absorption, severe toxicity can lead to hypercalcemia, including calcification of soft tissues, as in the heart, aorta, and renal tubules. Lethargy, confusion, and coma may accompany severe hypercalcemia.

Diagnosis

Thorough patient history suggests hypervitaminosis A; elevated serum vitamin A levels (more than 90 mcg/100 ml) confirm it. Patient history and elevated serum calcium levels (more than 10.1 mg/100 ml) suggest hypervitaminosis D; elevated serum vitamin D levels confirm it; in children, X-rays showing calcification of tendons, ligaments, and subperiosteal tissues support this diagnosis. Elevated serum carotene levels of 250 mcg/100 ml confirm hypercarotenemia.

Treatment

Withholding vitamin supplements usually corrects hypervitaminosis A quickly and hypervitaminosis D gradually. Hypercalcemia may persist for weeks or months after the patient stops taking vitamin D. Treatment for severe hypervitaminosis D may include glucocorticoids to control hypercalcemia and prevent renal damage. In the acute stage, diuretics or other emergency measures for severe hypercalcemia may be necessary. Hypercarotenemia responds well to dietary exclusion of foods high in carotene.

Additional considerations

- The patient should be kept comfortable, and reassured that symptoms will subside after he stops taking the vitamin.
- The patient or the parents of a child with these conditions must understand that vitamins aren't innocuous. They should be taught the hazards associated with excessive vitamin intake and that vitamin A and D requirements can easily be met with a diet containing dark green leafy vegetables, fruits, and fortified milk or milk products.
- To prevent hypervitaminosis A or D, serum vitamin A levels should be monitored in patients receiving doses above the recommended daily dietary allowance, and serum calcium levels should be monitored in patients receiving pharmacologic doses of vitamin D.

Iodine Deficiency

Iodine deficiency is the absence of sufficient levels of iodine to satisfy daily metabolic requirements. Because the thyroid gland uses most of the body's iodine stores, iodine deficiency is apt to cause hypothyroidism and thyroid gland hypertrophy (endemic goiter). Other effects of deficiency range from dental caries to cretinism in infants born to iodine-deficient mothers. Iodine deficiency is most common in pregnant or lactating women due to their exaggerated metabolic need for this element. Iodine deficiency is readily responsive to treatment with iodine supplements.

Causes

Iodine deficiency usually results from insufficient ingestion of dietary sources of iodine, mostly iodized table salt, seafood, and dark green leafy vegetables. (Normal iodine requirements range from 35 mcg/day for infants to 150 mcg/day for lactating women; the average adult needs 1 mcg/kg of body weight.) Iodine deficiency may also result from errors of metabolism:

• *failure to trap iodine in the thyroid gland,* due to the loss of certain enzymes necessary to iodize the amino acids needed for thyroid hormone synthesis

• *decrease in anterior pituitary function,* which results in a deficiency of thyroid-stimulating hormone (TSH), which is necessary for iodine uptake

• *failure to convert inorganic iodine into organic iodine*

• *increase in metabolic demands* during pregnancy, lactation, and adolescence.

Signs and symptoms

Clinical features of iodine deficiency depend on the degree of hypothyroidism that develops (in addition to the development of a goiter). Mild deficiency may produce only lassitude, fatigue, and loss of motivation. Severe deficiency generates overt and often unmistakable features of hypothyroidism: bradycardia, decreased pulse pressure and cardiac output, weakness, hoarseness, thick tongue, delayed relaxation phase in deep tendon reflexes, poor memory, hearing loss, chills, anorexia, and dry, cold skin. In women, this disorder may also cause menorrhagia and amenorrhea.

Diagnosis

 Abnormal laboratory test results include low T_4 with high ^{131}I uptake, low 24-hour urine iodine, and high TSH. Radioiodine uptake test traces ^{131}I in the thyroid 24 hours after administration; T_3- or T_4-resin uptake test shows values 25% below normal.

Treatment and additional considerations

Severe iodine deficiency necessitates administration of iodine supplements (potassium iodide [SSKI]). Mild deficiency may be corrected by increasing iodine intake through the use of iodized table salt and consumption of iodine-rich foods (seafood and green leafy vegetables).

When treating a patient with iodine deficiency, the hospital staff member should:

• administer SSKI preparation in milk or juice to reduce gastric irritation and mask its metallic taste; tell the patient to drink the solution through a straw, to prevent tooth discoloration; store the solution in a light-resistant container.

• recommend use of iodized salt and consumption of iodine-rich foods to prevent iodine deficiency in high-risk patients—especially pregnant or lactating women, and adolescents; advise pregnant women that severe iodine deficiency may produce cretinism in newborns, and instruct them to watch for early signs of iodine deficiency, such as fatigue, lassitude, weakness, and decreased mental function.

Zinc Deficiency

Zinc, an essential trace element that is present in the bones, teeth, hair, skin, testes, liver, and muscles, is also a vital component of many enzymes. Zinc promotes synthesis of DNA, RNA, and ultimately, protein, and maintains normal blood concentrations of vitamin A by mobilizing it from the liver.

Zinc deficiency is most common in persons from underdeveloped countries, especially the Middle East. Children are most susceptible to this deficiency during periods of rapid growth. Prognosis is good with correction of the deficiency.

Causes

Zinc deficiency almost invariably results from excessive intake of foods that bind zinc and prevent its absorption from the intestine, such as those containing calcium, vitamin D, and phytase found in unleavened bread. Occasionally, it results from blood loss due to parasitism and inadequate dietary intake of foods containing zinc. Alcohol and corticosteroids increase renal excretion of zinc.

Signs and symptoms

Zinc deficiency produces hepatosplenomegaly, sparse hair growth, soft and misshapen nails, poor wound healing, anorexia, hypogeusesthesia (decreased taste acuity), dysgeusia (unpleasant taste), hyposmia (decreased odor acuity), dysosmia (unpleasant odor in nasopharynx), severe iron deficiency anemia, bone deformities, and when chronic, hypogonadism, dwarfism, and hyperpigmentation.

Diagnosis

 Serum zinc levels below 121 (±19) mcg/100 ml confirm zinc deficiency and indicate altered phosphate metabolism, imbalance between aerobic and anerobic metabolisms, and decreased pancreatic enzyme levels.

Treatment and additional considerations

Treatment consists of correcting the underlying cause of the zinc deficiency and administering zinc supplements, as necessary. Prevention of the deficiency requires the patient eating a balanced diet that includes foods high in zinc, such as seafood, oatmeal, wheat bran, meat, eggs, and dry yeast; and avoiding the chronic use of calcium supplements. The patient can take zinc supplements with milk or meals to prevent gastric distress and vomiting.

Obesity

Obesity is an excess of body fat, generally 20% above ideal body weight. Prognosis for correction of obesity is poor: fewer than 30% of patients succeed in losing 20 lb (9 kg), and only half of these maintain the loss over a prolonged period.

Causes and incidence

Obesity results from excessive calorie intake and inadequate expenditure of energy. Theories to explain this condition include hypothalamic dysfunction of hunger and satiety centers, genetic predisposition, abnormal absorption of nutrients, and impaired action of gastrointestinal and growth hormones, and of hormonal regulators, such as insulin. An inverse relationship between socioeconomic status and the prevalence of obesity has been documented, especially in women. Obesity in parents increases the probability of obesity in children, from genetic or environmental factors, such as activity levels and learned patterns of eating. Psychologic factors may also contribute to obesity.

Diagnosis

Observation and comparison of height and weight to a standard table indicate obesity. Measurement of the thickness of subcutaneous fat folds with calipers provides an approximation of total body fat. Although this measurement is reliable and isn't subject to daily fluctuations, it has little meaning for the patient in monitoring subsequent weight loss. Obesity may lead to serious complications, such as respiratory difficulties, hypertension, cardiovascular disease, diabetes mellitus, renal disease, gallbladder disease, and psychosocial difficulties.

Treatment

Successful management of obesity must

decrease the patient's daily calorie intake, while increasing his activity level. To achieve long-term benefits, lifelong maintenance of these improved patterns is necessary. Treatment usually consists of a balanced, low-calorie diet that eliminates foods high in fat or sugar.

The popular low-carbohydrate diets offer no long-term advantage; rapid early weight reduction is due to loss of water, not fat. These and other crash or fad diets have the overwhelming drawback that they don't teach long-term modification of eating patterns and often lead to the yo-yo syndrome—episodes of repeated weight loss followed by weight gain.

Total fasting is an effective method of rapid weight reduction but requires close monitoring and supervision to minimize risks of ketonemia, electrolyte imbalance, hypotension, and loss of lean body mass. Prolonged fasting, or liquid protein diets have been associated with sudden death, possibly resulting from cardiac arrhythmias caused by electrolyte abnormalities. A better method is protein-sparing modified fasting, in which the patient eats 1 to 1.5 g protein/kg of body weight/day. However, these methods also neglect patient reeducation, which is necessary for long-term weight maintenance.

Treatment may also include hypnosis and behavior modification, which promote fundamental changes in eating habits and activity patterns. Psychotherapy may also be desirable for some patients, since weight reduction may cause depression or even psychosis.

Amphetamines have been used to aid adherence to a prescribed diet by temporarily suppressing the appetite and creating a feeling of well-being. However, because their value in long-term weight control is questionable, and they have a significant potential for dependence and abuse, their use is generally avoided. If amphetamines are used at all, they should be prescribed only for short-term therapy and should be monitored carefully.

As a last resort, *morbid* obesity may be treated surgically with jejunoileal bypass, which induces a permanent malabsorption syndrome. Postoperatively, the patient continues to lose weight until he reaches a plateau, in 12 to 18 months. Complications include a 2% to 10% mortality from electrolyte imbalance, malnutrition, urinary calculi, hepatic disorders, pancreatitis, gallstones, and arthritis. A new surgical technique, gastric stapling (gastric plication), decreases the volume of food necessary to produce satiety. This causes fewer complications than the bypass procedure.

Additional considerations

Health care for a patient being treated for obesity includes:

• obtaining an accurate diet history to identify eating patterns and the importance of food to the patient's life-style; asking the patient to keep a careful record of what and where he eats to identify situations that provoke overeating.

• explaining the prescribed diet carefully, and encouraging compliance to improve health status; promoting increased physical activity, including an exercise program, to increase calorie expenditure; recommending activity levels according to the patient's general condition and cardiovascular status.

• watching for signs of dependence if the patient is taking appetite-suppressing drugs, and for side effects, such as insomnia, excitability, dry mouth, and gastrointestinal disturbances.

• teaching the patient who is grossly obese the importance of good skin care to prevent breakdown in moist skin folds. Powder is recommended to keep skin dry.

• teaching parents to help prevent obesity by avoiding overfeeding their infants and by familiarizing themselves with real nutritional needs and optimum growth rate; discouraging them from using food to reward or console children, from emphasizing the importance of "clean plates," and from allowing eating to prevent hunger rather than satisfy it; encouraging physical activity and exercise to establish lifelong patterns; suggesting low-calorie snacks, such as raw vegetables.

Protein-calorie Malnutrition

One of the most prevalent and serious depletion disorders, protein-calorie malnutrition (PCM) occurs as marasmus (protein-calorie deficiency), characterized by growth failure and wasting, and as kwashiorkor (protein deficiency), characterized by tissue edema and damage. Both forms vary from mild to severe and may be fatal, depending on accompanying stress (particularly sepsis or injury) and duration of deprivation. PCM increases the risk of death from pneumonia, chickenpox, or measles.

Causes and incidence

Both marasmus (nonedematous PCM) and kwashiorkor (edematous PCM) are common in underdeveloped countries and in areas where dietary amino acid content is insufficient to satisfy growth requirements. Kwashiorkor typically occurs at about age 1, after infants are weaned from breast milk to a protein-deficient diet of starchy gruels or sugar water, but it can develop at any time during the formative years. Marasmus affects infants aged 6 to 18 months as a result of breast-feeding failure or a debilitating condition, such as chronic diarrhea.

In industrialized countries, PCM may occur secondary to chronic metabolic disease that decreases protein and calorie intake or absorption, or trauma that increases protein and calorie requirements. In the United States, PCM is estimated to occur to some extent in 50% of surgical and 48% of medical patients. Those who are not allowed anything by mouth for an extended period are at high risk of developing PCM. Conditions that increase protein-calorie requirements include severe burns and injuries, systemic infections, and cancer (accounts for the largest group of hospitalized patients with PCM). Conditions that cause defective utilization of nutrients include malabsorption syndrome, short-bowel syndrome, and Crohn's disease.

Signs and symptoms

Children with chronic PCM are small for their chronologic age and tend to be physically inactive, mentally apathetic, and susceptible to frequent infections. Anorexia and diarrhea are common. In acute PCM, children are small, gaunt, and emaciated, with no adipose tissue. Skin is dry and "baggy," and hair is sparse and dull brown or reddish yellow. Temperature is low; pulse rate and respirations, slowed. Such children are weak, irritable, and usually hungry, although they may have anorexia, with nausea and vomiting.

Unlike marasmus, chronic kwashiorkor allows the patient to grow in height, but adipose tissue diminishes as fat metabolizes to meet energy demands. Edema often masks severe muscle wasting; dry, peeling skin and hepatomegaly are common. Patients with secondary PCM show signs similar to marasmus, primarily loss of adipose tissue and lean body mass, lethargy, and edema. Severe secondary PCM may cause loss of immunocompetence.

Diagnosis

 Clinical appearance, dietary history, and anthropometry confirm PCM. If the patient does not suffer from fluid retention, weight change over time is the best index of nutritional status. Other factors support the diagnosis:
• height and weight less than 80% of standard for the patient's age and sex, and below standard arm circumference and triceps skinfold
• serum albumin less than 2.8 g/100 ml (normal 3.3 to 4.3 g/100 ml)
• urinary creatinine (24-hour), which shows lean body mass status by relating

CLINICAL FEATURES OF MALNUTRITION

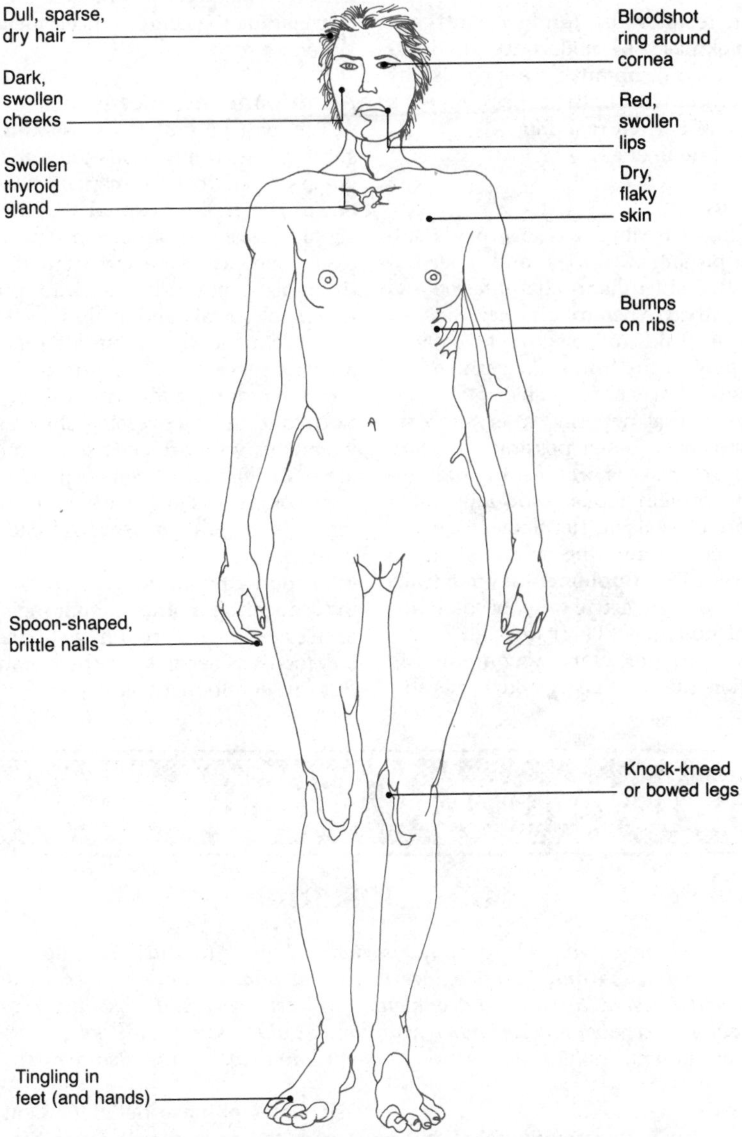

Dull, sparse, dry hair

Dark, swollen cheeks

Swollen thyroid gland

Spoon-shaped, brittle nails

Tingling in feet (and hands)

Bloodshot ring around cornea

Red, swollen lips

Dry, flaky skin

Bumps on ribs

Knock-kneed or bowed legs

The generalized body reaction to prolonged states of malnourishment produces a characteristic clinical picture of reduced body mass and abnormalities in rapidly regenerating body tissues. In addition, CNS effects cause behavioral modifications: mental apathy; anorexia; lethargy; and in order to preserve the delicate energy balance, chronically limited energy expenditure. Immunologic competence is severely compromised, and mortality from common infectious diseases is abnormally high.

creatinine excretion to height and ideal body weight, to yield creatinine height index
• skin tests with standard antigens (streptokinase-streptodornase) to indicate degree of immune compromise by determining reactivity expressed as a percent of normal reaction
• moderate anemia.

Treatment
The aim of treatment is to provide sufficient proteins, calories, and other nutrients for nutritional rehabilitation and maintenance. When treating severe PCM, restoring fluid and electrolyte balance parentally is the initial concern. A patient who shows normal absorption may receive enteral nutrition after anorexia has subsided. When possible, the preferred treatment is oral feeding of high-quality protein foods, especially milk, and protein-calorie supplements. A patient who is unwilling or unable to eat may require supplementary feedings through a nasogastric tube, or total parenteral nutrition (TPN) through a central venous catheter. Accompanying infection must also be treated, preferably with antibiotics that do not inhibit protein synthesis. Cautious realimentation is essential to prevent complications from overloading the compromised metabolic system.

Additional considerations
• The patient with PCM should consume as much nutritious food and beverage as possible (he can be "cheered on" as he eats). A hospital staff member should assist the patient to eat, if necessary, cooperate closely with the dietitian to monitor intake, and provide acceptable meals and snacks.
• If TPN is necessary, the staff member must observe strict aseptic technique when handling catheters, tubes, solutions, and during dressing changes.
• Patients who are susceptible to PCM are those who have been hospitalized for a prolonged period, have had no oral intake for several days, or have cachectic disease.
• Encouraging prolonged breast feeding, educating mothers about their children's needs, and providing supplementary foods, as needed, may help eradicate PCM in developing countries.

METABOLIC DISORDERS

Galactosemia

Galactosemia is any disorder of galactose metabolism. It produces symptoms ranging from cataracts and liver damage to mental retardation, and occurs in two forms: classic galactosemia and galactokinase deficiency galactosemia. Although a galactose-free diet relieves most symptoms, galactosemia-induced mental impairment is irreversible; some residual vision impairment may also persist.

Causes
Both forms of galactosemia are inherited as autosomal recessive defects, and occur in about 1 in 50,000 births in the United States. Up to 1.25% of the population is heterozygous for the classic galactosemia gene. Classic galactosemia results from a defect in the enzyme galactose-1-phosphate uridyl transfer-ase. Galactokinase deficiency galactosemia, the rarer form of this disorder, stems from a deficiency of the enzyme galactokinase. In both forms of galactosemia, inability to normally metabolize the sugar galactose (mainly formed by digestion of the disaccharide lactose present in milk) causes galactose accumulation.

Signs and symptoms

In children who are homozygous for the classic galactosemia gene, signs are evident at birth or begin within a few days after milk ingestion, and include failure to thrive, vomiting, and diarrhea. Other clinical effects include liver damage (which causes jaundice, hepatomegaly, cirrhosis, ascites), splenomegaly, galactosuria, proteinuria, and aminoaciduria. Cataracts may also be present at birth or develop later. Pseudotumor cerebri may occur.

Continued ingestion of galactose or lactose-containing foods may cause mental retardation, malnourishment, progressive hepatic failure, and death—from the still unknown process of galactose metabolites accumulating in body tissues. Although treatment may prevent mental impairment, galactosemia can produce a short attention span, difficulty with spatial and mathematical relationships, and apathetic, withdrawn behavior. Cataracts may be the only sign of galactokinase deficiency, resulting from the accumulation of galactitol, a metabolic by-product of galactose, in the lens.

Diagnosis

Deficiency of the enzyme galactose-1-phosphate uridyl transferase in RBCs confirms classic galactosemia; decreased RBC levels of galactokinase confirm galactokinase deficiency. Other related laboratory results include increased galactose levels in blood (normal value in children is less than 20 mg/dl) and urine (must use galactose oxidase to avoid confusion with other reducing sugars). Galactose measurements in blood and urine must be interpreted carefully, because some children who consume large amounts of milk have elevated plasma galactose concentrations and galactosuria but are not galactosemic. Also, newborns excrete galactose in their urine for about a week after birth; premature infants, even longer. Other test results include:

- *liver biopsy:* typical acinar formation
- *liver enzymes (SGOT, SGPT):* elevated
- *urinalysis:* albumin in urine
- *ophthalmoscopy:* punctate lesions in the fetal lens nucleus (with treatment, cataracts regress)
- *amniocentesis:* prenatal diagnosis of galactosemia (recommended for heterozygous and homozygous parents).

Treatment and additional considerations

Elimination of galactose and lactose from the diet causes most effects to subside. The infant gains weight; liver anomalies, nausea, vomiting, galactosemia, proteinuria, and aminoaciduria disappear; and cataracts regress. To eliminate galactose and lactose from an infant's diet, cow's milk formula or breast milk should

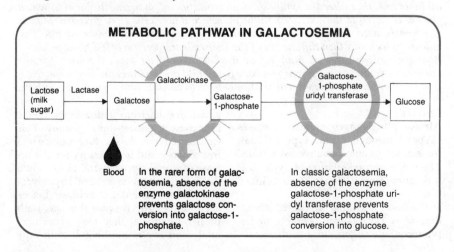

METABOLIC PATHWAY IN GALACTOSEMIA

In the rarer form of galactosemia, absence of the enzyme galactokinase prevents galactose conversion into galactose-1-phosphate.

In classic galactosemia, absence of the enzyme galactose-1-phosphate uridyl transferase prevents galactose-1-phosphate conversion into glucose.

PARENT TEACHING AID

DIET FOR GALACTOSEMIA

If your child has galactosemia, make sure he follows a diet free of lactose. He may eat:
- fish and animal products (except brains and mussels)
- fresh fruits and vegetables (except peas and lima beans).
- only bread and rolls made from

cracked wheat.
He should avoid:
- dairy products
- puddings, cookies, cakes, pies
- food coloring
- instant potatoes
- canned and frozen foods (if lactose is listed as an ingredient).

This patient teaching aid is intended for distribution to patients by doctors and nurses.
It should not be used without a doctor's approval.

---

be replaced with a meat-base or soybean formula. As the child grows, a balanced, galactose-free diet must be maintained. A pregnant woman who is heterozygous or homozygous for galactosemia should also follow a galactose-restricted diet. Such a diet supports normal growth and development, and may delay symptoms in the newborn.

• Parents must understand the necessity of strict compliance with dietary restric-tions. They should read all medication labels carefully and avoid giving any that contain lactose fillers.

• If the child has a learning disability, parents will need help securing appro-priate educational assistance. Parents who want to have other children should be referred for genetic counseling. In some states, the screening of all new-borns for galactosemia is required by law.

Glycogen Storage Diseases

Glycogen storage diseases consist of at least eight distinct errors of metabolism, all inherited, that alter the synthesis or degradation of glycogen, the form in which glucose is stored in the body. Normally, muscle and liver cells store glycogen. Muscle glycogen is used in muscle contraction; liver glycogen can be converted into free glucose, which can then diffuse out of the liver cells to increase blood glucose levels. Glycogen storage diseases manifest as dysfunctions of the liver, the heart, or the musculoskeletal system. Symptoms vary from mild and easily controlled hypoglyce-mia to severe organ involvement that may lead to cardiac and respiratory failure.

Causes

Almost all glycogen storage diseases (Types I through V and Type VII) are transmitted as autosomal recessive traits. The mode of transmission of Type VI is unknown; Type VIII may be an X-linked trait.

The most common glycogen storage disease is Type I—von Gierke's, or he-patorenal glycogen storage disease— which results from a deficiency of the liver enzyme glucose-6-phosphatase. This enzyme converts glucose-6-phosphate into free glucose and is necessary for the re-lease of stored glycogen and glucose into the bloodstream, to relieve hypoglyce-mia. Infants may die of acidosis before age 2; if they survive past this age, with proper treatment, they may grow nor-mally and live to adulthood, with only

RARE FORMS OF GLYCOGEN STORAGE DISEASE

TYPE	CLINICAL FEATURES	DIAGNOSTIC TEST RESULTS
II (*Pompe's*) Absence of alpha-1,4-glucosidase (acid maltase)	• *Infants:* cardiomegaly, profound hypotonia, and occasionally, endocardial fibroelastosis (usually fatal before age 1 due to cardiac or respiratory failure) • *Some infants and young children:* muscular weakness and wasting, variable organ involvement (slower progression, usually fatal by age 19) • *Adults:* muscle weakness without organomegaly (slowly progressive but not fatal)	• *Muscle biopsy:* increased concentration of glycogen with normal structure; alpha 1,4-glucosidase deficiency • *EKG* (in infants): large QRS complexes in all leads; inverted T waves; shortened P-R interval • *Electromyography* (in adults): muscle fiber irritability; myotonic discharges • *Amniocentesis:* alpha-1,4-glucosidase deficiency • *Placenta or umbilical cord examination:* alpha-1,4-glucosidase deficiency
III (*Cori's*) Absence of debranching enzyme (amylo-1,6-glucosidase) (*Note:* predominant cause of glycogen storage disease in Israel)	• *Young children:* massive hepatomegaly, which may disappear by puberty; growth retardation; moderate splenomegaly • *Adults:* progressive myopathy • Occasionally, moderate cardiomegaly, cirrhosis, muscle weakness and wasting, severe hypoglycemia, and convulsions	• *Liver biopsy:* deficient debranching activity; increased glycogen concentration • *Lab tests* (in children only): elevated SGOT and SGPT; increased erythrocyte glycogen
IV (*Andersen's*) Deficiency of branching enzyme (alpha-1,4-glucan-6-glycosyl transferase) (*Note:* extremely rare)	• *Infants:* hepatosplenomegaly, ascites, muscle hypotonia; usually fatal before age 2 from progressive cirrhosis	• *Liver biopsy:* deficient branching enzyme activity; glycogen molecule has longer outer branches.
V (*McArdle's*) Deficiency of muscle phosphorylase enzyme	• *Children:* mild or no symptoms • *Adults:* muscle cramps and pain during strenuous exercise, possibly resulting in myoglobinuria and renal failure • *Older patients:* significant muscle weakness and wasting	• *Serum lactate:* no increase in venous levels in sample drawn from extremity after ischemic exercise • *Muscle biopsy:* lack of phosphorylase activity; increased glycogen content
VI (*Hers'*) Possible deficiency of hepatic phosphorylase	• Mild symptoms (similar to those of Type I), requiring no treatment	• *Liver biopsy:* decreased phosphorylase b activity, increased glycogen concentrations
VII Deficiency of muscle phosphofructokinase	• Muscle cramps during strenuous exercise, resulting in myoglobinuria and possible renal failure • Reticulocytosis	• *Serum lactate:* no increase in venous levels in sample drawn from extremity after ischemic exercise • *Muscle biopsy:* deficient phosphofructokinase; marked rise in glycogen concentration • *Blood studies:* low erythrocyte phosphofructokinase activity; reduced half-life of RBCs
VIII Deficiency of hepatic phosphorylase kinase	• Mild hepatomegaly • Mild hypoglycemia	• *Liver biopsy:* deficient phosphorylase b kinase activity; increased liver glycogen • *Blood:* deficient phosphorylase b kinase in leukocytes

minimal hepatomegaly. However, there is a danger of adenomatous liver nodules, which may be premalignant.

Signs and symptoms
Primary clinical features of the liver glycogen storage diseases (Types I, III, IV, VI, and VIII) are hepatomegaly, and rapid onset of hypoglycemia and ketosis when food is withheld. Symptoms of the muscle glycogen storage diseases (Types II, V, and VII) include poor muscle tone; Type II may result in death from heart failure.

In addition, Type I may produce the following symptoms in...
• *infants:* acidosis, gastrointestinal bleeding, coma
• *children:* low resistance to infection and, without proper treatment, short stature
• *adolescents:* gouty arthritis and nephropathy; chronic tophaceous gout; bleeding (especially epistaxis); small superficial vessels visible in skin, due to impaired platelet function; fat deposits in cheeks, buttocks, and subcutaneous tissues; poor muscle tone; enlarged kidneys; xanthomas over extensor surfaces of arms and legs; steatorrhea; multiple, bilateral, yellow lesions in fundi; and osteoporosis, probably secondary to negative calcium balance. Correct treatment of glycogen storage disease should prevent all of these effects.

Diagnosis
Liver and muscle biopsies are the key tests in diagnosing Type I glycogen storage disease:
• *Liver biopsy* confirms diagnosis by showing normal glycogen synthetase and phosphorylase enzyme activities but reduced or absent glucose-6-phosphatase activity. Glycogen structure is normal, but amounts are elevated.
• *Laboratory studies* of plasma demonstrate low glucose levels but high levels of free fatty acids, triglycerides, cholesterol, and uric acid. Serum analysis reveals high pyruvic levels and high lactic acid levels.
• *Injection of glucagon or epinephrine* increases pyruvic and lactic acid levels but does not increase blood glucose levels. Glucose tolerance test curve typically shows depletional hypoglycemia and reduced insulin output. Intrauterine diagnosis is possible.

Treatment
For Type I, the aims of treatment are to maintain glucose homeostasis and prevent secondary consequences of hypoglycemia through frequent feedings and constant nocturnal nasogastric drip with Polycose, dextrose, or Vivonex. Treatment includes a low-fat diet, with normal amounts of protein and calories; carbohydrates should contain glucose or glucose polymers only.

Therapy for Type III includes frequent feedings and a high-protein diet. Type IV requires a high-protein, high-calorie diet; bed rest; diuretics; sodium restriction; and paracentesis, if necessary, to relieve ascites. Types V and VII require no treatment except avoidance of strenuous exercise. No treatment is necessary for Types VI and VIII, and no effective treatment exists for Type II.

Additional considerations
When managing a patient with Type I disease, the hospital staff member should:
• advise the patient or parents to include carbohydrate foods containing mainly starch in his diet and to sweeten foods with glucose only (not galactose, fructose, or sucrose).
• teach the patient or parents before discharge how to pass a nasogastric tube, use a pump with alarm capacity, monitor blood glucose with Dextrostix, and recognize symptoms of hypoglycemia.
• watch for and report signs of infection (fever, chills, myalgia) and of hepatic encephalopathy (mental confusion, stupor, asterixis, coma) due to increased blood ammonia levels.

Primary intervention by a health care professional for other types of glycogen storage disease includes:
• *Type II:* explaining test procedures,

such as electromyography, thoroughly.
- *Type III:* instructing the patient to eat a high-protein diet (eggs, nuts, fish, meat, poultry, and cheese).
- *Type IV:* watching for signs of hepatic failure (nausea, vomiting, irregular bowel function, clay-colored stools, upper right quadrant pain, jaundice, dehydration, electrolyte imbalance, edema, and changes in mental status, progressing to coma).

- *Types V through VIII:* explaining the disorder to the patient and family, and helping them accept the limitations imposed by this particular type of glycogen storage disease—care is minimal.

Parents of patients with Types II, III, and IV glycogen storage disease will need reassurance and emotional support. They may also need help in arranging for genetic counseling, if this is appropriate.

Hereditary Fructose Intolerance

Hereditary fructose intolerance is an inability to metabolize fructose. After eliminating fructose from the diet, symptoms subside within weeks. Older children and adults with hereditary fructose intolerance have normal intelligence and apparently normal liver and kidney function.

Causes
Transmitted as an autosomal recessive trait, hereditary fructose intolerance results from a deficiency in the enzyme fructose-1-phosphate aldolase. The enzyme operates at 1% to 10% of its normal biologic activity, thus preventing rapid uptake of fructose by the liver after ingestion of fruit or foods containing cane sugar.

Signs and symptoms
Typically, clinical features of hereditary fructose intolerance appear shortly after dietary introduction of foods containing fructose or sucrose. Symptoms are more severe in infants than in older persons, and include hypoglycemia, nausea, vomiting, pallor, excessive sweating, cyanosis, and tremor. In newborns and young children, continuous ingestion of foods containing fructose may result in failure to thrive, hypoglycemia, jaundice, hyperbilirubinemia, ascites, hepatomegaly, vomiting, dehydration, hypophosphatemia, albuminuria, aminoaciduria, seizures, convulsions, coma, febrile episodes, substernal pain, and anemia.

Diagnosis
 Although a dietary history often suggests hereditary fructose intolerance, a fructose tolerance test (using glucose oxidase or paper chromatography to measure glucose levels) usually confirms it. However, liver biopsy showing a deficiency in fructose-1-phosphate aldolase may be necessary for definitive diagnosis. Supportive values may include decreased serum inorganic phosphorus levels. Urine studies may show fructosuria and albuminuria.

Treatment and additional considerations
Treatment of hereditary fructose intolerance consists of exclusion of fructose and sucrose (cane sugar or table sugar) from the diet. The patient should avoid fruits containing fructose and vegetables containing sucrose (sugar beets, sweet potatoes, and peas), because sucrose is digested to fructose and glucose in the intestine.

The patient and family should be referred for genetic and dietary counseling, as appropriate.

Hyperlipoproteinemia

Hyperlipoproteinemia occurs as five distinct metabolic disorders, all of which may be inherited. Types I through IV are transmitted as autosomal dominant traits; Type V is transmitted as an autosomal recessive trait. About one in five persons with elevated plasma lipids and lipoproteins has hyperlipoproteinemia. It is marked by increased plasma concentrations of one or more lipoproteins. Hyperlipoproteinemia may also occur secondary to other conditions, such as diabetes, pancreatitis, hypothyroidism, or renal disease. This disorder affects lipid transport in serum and produces varied clinical changes, from relatively mild symptoms that can be corrected by dietary management to potentially fatal pancreatitis.

Signs and symptoms

• *Type I:* recurrent attacks of severe abdominal pain similar to pancreatitis, usually preceded by fat intake; abdominal spasm, rigidity, or rebound tenderness; hepatosplenomegaly, with liver or spleen tenderness; papular or eruptive xanthomas (pinkish-yellow cutaneous deposits of fat) over pressure points and extensor surfaces; lipemia retinalis (reddish-white retinal vessels); malaise; anorexia; and fever

• *Type II:* tendinous xanthomas (firm masses) on the Achilles tendons and tendons of the hands and feet, tuberous xanthomas, xanthelasma, juvenile corneal arcus (opaque ring surrounding the corneal periphery), accelerated atherosclerosis and premature coronary artery disease, and recurrent polyarthritis and tenosynovitis.

• *Type III:* peripheral vascular disease manifested by claudication or tuboeruptive xanthomas (soft, inflamed, pedunculated lesions) over the elbows and knees; palmar xanthomas on the hands, particularly fingertips; premature atherosclerosis

• *Type IV:* predisposition to atherosclerosis and early coronary artery disease, exacerbated by excessive calorie intake, obesity, diabetes, and hypertension

• *Type V:* abdominal pain (most common), pancreatitis, peripheral neuropathy, eruptive xanthomas on extensor surfaces of the arms and legs, lipemia retinalis, and hepatosplenomegaly.

Papular xanthomas, cutaneous deposits of fat, are characteristic of Type I hyperlipoproteinemia.

Treatment and prognosis

The first goal is to identify and treat any underlying problem, such as diabetes. If no underlying problem exists, then primary treatment for Types II, III, and IV is dietary management, especially restriction of cholesterol intake, possibly supplemented by drug therapy (cholestyramine, clofibrate, niacin) to lower plasma triglyceride or cholesterol level when diet alone is ineffective.

Type I hyperlipoproteinemia requires long-term weight reduction, with fat intake restricted to less than 40 to 60 g/day. A 20 to 40 g/day medium-chain triglyceride diet may be ordered to supplement calorie intake. The patient should also avoid alcoholic beverages, to de-

TYPES OF HYPERLIPOPROTEINEMIA

TYPE	CAUSES AND INCIDENCE	DIAGNOSTIC FINDINGS
I (Frederickson's, fat-induced hyperlipemia, idiopathic familial)	• Deficient or abnormal lipoprotein lipase, resulting in decreased or absent post-heparin lipolytic activity • Relatively rare	• Chylomicrons, very low density lipoproteins [VLDL], low density lipoproteins [LDL], high density lipoproteins [HDL], in plasma 14 hours or more after last meal • High serum chylomicrons and triglycerides; slightly elevated serum cholesterol; lower serum lipoprotein lipase • Leukocytosis
II (familial hyperbetalipoprotein-emia, essential familial hypercho-lesterolemia)	• Deficient cell surface receptor that regulates LDL degradation and cholesterol synthesis, resulting in increased levels of plasma LDL over joints and pressure points • Onset between ages 10 and 30	• Increased plasma concentrations of LDL • Increased serum cholesterol and triglycerides • Amniocentesis shows increased LDL
III (familial "broad beta" disease, xanthoma tuberosum)	• Unknown underlying defect results in deficient conversion of triglyceride-rich VLDL to LDL • Uncommon; usually occurs after age 20 but can occur earlier in men	• Abnormal serum beta-lipoprotein • Elevated cholesterol and triglycerides • Slightly elevated glucose tolerance • Hyperuricemia
IV (endogenous hypertriglyceridemia, hyperbetalipoprotein-emia)	• Usually occurs secondary to obesity, alcoholism, diabetes, or emotional disorders • Relatively common, especially in middle-aged men	• Elevated VLDL • Abnormal levels of triglycerides in plasma; variable increase in serum • Normal or slightly elevated serum cholesterol • Mildly abnormal glucose tolerance • Family history • Early coronary artery disease
V (mixed hypertriglyceridemia, mixed hyperlipidemia)	• Defective triglyceride clearance causes pancreatitis; usually secondary to another disorder, such as obesity or nephrosis • Uncommon; onset usually occurs in late adolescence or early adulthood	• Chylomicrons in plasma • Elevated plasma VLDL • Elevated serum cholesterol and triglycerides

crease plasma triglycerides. Prognosis is good, with treatment; without treatment, death can result from pancreatitis.

For Type II, dietary management to restore normal lipid levels and decrease the risk of atherosclerosis includes restriction of cholesterol intake to less than 300 mg/day for adults and less than 150 mg/day for children; triglycerides must be restricted to less than 100 mg/day for children and adults. Diet should also be high in polyunsaturated fats. Short-term drug therapy using cholestyramine may lower serum cholesterol levels. For severely affected children, portacaval shunt is a last resort to reduce plasma choles-

terol levels. Prognosis remains poor regardless of treatment; in homozygotes, myocardial infarction usually causes death before age 30.

For Type III, dietary management includes restriction of cholesterol intake to less than 300 mg/day; carbohydrates must also be restricted, while polyunsaturated fats are increased. Clofibrate and niacin help lower blood lipid levels. Weight reduction is helpful. With strict adherence to prescribed diet, prognosis is good.

For Type IV, weight reduction may normalize blood lipid levels without additional treatment. Long-term dietary management includes restricted cholesterol intake, increased polyunsaturated fats, and avoidance of alcoholic beverages. Clofibrate and niacin may lower plasma lipid levels. Prognosis remains uncertain, however, because of predisposition to premature coronary artery disease.

The most effective treatment for Type V is weight reduction and long-term maintenance of a low-fat diet. Alcoholic beverages must be avoided. Niacin (the drug of choice), clofibrate, and a 20 to 40 g/day medium-chain triglyceride diet may prove helpful. Prognosis is uncertain because of the risk of pancreatitis. Increased fat intake may cause recurrent bouts of illness, possibly leading to pseudocyst formation, hemorrhage, and death.

Additional considerations

Care for hyperlipoproteinemia emphasizes careful monitoring for drug side effects and teaching the importance of long-term dietary management. The health care professional should:
• administer cholestyramine before meals or before bedtime (this drug must not be given with other medications); watch for side effects, such as nausea, vomiting, constipation, steatorrhea, rashes, and hyperchloremic acidosis; also watch for malabsorption of other medications and fat-soluble vitamins.
• give clofibrate, as ordered, and watch for side effects, such as cholelithiasis, cardiac arrhythmias, intermittent claudication, thromboembolism, nausea, weight gain (from fluid retention), and myositis.
• *never* administer niacin to patients with active peptic ulcers or hepatic disease, and use with caution in patients with diabetes; watch for side effects in other patients, such as flushing, pruritus, hyperpigmentation, and exacerbation of inactive peptic ulcers.
• urge the patient to adhere to his diet (usually 1,000 to 1,500 calories/day), avoid excess sugar and alcoholic beverages, minimize intake of saturated fats (higher in meats, coconut oil), and increase intake of polyunsaturated fats (vegetable oils).
• instruct the patient, for the 2 weeks preceding serum cholesterol and serum triglyceride tests, to maintain a steady weight and to adhere strictly to the prescribed diet. He should also fast for 12 hours preceding the test.
• instruct women with elevated serum lipids to avoid oral contraceptives or drugs that contain estrogen.

Gaucher's Disease

Gaucher's disease, the most common lipidosis, causes an abnormal accumulation of glucocerebrosides in reticuloendothelial cells. It occurs in three forms: Type I (adult); Type II (infantile); and Type III (juvenile). Type II can prove fatal within 9 months of onset, usually from pulmonary involvement.

Causes and incidence

Gaucher's disease results from an autosomal recessive inheritance, which causes decreased activity of the enzyme glucocerebrosidase. Type I is 30 times more prevalent in eastern Europeans of Jewish ancestry. Types II and III are less common.

Signs and symptoms

Key signs of all types of Gaucher's disease are hepatosplenomegaly and bone lesions. In Type I, bone lesions lead to thinning of cortices, pathologic fractures, collapsed hip joints, and eventually, vertebral compression. Severe episodic pain may develop in the legs, arms, and back but usually not until adolescence. (The adult form of Gaucher's disease is generally diagnosed while the patient is in his teens; the word adult is used loosely here.) Other clinical effects of Type I are fever, abdominal distention (from hypotonicity of the large bowel), respiratory problems (pneumonia or, rarely, cor pulmonale), and easy bruising and bleeding. Anemia and, rarely, pancytopenia may occur. Older patients may develop a yellow pallor and a brown-yellow pigment on the face and legs.

In Type II, motor dysfunction and spasticity occur at age 6 to 7 months. Other signs of the infantile form of Gaucher's disease include abdominal distention, strabismus, muscular hypertonicity, retroflexion of the head, neck rigidity, dysphagia, laryngeal stridor, hyperreflexia, seizures, respiratory distress, and easy bruising and bleeding.

Clinical effects of Type III, after infancy, include convulsions, hypertonicity, strabismus, poor coordination and mental ability, and possibly, easy bruising and bleeding.

Diagnosis

Bone marrow aspiration showing Gaucher's cells, and direct assay of glucocerebrosidase activity, which can be performed on venous blood, confirm this diagnosis. Supportive lab-

oratory results include increased serum acid phosphatase level, decreased platelets and serum iron level, and in Type III, abnormal EEG after infancy.

Treatment and additional considerations

Treatment is mainly supportive, and consists of vitamins, supplemental iron or liver extract to prevent anemia caused by iron deficiency and to alleviate other hematologic problems, blood transfusions for anemia, splenectomy for thrombocytopenia, and strong analgesics for bone pain. Enzyme replacement therapy is still experimental but looks promising. Other treatment includes:

• preventing pathologic fractures in the patient confined to bed by turning him carefully; seeing that he is assisted when getting out of bed or walking if he is ambulatory.

• observing closely for changes in pulmonary status.

• explaining all diagnostic tests and procedures to the patient and/or his parents; helping the patient accept the limitations imposed by this disorder.

• recommending genetic counseling for parents who want to have another child.

Fabry's Disease

Fabry's disease is a rare systemic disorder characterized by glycolipid accumulations in body tissues. Males with this disease usually die of progressive renal failure between ages 30 and 50.

Causes and incidence

Fabry's disease is inherited in an X-linked recessive pattern, which causes a deficiency in the enzyme alphagalactosidase. It affects males most severely; females are carriers but may also get a less virulent form of this disease, characterized by corneal opacities.

Signs and symptoms

In Fabry's disease, purplish telangiectases may appear bilaterally. They usually develop slowly in superficial skin

layers, most conspicuously between the umbilicus and the knees. The key symptom is agonizing, burning pain, which may localize in the palms and soles, often radiating to the thighs, upper arms, and other parts of the body. Exercise, fatigue, stress, or a rapid change in climate usually triggers such pain. Severity of pain may increase with age. Associated abnormalities may be:

• *cardiovascular:* cardiomegaly, congestive heart failure, angina, myocardial ischemia and infarction, and thromboses that may lead to cerebrovascular accident

• *ophthalmic:* corneal opacities, conjunctival and retinal vascular tortuosity, and upper eyelid edema

• *respiratory:* wheezing, chronic bronchitis, and dyspnea, with alveolar capillary block (from abnormal lipid deposits)

• *gastrointestinal:* recurrent abdominal pain, with postprandial cramping; chronic diarrhea, or alternating diarrhea and constipation

• *renal:* polyuria and chronic renal failure that may lead to hypertension

• *other:* in adults, lymphedema of the legs.

Death usually results from renal, cardiac, or cerebral complications, or from other vascular diseases.

Diagnosis

Diagnosis is based on a positive family history and typical skin lesions, when present. Bone marrow biopsy may show foamy, lipid-laden macrophages. Slit-lamp examination reveals corneal opacities. Low plasma alpha-galactosidase levels support the diagnosis.

Treatment and additional considerations

Treatment is symptomatic, with low maintenance dosages of phenytoin or carbamazepine for pain relief. Renal transplantation is sometimes effective. Parents of children with Fabry's disease will need emotional support; they may want genetic counseling, and should consider prenatal studies during future pregnancies.

Amyloidosis

Amyloidosis is a rare, chronic disease resulting in the accumulation of an abnormal fibrous protein (amyloid), which infiltrates body organs and soft tissues. Amyloidosis occurs in two forms: primary amyloidosis occurs in the absence of an underlying disorder and most often affects the tongue, heart, gastrointestinal tract, and nerves; secondary amyloidosis coexists with other disorders—often those that produce chronic inflammation—and frequently affects the kidneys, liver, and spleen. Although prognosis varies with the site of involvement, amyloidosis results in permanent—even life-threatening—organ damage.

Causes and incidence

Primary amyloidosis is sometimes familial, especially in persons of Portuguese ancestry. Secondary amyloidosis usually occurs in conjunction with tuberculosis, chronic infection, rheumatoid arthritis, multiple myeloma, Hodgkin's disease, paraplegia, and familial Mediterranean fever (brucellosis). It may also accompany the aging process.

In amyloidosis, accumulation and infiltration of amyloid, a pathologic protein distinct from any other known mammalian protein, leads to organ and soft-tissue damage by producing pressure and causing atrophy of nearby cells. Reticuloendothelial cell dysfunction and abnormal immunoglobulin synthesis occur in some types of amyloidosis. In the United States, evidence of amyloidosis on autopsy is 0.5%, but true incidence is difficult to determine.

Signs and symptoms

Amyloidosis produces dysfunction, primarily of the kidneys, heart, and gastrointestinal tract, and occasionally, the liver.

• *Kidneys:* Renal involvement appears in most patients with secondary amyloidosis and in about half with the primary form. The primary symptom is proteinuria, leading to the nephrotic syndrome and eventual renal failure. Hypertension usually does not develop.

• *Heart:* Cardiac involvement occurs in

primary amyloidosis, in certain familial forms, and in elderly patients. Amyloidosis often causes intractable congestive heart failure.

• *Gastrointestinal tract:* Gastrointestinal amyloidosis may produce stiffness and enlargement of the tongue, making enunciation difficult. In addition, it may decrease intestinal motility, and produce malabsorption, bleeding, infiltration of blood vessel walls, abdominal pain, constipation, and diarrhea. Tumorlike amyloid deposits may occur in all portions of this system. Chronic malabsorption may lead to malnutrition and predispose to infection.

• *Liver:* Hepatic amyloidosis is rare and usually coexists with other forms of this disease. It generally produces liver enlargement, often with azotemia, anemia, albuminuria, and mild jaundice.

Diagnosis

Since most test results are nonspecific, diagnosis depends on histologic examination of tissue biopsy specimen, using a polarizing or electron microscope. In suspected amyloidosis, rectal mucosa biopsy is the best screening test, since it's less hazardous than kidney or liver biopsy. Depending on the location of amyloid deposits, other biopsy sites include the gingiva, skin, and nerves.

In cardiac amyloidosis, other findings include faint heart sounds, and an EKG demonstrating low voltage and conduction or rhythm abnormalities that may resemble those of a myocardial infarction. In hepatic amyloidosis, liver function studies are generally normal, except for slightly elevated serum alkaline phosphatase levels.

Treatment

In secondary amyloidosis, the goal of therapy is correction of the underlying disorder. Treatment is mainly supportive, but may include corticosteroids and other immunosuppressives to minimize inflammation. Transplantation may be useful for amyloidosis-induced renal

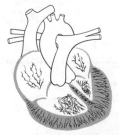

AMYLOIDOSIS OF THE HEART

Amyloid deposits in the subendocardium, endocardium, and myocardium often cause congestive heart failure.

failure. Patients with cardiac amyloidosis require conservative treatment; digitalis must be given with caution, since these patients are apt to develop dangerous arrhythmias. Malnutrition caused by malabsorption in end-stage gastrointestinal involvement may require total parenteral nutrition (TPN).

Additional considerations

The health care professional caring for a patient with amyloidosis should:

• maintain nutrition and fluid balance parenterally, if necessary; give analgesics, as ordered, to relieve intestinal pain; control constipation or diarrhea, as ordered; manage infection and fever, as indicated.

• provide good mouth care for the patient with tongue involvement; refer the patient for speech therapy, if needed, and provide an alternate method of communication if he can't talk.

• assess airway patency when the tongue is involved; prevent respiratory tract compromise by gentle and adequate suctioning; keep a tracheotomy tray at bedside in case of respiratory arrest.

• properly position the patient when long-term bed rest is necessary, and turn him often to prevent decubitus ulcers; perform range-of-motion exercises to prevent contractures.

• provide psychologic support. Patience and understanding will help the patient cope with this chronic illness.

Niemann-Pick Disease

Niemann-Pick disease is a rare disorder resulting in abnormal accumulation of sphingomyelin in reticuloendothelial cells. It occurs in five different phenotypes (Types A, B, C, D, and E), each characterized by slightly different symptoms. Except for Type B, each type results in progressive and eventually fatal CNS involvement. Type A (the most common) is generally fatal by age 3; Type C is usually fatal between ages 5 and 15.

Causes and incidence

Niemann-Pick disease is an autosomal recessive disorder. Types A, B, C, and E result from an inherited defect in sphingomyelinase activity; the highest incidence occurs among persons of eastern European Jewish ancestry. Type D occurs most often in western Nova Scotia; the cause is unknown.

Signs and symptoms

• *Type A* becomes clinically apparent at about age 6 months, with hepatosplenomegaly, abdominal distention, thin arms and legs, feeding difficulties, brownish-yellow skin coloration, cherry spots in the macula of the eye, motor function loss, and progressive intellectual impairment. It rapidly progresses to motor deterioration and death.

• *Type B* manifests as early as age 6 months, with hepatosplenomegaly and, from accumulation of sphingomyelin in lung tissue, pneumonia. CNS involvement does not occur, and prognosis is good.

• *Type C* appears after age 2, with progressive loss of mental function, moderate ataxia, grand mal seizures, loss of coordination, hypertonia, and hyperactive reflexes. It is usually fatal by age 15.

• *Type D* commonly begins between ages 2 and 4, with hepatomegaly, impaired coordination and intellectual function, grand mal and petit mal seizures, and jaundice.

• *Type E,* the rarest form, occurs in adults, and is marked by cherry spots in the macula of the eye, and hepatosplenomegaly.

Diagnosis

Diagnosis is based on the presence of hepatosplenomegaly, and the results of enzyme studies or bone marrow biopsy. Test results vary according to type:

• *Types A, B, and C:* Skin biopsy shows low sphingomyelinase activity in cultured skin fibroblasts, while *Types D and E* have normal levels. *Type E* also has an altered isoenzyme pattern of sphingomyelinase.

• *Type A:* Bone marrow and tissue biopsies demonstrate enlarged foamy Niemann-Pick cells in bone marrow, spleen, lymph nodes, adrenal medulla, and lung alveoli.

• *Type B:* Chest X-ray reveals diffusely infiltrative lung fields; bone marrow biopsy discloses birefractory foam cells in bone marrow.

• *Types C and E:* Bone marrow biopsy shows foamy histiocytes in bone marrow.

• *Type D:* Tissue biopsy shows foam cells in spleen and lymph nodes.

Prenatal diagnosis is possible with amniocentesis.

Treatment and additional considerations

Treatment is supportive and symptomatic. Signs of pneumonia are important. Antibiotic therapy for classic Niemann-Pick pneumonia is usually ineffective, because such pneumonia stems from extensive infiltration of Niemann-Pick cells, not from bacterial invasion. Parents of a child with Niemann-Pick disease should receive genetic counseling before having another child.

Porphyrias

Porphyrias are metabolic disorders that affect the biosynthesis of heme (a component of hemoglobin) and cause excessive production and excretion of porphyrins or their precursors. Porphyrins, which are present in all protoplasm, figure prominently in energy storage and utilization. Porphyrias are marked by skin lesions, neuropathy, acute abdominal pain, and extreme sensitivity to sunlight. Classification of porphyrias depends on the site of excessive porphyrin production, and may be erythropoietic (erythroid cells in bone marrow), hepatic (in the liver), or erythrohepatic (in bone marrow and liver). An acute episode of intermittent hepatic porphyria may cause fatal respiratory paralysis. In the other forms of porphyrias, prognosis is good with proper treatment.

Causes

Porphyrias are inherited as autosomal dominant traits, except for Günther's disease (autosomal recessive trait) and toxic-acquired porphyria (usually from ingestion of or exposure to lead).

Signs and symptoms

Porphyrias are generally marked by photosensitivity, acute abdominal pain, and neuropathy. Photosensitivity results from the photodynamic action of porphyrins deposited in the skin. Abdominal pain and neuropathy result from systemic accumulation of porphyrin precursors.

Hepatic porphyrias may produce a complex syndrome marked by distinct neurologic and hepatic dysfunction.

• Neurologic symptoms include chronic brain syndrome, peripheral neuropathy and autonomic effects, tachycardia, labile hypertension, severe colicky lower abdominal pain, and constipation.

• During an acute attack, fever, leukocytosis, and fluid and electrolyte imbalance may occur.

• Structural hepatic effects include fatty infiltration of the liver, hepatic siderosis, and focal hepatocellular necrosis.

• Skin lesions (not present in all patients) may cause itching and burning, erythema, and altered pigmentation and edema in areas exposed to light. Some chronic skin changes include milia (white papules on the dorsal aspects of the hands), and hirsutism on the upper cheeks and periorbital areas.

Diagnosis

 Generally, diagnosis requires screening tests for porphyrins or their precursors (such as aminolevulinic acid [ALA] and porphobilinogen [PBG]) in urine, stool, or blood, or occasionally, skin biopsy. Urinary lead level of 0.2 mg/ liter confirms toxic-acquired porphyria.

Other laboratory values may include increased serum iron levels in porphyria cutanea tarda; leukocytosis, SIADH, and elevated bilirubin and alkaline phosphatase in acute intermittent porphyria.

Treatment and additional considerations

Effective treatment must relieve pain, manage skin lesions, reduce photosensitivity, minimize acute exacerbations, and reduce excretion of porphyrins and their precursors. To minimize the effects of porphyrias and control flare-ups, the health care professional should:

• warn against exposure to the sun; suggest protective clothing, and a sunscreen, such as 10% *p*-aminobenzoic acid; administer beta-carotene to reduce photosensitivity.

• encourage a high-carbohydrate diet (the "glucose effect") to decrease urinary excretion of ALA and PBG, with restricted fluid intake (to inhibit release of ADH).

• warn the patient to avoid precipitating factors, especially alcohol, barbiturates, estrogens, and fasting.

CLINICAL VARIANTS OF PORPHYRIA

PORPHYRIA	SIGNS AND SYMPTOMS	TREATMENT
ERYTHROPOIETIC PORPHYRIA		
Günther's disease • Usual onset before age 5	• Red urine (earliest, most characteristic sign); severe cutaneous photosensitivity, leading to vesicular or bullous eruptions on exposed areas, and eventual scarring and ulceration • Hypertrichosis • Brown or red-stained teeth • Splenomegaly, hemolytic anemia	• Anti-inflammatory ointments, such as 1% hydrocortisone, for dermatitis • Prednisone to reverse anemia • Transfusion of packed red cells to inhibit erythropoiesis and reduce level of excreted porphyrins • Beta-carotene to reduce photosensitivity • Splenectomy for hemolytic anemia
ERYTHROHEPATIC PORPHYRIA		
Protoporphyria • Usually affects children • Occurs most often in males	• Photosensitive dermatitis • Hemolytic anemia • Chronic hepatic disease	• Avoidance of precipitating factors
Toxic-acquired porphyria • Usually affects children • Significant mortality	• Acute colicky pain • Anorexia, nausea, vomiting • Neuromuscular weakness • Behavioral changes • Convulsions, coma	• Chlorpromazine I.M. (25 mg every 4 to 6 hours during an acute attack) to relieve pain and G.I. symptoms • Avoidance of further exposure to lead
HEPATIC PORPHYRIA		
Acute intermittent porphyria • Most common form • Affects females most often, usually between ages 15 and 40	• Colicky abdominal pain with fever, general malaise, and hypertension • Peripheral neuritis, behavioral changes, possibly leading to frank psychosis • Respiratory paralysis can occur.	• Chlorpromazine I.M. (25 mg every 4 to 6 hours) to relieve abdominal pain, and control psychic abnormalities • Avoidance of barbiturates, infections, alcohol, and fasting • High-carbohydrate diet
Variegate porphyria • Usual onset between ages 30 and 50 • Occurs almost exclusively among South African Caucasians • Affects males and females equally	• Skin lesions, extremely fragile skin in exposed areas • Hypertrichosis • Hyperpigmentation • Abdominal pain during acute attack • Neuropsychiatric manifestations	• High-carbohydrate diet • Cholestyramine P.O. (4 g, three times a day) to relieve skin lesions • Avoidance of sunlight; wearing protective clothing when avoidance isn't possible
Porphyria cutanea tarda • Most frequent in men aged 40 to 60 • Highest incidence in South Africans	• Facial pigmentation • Red-brown urine • Photosensitive dermatitis • Hypertrichosis	• Avoidance of precipitating factors, such as alcohol and estrogens • Phlebotomy at 2-week intervals to lower serum iron level
Hereditary coproporphyria • Rare • Affects males and females equally	• Asymptomatic or mild neurologic, abdominal, or psychiatric symptoms	• High-carbohydrate diet • Avoidance of barbiturates

HOMEOSTATIC IMBALANCE

Potassium Imbalance

Potassium, a cation that is the dominant cellular electrolyte, facilitates contraction of both skeletal and smooth muscles—including myocardial contraction—and figures prominently in nerve impulse conduction, acid-base balance, enzyme action, and cell membrane function. Because serum potassium level has such a narrow range (3.5 to 5.5 mEq/liter), a slight deviation in either direction can produce profound clinical consequences. Paradoxically, both hypokalemia (potassium deficiency) and hyperkalemia (potassium excess) can lead to muscle weakness and flaccid paralysis, because both create an ionic imbalance in neuromuscular tissue excitability. Both conditions also diminish excitability and conduction rate of the heart muscle, which may lead to cardiac arrest.

Causes

Since many foods contain potassium, hypokalemia rarely results from a dietary deficiency. Instead, potassium loss results from:

• *excessive gastrointestinal or urinary losses,* such as vomiting, gastric suction, diarrhea, dehydration, anorexia, or chronic laxative abuse.

• *trauma* (injury, burns, or surgery), in which damaged cells release potassium, which enters serum or extracellular fluid, to be excreted in the urine.

• *chronic renal disease,* with tubular potassium wasting, and potassium-wasting diuretics and steroids, such as cortisone.

• *acid-base imbalances,* which cause potassium shifting into cells without true depletion. Prolonged acidosis or alkalosis results in urinary losses and leads to hypokalemia.

• *potassium-free I.V. therapy.*

• *hyperglycemia,* causing osmotic diuresis and glycosuria.

• *Cushing's syndrome, primary hyperaldosteronism,* and *excessive ingestion of licorice* (contains glyceric acid, a substance capable of an aldosterone effect).

Hyperkalemia results from the kidneys' inability to excrete excessive amounts of potassium infused intravenously or administered orally; from decreased urine output, renal dysfunction or failure; or the use of potassium-sparing diuretics, such as triamterene, by patients with renal disease. It may also result from any injuries or conditions that release cellular potassium or favor its retention, such as burns, crushing injuries, failing renal function, adrenal gland insufficiency, dehydration, or diabetic acidosis.

Diagnosis

• *Hypokalemia:* serum potassium levels < 3.5 mEq/liter; urine potassium levels > 100 mEq/24 hours.

• *Hyperkalemia:* serum potassium levels > 5.5 mEq/liter; urine potassium levels < 40 mEq/24-hour urine.

Additional tests may be necessary to determine the underlying cause.

Treatment

For hypokalemia, replacement therapy with potassium chloride (I.V. or P.O.) is the primary treatment. When diuresis is necessary, spironolactone, a potassium-sparing diuretic, may be administered concurrently with a potassium-wasting diuretic to minimize potassium loss. Hypokalemia can be prevented by giving a maintenance dose of potassium I.V. to patients who may not take anything by mouth and to others predisposed to potassium loss.

For hyperkalemia, rapid infusion of 10% calcium gluconate decreases myocardial irritability and temporarily prevents cardiac arrest but doesn't correct serum potassium excess; it's also contraindicated in patients receiving digitalis. As an emergency measure, sodium bicarbonate I.V. increases pH and causes potassium to shift back into the cells. Insulin and 10% to 50% glucose I.V. also move potassium back into cells, but their effect lasts only 6 hours; repeated use is less effective. Sodium polystyrene sulfonate with 70% sorbitol produces exchange of sodium ions for potassium ions in the intestine. Hemodialysis or peritoneal dialysis also aids in removal of excess potassium.

Additional considerations

When managing the patient with hypokalemia, the hospital staff member should:
• check serum potassium and other electrolyte levels often in patients apt to develop potassium imbalance and in those requiring potassium replacement—they are vulnerable to overcorrection to hyperkalemia.
• assess intake and output carefully (the kidneys excrete 80% to 90% of ingested potassium); never give supplementary potassium to a patient whose urinary output is below 600 ml/day; measure gastrointestinal loss from suctioning or vomiting.
• dilute oral potassium supplements in 4 oz (120 ml) or more of water or fluid to reduce irritation of gastric and small bowel mucosa; determine the patient's chloride level; give a potassium chloride supplement, as ordered, if the level is low; administer potassium gluconate, as ordered, if it's normal.
• give potassium I.V. only after it is diluted in solution—potassium is very irritating to vascular, subcutaneous, and fatty tissues, and may cause phlebitis or tissue necrosis if it infiltrates; infuse potassium slowly (no more than 20 mEq/liter/hour) to prevent hyperkalemia; *never* administer by I.V. push or bolus—it may cause cardiac arrest.

CLINICAL FEATURES OF POTASSIUM IMBALANCE

DYSFUNCTION	HYPOKALEMIA	HYPERKALEMIA
Cardiovascular	• Dizziness, hypotension, arrhythmias, EKG changes (flattened T waves, elevated U waves, depressed ST segment), cardiac arrest (with serum potassium levels < 2.5 mEq/liter)	• Tachycardia and later bradycardia, EKG changes (tented and elevated T waves, widened QRS, prolonged PR interval, flattened or absent P waves, depressed ST segment), cardiac arrest (with levels > 7.0 mEq/liter)
Gastrointestinal	• Nausea and vomiting, anorexia, diarrhea, abdominal distention, paralytic ileus or decreased peristalsis	• Nausea, diarrhea, abdominal cramps
Musculoskeletal	• Muscle weakness and fatigue, leg cramps	• Muscle weakness, flaccid paralysis
Genitourinary	• Polyuria	• Oliguria, anuria
CNS	• Malaise, irritability, confusion, mental depression, speech changes, decreased reflexes, respiratory paralysis	• Hyperreflexia progressing to weakness, numbness, tingling, and flaccid paralysis
Acid-base balance	• Metabolic alkalosis	• Metabolic acidosis

EKG CHANGES IN POTASSIUM IMBALANCE

HYPOKALEMIA

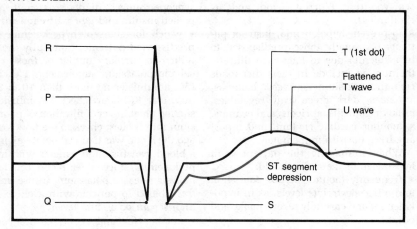

KEY

■ EKG tracing in hypo- and hyperkalemia

■ EKG tracing in normal potassium balance

HYPERKALEMIA

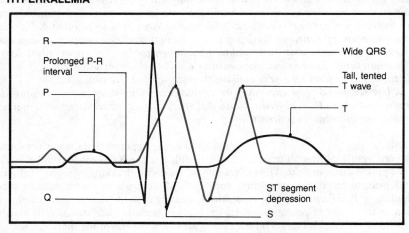

• carefully monitor patients receiving digitalis, since hypokalemia enhances the action of digitalis and may produce signs of digitalis toxicity (anorexia, nausea, vomiting, blurred vision, and arrhythmias).

• to prevent hypokalemia, instruct patients (especially those predisposed to hypokalemia due to long-term diuretic therapy) to include in their diet foods rich in potassium—oranges, bananas, tomatoes, dark green leafy vegetables, milk, dried fruits, apricots, and peanuts.

• monitor cardiac rhythm, and report any irregularities immediately.

When managing the patient with hyperkalemia, the staffer should:

• frequently monitor serum potassium and other electrolyte levels, as in hypokalemia, and carefully record intake and output.

• administer sodium polystyrene sulfonate orally or rectally (by retention enema); watch for signs of hypokalemia with prolonged use and for clinical effects of hypoglycemia (muscle weakness, syncope, hunger, diaphoresis) with repeated insulin and glucose treatment.

• watch for signs of hyperkalemia in predisposed patients, especially those with poor urinary output or those receiving potassium supplements P.O. or I.V.; administer no more than 10 to 20 mEq/liter KCl/hour; check I.V. infusion site for phlebitis or infiltration of potassium into tissues; check to see how long ago the blood was donated before giving a blood transfusion to patients with hyperkalemia, since older blood cell hemolysis releases potassium; infuse only *fresh* blood to patients with average to high serum potassium levels.

• monitor for and report cardiac arrhythmias.

Sodium Imbalance

Sodium is the major cation (90%) in extracellular fluid; potassium, the major cation in intracellular fluid. During repolarization, the sodium-potassium pump continually shifts sodium into the cells and potassium out of the cells; during depolarization, it does the reverse. Sodium cation functions include maintaining tonicity and concentration of extracellular fluid, acid-base balance (reabsorption of sodium ion and excretion of hydrogen ion), nerve conduction and neuromuscular function, glandular secretion, and water balance. Although the body requires only 2 to 4 g of sodium daily, most Americans consume 6 to 10 g daily (mostly sodium chloride, as table salt), excreting excess sodium through the kidneys and skin.

A low-sodium diet or excessive use of diuretics may induce hyponatremia (decreased serum sodium concentration); dehydration may induce hypernatremia (increased serum sodium concentration).

Causes
Hyponatremia can result from:

• excessive gastrointestinal loss of water and electrolytes due to vomiting, suctioning, or diarrhea; excessive perspiration or fever; use of potent diuretics; or tap-water enemas. When such losses decrease circulating fluid volume, increased secretion of antidiuretic hormone (ADH) promotes maximum water reabsorption, which further dilutes serum sodium. These factors are especially likely to cause hyponatremia when combined with too much free-water intake.

• excessive drinking of water, infusion of I.V. dextrose in water without other solutes, malnutrition or starvation, and a low-sodium diet, usually in combination with one of the other causes.

• trauma, surgery (wound drainage), or burns, which cause sodium to shift into damaged cells.

• adrenal gland insufficiency (Addison's disease) or hypoaldosteronism.

CLINICAL EFFECTS OF SODIUM IMBALANCE

DYSFUNCTION	HYPONATREMIA	HYPERNATREMIA
CNS	• Anxiety, headaches, muscle twitching and weakness, convulsions	• Fever, agitation, restlessness, convulsions
Cardiovascular	• Hypotension; tachycardia; with severe deficit, vasomotor collapse, thready pulse	• Hypertension, tachycardia, pitting edema, excessive weight gain
Gastrointestinal	• Nausea, vomiting, abdominal cramps	• Rough, dry tongue; intense thirst
Genitourinary	• Oliguria or anuria	• Oliguria
Respiratory	• Cyanosis with severe deficiency	• Dyspnea, respiratory arrest, and death (from dramatic rise in osmotic pressure)
Cutaneous	• Cold clammy skin, decreased skin turgor	• Flushed skin; dry, sticky mucous membranes

• syndrome of inappropriate antidiuretic hormone (SIADH) from brain tumor, cerebrovascular accident, pulmonary disease, or neoplasm with ectopic ADH production. Certain drugs such as chlorpropamide and clofibrate may produce an SIADH-like syndrome.

Causes of hypernatremia include:
• decreased water intake. When severe vomiting and diarrhea cause water loss that exceeds sodium loss, serum sodium levels rise, but overall extracellular fluid volume decreases.
• excess adrenocortical hormones, as in Cushing's syndrome.
• ADH deficiency (diabetes insipidus).
• salt intoxication (less common), which may follow excessive ingestion of table salt or seawater (as in near-drowning).

Signs and symptoms
Sodium imbalance has profound physiologic effects and can induce severe CNS, cardiovascular, and gastrointestinal abnormalities. For example, hyponatremia may cause renal dysfunction or, if serum sodium loss is abrupt or severe, may result in seizures; hypernatremia may produce pulmonary edema, circulatory disorders, and decreased level of consciousness.

Diagnosis
Hyponatremia is defined as serum sodium level less than 135 mEq/liter; hypernatremia, as serum sodium level greater than 145 mEq/liter. However, serum sodium values alone do not necessarily confirm true sodium excess or deficit. Additional laboratory studies determine etiology and differentiate between a real deficit and an apparent deficit due to sodium shift or to hyper- or hypovolemia. In true hyponatremia, supportive values include urine sodium greater than 100 mEq/24 hours, with low serum osmolality and extracellular fluid retention; in true hypernatremia, urine sodium is less than 40 mEq/24 hours, with high serum osmolality.

Treatment
Therapy for mild hyponatremia usually consists of restricted free-water intake when it is due to hemodilution, SIADH, or conditions such as congestive heart failure, cirrhosis of the liver, and renal failure. If fluid restriction alone fails to normalize serum sodium levels, demeclocycline or lithium, which blocks ADH action in the renal tubules, can be used to promote water excretion. In extremely rare instances of severe symptomatic hyponatremia, when serum sodium levels fall below 110 mEq/liter, treatment may include infusion of 3% or 5% saline solution and concomitant furosemide. Treatment with saline infusion requires

careful monitoring of venous pressure to prevent potentially fatal circulatory overload. The aim of treatment of secondary hyponatremia is to correct the underlying disorder.

Primary treatment of hypernatremia is administration of saltfree solutions (such as dextrose in water) to return serum sodium levels to normal, followed by infusion of 0.45% sodium chloride to prevent hyponatremia. Other measures include a sodium-restricted diet and discontinuation of drugs that promote sodium retention.

Additional considerations

When managing the patient with hyponatremia, the hospital staff member should:
• watch for and report extremely low serum sodium and accompanying serum chloride levels; monitor urine specific gravity and other laboratory results; record fluid intake and output accurately, and weigh the patient daily.
• watch closely for signs of hypervolemia (dyspnea, rales, engorged neck or hand veins) during administration of isosmolar or hyperosmolar saline solution; report conditions that may cause excessive sodium loss—diaphoresis or prolonged diarrhea or vomiting, and severe burns.
• refer the patient on maintenance dosage of diuretics to a dietitian for instruction about dietary sodium intake.
• administer isosmolar solutions to prevent hyponatremia.

When managing the patient with hypernatremia, the staffer should:
• measure serum sodium levels every 6 hours or at least daily; monitor vital signs for changes, especially for rising pulse rate; watch for signs of hypervolemia, especially in the patient receiving I.V. fluids.
• record fluid intake and output accurately, checking for body fluid loss; weigh the patient daily.
• obtain a drug history to check for drugs that promote sodium retention.
• explain the importance of sodium restriction, and teach the patient how to plan a low-sodium diet; closely monitor the serum sodium levels of high-risk patients.

Calcium Imbalance

Calcium plays an indispensable role in cell permeability, formation of bones and teeth, blood coagulation, transmission of nerve impulses, and normal muscle contraction. Nearly all (99%) of the body's calcium is found in the bones. The remaining 1% exists in ionized form in serum, and it is the maintenance of the 1% of ionized calcium in the serum that is critical to healthy neurologic function. The parathyroid glands regulate ionized calcium and determine its resorption into bone, absorption from the gastrointestinal mucosa, and excretion in urine and feces. Severe calcium imbalance requires emergency treatment, since a deficiency (hypocalcemia) can lead to tetany and convulsions; excess (hypercalcemia), to cardiac arrhythmias.

Causes

Common causes of hypocalcemia include:
• *inadequate intake of calcium and vitamin D*, in which inadequate levels of vitamin D inhibit intestinal absorption of calcium.
• *hypoparathyroidism* as a result of injury, disease, or surgery that decreases or eliminates secretion of parathyroid hormone (PTH), which is necessary for calcium absorption and normal serum calcium levels.
• *malabsorption or loss of calcium from the gastrointestinal tract,* caused by increased intestinal motility from severe diarrhea or laxative abuse. Malabsorption of calcium from the gastrointestinal

tract can also result from inadequate levels of vitamin D or PTH, or a reduction in gastric acidity, decreasing the solubility of calcium salts.

• *severe infections or burns,* in which diseased and burned tissue traps calcium from the extracellular fluid.

• *overcorrection of acidosis,* resulting in alkalosis, which causes decreased ionized calcium and induces symptoms of hypocalcemia.

• *pancreatic insufficiency,* which may cause malabsorption of calcium and subsequent calcium loss in feces. In pancreatitis, participation of calcium ions in saponification contributes to calcium loss.

• *renal failure,* resulting in excessive excretion of calcium secondary to increased retention of phosphate.

• *hypomagnesemia,* which causes decreased PTH secretion and blocks the peripheral action of that hormone.

Causes of hypercalcemia include:

• *Hyperparathyroidism* increases serum calcium levels by promoting calcium absorption from the intestine, resorption from bone, and reabsorption from the kidneys.

• *Hypervitaminosis D* can promote increased absorption of calcium from the intestine.

• *Tumors* raise serum calcium levels by destroying bone or by releasing PTH or a PTH-like substance, osteoclast-activating factor, prostaglandins, and perhaps, a vitamin D–like sterol.

• *Multiple fractures and prolonged immobilization* release bone calcium and raise the serum calcium level.

• *Multiple myeloma* promotes loss of calcium from bone.

Other causes include milk-alkali syndrome, sarcoidosis, hyperthyroidism, adrenal insufficiency, thiazide diuretics, and loss of serum albumin secondary to renal disease.

Signs and symptoms

Calcium deficit causes nerve fiber irritability and repetitive muscle spasms. Consequently, characteristic symptoms of hypocalcemia include perioral paresthesia, twitching, carpopedal spasm, tetany, seizures, and possibly, cardiac arrhythmias. Chvostek's sign and Trousseau's sign are reliable indicators of hypocalcemia.

SYMPTOMS OF CALCIUM IMBALANCE

DYSFUNCTION	HYPOCALCEMIA	HYPERCALCEMIA
CNS	• Anxiety, irritability, twitching around mouth, laryngospasm, convulsions, Chvostek's sign, Trousseau's sign	• Drowsiness, lethargy, headaches, depression or apathy, irritability, confusion
Musculoskeletal	• Paresthesia (tingling and numbness of the fingers), tetany or painful tonic muscle spasms, facial spasms, abdominal cramps, muscle cramps, spasmodic contractions	• Weakness, muscle flaccidity, bone pain, pathologic fractures
Cardiovascular	• Arrhythmias, hypotension	• Signs of heart block, cardiac arrest in systole, hypertension
Gastrointestinal	• Increased GI motility, diarrhea	• Anorexia, nausea, vomiting, constipation, dehydration, polydipsia
Other	• Blood-clotting abnormalities	• Renal polyuria, flank pain, and eventually, azotemia

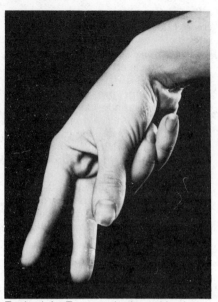

To check for Trousseau's sign, a blood pressure cuff is applied to the patient's arm. A carpopedal spasm that causes thumb adduction and phalangeal extension, as shown, confirms tetany.

Clinical effects of hypercalcemia include lethargy, anorexia, constipation, nausea, vomiting, dehydration, polydipsia, and polyuria. Severe hypercalcemia (serum levels that exceed 5.7 mEq/liter) may produce cardiac arrhythmias and, eventually, coma.

Diagnosis

Serum calcium level less than 4.5 mEq/liter confirms hypocalcemia; more than 5.5 mEq/liter, hypercalcemia. (However, since one half of serum calcium is bound to albumin, changes in serum protein must be considered when interpreting serum calcium levels.) The Sulkowitch urine test shows increased calcium precipitation in hypercalcemia. In hypocalcemia, EKG reveals lengthened Q-T interval, prolonged ST segment, and arrhythmias; in hypercalcemia, it may reveal shortened Q-T interval, and heart block.

Treatment

Treatment varies, and requires correction of the acute imbalance, followed by maintenance therapy and correction of the underlying cause. Mild hypocalcemia may require nothing more than an adjustment in diet to allow adequate intake of calcium, vitamin D, and protein, possibly with oral calcium supplements. Acute hypocalcemia is an emergency that needs immediate correction by I.V. administration of calcium gluconate or calcium chloride. Chronic hypocalcemia also requires vitamin D supplements to facilitate gastrointestinal absorption of calcium. To correct mild deficiency states, the amounts of vitamin D in most multivitamin preparations are adequate. For severe deficiency, vitamin D is used in three forms: ergocalciferol (vitamin D_2), cholecalciferol (vitamin D_3), and dihydrotachysterol, a synthetic form of vitamin D_3.

Treatment of hypercalcemia primarily eliminates serum calcium excess through hydration with normal saline solution, which promotes calcium excretion in urine. Loop diuretics, such as ethacrynic acid and furosemide, also promote calcium excretion. (Thiazide diuretics are contraindicated in hypercalcemia, because they inhibit calcium excretion.) Corticosteroids, such as prednisone and hydrocortisone, are helpful in treating sarcoidosis, hypervitaminosis D, and certain tumors. Mithramycin can also lower serum calcium level and is especially effective against hypercalcemia secondary to certain tumors. Calcitonin may also be helpful in certain instances. Sodium phosphate solution administered P.O. or by retention enema promotes deposition of calcium in bone and inhibits its absorption from the gastrointestinal tract.

Additional considerations

Patients at risk for hypocalcemia include those receiving massive transfusions of citrated blood, and those with chronic diarrhea, severe infections, and insufficient dietary intake of calcium and protein (especially the elderly).

When treating a patient with hypocalcemia, the hospital staff member should:
• monitor serum calcium levels every 12 to 24 hours, and report a calcium deficit less than 4.5 mEq/liter immediately; check pH level frequently when giving calcium supplements, since an alkalotic state that exceeds 7.45 pH inhibits calcium ionization; check for Trousseau's and Chvostek's signs.
• administer calcium gluconate in 5% dextrose in water (*never* in saline solution, which encourages renal calcium loss); avoid adding calcium gluconate to solutions containing bicarbonate, since it will precipitate; watch for anorexia, nausea, and vomiting when administering calcium solutions—possible signs of overcorrection to hypercalcemia.
• watch for abdominal discomfort if the patient is receiving calcium chloride.
• monitor the patient closely for a possible drug interaction if he's receiving digitalis with large doses of oral calcium supplements; watch for signs of digitalis toxicity (anorexia, nausea, vomiting, yellow vision, and cardiac arrhythmias); administer oral calcium supplements 1 to 1½ hours after meals or with milk.

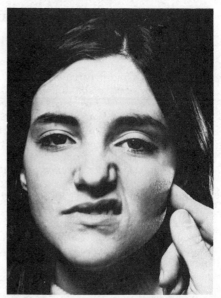

To check for Chvostek's sign, the facial nerve above the manibular angle, adjacent to the ear lobe, is tapped. A facial muscle spasm that causes the patient's upper lip to twitch, as shown, confirms tetany.

• provide a quiet, stress-free environment for the patient with tetany; observe seizure precautions for patients with severe hypocalcemia that may lead to convulsions.
• advise all patients—especially the elderly—to prevent hypocalcemia by eating foods rich in calcium, vitamin D, and protein, such as fortified milk and cheese; explain how important calcium is for normal bone formation and blood coagulation; discourage chronic use of laxatives; warn hypocalcemic patients not to overuse antacids, since these may aggravate the condition.

If the patient has hypercalcemia, the staffer should:
• monitor serum calcium levels frequently; watch for cardiac arrhythmias if serum calcium level exceeds 5.7 mEq/liter; increase fluid intake to dilute calcium in serum and urine, and to prevent renal damage and dehydration; watch for signs of congestive heart failure in patients receiving normal saline solution

diuresis therapy.
• administer loop diuretics (not thiazide diuretics), as ordered; monitor intake and output, and check urine for renal calculi and acidity; provide acid-ash drinks, such as cranberry or prune juice, since calcium salts are more soluble in acid than in alkali.
• check EKG and vital signs frequently; watch for signs of toxicity in the patient receiving digitalis, such as anorexia, nausea, vomiting, and bradycardia (often with arrhythmia).
• ambulate the patient as soon as possible; handle the patient with chronic hypercalcemia *gently* to prevent pathologic fractures; reposition the patient frequently if he is bedridden, and encourage range-of-motion exercises to promote circulation and prevent urinary stasis and calcium loss from bone.
• suggest a low-calcium diet, with increased fluid intake, to prevent recurrence.

Chloride Imbalance

Hypochloremia and hyperchloremia are, respectively, conditions of deficient or excessive serum levels of the anion chloride. A predominantly extracellular anion, chloride accounts for two thirds of all serum anions. Secreted by stomach mucosa as hydrochloric acid, it provides an acid medium conducive to digestion and activation of enzymes. Chloride also participates in maintaining acid-base and body water balances, influences the osmolality or tonicity of extracellular fluid, plays a role in the exchange of oxygen and carbon dioxide in RBCs, and helps activate salivary amylase (which, in turn, activates the digestive process).

Causes

Hypochloremia may result from:
• decreased chloride intake or absorption, as in low dietary sodium intake, sodium deficiency, potassium deficiency, metabolic alkalosis; prolonged use of mercurial diuretics; or administration of dextrose I.V. without electrolytes.
• excessive chloride loss, resulting from prolonged diarrhea or diaphoresis; loss of hydrochloric acid in gastric secretions, due to vomiting, gastric suctioning, or gastric surgery.

Hyperchloremia may result from:
• excessive chloride intake or absorption—as in hyperingestion of ammonium chloride, or ureterointestinal anastomosis—allowing reabsorption of chloride by the bowel.
• hemoconcentration, caused by dehydration.
• compensatory mechanisms for other metabolic abnormalities, as in metabolic acidosis, brain stem injury causing neurogenic hyperventilation, and hyperparathyroidism.

Signs and symptoms

Hypochloremia is usually associated with hyponatremia and its characteristic muscular weakness and twitching, since renal chloride loss always accompanies sodium loss, and sodium reabsorption is not possible without chloride. However, if chloride depletion results from metabolic alkalosis secondary to loss of gastric secretions, chloride is lost independently from sodium; typical symptoms are muscle hypertonicity, tetany,

and shallow, depressed breathing.

Because of the natural affinity of sodium and chloride ions, hyperchloremia usually produces clinical effects associated with hypernatremia and resulting extracellular fluid volume excess (agitation, tachycardia, hypertension, pitting edema, dyspnea). Hyperchloremia associated with metabolic acidosis is due to excretion of base bicarbonate by the kidneys, and induces deep, rapid breathing; weakness; diminished cognitive ability; and ultimately, coma.

Diagnosis

 Serum chloride level < 98 mEq/liter confirms hypochloremia; supportive values with metabolic alkalosis include serum pH > 7.45 and serum CO_2 > 32 mEq/liter.

Serum chloride level > 108 mEq/liter confirms hyperchloremia; with metabolic acidosis, serum pH is < 7.35 and serum CO_2 is < 22 mEq/liter.

Treatment

The aims of treatment for hypochloremia are to correct the condition that causes excessive chloride loss and to give oral replacement, such as salty broth. When oral therapy is not possible or when emergency measures are necessary, treatment may include normal saline solution I.V. (if hypovolemia is present) or chloride-containing drugs, such as ammonium chloride, to increase serum chloride levels, and potassium chloride for metabolic alkalosis. For severe hyperchloremic acidosis, treatment consists of sodium bicarbonate I.V. to raise serum bicarbonate level and permit renal excretion of the chloride anion, since bicarbonate and chloride compete for combination with sodium. In patients with mild hyperchloremia, Ringer's lactate solution is administered and converted to bicarbonate in the liver, thus increasing base bicarbonate to correct acidosis.

In either kind of chloride imbalance, treatment must correct the underlying disorder.

Additional considerations

When managing the patient with hypochloremia, the hospital staff member should:

• monitor serum chloride levels frequently, particularly during I.V. therapy.

• watch for signs of hyper- or hypochloremia; be alert for respiratory difficulty.

• monitor laboratory results (serum electrolytes and blood gases) and fluid intake and output to prevent hypochloremia in patients who are vulnerable to chloride imbalance, particularly those recovering from gastric surgery; record and report excessive or continuous loss of gastric secretions; also report prolonged infusion of dextrose in water without saline.

When managing the patient with hyperchloremia, the staff member should:

• check serum electrolyte levels every 3 to 6 hours; if the patient is receiving high doses of sodium bicarbonate, watch for signs of overcorrection (metabolic alkalosis, respiratory depression) or lingering signs of hyperchloremia, which indicate inadequate treatment.

• check laboratory results for elevated serum chloride or potassium imbalance to prevent hyperchloremia if the patient is receiving I.V. solutions containing sodium chloride, and monitor fluid intake and output; watch for signs of metabolic acidosis; monitor flow rate when administering I.V. fluids containing Ringer's lactate solution according to the patient's age, physical condition, and bicarbonate level; report any irregularities promptly.

Magnesium Imbalance

Approximately one third of magnesium taken into the body is absorbed through the small intestine and is eventually excreted in urine; the remaining unabsorbed magnesium is excreted in stool.

Since many common foods contain magnesium, a dietary deficiency is rare. Magnesium deficiency (hypomagnesemia) generally follows impaired absorption or too rapid excretion of magnesium. It frequently coexists with other electrolyte imbalances, especially low calcium and potassium levels. Magnesium excess (hypermagnesemia) is common in patients with renal failure and excessive intake of magnesium-containing antacids.

Magnesium is the second most common cation in intracellular fluid. Although its major function is to enhance neuromuscular integration, it also stimulates parathyroid hormone (PTH) secretion, thus regulating intracellular fluid calcium levels. Therefore, hypomagnesemia may result in transient hypoparathyroidism and/or interference with the peripheral action of PTH. Magnesium may also regulate skeletal muscles through its influence on calcium utilization by depressing acetylcholine release at synaptic junctions. In addition, magnesium activates many enzymes for proper carbohydrate and protein metabolism, aids in cell metabolism and the transport of sodium and potassium across cell membranes, and influences sodium, potassium, calcium, and protein levels.

Causes

Hypomagnesemia usually results from impaired absorption of magnesium in intestines or excessive excretion in urine or stool. Possible causes include:

• **decreased magnesium intake or absorption,** as in malabsorption syndrome, chronic diarrhea, or postoperative complications after bowel resection; chronic alcoholism; prolonged diuretic therapy, nasogastric suctioning, or administration of parenteral fluids without magnesium salts; starvation or malnutrition.

• **excessive loss of magnesium,** as in severe dehydration and diabetic acidosis; hyperaldosteronism and hypoparathyroidism, which result in hypokalemia and hypocalcemia; hyperparathyroidism and hypercalcemia; excessive release of adrenocortical hormones; diuretic therapy.

Hypermagnesemia results from the kidneys' inability to excrete magnesium that was either absorbed from the intestines or infused. Common causes of hypermagnesemia include:

• chronic renal insufficiency.

• use of laxatives (magnesium sulfate, milk of magnesia, and magnesium citrate solutions), especially with renal insufficiency.

• overuse of magnesium-containing antacids.

• severe dehydration (resulting oliguria can cause magnesium retention).

• overcorrection of hypomagnesemia.

Signs and symptoms

Hypomagnesemia causes neuromuscular irritability and cardiac arrythmias. Hypermagnesemia causes CNS and respiratory depression, in addition to neuromuscular and cardiac effects.

Diagnosis

 Decreased serum magnesium levels (less than 1.5 mEq/liter) confirm hypomagnesemia; increased levels (greater than 2.5 mEq/liter), hypermagnesemia. Low levels of other serum electrolytes (especially potassium and calcium) often coexist with hypomagnesemia. In fact, unresponsiveness to correct treatment for hypokalemia strongly suggests hypomagnesemia. Similarly, elevated levels of other serum electrolytes are associated with hypermagnesemia.

Treatment

The aim of therapy for magnesium imbalance is identification and correction of the underlying cause.

Treatment of mild hypomagnesemia consists of daily magnesium supplements I.M. or P.O.; of severe hypomagnesemia, magnesium sulfate I.V. (10 to 40 mEq/liter diluted in I.V. fluid). Magnesium intoxication (a possible side effect) requires calcium gluconate I.V.

SIGNS AND SYMPTOMS OF MAGNESIUM IMBALANCE

DYSFUNCTION	HYPOMAGNESEMIA	HYPERMAGNESEMIA
Neuromuscular	• Hyperirritability, tetany, leg and foot cramps, Chvostek's sign (facial muscle spasms induced by tapping the branches of the facial nerve)	• Diminished reflexes, muscle weakness, flaccid paralysis, respiratory muscle paralysis that may cause respiratory embarrassment
CNS	• Confusion, delusions, hallucinations, convulsions	• Drowsiness, flushing, lethargy, confusion, diminished sensorium
Cardiovascular	• Arrhythmias, vasomotor changes (vasodilation and hypotension), occasionally, hypertension	• Bradycardia, weak pulse, hypotension, heart block, cardiac arrest (common with serum levels of 25 mEq/liter)

Therapy for hypermagnesemia includes increased fluid intake, and loop diuretics, such as furosemide, with impaired renal function; calcium gluconate (10%), a magnesium antagonist, for temporary relief of symptoms in an emergency; and peritoneal dialysis or hemodialysis if renal function fails or if excess magnesium can't be eliminated.

Additional considerations
Treatment for patients with hypomagnesemia includes:
- monitoring serum electrolytes daily for mild deficits and every 6 to 12 hours during replacement therapy; reporting abnormal levels immediately.
- measuring intake and output frequently (urinary output shouldn't fall below 25 ml/hour or 600 ml/day since the kidneys excrete excess magnesium, and hypermagnesemia could occur with renal insufficiency).
- assessing vital signs often during I.V. therapy; infusing magnesium replacement slowly, and watching for bradycardia, heart block, and decreased respirations.
- having calcium gluconate I.V. available to reverse hypermagnesemia from overcorrection.
- advising patients to eat foods high in

magnesium (fish and green vegetables).
- watching for and reporting signs of hypomagnesemia in patients with predisposing diseases, especially those not permitted anything by mouth or those receiving I.V. fluids without magnesium.

Treatment for patients with hypermagnesemia includes:
- assessing level of consciousness, muscle activity, and vital signs.
- keeping accurate intake and output records; providing adequate fluids for hydration and maintenance of renal function.
- reporting abnormal serum electrolyte levels immediately.
- monitoring and reporting EKG changes (peaked T waves, increased P-R intervals, widened QRS complex).
- watching patients receiving digitalis and calcium gluconate simultaneously, since calcium excess enhances digitalis action, predisposing the patient to digitalis intoxication.
- advising patients to avoid continual use of laxatives and antacids containing magnesium, particularly the elderly or patients with compromised renal function.
- watching for signs of hypermagnesemia in predisposed patients; observing for respiratory distress if magnesium serum levels rise above 10 mEq/liter.

Phosphorus Imbalance

Phosphorus, the principal intracellular anion, exists primarily in inorganic combination with calcium in teeth and bones. In extracellular fluid, the phosphate ion supports several metabolic functions: utilization of B vitamins, acid-base homeostasis, bone formation, nerve and muscle activity, cell division, transmission of hereditary traits, and metabolism of carbohydrates, proteins, and fats. Renal tubular reabsorption of phosphate is inversely regulated by calcium levels—an increase in phosphorus causes a decrease in calcium. An imbalance causes hypophosphatemia (low serum phosphorus level) or hyperphosphatemia (high serum phosphorus level). Incidence of hypophosphatemia varies with the underlying cause; hyperphosphatemia occurs most often in children, who tend to consume more phosphorus-rich foods and beverages than adults, and in children and adults with renal insufficiency. Prognosis for both conditions depends on the underlying cause.

Causes
Hypophosphatemia is usually the result

of inadequate dietary intake; it is often related to malnutrition from a prolonged

FOODS HIGH IN PHOSPHORUS (P)		
FOOD	PORTION	P (mg)
Almonds	⅔ cup	475
Beef liver (fried)	3½ oz	476
Broccoli (cooked)	⅔ cup	62
Carbonated beverage	12 oz	up to 500
Milk (whole)	8 oz	93
Turkey (roasted)	3½ oz	251

catabolic state or chronic alcoholism. It may also stem from intestinal malabsorption, chronic diarrhea, hyperparathyroidism with resultant hypercalcemia, hypomagnesemia, or deficiency of vitamin D, which is necessary for intestinal phosphorus absorption. Other important causes include chronic use of antacids containing aluminum hydroxide, use of hyperalimentation solution with inadequate phosphate content, renal tubular defects, tissue damage in which phosphorus is released by injured cells, and diabetic acidosis.

Hyperphosphatemia is generally secondary to hypocalcemia, hypervitaminosis D, hypoparathyroidism, or renal failure (often due to stress or injury). It may also result from overuse of laxatives or phosphate enemas.

Signs and symptoms
Hypophosphatemia produces anorexia, muscle weakness, tremor, paresthesia, and when persistent, osteomalacia, causing bone pain. Impaired RBC functions may occur in hypophosphatemia due to alterations in oxyhemoglobin dissociation, which may result in peripheral hypoxia. Hyperphosphatemia usually remains asymptomatic unless it results in hypocalcemia, with tetany and convulsions.

Diagnosis

Serum phosphorus level less than 1.7 mEq/liter confirms hypophosphatemia. Urine phosphorus level more than 1.3 g/24 hours supports this diagnosis.

Serum phosphorus level over 2.6 mEq/liter confirms hyperphosphatemia. Supportive values include decreased levels of serum calcium (less than 9 mg/100 ml) and urine phosphorus (less than 0.9 g/24 hours).

Treatment
The goal of treatment is correction of the underlying cause of hypo- or hyperphosphatemia. Until this is done, management of hypophosphatemia consists of phosphorus replacement, with a high-phosphorus diet and P.O. administration of phosphate salt tablets or capsules. Severe hypophosphatemia requires I.V. infusion of potassium phosphate. Severe hyperphosphatemia may require peritoneal dialysis or hemodialysis to lower the serum phosphorus level.

Additional considerations
All serum electrolyte, and calcium, magnesium, and phosphorus levels should be carefully monitored and any changes reported immediately.

Hypophosphatemia care includes:
• recording intake and output accurately; administering potassium phosphate by slow I.V. to prevent overcorrection to hyperphosphatemia; assessing renal function and being alert for hypocalcemia when giving phosphate supplements; using capsules of phosphate salt if tablets cause nausea.
• advising the patient to follow a high-phosphorus diet containing milk and milk products, kidney, liver, turkey, and dried fruits to prevent recurrence.

Hyperphosphatemia care includes:
• monitoring intake and output; notifying the doctor if urinary output falls below 25 ml/hour or 600 ml/day, since decreased output can seriously affect renal clearance of excess serum phosphorus.
• watching for signs of hypocalcemia, such as muscle twitching and tetany, which often accompany hyperphosphatemia.
• advising the patient to eat foods with low phosphorus content, such as vegetables; obtaining a special diet if chronic renal insufficiency is the cause.

Syndrome of Inappropriate Antidiuretic Hormone Secretion

Syndrome of inappropriate antidiuretic hormone (SIADH) secretion is marked by excessive release of ADH that disturbs fluid and electrolyte balance. Such disturbances result from inability to excrete dilute urine, retention of free water, expansion of extracellular fluid volume, and hyponatremia. SIADH occurs secondary to diseases that affect the osmoreceptors (supraoptic nucleus) of the hypothalamus. Prognosis depends on severity of the underlying disorder and response to treatment.

Causes
The most common cause of SIADH (80% of patients) is oat cell carcinoma of the lung, which secretes excessive ADH or vasopressorlike substances. Other neoplastic diseases—such as pancreatic and prostatic cancer, Hodgkin's disease, and thymoma—may also trigger SIADH. Less common causes include:

• *CNS disorders:* brain tumor or abscess, cerebrovascular accident, head injury, Guillain-Barré syndrome, and lupus erythematosus
• *pulmonary disorders:* pneumonia, tuberculosis, lung abscess, and positive-pressure ventilation
• *drugs:* chlorpropamide, vincristine, cyclophosphamide, carbamazepine, and clofibrate
• *miscellaneous conditions:* myxedema and psychosis.

Signs and symptoms
SIADH may produce weight gain despite anorexia, nausea, and vomiting; muscle weakness, restlessness, or irritability, possibly progressing to coma and convulsions, may also occur. Edema is rare unless water overload exceeds 4 liters, since much of the free water excess is within cellular boundaries.

Diagnosis

Complete medical history revealing positive water balance may suggest SIADH, but urine osmolality more than 150 mOsm/kg of water and serum osmolality less than 280 mOsm/kg of water confirm it (normal urine osmolality is one and a half times serum values). Supportive laboratory values include BUN less than 8 mg% (or less than 10 mg% with concurrent hyponatremia); low serum creatinine and albumin; high urine sodium concentration (more than 20 mEq/liter).

Treatment
Treatment for SIADH is symptomatic and begins with restricted water intake (500 to 1,000 ml/day). With severe water intoxication, administration of 200 to 300 ml of 5% saline may be necessary to raise serum sodium level. Therapy may also include simultaneous administration of furosemide to prevent circulatory overload. When possible, treatment should include correction of the underlying cause of SIADH, such as surgery or chemotherapy for neoplasms. If fluid restriction is ineffective, demeclocycline or lithium may be helpful by blocking the renal response to ADH.

Additional considerations
The health care professional caring for a patient with SIADH should:
• closely monitor and record intake and output, vital signs, and daily weight; watch for hyponatremia.
• observe for restlessness, irritability, convulsions, congestive heart failure, and unresponsiveness due to hyponatremia and water toxicity.
• explain to the patient and his family why he *must* restrict his intake to prevent water intoxication.

Metabolic Acidosis

Metabolic acidosis is a physiologic state of excess acid accumulation and deficient base bicarbonate produced by an underlying pathologic disorder. Symptoms result from the body's attempts to correct the acidotic condition through compensatory mechanisms in the lungs, kidneys, and cells. Metabolic acidosis is more prevalent among children, who are vulnerable to acid-base imbalance because their metabolic rates are faster and their ratios of water to total-body weight are lower. Severe or untreated metabolic acidosis can be fatal.

Causes

Metabolic acidosis usually results from excessive burning of fats in the absence of usable carbohydrates. This can be caused by diabetic ketoacidosis, chronic alcoholism, malnutrition, or a low-carbohydrate, high-fat diet—all of which produce more keto acids than the metabolic process can handle. Other causes include:

• *anaerobic carbohydrate metabolism:* a decrease in tissue oxygenation or perfusion, as occurs with pump failure after myocardial infarction, or with pulmonary or hepatic disease, shock, or anemia forces a shift from aerobic to anaerobic metabolism, causing a corresponding rise in lactic acid level.

• *renal insufficiency and failure (renal acidosis):* underexcretion of metabolized acids or inability to conserve base.

• *diarrhea and intestinal malabsorption:* loss of sodium bicarbonate from the intestines, causing the bicarbonate buffer system to shift to the acidic side. For example, ureteroenterostomy and Crohn's disease can also induce metabolic acidosis.

Less frequently, metabolic acidosis results from salicylate intoxication (overuse of aspirin), exogenous poisoning, or Addison's disease (due to increased excretion of sodium and chloride, and retention of potassium ions).

Signs and symptoms

In mild acidosis, symptoms of the underlying disease may obscure any direct clinical evidence. Metabolic acidosis typically begins with headache and lethargy, progressing to drowsiness, CNS depression, Kussmaul's respirations (as the lungs attempt to compensate by "blowing off" CO_2), stupor, and if the condition is severe and goes untreated, coma and death. Associated gastrointestinal distress usually produces anorexia, nausea, vomiting, and diarrhea, and

---

ANION GAP (THE DELTA)

The anion gap is the difference between concentrations of serum cations and anions—determined by measuring one cation (sodium) and two anions (chloride and bicarbonate). The normal concentration of sodium is 140 mEq/liter; of chloride, 102 mEq/liter; and of bicarbonate, 26 mEq/liter. Thus, the anion gap between *measured* cations (actually sodium alone) and *measured* anions is about 12 mEq/liter (140 minus 128).

Concentrations of potassium, calcium, and magnesium (*unmeasured* cations), or proteins, phosphate, sulfate, and organic acids (*unmeasured* anions) are not needed to measure the anion gap. Added together, the concentration of unmeasured cations would be about 11 mEq/liter; of unmeasured anions, about 23 mEq/liter. Thus, the normal anion gap between unmeasured cations and anions is about 12 mEq/liter (23 minus 11)—give or take 2 mEq/liter for normal variation. An anion gap over 14 mEq/liter indicates *metabolic acidosis*. It may result from accumulation of excess organic acids or from retention of hydrogen ions, which chemically bond with bicarbonate and decrease bicarbonate levels.

may lead to dehydration. Underlying diabetes mellitus may cause fruity breath from catabolism of fats and excretion of accumulated ketones, such as acetone, through the lungs.

Diagnosis

Arterial pH below 7.35 confirms metabolic acidosis. In severe acidotic states, pH may fall to 7.10 and arterial blood gas PCO_2 may be normal or < 34 mmHg as compensatory mechanisms take hold. HCO_3^- may be < 22 mEq/liter. Supportive findings include the following:

• urine pH: < 4.5 in the absence of renal disease
• serum potassium levels: > 5.5 mEq/liter from chemical buffering
• glucose: > 150 mg/100 ml in diabetes
• serum ketone bodies: elevated in diabetes mellitus
• plasma lactic acid: elevated in lactic acidosis
• anion gap: > 14 indicates metabolic acidosis.

Treatment

Treatment for metabolic acidosis includes sodium bicarbonate I.V. to neutralize blood acidity, careful evaluation and correction of electrolyte imbalances, and ultimately, correction of the underlying cause. For example, in diabetic ketoacidosis, low-dose continous I.V. insulin infusion is recommended.

Additional considerations

• Sodium bicarbonate ampules should be kept handy for emergency administration. The patient's vital signs and levels of consciousness must be frequently monitored, as well as the laboratory results.
• In diabetic acidosis, secondary changes due to hypovolemia, such as decreasing blood pressure, must be watched for.
• The patient's intake and output must be recorded accurately to monitor renal function. He should be watched for signs of excessive serum potassium—weakness, flaccid paralysis, and arrhythmias, possibly leading to cardiac arrest. After treatment, as potassium moves back into the cells, the patient should be checked for overcorrection to hypokalemia.
• The patient should be positioned in a way that will prevent aspiration, because metabolic acidosis commonly causes vomiting. Since convulsions are possible, seizure precautions are necessary.
• Good oral hygiene can be provided by using sodium bicarbonate washes to neutralize mouth acids, and lubricating the patient's lips with lemon and glycerine swabs.
• Patients receiving I.V. therapy or who have intestinal tubes in place, as well as those suffering from shock, hyperthyroidism, hepatic disease, and circulatory failure, or dehydration must be watched carefully to prevent metabolic acidosis. The diabetes patient should know how to routinely test urine for sugar and acetone, and must strictly adhere to therapy.

Metabolic Alkalosis

A clinical state marked by decreased amounts of acid or increased amounts of base bicarbonate, metabolic alkalosis causes metabolic, respiratory, and renal responses, producing characteristic symptoms—most notably, hypoventilation. This condition is always secondary to an underlying cause. With early diagnosis and prompt treatment, prognosis is good; however, untreated metabolic alkalosis may lead to coma and death.

Causes

Metabolic alkalosis results from loss of acid, retention of base, or renal mechanisms associated with decreased serum levels of potassium and chloride.

Causes of critical acid loss include

vomiting, nasogastric tube drainage or gavage without adequate electrolyte replacement, fistulas, and the use of steroids and certain diuretics (furosemide, thiazides, and ethacrynic acid). Hyperadrenocorticism is another cause of severe acid loss. Cushing's disease, primary hyperaldosteronism, and Bartter's syndrome, for example, all lead to retention of sodium and chloride, and urinary loss of potassium and hydrogen.

Excessive retention of base can result from excessive intake of bicarbonate of soda or other antacids (usually for treatment of gastritis or peptic ulcer), excessive intake of absorbable alkali (as in milk-alkali syndrome, often seen in patients with peptic ulcers), administration of excessive amounts of I.V. fluids with high concentrations of bicarbonate or lactate, or respiratory insufficiency— all of which cause chronic hypercapnia, from high levels of plasma bicarbonate.

Signs and symptoms
Clinical features of metabolic alkalosis result from the body's attempt to correct the acid-base imbalance, primarily through hypoventilation. Other manifestations include irritability, picking at bedclothes (carphology), twitching, confusion, nausea, vomiting, and diarrhea (which aggravates alkalosis). Cardiovascular abnormalities—such as atrial tachycardia—and respiratory disturbances—such as cyanosis and apnea— also occur. In the alkalotic patient, diminished peripheral blood flow during repeated blood pressure checks may provoke carpopedal spasm in the hand—a possible sign of impending tetany (Trousseau's sign). Uncorrected metabolic alkalosis may progress to convulsions and coma.

Diagnosis

Blood pH level > 7.45 and HCO_3 > 29 mEq/liter confirm diagnosis. A PCO_2 > 45 mmHg indicates attempts at respiratory compensation. Serum electrolyte levels show potassium 3.5 mEq/liter and chloride 98 mEq/liter.

Other characteristic laboratory findings include:
• *Urine pH* is usually about 7.
• *Urinalysis* reveals alkalinity after the renal compensatory mechanism begins to excrete bicarbonate.
• *EKG* may show low T wave, merging with a P wave, and atrial tachycardia.

Treatment
The goal of treatment is to correct the underlying cause of metabolic alkalosis. Therapy for severe alkalosis may include cautious administration of ammonium chloride I.V. to release hydrogen chloride and restore concentration of extracellular fluid and chloride levels. Potassium chloride and normal saline solution (except in the presence of congestive heart failure) are usually sufficient to replace losses from gastric drainage. Electrolyte replacement with potassium chloride and discontinuing diuretics correct metabolic alkalosis resulting from potent diuretic therapy.

Additional considerations
Care of the metabolic alkalosis patient is structured around cautious I.V. therapy, keen observation, and strict monitoring of the patient's status. The health care professional should:
• dilute potassium when giving I.V. containing potassium salts; monitor the infusion rate to prevent damage to blood vessels and watch for signs of phlebitis; limit the infusion rate of ammonium chloride 0.9% to 1 liter in 4 hours, since faster administration may cause hemolysis of RBCs; avoid overdosage, since it may cause overcorrection to metabolic acidosis; not give ammonium chloride with signs of hepatic or renal disease.
• watch closely for signs of muscle weakness, tetany, or decreased activity; monitor vital signs frequently, and record intake and output to evaluate respiratory, fluid, and electrolyte status. Respiratory rate usually decreases in an effort to compensate for alkalosis. Hypotension and tachycardia may indicate electrolyte imbalance, especially hypokalemia.

- observe seizure precautions.
- warn patients against overdosing with alkaline agents, such as sodium bicarbonate; irrigate nasogastric tubes with isotonic saline solution instead of plain water to prevent excessive loss of gastric electrolytes; monitor I.V. fluid concentrations of bicarbonate or lactate; teach patients with ulcers to recognize signs of milk-alkali syndrome (a distaste for milk, anorexia, weakness, and lethargy).

Selected References

Adlard, John M., and Jack M. George. *Hyponatremia,* HEART AND LUNG. 7:537-593, July/August 1978.

Bondy, Philip K., and Leon E. Rosenberry, eds. DUNCAN'S DISEASES OF METABOLISM, 8th ed. Philadelphia: W.B. Saunders Co., 1979.

Brenner, Barry M., and Jay H. Stein, eds. ACID BASE AND POTASSIUM HOMEOSTASIS. New York: Churchill Livingston, Inc., 1978.

Burch, Robert E., and James F. Sullivan. *Diagnosis of Zinc, Copper and Manganese Abnormalities in Man,* MEDICAL CLINICS OF NORTH AMERICA. 655-660, July 1976.

Burgess, Audrey. NURSE'S GUIDE TO FLUID AND ELECTROLYTE BALANCE, 2nd ed. New York: McGraw-Hill Book Co., 1979.

Cohen, A.S., et al. *Amyloidosis, Current Trends in Its Investigation,* ARTHRITIS AND RHEUMATISM. February 1978.

Goodhart, Robert S., and Maurice E. Shils, eds. MODERN NUTRITION IN HEALTH AND DISEASE: DIETOTHERAPY, 6th ed. Philadelphia: Lea & Febiger, 1980.

Greenberg, B.H., et al. *Primary Type V Hyperlipoproteinemia,* ANNALS OF INTERNAL MEDICINE. 87:526-534, 1977.

Howell, R. Rodney. *The Glycogen Storage Disease,* in John B. Stanbury and James B. Wyngaarden, eds. THE METABOLIC BASIS OF INHERITED DISEASE, 4th ed. New York: McGraw-Hill Book Co., 1978.

Hsia, David Yi-Yung. GALACTOSEMIA. Springfield, Ill.: Charles C. Thomas, 1969.

Kee, Joyce L. FLUIDS AND ELECTROLYTES WITH CLINICAL APPLICATIONS: A PROGRAMMED APPROACH, 2nd ed. New York: John Wiley & Sons, Inc., 1978.

Krause, Marie V., and Kathleen L. Mahan. FOOD, NUTRITION, AND DIET THERAPY, 6th ed. Philadelphia: W.B. Saunders Co., 1979.

Kubo, Winifred, et al. *Fluid and Electrolyte Problems of Tube-fed Patients,* AMERICAN JOURNAL OF NURSING. 76:912-916, June 1976.

Metheny, Norma M., and W.D. Snively, Jr. NURSES' HANDBOOK OF FLUID BALANCE, 3rd ed. Philadelphia: J.B. Lippincott Co., 1979.

MONITORING FLUIDS AND ELECTROLYTES PRECISELY. Nursing Skillbook™ Series. Springhouse, Pa: Intermed Communications, Inc., 1978.

Pestana, Carlos. FLUIDS AND ELECTROLYTES IN THE SURGICAL PATIENT. Baltimore: Williams & Wilkins Co., 1977.

Robinson, Corinne H., and Marilyn R. Lawler. NORMAL AND THERAPEUTIC NUTRITION, 15th ed. New York: Macmillan Publishing Co., 1977.

Segal, Stanton. *Disorders of Galactose Metabolism,* in John B. Stanbury and James B. Wyngaarden, eds. THE METABOLIC BASIS OF INHERITED DISEASE, 4th ed. New York: McGraw-Hill Book Co., 1978.

Stanbury, John B., and James B. Wyngaarden, eds. THE METABOLIC BASIS OF INHERITED DISEASE, 4th ed., New York: McGraw-Hill Book Co., 1978.

Steinberg, D., and S.M. Grundy. *Management of Hyperlipidemia,* ARCHIVES OF SURGERY. 113:55-60, January 1978.

Stroot, Violet R., et al. FLUIDS AND ELECTROLYTES: A PRACTICAL APPROACH, 2nd ed. Philadelphia: F.A. Davis Co., 1977.

Thiele, Victoria F. CLINICAL NUTRITION. St. Louis: C.V. Mosby Co., 1976.

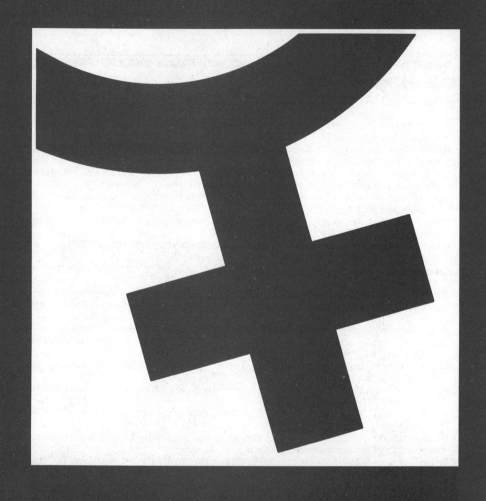

15 Obstetric and Gynecologic Disorders

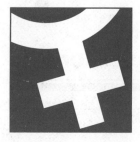

Obstetric and Gynecologic Disorders

Introduction

Clinical care of the obstetric or gynecologic patient reflects a growing interest in improving the quality of health care for females. Today, the health care professional must be able to assess, counsel, teach, and refer these patients, while weighing such relevant factors as the desire to have children, problems of sexual adjustment, and self-image. Frequently, the situation is further complicated by the fact that multiple obstetric and gynecologic abnormalities occur simultaneously. For example, a patient with dysmenorrhea may also have trichomonal vaginitis, dysuria, and unsuspected infertility. Her condition may be further complicated by associated urologic disorders, due to the proximity of the urinary and reproductive systems. This tendency to multiple and complex disorders is readily understandable upon review of the anatomic structure of the female genitalia.

External structures

Female genitalia include the following external structures, collectively known as the *vulva:* mons pubis (or mons veneris), labia majora, labia minora, clitoris, vestibule, urethral meatus, hymen, Bartholin's glands and Skene's glands (paraurethral glands), fourchette, and perineum. The size, shape, and color of these structures—as well as pubic hair distribution, and skin texture and pigmentation—vary from person to person

and race to race. Furthermore, these external structures undergo distinct changes during the life cycle.

The *mons pubis* is the pad of fat over the symphysis pubis (pubic bone), which is usually covered by the base of the inverted triangular patch of pubic hair that grows over the vulva after puberty.

The *labia majora* are the two thick, longitudinal folds of fatty tissue that extend from the mons pubis to the perineum. The labia majora protect the perineum and contain large sebaceous glands that help maintain lubrication. Virtually absent in the young child, their development is a characteristic sign of onset of puberty. The skin of the more prominent parts of the labia majora is pigmented, and darkens after puberty.

The *labia minora* are the two thin, longitudinal folds of skin that border the vestibule. Firmer than the labia majora, they extend from the clitoris to the fourchette.

The *clitoris* is the small, protuberant organ located just beneath the arch of the mons pubis. The clitoris contains erectile tissue, venous cavernous spaces, and specialized sensory corpuscles that are stimulated during coitus.

The *vestibule* is the oval space bordered by the clitoris, labia minora, and fourchette. The *urethral meatus* is located in the anterior portion of the vestibule; the *vaginal meatus,* in the posterior portion. The *hymen* is the elastic membrane that partially obstructs the vaginal meatus in virgins.

Several glands lubricate the vestibule. *Skene's glands* open on both sides of the urethral meatus; *Bartholin's glands*, on both sides of the vaginal meatus.

The *fourchette* is the posterior junction of the labia majora and labia minora. The *perineum*, which includes the underlying muscles and fascia, is the external surface of the floor of the pelvis,

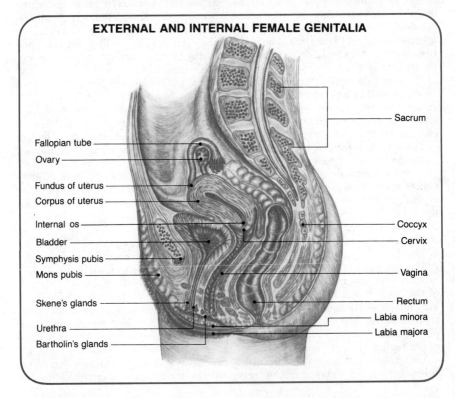

EXTERNAL AND INTERNAL FEMALE GENITALIA

- Fallopian tube
- Ovary
- Fundus of uterus
- Corpus of uterus
- Internal os
- Bladder
- Symphysis pubis
- Mons pubis
- Skene's glands
- Urethra
- Bartholin's glands
- Sacrum
- Coccyx
- Cervix
- Vagina
- Rectum
- Labia minora
- Labia majora

extending from the fourchette to the anus.

Internal structures

The following internal structures are included in the female genitalia: vagina, cervix, uterus, fallopian tubes (or oviducts), and ovaries.

The *vagina* occupies the space between the bladder and the rectum. A muscular, membranous tube approximately 3" (7.5 cm) long, the vagina connects the uterus and the vestibule of the external genitalia. It serves as a passageway for sperm to the fallopian tubes, for the discharge of menstrual fluid, and for childbirth.

The *cervix,* or neck of the uterus, protrudes at least ¾" (2 cm) into the proximal end of the vagina. A rounded, conical structure, the cervix joins the uterus and the vagina at a 45° to 90° angle.

The *uterus* is the hollow, pear-shaped organ in which the conceptus grows during pregnancy. The part of the uterus above the junction of the fallopian tubes is called the *fundus;* the part below this junction is called the *corpus.* The junction of the corpus and cervix forms the *internal cervical os.*

The thick uterine wall consists of mucosal, muscular, and serous layers. The inner mucosal lining—the *endometrium*—undergoes cyclic changes to facilitate and maintain pregnancy.

The smooth muscular middle layer—the *myometrium*—interlaces the uterine and ovarian arteries and veins that circulate blood through the uterus. During pregnancy, this vascular system expands dramatically. After abortion or childbirth, the myometrium contracts to constrict the vasculature and control the loss of blood.

The outer serous layer—the *parietal peritoneum*—covers all the fundus, part of the corpus, but none of the cervix. This incompleteness allows surgical entry into the uterus without incision of the peritoneum, thereby reducing the risk of peritonitis.

The *fallopian tubes* extend from the sides of the fundus and terminate near the ovaries. Through ciliary and muscular action, these small tubes (3¼" to 5½" [8 to 14 cm] long) carry ova from the ovaries to the uterus, and facilitate the movement of sperm from the uterus toward the ovaries. Fertilization of the ovum normally occurs in a fallopian tube. The same ciliary and muscular action helps move a *zygote* (fertilized ovum) down to the uterus, where it implants in the uterine wall.

The *ovaries* are two almond-shaped organs, one on either side of the fundus, situated behind and below the fallopian tubes. The ovaries produce ova and two primary hormones—estrogen and progesterone—in addition to small amounts of androgen. These hormones, in turn, produce and maintain secondary sex characteristics, prepare the uterus for pregnancy, and stimulate mammary gland development.

The ovaries are connected to the uterus by the utero-ovarian ligament, and are divided into two parts: the *cortex,* which contains primordial and graafian follicles in various stages of development; and the *medulla,* which consists primarily of vasculature and loose connective tissue.

A normal female is born with at least 400,000 primordial follicles in the ovaries. Following puberty, these ova precursors become graafian follicles, in response to the effects of pituitary gonadotropic hormones—follicle-stimulating hormone (FSH) and luteinizing hormone (LH). In the life cycle of a female, however, less than 500 ova eventually mature and develop the potential for fertilization.

The menstrual cycle

Maturation of the hypothalamus and the resultant increase in hormone levels initiate puberty. In the young girl, breast development—the first sign of puberty—is followed by the appearance of pubic and axillary hair and the characteristic adolescent growth spurt. The reproductive system begins to undergo a series of hormone-induced changes that result in *menarche,* onset of menstruation (or

PHASES OF
THE MENSTRUAL CYCLE

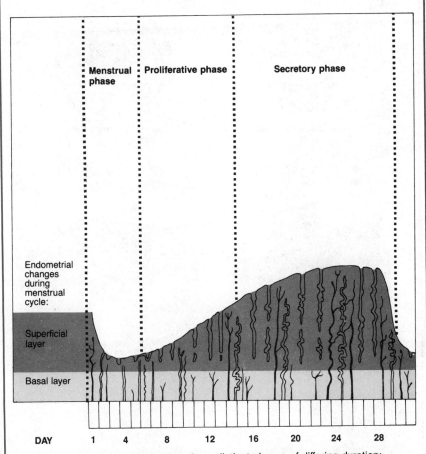

The menstrual cycle is divided into three distinct phases of differing duration:
• The first phase, the menstrual phase, starts on the first day of menstruation, and lasts about six days. The flow which occurs at this time is called the menses. It consists of blood, mucus, and unneeded tissue resulting from the breakdown of the top layer of the endometrium (the material lining the uterus). This phase is caused by decreased levels of estrogen and progesterone.
• The second phase, the proliferative phase, begins when the menses stop, lasts approximately eight days, and ends with ovulation. During this phase the endometrium begins to thicken and revascularize. Estrogen levels rise during this phase.
• The third phase, the secretory phase, starts on the day of ovulation (about day 14), and lasts approximately 14 days. During this phase the endometrium continues to thicken to nourish an embryo in case fertilization occurs. Without fertilization, the top layer of the endometrium breaks down, and the menstrual phase of the cycle begins again. Hormonal levels depend on whether or not fertilization has taken place.

FOLLICULAR CYCLE
(Corresponding to days of the menstrual cycle)

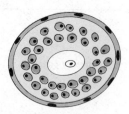

1. Early follicular phase
Days 1 to 5

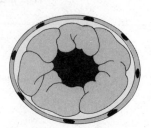

4. Early luteal phase
Days 16 to 20

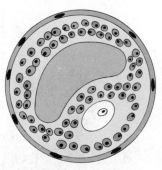

2. Late follicular phase
Days 6 to 10

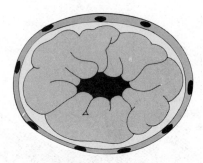

5. Midluteal phase
Days 21 to 25

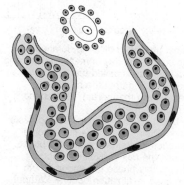

3. Ovulatory phase
Days 11 to 15

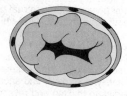

6. Late luteal phase
Days 26 to 28

menses). In North American females, menarche usually occurs at about age 13 but may occur anytime between ages 9 and 18. Usually, initial menstrual periods are irregular and anovulatory, but after a year or so, periods generally are more regular.

The menstrual cycle is made up of three different phases: menstrual, proliferative (estrogen-dominated), and secretory (progesterone-dominated). These phases correspond to the phases of ovarian function. The menstrual and proliferative phases correspond to the follicular ovarian phase; the secretory phase, to the luteal ovarian phase.

The *menstrual phase* begins with day 1 of menstruation. During this phase, decreased estrogen and progesterone levels provoke shedding of most of the endometrium. When these hormone levels are low, positive feedback causes the hypothalamus to produce LH-releasing factor and FSH-releasing factor. These two factors, in turn, stimulate pituitary secretion of FSH and LH. FSH stimulates the growth of ovarian follicles; LH stimulates these follicles to secrete estrogen.

The *proliferative phase* begins with the cessation of the menstrual period and ends with ovulation. During this phase, the increased amount of estrogen secreted by the developing ovarian follicles causes the endometrium to proliferate in preparation for possible pregnancy. Around day 14 of a 28-day menstrual cycle (the average length), these high estrogen levels trigger ovulation—the rupture of one of the developing follicles and subsequent release of an ovum.

The *secretory phase* extends from the day of ovulation to about 3 days before the next menstrual period (premenstrual phase). In most women, this final phase of the menstrual cycle lasts 13 to 15 days (its length varies less than those of the menstrual and proliferative phases). After ovulation, the ruptured follicle that released the ovum remains under the influence of LH. It then becomes the *corpus luteum* and starts secreting progesterone, in addition to estrogen.

In the nonpregnant female, LH controls the secretions of the corpus luteum; in the pregnant female, human chorionic gonadotropin (HCG) controls them. At the end of the secretory phase, the uterine lining is ready to receive and nourish a zygote. If fertilization doesn't occur, increasing estrogen and progesterone levels decrease LH and FSH production. Since LH is necessary to maintain the corpus luteum, a decrease in LH production causes the corpus luteum to atrophy and stop secreting estrogen and progesterone. The thickened uterine lining then begins to slough off, and menstruation begins again, renewing the cycle.

However, if fertilization and pregnancy do occur, the endometrium grows even thicker. After implantation of the zygote (about 5 or 6 days after fertilization), the endometrium becomes the *decidua*. Chorionic villi produce HCG soon after implantation, stimulating the corpus luteum to continue secreting estrogen and progesterone, a process that prevents further ovulation and menstruation.

HCG continues to stimulate the corpus luteum until the placenta—the vascular organ that develops to transport materials to and from the fetus—forms and starts producing its own estrogen and progesterone. After the placenta takes over hormonal production, secretions of the corpus luteum are no longer needed to maintain the pregnancy, and the corpus luteum gradually decreases its function and begins to degenerate.

Pregnancy

Cell multiplication and differentiation begin in the zygote at the moment of conception. By about 17 days after conception, the placenta has established circulation to what is now an *embryo* (the term used for the conceptus between the 2nd and 7th weeks of pregnancy). By the end of the embryonic stage, fetal structures are formed. Further development now consists primarily of growth and maturation of already formed structures. From this point until birth, the conceptus is called a *fetus*.

First trimester

The length of a normal pregnancy ranges from 240 to 300 days. Although pregnancies vary in duration, they're conveniently divided into three trimesters.

During the first trimester, a female usually experiences physical changes, such as amenorrhea, urinary frequency, nausea and vomiting (more severe in the morning or when the stomach is empty), breast swelling and tenderness, fatigue, increased vaginal secretions, and constipation.

Within 3 weeks after the last menstrual period, pregnancy tests, which detect HCG in the urine and serum, are usually positive. Although positive tests strongly suggest pregnancy, a pelvic examination helps confirm it by showing Hager's sign (cervical and uterine softening), Chadwick's sign (a bluish tone to the vagina and cervix from increased venous blood circulation), and an enlarged uterus.

The first trimester is a critical time during pregnancy. Rapid cell differentiation makes the developing embryo or fetus highly susceptible to the teratogenetic effects of viruses, alcohol, cigarettes, caffeine, and drugs.

Second trimester

From the 13th to the 26th week of pregnancy, uterine and fetal size increase substantially, causing weight gain, a thickening waistline, abdominal enlargement, and possibly, reddish streaks as abdominal skin stretches (striation). In addition, pigment changes may cause skin alterations, such as linea nigra, melasma (mask of pregnancy), and a darkening of the areolae of the nipples.

Other physical changes may include diaphoresis, increased salivation, indigestion, continuing constipation, hemorrhoids, nosebleeds, and some dependent edema. The breasts become larger and heavier, and approximately 19 weeks after the last menstrual period, they may secrete colostrum. By about the 16th to 18th week of pregnancy, the fetus is large enough for the mother to feel it move (quickening).

Third trimester

During this period, the mother feels Braxton Hicks contractions—sporadic episodes of painless uterine tightening—which help strengthen uterine muscles in preparation for labor. Increasing uterine size may displace pelvic and intestinal structures, causing indigestion, protrusion of the umbilicus, shortness of breath, and insomnia. The mother may experience backaches because she walks with a swaybacked posture to counteract her frontal weight. By lying down, she can help minimize the development of varicose veins, hemorrhoids, and ankle edema.

Labor and delivery

About 2 to 3 weeks before birth, lightening—the descent of the fetal head into the pelvis—shifts the uterine position. This relieves pressure on the diaphragm and enables the mother to breathe more easily.

Onset of labor characteristically produces low back pain and passage of a small amount of bloody "show," a brownish or blood-tinged plug of cervical mucus. As labor progresses, the cervix becomes soft, then effaces and dilates; the amniotic membranes may rupture spontaneously, causing a gush or leakage of amniotic fluid. Uterine contractions become increasingly regular, frequent, intense, and longer.

Labor is usually divided into four stages:

• *Stage I*, the longest stage, lasts from onset of regular contractions until full cervical dilation (4″ [10 cm]). Average duration of this stage is about 12 hours for a primigravida and 6 hours for a multigravida.

• *Stage II* lasts from full cervical dilation until delivery of the infant—about 1½ hours for a primigravida, 30 minutes for a multigravida.

• *Stage III*, the time between delivery and expulsion of the placenta, usually lasts 3 to 4 minutes for a primigravida and 4 to 5 minutes for a multigravida, but may last an hour.

• *Stage IV* constitutes a period of recov-

STAGES OF LABOR

LIGHTENING

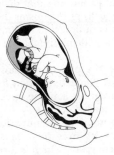

Descent of the fetal head into the pelvis

STAGE I

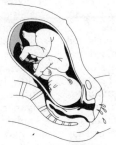

Onset of regular contractions and breaking of the amniotic sac

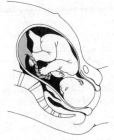

Full cervical dilation

STAGE II

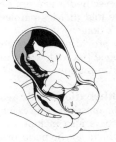

Delivering the head

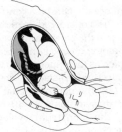

Rotating the head

STAGE III

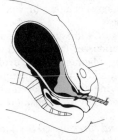

Uterine contractions

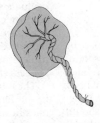

Expulsion of the placenta

STAGE IV

Reestablishment of homeostasis during this stage includes recuperation from anesthetic (if used), normalization of vital signs, cessation of bleeding, and return of muscle tone.

ery during which homeostasis is reestablished. This final stage lasts 1 to 4 hours after expulsion of the placenta.

Sources of pathology

In no other part of the body do so many interrelated physiologic functions occur in such proximity as in the area of the female reproductive tract. Besides the internal genitalia already discussed, the female pelvis contains the organs of the urinary and the gastrointestinal systems (bladder, ureters, urethra, sigmoid colon, and rectum). The reproductive tract and its surrounding area are thus the site of urination, defecation, menstruation, ovulation, copulation, impregnation, and parturition. It's easy to understand how an abnormality in one pelvic organ can readily induce abnormality in another.

When conducting a pelvic examination, all possible sources of pathology must be considered—serious abnormalities of the pelvic organs can be asymptomatic. Also to be considered is that abnormal findings in the pelvic area may result from pathologic changes in other organ systems, such as the upper urinary and the gastrointestinal tracts, the endocrine glands, and the neuromusculoskeletal system. Pain symptoms are often associated with the menstrual cycle; therefore, in many common diseases of the female reproductive tract, such pain follows a cyclic pattern. A patient with pelvic inflammatory disease, for example, may complain of increasing premenstrual pain that is relieved by onset of menstruation.

Pelvic examination

A pelvic examination, accompanied by a thorough patient history, is essential for any patient with symptoms related to the reproductive tract or adjacent body systems. The patient's history of pregnancy, miscarriage and abortion should be documented. The patient should be asked if she has experienced any recent changes in her urinary habits or menstrual cycle, what method of birth control she uses, if any, and whether she has

experienced any side effects from her birth control method.

Preparing the patient for the pelvic examination includes:
• asking if she's douched within the last 24 hours and explaining that douching washes away cells or organisms that the examination is designed to evaluate.
• checking the patient's weight and blood pressure.
• instructing the patient to empty her bladder before the examination for her comfort; providing a urine specimen container, if needed.
• explaining what the examination entails and why it's necessary. This will help the patient relax, which is essential for a thorough pelvic examination.
• informing the patient scheduled for a Papanicolaou (Pap) smear that another smear may have to be taken later, and reassuring her that this is done to confirm the results of the first test. If she has never had a Pap test before, she should be told that it's painless, and also why it's done.
• providing the patient with premoistened tissues to clean the vulva after the examination.

Other diagnostic tests

Diagnostic measures for gynecologic disorders also include the following tests, which can be performed in the doctor's office:
• *wet smear* to examine vaginal secretions for specific organisms, such as *Trichomonas vaginalis, Candida albicans,* or *Hemophilus vaginalis,* or to evaluate semen specimens in rape or infertility cases
• *endometrial biopsy* to assess hormonal secretions of the corpus luteum, to determine whether normal ovulation is occurring, and to check for neoplasia.

The following surgical procedures can be performed only in a hospital under anesthesia:
• *dilation and curettage* (D & C) to evaluate atypical bleeding
• *laparoscopy* to evaluate infertility, dysmenorrhea, and pelvic pain, and as a means of sterilization.

GYNECOLOGIC DISORDERS

Premenstrual Tension

Premenstrual tension is characterized by a varying syndrome that appears 7 to 14 days before menses and usually subsides with its onset. The effects of premenstrual tension range from minimal discomfort to severe, disruptive symptoms (premenstrual tension syndrome) and often include nervousness, irritability, and abdominal bloating. This disorder occurs in 30% to 50% of women, usually between ages 25 and 40. Incidence seems to rise with age and parity.

Causes

Although the direct cause of premenstrual tension is unknown, a known precipitating factor is the loss of intravascular fluid into body tissues, which triggers an increase in antidiuretic hormone and aldosterone secretion. This causes transient water retention, which in turn produces characteristic symptoms such as edema, bloating, weight gain, and breast tenderness. Edema induces CNS changes, resulting in headaches and mood shifts.

Other conditions that possibly contribute to premenstrual tension include estrogen-progesterone imbalance, progesterone allergy, and hypoglycemia, as well as psychogenic factors.

Signs and symptoms

Clinical effects vary widely and may include any combination of the following:
• *behavioral:* mild to severe personality changes, nervousness, irritability, agitation, sleep disturbances, fatigue, lethargy, and depression
• *neurologic:* headache, vertigo, syncope, paresthesia of the arms and legs, exacerbation of epilepsy
• *respiratory:* increased incidence of colds, exacerbation of allergic rhinitis and asthma
• *gastrointestinal:* abdominal bloating (most common symptom), diarrhea or constipation, change in appetite, exacerbation of spastic colitis
• *other:* edema, temporary weight gain, palpitations, backache, exacerbation of

skin problems (such as acne), breast changes (such as enlargement and tenderness), oliguria, easy bruising (due to capillary fragility), and eye disorders (such as conjunctivitis).

Diagnosis

Patient history shows typical menstrually related symptoms. Estrogen and progesterone blood levels may be evaluated to rule out hormonal imbalance.

Treatment

Treatment is primarily symptomatic, and may include tranquilizers and sedatives to relieve behavioral symptoms, and diuretics and decreased salt intake to relieve bloating and edema. Since the precipitative cause of premenstrual tension is often unknown, drug therapy should be avoided, when possible. Some doctors consider salt restriction or the use of diuretics unnecessary.

Additional considerations

• Women should know that premenstrual tension is not a serious disorder.
• Measures which may help relieve symptoms include restricting salt intake for 10 days before menses to minimize fluid retention, and avoiding or restricting the use of stimulants, such as caffeine, nicotine, and alcoholic beverages.
• A complete history will help identify any emotional problems that may contribute to premenstrual tension. If necessary, the woman should be referred for psychologic counseling.

- Various life-style changes might help alleviate symptoms by reducing stress and anxiety, and allowing more relaxation.

- If manifestations of premenstrual tension are severe enough to disrupt normal life-style, medical help may be necessary.

Dysmenorrhea

Dysmenorrhea—painful menstruation—is the most common gynecologic complaint and a leading cause of absenteeism from school (affects 10% of high school girls each month) and work (estimated 140 million work hours lost annually). Dysmenorrhea can occur as a primary disorder or secondary to an underlying disease. Since primary dysmenorrhea is self-limiting, prognosis is generally good. Prognosis for secondary dysmenorrhea depends on the underlying disorder.

Causes and incidence

Although primary dysmenorrhea is unrelated to any identifiable cause, possible contributing factors include hormonal imbalances and psychogenic factors. The pain of dysmenorrhea probably results from increased prostaglandin secretion, which intensifies uterine contractions. Dysmenorrhea may also be secondary to endometriosis, cervical stenosis, uterine leiomyomas, uterine malposition, pelvic inflammatory disease, pelvic tumors, or adenomyosis.

Since dysmenorrhea almost always follows an ovulatory cycle, both the primary and secondary forms are rare during the first 2 years of menses, which are usually anovulatory. After age 20, dysmenorrhea is generally secondary.

Signs and symptoms

Dysmenorrhea produces sharp, intermittent, cramping, lower abdominal pain, which usually radiates to the back, thighs, groin, and vulva. Such pain—sometimes compared to labor pains—typically starts with or immediately before menstrual flow and peaks within 24 hours. Dysmenorrhea may be associated with symptoms of premenstrual tension (urinary frequency, nausea, vomiting, diarrhea, headache, chills, abdominal bloating, painful breasts, depression, and irritability).

Diagnosis

Pelvic examination, a detailed patient history, and if necessary, psychiatric evaluation may suggest the cause of dysmenorrhea.

 A uterine sound passed through the internal cervical os reproduces the typical pain and confirms primary dysmenorrhea. Appropriate tests (such as laparoscopy, dilation and cu-

---

CAUSES OF PELVIC PAIN

The characteristic pelvic pain of dysmenorrhea must be distinguished from the acute pain caused by many other disorders, such as:
- *gastrointestinal disorders:* appendicitis, acute diverticulitis, acute or chronic cholecystitis, chronic cholelithiasis, acute pancreatitis, peptic ulcer perforation, intestinal obstruction
- *urinary tract disorders:* cystitis, renal calculi
- *reproductive disorders:* acute salpingitis, chronic inflammation, degenerating fibroid, ovarian cyst torsion
- *pregnancy disorders:* impending abortion (pain and bleeding early in pregnancy), ectopic pregnancy, abruptio placentae, uterine rupture, leiomyoma degeneration, toxemia
- *emotional conflicts:* psychogenic (functional) pain.

Various conditions may mimic dysmenorrhea. These include ovulation and normal uterine contractions in pregnancy.

rettage, and X-rays) are used to diagnose underlying disorders in secondary dysmenorrhea.

Treatment
Treatment to relieve pain may include:
• *analgesics,* such as aspirin, for mild to moderate pain (most effective when taken 24 to 48 hours before onset of menses). Aspirin is especially effective because it also inhibits prostaglandin activity.
• *narcotics* if pain is severe (infrequently used).
• *prostaglandin inhibitors* (such as mefenamic acid and ibuprofen) to relieve pain by decreasing uterine contractions.
• *heat* applied locally to the lower abdomen (may relieve discomfort in women but is not recommended in young girls because appendicitis may mimic dysmenorrhea).

For *primary dysmenorrhea,* sex steroid therapy is an alternative to treatment with analgesics. Such therapy usually consists of oral contraceptives, but may include estrogen alone, to relieve pain by suppressing ovulation (effective in 90% of patients). A single trial dose, which may suppress ovulation for three to five menstrual cycles, cures 10% of patients. Most patients, however, require repeated doses for more than 6 months. Persistently severe dysmenorrhea may have a psychogenic cause.

In *secondary dysmenorrhea,* treatment is designed to identify and correct the underlying cause. This may include surgical treatment of underlying disorders, such as endometriosis or uterine leiomyomas, but only after conservative therapy fails. Rarely, severe and disabling dysmenorrhea may require insertion of a stem pessary into the cervical os, transection of the uterosacral ligaments (Doyce operation), or presacral neurectomy (Cotte's operation).

Additional considerations
Management focuses on relief of symptoms, emotional support, and patient teaching, especially for the adolescent. This includes:
• obtaining a complete patient history, including information on possible symptoms of pelvic disease, such as excessive bleeding, changes in bleeding pattern, vaginal discharge, and dyspareunia.
• explaining normal anatomy and physiology to the patient, as well as the nature of dysmenorrhea (this may be a good opportunity, if warranted, to provide the adolescent patient with information on pregnancy and contraception).
• encouraging the patient to seek medical care if her symptoms persist.

Vulvovaginitis

Vulvovaginitis is inflammation of the vulva (vulvitis) and vagina (vaginitis). Because of the proximity of these two structures, inflammation of one usually precipitates inflammation of the other. Vulvovaginitis may occur at any age and affects most females at some time. Prognosis is good with treatment.

Causes
Common causes of vaginitis (with or without consequent vulvitis) include:
• infection with *Trichomonas vaginalis,* a protozoan flagellate, usually transmitted through sexual intercourse.
• infection with *Candida albicans (Monilia),* a fungus that requires glucose for growth. Incidence rises during the secretory phase of the menstrual cycle. Such infection occurs twice as often in pregnant females as in nonpregnant females. It also commonly affects users of oral contraceptives, diabetics, and patients receiving systemic therapy with broad-spectrum antibiotics (incidence may reach 75%).
• infection with *Hemophilus vaginalis,*

a gram-negative bacillus.

• venereal infection with *Neisseria gonorrhoeae* (gonorrhea), a gram-negative diplococcus.

• viral infection with venereal warts (condylomata acuminata) or herpesvirus Type II, usually transmitted by sexual intercourse.

• vaginal mucosa atrophy in menopausal women due to decreasing levels of estrogen, which predisposes to bacterial invasion.

Common causes of vulvitis include:

• parasitic infection (*Phthirus pubis* [crab louse]).

• trauma (skin breakdown may lead to secondary infection).

• poor personal hygiene, especially from contamination with urine, feces, or vaginal secretions.

• chemical irritations, or allergic reactions to feminine hygiene sprays, douches, detergents, clothing, or toilet paper.

• vulval atrophy in menopausal women due to decreasing estrogen levels.

Signs and symptoms

In trichomonal vaginitis, vaginal discharge is thin, bubbly, green-tinged, and malodorous. This infection causes marked irritation and itching, and urinary symptoms, such as burning and frequency. Monilia vaginitis produces a thick, white, cottage-cheese–like discharge and red, edematous mucous membranes, with white flecks adhering to the vaginal wall, and is often accompanied by intense itching. Hemophilus vaginitis produces a gray, foul-smelling discharge. Gonorrhea may produce no symptoms at all, or a profuse, purulent discharge and dysuria.

Acute vulvitis causes a mild to severe inflammatory reaction, including edema, erythema, burning, and pruritus. Severe pain on urination and dyspareunia may necessitate immediate treatment. Herpes infection may cause painful ulceration or vesicle formation during the active phase. Chronic vulvitis generally causes relatively mild inflammation, possibly associated with severe edema that may involve the entire perineum.

Diagnosis

Diagnosis of vaginitis requires identification of the infectious organism during microscopic examination of vaginal exudate on a wet slide preparation (a drop of vaginal exudate placed in normal saline solution).

• In trichomonal infections, the presence of motile, flagellated trichomonads confirms the diagnosis.

• In monilia vaginitis, 10% potassium hydroxide is added to the slide, and microscopic examination seeks "clue cells" (granular epithelial cells); however, diagnosis requires identification of *C. albicans* fungi.

• Gonorrhea necessitates culture of vaginal exudate on Thayer-Martin or Transgrow medium to confirm diagnosis.

Diagnosis of vulvitis or suspected venereal disease may require CBC, urinalysis, cytology screening, biopsy of chronic lesions to rule out malignancy, and culture of exudate from acute lesions.

Treatment

Common therapeutic measures include the following:

• metronidazole P.O. for the patient with trichomonal vaginitis, and all sexual partners (if possible), since recurrence often results from reinfection by an asymptomatic male.

• vaginal ointments and suppositories, such as nystatin, for monilia vaginitis.

• local antibiotic therapy for hemophilus vaginitis.

• systemic antibiotic therapy (penicillin and probenicid) for the patient with gonorrhea, and all sexual partners.

Cold compresses or cool sitz baths may provide relief from pruritus in acute vulvitis; severe inflammation may require warm compresses. Other therapy includes avoiding drying soaps, wearing loose clothing to promote air circulation, and applying topical corticosteroids to reduce inflammation. Chronic vulvitis may respond to topical hydrocortisone or antipruritics and good hygiene (especially in elderly or incontinent patients). Topical estrogen ointments may be used to treat atrophic vulvovaginitis. No treatment currently exists for herpesvirus infections; however, the investigational drug 2-deoxy-d-glucose shows promise.

Additional considerations
Management of vulvovaginitis includes:
• asking the patient if she has any drug allergies; stressing the importance of taking the medication for the length of time prescribed, even if symptoms subside.
• teaching the patient how to insert vaginal ointments and suppositories; telling her to remain prone for at least 30 minutes after insertion to promote absorption (insertion at bedtime is ideal); suggesting that she wear a pad to prevent staining her underclothing.
• encouraging good hygiene; advising the patient with a history of recurrent vulvovaginitis to wear all-cotton underpants; advising her to avoid wearing clothing that increases moisture in the genital area (such as tight-fitting pants and panty hose), thereby favoring the growth of the infecting organisms.
• reporting cases of venereal disease to the local public health authorities.
• advising the patient of the correlation between sexual contact and the spread of vaginal infections.

Ovarian Cysts

Ovarian cysts are usually nonneoplastic sacs on an ovary that contain fluid or semisolid material. Although these cysts are usually small and produce no symptoms, they require thorough investigation as possible sites of malignant change. Common ovarian cysts include follicular cysts, lutein cysts (granulosa-lutein [corpus luteum] and theca-lutein cysts), and polycystic (or sclerocystic) disease. Ovarian cysts can develop any time between puberty and menopause, including during pregnancy. Granulosa-lutein cysts occur infrequently, usually during early pregnancy. Prognosis for nonneoplastic ovarian cysts is excellent.

Causes
Follicular cysts are generally very small and arise from follicles that overdistend instead of going through the atretic stage of the menstrual cycle. When such cysts persist into menopause, they secrete excessive amounts of estrogen in response to the hypersecretion of follicle-stimulating hormone and luteinizing hormone that normally occurs during menopause.

Granulosa-lutein cysts, which occur within the corpus luteum, are functional, nonneoplastic enlargements of the ovaries, caused by excessive accumulation of blood during the hemorrhagic phase of the menstrual cycle. *Theca-lutein cysts* are commonly bilateral and filled with clear, straw-colored fluid; they are often associated with hydatidiform mole, choriocarcinoma, or hormone therapy (with human chorionic gonadotropin [HCG] or clomiphene citrate).

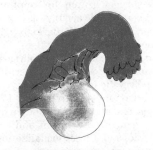

FOLLICULAR CYST

A common type of ovarian cyst, a follicular cyst is usually semi-transparent and overdistended with watery fluid that is visible through its thin walls.

Polycystic ovarian disease is part of the Stein-Leventhal syndrome and stems from endocrine abnormalities.

Signs and symptoms

Small ovarian cysts (such as follicular cysts) usually don't produce symptoms unless torsion or rupture causes signs of an acute abdomen (abdominal tenderness, distention, and rigidity). Large or multiple cysts may induce mild pelvic discomfort, low back pain, dyspareunia, or abnormal uterine bleeding secondary to a disturbed ovulatory pattern. Ovarian cysts with torsion induce acute abdominal pain similar to that of appendicitis.

Granulosa-lutein cysts that appear early in pregnancy may grow as large as 2″ to 2½″ (5 to 6 cm) in diameter and produce unilateral pelvic discomfort and, if rupture occurs, massive intraperitoneal hemorrhage. In nonpregnant women, these cysts may cause delayed menses, followed by prolonged or irregular bleeding. Polycystic ovarian disease may also produce secondary amenorrhea, oligomenorrhea, or infertility.

Diagnosis

Generally, characteristic clinical features suggest ovarian cysts.

 Visualization of the ovary through pelvic pneumoroentgenography, culdoscopy, culdotomy, laparoscopy, or surgery (often for another condition) confirms ovarian cysts.

Extremely elevated HCG titers strongly suggest theca-lutein cysts.

In polycystic ovarian disease, physical examination demonstrates bilaterally enlarged polycystic ovaries. Tests reveal slight elevation of urinary 17-ketosteroids, and anovulation (shown by basal body temperature graphs and endometrial biopsy). Direct visualization must rule out paraovarian cysts of the broad ligament, salpingitis, endometriosis, and neoplastic cysts.

Treatment

Follicular cysts generally don't require treatment, since they tend to disappear spontaneously within 60 days. However, if they interfere with daily activities, clomiphene citrate P.O. for 5 days or progesterone I.M. (also for 5 days) re-establishes the ovarian hormonal cycle and induces ovulation. Oral contraceptives may also accelerate involution of functional cysts (including both types of lutein cysts and follicular cysts).

Treatment for granulosa-lutein cysts that occur during pregnancy is symptomatic, since these cysts diminish during the third trimester and rarely require surgery. Theca-lutein cysts disappear spontaneously after elimination of the hydatidiform mole, destruction of choriocarcinoma, or discontinuation of HCG or clomiphene citrate therapy.

Treatment for polycystic ovarian disease varies and may include drugs, such as hydrocortisone or clomiphene citrate, to induce ovulation, or surgical wedge resection of one half to one third of the ovary if drug therapy fails to induce ovulation.

Treatment for ovarian cysts, in general, consists primarily of observation, if the cyst is known to be nonmalignant. However, because a doubt often exists, surgery frequently becomes necessary for both diagnosis and treatment.

Additional considerations

Thorough patient teaching is a primary consideration. The nature of the particular cyst should be explained to the patient, as well as the type of discomfort—if any—she is apt to experience, and how long the condition is expected to last. The hospital staff member should:
• preoperatively, watch for signs of cyst rupture, such as increasing abdominal pain, distention, and rigidity; monitor vital signs for fever, tachypnea, or hypotension, a sign of possible peritonitis or intraperitoneal hemorrhage; administer sedatives, as ordered, to assure adequate preoperative rest and minimize the patient's fear of surgery.
• postoperatively, encourage frequent movement in bed and early ambulation, as ordered, to prevent pulmonary embo-

lism.
• provide emotional support; offer appropriate reassurance if the patient fears cancer or infertility; assure the patient worried about the possibility of recurrence that it is unlikely.

• advise the patient before discharge to increase her at-home activity gradually—preferably over 4 to 6 weeks; tell her to abstain from intercourse, and to avoid using tampons and douching during this time.

Endometriosis

Endometriosis is the presence of endometrial tissue outside the lining of the uterine cavity. Such ectopic tissue is generally confined to the pelvic area, most commonly around the ovaries, uterovesical peritoneum, uterosacral ligaments, and the cul-de-sac, but it can appear anywhere in the body. Active endometriosis usually occurs between ages 30 and 40, especially in women who postpone childbearing; it's uncommon before age 20. Severe symptoms of endometriosis may have an abrupt onset or may develop over many years. Generally, this disorder becomes progressively severe during the menstrual years; after menopause, it tends to subside.

Causes
The direct cause is unknown, but familial susceptibility or recent surgery that necessitated opening the uterus (such as a cesarean section) may predispose a woman to endometriosis. Although neither of these possible predisposing factors explains all the lesions in endometriosis or their location, research focuses on the following possible causes:
• *Transportation:* During menstruation, the fallopian tubes expel endometrial fragments that implant on the ovaries or pelvic peritoneum.
• *Formation in situ:* Inflammation or a hormonal change triggers metaplasia (differentiation of coelomic epithelium to endometrial epithelium).
• *Induction* (a combination of transportation and of formation in situ): The endometrium chemically induces undifferentiated mesenchyma to form endometrial epithelium. (This is the most likely cause.)

Signs and symptoms
The classic symptom of endometriosis is acquired dysmenorrhea, which produces constant pain in the lower abdomen, and in the vagina, posterior pelvis, and back. This pain usually begins from 5 to 7 days before menses reaches its

peak and lasts for 2 to 3 days. It differs from primary dysmenorrheal pain, which is more cramplike and concentrated in the abdominal midline. However, the severity of pain doesn't necessarily indicate the extent of the disease.

Other clinical features, and pain severity depend on the location of the ectopic tissue:
• *ovaries and oviducts:* infertility and

STAGING OF ENDOMETRIOSIS

Stage I: One or more small superficial implants on the pelvic peritoneum

Stage II: Larger superficial implants on uterosacral ligaments, rectovaginal septum, or ovaries

Stage III: Endometriomas of the ovary (more than 5 mm in diameter), with possible superficial implants on broad ligaments and adjacent organs

Stage IV: Penetration of vagina, bowel, or urinary tract, and distant metastases (lymph nodes, umbilicus, surgical wounds)

Stage V: Endometriomas become adenocarcinomas.

Adapted with permission from R.C. Benson, ed., CURRENT OBSTETRIC AND GYNECOLOGIC DIAGNOSIS AND TREATMENT (Los Altos, Calif. Lange Medical Publications, 1980).

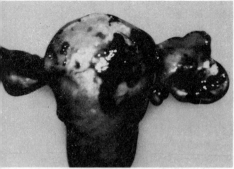

This photo shows endometrial deposits on the outer uterine wall, fallopian tubes, and ovaries. These deposits can also occur anywhere on the peritoneal surface of the pelvis and occasionally in extraperitoneal locations, such as postoperative scar endometriosis.

profuse menses
• *ovaries or cul-de-sac:* deep-thrust dyspareunia
• *bladder:* menstrual hematuria
• *rectovaginal septum and colon:* painful defecation, rectal bleeding with menses, pain in the coccyx or sacrum
• *small bowel and appendix:* nausea and vomiting, which worsen before menses; and abdominal cramps
• *cervix, vagina, and perineum:* bleeding from endometrial deposits in these areas during menses.

The primary complication of endometriosis is infertility, which occurs in 34% of patients (as opposed to 12% of the general female population).

Diagnosis

Pelvic examination suggests endometriosis. Palpation may detect multiple tender nodules on uterosacral ligaments or in the rectovaginal septum of the posterior fornix of the vagina. These nodules enlarge and become more tender during menses. Palpation may also uncover ovarian enlargement in the presence of endometrial cysts on the ovaries or thickened, nodular adnexa (as in pelvic inflammatory disease).

Laparoscopy may confirm diagnosis and determine the stage of the disease.

Cul-de-sac aspiration revealing abdominal bleeding indicates endometrial cyst rupture. Barium enema rules out malignant or inflammatory bowel disease.

Endometriosis is uncovered in 20% of patients undergoing gynecologic surgery for other disorders. In about one third of these patients, the disorder is in an advanced stage.

Treatment and additional considerations

Treatment varies according to the stage of the disease, and the patient's age and desire to have children. Conservative therapy for young women who want to have children includes androgens, such as danazol, which produce a temporary remission in Stages I and II. Continuous progesterone therapy may induce a similar remission in Stages I and II by gradually producing pseudopregnancy, which results in prolonged amenorrhea and, possibly, relief of symptoms. Mild analgesics may alleviate pain, especially if the disease is not severe.

When ovarian masses are present (Stages III to V), surgery must rule out malignancy. Conservative surgery may include resection of cysts and lysis of adhesions. However, treatment of choice for women who don't want to bear children or for extensive disease (Stages III to V) is a total abdominal hysterectomy with bilateral salpingo-oophorectomy.

• Minor gynecologic procedures are contraindicated immediately before and during menstruation.

• Adolescents should use sanitary napkins instead of tampons; this can help prevent retrograde flow in girls with a narrow vagina or small introitus.

• The patient needs reassurance that endometriosis is not a life-threatening condition.

• Since infertility is a possible complication, the patient who wants to have children should not postpone childbearing.

• All patients should have an annual pelvic examination and Pap smear for earlier diagnosis and more effective treatment.

Uterine Leiomyomas

(Myomas, fibromyomas, fibroids)

The most common benign tumors in women, uterine leiomyomas are smooth-muscle tumors. They are usually multiple and generally occur in the uterine corpus, although they may appear on the cervix or on the round or broad ligament. Uterine leiomyomas are often called fibroids, but this term is misleading, since these tumors consist of muscle cells and not fibrous tissue. "Myoma" is sometimes used as a shortened form of leiomyoma.

Uterine leiomyomas occur in approximately 20% of all women over age 35, and affect Blacks three times more often than Caucasians. Malignancy (leiomyosarcoma) develops in only 0.1% of patients.

Causes and incidence

The cause of uterine leiomyomas is unknown, but estrogen and human growth hormone (HGH) may influence tumor formation by stimulating susceptible fibromuscular elements. This theory seems likely, since large doses of estrogen and the later stages of pregnancy increase both tumor size and HGH levels. Also, leiomyomas usually shrink or disappear after menopause, when estrogen production decreases.

Signs and symptoms

Usually, hypermenorrhea is the cardinal sign of uterine leiomyomas, although other forms of abnormal endometrial bleeding, as well as dysmenorrhea or leukorrhea are possible. Pain may occur if the tumors twist or degenerate after circulatory occlusion or infection, or if the uterus contracts in an attempt to expel a pedunculated submucous leiomyoma. Large tumors may produce a feeling of heaviness in the abdomen; pressure on surrounding organs may cause secondary pain, backache, intestinal obstruction, constipation, and urinary frequency or urgency. Also, irregular uterine enlargement may occur, often asymptomatically.

Diagnosis

Clinical findings and a thorough patient history suggest uterine leiomyomas. Blood studies showing anemia from abnormal bleeding support the diagnosis, but palpation of the tumor, revealing a round mass, helps to confirm it. Results of radioimmunoassays of plasma HGH and estrogen in patients with leiomyomas are inconclusive. Other diagnostic procedures include dilation and curettage (D & C) to detect submucous leiomyomas in the endometrial cavity, or laparoscopy to visualize subserous leiomyomas on the uterine surface. Barium enema X-rays may rule out colonic tumors.

Treatment

Treatment depends on the severity of symptoms, size and location of the tumors, and the patient's age, parity, pregnancy status, desire to have children, and general health.

To monitor tumor growth patterns in a nonpregnant, asymptomatic woman, only a pelvic examination every 6 to 12 months is required. If they have caused problems in the past, or if they are likely to threaten a future pregnancy, small leiomyomas may be surgically removed. This is the treatment of choice for a young woman who wants to have children.

Tumors that twist or grow large enough to cause intestinal obstruction require a hysterectomy, with preservation of the ovaries, if possible. Anemia caused by excessive bleeding may necessitate blood transfusions.

If the patient is pregnant, but her uterus is no larger than a 6-month normal uterus by the 16th week of preg-

BENIGN UTERINE TUMOR

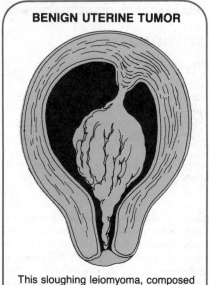

This sloughing leiomyoma, composed of smooth muscle cells, is attached to the myometrium by an elongated pedicle. The tumor's smooth surface is interrupted by fibrous bands, bloody discharge, and necrotic tissue.

has a leiomyomatous uterus the size of a 5- to 6-month normal uterus by the 9th week of pregnancy, spontaneous abortion will probably occur, especially with a cervical leiomyoma. If surgery becomes necessary, a hysterectomy is usually performed 5 to 6 months after delivery, when involution is complete, with preservation of the ovaries, if possible.

Additional considerations
• The patient must report any abnormal bleeding or pelvic pain immediately.
• If a hysterectomy or oophorectomy is indicated, the effects of the operation on menstruation, menopause, and sexual activity should be explained to the patient and her husband.
• The patient will need reassurance that she won't experience premature menopause if the ovaries are left intact.
• If a multiple myomectomy is necessary, the patient must understand that pregnancy is still possible; however, if the uterine cavity is entered during surgery, a cesarean delivery may be necessary when she is pregnant.
• In a patient with severe anemia due to excessive bleeding, iron and blood transfusions should be given, as ordered, and their importance explained.

nancy, the outcome for the pregnancy is favorable, and surgery is usually unnecessary. However, if a pregnant woman

Precocious Puberty in Females

In females, precocious puberty is onset of pubertal changes (breast development, pubic and axillary hair, and menarche) before age 9 (normally, the mean age for menarche is 13). In true precocious puberty, the ovaries mature and pubertal changes progress in an orderly manner. In pseudoprecocious puberty, the genitalia mature and secondary sex characteristics appear without corresponding ovarian maturation.

Causes
About 85% of all true precocious puberty in females is constitutional, resulting from early development and activation of the endocrine glands without corresponding abnormality. Other causes of true precocious puberty are pathologic, and include CNS disorders resulting from tumors, trauma, infection, or other le-

sions. These CNS disorders include hypothalamic tumors, intracranial tumors (pinealoma, granuloma, hamartoma), hydrocephaly, degenerative encephalopathy, tuberous sclerosis, neurofibromatosis, encephalitis, skull injuries, meningitis, and peptic arachnoiditis. Albright's syndrome, Silver's syndrome, and juvenile hypothyroidism are conditions often associated with female precocity.

Pseudoprecocious puberty may result from increased levels of sex hormones due to ovarian and adrenocortical tumors, adrenal cortical virilizing hyperplasia, and ingestion of estrogens or androgens. It may also result from increased end-organ sensitivity to low levels of circulating sex hormones, whereby estrogens promote premature breast development and androgens promote premature pubic and axillary hair growth.

Signs and symptoms

The usual pattern of precocious puberty in females is a rapid growth spurt, thelarche (breast development), pubarche (pubic hair development), and menarche—all before age 9. These changes may occur independently or simultaneously.

Diagnosis

Diagnosis requires a complete patient history, a thorough physical examination, and special tests to differentiate between true and pseudoprecocious puberty and to indicate what treatment may be necessary. X-rays of hands, wrists, knees, and hips determine bone age, and possible premature epiphyseal closure. Other tests detect abnormally high hormonal levels for the patient's age: vaginal smear for estrogen secretion, urinary tests for gonadotropic activity and excretion of 17-ketosteroids, and radioimmunoassay for both luteinizing and follicle-stimulating hormones.

As indicated, laparoscopy or exploratory laparotomy may verify a suspected abdominal lesion; electroencephalography, ventriculography, pneumoencephalography, CAT scan, or angiography can detect CNS disorders.

Treatment

Although still controversial, treatment of constitutional true precocious puberty may include medroxyprogesterone to reduce secretion of gonadotropins and prevent menstruation. Other therapy depends on the cause of precocious puberty

and its stage of development:

• *Adrenogenital syndrome* necessitates cortical or adrenocortical steroid replacement.

• *Abdominal tumors* necessitate surgery to remove ovarian and adrenal tumors. Regression of secondary sex characteristics may follow such surgery, especially in young children.

• *Choriocarcinomas* require surgery and chemotherapy.

• *Hypothyroidism* requires thyroid extract or levothyroxine to decrease gonadotropic secretions.

• *Drug ingestion* requires that the medication be discontinued.

In precocious thelarche and pubarche, no treatment is necessary.

Additional considerations

The dramatic physical changes produced by precocious puberty can be upsetting and alarming for the child and her family. The patient and family should be encouraged to express their feelings about these changes in a calm, supportive atmosphere. The patient and family should be given a clear explanation of all diagnostic procedures, and must know that surgery may be necessary.

• Explaining her condition to the child in terms she can understand can prevent psychologic damage stemming from feelings of shame and loss of self-esteem. The patient will need appropriate sex education, including information on menstruation and related hygiene.

• Parents should understand that although their daughter seems physically mature, she is not psychologically mature, and the discrepancy between physical appearance and psychologic and psychosexual maturation may create problems. They must be warned against expecting more of her than they would expect of other children her age.

• Parents should continue to dress their daughter in clothes that are appropriate for her age and in styles that don't call attention to her physical development.

• Parents should be reassured that precocious puberty *doesn't* usually precipitate precocious sexual behavior.

Menopause

Menopause is the gradual decline and eventual cessation of menstruation and of the physiologic mechanisms that cause it. Menopause includes a complex syndrome of physiologic and psychosocial changes—the climacteric—caused by declining ovarian function.

Causes and incidence

Menopause occurs in three forms:
- *Physiologic menopause,* the normal decline in ovarian function due to aging, begins in most women between ages 40 and 50, and results in infrequent ovulation, decreased menstrual function, and eventually, cessation of menstruation (usually between ages 45 and 55).
- *Pathologic menopause* (premature menopause), the gradual or abrupt cessation of menstruation before age 40, occurs idiopathically in about 5% of women in the United States. However, certain diseases, especially severe infections and reproductive tract tumors, may cause pathologic menopause by seriously impairing ovarian function. Other factors that may precipitate pathologic menopause include malnutrition, debilitation, extreme emotional stress, excessive radiation exposure, and surgical procedures that impair ovarian blood supply.
- *Artificial menopause* is the cessation of ovarian function following radiation therapy or surgical procedures, such as oophorectomy.

Signs and symptoms

The decline in ovarian function and consequent decreased estrogen level that characterize all forms of menopause produce various menstrual cycle irregularities: a decrease in the amount and duration of menstrual flow, spotting, and episodes of amenorrhea and polymenorrhea (possibly with hypermenorrhea). These irregularities may last only a few months or may persist for several years before menstruation ceases permanently.

The following changes may occur in the body's systems but usually not until after the permanent cessation of menstruation:

- *reproductive system:* shrinkage of vulval structures and loss of subcutaneous fat, possibly leading to atrophic vulvitis; atrophy of vaginal mucosa and flattening of vaginal rugae, possibly causing bleeding after coitus or douching; vaginal itching, and discharge from bacterial invasion; and loss of capillaries in the atrophying vaginal wall, causing the pink, rugal lining to become smooth and white. Menopause may also produce excessive vaginal dryness and dyspareunia due to decreased lubrication from the vaginal walls and decreased secretion from Bartholin's glands; a reduction in the size of the ovaries and oviducts; and progressive pelvic relaxation, as the supporting structures of the reproductive tract lose their tone due to the absence of estrogen.
- *urinary system:* atrophic cystitis due to the deleterious effects of decreased estrogen levels on bladder mucosa and related structures, causing pyuria, dysuria, urinary frequency, urgency, and incontinence. Urethral carbuncles from loss of urethral tone and thinning of the mucosa may cause dysuria, meatal tenderness, and occasionally, hematuria.
- *mammary system:* reduction in breast size
- *integumentary system:* loss of skin elasticity and turgor due to estrogen deprivation, loss of pubic and axillary hair, and occasionally, slight alopecia
- *autonomic nervous system:* hot flashes and night sweats (in 60% of women), vertigo, syncope, tachycardia, dyspnea, tinnitus, emotional disturbances (such as irritability, nervousness, crying spells,

fits of anger), and exacerbation of preexisting neurotic disorders (such as depression, anxiety, and compulsive, manic, or schizoid behavior).

Menopause may also induce atherosclerosis and osteoporosis. The role of estrogen deficiency in causing atherosclerosis is unclear. However, a decrease in estrogen level is known to contribute to osteoporosis, or bone loss caused by increased bone resorption and decreased bone formation, which may lead to long-bone fractures. Maximum bone loss occurs in weight-bearing bones, commonly producing kyphosis and, possibly, severe pain.

Artificial menopause, without estrogen replacement, produces symptoms within 2 to 5 years in 95% of women. Since the cessation of menstruation in both pathologic and artificial menopause is often abrupt, severe vasomotor and emotional disturbances may result. Menstrual bleeding after 1 year of amenorrhea may indicate organic disease.

Diagnosis
Patient history and typical clinical features suggest menopause. A Pap smear may support the diagnosis by showing the influence of estrogen deficiency on vaginal mucosa. In addition, radioimmunoassay reveals the following blood hormone levels:
- estrogen: 0 to 14 ng/dl
- plasma estradiol: 15 to 40 pg/ml
- estrone: 25 to 50 pg/ml.

Radioimmunoassay also shows the following urine values:
- estrogen: 6 to 28 mcg/24 hours
- pregnanediol (urinary secretion of progesterone): 0.3 to 0.9 mg/24 hours.

The most striking endocrine change occurs in the secretion of pituitary gonadotropins. Follicle-stimulating hormone production may increase as much as 15 times its normal level; luteinizing hormone production, as much as 5 times.

X-rays of the spine, femurs, or metacarpals may show osteopenia or osteoporosis. Pelvic examination, endometrial biopsy, and dilation and curettage may be performed to rule out suspected organic disease in the presence of abnormal menstrual bleeding.

THE ESTROGEN CONTROVERSY

Estrogen replacement therapy (ERT) to counteract decreasing estrogen levels during menopause persists as one of the hottest controversies in modern medicine. Those in favor of ERT claim that it successfully controls the physical and emotional symptoms of menopause; opponents argue that ERT produces undesirable side effects, such as vaginal bleeding, breast tenderness, nausea, vomiting, abdominal bloating, and uterine cramps. At the heart of the controversy, however, is the increased risk of endometrial cancer in women who take supplemental estrogen.

According to recent studies, these are the facts concerning estrogen use:
- ERT has proven to be an effective treatment for only two complaints associated with menopause—hot flashes and atrophic vaginitis.
- The increased risk of cancer is directly linked to the duration of ERT. Use of supplemental estrogen for more than 5 years multiplies the risk by as much as 15 times in the general population; its use for less than 1 year only doubles the risk.
- The risk of cancer does not significantly decrease with the use of cyclic therapy or of progestins for 7 days each month.
- To minimize the risk of cancer, estrogen should be prescribed in the lowest possible dosage.
- Women who experience menopause prematurely or as a result of surgery may need ERT to prevent osteoporosis.
- Smoking greatly increases the risk of thromboembolic disease in users of exogenous estrogen.
- Women with strong family histories of genital and breast carcinoma should not use exogenous estrogen.

Treatment and additional considerations
Since physiologic menopause is a normal process, it may not require treatment. Atypical or adenomatous hyperplasia

necessitates the administration of drugs such as medroxyprogesterone or norethindrone, which cause the endometrium to "shed," followed by methyltestosterone to suppress endometrial growth. Cyclic endometrial hyperplasia does not require treatment. If osteoporosis occurs, estrogen therapy may be necessary.

Controversy continues over the efficacy of estrogen replacement therapy (ERT). A patient or family history of cancer definitely contraindicates the use of ERT. Women who take estrogen must be monitored regularly to detect possible cancer in its earliest, asymptomatic stages.

Management of a menopausal woman includes:

• providing the patient who is considering ERT with all the facts about this controversial therapy—both pro and con—so she can make an informed decision; making sure the patient on ERT realizes the importance of regular monitoring to detect cancer.

• advising the patient not to discontinue contraceptive measures until confirmation that menstruation has ceased.

• reassuring the patient experiencing physiologic menopause that current body changes are normal and predictable.

• reassuring the patient who considers menopause a threat to her femininity that she is still capable of enjoying an active sex life; suggesting counseling if the patient is unusually distressed.

• telling the patient to immediately report vaginal bleeding or spotting after cessation of menstruation.

Female Infertility

Infertility, the inability to conceive after regular intercourse for at least 1 year without contraception, affects approximately 10% to 15% of all couples in the United States. About 40% to 50% of all infertility is attributed to the female. (See also MALE INFERTILITY *in Chapter 16.) Following extensive investigation and treatment, approximately 50% of these infertile couples achieve pregnancy. Of the 50% who do not, 10% have no pathologic basis for infertility; the prognosis in this group becomes extremely poor if pregnancy is not achieved after 3 years.*

Causes

The causes of female infertility may be functional, anatomic, or psychologic:

• *Functional:* complex hormonal interactions determine the normal function of the female reproductive tract and require an intact hypothalamic-pituitary-ovarian axis, a system that stimulates and regulates the production of hormones necessary for normal sexual development and function. Any defect or malfunction of this system axis can cause infertility, due to insufficient gonadotropin secretions (both luteinizing and follicle-stimulating hormones). The ovary controls, and is controlled by, the hypothalamus through a system of negative and positive feedback mediated by estrogen production. Insufficient gonadotropin levels may result from infections, tumors, or neurologic disease of the hypothalamus or pituitary gland. Hypothyroidism also impairs fertility.

• *Anatomic causes are the following:*

—*Ovarian factors* are related to anovulation and oligo-ovulation (infrequent ovulation), and are a major cause of infertility. Pregnancy or direct visualization provides irrefutable evidence of ovulation. Presumptive signs of ovulation include regular menses, cyclic changes reflected in basal body temperature readings, postovulatory progesterone levels, and endometrial changes due to the presence of progesterone. Absence of presumptive signs suggests anovulation. Ovarian failure, in which no ova are produced by the ovaries, may result from ovarian dysgenesis or premature menopause. Amenorrhea is often associated with ovarian failure. Oligo-ovulation may be due to a mild hormonal imbalance in gonadotropin production and regulation, and may be caused by polycystic disease of the ovary or abnormalities in the adrenal or thyroid gland that adversely affect hypothalamic-pituitary functioning.

—*Uterine abnormalities* may include congenitally absent uterus, bicornuate or double uterus, leiomyomas, or Asherman's syndrome, in which the anterior and posterior uterine walls adhere because of scar tissue formation.

—*Tubal and peritoneal factors* are due to faulty tubal transport mechanisms and unfavorable environmental influences affecting the sperm, ova, or recently fertilized ovum. Frequently, they result from anatomic abnormalities: bilateral occlusion of the tubes due to salpingitis (resulting from gonorrhea, tuberculosis, or puerperal sepsis), peritubal adhesions (resulting from endometriosis, diverticulosis, or childhood rupture of the appendix), and uterotubal obstruction due to tubal spasm.

—*Cervical factors* may include malfunctioning cervix that produces deficient or excessively viscous mucus and is impervious to sperm, preventing entry into the uterus. In cervical infection, viscous mucus may contain spermicidal macrophages. The possible existence of cervical antibodies that immobilize sperm is also under investigation.

• *Psychologic problems* probably account for relatively few cases of infertility. Occasionally, ovulation may stop under stress due to failure of LH release. Marital discord may affect the frequency of intercourse. More often, however, psychologic problems result from infertility, instead of causing it.

Symptoms and diagnosis

The inability to achieve pregnancy after having regular intercourse without contraception for at least 1 year suggests infertility.

Diagnosis requires a complete physical examination and health history, including specific questions on the patient's reproductive and sexual function, past diseases, mental state, previous surgery, types of contraception used in the past, and family history. Irregular, painless menses may indicate anovulation. A history of pelvic inflammatory disease may suggest fallopian tube blockage.

The following tests assess ovulation:
• *Basal body temperature graph* shows a sustained elevation in body temperature postovulation until just before onset of menses, indicating the approximate time of ovulation.
• *Endometrial biopsy*, done on or about day 5 after the basal body temperature elevates, provides histologic evidence that ovulation has occurred.
• *Progesterone blood levels*, measured when they should be highest, can show a luteal phase deficiency.

The following procedures assess structural integrity of the tubes, the ovaries, and the uterus:
• *Rubin's insufflation test* determines tubal patency by the uterotubal insufflation of CO_2. If one or both tubes are patent, the passage of CO_2 into the peritoneal cavity irritates the phrenic nerve, producing referred pain to the shoulder; if the patient feels no pain, the fallopian tubes aren't patent, and intrauterine pressure of CO_2 rises rapidly.
• *Hysterosalpingography* provides radiologic evidence of tubal obstruction and abnormalities of the uterine cavity by injecting radiopaque contrast fluid through the cervix.
• *Endoscopy* confirms the results of hysterosalpingography and visualizes the endometrial cavity by hysteroscopy or explores the posterior surface of the uterus, fallopian tubes, and ovaries by culdoscopy. Laparoscopy allows visualization of the abdominal and pelvic areas.

Male-female interaction studies include the following:
• *Postcoital test* (Sims-Huhner test) examines the cervical mucus for motile sperm cells following intercourse at midcycle (as close to ovulation as possible).
• *Immunologic or antibody testing* detects spermicidal antibodies in the sera

of the female. Further research is being conducted in this area.

Treatment

Treatment depends on identifying the underlying abnormality or dysfunction within the hypothalamic-pituitary-ovarian complex. In hyper- or hypoactivity of the adrenal or thyroid gland, hormone therapy is necessary; progesterone deficiency requires progesterone replacement. Anovulation necessitates treatment with clomiphene, human menopausal gonadotropins, or human chorionic gonadotropin; ovulation usually occurs several days after such administration. If mucus production decreases (a side effect of clomiphene), small doses of estrogen to improve the quality of cervical mucus may be given concomitantly.

Surgical restoration may correct certain anatomic causes of infertility, such as fallopian tube obstruction. Surgery may also be necessary to remove tumors located within or near the hypothalamus or pituitary gland. Endometriosis requires drug therapy (danazol or me-droxyprogesterone, or noncyclic administration of oral contraceptives), surgical removal of areas of endometriosis, or a combination of both.

In vitro (test tube) fertilization has been successful in a few instances and has been widely publicized. However, this procedure is still experimental.

Additional considerations

Management includes providing the infertile couple with emotional support and information about diagnostic and treatment techniques. An infertile couple may suffer loss of self-esteem; they may feel angry, guilty, or inadequate, and the diagnostic procedures for this disorder may intensify their fear and anxiety. The health care professional can help by explaining these procedures thoroughly. Above all, the patient should be encouraged to talk about her feelings, and the professional should listen to her with a nonjudgmental attitude.

If the patient requires surgery, she should know what to expect postoperatively; this, of course, depends on which procedure is to be performed.

Pelvic Inflammatory Disease

Pelvic inflammatory disease (PID) is any acute, subacute, recurrent, or chronic infection of the oviducts and ovaries, with adjacent tissue involvement. It includes inflammation of the cervix (cervicitis), uterus (endometritis), fallopian tubes (salpingitis), and ovaries (oophoritis), which can extend to the connective tissue lying between the broad ligaments (parametritis). Early diagnosis and treatment prevents damage to the reproductive system. Untreated PID may cause infertility and may lead to potentially fatal septicemia, pulmonary emboli, and shock.

Causes

PID can result from infection with aerobic or anaerobic organisms. The aerobic organism *Neisseria gonorrhoeae* is its most common cause, because it most readily penetrates the bacteriostatic barrier of cervical mucus.

Normally, cervical secretions have a protective and defensive function. Therefore, conditions or procedures that alter or destroy cervical mucus impair this bacteriostatic mechanism and allow bacteria present in the cervix or vagina to ascend into the uterine cavity; such procedures include conization or cauterization of the cervix.

Uterine infection can also follow the transfer of contaminated cervical mucus into the endometrial cavity by instrumentation. Consequently, PID can follow insertion of an intrauterine device, use of a biopsy curet or of an irrigation cath-

FORMS OF PELVIC INFLAMMATORY DISEASE

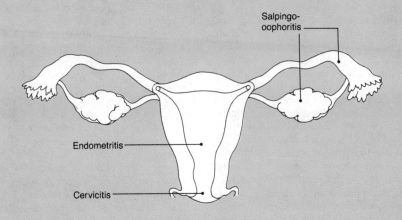

Salpingo-oophoritis

Endometritis

Cervicitis

CLINICAL FEATURES

Salpingo-oophoritis
- *Acute:* sudden onset of lower abdominal and pelvic pain, usually following menses; increased vaginal discharge; fever; malaise; lower abdominal pressure and tenderness; tachycardia; pelvic peritonitis
- *Chronic:* recurring acute episodes

Cervicitis
- *Acute:* purulent, foul-smelling vaginal discharge; vulvovaginitis, with itching or burning; red, edematous cervix; pelvic discomfort; sexual dysfunction; metrorrhagia; infertility; spontaneous abortion
- *Chronic:* cervical dystocia, laceration or eversion of the cervix, ulcerative vesicular lesion (when cervicitis results from herpes simplex virus II)

Endometritis (generally postpartum or postabortion)
- *Acute:* mucopurulent or purulent vaginal discharge oozing from the cervix; edematous, hyperemic endometrium, possibly leading to ulceration and necrosis (with virulent organisms); lower abdominal pain and tenderness; fever; rebound pain; abdominal muscle spasm; thrombophlebitis of uterine and pelvic vessels (in severe forms)
- *Chronic:* recurring acute episodes (increasingly common because of widespread use of IUDs)

DIAGNOSTIC FINDINGS

- Blood studies show leukocytosis or normal WBC.
- X-ray may show ileus.
- Pelvic exam reveals extreme tenderness.
- Smear of cervical or periurethral gland exudate shows gram-negative intracellular diplococci.

- Cultures for *N. gonorrhoeae* are positive (> 90% of patients).
- Cytologic smears may reveal severe inflammation.
- If cervicitis is not complicated by salpingitis, WBC normal or slightly elevated; ESR elevated.
- In *acute cervicitis*, cervical palpation reveals tenderness.
- In *chronic cervicitis*, causative organisms are usually staphylococcus or streptococcus.

- In severe infection, palpation may reveal boggy uterus.
- Uterine and blood samples positive for causative organism, usually staphylococcus.
- WBC and ESR are elevated.

eter, or tubal insufflation. Other predisposing factors include abortion, pelvic surgery, and infection during or after pregnancy.

Bacteria may also enter the uterine cavity through the bloodstream or from drainage from a chronically infected fallopian tube, a pelvic abscess, a ruptured appendix, diverticulitis of the sigmoid colon, or other infectious foci.

The most common bacteria found in cervical mucus are staphylococci, streptococci, diphtheroids, and coliforms, including *Pseudomonas* and *Escherichia coli*. Uterine infection can result from any one or several of these organisms, or may follow the multiplication of normally nonpathogenic bacteria in an altered endometrial environment. Bacterial multiplication is most common during parturition, because the endometrium is atrophic, quiescent, and not stimulated by estrogen.

Symptoms and diagnosis

Clinical features of PID vary with the affected area but generally include a profuse, purulent vaginal discharge, sometimes accompanied by low-grade fever and malaise (particularly if gonorrhea is the cause). The patient experiences lower abdomen pain; movement of the cervix or palpation of the adnexa may be extremely painful.

Diagnostic tests generally include:
• *Gram's stain* of secretions from the endocervix or cul-de-sac. Culture and sensitivity testing aids selection of the appropriate antibiotic. Urethral and rectal secretions may also be cultured.
• *ultrasonography* to identify an adnexal or uterine mass. (X-rays seldom identify pelvic masses.)
• *culdocentesis* to obtain peritoneal fluid or pus for culture and sensitivity testing.

In addition, patient history is significant. In general, PID is associated with recent sexual intercourse, IUD insertion, childbirth, or abortion.

Treatment

To prevent progression of PID, antibiotic therapy begins immediately after culture specimens are obtained. Such therapy can be reevaluated as soon as laboratory results are available (usually after 24 to 48 hours). Infection may become chronic if treated inadequately.

The preferred antibiotic therapy for PID resulting from gonorrhea is penicillin G procaine I.M. in two injection sites, combined with probenecid P.O. If the patient is allergic to penicillin, tetracycline may be used. (A patient with gonorrhea may also require therapy for syphilis.) Supplemental treatment of PID may include bed rest, analgesics, and I.V. therapy.

Development of pelvic abscess necessitates adequate drainage. A ruptured pelvic abscess is a life-threatening condition. If this complication develops, the patient may need a total abdominal hysterectomy, with bilateral salpingo-oophorectomy.

Additional considerations

• Antibiotics and analgesics should be administered after patient allergies are determined.
• The patient should be checked for elevated temperature; if fever persists, her fluid intake and output must be carefully monitored for signs of dehydration.
• Abdominal rigidity and distention in the patient are possible signs of developing peritonitis. Frequent perineal care should be provided if vaginal drainage occurs.
• To prevent recurrence, the patient must comply with treatment, and must understand the nature and seriousness of PID.
• The patient's sexual partner needs to be examined and, if necessary, treated for infection.
• Pelvic inflammation can cause painful intercourse. If the patient frequently feels pain during sexual activity, she should contact her doctor.
• To prevent major infection after minor gynecologic procedures, the patient should immediately report signs of inflammation (fever, increased vaginal discharge, pain). After such procedures, the patient must avoid douching or intercourse for at least 7 days.

UTERINE BLEEDING DISORDERS

Amenorrhea

Amenorrhea is the abnormal absence or suppression of menstruation. Primary amenorrhea is the absence of menarche in an adolescent (by age 18). Secondary amenorrhea is the failure of menstruation for at least 3 months after normal onset of menarche.

Causes

Amenorrhea is normal before puberty, after menopause, or during pregnancy and lactation; it is pathologic at any other time. As a disorder, it usually results from anovulation due to hormonal abnormalities, such as decreased secretion of estrogen, gonadotropins, luteinizing hormone, and follicle-stimulating hormone; lack of ovarian response to gonadotropins; or constant presence of progesterone or other endocrine abnormalities.

Amenorrhea may also result from the absence of a uterus, endometrial damage, or from ovarian, adrenal, or pituitary tumors. It is also linked to emotional disorders, and is common in patients with severe disorders such as depression and anorexia nervosa. Mild emotional disturbances tend merely to distort the ovulatory cycle, while severe psychic trauma may abruptly change the bleeding pattern or may completely suppress one or more full ovulatory cycles. Amenorrhea may also result from malnutrition and, occasionally, from prolonged use of oral contraceptives.

Symptoms and diagnosis

A history of failure to menstruate in a female over age 18 confirms primary amenorrhea. Secondary amenorrhea can be diagnosed when a change is noted in a previously established menstrual pattern (absence of menstruation for 3 months). A thorough physical and pelvic examination rules out pregnancy, as well as anatomic abnormalities (such as cervical stenosis) that may cause false amenorrhea (cryptomenorrhea), in which menstruation occurs without external bleeding.

Onset of menstruation within 1 week after administration of pure progestational agents, such as medroxyprogesterone and progesterone, indicates a functioning uterus. If menstruation does not occur, special diagnostic studies are appropriate.

Blood and urine studies may reveal hormonal imbalances—such as lack of ovarian response to gonadotropins (elevated pituitary gonadotropins) and failure of gonadotropin secretion (low pituitary gonadotropin levels). Tests for identification of dominant or missing hormones include cervical mucus ferning, vaginal cytologic examinations, basal body temperature, endometrial biopsy (during dilation and curettage), urinary 17-ketosteroids, and plasma progesterone, testosterone, and androgen levels. A complete medical workup, including appropriate X-rays, laparoscopy, and a biopsy, may determine ovarian, adrenal, and pituitary tumors.

Treatment and additional considerations

Generally, appropriate hormone replacement reestablishes menstruation. Treatment of amenorrhea not related to hormone deficiency depends on the underlying cause. For example, amenorrhea that results from a tumor usually requires surgery.

Care for an amenorrheic patient includes: explaining all diagnostic procedures; providing emotional support; and encouraging the patient to verbalize her fears, since amenorrhea may cause profound psychologic distress. Psychiatric counseling may be necessary if amenor- rhea results from emotional disturbances.

After treatment, the patient must be taught how to keep an accurate record of her menstrual cycles to aid early detection of recurrent amenorrhea.

Abnormal Premenopausal Bleeding

Abnormal premenopausal bleeding refers to any bleeding that deviates from the normal menstrual cycle before menopause. These deviations include menstrual bleeding that is abnormally infrequent (oligomenorrhea), abnormally frequent (polymenorrhea), excessive (menorrhagia or hypermenorrhea), deficient (hypomenorrhea), or irregular (metrorrhagia [uterine bleeding between menses]). Rarely, symptoms of menstruation are not accompanied by external bleeding (cryptomenorrhea). Premenopausal bleeding may merely be troublesome or can result in severe hemorrhage; however, prognosis depends on the underlying cause. Abnormal patterns of bleeding often respond to hormonal or other therapy.

Causes and incidence

Causes of abnormal premenopausal bleeding vary with the type of bleeding.

• *Oligomenorrhea* and *polymenorrhea* usually result from anovulation due to an endocrine or systemic disorder.

• *Menorrhagia* usually results from local lesions, such as uterine leiomyomas, endometrial polyps, and endometrial hyperplasia. It may also result from endometritis, salpingitis, and anovulation.

• *Hypomenorrhea* results from local, endocrine, or systemic disorders, or from blockage due to partial obstruction by the hymen or to cervical obstruction.

• *Cryptomenorrhea* may result from an imperforate hymen or cervical stenosis.

• *Metrorrhagia* usually results from slight physiologic bleeding from the endometrium during ovulation but may also result from local disorders, such as uterine malignancy, cervical erosions, polyps (which tend to bleed after intercourse), or inappropriate estrogen therapy. Complications of pregnancy can also cause premenopausal bleeding. Such bleeding may be as mild as spotting or as severe as menorrhagia.

Signs and symptoms

Bleeding not associated with abnormal pregnancy is usually painless, but it may be severely painful. When bleeding is associated with abnormal pregnancy, other symptoms include nausea, breast tenderness, bloating, and fluid retention. Severe or prolonged bleeding causes anemia, especially in patients with underlying disease (such as blood dyscrasias) and in patients receiving anticoagulants.

Diagnosis

Typical clinical picture confirms abnormal premenopausal bleeding. Special tests are appropriate to identify the underlying cause:

• *Serum hormone levels* reflect adrenal, pituitary, or thyroid dysfunction.

• *Urinary 17-ketosteroids* reveal adrenal hyperplasia, hypopituitarism, or polycystic ovarian disease.

• *Basal body temperatures and endometrial sampling at onset of bleeding* check for anovulation.

• *Pelvic examination, Pap smear, and history* rule out local or malignant causes.

• *CBC* rules out anemia.

If testing rules out pelvic and hormonal causes of abnormal bleeding, a complete hematologic survey (including platelet count and bleeding time) is appropriate to determine clotting abnormalities.

Treatment

Treatment depends on the type of bleeding abnormality and its cause. Menstrual irregularity alone may not require therapy unless it interferes with the patient's attempt to achieve or avoid conception, or leads to anemia. When it does require treatment, clomiphene induces ovulation. Electrocautery, chemical cautery, or cryosurgery can remove cervical polyps; dilation and curettage, uterine polyps. Organic disorders—such as cervical or uterine malignancy, or leiomyoma—may necessitate hysterectomy, radium or X-ray therapy, or a combination of these treatments, depending on the site and extent of the disease. And, of course, anemia and infections require appropriate treatment.

Additional considerations

• If a patient complains of abnormal bleeding, she should start recording the dates of the bleeding and the number of tampons or pads she uses per day. This will help the doctor to assess the cyclic pattern and the amount of bleeding. She must also report abnormal bleeding immediately to help rule out major hemorrhagic disorders, such as occur in abnormal pregnancy.

• To prevent abnormal bleeding due to organic causes, and for early detection of malignancy, the patient should have a Pap smear and a pelvic examination annually.

• Since the patient may be particularly anxious about excessive or frequent blood loss and the passage of clots, she will need reassurance and support. She can minimize blood flow by avoiding strenuous activity and occasionally lying down with her feet elevated. She should also try to relax.

CAUSES OF ABNORMAL PREMENOPAUSAL BLEEDING

	OLIGOMENORRHEA	HYPOMENORRHEA	POLYMENORRHEA	METRORRHAGIA	MENORRHAGIA
Malnutrition	•	•			
Hyperthyroidism	•	•			
Hypothyroidism				•	•
Severe psychic trauma		•	•		•
Blood dyscrasias					•
Severe infections	•	•			
Hepatic disease			•		
Cardiovascular disease					•
Drugs (such as digitalis, corticosteroids, anticoagulants)					•
Uterine tumors			•		•

Dysfunctional Uterine Bleeding

Dysfunctional uterine bleeding (DUB) refers to abnormal endometrial bleeding without recognizable organic lesions. Prognosis varies with the cause. DUB is the indication for almost 25% of gynecologic surgery.

Causes

DUB usually results from an imbalance in the hormonal-endometrial relationship, where persistent and unopposed stimulation of the endometrium by estrogen occurs. Disorders that cause sustained high estrogen levels are polycystic ovary syndrome, obesity, immaturity of the hypothalamic-pituitary-ovarian mechanism (in postpubertal teenagers), and anovulation (in women in their late 30s or early 40s).

In most cases of DUB, the endometrium shows no pathologic changes. However, in chronic unopposed estrogen stimulation (as from a hormone-producing ovarian tumor), the endometrium may show hyperplastic or malignant changes.

Signs and symptoms
DUB usually occurs as metrorrhagia (episodes of vaginal bleeding between menses); it may also occur as hypermenorrhea (heavy or prolonged menses, longer than 8 days) or chronic polymenorrhea (menstrual cycle of less than 18 days). Such bleeding is unpredictable and can cause anemia.

Diagnosis
Diagnostic studies must rule out other causes of excessive vaginal bleeding, such as organic, systemic, psychogenic, and endocrine causes, including malignancy, polyps, incomplete abortion, pregnancy, and infection.

 Dilation and curettage (D & C), and biopsy results confirm the diagnosis by revealing endometrial hyperplasia. Hematocrit and hemoglobin levels determine the need for blood or iron replacement.

Treatment
High-dose estrogen-progestogen combination therapy (oral contraceptives), the primary treatment, is designed to control endometrial growth and reestablish a normal cyclical pattern of menstruation. These drugs are usually administered four times daily for 5 to 7 days, even though bleeding usually stops in 12 to 24 hours. (The patient's age and the cause of bleeding help determine the drug choice and dosage.) In patients over age 35, endometrial biopsy is necessary before the start of estrogen therapy to rule out endometrial adenocarcinoma. Progestogen therapy is a necessary alternative in some women, such as those susceptible to the adverse effects of estrogen (thrombophlebitis, for example).

If drug therapy is ineffective, a D & C can rule out other causes and serves as a supplementary treatment, through removal of a large portion of the bleeding endometrium. Also, a D & C can help determine the original cause of hormonal imbalance and can aid in planning further therapy. Regardless of the primary treatment, the patient may need iron replacement, or transfusions of packed cells or whole blood, as indicated, because of anemia caused by recurrent bleeding.

Additional considerations
The patient must understand the importance of adhering to the prescribed hormonal therapy. If a D & C is ordered, this procedure and its purpose should be explained to her.

She must also understand the need for regular checkups to assess treatment.

Postmenopausal Bleeding

Postmenopausal bleeding is defined as bleeding from the reproductive tract that occurs 1 year or more after cessation of menses. Sites of bleeding include the vulva, vagina, cervix, and endometrium. Prognosis varies with the cause.

Causes
Postmenopausal bleeding may result from:
• *exogenous estrogen,* when administration is excessive or prolonged, or when small amounts are given in the presence of a hypersensitive endometrium.
• *endogenous estrogen production,* especially when levels are high, as in persons with estrogen-producing ovarian tumor; however, in some persons, even

slight fluctuation in estrogen levels may cause bleeding.

• *atrophic vaginitis,* which is usually triggered by trauma during coitus, in the absence of estrogen administration or production.

• *aging,* which increases vascular vulnerability by thinning epithelial surfaces, increasing vascular fragility, producing degenerative tissue changes, and decreasing local resistance to infections.

• *cervical or endometrial cancer* (more common after age 60).

• *adenomatous hyperplasia or atypical adenomatous hyperplasia* (usually considered a premalignant lesion).

Signs and symptoms

Vaginal bleeding, the predominant symptom, ranges from brownish spotting to outright hemorrhage; its duration also varies. Other symptoms depend on the cause. Excessive estrogen stimulation, for example, may also produce copious cervical mucus; estrogen deficiency may cause vaginal mucosa to atrophy.

Diagnosis

Diagnostic evaluation of the patient with postmenopausal bleeding should include physical examination (especially pelvic examination), a detailed history, standard laboratory tests (such as CBC), and cytologic examination of smears from the cervix and the endocervical canal. Dilation and curettage (D & C) shows pathologic findings in the lining of the endometrial cavity.

Diagnosis must rule out underlying degenerative or systemic disease. For instance, evidence of elevated levels of endogenous estrogen may suggest an ovarian tumor. Before testing for estrogen levels, the patient must stop all sources of exogenous estrogen intake—including face and body creams that contain estrogen—to rule out excessive exogenous estrogen as a cause.

Treatment

Emergency treatment to control massive hemorrhage is rarely necessary, except in advanced malignancy. Treatment may include D & C to relieve bleeding. Other therapy varies according to the underlying cause. Estrogen creams and suppositories are usually very effective in correcting estrogen deficiency, since they are rapidly absorbed. Hysterectomy is indicated only for repeated episodes of postmenopausal bleeding from the endometrial cavity. Such bleeding may indicate endometrial cancer.

Additional considerations

The health care professional should: obtain a detailed patient history to rule out excessive exogenous estrogen as a cause of bleeding; ask the patient about use of cosmetics (especially face and body creams), drugs, and other products that may contain estrogen; discuss the risks and benefits of estrogen replacement therapy with her.

The patient will need emotional support, and will probably be afraid that the bleeding indicates cancer.

Periodic gynecologic examinations are necessary to prevent disorders that cause postmenopausal bleeding. The patient must realize that these examinations are as important after menopause as they were before.

DISORDERS OF PREGNANCY

Abortion

Abortion is the spontaneous or induced (therapeutic) expulsion of the products of conception from the uterus before fetal viability (fetal weight of less than 17½ oz

[500 g] and gestation of less than 20 weeks). Up to 15% of all pregnancies and approximately 30% of first pregnancies end in spontaneous abortion (miscarriage). At least 75% of miscarriages occur during the first trimester. Incidence of legal therapeutic abortions is rising in the United States. Roughly 25% of all pregnancies end in elective abortions, usually during the first trimester.

Causes

Spontaneous abortion may result from fetal, placental, or maternal factors. Fetal factors usually cause such abortions at 9 to 12 weeks of gestation, and include:

• defective embryologic development due to abnormal chromosome division (most common cause of fetal death).
• faulty implantation of fertilized ovum.
• failure of the endometrium to accept the fertilized ovum.

Placental factors usually cause abortion around the 14th week of gestation, when the placenta takes over the hormone production necessary to maintain the pregnancy, and include:

• premature separation of the normally implanted placenta.
• abnormal placental implantation.
• abnormal platelet function.

Maternal factors usually cause abortion between 11 and 19 weeks of gestation, and include:

• maternal infection, severe malnutrition, abnormalities of the reproductive organs (especially incompetent cervix, in which the cervix dilates painlessly and bloodlessly in the second trimester).
• endocrine problems, such as thyroid dysfunction or lowered estriol secretion.
• trauma, including any type of surgery that necessitates manipulation of the pelvic organs.
• blood group incompatibility and Rh isoimmunization (still under investigation as a possible cause).
• drug ingestion.

The goal of *therapeutic abortion* is to preserve the mother's mental or physical health in cases of rape, unplanned pregnancy, or medical conditions, such as moderate or severe cardiac dysfunction.

Signs and symptoms

Prodromal symptoms of spontaneous abortion may include a pink discharge for several days or a scant brown discharge for several weeks before onset of cramps and increased vaginal bleeding. For a few hours the cramps intensify and occur more frequently; then the cervix dilates for expulsion of uterine contents. If the entire contents are expelled, cramps and bleeding subside. However, if any contents remain, cramps and bleeding continue.

Diagnosis

Diagnosis of spontaneous abortion is based on clinical evidence of expulsion of uterine contents, pelvic examination, and laboratory studies. Human chorionic gonadotropin in the blood or urine confirms pregnancy. Pelvic examination determines the size of the uterus and whether this size is consistent with the length of the pregnancy. Tissue cytology indicates evidence of products of conception. Laboratory tests reflect decreased hematocrit and hemoglobin levels due to blood loss.

Treatment

An accurate evaluation of uterine contents is necessary before planning treatment. Spontaneous abortion usually requires bed rest for 24 hours after spotting, or complete bed rest as long as spotting continues. The progression of spontaneous abortion cannot be prevented, except in those cases caused by an incompetent cervix. Hospitalization is necessary, to control severe hemorrhage. Severe bleeding requires transfusion with packed RBCs or whole blood. Initially, I.V. administration of an oxytocin stimulates uterine contractions. If remnants remain in the uterus, dilation and curettage (D & C) or dilation and evacuation (D & E) should be performed.

A D & E is also used in first-trimester therapeutic abortions. In second-trimester therapeutic abortions, an injection of hypertonic saline solution into the amniotic sac, or a prostaglandin vaginal suppository induces expulsion.

After an abortion, spontaneous or induced, an Rh-negative female with a negative indirect Coombs' test should receive Rh_o (D) immune human globulin to prevent future Rh isoimmunization.

In a habitual aborter, spontaneous abortion can result from an incompetent cervix. Treatment, therefore, involves surgical reinforcement of the cervix (Shirodkar-Barter procedure) about 14 to 16 weeks after the last menstrual period. A few weeks before the estimated delivery date, the sutures are removed, and the patient remains hospitalized and is monitored carefully for onset of labor. An alternative procedure, especially for the woman who wants to have more children, is to leave the sutures in place, and to deliver the infant by cesarean section.

Additional considerations

The patient should be prepared as thoroughly as possible before spontaneous or elective abortion. The patient should *not* have bathroom privileges, because she may expel uterine contents without knowing it. After she uses the bedpan, the contents must be carefully inspected for intrauterine material.

Health care following spontaneous or elective abortion includes:
• noting the amount, color, and odor of vaginal bleeding; saving all the pads the patient uses for evaluation.
• administering analgesics and oxytocin, as ordered.
• giving good perineal care.
• obtaining vital signs every 4 hours for 24 hours.
• monitoring urinary output.

Care of the patient who has had a spontaneous abortion includes emotional support and counseling during the grieving process. The patient and her husband should be encouraged to express their feelings. Some couples may want to talk to a member of the clergy or, depending on their religion, may wish to have the fetus baptized.

The patient who has had a therapeutic

TYPES OF SPONTANEOUS ABORTION

• *Threatened abortion:* Bloody vaginal discharge occurs during the first half of pregnancy. Approximately 20% of pregnant women have vaginal spotting or actual bleeding early in pregnancy; of these, about 50% abort.
• *Inevitable abortion:* Membranes rupture and the cervix dilates. As labor continues, the uterus expels the products of conception.
• *Incomplete abortion:* Uterus retains part or all of the placenta. Before the 10th week of gestation, the fetus and placenta usually are expelled together; after the 10th week, separately. Because part of the placenta may adhere to the uterine wall, bleeding continues. Hemorrhage is possible because the uterus doesn't contract and seal the large vessels that fed the placenta.
• *Complete abortion:* Uterus passes all the products of conception. Minimal bleeding usually accompanies complete abortion because the uterus contracts and compresses the maternal blood vessels that fed the placenta.
• *Missed abortion:* Uterus retains the products of conception for 2 months or more after the death of the fetus. Uterine growth ceases; uterine size may even seem to decrease. Prolonged retention of the dead products of conception may cause coagulation defects, such as disseminated intravascular coagulation (DIC).
• *Habitual abortion:* Spontaneous loss of three or more consecutive pregnancies constitutes habitual abortion.
• *Septic abortion:* Infection accompanies abortion. This may occur with spontaneous abortion but usually results from an illegal abortion.

---

abortion will also benefit from support. She should verbalize her feelings, since she may feel ambivalent about the procedure—intellectual acceptance of abortion and gut acceptance are not the same. She should be referred for counseling, if necessary.

To prepare the patient for discharge,

the hospital staff member should:

• tell the patient to expect vaginal bleeding or spotting, and report bleeding that lasts longer than 8 to 10 days or excessive, bright-red blood immediately.

• advise the patient to watch for signs of infection, such as a temperature higher than 100° F. (37.8° C.), and foul-smelling vaginal discharge.

• encourage the gradual increase of daily activities to include whatever tasks the patient feels comfortable doing (cooking, sewing, cleaning, for example), as long as these activities don't increase vaginal bleeding or cause fatigue. Most patients return to work within 2 to 4 weeks.

• urge 2 to 3 weeks' abstinence from intercourse.

• instruct the patient to avoid using tampons for 2 to 4 weeks.

• be sure to inform the patient who desires an elective abortion of all the available alternatives—she needs to know what the procedure involves, what the risks are, and what to expect during and after the procedure, both emotionally and physically; be sure to ascertain whether the patient is comfortable with her decision to have an elective abortion; encourage her to verbalize her thoughts both when the procedure is performed and at a follow-up visit, usually 2 weeks later; refer the patient for professional counseling if she is using an inappropriate coping response.

• tell the patient to see her doctor in 2 to 4 weeks for a follow-up examination.

To help prevent unwanted pregnancies, medical and health care personnel need to make contraceptive information available. An educated population motivated to utilize contraception would have little need for elective abortion.

To minimize the risk of future spontaneous abortions, the pregnant woman should understand the importance of good nutrition and the need to exclude alcohol, cigarettes, and drugs. Most clinicians recommend that the couple wait two or three normal menstrual cycles after a spontaneous abortion has occurred before attempting conception. If the patient has a history of habitual spontaneous abortions, she and her husband should have thorough examinations. For the woman, this can include premenstrual endometrial biopsy, a hormone assessment (estrogen, progesterone, and thyroid, follicle-stimulating, and luteinizing hormones), and hysterosalpingography and laparoscopy to detect anatomic abnormalities. Genetic counseling is also indicated.

Ectopic Pregnancy

Ectopic pregnancy is the implantation of the fertilized ovum outside the uterine cavity. The most common site is the fallopian tube (more than 90% of ectopic implantations occur in the fimbria, ampulla, or isthmus), but other possible sites may include the interstitium, tubo-ovarian ligament, ovary, abdominal viscera, and external cervical os. In Caucasians, ectopic pregnancy occurs in 1 in 200 pregnancies; in non-Caucasians, in 1 in 120. Prognosis is good with prompt diagnosis, appropriate surgical intervention, and control of bleeding; rarely, in cases of abdominal implantation, the fetus may survive to term. Usually, subsequent intrauterine pregnancy is achieved.

Causes

Conditions that prevent or retard the passage of the fertilized ovum through the fallopian tube and into the uterine cavity include:

• *endosalpingitis,* an inflammatory action that causes folds of the tubal mucosa to agglutinate, narrowing the tube.

• *diverticula,* the formation of blind pouches that cause tubal abnormalities.

• *tumors* pressing against the tube.

• *previous surgery* (tubal ligation or

IMPLANTATION SITES OF ECTOPIC PREGNANCY

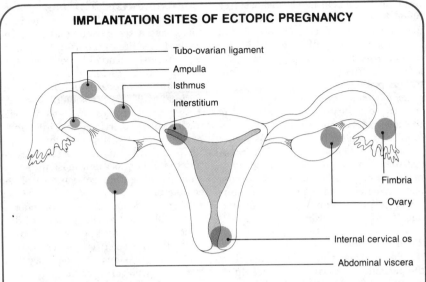

- Tubo-ovarian ligament
- Ampulla
- Isthmus
- Interstitium
- Fimbria
- Ovary
- Internal cervical os
- Abdominal viscera

In 90% of patients with ectopic pregnancy, the ovum implants in the fallopian tube, either in the fimbria, ampulla, or isthmus. Other possible sites of implantation include the interstitium, tubo-ovarian ligament, ovary, abdominal viscera, and internal cervical os.

resection, or adhesions from previous abdominal or pelvic surgery).

- *transmigration of the ovum* (from one ovary to the opposite tube), resulting in delayed implantation.

Rarely, ectopic pregnancy may result from congenital defects in the reproductive tract or ectopic endometrial implants in the tubal mucosa. Ectopic pregnancy may also be related to use of an intrauterine device (IUD). Such use may exaggerate the risk of ectopic pregnancy, because an IUD causes localized action on the cellular lining of the uterus, extending into the fallopian tubes.

Signs and symptoms

Ectopic pregnancy sometimes produces symptoms of normal pregnancy or no symptoms other than mild abdominal pain (the latter is especially likely in abdominal pregnancy), making diagnosis difficult. Characteristic clinical effects after fallopian tube implantation include amenorrhea or abnormal menses, followed by slight vaginal bleeding, and unilateral pelvic pain over the mass. Rupture of the tube causes life-threatening complications, including hemorrhage, shock, and peritonitis. The patient experiences sharp lower abdominal pain, possibly radiating to the shoulders and neck, often precipitated by activities that increase abdominal pressure, such as a bowel movement; she feels extreme pain upon motion of the cervix and palpation of the adnexa during a pelvic examination. She has a tender, boggy uterus.

Diagnosis

Clinical features, patient history, and the results of a pelvic examination suggest ectopic pregnancy. The following tests confirm it:

- *Serum pregnancy test* shows presence of human chorionic gonadotropin.
- *Gray scale ultrasonography* determines intrauterine pregnancy or ovarian cyst (performed if blood pregnancy test is positive).
- In *culdocentesis,* fluid is aspirated

from the vaginal cul-de-sac to detect free blood in the peritoneum (performed if ultrasonography detects the absence of a gestational sac in the uterus).

• *Laparoscopy* reveals pregnancy outside the uterus (performed if culdocentesis is positive).

• *Exploratory laparotomy* confirms and treats the ectopic pregnancy by removing the affected fallopian tube (salpingectomy) and controlling bleeding.

Decreased hemoglobin and hematocrit due to blood loss support the diagnosis. Differential diagnosis must rule out uterine abortion, appendicitis, ruptured corpus luteum cyst, salpingitis, and torsion of the ovary.

Treatment

If culdocentesis is positive for blood in the peritoneum, laparotomy and salpingectomy are indicated, possibly preceded by laparoscopy. The ovary is saved, if possible; however, ovarian pregnancy necessitates oophorectomy. Interstitial pregnancy may require hysterectomy; abdominal pregnancy requires a laparotomy to remove the fetus, except in rare cases, when the fetus survives to term or calcifies undetected in the abdominal cavity. Supportive treatment includes transfusion with whole blood or packed red cells to replace excessive blood loss, broad-spectrum antibiotics I.V. for septic infection, supplemental iron P.O. or I.M., and a diet high in protein.

Additional considerations

Supportive care includes careful monitoring and assessment of vital signs and vaginal bleeding, preparing the patient with excessive blood loss for emergency surgery, and providing blood replacement and emotional support. Also, the hospital staff member should:

• frequently assess vital signs to check for internal hemorrhage and infection.

• record the location and character of the pain, and administer analgesics, as ordered (analgesics may mask the symptoms of intraperitoneal rupture of the ectopic pregnancy.)

• check the amount, color, and odor of vaginal bleeding; ask the patient the date of her last menstrual period, and to describe the character of this period.

• observe for signs of pregnancy (enlarged breasts, soft cervix).

• provide a quiet, relaxing environment, and encourage the patient to freely express her feelings of fear, loss, and grief.

Ectopic pregnancy can be prevented by:

• advising prompt treatment of pelvic infections to prevent diseases of the fallopian tubes; informing patients who have undergone surgery involving the fallopian tubes, or those with confirmed pelvic inflammatory disease that they have an increased risk of ectopic pregnancy.

• telling the patient vulnerable to ectopic pregnancy to delay using an IUD until she has completed her family.

Hyperemesis Gravidarum

Unlike the transient nausea and vomiting normally experienced between the sixth and twelfth weeks of pregnancy, hyperemesis gravidarum is severe and unremitting nausea and vomiting that persists after the first trimester. If untreated, it produces substantial weight loss; starvation; dehydration, with subsequent fluid and electrolyte imbalance (hypokalemia); and acid-base disturbances (acidosis and alkalosis). This syndrome occurs in approximately 1 in 200 pregnancies. Prognosis is good with appropriate treatment.

Causes

Although its cause is unknown, hyperemesis gravidarum often affects pregnant females with conditions that produce high levels of human chorionic gonadotropin, such as hydatidiform mole or multiple pregnancy. This disorder also may be a symptom of pancreatitis, since many of these patients have elevated serum amylase levels. Its other possible causes include biliary tract disease, drug toxicity, inflammatory obstructive bowel disease, and vitamin deficiency (especially B_6). In some patients, hyperemesis gravidarum may be related to psychologic factors, such as ambivalence toward pregnancy.

Signs and symptoms

The cardinal symptoms of hyperemesis gravidarum are unremitting nausea and vomiting. The vomitus initially contains undigested food, mucus, and small amounts of bile; later, it contains only bile and mucus; and finally, blood and what resembles coffee-ground material. Persistent vomiting causes the patient to lose a substantial amount of weight, and she eventually becomes emaciated. Her skin turns pale, dry, and waxy, and may appear jaundiced; temperature may be subnormal or elevated; pulse rate may exceed 90 beats per minute; acidosis gives her breath a fetid, fruity odor. Associated CNS symptoms include confusion, delirium, headache, lassitude, somnolence, and stupor; these symptoms may progress to coma.

Diagnosis

Diagnosis depends on a history of uncontrolled nausea and vomiting that persists beyond the first trimester, evidence of substantial weight loss, and other characteristic clinical features. Serum analysis shows decreased protein, chloride, sodium, and potassium levels, and increased BUN. Other laboratory tests reveal ketonuria, slight proteinuria, and elevated hemoglobin and WBC levels. Diagnosis must rule out other conditions with similar clinical effects.

Treatment

Hyperemesis gravidarum may necessitate hospitalization to correct electrolyte imbalance and prevent starvation. Intravenous infusions maintain nutrition until the patient can tolerate oral feedings.

She progresses slowly to a clear liquid diet, then a full liquid diet, and finally, small, frequent meals of high-protein solid foods. A midnight snack helps stabilize blood glucose levels; vitamin B supplements help correct vitamin deficiency.

If vomiting continues, a combination of doxylamine succinate and pyridoxine administered P.O. at bedtime and in the morning may help control it. These drugs reduce gastrointestinal spasms and produce few side effects. If these drugs are ineffective, therapy may include promethazine rectal suppositories at bedtime and in the morning, or prochlorperazine two to three times daily; the latter drugs should be used with extreme caution in the first trimester. The safest possible drug should be used in the lowest possible dose to minimize any harmful effect to the fetus.

When vomiting stops and electrolyte balance has been restored, the pregnancy usually continues without recurrence of hyperemesis gravidarum. Most patients feel better as they begin to regain normal weight, but some continue to vomit throughout the pregnancy, requiring extended treatment. If appropriate, patients may benefit from consultations with clinical nurse specialists, psychologists, or psychiatrists.

Additional considerations

• The patient should be encouraged to eat. Dry foods and decreased liquid intake during meals may help reduce subsequent nausea. Company and diversionary conversation at mealtime may also be beneficial.
• The patient's environment should be kept as neat, clean, and odorfree as possible; the emesis basin should be kept out of sight.
• The patient should remain upright for 45 minutes after eating to decrease reflux.
• Reassurance and a calm, restful atmosphere will help. The patient should discuss her feelings regarding her pregnancy.
• Before discharge, the patient should receive nutritional counseling.

Toxemia of Pregnancy

Toxemia of pregnancy, a potentially life-threatening hypertensive disorder, usually develops late in the second trimester, or in the third trimester. Preeclampsia, the nonconvulsive form of toxemia, develops in about 7% of pregnancies. It is mild or severe, and the incidence is significantly higher in low socioeconomic groups. Eclampsia is the convulsive form of toxemia. About 5% of females with preeclampsia develop eclampsia; of these, about 15% die from toxemia itself or its complications. Fetal mortality is high due to the increased incidence of premature delivery.

Causes
The cause of toxemia of pregnancy is unknown, but it appears to be related to inadequate prenatal care (especially poor nutrition), parity (more prevalent in primigravidas), multiple pregnancies, preexisting diabetes mellitus or hypertension, hydramnios, or hydatidiform mole. Other theories postulate a long list of potential toxic sources, such as autolysis of placental infarcts, autointoxication, uremia, maternal sensitization to total proteins, and pyelonephritis.

Signs and symptoms
Mild preeclampsia produces hypertension, proteinuria, generalized edema (especially of the hands, face, and feet), and sudden weight gain of more than 3 lb (1.25 kg) a week during the second trimester, or more than 1 lb (0.45 kg) a week during the third trimester.

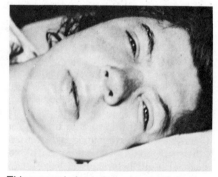

This woman's face shows some of the classic symptoms of preeclampsia—edema of the face and eyelids, and coarsening of the features.

Severe preeclampsia is marked by increased hypertension and proteinuria, eventually leading to oliguria. Other signs that may indicate worsening preeclampsia include blurred vision due to retinal arteriolar spasms, epigastric pain or heartburn, irritability, emotional tension, and severe frontal headache.

In eclampsia, all the clinical manifestations of preeclampsia are magnified, and are associated with convulsions and, possibly, coma. Complications of persistent convulsions include cerebral hemorrhage, blindness, abruptio placentae, premature labor, stillbirth, renal failure, and hepatic damage.

Diagnosis
The following findings suggest mild preeclampsia:
• *high blood pressure readings:* 140 systolic, or a rise of 30 mmHg or more above the patient's normal systolic pressure, on two occasions, 6 hours apart; 90 diastolic, or a rise of 15 mmHg or more above the patient's normal diastolic pressure, on two occasions, 6 hours apart
• *proteinuria:* more than 500 mg/ 24 hours

These findings suggest severe preeclampsia:
• *higher blood pressure readings:* 160/ 110 mmHg or higher on two occasions, 6 hours apart, at bed rest
• *increased proteinuria:* 5 g/24 hours or more
• *oliguria:* urine output less than or equal to 400 ml/24 hours
• *deep tendon reflexes:* possibly hyperactive as CNS irritability increases.

Typical clinical features—especially convulsions—with typical findings for severe preeclampsia, strongly suggest eclampsia. In addition, ophthalmoscopic examination may reveal vascular spasm, papilledema, retinal edema or detachment, and arteriovenous nicking or hemorrhage.

Urinary estriols, and stress and nonstress tests evaluate fetal well-being. In the stress test, oxytocin stimulates contractions; fetal heart tones are then monitored electronically. In the nonstress test, fetal heart tones are monitored electronically during periods of fetal activity, without oxytocin stimulation.

Treatment

Therapy for preeclampsia is designed to halt the disorder's progress—specifically, signs of eclampsia, such as convulsions, residual hypertension, and renal shutdown—and to ensure fetal survival. Some doctors advocate prompt induction of labor, especially if the patient is near term; others follow a more conservative approach. Therapy may include sedatives, such as phenobarbital, along with complete bed rest, to relieve anxiety, reduce hypertension, and evaluate response to therapy. If renal function is adequate, a high-protein, low-sodium, low-carbohydrate diet with increased fluid intake is recommended.

If the patient's blood pressure fails to respond to bed rest and sedation, and persistently rises above 160/100 mmHg, or if CNS irritability increases, magnesium sulfate may produce general sedation, promote diuresis, reduce blood pressure, and prevent convulsions. If these measures fail to improve the patient's condition, or if fetal life is endangered (as determined by stress or nonstress tests), cesarean section or oxytocin induction may be required to terminate the pregnancy.

Emergency treatment of eclamptic convulsions consists of immediate administration of diazepam I.V., followed by magnesium sulfate (I.V. drip), oxygen administration, and electronic fetal monitoring. After the patient's condition stabilizes, a cesarean section may be performed.

Adequate nutrition, good prenatal care, and control of preexisting hypertension during pregnancy decrease the incidence and severity of preeclampsia. Early recognition and prompt treatment of preeclampsia can prevent eclampsia.

Additional considerations

When treating a patient with preeclampsia or eclampsia, the hospital staff member should:

• monitor the patient regularly for changes in blood pressure, pulse rate, respiration, fetal heart tones, vision, level of consciousness, and deep tendon reflexes, and for headache unrelieved by medication; report changes immediately; assess these signs before administering medications; watch for signs of magnesium sulfate toxicity (absence of patellar reflexes).

• assess fluid balance by measuring intake and output, and daily weight.

• observe for signs of fetal distress by closely monitoring the results of stress and nonstress tests.

• instruct the patient to lie in a left lateral position to increase venous return, cardiac output, and renal blood flow.

• keep emergency resuscitative equipment and drugs (including diazepam and magnesium sulfate) available in case of convulsions and cardiac or respiratory arrest; keep calcium gluconate at the bedside, since it counteracts the toxic effects of magnesium sulfate.

• maintain seizure precautions to protect the patient from injury during a convulsion; never leave an unstable patient unattended.

• assist with emergency medical treatment for the convulsive patient; provide a quiet, darkened room until the patient's condition stabilizes, and enforce absolute bed rest; carefully monitor administration of magnesium sulfate; give oxygen, as ordered; never administer anything by mouth; insert a Foley catheter for accurate measurement of output.

• provide emotional support for the patient and family; point out, if the patient must give birth prematurely, that infants of mothers with toxemia are usually small for gestational age, but sometimes fare better than other premature babies, possibly because they have developed adaptive responses to stress in utero.

Hydatidiform Mole

Hydatidiform mole is an uncommon chorionic tumor of the placenta. Its early signs—amenorrhea and uterine enlargement—mimic normal pregnancy; however, it eventually causes vaginal bleeding. Hydatidiform mole occurs in 1 in 1,500 to 2,000 pregnancies, most commonly in women over age 45. Incidence is highest in Oriental women. With prompt diagnosis and appropriate treatment, prognosis is excellent; however, approximately 10% of patients with these moles develop chorionic malignancy. Recurrence is possible in about 2% of cases.

Causes
The cause of hydatidiform mole is unknown, but death of the embryo and loss of fetal circulation seem to precede formation of the mole. Despite embryo death, maternal circulation continues to nourish the trophoblast, but loss of fetal circulation causes abnormal accumulation of fluid within the villi. This converts some or all of the chorionic villi into a mass of clear vesicles, resembling a bunch of grapes.

Signs and symptoms
The early stages of a pregnancy in which a hydatidiform mole develops seem normal, except that the uterus grows more rapidly than usual. The first obvious signs of trouble—vaginal bleeding (ranging from spotting to hemorrhage) and lower abdominal cramps—mimic spontaneous abortion. The blood may contain hydatid vesicles; hyperemesis is likely, and signs of preeclampsia are possible. Other possible complications include anemia, infection, spontaneous abortion, uterine rupture, and choriocarcinoma.

Diagnosis
Persistent bleeding and an abnormally enlarged uterus suggest hydatidiform mole. Diagnosis is based on the passage of hydatid vesicles that allow histologic confirmation. Without identification of hydatid vesicles, it's difficult to differentiate hydatidiform mole from other complications of pregnancy, particularly threatened abortion; then confirmation requires dilation and curettage (D & C).

The following information also supports a diagnosis of hydatidiform mole:
• *Ultrasound* assesses uterine contents; the Doppler technique demonstrates the absence of fetal heart tones.
• *Pregnancy test* shows elevated human chorionic gonadotropin (HCG) serum levels 100 or more days after the last menstrual period.
• Evidence of preeclampsia develops earlier in pregnancy than usual.
• *Hemoglobin* is decreased as a result of blood loss.
• *Chest X-ray* is negative for evidence of choriocarcinoma metastasis.

Uterine contents show grape-clustered chorionic villi and hyperplastic placental tissue characteristic of hydatidiform mole.

• *Arteriography* shows typical early venous shadows.

Treatment

Hydatidiform mole necessitates uterine evacuation via D & C, or, if this is ineffective, abdominal hysterectomy or suction curettage. Before evacuation, oxytocin I.V. promotes uterine contractions. Postoperative treatment varies, depending on the amount of blood lost, and complications. If no complications develop, hospitalization is usually brief, and normal activities can be resumed, as tolerated.

Because of the possibility of choriocarcinoma following hydatidiform mole, follow-up care is essential. Such care includes monitoring HCG levels until they return to normal, and chest X-rays to check for lung metastasis. Most doctors advise postponing another pregnancy until a year after HCG levels return to normal.

Additional considerations

• Preoperatively, the patient should be observed for signs of complications, such as hemorrhage and uterine infection, and vaginal passage of hydatid vesicles. Any expelled tissue must be saved for laboratory analysis.
• Postoperatively, vital signs, especially blood pressure, should be monitored and the patient checked for blood loss.
• Patient and family teaching, and emotional support are important. The patient should be encouraged to express her feelings, and helped through the grieving for her lost infant.
• Any new symptoms (for example, hemoptysis, cough, suspected pregnancy, nausea, vomiting, and vaginal bleeding) must be reported.
• Regular follow-up by HCG and chest X-ray monitoring is important for early detection of possible malignant changes.
• The patient should understand why she must use contraceptives to prevent pregnancy for at least 1 year after HCG levels return to normal, and regular ovulation and menstrual cycles are reestablished.

TYPES OF HYSTERECTOMY

There are three types of hysterectomy: subtotal hysterectomy, total hysterectomy, and total hysterectomy with a salpingo-oophorectomy. The excised portion (which is shaded) varies in each one. In each of these procedures, however, the external genitalia and the vagina are left intact, and the woman is able to resume sexual relations.

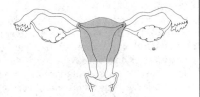

In a *subtotal hysterectomy*, all but the distal portion of the uterus is removed. The cervix is left in place. If the woman is not menopausal, she will continue to menstruate.

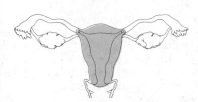

In a *total hysterectomy*, the entire uterus and the cervix are removed. This woman will no longer menstruate.

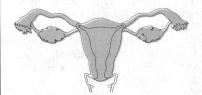

In a *total hysterectomy with a salpingo-oophorectomy*, the uterus, the cervix, the fallopian tubes, and the ovaries are removed. This woman will no longer menstruate.

Placenta Previa

In placenta previa, the placenta is implanted in the lower uterine segment, where it encroaches on the internal cervical os. This disorder, one of the most common causes of bleeding during the second half of pregnancy, occurs in approximately 1 in 200 pregnancies, more commonly in multigravidas than in primigravidas. Generally, termination of pregnancy is necessary when placenta previa is diagnosed in the presence of heavy maternal bleeding. Maternal prognosis is good if hemorrhage can be controlled; fetal prognosis depends on gestational age and amount of blood lost.

Causes
In placenta previa, the placenta may cover all (total, complete, or central), part (partial or incomplete), or a fraction (marginal or low-lying) of the internal cervical os. The degree of placenta previa depends largely on the extent of cervical dilation at the time of examination, because the dilating cervix gradually uncovers the placenta. Although the specific cause of placenta previa is unknown, factors that may affect the site of the placenta's attachment to the uterine wall include:
• early or late fertilization.
• receptivity and adequacy of the uterine lining.
• multiple pregnancy (the placenta requires a larger surface for attachment).
• previous uterine surgery.
• multiparity.
• advanced maternal age.

In placenta previa, the lower segment of the uterus fails to provide as much nourishment as the fundus. The placenta tends to spread out, seeking the blood supply it needs, and becomes larger and thinner than normal. Eccentric insertion of the umbilical cord often develops, for unknown reasons. Hemorrhage occurs as the internal cervical os effaces and dilates, tearing the uterine vessels.

Signs and symptoms
Placenta previa usually produces painless third trimester bleeding (often the first complaint). Various malpresentations occur because of the placenta's location, and interfere with proper descent of the fetal head. (The fetus remains active, however, with good heart tones.) Complications of placenta previa include shock, or maternal and fetal death.

Diagnosis
Special diagnostic measures that confirm placenta previa include:
• *ultrasound scanning* for placental position.
• *pelvic examination* (under a double setup because of the likelihood of hemorrhage), performed only immediately before delivery, to confirm diagnosis. In most cases, only the cervix is visualized.

Findings that may support the diagnosis of placenta previa include:
• degree of descent of the fetal head.
• decreased hemoglobin (due to blood loss).
• radiologic testing (soft-tissue X-rays, femoral arteriography, retrograde catheterization, or radioisotope scanning or localization) to locate the placenta. However, these tests have limited value, are very risky, and are usually performed only when ultrasound is unavailable.

Treatment
Treatment of placenta previa is designed to assess, control, and restore blood loss; to deliver a viable infant; and to prevent coagulation disorders. Immediate therapy includes starting an I.V. using a large-bore catheter; drawing blood for hemoglobin and hematocrit, as well as type and cross match; initiating external electronic fetal monitoring; monitoring maternal blood pressure, pulse rate, and

respirations; and assessing the amount of vaginal bleeding.

If the fetus is premature, following determination of the degree of placenta previa and necessary fluid and blood replacement, treatment consists of careful observation to allow the fetus more time to mature. If clinical evaluation confirms complete placenta previa, the patient is usually hospitalized due to the increased risk of hemorrhage. As soon as the fetus is sufficiently mature, or in case of intervening severe hemorrhage, immediate delivery by cesarean section may be necessary. Vaginal delivery is sometimes chosen to provide tamponade by compressing the detached placenta against the implantation site during labor. Because of the possibility of fetal blood loss through the placenta, a pediatric team should be on hand during such delivery to immediately assess and treat neonatal shock, blood loss, and hypoxia.

Complications of placenta previa necessitate appropriate and immediate intervention.

Additional considerations

If the patient shows active bleeding because of placenta previa, a health care professional should be assigned for continuous monitoring of maternal blood pressure, pulse rate, respirations, central venous pressure, intake and output, amount of vaginal bleeding, and fetal heart tones (electronically, every 10 to 15 minutes).

The professional should also:
• prepare the patient and family for a possible cesarean section and a premature infant; thoroughly explain postpartum care, so the patient and family know what to expect.
• provide emotional support during labor (because of the infant's prematurity, the patient won't be given analgesics, so labor pain may be intense); reassure her of her progress throughout labor, and keep her informed of the fetus' condition.

Although neonatal death is a possibility, frequent monitoring and prompt management reduce this prospect.

THREE TYPES OF PLACENTA PREVIA

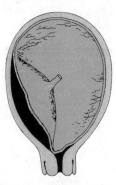

Low marginal implantation—A small placental edge can be felt through the internal os.

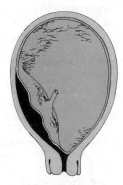

Partial placenta previa—Placenta partially caps the internal os.

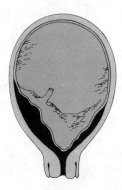

Total placenta previa—The internal os is covered entirely.

Abruptio Placentae
(Placental abruption)

In abruptio placentae, the placenta separates from the uterine wall prematurely, usually after the 20th week of gestation, producing hemorrhage. Abruptio placentae occurs most often in multigravidas—usually in women over age 35—and is a common cause of bleeding during the second half of pregnancy. Firm diagnosis, in the presence of heavy maternal bleeding, generally necessitates termination of pregnancy. Fetal prognosis depends on gestational age and amount of blood lost; maternal prognosis is good if hemorrhage can be controlled.

Causes

The cause of abruptio placentae is unknown. Predisposing factors include trauma—such as a direct blow to the uterus—placental site bleeding from a needle puncture during amniocentesis, chronic hypertension (which raises pressure on the maternal side of the placenta), acute toxemia, and pressure on the vena cava from an enlarged uterus.

In abruptio placentae, blood vessels at the placental bed rupture spontaneously, due to a lack of resiliency or changes in uterine vasculature. Hypertension complicates the situation, as does an enlarged uterus, which can't contract to seal off the torn vessels. Consequently, bleeding continues unchecked, possibly shearing off the placenta partially or completely. Bleeding is external or marginal (in 80% of patients) if a peripheral portion of the placenta separates from the uterine wall. Bleeding is internal or concealed (in the remaining 20%) if the central portion of the placenta becomes detached, in which case the still-intact peripheral portions trap the blood. As blood enters the muscle fibers, complete relaxation of the uterus becomes impossible, causing increased uterine tone and irritability. If bleeding into the muscle fibers is profuse, the uterus turns blue or purple, and the bleeding prevents it from contracting normally after delivery (Couvelaire uterus, or uteroplacental apoplexy).

Signs and symptoms

Abruptio placentae produces a wide range of clinical effects, depending on the extent of placental separation and the amount of blood lost from maternal circulation. Mild abruptio placentae (marginal separation) develops gradually and produces mild to moderate bleeding, vague lower abdominal discomfort, mild to moderate abdominal tenderness, and uterine irritability. Fetal heart tones remain strong and regular.

Moderate abruptio placentae (about 50% placental separation) may develop gradually or abruptly, and produces continuous abdominal pain, moderate dark red vaginal bleeding, a very tender uterus that remains firm between contractions, barely audible or irregular and bradycardic fetal heart tones, and possibly, signs of shock. Labor usually starts within 2 hours and often proceeds rapidly.

Severe abruptio placentae (nearly 70% placental separation) usually develops abruptly, and causes agonizing, unremitting uterine pain (often described as tearing or knifelike); a boardlike, tender uterus; moderate vaginal bleeding; rapidly progressive shock; and absence of fetal heart tones.

In addition to hemorrhage and shock, complications of abruptio placentae may include renal failure, disseminated intravascular coagulation (DIC), and maternal and fetal death.

Diagnosis

Diagnostic measures for abruptio placentae include observation of clinical features, pelvic examination (under double setup), and ultrasonography to rule out placenta previa. Decreased hemoglobin and platelet counts support the diagnosis. Periodic assays for fibrin split products aid in monitoring the progression of abruptio placentae and detect the development of DIC.

Treatment

Treatment of abruptio placentae is designed to assess, control, and restore the amount of blood lost; to deliver a viable infant; and to prevent coagulation disorders. Immediate measures for the patient with abruptio placentae include starting I.V. infusion (via large-bore catheter) of appropriate fluids (lactated Ringer's solution) to combat hypovolemia; drawing blood for hemoglobin and hematocrit determination and for type and cross match; initiating external electronic fetal monitoring; monitoring maternal blood pressure, pulse rate, and respirations; and assessing the amount of vaginal bleeding.

After determination of the severity of abruption and appropriate fluid and blood replacement, prompt delivery of the fetus by cesarean section is necessary if the fetus is alive but in distress. If the fetus is not in distress, monitoring continues; delivery is usually performed at the earliest sign of fetal distress. Because of the possibility of fetal blood loss through the placenta, a pediatric team should be on hand at delivery to immediately assess and treat the newborn for shock, blood loss, and hypoxia. If placental separation is severe and there are no signs of fetal life, vaginal delivery may be performed unless uncontrolled hemorrhage or other complications contraindicate it.

Complications of abruptio placentae require appropriate treatment. For example, DIC requires immediate intervention with heparin, platelets, and whole blood to prevent exsanguination.

Additional considerations

When treating a patient with abruptio placentae, the hospital staff member should:
• check maternal blood pressure, pulse rate, respirations, central venous pressure, intake and output, and amount of

DEGREES OF PLACENTAL SEPARATION IN ABRUPTIO PLACENTAE

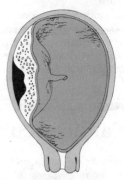

Mild separation with internal bleeding between placenta and uterine wall

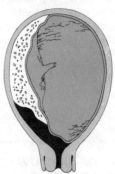

Moderate separation with external hemorrhage through the vagina

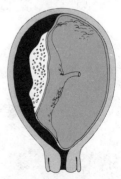

Severe separation with external hemorrhage

vaginal bleeding every 10 to 15 minutes; monitor fetal heart tones electronically.
• prepare the patient and family for cesarean section; thoroughly explain postpartum care.
• provide emotional support during labor if vaginal delivery is scheduled (because of the infant's prematurity, the mother will not receive analgesics during labor and may experience intense pain); reassure the patient of her progress through labor, and keep her informed of the fetus' condition.
• tactfully suggest the possibility of neonatal death; tell the mother the infant's survival depends primarily on gestational age, blood loss, and associated hypertensive disorders; assure her that frequent monitoring and prompt management greatly reduce risk of fatality.

Cardiovascular Disease in Pregnancy

Cardiovascular disease ranks fourth (after infection, toxemia, and hemorrhage) among the leading causes of maternal death. The physiologic stress of pregnancy and delivery is often more than a compromised heart can tolerate and often leads to maternal and fetal mortality. Approximately 1% to 2% of pregnant females have cardiac disease, but the incidence is rising because medical treatment today allows more females with rheumatic heart disease and congenital defects to reach childbearing age. Prognosis for the pregnant patient with cardiovascular disease is good, with careful management. Decompensation is the leading cause of maternal death. Infant mortality increases with decompensation, since uterine congestion, insufficient oxygenation, and the elevated carbon dioxide content of the blood not only compromise the fetus, but frequently cause premature labor and delivery.

Causes

Rheumatic heart disease is present in more than 80% of patients who develop cardiovascular complications. In the rest, these complications stem from congenital defects (10% to 15%) and coronary artery disease (2%).

The diseased heart is sometimes unable to meet the normal demands of pregnancy: 25% increase in cardiac output, 40% to 50% increase in plasma volume, increased oxygen requirements, retention of salt and water, weight gain, and alterations in hemodynamics during delivery. This physiologic stress often leads to the heart's failure to maintain adequate circulation (decompensation). The degree of decompensation depends on the patient's age, the duration of cardiac disease, and the functional capacity of the heart at the outset of pregnancy.

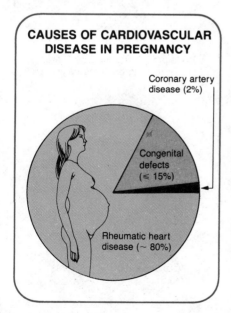

CAUSES OF CARDIOVASCULAR DISEASE IN PREGNANCY

Coronary artery disease (2%)

Congenital defects (≤ 15%)

Rheumatic heart disease (~ 80%)

Signs and symptoms

Typical clinical features of cardiovascular disease during pregnancy include distended neck veins, diastolic murmurs, moist basilar pulmonary rales, cardiac enlargement (discernible on percussion or as a cardiac shadow on chest X-ray), and cardiac dysrhythmias (other than sinus or paroxysmal atrial tachycardia). Other characteristic abnormalities may include cyanosis, pericardial friction rub, pulse delay, and pulsus alternans.

Decompensation may develop suddenly or gradually, with persistent rales at the lung bases. As it progresses, edema, increasing dyspnea on exertion, palpitations, a smothering sensation, and hemoptysis may occur.

Diagnosis
A diastolic murmur, cardiac enlargement, a systolic murmur of grade 3/6 intensity, and severe arrhythmia suggest cardiovascular disease. Determination of the extent and cause of the disease may necessitate electrocardiography, echocardiography (for valvular disorders, such as rheumatic heart disease), or phonocardiography. X-rays show cardiac enlargement and pulmonary congestion. Cardiac catheterization should be postponed until after delivery, unless surgery is necessary.

Treatment
The goal of antepartum management is to prevent complications and minimize the strain on the mother's heart, primarily through rest. This may require periodic hospitalization for patients with moderate cardiac dysfunction or with symptoms of decompensation, toxemia, or infection. Older women or those with previous decompensation may require hospitalization and bed rest throughout the pregnancy.

Drug therapy is often necessary and should always include the safest possible drug in the lowest possible dosage to minimize harmful effects to the fetus. Diuretics and drugs that increase blood pressure, blood volume, or cardiac output should be used with extreme caution. If an anticoagulant is needed, heparin is the drug of choice. Digitalis and common antiarrhythmics, such as quinidine and procainamide, are often

required. The prophylactic use of antibiotics is reserved for patients who are susceptible to endocarditis.

A therapeutic abortion may be considered for patients with severe cardiac dysfunction, especially if decompensation occurs during the first trimester. Patients hospitalized with heart failure usually follow a regimen of digitalis, oxygen, rest, sedation, diuretics, and restricted intake of sodium and fluids. Patients in whom symptoms of heart failure do not improve after treatment with bed rest and digitalis may require cardiac surgery, such as valvotomy and commissurotomy. During labor, the patient may require oxygen and an analgesic, such as meperidine or morphine, for relief of pain and apprehension without undue depression of the fetus or herself. Depending on which procedure promises to be less stressful for the patient's heart, delivery may be vaginal or by cesarean section.

Bed rest and medications already instituted should continue for at least 1 week after delivery because of a high incidence of decompensation, cardiovascular collapse, and maternal death during the early puerperal period. These complications may result from the sudden release of intra-abdominal pressure at delivery and the mobilization of extracellular fluid for excretion, which increase the strain on the heart, especially if excessive interstitial fluid has accumulated. Breast-feeding is undesirable for patients with severely compromised cardiac dysfunction, because it increases fluid and metabolic demands on the heart.

Additional considerations
• During pregnancy, rest and weight control is important to decrease the strain on the heart. Limited fluid and sodium intake will prevent vascular congestion. The patient should take supplementary folic acid and iron to prevent anemia.
• During labor, the patient must be watched for signs of decompensation. Pulse rate, respirations, and blood pressure must be monitored. She should be auscultated

for rales every 30 minutes during the first phase of labor and every 10 minutes during the active and transition phases. She should be checked carefully for edema and cyanosis, and her intake and output assessed. Oxygen may be needed to relieve respiratory difficulty.

• Electronic fetal monitoring can be used to detect early signs of fetal distress.

• The patient should be kept in a semirecumbent position. Her efforts to bear down during labor must be limited, because they significantly raise blood pressure and stress the heart.

• After delivery, the patient will need reassurance, and encouragement to adhere to her program of treatment. The need for rest must be emphasized.

Megaloblastic Anemia

An uncommon complication of pregnancy, megaloblastic anemia results from a folic acid deficiency that alters the nucleic acid production necessary for erythrocyte maturation in bone marrow. Although this disorder can affect females of any age or parity, it's most common among multiparas over age 30, especially those who are malnourished. Megaloblastic anemia is rare in the United States, occurring in only 0.5% to 2% of all pregnancies.

Causes
Although megaloblastic anemia isn't unique to pregnancy, the increased demand for folic acid and possible interference with its utilization during pregnancy significantly increase susceptibility to folic acid deficiency and, consequently, to megaloblastic anemia. The normal folic acid requirement in nonpregnant females is 50 mcg/day. The requirement during pregnancy has not been established but may rise to 400 mcg/day. Other predisposing factors include inadequate dietary intake of fresh, leafy, green vegetables and of foods high in animal protein, and excessive cooking, which destroys the folic acid content of many foods. (For other causes of folic acid deficiency anemia, see Chapter 18, HEMATOLOGIC DISORDERS.).

Signs and symptoms
Severe anemia despite sufficient iron intake, near term or postpartum, may indicate megaloblastic anemia. Its characteristic signs include weakness, fatigue, palpitations, light-headedness, glossitis, extreme pallor, dyspnea, and slight jaundice. Progressive anorexia, nausea, and vomiting further jeopardize nutritional status.

Diagnosis
 Progressively decreasing hemoglobin levels, CBC showing decreased RBCs (less than 3,000,000/mm³), and hypersegmentation of neutrophilic leukocytes suggest megaloblastic anemia; bone marrow analysis revealing hyperplastic or megaloblastic cells confirms the disorder. Decreased serum folic acid and total iron-binding capacity support the diagnosis.

Treatment and additional considerations
Treatment requires administration of folic acid (1 mg/day), with iron supplements and a diet high in vitamins and protein. Normal hemoglobin levels return within 4 weeks if infection doesn't occur. Severe anemia near term may necessitate blood transfusions.

• The patient should adhere to the prescribed diet and take the necessary vitamin supplements.

• Patients with megaloblastic anemia are vulnerable to infection. They must be taught to watch for early signs of infection, such as fever, chills and malaise, and should contact their doctor if such symptoms develop.

Adolescent Pregnancy

In the United States, an estimated 1 million adolescents become pregnant each year. Since up to 70% of them don't receive early prenatal care (some receive none at all), they are apt to develop special problems, and are known to have a significantly higher incidence of anemia, toxemia, and perinatal mortality. For example, pregnant adolescents are known to have a higher suicide rate; they're also more likely to have premature babies of low birth weight with a higher neonatal mortality, and who are predisposed to injury at birth, childhood illness, and retardation or other neurologic defects. As a rule, the younger the mother, the greater the health risk for both mother and infant. Adolescents account for one third of all abortions performed in the United States.

Causes

Adolescent pregnancy is prevalent in all socioeconomic levels, and its contributing factors vary. Such factors may include ignorance about sexuality and contraception, increasing sexual activity at a young age, rebellion against parental influence, and a need to escape an unhappy family situation.

Signs and symptoms

Clinical manifestations of adolescent pregnancy are the same as those of adult pregnancy (amenorrhea, nausea, vomiting, breast tenderness, fatigue). However, the pregnant adolescent is much more likely to develop complications such as prematurity, preeclampsia, and—if she is younger than 15—contracted pelvis. Some of these complications are related to physical immaturity; others to her need to deny her condition or to her ignorance of early signs of pregnancy that often delays proper prenatal care.

Diagnosis

 A pregnancy test showing human chorionic gonadotropin in the blood or urine, and a pelvic examination confirm pregnancy. Auscultation of fetal heart sounds with a Doppler or fe-

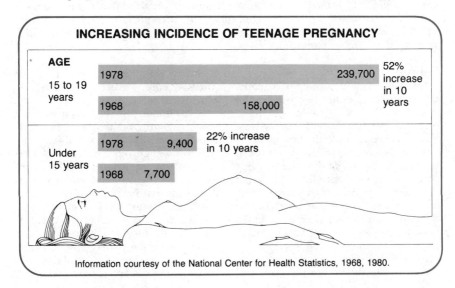

INCREASING INCIDENCE OF TEENAGE PREGNANCY

AGE

15 to 19 years
1978 — 239,700
1968 — 158,000

52% increase in 10 years

Under 15 years
1978 — 9,400
1968 — 7,700

22% increase in 10 years

Information courtesy of the National Center for Health Statistics, 1968, 1980.

toscope and ultrasonography assess fetal gestational age.

Treatment and additional considerations

The pregnant adolescent requires the standard prenatal care that is appropriate for an adult. However, she needs close observation for signs of complications, and psychologic support.

The health care professional *must* help motivate the pregnant adolescent to follow medical advice without being judgmental or condescending. Adhering to a strict diet, getting plenty of rest, and taking prescribed vitamin and iron supplements are very important. Understanding and support can ensure proper health care during the pregnancy for both mother and infant. The patient may need encouragement to ask questions and express her feelings about the pregnancy. Any questions should be answered as fully as possible.

If possible, the patient should be referred to a school or clinic for pregnant adolescents, where she can continue her education while receiving proper prenatal care. Pregnancy is the most common reason adolescent girls drop out of school.

Statistics show that almost half of all pregnant adolescents become pregnant again within a year after delivery. To prevent recurrence, the pregnant adolescent should receive comprehensive information on contraception, including charts, simplified explanations, and take-home pamphlets. The patient can be referred to a family planning counselor.

Diabetic Complications During Pregnancy

Pregnancy places special demands on carbohydrate metabolism and causes the insulin requirement to increase, even in a healthy female. Consequently, pregnancy may lead to a prediabetic state, to the conversion of an asymptomatic subclinical diabetic state to a clinical one (gestational diabetes occurs in about 1% to 2% of all pregnancies), or to complications in a previously stable diabetic state.

Prevalence of diabetes mellitus increases with age. Maternal and fetal prognoses can be equivalent to those in nondiabetic females if maternal blood glucose is well controlled and ketosis and other complications are prevented. Infant morbidity and mortality depend on recognizing and successfully controlling hypoglycemia, which may develop within hours after delivery.

Causes

In diabetes mellitus, glucose is inadequately utilized either because insulin is not synthesized (as in a Type I, insulin-dependent diabetic) or because tissues are resistant to the hormonal action of endogenous insulin (as in a Type II, noninsulin-dependent diabetic). During pregnancy, the fetus relies on maternal glucose as a primary fuel source. Pregnancy triggers protective mechanisms that have anti-insulin effects: increased hormone production (placental lactogen, estrogen, and progesterone), which antagonizes the effects of insulin; degradation of insulin by the placenta; and prolonged elevation of stress hormones (cortisol, epinephrine, and glucagon), which raise blood glucose levels.

In a normal pregnancy, an increase in anti-insulin factors is counterbalanced by an increase in insulin production to maintain normal blood glucose levels. However, females who are prediabetic or diabetic are unable to produce sufficient insulin to overcome the insulin antagonist mechanisms of pregnancy, or their tissues are insulin-resistant. As insulin requirements rise toward term, the patient who is prediabetic may develop gestational diabetes, necessitating dietary management and, possibly, exogenous insulin to achieve glycemic control, while the patient who is insulin-dependent may need increased insulin dosage.

Signs and symptoms
Indications for diagnostic screening for maternal diabetes mellitus during pregnancy include obesity, excessive weight gain, excessive hunger or thirst, polyuria, recurrent monilial infections, previous delivery of a large infant, hydramnios, maternal hypertension, and a family history of diabetes.

Uncontrolled diabetes in a pregnant female can cause stillbirth, fetal anomalies, premature delivery, and birth of an infant who is large or small for gestational age. Such infants are predisposed to severe episodes of hypoglycemia shortly after birth. These infants may also develop hypocalcemia, hyperbilirubinemia, and respiratory distress syndrome.

Diagnosis
The prevalence of gestational diabetes makes careful screening for hyperglycemia appropriate in all pregnancies in each trimester. Abnormal fasting or postprandial blood glucose levels, and clinical signs and history suggest diabetes in patients not previously diabetic.

 A 3-hour glucose tolerance test confirms diabetes mellitus when two or more values are above normal.

Procedures to assess fetal status include stress and nonstress tests, ultrasonography to determine fetal age and growth, measurement of urinary estriols, and determination of the lecithin-sphingomyelin ratio from amniotic fluid to predict pulmonary maturity.

Treatment
Treatment of both the newly diagnosed and the established diabetic is designed to maintain blood glucose levels within acceptable limits through dietary management and insulin administration. Most females with overt diabetes mellitus require hospitalization at the beginning of pregnancy to assess physical status, to check for associated cardiac and renal disease, and to regulate diabetes.

For pregnant patients with diabetes, therapy includes:

• bimonthly visits to the obstetrician and the internist during the first 6 months of pregnancy. Weekly visits may be necessary during the third trimester.

• maintenance of blood sugar levels appropriate for the week of gestation.

• frequent monitoring for glycosuria and ketonuria (ketosis presents a grave threat to the fetal central nervous system).

• weight control (gain not to exceed 3 to 3½ lb [1.36 to 1.59 kg] per month during the last 6 months of pregnancy).

• high-protein diet of 2 g/day/kg of body weight, or a minimum of 80 g/day during the second half of pregnancy; daily calorie intake of 30 to 40 calories/kg of body weight; daily carbohydrate intake of 200 g; and enough fat to provide 36% of total calories. However, vigorous calorie restriction is not recommended, since it can cause starvation ketosis.

• exogenous insulin if diet doesn't control blood sugar levels. Insulin requirements can change from one trimester to the next and immediately postpartum. Oral hypoglycemic agents are contraindicated during pregnancy, because they may cause fetal hypoglycemia and abnormalities.

Generally, the optimal time for delivery is between 37 and 39 weeks' gestation. The insulin-dependent diabetic requires hospitalization for at least 1 week before delivery, because bed rest promotes uteroplacental circulation and myometrial tone. In addition, hospitalization permits frequent monitoring of blood glucose levels and prompt intervention if complications develop.

Depending on fetal status and obstetrical history, the obstetrician may induce labor or perform a cesarean delivery. During labor and delivery, the patient with diabetes should have an I.V. infusion of dextrose in water. Maternal and fetal status must be monitored closely throughout labor. The patient may benefit from half her prepregnancy dosage of insulin before a cesarean delivery. Her insulin requirement will fall markedly after delivery.

Additional considerations
• The newly diagnosed patient must be taught about diabetes, including dietary management, insulin administration, home monitoring of blood glucose or urine testing for glucose and ketones as an alternative, and skin and foot care. She should report ketonuria immediately.
• The diabetic patient's knowledge about this disease should be evaluated, and supplementary teaching provided, as needed.

She should know that frequent monitoring and adjustment of insulin dosage are necessary throughout pregnancy.
• The patient will need reassurance that with strict compliance to prescribed therapy, the outcome of the pregnancy should be favorable.
• The patient should be referred to an appropriate social service agency if financial assistance is necessary because of prolonged hospitalization.
• The patient should get medical counseling regarding the prognosis of future pregnancies.

ABNORMALITIES OF PARTURITION

Premature Labor
(Preterm labor)

Premature labor is onset of rhythmic uterine contractions that produce cervical change after fetal viability but before fetal maturity. It usually occurs between the 26th and 37th weeks of gestation. Approximately 5% to 10% of pregnancies end prematurely; about 75% of neonatal deaths and a great many birth defects stem from this disorder. Fetal prognosis depends on birth weight and length of gestation: infants weighing less than 1 lb 10 oz (750 g) and of less than 26 weeks' gestation have a survival rate of about 10%; infants weighing 1 lb 10 oz to 2 lb 3 oz (750 to 1,000 g) and of 27 to 28 weeks' gestation have a survival rate of more than 50%; those weighing 2 lb 3 oz to 2 lb 11 oz (1,000 to 1,250 g) and of more than 28 weeks' gestation have a 70% to 90% survival rate.

Causes
The possible causes of premature labor are many; they may include premature rupture of the membranes (occurs in 30% to 50% of premature labors), preeclampsia, chronic hypertensive vascular disease, hydramnios, multiple pregnancy, placenta previa, abruptio placentae, incompetent cervix, abdominal surgery, trauma, structural anomalies of the uterus, infections (such as rubella or toxoplasmosis), congenital adrenal hyperplasia, and fetal death.

Other important provocative factors:
• *Fetal stimulation:* Genetically imprinted information tells the fetus that nutrition is inadequate and that a change in environment is required for well-

being; this provokes onset of labor.
• *Progesterone deficiency:* Decreased placental production of progesterone—thought to be the hormone that maintains pregnancy—triggers labor.
• *Oxytocin sensitivity:* Labor begins because the myometrium becomes hypersensitive to oxytocin, the hormone that normally induces uterine contractions.
• *Myometrial oxygen deficiency:* The fetus becomes increasingly proficient in obtaining oxygen, depriving the myometrium of the oxygen and energy it needs to function normally, thus making the myometrium irritable.
• *Maternal genetics:* A genetic defect in the mother shortens gestation and precipitates premature labor.

Signs and symptoms

Like labor at term, premature labor produces rhythmic uterine contractions, cervical dilation and effacement, possible rupture of the membranes, expulsion of the cervical mucous plug, and a bloody discharge.

Diagnosis

Premature labor is confirmed by the combined results of prenatal history, physical examination, presenting signs and symptoms, and ultrasonography (if available) showing the position of the fetus in relation to the mother's pelvis. Vaginal examination confirms progressive cervical effacement and dilation.

Treatment

Treatment is designed to suppress premature labor when tests show immature fetal pulmonary development, cervical dilation of less than 2″ (5 cm), and the absence of factors that contraindicate continuation of pregnancy. Such treatment consists of bed rest and, when necessary, drug therapy.

The following pharmacologic agents can suppress premature labor:
• *Ethyl alcohol:* A 10% solution in dextrose 5% in water, administered I.V., directly depresses the myometrium, and theoretically decreases uterine activity by interfering with oxytocin secretion. It also produces signs of alcohol intoxication (light-headedness, incoherence, nausea, and vomiting) in the mother and may harm the fetus. If labor suppression is unsuccessful, neonatal alcohol blood levels should be monitored with resuscitative equipment available.
• *Beta-adrenergic stimulants* (isoxsuprine or ritodrine): Stimulation of the beta$_2$ receptors inhibits contractility of uterine smooth muscle. Side effects include maternal tachycardia and hypotension, and fetal tachycardia.

Maternal factors that jeopardize the fetus, making premature delivery the lesser risk, include intrauterine infection, abruptio placentae, placental insufficiency, and severe preeclampsia. Among the fetal problems that become more perilous as pregnancy nears term are severe isoimmunization and congenital anomalies.

Ideally, treatment for active premature labor should take place in a regional perinatal intensive care center, where the staff is specially trained to handle this situation. In such settings, the infant can remain close to his parents. (Community hospitals commonly lack the facilities for special neonatal care and transfer the infant alone to a perinatal center.)

Treatment and delivery necessitate intensive team effort, focusing on:
• continuous assessment of the infant's health through fetal monitoring.
• avoidance of sedatives and narcotics that might harm the infant. Morphine or meperidine may be required to minimize pain; these drugs have little effect on uterine contractions, but depress CNS function and may cause fetal respiratory depression. These agents should be administered in the smallest dose possible and only when extremely necessary.
• avoidance of amniotomy, if possible, to prevent cord prolapse or damage to the infant's tender skull.
• maintenance of adequate hydration through I.V. fluids.

Prevention of premature labor requires good prenatal care, adequate nutrition, and proper rest. Insertion of a pursestring suture (cerclage) to reinforce an incompetent cervix at 14 to 18 weeks' gestation may prevent premature labor in patients with histories of this disorder.

Additional considerations

Premature labor requires close observation for signs of fetal or maternal distress, and comprehensive supportive care. The hospital staff member should:
• maintain bed rest and administer medications, as ordered, during attempts to suppress premature labor; give sedatives and analgesics sparingly, mindful of their potentially harmful effect on the fetus; minimize the need for these drugs by providing comfort measures, such as frequent repositioning,

and good perineal and back care.

• monitor blood pressure, pulse rate, respirations, fetal heart rate, and uterine contraction pattern when ethyl alcohol is given; titrate alcohol infusion rate to achieve the blood level ordered; help the patient cope with distressing side effects of alcohol intoxication; keep her in a right or left lateral recumbent position, if possible, to prevent aspiration of vomitus, which can occur if her level of consciousness is reduced; keep suctioning equipment at the bedside.

• monitor blood pressure, pulse rate, respirations, fetal heart rate, and uterine contraction pattern when administering beta-adrenergic stimulants, sedatives, and narcotics; minimize side effects by keeping the patient in a lateral recumbent position as much as possible; provide adequate hydration.

• offer emotional support to the patient and family; encourage the parents to express their fears concerning the infant's survival and health.

• remember during active premature labor that the premature infant has a lower tolerance for the stress of labor and is much more likely to become hypoxic than the term infant; administer oxygen, if necessary, through a nasal cannula; encourage the patient to lie on her left side or sit up during labor (this position prevents caval compression, which can cause supine hypotension and subsequent fetal hypoxia); observe fetal response to labor through continuous fetal monitoring; avoid maternal hyperventi-lation—a rebreathing bag may be necessary; continually reassure the patient to reduce her anxiety.

• help the patient get through labor with as little analgesic and anesthetic as possible; avoid administering analgesics when delivery seems imminent to minimize fetal CNS depression; monitor fetal and maternal response to local and regional anesthetics.

• explain all procedures; keep the patient informed of her progress and the condition of the fetus. If the father is present during labor, the parents should have some time together to share their feelings.

• instruct the patient during delivery to push only during contractions and only as long as she is told. Pushing between contractions is not only ineffective but can damage the premature infant's soft skull. A neonatal clinician and nurse should be in attendance to take care of the newborn immediately. Resuscitative equipment should be available in case of neonatal respiratory distress.

• inform the parents of their child's condition; describe his appearance, and explain the purpose of any supportive equipment; help them gain confidence in their ability to care for their child through demonstration and instruction; provide privacy, and encourage them to hold and feed the infant, when possible.

• refer the parents before they leave the hospital with the baby to a community health nurse who can help them adjust to caring for a premature infant.

Premature Rupture of the Membranes

Premature rupture of the membranes (PROM) is a spontaneous break or tear in the amniochorial sac before onset of regular contractions, resulting in progressive cervical dilation. PROM occurs in nearly 10% of all pregnancies over 20 weeks' gestation, and labor usually starts within 24 hours; more than 80% of these infants are mature. The latent period (between membrane rupture and onset of labor) is generally brief when the membranes rupture near term; when the infant is premature, this period is prolonged, which increases the risk of mortality from maternal infection (amnionitis, endometritis), fetal infection (pneumonia, septicemia), and prematurity.

Causes

Although the cause of PROM is unknown, malpresentation and contracted pelvis commonly accompany the rupture. Predisposing factors may include:
• poor nutrition and hygiene, and lack of proper prenatal care.
• incompetent cervix (perhaps as a result of abortions).
• increased intrauterine tension resulting from multiple pregnancies, or hydramnios.
• defects in the membranes' tensile strength.

Signs and symptoms

Typically, PROM causes blood-tinged amniotic fluid containing vernix particles to gush or leak from the vagina. Maternal fever, fetal tachycardia, and foul-smelling vaginal discharge indicate infection.

Diagnosis

Characteristic passage of amniotic fluid confirms PROM. Physical examination shows amniotic fluid in the vagina. Examination of this fluid helps determine appropriate management. For example, aerobic and anaerobic cultures, and a Gram's stain from the cervix reveal pathogenic organisms and indicate uterine or systemic infection.

 Alkaline pH of fluid collected from the posterior fornix turns nitrazine paper deep blue. If a smear of fluid is placed on a slide and allowed to dry, it takes on a fernlike pattern due to a high sodium and protein content of amniotic fluid. Staining the fluid with Nile blue sulfate reveals two categories of cell bodies. Blue-stained bodies represent shed fetal epithelial cells, while orange-stained bodies originate in sebaceous glands. Incidence of prematurity is low when more than 20% of cells stain orange.

Physical examination also determines multiple pregnancies. Fetal presentation and size should be assessed by abdominal palpation (Leopold's maneuvers). Other data determine the fetus' gestational age:

• *historical:* date of last menstrual period, quickening
• *physical:* initial detection of unamplified fetal heart rate, measurement of fundal height above the symphysis, ultrasound measurements of fetal biparietal diameter
• *chemical:* tests on amniotic fluid, such as the lecithin-sphingomyelin ratio (an L/S ratio greater than 2.0 indicates pulmonary maturity); foam stability (shake test) also indicates pulmonary maturity.

Treatment

Treatment for PROM depends on fetal age and the risk of infection. If spontaneous labor and vaginal delivery are not achieved within a relatively short time (usually within 24 hours of the time membranes rupture), a term pregnancy usually requires induction of labor with oxytocin or, if induction fails, cesarean delivery. Cesarean hysterectomy is recommended when gross uterine infection is present.

A preterm pregnancy of less than 28 weeks also necessitates induction to terminate pregnancy, since fetal mortality is almost certain, and carrying the fetus in a ruptured amniotic sac exposes the mother to infection. With a preterm pregnancy of 28 to 35 weeks, treatment includes hospitalization and observation for signs of infection (maternal leukocytosis or fever, and fetal tachycardia) while awaiting fetal maturation. If clinical status suggests infection, baseline cultures and sensitivity tests are appropriate. If these tests confirm infection, labor must be induced, followed by I.V. administration of antibiotics. A culture should also be made of gastric aspirate or a swabbing from the infant's ear, as antibiotic therapy may be indicated for the newborn as well. At such delivery, resuscitative equipment should be available to treat neonatal distress.

Additional considerations

• The patient should be taught in the early stages of pregnancy how to recognize PROM. She must understand that amniotic fluid doesn't always gush; it

sometimes leaks slowly.
• The patient *must* report PROM immediately, since prompt treatment may prevent dangerous infection.
• The patient must not engage in sexual intercourse or douche after the membranes rupture.
• Before physical examination in suspected PROM, all diagnostic tests should be explained and any misunderstandings the patient may have should be clarified. During the examination, the patient will need reassurance. Such examination requires sterile gloves and sterile lubricating jelly. Iodophor antiseptic solution should not be used, since it discolors nitrazine paper and makes pH determination impossible.
• After the examination, proper perineal care is needed. Fluid samples should go to the laboratory promptly, since bacteriologic studies need immediate evaluation to be valid. If labor starts, the mother's contractions should be observed, and her vital signs monitored every 2 hours. The patient must be watched for signs of maternal infection (fever, abdominal tenderness, and changes in amniotic fluid, such as foul odor or purulence) and fetal tachycardia. (Fetal tachycardia may precede maternal fever.)

Cesarean Birth
(Cesarean section)

Cesarean birth is delivery of an infant by surgical incision through the abdomen and uterus. It can be performed as elective surgery, or as an emergency procedure when conditions prohibit vaginal delivery. The rising incidence of cesarean birth coincides with recent medical and technologic advances in fetal and placental surveillance and care. In the United States, 9% to 16% of all pregnancies terminate in cesarean births, rising to 17% to 20% in perinatal centers that handle high-risk deliveries.

Causes
The most common reasons for cesarean birth are malpresentation (such as shoulder or face presentation), fetal distress, cephalopelvic disproportion ([CPD] the pelvis is too small to accommodate the fetal head), certain cases of toxemia, previous cesarean birth, and inadequate progress in labor (failure of induction).

Conditions causing fetal distress that indicate a need for cesarean birth include prolapsed cord with a live fetus, fetal hypoxia, abnormal fetal heart rate patterns, unfavorable intrauterine environment (from infection), and moderate to severe Rh isoimmunization. Less common maternal conditions that may necessitate cesarean birth include complete placenta previa, abruptio placentae, placenta accreta, malignant tumors, and chronic diseases in which delivery is indicated before term.

Cesarean birth may also be necessary if induction is contraindicated or difficult, or if advanced labor increases the risk of morbidity and mortality.

In the case of a previous cesarean delivery, some doctors allow a subsequent vaginal delivery if the cesarean wasn't classic or due to CPD, or if the original reason for the cesarean no longer exists. However, vaginal delivery risks uterine rupture if the uterus is scarred.

Diagnosis
Special tests and monitoring procedures provide early indications of the need for cesarean birth:
• *X-ray pelvimetry* reveals CPD and malpresentation.
• *Ultrasonography* shows pelvic masses that interfere with vaginal delivery and fetal position.
• *Amniocentesis* determines fetal ma-

turity, Rh isoimmunization, fetal distress, and fetal genetic abnormalities.

• Auscultation of *fetal heart rate* (fetoscope or Doppler unit) determines acute fetal distress.

Treatment

The most common type of cesarean birth is the *lower segment cesarean,* in which a transverse incision across the lower abdomen opens the visceral peritoneum over the uterus. The lower anterior uterine wall is then incised (transversely or longitudinally) behind the bladder. Since the peritoneum completely covers this part of the uterus, uterine seepage is reduced and, consequently, so is the risk of postpartum infection.

The *classic cesarean*—in which a longitudinal incision is made into the body of the uterus, extending into the fundus and opening the top of the uterus—is rarely performed, because it exaggerates the risk of infection and of uterine rupture in subsequent pregnancies. *Cesarean hysterectomy* removes the entire uterus and is reserved for cases such as malignant tumors, severe infection, and placenta accreta.

Patients may have general or spinal anesthetic for surgery, depending on the extent of maternal or fetal distress. Possible maternal complications of cesarean delivery include respiratory tract infection, wound dehiscence, thromboembolism, paralytic ileus, hemorrhage, and genitourinary tract infection.

Additional considerations

Before cesarean delivery, the hospital staff member should:

• explain cesarean birth to the patient and her husband, and answer any questions they may have; provide reassurance and emotional support. Cesarean birth often is performed after hours of labor have exhausted the patient.

• administer preoperative medications as ordered.

• prepare the patient by shaving her from below the breasts to the pubic region and the upper quarter of the anterior thighs; make sure her bladder is empty, using a

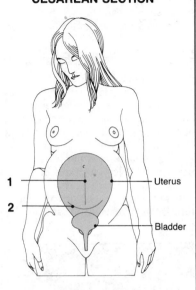

UTERINE INCISIONS FOR CESAREAN SECTION

1 — Uterus

2 — Bladder

1. In *classic cesarean,* a vertical incision extends from the uterine fundus through the body, stopping above the level of the bladder.

2. In *lower segment cesarean,* the preferred method, a transverse incision is made across the lower abdomen and along the lower anterior uterine wall behind the bladder. This avoids incision of the peritoneum, reducing the risk of peritonitis.

Foley catheter, as ordered; insert an I.V. line for fluid replacement therapy, as ordered; assess maternal temperature, pulse rate, respirations, blood pressure, and fetal heart rate.

• place the patient in a slight lateral position in the operating room; a 15° wedge to reduce caval compression (supine hypotension) and subsequent fetal hypoxia.

After cesarean delivery, the staff member should:

• check vital signs every 15 minutes until they stabilize; maintain a patent airway; remain with the patient until she's responsive if general anesthetic was used;

monitor the return of sensation to the legs if spinal anesthetic was used.
• encourage parent-infant bonding as soon as practical.
• gently assess the fundus; check the incision and lochia for signs of infection, such as a foul odor; check frequently for bleeding, and report it immediately; keep the incision clean and dry.
• observe the infant for signs of respiratory distress (tachypnea, retractions, and cyanosis) until there is evidence of physiologic stability; keep resuscitative equipment available.
• assess intake and output (some patients have Foley catheters in place up to 48 hours postoperative); observe the patient closely for indications of bladder fullness or urinary tract infection.

• administer pain medication, as ordered, and comfort measures for breast engorgement, as appropriate; offer reassurance and reduce anxiety by answering any questions; offer encouragement and help if the mother wishes to breast-feed; recognize after-pains in multiparas.
• promote early ambulation to prevent cardiovascular and pulmonary complications.
• provide psychologic support. If the patient seems anxious about having had a cesarean delivery, she should be encouraged to share her feelings. If appropriate, she may want to participate in a cesarean birth sharing group. Support from family members should be encouraged.

POSTPARTUM DISORDERS

Puerperal Infection

A common cause of childbirth-related death, puerperal infection is an inflammation of the birth canal during the postpartum period or after abortion. It can occur as localized lesions of the perineum, vulva, and vagina, or it may spread, causing endometritis, parametritis, pelvic and femoral thrombophlebitis, and peritonitis. In the United States, puerperal infection develops in about 6% of maternity patients. Prognosis is good with treatment.

Causes
Microorganisms that commonly cause puerperal infection include streptococci, coagulase-negative staphylococci, *Clostridium perfringens*, *Bacteroides fragilis*, and *Escherichia coli*. Most of these organisms are considered normal vaginal flora but are known to cause puerperal infection in the presence of certain predisposing factors, which include:
• prolonged and premature rupture of the membranes.
• prolonged (more than 24 hours) or traumatic labor.
• frequent or unsanitary vaginal examinations, or unsanitary delivery.
• invasive techniques, such as application of a fetal scalp electrode.

• intercourse after rupture of the membranes.
• retained products of conception.
• hemorrhage.
• preexisting maternal conditions, such as anemia or debilitation from malnutrition.

Signs and symptoms
A characteristic sign of puerperal infection is fever (100.4° F. [38° C.]) that occurs after the first 24 hours postpartum on any 2 consecutive days up to the 11th day. This fever can spike as high as 105° F. (40.6° C.), and is commonly associated with chills, headache, malaise, restlessness, and anxiety. Accompanying symptoms depend on the site of

infection, and may include:
- *local lesions of the perineum, vulva, and vagina:* pain, inflammation, edema of the affected area, dysuria, profuse purulent discharge.
- *endometritis:* heavy, sometimes foul-smelling lochia; tender, enlarged uterus; backache; severe uterine contractions persisting after childbirth.
- *parametritis (pelvic cellulitis):* vaginal tenderness, and abdominal pain and tenderness (pain may become more intense as infection spreads).

The inflammation may remain localized, may lead to abscess formation, or may spread through the blood or lymph. Widespread inflammation may cause:
- *pelvic thrombophlebitis:* severe, repeated chills and dramatic swings in temperature; lower abdominal or flank pain; and possibly, a palpable tender mass over the affected area that usually occurs near the second postpartum week.
- *femoral thrombophlebitis:* pain, stiffness, or swelling in a leg or the groin; inflammation or shiny, white appearance of the affected leg; malaise; fever; and chills, usually beginning 10 to 20 days postpartum. These signs may precede pulmonary embolism.
- *peritonitis:* temperature usually high, tachycardia (more than 140 beats per minute), weak pulse, hiccups, nausea, vomiting, and diarrhea; abdominal pain is constant and, possibly, excruciating.

Diagnosis
Clinical features, especially fever within 48 hours after delivery, suggest puerperal infection.

 A culture of lochia, blood, incisional exudate (from cesarean incision or episiotomy), uterine tissue, or material collected from the vaginal cuff, revealing the causative organism, confirms it. WBC count usually demonstrates leukocytosis (15,000 to 30,000/mm^3).

Typical clinical features usually suffice for diagnosis of endometritis and peritonitis. In parametritis, pelvic examination shows induration without

---

PUERPERAL INFECTION AND DR. IGNAZ SEMMELWEISS

Puerperal infection was well known throughout recorded history. Hippocrates, for example, wrote that puerperal infection resulted from the suppression of vaginal discharge. Its true cause remained unknown until Louis Pasteur's discoveries in microbiology, and puerperal infection persisted as a common cause of maternal death well into the 19th century.

In 1847, Dr. Ignaz Semmelweiss, while working at a maternity hospital in Vienna, observed the dramatically low mortality from puerperal infection in a ward managed by midwives, compared to the high mortality in a ward managed by doctors. In the Vienna of his time, Dr. Semmelweiss' colleagues went directly from dissecting cadavers to examining patients who were recovering from childbirth. He concluded that the doctors were spreading this fatal infection via their unwashed hands. He got dramatic proof of his theory when he saw a co-worker die of septicemia after accidentally cutting himself with a scalpel used during autopsy of a woman who had died of puerperal infection. As a result, Semmelweiss required his staff to wash their hands with an antiseptic solution before examining maternity patients. During the first year of the hand-washing mandate, mortality from puerperal infection at Semmelweiss' hospital dropped sharply from almost 12% to 3.8%.

Despite such dramatic results, Semmelweiss' colleagues did not accept his theory for another 20 years—not until Pasteur's microbiologic theories and Lister's application of aseptic technique made Semmelweiss' theory indisputable.

Almost coincidentally with Semmelweiss' discovery, similar progress began in the United States. In an article published in 1843 in the *New England Journal of Medicine,* Oliver Wendell Holmes stressed the importance of adequate precautions by doctors and nurses to prevent puerperal infection.

purulent discharge; culdoscopy shows pelvic adnexal induration and thickening. Red, swollen abscesses on the broad ligaments are even more serious indications, since rupture leads to peritonitis.

Diagnosis of pelvic or femoral thrombophlebitis is suggested by characteristic clinical signs, venography, Doppler ultrasonography, Rielander's sign (palpable veins inside the thigh and calf), Payr's sign (pain in the calf when pressure is applied on the inside of the foot), and Homans' sign (pain on dorsiflexion of the foot with the knee extended).

Treatment

Treatment begins with I.V. infusion of a broad-spectrum antibiotic to control the infection and prevent its spread while awaiting culture results. After identification of the infecting organism, a more specific antibiotic should be administered. (An oral antibiotic may be prescribed after hospital discharge.)

Ancillary measures include analgesics for pain; anticoagulants, such as heparin I.V., for thrombophlebitis and endometritis (after clotting time and partial thromboplastin time determine dosage); antiseptics for local lesions; and antiemetics for nausea and vomiting from peritonitis. Isolation or patient transfer from the maternity unit also may be indicated.

Supportive care includes bed rest, adequate fluid intake, I.V. fluids when necessary, and measures to reduce fever. Sitz baths and heat lamps may relieve discomfort from local lesions.

Surgery may be necessary to remove any remaining products of conception or to drain local lesions, such as an abscess in parametritis.

Management of femoral thrombophlebitis requires warm soaks, elevation of the affected leg to promote venous return, and observation for signs of pulmonary embolism. Rarely, recurrent pulmonary emboli from pelvic thrombophlebitis require laparotomy for plication of the inferior vena cava and ovarian vein ligation.

Additional considerations

The hospital staff member caring for a patient with puerperal infection should:
• monitor vital signs every 4 hours (more frequently if peritonitis has developed), and intake and output; enforce strict bed rest.
• frequently inspect the perineum; assess the fundus, and palpate for tenderness (subinvolution may indicate endometritis); note and document the amount, color, and odor of vaginal drainage.
• administer antibiotics and analgesics, as ordered; assess and document the type, degree, and location of pain, as well as the patient's response to analgesics; give an antiemetic to relieve nausea and vomiting, as necessary.
• provide sitz baths and a heat lamp for local lesions; change bed linen and perineal pads and underpads frequently; keep the patient warm.
• elevate the thrombophlebitic leg about 30°; never rub or manipulate it, or compress it with bed linen; provide warm soaks for the leg; watch for signs of pulmonary embolism, such as cyanosis, dyspnea, and chest pain.
• offer emotional support; thoroughly explain all procedures to the patient and family.
• provide frequent reassurance about the infant's progress if the mother is separated from him; encourage the father to reassure her about the infant's condition.

To prevent puerperal infection, care includes:
• maintaining aseptic technique when performing a vaginal examination; limiting the number of vaginal examinations performed during labor; washing hands thoroughly after each patient contact.
• instructing all pregnant women to call their doctors immediately when their membranes rupture; warning them to avoid intercourse after rupture or leak of the amniotic sac.
• keeping the episiotomy site clean, and teaching the patient how to ensure good perineal hygiene.
• screening personnel and visitors to keep persons with active infections away from maternity patients.

Mastitis and Breast Engorgement

Mastitis (parenchymatous inflammation of the mammary glands) and breast engorgement (congestion) are disorders that may affect lactating females. Mastitis occurs postpartum in about 1%, mainly in primiparas who are breast-feeding. It occurs occasionally in nonlactating females and rarely in males. All breast-feeding mothers develop some degree of engorgement, but it's especially likely to be severe in primiparas. Prognosis for both disorders is good.

Causes

Mastitis develops when a pathogen that typically originates in the nursing infant's nose or pharynx invades breast tissue through a fissured or cracked nipple and disrupts normal lactation. The most common pathogen of this type is *Staphylococcus aureus*; less frequently,

PHYSIOLOGY OF LACTATION

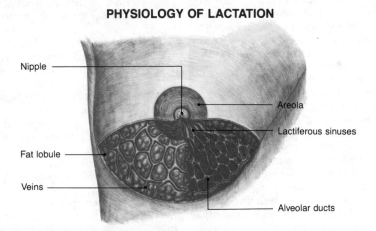

During pregnancy, progesterone and estrogen normally interact to suppress milk secretion while developing the breasts for lactation. Estrogen causes the breasts to grow by increasing their fat content; progesterone causes lobule growth and develops the alveolar cells' secretory capacity.

After childbirth, the mother's anterior pituitary gland secretes prolactin (suppressed during pregnancy), which helps the alveolar epithelium produce and release colostrum. Usually, within 3 days of prolactin release, the breasts secrete large amounts of milk rather than colostrum. The infant's sucking stimulates nerve endings at the nipple, initiating the let-down reflex that allows the expression of milk from the mother's breasts. Sucking also stimulates the release of another pituitary hormone, oxytocin, into the mother's bloodstream. This hormone causes alveolar contraction, which forces milk into the ducts and the lactiferous sinuses beneath the alveolar surface, making milk available to the infant. (It also promotes normal involution of the uterus.)

The infant's suckling provides the stimulus for both milk production and milk expression. Consequently, the more the infant breast-feeds, the more milk the breast produces. Conversely, the less sucking stimulation the breast receives, the less milk it produces.

it's *Staphylococcus epidermidis* or *beta-hemolytic streptococcus*. Rarely, mastitis may result from disseminated tuberculosis or the mumps virus. Predisposing factors include a fissure or abrasion on the nipple; blocked milk ducts; and an incomplete let-down reflex, usually due to emotional trauma. Blocked milk ducts can result from a tight bra or prolonged intervals between breast-feedings.

Causes of breast engorgement include venous and lymphatic stasis, and alveolar milk accumulation.

Signs and symptoms
Mastitis may develop anytime during lactation but usually begins 3 to 4 weeks postpartum, with fever (101° F. [38.3° C.], or higher in acute mastitis), malaise, and flulike symptoms. The breasts (or, occasionally, one breast) become tender, hard, swollen, and warm. Unless mastitis is treated adequately, it may progress to breast abscess.

Breast engorgement generally starts with onset of lactation (day 2 to day 5 postpartum). The breasts undergo changes similar to those in mastitis, and body temperature may be elevated. Engorgement may be mild, causing only slight discomfort, or severe, causing considerable pain. A severely engorged breast can interfere with the infant's capacity to feed due to his inability to position his mouth properly on the swollen, rigid breast.

Diagnosis
In a lactating female with breast discomfort or other signs of inflammation, cultures of expressed milk confirm generalized mastitis; cultures of breast skin surface confirm localized mastitis. Such cultures also determine appropriate antibiotic treatment. Obvious swelling of lactating breasts confirms engorgement.

Treatment
Antibiotic therapy, the primary treatment for mastitis, generally consists of penicillin G to combat staphylococcus; erythromycin or kanamycin is used for penicillin-resistant strains. Although symptoms usually subside 2 to 3 days after treatment begins, antibiotic therapy should continue for 10 days. Other appropriate measures include analgesics for pain and, rarely, when antibiotics fail to control the infection and mastitis progresses to breast abscess, incision and drainage of the abscess.

The goal of treatment of breast engorgement is to relieve discomfort and control swelling, and may include analgesics to alleviate pain, and ice packs and an uplift support to minimize edema. Rarely, oxytocin nasal spray may be necessary to release milk from the alveoli into the ducts. To facilitate breast-feeding, the mother may manually express excess milk before a feeding so the infant can grasp the nipple properly.

Additional considerations
If the patient has mastitis, care includes:
• isolating the patient and infant to prevent the spread of infection to other nursing mothers; explaining mastitis to the patient and why isolation is necessary.
• obtaining a complete patient history, including a drug history, especially allergy to penicillin.
• assessing and recording the cause and amount of discomfort; giving analgesics, as needed.
• reassuring the mother that breast-feeding during mastitis won't harm her infant, since he's the source of infection; telling her to offer the affected breast first to promote complete emptying of the breast and prevent clogged ducts. (However, if an open abscess develops, she must stop breast-feeding with this breast and use a breast pump until the abscess heals. She should continue to breast-feed on the unaffected side. Applying a warm, wet towel to the affected breast or taking a warm shower will help her relax and improve her ability to breast-feed.)
• teaching the patient good health care, breast care, and breast-feeding habits to prevent mastitis and relieve its symptoms; advising her to always wash her hands before touching her breasts.
• instructing the patient to combat fever by getting plenty of rest, drinking suf-

PATIENT TEACHING AID

Tips for Effective Breast-Feeding

During pregnancy and lactation, good health care, breast care, and breast-feeding habits are essential.

- Maintain good nutrition, and get plenty of rest and sleep. Limit stress factors, which can inhibit your ability to breast-feed your infant.
- Don't use soap or other irritating substances on your breasts during the last trimester of pregnancy. These agents remove protective oils. Toughen nipples during pregnancy by rolling them between your fingertips twice daily and rubbing them with a washcloth. Wear a comfortable support bra (not lowcut or tight) with protective pads to prevent staining clothing. Keep your breasts dry and, when possible, open to the air.
- If you plan to breast-feed, begin as soon as your child is born. Breast-feed at regular intervals, including at least once during the night. Alternate breasts at each feeding. Relax in a comfortable position so the infant can suck effectively. If your breasts feel engorged, express excess milk manually. You may find that applying warm wet towels or taking a relaxing shower may help you to express milk more easily; or, you may find it helpful to use a hand or electric breast pump. Avoid sleeping on your stomach, since this may cause mechanical milk stasis.
- If your nipples become dry and

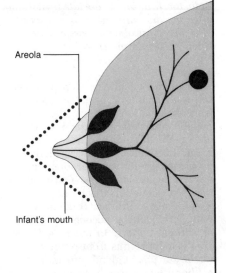

Areola

Infant's mouth

For effective breast-feeding, place the infant's mouth around but not directly on the areola.

cracked, apply pure lanolin. Vitamins A and D ointment is sometimes recommended; if you use this, be sure to apply it only around the nipples and not to the duct openings.

- Wash your nipples thoroughly before breast-feeding.

ficient fluids, and following prescribed antibiotic therapy.

If the patient has breast engorgement, care includes:

- assessing and recording the level of discomfort; giving analgesics, and applying ice packs, as needed.
- teaching the patient how to express excess breast milk manually just before nursing to enable the infant to get the swollen areola into his mouth; cautioning against excessive expression of milk between feedings, as this stimulates milk production and prolongs engorgement.
- explaining that because breast engorgement is due to the physiologic processes of lactation, breast-feeding is the best remedy for engorgement; suggesting breast-feeding every 2 to 3 hours and at least once during the night.
- ensuring that the mother wears a well-fitted nursing bra, usually a size larger than she normally wears, to minimize edema.

Galactorrhea

(Hyperprolactinemia)

Galactorrhea, inappropriate breast milk secretion, generally occurs 3 to 6 months after the discontinuation of breast-feeding (usually after a first delivery). It may also follow an abortion or may develop in a female who hasn't been pregnant; it rarely occurs in males.

Causes

Galactorrhea usually develops in a person with increased prolactin secretion from the anterior pituitary gland, with possible abnormal patterns of secretion of growth, thyroid, and adrenocorticotropic hormones. However, increased prolactin serum concentration doesn't always cause galactorrhea. Other factors may precipitate this disorder:

• *endogenous:* pituitary (high incidence with chromophobe adenoma), ovarian, or adrenal tumors. In males, galactorrhea usually results from pituitary, testicular, or pineal gland tumors.

• *idiopathic:* possibly from stress or anxiety, which causes neurogenic depression of the prolactin-inhibiting factor

• *exogenous:* breast stimulation, intercourse, or drugs (such as oral contraceptives, meprobamate, phenothiazines).

Signs and symptoms

In the female with galactorrhea, milk continues to flow after the 21-day period that is normal after weaning. Galactorrhea may also be spontaneous and unrelated to normal lactation, or due to manual expression. Such abnormal flow is usually bilateral and may be accompanied by amenorrhea.

Diagnosis

Characteristic clinical features and patient history (including drug and sex histories) confirm galactorrhea. Urinary excretion of 17-ketosteroids may be normal, but urinary excretion of estrogen and gonadotropins is usually low. Other tests to help determine the cause include measurement of serum levels of prolactin, cortisol, growth hormone, thyroid-stimulating hormone, triiodothyronine, and thyroxine. Skull X-rays and, possibly, mammography may be indicated.

Treatment

Treatment varies according to the underlying cause, and ranges from simple avoidance of precipitating exogenous factors, such as drugs, to treatment of tumors with surgery, radiation, or chemotherapy. Therapy for idiopathic galactorrhea depends on whether or not the patient plans to have more children. If she does, treatment usually consists of bromocriptine or, less frequently, clomiphene, gonadotropin, or levodopa; if she doesn't, oral estrogens (such as ethinyl estradiol) and progestins (such as progesterone). Idiopathic galactorrhea may recur after discontinuation of therapy.

Additional considerations

• The patient should keep her breasts and nipples clean.

• She should watch for and report CNS abnormalities, such as headache, failing vision, and dizziness.

• Maintaining adequate fluid intake is important, especially if the patient has a fever. However, she should avoid tea, coffee, and some tranquilizers that may aggravate engorgement.

• The patient who is taking levodopa should watch for and report nausea, vomiting, loss of appetite, and hypotension. To prevent gastrointestinal upset, she should eat small meals frequently and take this drug with dry toast or crackers.

• The patient who is taking bromocriptine should watch for and report nausea, dizziness, fatigue, numbness, and dyspepsia. After treatment with this drug, milk secretion usually stops in 1 to 2 months, and menstruation recurs after 6 to 24 weeks.

HEMOLYTIC DISEASES OF THE NEWBORN

Hyperbilirubinemia
(Neonatal jaundice)

Hyperbilirubinemia, the result of hemolytic processes in the newborn, is marked by elevated serum bilirubin levels and mild jaundice. It can be physiologic (with jaundice the only symptom) or pathologic (resulting from an underlying disease). Physiologic jaundice is very common, and tends to be more common and more severe in certain ethnic groups (Chinese, Japanese, Koreans, American Indians), whose mean peak of unconjugated bilirubin is approximately twice that of the rest of the population. Physiologic jaundice is self-limiting; prognosis for pathologic jaundice varies, depending on the cause. Untreated, severe hyperbilirubinemia may result in kernicterus, a neurologic syndrome resulting from deposition of unconjugated bilirubin in the brain cells and characterized by severe neural symptoms. Survivors may develop cerebral palsy, epilepsy, or mental retardation, or have only minor sequelae, such as perceptual-motor handicaps and learning disorders.

Causes

As erythrocytes break down at the end of their neonatal life cycle, hemoglobin separates into globin (protein) and heme (iron) fragments. Heme fragments form unconjugated (indirect) bilirubin, which binds with albumin for transport to liver cells to conjugate with glucuronide, forming direct bilirubin. Because unconjugated bilirubin is fat-soluble and cannot be excreted in the urine or bile, it may escape to extravascular tissue, especially fatty tissue and the brain, resulting in hyperbilirubinemia.

This pathophysiologic process may develop when...
- Factors that disrupt conjugation and usurp albumin-binding sites include drugs such as aspirin, tranquilizers, and sulfonamides, and conditions such as hypothermia, anoxia, hypoglycemia, and hypoalbuminemia.
- Decreased hepatic function results in reduced bilirubin conjugation.
- Increased erythrocyte production or breakdown results from hemolytic disorders, or Rh or ABO incompatibility.
- Biliary obstruction or hepatitis results in blockage of normal bile flow.
- Maternal enzymes present in breast milk inhibit the infant's glucuronyl transferase-conjugating activity.

Signs and symptoms

The predominant sign of hyperbilirubinemia is jaundice, which does not become clinically apparent until serum bilirubin levels reach about 7 mg/100 ml. Physiologic jaundice develops 24 hours after delivery in 50% of term infants (usually day 2 to day 3) and 48 hours after delivery in 80% of premature infants (usually day 3 to day 5). It generally disappears by day 7 in term infants and by day 9 or day 10 in premature infants. Throughout physiologic jaundice, serum unconjugated bilirubin does not exceed 12 mg/100 ml. Pathologic jaundice may appear anytime after the first day of life, and persists beyond 7 days with serum bilirubin levels greater than 12 mg/100 ml in a term infant, 15 mg/100 ml in a premature infant, or increasing more than 5 mg/100 ml in 24 hours.

UNDERLYING CAUSES OF HYPERBILIRUBINEMIA

When jaundice occurs during the first day of life:
• Blood type incompatibility (Rh, ABO, other minor blood groups)
• Intrauterine infection (rubella, cytomegalic inclusion body disease, toxoplasmosis, syphilis, and occasionally, bacteria such as *Escherichia coli*, staphylococcus, *Pseudomonas*, *Klebsiella*, *Proteus*, and streptococcus)

When jaundice occurs during the second or third day of life:
• Infection (usually from gram-negative bacteria)
• Polycythemia
• Enclosed hemorrhage (skin bruises, subdural hematoma)
• Respiratory distress syndrome (hyaline membrane disease)
• Heinz body anemia from drugs and toxins (vitamin K₃, sodium nitrate)
• Transient neonatal hyperbilirubinemia
• Abnormal RBC morphology
• Red cell enzyme deficiencies (glucose 6-phosphate dehydrogenase, hexokinase)
• Physiologic jaundice
• Blood group incompatibilities

When jaundice occurs during the fourth and fifth days of life:
• Breast-feeding, respiratory distress syndrome, maternal diabetes
• Crigler-Najjar syndrome (congenital nonhemolytic icterus)
• Gilbert syndrome

When jaundice occurs after one week of life:
• Herpes simplex
• Pyloric stenosis
• Hypothyroidism
• Neonatal giant cell hepatitis
• Infection (usually acquired in neonatal period)
• Bile duct atresia
• Galactosemia
• Choledochal cyst

Diagnosis

 Jaundice and elevated levels of serum bilirubin confirm hyperbilirubinemia. Inspection of the infant in a well-lit room (without yellow or gold lighting) reveals a yellowish skin coloration, particularly in the sclerae. Jaundice can be verified by pressing the skin on the cheek or abdomen lightly with one finger, then releasing pressure and observing skin color immediately. Signs of jaundice necessitate measuring and charting serum bilirubin levels every 4 hours. Testing may include direct and indirect bilirubin levels, particularly for pathologic jaundice. Bilirubin levels that are excessively elevated or vary daily suggest a pathologic process.

Identifying the underlying cause of hyperbilirubinemia requires a detailed patient history (including prenatal history), family history (paternal Rh factor, inherited red cell defects), present infant status (immaturity, infection), and blood testing of the infant and mother (blood group incompatibilities, hemoglobin level, direct Coombs' test, hematocrit).

Treatment

Depending on the underlying cause, treatment may include phototherapy, exchange transfusions, albumin infusion, and possibly, drug therapy. Phototherapy is the treatment of choice for physiologic jaundice, and pathologic jaundice due to erythroblastosis fetalis (after the initial exchange transfusion). Phototherapy uses fluorescent light to decompose bilirubin in the skin by oxidation, and is usually discontinued after bilirubin levels fall below 10 mg/100 ml and continue to decrease for 24 hours. However, phototherapy is rarely the only treatment for jaundice due to a pathologic cause.

An exchange transfusion replaces the infant's blood with fresh blood (less than 48 hours old), removing some of the unconjugated bilirubin in serum. Possible indications for exchange transfusions include hydrops fetalis, polycythemia, erythroblastosis fetalis, marked reticulocytosis, drug toxicity, and jaundice that develops within the first 6 hours after birth.

Other therapy for excessive bilirubin levels may include albumin administration (1 g/kg of 25% salt-poor albumin), which provides additional albumin for binding unconjugated bilirubin. This may be done 1 to 2 hours before exchange or as a substitute for a portion of the plasma in the transfused blood.

Drug therapy, which is rare, usually consists of phenobarbital administered to the mother before delivery and to the newborn several days after delivery. This drug stimulates the hepatic glucuronide-conjugating system.

Additional considerations

The infant's jaundice must be assessed and recorded; the time it began should be noted. Jaundice and serum bilirubin levels must be reported immediately.

For the infant receiving phototherapy, the hospital staff member should:
• keep a record of how long each bilirubin light bulb is in use, since these bulbs require frequent changing for optimum effectiveness.
• undress the infant, so his entire body surface is exposed to the light rays; keep him 18" to 30" (45 to 75 cm) from the light source; protect his eyes with shields that filter the light.
• monitor and maintain the infant's body temperature—high and low temperatures predispose to kernicterus; remove him from the light source every 3 to 4 hours, and take off the eye shields; allow his parents to visit and feed him.
• discontinue phototherapy, as ordered, when the infant's bilirubin level is less than 10 mg/100 ml and has been decreasing for 24 hours (the infant usually shows a decrease in serum bilirubin level 1 to 12 hours after the start of phototherapy); resume therapy, as ordered, if serum bilirubin increases several milligrams per 100 ml, as it often does, due to a rebound effect.

For the infant receiving exchange transfusions, the staffer should:
• prepare infant warmer and tray before the transfusion; give him nothing by mouth for 3 to 4 hours before the procedure.
• check the blood to be used for the exchange—type, Rh, age; keep emergency equipment (resuscitative and intubation equipment, and oxygen) available; monitor respiratory and heart rates every 15 minutes and check the infant's temperature every 30 minutes during the procedure; continue to monitor vital signs every 15 to 30 minutes for 2 hours.
• measure intake and output; observe for cord bleeding and complications, such as hemorrhage, hypocalcemia, sepsis, and shock; report serum bilirubin and hemoglobin levels. Bilirubin levels may rise, due to a rebound effect, within 30 minutes after transfusion, necessitating repeat transfusions.

To prevent hyperbilirubinemia, the staffer should:
• maintain oral intake; not skip any feedings, since fasting stimulates the conversion of heme to bilirubin.
• administer Rh_0 (D) immune human globulin, as ordered, to an unsensitized Rh-negative mother after the birth of an Rh-positive infant, or to an Rh-negative mother after spontaneous or elective abortion, so that subsequent infants aren't subject to hemolytic disease.

Parents must realize that most infants experience some degree of jaundice. They should be taught about hyperbilirubinemia, its causes, diagnostic laboratory tests, and its treatment. They should also know that the infant's stool contains some bile and therefore may be greenish.

Erythroblastosis Fetalis

Erythroblastosis fetalis, a hemolytic disease of the fetus and newborn, stems from an incompatibility of fetal and maternal blood, resulting in maternal antibody activity against fetal red cells. Intrauterine transfusions can save 40% of fetuses with erythroblastosis. However, in severe, untreated erythroblastosis fetalis, prognosis is poor, especially if kernicterus develops. About 70% of these infants die, usually within the first week of life; survivors inevitably develop pronounced neu-

rologic damage (sensory impairment, mental deficiencies, cerebral palsy). Severely affected fetuses who develop hydrops fetalis—the most severe form of this disorder, associated with profound anemia and edema—are commonly stillborn; even if they are delivered live, they rarely survive longer than a few hours.

Causes and incidence

Although over 60 red cell antigens can stimulate antibody formation, erythroblastosis fetalis usually results from Rh isoimmunization—a condition that develops in approximately 7% of all pregnancies in the United States. Before the development of $Rh_o(D)$ immune human globulin, this condition was an important cause of kernicterus and neonatal death.

During her first pregnancy, an Rh-negative female becomes sensitized (during delivery or abortion) by exposure to Rh-positive fetal blood antigens inherited from the father. A female may also become sensitized from receiving blood transfusions with alien Rh antigens, causing agglutins to develop; from inadequate doses of $Rh_o(D)$; or from failure to receive $Rh_o(D)$ after significant fetal-maternal leakage from abruptio placentae. Subsequent pregnancy with an Rh-positive fetus provokes increasing amounts of maternal agglutinating antibodies to cross the placental barrier, attach to Rh-positive cells in the fetus, and cause hemolysis and anemia. To

---

ABO INCOMPATIBILITY

ABO incompatibility—a form of fetomaternal incompatibility—occurs between mother and fetus in about 25% of all pregnancies, with highest incidence among Blacks. In about 1% of this number, it leads to hemolytic disease of the newborn. Although ABO incompatibility is more common than Rh isoimmunization, it is fortunately less severe. Low antigenicity of fetal or newborn ABO factors may account for the milder clinical effects.

Each blood group has specific antigens on RBCs and specific antibodies in serum. Maternal antibodies form against fetal cells when blood groups differ. Infants with group A blood, born of group O mothers, account for approximately 50% of all ABO incompatibilities. Unlike Rh isoimmunization, which always follows sensitization during a previous pregnancy, ABO incompatibility is likely to develop in a firstborn infant.

Blood Group	Antigens on RBCs	Antibodies in Serum	Most Common Incompatible Groups
A	A	Anti-B	Mother A, infant B or AB
B	B	Anti-A	Mother B, infant A or AB
AB	A and B	No antibodies	Mother AB, infant (no incompatibility)
O	No antigens	Anti-A and B	Mother O, infant A or B

Clinical effects of ABO incompatibility include jaundice, which usually appears in the newborn in 24 to 48 hours, mild anemia, and mild hepatosplenomegaly.

Diagnosis is based on clinical symptoms in the newborn, the presence of ABO incompatibility, a weak to moderately positive Coombs' test, and elevated serum bilirubin levels. Cord hemoglobin, and indirect bilirubin levels indicate the need for exchange transfusion. An exchange transfusion is done with blood of the same group and Rh type as that of the mother. Fortunately, because infants with ABO incompatibility respond so well to phototherapy, exchange transfusion is seldom necessary.

compensate for this, the fetus steps up the production of RBCs, and erythroblasts (immature RBCs) appear in the fetal circulation. Extensive hemolysis results in the release of large amounts of unconjugated bilirubin, which the liver is unable to conjugate and excrete, causing hyperbilirubinemia and hemolytic anemia.

Signs and symptoms

Jaundice usually isn't present at birth but may appear as soon as 30 minutes later or within 24 hours. The mildly affected infant shows mild to moderate hepatosplenomegaly and pallor. In severely affected infants who survive birth, erythroblastosis fetalis usually produces pallor, edema, petechiae, hepatosplenomegaly, grunting respirations, pulmonary rales, poor muscle tone, neurologic unresponsiveness, possible heart murmurs, a bile-stained umbilical cord, and yellow or meconium-stained amniotic fluid. Approximately 10% of untreated infants develop kernicterus from hemolytic disease and show symptoms such as anemia, lethargy, poor sucking ability, retracted head, stiff extremities, squinting, a high-pitched cry, and convulsions.

Hydrops fetalis causes extreme hemolysis, fetal hypoxia, heart failure (with possible pericardial effusion and circulatory collapse), edema (ranging from mild peripheral edema to anasarca), peritoneal and pleural effusions (with dyspnea and pulmonary rales), and green- or brown-tinged amniotic fluid (usually indicating a stillbirth).

Other distinctive characteristics of the infant with hydrops fetalis include enlarged placenta, marked pallor, hepatosplenomegaly, cardiomegaly, and ascites. Petechiae and widespread ecchymoses are present in severe cases, indicating concurrent disseminated intravascular coagulation. This disorder retards intrauterine growth, so the infant's lungs, kidneys, brain, and thymus are small, and despite edema, his body size is smaller than that of infants of comparable gestational age.

PREVENTION OF RH ISOIMMUNIZATION

Administration of Rh_o(D) immune human globulin to an unsensitized Rh-negative mother as soon as possible after the birth of an Rh-positive infant, or after a spontaneous or elective abortion prevents complications in subsequent pregnancies.

The following patients should be screened for Rh isoimmunization or irregular antibodies:
• all Rh-negative mothers during their first prenatal visit, and at 24, 28, 32, and 36 weeks' gestation.
• all Rh-positive mothers with histories of transfusion; a jaundiced baby; stillbirth; cesarean birth; induced abortion; placenta previa; or abruptio placentae.

Diagnosis

Diagnostic evaluation takes into account both prenatal and neonatal findings:
• maternal history (for erythroblastotic stillbirths, abortions, previously affected children, previous anti-Rh titers)
• blood typing and screening (titers should be taken frequently to determine changes in the degree of maternal immunization)
• paternal blood test (for Rh, blood group, and Rh zygosity)
• history of blood transfusion.

In addition, amniotic fluid analysis may show an increase in bilirubin (indicating possible hemolysis) and elevations in anti-Rh titers. Radiologic studies may show edema and, in hydrops fetalis, the halo sign (edematous, elevated, subcutaneous fat layers) and the Buddha position (fetus' legs are crossed).

Neonatal findings indicating erythroblastosis fetalis include:
• direct Coombs' test of umbilical cord blood to measure RBC (Rh-positive) antibodies in the newborn (positive only when the mother is Rh-negative and the fetus is Rh-positive).
• decreased cord hemoglobin count (less than 10 g), signaling severe disease.
• many nucleated peripheral RBCs.

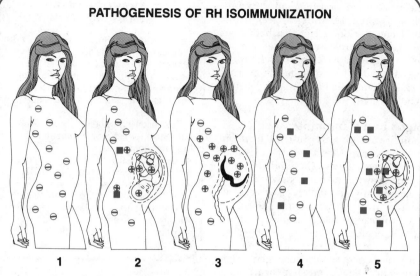

PATHOGENESIS OF RH ISOIMMUNIZATION

Fig. 1) Rh-negative woman prepregnancy. Fig. 2) Pregnancy with Rh-positive fetus. Fig. 3) Placental separation. Fig. 4) Postdelivery, mother becomes sensitized to Rh-positive blood and develops anti–Rh-positive antibodies (darkened squares). Fig. 5) During the next pregnancy with Rh-positive fetus, maternal anti–Rh-positive antibodies enter fetal circulation and attach to Rh-positive RBCs, subjecting them to hemolysis.

Treatment

Treatment depends on the degree of maternal sensitization and the effects of hemolytic disease on the fetus or newborn.

• *Intrauterine-intraperitoneal transfusion* is performed when amniotic fluid analysis suggests the fetus is severely affected and delivery is inappropriate due to fetal immaturity. A transabdominal puncture under fluoroscopy into the fetal peritoneal cavity allows infusion of group O, Rh-negative blood. This may be repeated every 2 weeks until the fetus is mature enough for delivery.

• *Planned delivery* is usually done 2 to 4 weeks before term date, depending on maternal history, serologic tests, and amniocentesis; labor may be induced from the 34th to 38th week of gestation. During labor, the fetus should be monitored electronically; capillary blood scalp sampling determines acid-base balance. Any indication of fetal distress necessi-

tates immediate cesarean delivery.

• *Phenobarbital* administered during the last 5 to 6 weeks of pregnancy may lower serum bilirubin levels in the newborn.

• An *exchange transfusion* removes antibody-coated RBCs and prevents hyperbilirubinemia through removal of the infant's blood and replacement with fresh group O, Rh-negative blood.

• *Albumin infusion* aids in the binding of bilirubin, reducing the chances of hyperbilirubinemia.

• *Phototherapy* by exposure to ultraviolet light reduces bilirubin levels.

Neonatal therapy for hydrops fetalis consists of maintaining ventilation by intubation, oxygenation, and mechanical assistance, when necessary; and removal of excess fluid to relieve severe ascites and respiratory distress. Other appropriate measures include an exchange transfusion and maintenance of the infant's body temperature.

Gamma globulin that contains anti–

Rh-positive antibody (Rh₀ [D]) can provide passive immunization, which prevents maternal Rh isoimmunization in Rh-negative females. However, it's ineffective if sensitization has already resulted from a previous pregnancy, abortion, or transfusion.

Additional considerations

The care plan is structured around close maternal and fetal observation, explanations of all diagnostic tests and therapeutic measures, and emotional support. The hospital staff member should:
• reassure the parents that they're not at fault in having a child with erythroblastosis fetalis; encourage them to express their fears concerning possible complications of treatment.
• explain the intrauterine transfusion procedure and its purpose; obtain a baseline fetal heart rate through electronic monitoring; carefully observe the mother afterward for uterine contractions and fluid leakage from the puncture site; monitor fetal heart rate for tachycardia or bradycardia.
• maintain the infant's body temperature during exchange transfusion by placing him under a heat lamp or overhead radiant warmer; keep resuscitative and monitoring equipment handy, and

warm the blood before administering it to the infant.
• watch for complications of transfusion, such as lethargy, muscular twitching, convulsions, dark urine, edema, and change in vital signs; watch for postexchange serum bilirubin levels that are usually 50% of preexchange levels (although these levels may rise to 70% to 80% of preexchange levels due to rebound effect); monitor for bilirubin rebound within 30 minutes of transfusion, which requires repeat exchange transfusions.
• measure intake and output; observe for cord bleeding and complications, such as hemorrhage, hypocalcemia, sepsis, and shock; report serum bilirubin and hemoglobin levels.
• encourage parents to visit to promote normal parental bonding, and to help care for the infant as often as possible.
• evaluate all pregnant females for possible Rh incompatibility to prevent hemolytic disease in the newborn; administer Rh₀ (D) I.M., as ordered, to all Rh-negative, antibody-negative females within 72 hours of uterine evacuation, transfusion reaction, or ectopic pregnancy, or during the second and third trimesters to patients with abruptio placentae.

Selected References

Aladjem, Silvio, and Audrey K. Brown, eds. PERINATAL INTENSIVE CARE. St. Louis: C.V. Mosby Co., 1977.

Benson, Ralph C., ed. CURRENT OBSTETRIC AND GYNECOLOGIC DIAGNOSIS AND TREATMENT, 2nd ed. Los Altos, Calif.: Lange Medical Pub., 1978.

Bolognese, Ronald. PERINATAL MEDICINE: CLINICAL MANAGEMENT OF THE HIGH RISK FETUS AND NEONATE. Baltimore: Williams & Wilkins Co., 1977.

Clark, Ann L., et al. CHILDBEARING: A NURSING PERSPECTIVE, 2nd ed. Philadelphia: F.A. Davis Co., 1979.

Jenson, Margaret D., et al. MATERNITY CARE: THE NURSE AND THE FAMILY. St. Louis: C.V. Mosby Co., 1977.

MacNall, Lee, ed. CURRENT PRACTICE IN OBSTETRIC AND GYNECOLOGIC NURSING, Vol. 3. St. Louis: C.V. Mosby Co., 1980.

Martin, Leonide L. HEALTH CARE OF WOMEN. Philadelphia: J.B. Lippincott Co., 1978.

Pritchard, Jack A., and Paul C. MacDonald. WILLIAMS OBSTETRICS, 15th ed. New York: Appleton-Century-Crofts, 1976.

Reeder, Sharon R., et al. MATERNITY NURSING, 13th ed. Philadelphia: J.B. Lippincott Co., 1976.

Tovey, L., and A. Robinson. *Reduced Severity of Rh-Hemolytic Disease after Anti-D Immunoglobulin*, BRITISH MEDICAL JOURNAL. 4:320, 1975.

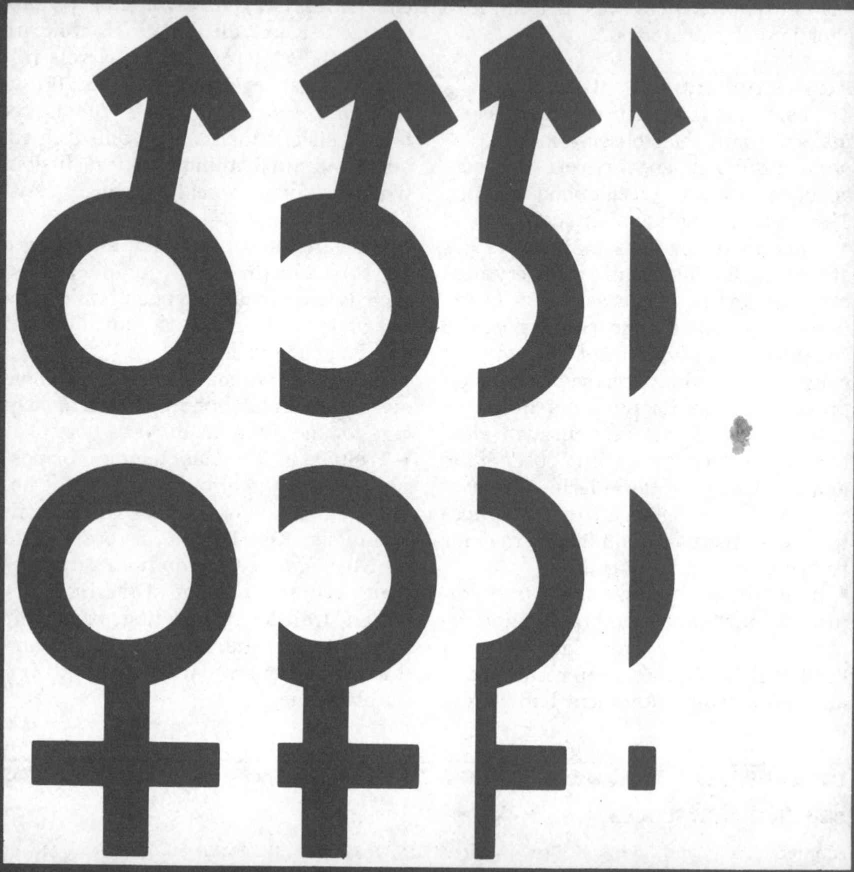

16 Sexual Disorders

Sexual Disorders

Sexuality is an integral human function that is inevitably colored and influenced by a host of interrelated factors. Its expression reflects the interaction of all the biologic, psychologic, and sociologic factors that affect a person's self-image and behavior.

Depending on these complex factors, human sexuality can be healthy and enriching, or it can be the source of mental and physical distress. J.W. Maddock, in *Postgraduate Medicine*,* defines a sexually healthy person as one who meets the following criteria:

• His behavior agrees with his gender identity (persistent feeling of oneself as male or female).

• He can participate in a potentially loving or committed relationship.

• He finds erotic stimulation pleasurable.

• He can make decisions about his sexual behavior that are compatible with his values and beliefs.

Hazards to sexual health

An important group of sexually related disorders results from infection that is transmitted through sexual contact: gonorrhea, syphilis, genital herpes, genital warts, trichomoniasis, chancroid, lymphogranuloma venereum, granuloma inguinale, balanitis, balanoposthitis, and

*"Sexual Health and Health Care," *Postgraduate Medicine*. 58:52-58, 1975.

nonspecific genitourinary infections. As a group, venereal diseases are among the most prevalent infections worldwide; gonorrhea is now reaching epidemic proportions in the United States.

Other sexually related disorders affect an individual's sexual ability or response, and can have physical or psychologic causes. In the female, such disorders are usually orgasmic dysfunction; in the male, erectile dysfunction.

Disorders of sexual preference are more properly classified as psychiatric problems. They include voyeurism, exhibitionism, transvestitism, fetishism, masochism, sadism, necrophilia, pedophilia, incest, and rape.

Physical assessment first

Physical assessment, primarily a diagnostic tool, can also serve as an excellent opportunity for patient teaching.

• During examination of the female, breast development (symmetry, contour, size), pubic hair distribution, and external genitalia development are evaluated, and the uterus and ovaries are palpated. A speculum is used to examine internal genitalia, including the cervix and vagina.

• During examination of the male, pubic and axillary hair distribution is checked. Then with a gloved hand, the penis, scrotum, prostate gland, and rectum are palpated. The penis (shaft, glans, urethral meatus) is inspected for lesions, swelling, inflammation, scars, or discharge. In the uncircumcised male, the foreskin must be retracted to visualize the glans. The scrotum is examined for size, shape, and abnormalities, such as nodules or inflammation, and for the presence of both testes (in many males, the left testis is lower than the right).

PRODUCTION OF SPERMATOZOA

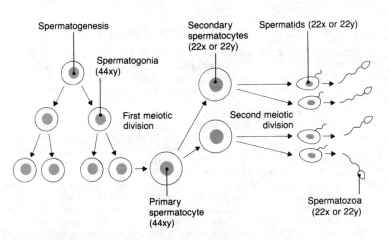

Spermatogenesis, the production of male gametes within the seminiferous tubules of the testes, is basically a five-step process: 1) Diploid spermatogonia, the cells forming the tubule's outer layer, divide mitotically to generate new cells used in spermatozoa production. 2) Some of the spermatogonia move toward the lumen of the tubule, and enlarge to primary spermatocytes. 3) Each primary spermatocyte divides meiotically, forming two secondary spermatocytes, one retaining the x chromosome and the other the y chromosome. 4) Each secondary spermatocyte also divides meiotically, becoming spermatids. 5) After a series of structural changes, the spermatids develop into mature spermatozoa.

MALE GENITALIA

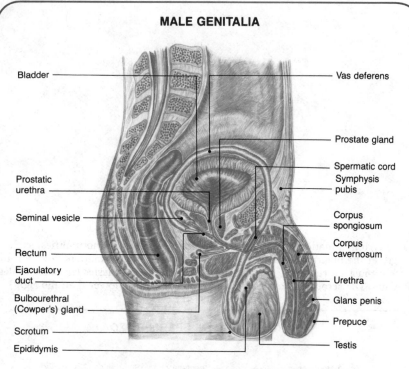

Bladder

Vas deferens

Prostate gland

Spermatic cord
Symphysis
pubis

Prostatic
urethra

Corpus
spongiosum

Seminal vesicle

Corpus
cavernosum

Rectum

Ejaculatory
duct

Urethra

Bulbourethral
(Cowper's) gland

Glans penis

Prepuce

Scrotum

Testis

Epididymis

REVIEW OF MALE SEXUAL ANATOMY

The *scrotum,* which contains the testes, epididymis, and lower spermatic cords, maintains the proper testicular temperature for spermatogenesis through relaxation and contraction. The *penis* consists of three cylinders of erectile tissue: two corpora cavernosa, and the corpus spongiosum, which contains the urethra.

The *testes* (gonads, testicles) produce sperm in the seminiferous tubules, with complete spermatogenesis developing in most males by age 15 or 16. In the fetus, the testes form in the abdominal cavity and descend into the scrotum during the seventh month of gestation. The testes also secrete hormones, especially testosterone, in the interstitial cells (Leydig's cells). Testosterone affects the development and maintenance of secondary sex characteristics and sex drive. It also regulates metabolism, stimulates protein anabolism (encouraging skeletal growth and muscular development), inhibits pituitary secretion of the gonadotropins (follicle-stimulating hormone and interstitial cell-stimulating hormone), promotes potassium excretion, and mildly influences renal sodium reabsorption.

The *vas deferens* connects the *epididymis,* in which sperm mature and ripen for up to 6 weeks, and the *ejaculatory ducts.* (Vasectomy achieves sterilization by severing the vas deferens.) The *seminal vesicles,* two convoluted membranous pouches, secrete a viscous liquid of fructose-rich semen and prostaglandins that probably facilitates fertilization. The *prostate gland* secretes the thin alkaline substance that comprises most of the seminal fluid; this fluid also protects sperm from acidity in the male urethra and in the vagina, increasing sperm motility.

The *bulbourethral* (Cowper's) *glands* secrete an alkaline preejaculatory fluid, probably similar in function to that produced by the prostate gland. The *spermatic cords* are cylindrical fibrous coverings in the inguinal canal, containing the vas deferens, blood vessels, and nerves.

Sexual assessment: The history

Careful assessment helps to identify the cause of a sexual problem as psychologic or physical. A sexual assessment provides the basis for clinical diagnosis and treatment. When a sexual assessment is performed, the following points should be considered:

• Privacy and a relaxed pace are important. The patient must be made to feel at ease and unrushed.

• Sexual health is relative, so objectivity is crucial. Making assumptions or judgments about the patient's sexual activities should be avoided.

• The level of sexual understanding varies from patient to patient. The assessment must be conducted using language the patient understands. Technical terms should be avoided, and so should talking down to the patient.

• The least threatening questions are best asked first. Discussing the patient's urologic history, for example, can be used to lead the conversation into his sexual history.

• The patient's life-style and nonverbal behavior often say more about his sexual problems than the assessment's questions and answers reveal. Between-the-lines information in the patient's statements should never be ignored. But interpreting them must be done cautiously. Snap judgments or overreaction must be avoided.

• Sexual practices can influence the treatment of some sexual disorders. For example, homosexual activity may affect the treatment of gonorrhea. This subject must be fully explored to compile a complete assessment picture.

• Current and past contraceptive practices should be investigated thoroughly.

• The assessment procedure itself may prove therapeutic and informative. The patient should be encouraged to express his anxieties and to ask questions himself. Such general discussion may help alleviate some of his fears and clear up any of his misconceptions.

Therapy varies

Sex therapy can be a vital therapeutic tool for treating sexual dysfunctions. Before psychotherapy begins, history, physical examination, and appropriate treatment must rule out organic causes of sexual dysfunction. The major forms of sex therapy include psychoanalysis, behavioral therapy, group therapy, classic (Masters and Johnson) therapy, and Kaplan's sex therapy. The sex therapy appropriate to the patient depends on his problems, needs, and finances.

SEXUALLY TRANSMITTED DISEASES

Gonorrhea

The most common venereal disease, gonorrhea is an infection of the genitourinary tract (especially the urethra and cervix) and, occasionally, the rectum, pharynx, and eyes. Untreated gonorrhea can spread through the blood to the joints, tendons, meninges, and endocardium; in females, it can also lead to chronic pelvic inflammatory disease (PID) and sterility. After adequate treatment, prognosis in both males and females is excellent, although reinfection is common. Incidence of gonorrhea is rising, with more than 3 million new cases reported annually in the United States; it's especially prevalent among unmarried persons and young people, particularly between ages 19 and 25.

Causes

Transmission of *Neisseria gonorrhoeae,* the organism that causes gonorrhea, almost exclusively follows sexual contact with an infected person. Children born of infected mothers can contract gonococcal ophthalmia neonatorum during passage through the birth canal. Children and adults with gonorrhea can contract gonococcal conjunctivitis by touching their eyes with contaminated hands.

Signs and symptoms

Although some infected males may be asymptomatic, after a 3- to 6-day incubation period, most develop symptoms of urethritis, including dysuria and purulent urethral discharge, with redness and swelling at the site of infection. Most infected females remain asymptomatic but may develop inflammation and a greenish-yellow discharge from the cervix—the most common gonorrheal symptoms in females. Other clinical features vary according to the site involved:
● *urethra:* dysuria, urinary frequency and incontinence, purulent discharge, itching, red and edematous meatus
● *vulva:* occasional itching, burning, and

pain due to exudate from an adjacent infected area. Vulval symptoms tend to be more severe before puberty or after menopause.
● *vagina* (most common site in children over age 1): engorgement, redness, swelling, and profuse purulent discharge
● *pelvis:* severe pelvic and lower abdominal pain, muscular rigidity, tenderness, and abdominal distention. As the infection spreads, nausea, vomiting, fever, and tachycardia may develop in patients with salpingitis or PID.
● *liver:* upper right quadrant pain in patients with perihepatitis.

Other possible symptoms include pharyngitis, tonsillitis, and rectal burning, itching, and bloody mucopurulent discharge.

Gonococcal septicemia is more common in females than in males. Its characteristic signs include tender papillary skin lesions on the hands and feet; these lesions may be pustular, hemorrhagic, or necrotic. Gonococcal septicemia may also produce migratory polyarthralgia,

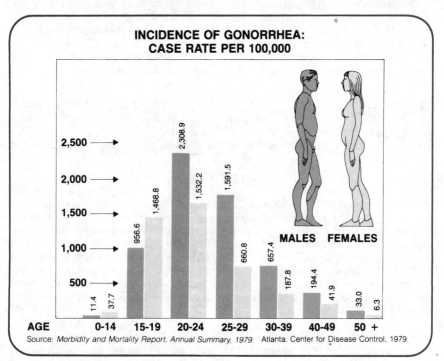

INCIDENCE OF GONORRHEA: CASE RATE PER 100,000

Source: *Morbidity and Mortality Report, Annual Summary, 1979.* Atlanta: Center for Disease Control, 1979.

and polyarthritis and tenosynovitis of the wrists, fingers, knees, or ankles. Untreated septic arthritis leads to progressive joint destruction.

Signs of gonococcal ophthalmia neonatorum include lid edema, bilateral conjunctival infection, and abundant purulent discharge 2 to 3 days after birth. Adult conjunctivitis, most common in men, causes unilateral conjunctival redness and swelling. Untreated gonococcal conjunctivitis can progress to corneal ulceration and blindness.

Diagnosis

A culture from the site of infection (urethra, cervix, rectum, or pharynx), grown on a Thayer-Martin or Transgrow medium, usually establishes diagnosis by isolating the organism. A Gram's stain showing gram-negative diplococci supports the diagnosis and may be sufficient to confirm gonorrhea in males.

Confirmation of gonococcal arthritis requires identification of gram-negative diplococci on smears made from joint fluid and skin lesions. Complement fixation and immunofluorescent assays of serum reveal antibody titers four times the normal rate. Culture of conjunctival scrapings confirms gonococcal conjunctivitis.

Treatment

Treatment of choice for uncomplicated gonorrhea (including gonorrhea during pregnancy) is probenecid P.O. to block penicillin excretion from the body, followed in 30 minutes by I.M. administration of 4.8 million units of aqueous procaine penicillin injected at two separate sites in a large muscle mass. If the patient is allergic to penicillin, tetracycline P.O. (contraindicated in pregnant women) or spectinomycin I.M. may be substituted.

Gonorrhea complicated by severe PID or septicemia requires I.V. antibiotic therapy with penicillin G or tetracycline. Outpatient therapy may consist of oral tetracycline or intramuscular penicillin

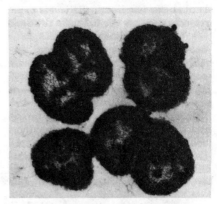

In gonorrhea, microscopic examination reveals gram-negative diplococcus—*Neisseria gonorrhoeae,* the causative organism.

G, each with probenecid, followed by continued antibiotic therapy for 10 days. Treatment of gonococcal conjunctivitis requires I.V. administration of penicillin G, accompanied by irrigation of the eye with penicillin G and saline solution.

To confirm cure of gonococcal infection, follow-up cultures are necessary 7 to 14 days after treatment and again in 6 months, or, in pregnant females, before delivery.

Routine instillation of 1% silver nitrate drops into the eyes of newborns has greatly reduced the incidence of gonococcal ophthalmia neonatorum.

Additional considerations

The patient must be tested, before treatment, for any drug sensitivities, especially to penicillin, and must be watched closely for drug reactions during therapy. The health care professional should be prepared to treat anaphylaxis after parenteral administration of penicillin.

The patient should know that until cultures prove negative, he is still infectious and can transmit gonococcal infection. Consequently, the professional should double bag all soiled dressings and contaminated instruments and wear gloves when handling contaminated material and giving patient care. The patient with a gonococcal eye infection should be isolated. If the patient is being treated as an outpatient, the family must take similar infection precautions.

For the patient with gonococcal arthritis, moist heat can be applied to ease pain in affected joints.

The patient should inform sexual partners of his infection so they can seek treatment also. All cases must be reported to the local public health authorities for follow-up on sexual contacts. All persons exposed to gonorrhea should be examined and tested.

Newborns of infected mothers should also be tested for signs of infection. This requires culturing specimens from the infant's eyes, pharynx, and rectum.

To prevent gonorrhea, patients should avoid anyone suspected of being infected, use condoms during intercourse, and avoid sharing washcloths or douche equipment.

Genital Herpes
(Venereal herpes)

Genital herpes is an acute, inflammatory disease of the genitalia, resulting from infection with herpes simplex II virus. This infection is one of the most common recurring disorders of the genitalia. Prognosis varies according to the patient's age, the strength of his immune defenses, and the infection site. Primary genital herpes is usually self-limiting but may cause painful local or systemic disease. In newborns, in patients with weak immune defenses, and in those with disseminated disease, genital herpes is often severe, with complications and a high mortality.

Causes
Genital herpes is usually transmitted through sexual contact, but contamination from infected toilet seats, towels, and bathtubs also occurs. Pregnant females may transmit the infection to newborns during vaginal delivery. Such transmitted infection may be localized (for instance, in the eyes) or disseminated, and may be associated with CNS involvement.

Signs and symptoms
After a 3- to 7-day incubation period, fluid-filled vesicles appear, usually on the cervix (the primary infection site) and, possibly, on the labia, perianal skin, vulva, or vagina of the female; on the glans penis, foreskin, or penile shaft of the male. Extragenital lesions may appear on the mouth or anus. In both males and females, the vesicles, usually painless at first, may rupture and develop into extensive, shallow, painful ulcers, creating redness, marked edema, and tender, inguinal lymph nodes.

Other features of initial mucocuta-neous infection include fever, malaise, dysuria, and in the female, leukorrhea. Rare complications—which generally arise from extragenital lesions—include herpetic keratitis, which may lead to blindness, and potentially fatal herpetic encephalitis.

Diagnosis
Diagnosis is based on physical examination and patient history. Helpful (but nondiagnostic) measures include laboratory data showing increased antibody titers, and smears of genital lesions showing atypical cells.

 Diagnosis can be confirmed by demonstration of herpes simplex II virus in vesical fluid, using tissue culture techniques.

Treatment and additional considerations
Most antiviral agents are ineffective against herpes infection. Medications such as Burow's solution (aluminum acetate) and, occasionally, sulfonamide

creams help reduce edema and may ease discomfort of painful lesions. Two new drugs, 2-deoxy-d-glucose and Acyclovir, promise to be beneficial by preventing multiplication of the virus. Antibacterial agents help combat secondary infections.

The patient must get adequate rest and nutrition, and keep the lesions dry, except for applying prescribed medications, as directed, using aseptic technique.

The patient may maintain normal activity but should avoid sexual intercourse during the active stage of this disease (while lesions are present). The patient's sexual partners should also seek medical examination for herpes.

The patient experiencing pain and fever should be on strict bed rest and heat therapy. He may also need to be hospitalized.

The infected pregnant patient risks her newborn's health if she has a vaginal delivery. She should consider cesarean delivery if lesions are active at term.

Herpetics Engaged in Living Productively (HELP), an American Social Health Association group located in Palo Alto, California, can provide information and emotional support to the patient with genital herpes.

Genital Warts
(Venereal warts, condylomata acuminata)

Genital warts consist of papillomas, with fibrous tissue overgrowth from the dermis and thickened epithelial coverings. They are uncommon before puberty or after menopause.

Causes
Genital warts are usually transmitted sexually and possibly result from the same human papillomavirus that causes the common wart (verruca vulgaris). Genital warts grow rapidly in the presence of heavy perspiration, poor personal hygiene, or pregnancy, and often accompany other infections, such as trichomoniasis, candidiasis, and gonorrhea.

Signs and symptoms
After a 1- to 6-month incubation period (usually 2 months), genital warts develop on moist surfaces: in males, on the subpreputial sac, within the urethral meatus, and less commonly, on the penile shaft; in females, on the vulva, and on vaginal and cervical walls; in both sexes, papillomas spread to the perineum and the perianal area. These painless warts start as tiny red or pink swellings that grow (sometimes to 4″ [10 cm]) and become pedunculated. Multiple swellings are common and give such warts a cauliflower appearance. If

these lesions are infected, they become malodorous.

Diagnosis
Dark-field examination of scrapings from wart cells shows marked vascularization of epidermal cells, which helps to differentiate genital warts from condylomata lata.

Treatment
The initial goal of treatment is to eradicate associated genital infections. If the warts do not cause discomfort, no therapy may be indicated, and the warts may resolve spontaneously. If treatment is necessary, topical drug therapy (20% podophyllum in tincture of benzoin, or trichloroacetic acid) removes small warts within 2 to 4 days. Warts larger than ¾″ (2 cm) are generally removed by surgery, cryosurgery, electrocautery, or 5-fluorouracil cream debridement. Rarely, the patient's warts are excised and made into a vaccine, which is then injected into the patient's body to try to create antibodies.

Additional considerations

- The patient must protect the tissue surrounding his wart by applying petrolatum before applying trichloroacetic acid.
- The patient must wash off podophyllum with soap and water 4 to 6 hours after application.
- The patient must make use of a condom during intercourse until healing is complete.
- Preventive measures for both sexes include: avoiding sex with an infected partner and regularly washing genitalia with soap and water.
- Preventive measures for the female include: avoiding feminine hygiene sprays and frequent douching, and not wearing tight pants, nylon underpants, or panty hose.

Syphilis

A chronic, infectious, venereal disease, syphilis begins in the mucous membranes and quickly becomes systemic, spreading to nearby lymph nodes and the bloodstream. This disease, when untreated, is characterized by progressive stages: primary, secondary, latent, and late (formerly called tertiary). About 25,000 cases of syphilis, in primary and secondary stages, are reported annually in the United States, making it the third most prevalent reportable infectious disease. Incidence is highest among urban populations, especially in persons between ages 15 and 39. Untreated syphilis leads to crippling or death, but prognosis is excellent with early treatment.

Causes

The spirochete *Treponema pallidum* causes syphilis. Transmission occurs primarily through sexual contact during the primary, secondary, and early latent stages of infection. Prenatal transmission from an infected mother to the fetus is also possible.

In syphilis, a dark-field examination that shows spiral-shaped bacterial organisms—*Treponema pallidum*—confirms diagnosis.

Signs and symptoms

Primary syphilis develops after an incubation period that generally lasts about 3 weeks. Initially, one or more chancres (small, fluid-filled lesions) erupt on the genitalia; others may erupt on the anus, fingers, lips, tongue, nipples, tonsils, or eyelids. These chancres, which are usually painless, start as papules and then erode; they have indurated, raised edges and clear bases. Even untreated chancres disappear after 3 to 6 weeks. They are usually associated with regional lymphadenopathy (unilateral or bilateral). In females, chancres are often overlooked because they often develop on the cervix or the vaginal wall.

Symmetric mucocutaneous lesions and general lymphadenopathy signal the start of *secondary syphilis*, which may develop within a few days or up to 8 weeks after the initial chancre. The rash of secondary syphilis can be macular, papular, pustular, or nodular. The lesions are of uniform size, well defined, and generalized. Macules often erupt between rolls of fat on the trunk and, proximally, on the arms, palms, soles, face, and scalp. In warm, moist areas (perineum, scrotum, vulva, between rolls of fat), the lesions enlarge and erode, producing highly contagious, pink, or grayish-white lesions (condylomata lata).

Mild constitutional symptoms of syphilis appear in the second stage, and may include headache, malaise, anorexia, weight loss, nausea, vomiting, sore throat, and possibly, slight fever. Alopecia may occur, with or without treatment, and is usually temporary. Nails become brittle and pitted.

Latent syphilis is characterized by an absence of clinical symptoms but a reactive serologic test for syphilis. Since infectious mucocutaneous lesions may reappear when infection is of less than 4 years' duration, early latent syphilis is considered contagious. Approximately two thirds of patients remain asymptomatic in the late latent stage, until death. The rest develop characteristic late-stage symptoms.

Late syphilis is the final, destructive but noninfectious stage of the disease. It has three subtypes, any or all of which may affect the patient: late benign syphilis, cardiovascular syphilis, and neurosyphilis. The lesions of late benign syphilis develop between 1 and 10 years after infection. They may appear on the skin, bones, mucous membranes, upper respiratory tract, liver, or stomach. The typical lesion is a gumma—a chronic, superficial nodule or deep, granulomatous lesion that is solitary, asymmetric, painless, and indurated. Gummas can be found on any bone—particularly the long bones of the legs—and in any organ. If late syphilis involves the liver, it can cause epigastric pain, tenderness, enlarged spleen, and anemia; if it involves the upper respiratory tract, it may cause perforation of the nasal septum or the palate. In severe cases, late benign syphilis results in destruction of bones or organs, which eventually causes death.

Cardiovascular syphilis develops about 10 years after the initial infection in approximately 10% of patients with late, untreated syphilis. It causes fibrosis of elastic tissue of the aorta and leads to aortitis, most often in the ascending and transverse sections of the aortic arch. Cardiovascular syphilis may be asymptomatic or may cause aortic regurgitation or aneurysm.

Symptoms of neurosyphilis develop in about 8% of patients with late, untreated syphilis and appear from 5 to 35 years after infection. These clinical effects consist of meningitis and widespread CNS damage that may include general paresis, personality changes, and arm and leg weakness.

Diagnosis

 Identifying *T. pallidum* from a lesion on dark-field examination provides immediate diagnosis of syphilis. This method is most effective when moist lesions are present, as in primary, secondary, and prenatal syphilis. The Fluorescent Treponemal Antibody-Absorption (FTA-ABS) test identifies antigens of *T. pallidum* in tissue, ocular fluid, CSF, tracheobronchial secretions, and exudates from lesions. This is the most sensitive test available for detecting syphilis in all stages. Once reactive, it remains so permanently. Other appropriate procedures include the following:

• *Venereal Disease Research Laboratory* (VDRL) *slide test* and *Rapid Plasma Reagin* (RPR) *test* detect nonspecific antibodies. Both tests, if positive, become reactive within 1 to 2 weeks after the primary lesion appears, or 4 to 5 weeks after the infection begins.

• *CSF examination* identifies neurosyphilis when total protein level is above 40 mg/100 ml, VDRL slide test is reactive, and cell count exceeds five mononuclear cells/mm³.

Treatment

Treatment of choice is administration of penicillin I.M. For early syphilis, treatment may consist of a single injection of penicillin G benzathine I.M. (2.4 million

PRENATAL SYPHILIS

A woman can transmit syphilis transplacentally to her unborn child throughout pregnancy. This type of syphilis is often called congenital, but prenatal is a more accurate term. Approximately 50% of infected fetuses die before or shortly after birth. Prognosis is better for infants who develop overt infection after age 2.

The infant with prenatal syphilis may appear healthy at birth, but usually develops characteristic lesions—vesicular, bullous eruptions, often on the palms and soles—3 weeks later. Shortly afterward, a maculopapular rash similar to that in secondary syphilis may erupt on the face, mouth, genitalia, palms, or soles. Condylomata lata often occur around the anus. Lesions may erupt on the mucous membranes of the mouth, pharynx, and nose. When the infant's larynx is affected, his cry becomes weak and forced. If the nasal mucous membranes are involved, he may also develop nasal discharge, which can be slight and mucopurulent or copious with blood-tinged pus. Visceral and bone lesions, liver or spleen enlargement with ascites, and nephrotic syndrome may also develop.

Late prenatal syphilis becomes apparent after age 2; it may be identifiable only through blood studies or may cause unmistakable syphilitic changes: screwdriver-shaped central incisors, deformed molars or cusps, thick clavicles, saber shins, bowed tibias, nasal septum perforation, eighth nerve deafness, and neurosyphilis.

In the infant with prenatal syphilis, VDRL titer, if reactive at birth, stays the same or rises, indicating active disease. The infant's titer drops in 3 months if the mother has received effective prenatal treatment. Absolute diagnosis necessitates dark-field examination of umbilical vein blood or lesion drainage.

An infant with abnormal CSF may be treated with aqueous crystalline penicillin G, I.M. or I.V., (50,000 units/kg of body weight/day divided in two doses for at least 10 days), or aqueous penicillin G procaine I.M. (50,000 units/kg of body weight/day for at least 10 days). An infant with normal CSF may be treated with a single injection of penicillin G benzathine (50,000 units/kg of body weight). Care of a child with prenatal syphilis includes: recording the extent of the rash, and watching for signs of systemic involvement, especially laryngeal swelling, jaundice, and decreasing urinary output.

units), or injections of aqueous penicillin G procaine I.M. (600,000 units/day for 8 days), or penicillin G procaine in oil with 2% aluminum monostearate (initially, 2.4 million units; then, 1.2 million units/dose for two subsequent doses given 3 days apart). Syphilis of more than 1 year's duration should be treated with penicillin G benzathine I.M. (2.4 million units/week for 3 weeks) or aqueous penicillin G procaine I.M. (600,000 units/day for 15 days).

Patients who are allergic to penicillin may be treated successfully with tetracycline or erythromycin (in either case, 500 mg P.O., four times a day for 15 days for early syphilis; 30 days, for late infections). Tetracycline is contraindicated in pregnant females.

Additional considerations
• The patient must adhere to the dosage schedule for medication. Before the first dose is administered, the patient's medical history will be checked for any record of drug sensitivity.
• In secondary syphilis, lesions must be kept clean and dry. If they're draining, contaminated materials must be disposed of carefully.
• In late syphilis, symptomatic care must be provided during prolonged treatment.
• In cardiovascular syphilis, decreased cardiac output (decreased urinary output, hypoxia, decreased sensorium) and pulmonary congestion also may occur.
• In neurosyphilis, the patient's level of consciousness should be watched. The patient may also experience ataxia.

- The patient should seek VDRL testing 1, 3, 9, and 12 months after treatment has ended, to detect possible relapse. The patient treated for latent or late syphilis should receive blood tests at 6-month intervals for 2 years.
- All cases of syphilis must be reported to local public health authorities. Sexual partners of patients with syphilis should receive treatment.

Trichomoniasis

A protozoal infection of the lower genitourinary tract, trichomoniasis affects about 15% of sexually active females and 10% of sexually active males. Incidence is worldwide. In females, the condition may be acute or chronic. Recurrence of trichomoniasis is minimized when sexual partners are treated concurrently.

Causes

Trichomonas vaginalis—a tetraflagellated, motile protozoan—causes trichomoniasis in females by infecting the vagina, the urethra, and possibly, the endocervix, Bartholin's glands, Skene's glands, or the bladder; in males, it infects the lower urethra and, possibly, the prostate gland, seminal vesicles, or the epididymis.

T. vaginalis grows best when the vaginal mucosa is more alkaline than normal (pH about 5.5 to 5.8). Therefore, factors that raise the vaginal pH—use of oral contraceptives, pregnancy, bacterial overgrowth, exudative cervical or vaginal lesions, or frequent douching, which disturbs lactobacilli that normally live in the vagina and maintain acidity—may predispose to trichomoniasis.

Trichomoniasis is usually transmitted by intercourse; less often, by contaminated douche equipment or moist washcloths. Occasionally, the newborn of an infected mother develops the condition through vaginal delivery.

Signs and symptoms

Approximately 70% of females—including those with chronic infections—and most males with trichomoniasis are asymptomatic. In females, acute infection may produce variable signs, such as a gray or greenish-yellow, and possibly profuse and frothy, malodorous vaginal discharge. Its other effects include severe itching, redness, swelling, tenderness, dyspareunia, dysuria, urinary frequency, and occasionally, postcoital spotting, menorrhagia, or dysmenorrhea.

Such symptoms may persist for a week to several months and may be more pronounced just after menstruation or during pregnancy. If trichomoniasis is untreated, symptoms may subside, although *T. vaginalis* infection persists, possibly associated with an abnormal cytologic smear of the cervix.

In males, trichomoniasis may produce mild to severe transient urethritis, possibly with dysuria and frequency.

Diagnosis

 Direct microscopic examination of vaginal or seminal discharge is decisive when it reveals *T. vaginalis*, a motile, pear-shaped organism. Examination of clear urine specimens may also reveal *T. vaginalis*.

Physical examination of symptomatic females shows vaginal erythema; edema; frank excoriation; a frothy, malodorous, greenish-yellow vaginal discharge; and rarely, a thin, gray pseudomembrane over the vagina. Cervical examination demonstrates punctate cervical hemorrhages, giving the cervix a strawberry appearance that is almost pathognomonic for this disorder.

Treatment

Metronidazole P.O., given to both sexual

partners, effectively cures trichomoniasis. Metronidazole may be given in small doses for 7 days, or in a single, large dose. For females, a mild douche with a vinegar and water solution may help acidify vaginal pH.

Acidifying or antiseptic douches are useful to relieve symptoms in pregnant females with trichomoniasis. Such douches may minimize the extent of infection if used promptly. Metronidazole P.O. hasn't proven safe during pregnancy, especially in the first trimester.

After treatment, both sexual partners require a follow-up examination to check for residual signs of infection.

Additional considerations
• To help prevent reinfection during treatment, the patient should abstain from intercourse, or make use of a condom.
• The patient must abstain from alcoholic beverages while taking metronidazole, since alcohol consumption may provoke a disulfiram-type reaction (confusion, headache, cramps, vomiting, convulsions). The patient should also know this drug may turn urine dark-brown.
• Since bacteria flourish in a warm, dark, moist environment, the female patient can reduce the risk of genitourinary bacterial growth by wearing loose-fitting cotton underwear that allows for ventilation.
• The female patient should not douche before being examined for trichomoniasis, but will be instructed to use an acidic douche each day of treatment. She should know, however, that chronic use of douches and vaginal sprays can predispose her reproductive system to infection by altering normal vaginal pH.
• If the patient's pregnant, she can prevent her newborn from contracting trichomoniasis by receiving adequate treatment before delivery.

Chancroid
(Soft chancre)

Chancroid is a venereal disease characterized by painful genital ulcers and inguinal adenitis. This infection occurs worldwide but is particularly common in tropical countries; it affects males more often than females. Chancroidal lesions may heal spontaneously, and usually respond well to treatment in the absence of secondary infections.

Causes
Chancroid results from *Hemophilus ducreyi*, a short, nonmotile, gram-negative streptobacillus. Poor personal hygiene may predispose males—especially those who are uncircumcised—to this disease. Chancroid is transmitted through sexual contact.

Signs and symptoms
After a 3- to 5-day incubation period, a small papule appears at the site of entry, usually the groin or inner thigh; in the male, it may appear on the penis; in the female, on the vulva, vagina, or cervix. Occasionally, this papule may erupt on the tongue, lip, breast, or navel. Such a papule (more than one may appear) rapidly ulcerates—becoming painful, soft, and malodorous—bleeds easily, and produces pus. It is gray and shallow, with irregular edges, and measures up to ¾" (2 cm) in diameter. Within 2 to 3 weeks, inguinal adenitis develops, creating suppurated, inflamed nodes that may rupture into large ulcers or buboes. Headache and malaise occur in 50% of patients. During the healing stage, phimosis may develop.

Diagnosis
Gram's stain smears of ulcer exudate or

bubo aspirate are 50% reliable; blood agar cultures are 75% reliable. Biopsy confirms diagnosis but is reserved for resistant cases or when malignancy is suspected. Dark-field examination and serologic testing rule out other venereal diseases (genital herpes, syphilis, lymphogranuloma venereum), which cause similar ulcers.

Treatment and additional considerations

Sulfonamides usually cure chancroid within 2 weeks. Alternatives to sulfonamides include kanamycin and tetracycline, but these may prevent detection of coexisting syphilis. Aspiration of fluid-filled nodes helps prevent infection from spreading.

• Prior to treatment, the patient must be confirmed as not allergic to sulfonamides or any other prescribed medication.

• The patient must not apply creams, lotions, or oils on or near genitalia or on other lesion sites.

• The patient should abstain from sexual contact until healing is complete (usually about 2 weeks after treatment begins) and should wash the genitalia

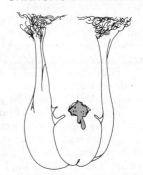

CHANCROIDAL LESION

Chancroid produces a soft, painful chancre, similar to that of syphilis. Without treatment, it may progress to inguinal adenitis and formation of buboes.

daily with soap and water. The uncircumcised male must retract his foreskin to thoroughly clean the glans penis.

• To prevent chancroid, the patient should avoid sexual contact with infected persons, use condoms during sexual activity, and wash his genitalia with soap and water after sexual activity.

Lymphogranuloma Venereum
(Lymphopathia venereum, Durand-Nicolas-Favre disease)

A highly contagious venereal disease characterized by inguinal lymphadenitis, lymphogranuloma venereum (LGV) occurs worldwide, mostly in the tropical and semitropical areas of South America, Africa, Asia, and in the southeastern United States. Incidence of LGV is highest among sexually active young adults. This infection develops more often in males than in females. With proper treatment, prognosis is excellent, in the absence of secondary bacterial infections and other venereal diseases.

Causes

Microorganisms of the *Chlamydia trachomatis* group cause LGV. In most cases, these microorganisms are transmitted through sexual intercourse; rarely, through nonsexual person-to-person contact or contact with contaminated objects.

Signs and symptoms

After a 1- to 3-week incubation period, a painless lesion appears on the genitalia, usually on the fourchette, urethral meatus, or medial surface of the labia in females, and on the glans penis or coronal sulcus in males. The lesion may range from a slight erosion to a small, macule or papule, and often goes un-detected because of its location. This lesion heals spontaneously in a few days.

Most patients show no other clinical symptoms initially but develop inguinal lymph node swelling about 2 weeks later. In males, these enlarged nodes may become fluctuant, tender masses. If the regional nodes draining the initial lesion become involved, they may enlarge and appear bilaterally as a series of buboes. Untreated buboes rupture and form sinus tracts that discharge a thick, yellow, granular secretion. Eventually, a scar forms or an indurated inguinal mass develops, which may persist for life.

Females may develop iliac and sacral lymphatic obstruction, causing perineal edema. Occasionally, females develop genitoanorectal syndrome—which may be complicated by secondary bacterial infection—characterized by mucopurulent rectal discharge and bloody diarrhea. The rectal mucosa becomes edematous, ulcerated, and friable. Healing leaves extensive cutaneous keloidal scarring and often causes rectovaginal fistulas, rectal strictures, and pararectal abscesses.

Systemic symptoms in both males and females include myalgia, headache, fever, chills, malaise, backache, and weight loss. These effects generally appear after the initial lesion has healed, coinciding with lymphadenopathy.

Diagnosis

The Frei test, positive in about 80% of infected patients, is helpful but not specific to LGV. An intradermal injection of 0.1 ml of prepared antigen in the forearm produces a red papule or pustule within 48 to 72 hours, if the test is positive. Serologic testing in dilution of 1:40 or higher aids diagnosis, as do complement fixation tests producing a titer of at least 1:16. The microimmunofluorescence (Micro IF) test reveals a high serum antibody titer in patients with LGV. Other testing methods show increased sedimentation rate and, possibly, increased IgA. Isolation of the organism from aspirated blood, pus, or CSF is the only conclusive diagnostic method, but this is not always practical.

Treatment

Tetracycline, oxytetracycline, or chlortetracycline given P.O. for 14 to 28 days, or sulfadiazine given P.O. for 14 days promptly relieves systemic symptoms, but buboes may take months to heal. Fluctuant buboes necessitate aspiration to lessen pain and swelling; complications, such as strictures or fistulas, may require corrective surgery.

Additional considerations

• Warm sitz baths three or four times a day will make the patient more comfortable and clean his lesions.
• Ruptured buboes should be covered with nonadherent dressings. Lotions, creams, sprays, or ointments should not be applied to the affected area.
• The female patient should get biannual pelvic examinations to detect possible malignant changes.
• The patient should not have sexual contact during the infectious period. In males, the infectious period lasts about 3 weeks. In females, the duration of the infectious period is unknown, but it may last for months.

Nonspecific Genitourinary Infections

Nonspecific genitourinary infections, including nongonococcal urethritis (NGU) in males and mild vaginitis or cervicitis in females, comprise a group of infections with similar manifestations that are not linked to a single organism. Such infections have become more prevalent since the mid-1960s and may be more widespread than gonorrhea. Prognosis is good if sexual partners are treated simultaneously.

Causes

In males, NGU often results from infection with *Chlamydia trachomatis* and *Ureaplasma urealyticum*. Such infection may also result from bacteria, such as staphylococci, diphtheroids, coliform organisms, and *Corynebacterium vaginale (Hemophilus vaginalis)*. Less often, it may be related to preexisting strictures, neoplasms, and chemical or traumatic inflammation. Such infection spreads primarily through sexual intercourse.

Although less is known about nonspecific genitourinary infections in females, chlamydial or corynebacterial organisms may also cause these infections. A thin vaginal epithelium may predispose prepubertal and postmenopausal females to nonspecific vaginitis.

Signs and symptoms

NGU occurs 1 week to 1 month after coitus, with scant or moderate mucopurulent urethral discharge, variable dysuria, and occasional hematuria. If untreated, NGU may lead to acute epididymitis. Subclinical urethritis may be found on physical examination, especially if the sex partner has a positive diagnosis.

Females with nonspecific genitourinary infections may experience persistent vaginal discharge, acute or recurrent cystitis for which no cause can be found, or cervicitis with inflammatory erosion. Both males and females may be asymptomatic but show signs of urethral, vaginal, or cervical infection on physical examination.

Diagnosis

In males, microscopic examination of smears of prostatic or urethral secretions shows excess polymorphonuclear leukocytes but few, if any, specific organisms. In females, cervical or urethral smears also reveal excess leukocytes and no specific organisms.

Treatment

Therapy for both sexes consists of oral tetracycline or erythromycin; or streptomycin followed by a sulfonamide.

Therapy for females may also include preparatory cleaning of the pubic area and application of a sulfa vaginal cream. Cervicitis occasionally necessitates cryosurgery.

Additional considerations

To prevent nonspecific genitourinary infections, these measures should be followed:

• The patient should abstain from sexual contact with infected partners, follow appropriate hygienic measures after sexual activity and void before and after intercourse.

• The male patient should use a condom during intercourse. The female patient should ask her partner to use a condom during intercourse.

• The patient should maintain adequate fluid intake.

• The female patient should avoid routine use of douches and hygiene sprays, and the insertion of foreign objects, including tampons, into her vagina. She should wear loose-fitting cotton underpants and remove them before going to bed.

Granuloma Inguinale

Granuloma inguinale is a chronic, mildly contagious infection of the genital or perianal skin, and the lymphatics. It spreads within the infected patient by autoinoculation, contiguous skin contact, or lymphatic extension. Incidence is highest in young men. Granuloma inguinale rarely occurs in Caucasians; it is most prevalent in tropical regions, such as South America, the West Indies, Central America, India, Indonesia, and the Pacific Islands. Prognosis is excellent with early diagnosis and prompt, adequate treatment.

Causes

The gram-negative bacillus *Calymmatobacterium granulomatis* (formerly called *Donovania granulomatis*) causes granuloma inguinale. The prevalence of primary lesions on the genital mucosa suggests transmission through intercourse.

Signs and symptoms

After a 1- to 12-week incubation period (usually 30 days), a single, painless macule or papule appears on external genitalia, ulcerating into a raised, clean, beefy-red lesion, with a granulated, friable border. In the initial stage of granuloma inguinale, other painless and possibly foul-smelling lesions develop and coalesce, often on the labia, vagina, or cervix in females, and on the glans, foreskin, or penile shaft in males. Extragenital lesions sometimes erupt on the nose, mouth, or pharynx.

In the second stage, ulcers become infected, painful, and foul-smelling. In females, regional lymph nodes enlarge and occasionally become tender; in males, pseudobuboes (subcutaneous swelling, with minimal lymph node involvement) develop. Systemic effects include fever, anemia, weight loss, malaise, and leukocytosis.

If the disease progresses to the third stage, fibrosis, keloidal scarring, and depigmentation of ulcerative sites may occur. Scar tissue may possibly cause lymphatic obstruction, resulting in elephantiasis and vaginal and anal stenoses. Long-term, inadequately treated chronic infection may spread to bones and joints and may lead to death.

Diagnosis

 Diagnosis depends on discovery of Donovan bodies in smears made from tissue scrapings of lesion borders. The Donovan body turns red with Giemsa stain. Tests for syphilis should also be done, as the two diseases often coexist.

Treatment

Tetracycline, oxytetracycline, or chlortetracycline for 10 to 21 days, or I.M. streptomycin for 8 to 10 days usually heals these lesions within 6 weeks. Follow-up evaluations should continue for 6 months after treatment.

Additional considerations

• To prevent secondary infections and promote comfort, the patient should be given warm sitz baths in a 1:10,000 solution of potassium permanganate three to four times daily.

• The patient must not use creams, lotions, or sprays on the affected area, or engage in sexual activity until lesions heal completely.

• The patient should seek out follow-up care, especially pelvic examinations and Pap smears for females, since a link may exist between granuloma inguinale and vulval cancer. The patient's sexual partner should also be examined.

• To prevent granuloma inguinale, the patient must avoid sexual contact with infected persons and observe good sexual hygiene, including washing genitalia with soap and water after sexual contact. The male patient should wear a condom during intercourse.

Balanitis and Balanoposthitis

Balanitis, a relatively uncommon penile disease, occurs in the uncircumcised male when the glans penis becomes inflamed and gradually develops an erosive and possibly gangrenous lesion that may extend to the penile shaft. Posthitis, an inflammation of the prepuce, usually occurs with balanitis, so balanoposthitis is most commonly seen. The inflammation is resolved with adequate medical treatment, but balanoposthitis often recurs.

Causes and incidence
Both balanitis and balanoposthitis are caused by many different organisms: the spirochete *Borrelia vincentii*, streptococci, staphylococci, *Neisseria gonorrhoeae*, and fungi (*Candida albicans*). Balanoposthitis is probably transmitted through sexual contact, and is likely to develop in males with long prepuces, especially those who improperly retract their prepuces and observe poor personal hygiene. These conditions may also occur in young boys, possibly due to poor personal hygiene, forceful manipulation of foreskin, or masturbation. Balanoposthitis often develops in males with phimosis and, when associated with this anatomic defect, often recurs.

Signs and symptoms
Two to three days after exposure to an infecting organism, irritation and soreness develop under the prepuce, followed by pain, foul discharge, edema, and ulcer formation (on the glans, foreskin, or penile shaft). Acute infection may produce fever, chills, malaise, dysuria, and possibly, inguinal adenitis. If untreated, the initial ulcer deepens and new ones form; eventually, the entire penis and scrotum may become gangrenous, producing overwhelming and possibly fatal sepsis.

Diagnosis

Cultures and Gram's stain of urethral and subpreputial secretions showing the infecting organism confirm balanitis and balanoposthitis.

Treatment
For mild cases of balanitis or balanoposthitis, treatment consists of saline washes if the prepuce can be retracted, or subpreputial irrigation if it can't. For moderate to severe infection, penicillin or tetracycline may be given for 5 to 7 days. Circumcision is indicated for recurrent balanoposthitis or phimosis.

Additional considerations
Mild soap and water soaks applied to the infected area will ease pain. The patient must abstain from intercourse until balanitis or balanoposthitis clears.

To prevent recurrence, the patient must practice good personal hygiene including: retraction of prepuce when washing; avoiding sexual contact with a known infected partner; using a condom during intercourse; and washing with soap and water afterward.

After circumcision, the patient will have to change the petrolatum dressing after each voiding. If excess bleeding occurs, he should notify his doctor.

FEMALE SEXUAL DYSFUNCTION

Arousal and Orgasmic Dysfunctions

Arousal dysfunction, one of the most severe forms of female sexual dysfunction, is an inability to experience sexual pleasure. Orgasmic dysfunction, the most common female sexual dysfunction, is an inability to achieve orgasm. Unlike the female with arousal dysfunction, the female with orgasmic dysfunction may have a desire for sexual activity and become aroused but feels inhibited as she approaches orgasm. Both arousal and orgasmic dysfunctions are considered primary if they exist in a female who has never experienced sexual pleasure; they are secondary when some physical, mental, or situational condition has inhibited or obliterated a previously normal sexual function. Prognosis is good for temporary or mild dysfunctions resulting from misinformation or situational stress, but is guarded for dysfunctions that result from intense anxiety, chronically discordant relationships, or psychologic disturbances.

Causes

Any of the following factors, alone or in combination, may cause arousal or orgasmic dysfunction:

• *drug use:* CNS depressants and oral contraceptives
• *disease:* general systemic illness, diseases of the endocrine or nervous system, or diseases that impair muscle tone or contractility
• *gynecologic factors:* chronic vaginal or pelvic infection, congenital anomalies, and genital malignancies
• *stress and fatigue*
• *inadequate or ineffective stimulation*
• *psychologic factors:* performance anxiety, guilt, depression, or unconscious conflicts about sexuality
• *discordant relationships:* poor communication, hostility or ambivalence toward the partner, fear of abandonment or of asserting independence, or boredom with sex.

All these factors may contribute to involuntary inhibition of the orgasmic reflex. Another crucial factor is the fear of losing control of feelings or behavior. Whether or not these factors produce sexual dysfunction and the type of dysfunction depend on how well the female copes with the resulting pressures. Physical factors alone rarely cause arousal or orgasmic dysfunction.

Signs and symptoms

The female with arousal dysfunction has limited or absent sexual desire and experiences little or no pleasure from sexual stimulation. Physical signs of this dysfunction include lack of vaginal lubrication or absence of signs of genital vasocongestion.

The female with orgasmic dysfunction reports an inability to achieve orgasm, either totally or under certain circumstances. Some females experience orgasm through masturbation or other means but not during intercourse. Others achieve orgasm with some partners but not with others.

Diagnosis

Thorough physical examination, laboratory tests, and medical history rule out physical causes of arousal or orgasmic dysfunction. In the absence of such causes, a complete psychosexual history is the most important tool for assessment. Such a history should include:

• detailed information concerning previous sexual response patterns.
• the patient's feelings during childhood and adolescence about sex in general and, specifically, about masturbation, incest, rape, sexual fantasies, and homo- or heterosexual practices.
• contraceptive practices and reproductive goals.
• the nature of the patient's present relationship, including her partner's attitude toward sex.
• assessment of the patient's self-esteem and body image.
• any history of psychotherapy.

Treatment

Arousal dysfunction is difficult to treat, especially if the female has never experienced sexual pleasure. Therapy is designed to help the patient relax, to become aware of her feelings about sex, and to eliminate guilt and the fear of rejection. Specific measures usually include sensate focus exercises similar to those developed by Masters and Johnson, which emphasize touching and awareness of sensual feelings over entire body—not just genital sensations—and minimize the importance of intercourse and orgasm. Psychoanalytic treatment consists of free association, dream analysis, and discussion of life patterns to achieve greater sexual awareness. One behavioral approach attempts to correct maladaptive patterns through systematic desensitization to situations that provoke anxiety, partially by encouraging the patient to fantasize about these situations.

The goal in treating orgasmic dysfunction is to decrease or eliminate involuntary inhibition of the orgasmic reflex. As with arousal dysfunction, treatment may include experiential therapy, psychoanalysis, or behavior modification.

Treatment of primary orgasmic dysfunction may involve teaching the patient self-stimulation. Also, the therapist may teach distraction techniques, such as focusing attention on fantasies, breathing patterns, or muscular contractions to relieve anxiety. Thus, the patient learns new behavior through exercises she does in the privacy of her own home between sessions. Gradually, the therapist involves the patient's sexual partner in the treatment sessions, although some therapists treat the couple as a unit from the outset.

Treatment of secondary orgasmic dysfunction is designed to decrease anxiety and promote the factors necessary for the patient to experience orgasm. Sensate focus exercises are often used. The therapist should communicate an accepting and permissive attitude, and help the patient understand that satisfactory sexual experiences don't always require coital orgasm.

Additional considerations

The professional dealing with such a patient should:

• be alert for clues to arousal or orgasmic dysfunction when discussing the patient's health history.

• maintain an open, nonjudgmental attitude; listen to the patient's problems sympathetically.

• answer questions and provide information about sexual anatomy and physiology, and sexual response patterns.

• refer the patient to a health care professional who's trained in sexual therapy. As a helpful guideline, inform the patient that the therapist's membership in the American Association of Sex Educators, Counselors, and Therapists, or in the American Society for Sex Therapy and Research usually assures quality treatment. If the therapist is not a member of these organizations, advise the patient to inquire about the therapist's training in sex counseling and therapy.

Dyspareunia

Dyspareunia is pain associated with intercourse. It may be mild, or severe enough to affect a female's enjoyment of intercourse. Dyspareunia is commonly associated with physical problems or, less commonly, with psychologically based sexual dysfunctions. Prognosis is good if the underlying disorder can be treated successfully.

Causes

Physical causes of dyspareunia include an intact hymen; deformities or lesions of the introitus or vagina; retroversion of the uterus; genital, rectal, or pelvic scar tissue; acute or chronic infections of the genitourinary tract; and disorders of the surrounding viscera (including residual effects of pelvic inflammatory disease or disease of the adnexal and broad ligaments). Among the many other possible physical causes are:

• endometriosis
• benign and malignant growths and tumors

• insufficient lubrication
• radiation to the area
• allergic reactions to diaphragms, condoms, or other contraceptives.

Psychologic causes include fear of pain or of injury during intercourse, recollection of a previous painful experience, guilt feelings about sex, fear of pregnancy or of injury to the fetus during pregnancy, anxiety caused by a new sexual partner or technique, and mental or physical fatigue.

Signs and symptoms

Dyspareunia produces discomfort, ranging from mild aches to severe pain before, during, or after intercourse. It also may be associated with vaginal itching or burning.

Diagnosis

Physical examination and laboratory tests, which vary with the suspected cause, help determine the underlying disorder. Diagnosis also depends on a detailed sexual history and the answers to such questions as: When does the pain occur? Does it occur with certain positions or techniques, or at certain times during the sexual response cycle? Where does the pain occur? What is its quality, frequency, and duration? What factors relieve or aggravate it?

Treatment and additional considerations

Treatment of physical causes may include creams and water-soluble jellies for inadequate lubrication, appropriate medications for infections, excision of hymenal scars, and gentle stretching of painful scars at the vaginal opening with a medium-sized Graves speculum. The patient may be advised to change her coital position to reduce pain on deep penetration.

Methods for treating psychologically based dyspareunia vary with the particular patient. Psychotherapy may uncover hidden conflicts that are creating fears concerning intercourse. Sensate focus exercises de-emphasize intercourse itself and teach appropriate foreplay techniques. Education concerning appropriate methods of contraception can reduce fear of pregnancy; education concerning sexual activity during pregnancy can relieve fear of harming the fetus.

Care for the patient with dyspareunia must include these points:
• The patient should be instructed in anatomy and physiology of the reproductive system, contraception, and the human sexual response cycle.
• The patient may want advice and information on drugs that affect her sexually, and on lubricating jellies and creams.
• The patient's complaints of sex-related pain should be listened to with sympathetic, nonjudgmental attitude. This will encourage her to express her feelings without embarrassment.

Vaginismus

Vaginismus is involuntary spastic constriction of the lower vaginal muscles, usually from fear of vaginal penetration. This disorder may coexist with dyspareunia and, if severe, may prevent intercourse (a common cause of unconsummated marriages). Vaginismus affects females of all ages and backgrounds. Prognosis is excellent for a motivated patient who doesn't have untreatable organic abnormalities.

Causes

Vaginismus may be physical or psychologic in origin. It may occur spontaneously as a protective reflex to pain or result from organic causes, such as hymenal abnormalities, genital herpes, obstetric trauma, and atrophic vaginitis.

Psychologic causes may include:
• childhood and adolescent exposure to rigid, punitive, and guilt-ridden attitudes toward sex.
• fears resulting from painful or traumatic sexual experiences, such as incest or rape.
• early traumatic experience with pelvic examinations.
• phobias of pregnancy, venereal disease, or cancer.

Signs and symptoms

The female with vaginismus typically experiences muscle spasm with constriction and pain on insertion of any object into the vagina, such as a vaginal tampon, diaphragm, or speculum. She may profess no interest in sex or may exhibit a normal level of sexual desire (often characterized by sexual activity without intercourse).

Diagnosis
Diagnosis depends on sexual history and pelvic examination to rule out physical disorders. Sexual history must include early childhood experiences and family attitudes toward sex, previous and current sexual responses, contraceptive practices and reproductive goals, feelings about her sexual partner, and specifics about pain on insertion of any object into the vagina.

 A carefully performed pelvic examination confirms diagnosis by showing involuntary constriction of the musculature surrounding the outer portion of the vagina.

Treatment
Treatment is designed to eliminate maladaptive muscular constriction and underlying psychologic problems. In Masters and Johnson therapy, the patient uses a graduated series of plastic dilators, which she inserts into her vagina while tensing and relaxing her pelvic muscles. The patient controls the time the dilator is left in place (if possible, she retains it for several hours) and the movement of the dilator. Together with her sexual partner, she begins sensate focus and counseling therapy to increase sexual responsiveness, improve communications skills, and resolve any underlying conflicts.

Kaplan therapy also uses progressive insertion of dilators or fingers (in vivo/desensitization therapy), with behavior therapy (imagining vaginal penetration until it can be tolerated) and, if necessary, psychoanalysis and hypnosis. Both Masters and Johnson, and Kaplan therapies report 100% cure; however, Kaplan states the patient and her partner may show other sexual dysfunctions that necessitate additional therapy.

Additional considerations
• The health care professional conducting a pelvic examination must remember that it may be painful for the patient with vaginismus and should proceed at the patient's own pace. The patient will need support throughout the examination. Each step should be explained before it is done. The patient should be encouraged to verbalize her feelings, and be given time to ask any questions.
• The patient may need to be taught about anatomy and physiology of the reproductive system, contraception, and human sexual response.
• The patient may be taking medications (antihypertensives, tranquilizers, steroids) that affect her sexual response. If she has insufficient lubrication for intercourse, she might find lubricating jellies and creams helpful.

MALE SEXUAL DYSFUNCTION

Erectile Dysfunction
(Impotence)

Erectile dysfunction refers to a male's inability to attain or maintain penile erection sufficient to complete intercourse. The patient with primary impotence has never achieved a sufficient erection; secondary impotence, which is more common and less serious than the primary form, implies that, despite present inability, the patient has succeeded in completing intercourse in the past. Transient periods of impotence are not considered dysfunction and probably occur in half of adult males. Erectile dysfunction affects all age-groups but increases in frequency with age. Prognosis depends on the severity and duration of impotence and the underlying cause.

Causes

Psychogenic factors are responsible for approximately 80% of erectile dysfunction; organic factors, for the rest. In some patients, psychogenic and organic factors coexist, making isolation of the primary cause difficult.

Psychogenic causes may be intrapersonal, reflecting personal sexual anxieties; or interpersonal, reflecting a disturbed sexual relationship. Intrapersonal factors generally involve guilt, fear, depression, or feelings of inadequacy resulting from previous traumatic sexual experience, rejection by parents or peers, exaggerated religious orthodoxy, abnormal mother-son intimacy, or homosexual experiences. Interpersonal factors may stem from differences in sexual preferences between partners, lack of communication, insufficient knowledge of sexual function, or nonsexual personal conflicts. Situational impotence, a temporary condition, may develop in response to stress.

Organic causes may include chronic diseases, such as cardiopulmonary disease, diabetes, multiple sclerosis, or renal failure; spinal cord trauma; complications of surgery; drug- or alcohol-induced dysfunction; and rarely, genital anomalies or CNS defects.

Signs and symptoms

Secondary erectile dysfunction is classified as follows:
• *Partial:* The patient is unable to achieve a full erection.
• *Intermittent:* The patient is sometimes potent with the same partner.
• *Selective:* The patient is potent only with certain females.

Some patients lose erectile function suddenly; others lose it gradually. If the cause is not organic, erection may still be achieved through masturbation.

Patients with psychogenic impotence may appear anxious, with sweating and palpitations; or they may become totally disinterested in sexual activity. Patients with psychogenic or drug-induced impotence may suffer extreme depression, which may cause the impotence or result from it.

Diagnosis

Personal sexual history provides the most useful clues in differentiating between organic and psychogenic factors, and between primary and secondary impotence: Does the patient have intermittent, selective, nocturnal, or early-morning erections? Can he achieve erections through other sexual activity, such as masturbation or fantasizing? When did his dysfunction begin, and what was his life situation at that time? Did erectile problems occur suddenly or gradually? Is he taking large quantities of prescription or nonprescription drugs?

Diagnosis must rule out chronic disease, such as diabetes and other vascular, neurologic, or urogenital problems.

Treatment

Sexual therapy, largely directed at reducing performance anxiety, may effectively cure psychogenic impotence. Such therapy should include both partners.

The course and content of sexual therapy for impotence depend on the specific cause of the dysfunction and the nature of the male-female relationship. Usually, therapy includes the concept of sensate focus, which restricts the couple's sexual activity and encourages them to become more attuned to the physical sensations of touching. Sexual therapy also includes improving verbal communication skills, eliminating unreasonable guilt, and reevaluating attitudes toward sex and sexual roles.

Treatment of organic impotence focuses on reversing the cause, if possible. If not, psychologic counseling may help the couple deal realistically with their situation and explore alternatives for sexual expression. Certain patients with organic impotence may benefit from surgically inserted inflatable or noninflatable penile implants.

Additional considerations
When a patient has impotence or a condition that may cause him to become impotent, he should be made to feel comfortable about discussing his sexuality. His sexual health should be assessed during the initial medical history. He may need to be referred for further evaluation or treatment.

After penile implant surgery, a patient must avoid intercourse until the incision heals, usually in 6 weeks.

To help prevent impotence, responsible health and sex education programs are needed at primary, secondary, and college levels. Additionally, information about resuming sexual activity should be included as part of every hospital's discharge instructions for any patient with a condition that requires modification of daily activities. Such patients include those with cardiac disease, diabetes, hypertension, COPD, and all postoperative patients.

Hypogonadism

Hypogonadism is a condition resulting from decreased androgen production in males, which may impair spermatogenesis (causing infertility) and inhibit the development of normal secondary sex characteristics. The clinical effects of androgen deficiency depend on age at onset.

Causes
Primary hypogonadism results directly from interstitial (Leydig's cell) cellular or seminiferous tubular damage due to faulty development or mechanical damage. This causes increased secretion of gonadotropins by the pituitary in an attempt to increase the testicular functional state, and is therefore termed hypergonadotropic hypogonadism. It includes the following: Klinefelter's syndrome, Reifenstein's syndrome, male Turner's syndrome, Sertoli-cell–only syndrome, anorchism, orchitis, and sequelae of irradiation. Secondary hypogonadism results from faulty interaction within the hypothalamic-pituitary axis, resulting in failure to secrete normal levels of gonadotropins, and is therefore termed hypogonadotropic hypogonadism. It includes the following: hypopituitarism, isolated follicle-stimulating hormone deficiency, isolated luteinizing hormone deficiency, Kallmann's syndrome, and Prader-Willi syndrome. Depending on the patient's age at onset, hypogonadism may cause eunuchism (complete gonadal failure) or eunuchoidism (partial failure).

Signs and symptoms
Although symptoms vary, depending on the specific cause of hypogonadism, some characteristic findings may include delayed closure of epiphyses and immature bone age; delayed puberty; infantile penis and small, soft testes; below-average muscle development and strength; fine, sparse facial hair; scant or absent axillary, pubic, and body hair; and a high-pitched, effeminate voice. In an adult, hypogonadism diminishes sex drive and potency, and causes regression of secondary sex characteristics.

Diagnosis
Accurate diagnosis necessitates a detailed patient history, physical examination, and hormonal studies. Serum and urinary gonadotropin levels increase in primary, or hypergonadotropic, hypogonadism but decrease in secondary, or hypogonadotropic, hypogonadism. Other relevant hormonal studies include assessment of neuroendocrine functions, such as thyrotropin, adrenocorticotropin, growth hormone, and vasopressin levels. Chromosomal analysis may determine the specific

causative syndrome. Testicular biopsy and semen analysis determine sperm production, identify impaired spermatogenesis, and assess low levels of testosterone.

Treatment

Treatment depends on the underlying cause and may consist of hormonal replacement, especially with testosterone, methyltestosterone, or human chorionic gonadotropin (HCG) for primary hypogonadism, and with HCG for secondary hypogonadism. Fertility cannot be restored after permanent testicular damage. However, eunuchism that results from hypothalamic-pituitary lesions can be corrected when administration of gonadotropins stimulates normal testicular function.

Additional considerations

The patient with hypogonadism tends to have multiple associated physical problems, so care should be tailored to meet his specific needs.

When the patient's an adolescent boy, effort must be made to promote his self-confidence. If he feels sensitive about his underdeveloped body, he should be given access to a private bathroom, if possible. His parents need to understand hypogonadism. They should be encouraged to express their concerns about their son's delayed development.

The parents and the patient need reassurance that effective treatment is available and should understand the therapy fully, including expected side effects, such as water retention and outbreaks of acne.

Undescended Testes
(Cryptorchidism)

In this congenital disorder, one or both testes fail to descend into the scrotum, remaining in the abdomen, inguinal canal, or at the external ring. Although this condition may be bilateral, it more commonly affects the right testis. True undescended testes remain along the path of normal descent, while ectopic testes deviate from that path. If bilateral cryptorchidism persists untreated into adolescence, it may result in sterility, make the testes more vulnerable to trauma, and significantly increase the risk of testicular malignancy.

Causes

The mechanism whereby the testes descend into the scrotum is still unexplained. Some evidence is available to implicate hormonal factors—most likely androgenic hormones from the placenta, maternal or fetal adrenals, or the fetal immature testis, and possibly, maternal progesterone or gonadotropic hormones from the maternal pituitary.

A popular but still unsubstantiated theory links undescended testes to the development of the gubernaculum. In the normal male fetus, testosterone stimulates the formation of a fibromuscular band (the gubernaculum), which connects the testes to the scrotal floor. This band probably helps pull the testes into the scrotum by shortening as the fetus grows. Thus, cryptorchidism may result from inadequate testosterone levels or a defect in the testes or the gubernaculum.

Since the testes normally descend into the scrotum during the eighth month of gestation, cryptorchidism most commonly affects premature newborns. It occurs in 30% of premature male newborns but in only 3% of those born at term. In about 80% of these infants with cryptorchidism, the testes descend spontaneously during the first year; in the rest, the testes may or may not descend later.

Signs and symptoms

In the young boy with unilateral cryptorchidism, the testis on the affected side isn't palpable in the scrotum, and his scrotum may appear underdeveloped. On the unaffected side, the scrotum occasionally appears enlarged, as a result of compensatory hypertrophy. After puberty, uncorrected bilateral cryptorchidism prevents spermatogenesis and results in infertility, although testosterone levels remain normal.

Diagnosis

 Physical examination confirms cryptorchidism after laboratory tests determine sex:
• *Buccal smear* determines genetic sex by showing a male sex chromatin pattern.
• *Serum gonadotropin* confirms the presence of testes by assessing the level of circulating hormone.

Treatment

If the testes don't descend spontaneously by age 1, surgical correction is generally indicated. Orchiopexy secures the testes in the scrotum and is commonly performed when the boy is between ages 1 and 6 (optimum age is 5 years). Orchiopexy prevents sterility, and excessive trauma from abnormal positioning. It also prevents harmful psychologic effects. Rarely, human chorionic gonadotropin (HCG) I.M. may stimulate descent. However, hormonal therapy with HCG is ineffective if the testes are located in the abdomen.

Additional considerations

The parents of the child with undescended testes should be encouraged to express their concern about his condition. They may want information about causes, available treatments, and ultimate effect on reproduction. They should know that, especially in premature infants, the testes may descend spontaneously.

If orchiopexy is necessary, the surgery should be explained to the child, using terms he understands. He should know that, following surgery:
• his scrotum may swell but should not be painful.
• he'll have to perform coughing and deep-breathing exercises.
• he must wipe from front to back after defecating to keep the surgical site clean.
• his testis may be held in place with a rubber band taped to his thigh for about 1 week.

Postoperatively, the patient's vital signs and fluid intake and output will be monitored, one of the objects being to guard against urinary retention.

Parents may want to participate in postoperative care, such as bathing or feeding the child. Of course, the child should be encouraged to do as much for himself as possible.

Premature Ejaculation

Premature ejaculation refers to a male's inability to control the ejaculatory reflex during intravaginal containment, resulting in persistently early ejaculation. This common sexual disorder affects all age-groups.

Causes

Premature ejaculation may result from anxiety and is often linked to immature sexual experiences. Other psychologic factors may include ambivalence toward or unconscious hatred of females, a negative sexual relationship in which the male unconsciously denies his partner sexual fulfillment, and guilty feelings about sex.

However, psychologic factors aren't always the cause of premature ejaculation, since this disorder can occur in emotionally healthy males with stable, positive relationships. Rarely, premature ejaculation may be linked to an underlying degenerative neurologic disorder, such as multiple sclerosis, or an inflammatory process, such as posterior urethritis or prostatitis.

Signs and symptoms
Premature ejaculation may have a devastating psychologic impact on some males, and they may exhibit signs of severe inadequacy or self-doubt, in addition to general anxiety and guilt. The patient may be unable to prolong foreplay, or he may have prolonged foreplay capacity but ejaculates as soon as intromission occurs. In other males, however, premature ejaculation may have little or no psychologic impact. In such cases, the complaint lies solely with the sexual partner, who may believe that the male is indifferent to her sexual needs.

Diagnosis
Physical examination and laboratory test results are usually normal, since most males with this complaint are quite healthy. However, detailed sexual history can aid immeasurably in diagnosis. A history of adequate ejaculatory control in the absence of precipitating psychic trauma should arouse suspicion of an organic cause.

Treatment
Masters and Johnson have developed a highly successful, intensive program synthesizing insight therapy, behavioral techniques, and experiential sessions involving both sexual partners. The program is designed to help the patient focus on sensations of impending orgasm. The sessions, which continue for 2 weeks or longer, include:

• *mutual physical examination*, which increases the couple's awareness of anatomy and physiology, while reducing shameful feelings about sexual parts of the body.

• *sensate focus*, which allows each partner, in turn, to caress the other's body, without intercourse, and to focus on the pleasurable sensations of touch.

• *Semans squeeze technique*, which helps the patient gain control of ejaculatory tension by having the woman squeeze his penis, with her thumb on the frenulum and her forefinger and middle finger on the dorsal surface, near the coronal ridge. At the male's direction, she applies and releases pressure every few minutes, during a touching exercise to delay ejaculation by keeping the male at an earlier phase of the sexual response cycle.

The *stop-and-start technique* helps delay ejaculation. With the female in the superior position, this method involves pelvic thrusting until orgasmic sensations start, then stopping and restarting to aid in control of ejaculation. Eventually, the couple is allowed to achieve orgasm.

Additional considerations
• The patient should be assured that premature ejaculation is readily treatable.
• The patient should also be assured that premature ejaculation is a common disorder that does not reflect on his masculinity.
• The patient should be given appropriate resources for therapy.

Testicular Torsion

Testicular torsion is an abnormal twisting of the spermatic cord, due to rotation of a testis or the mesorchium (a fold in the area between the testis and epididymis), which causes strangulation and, if untreated, eventual infarction of the testis. This condition is almost always (90%) unilateral. Testicular torsion is most common between ages 12 and 18, but it may occur at any age. Prognosis is good with early detection and prompt treatment.

Causes

Normally, the tunica vaginalis envelops the testis and attaches to the epididymis and spermatic cord. In *intravaginal torsion* (the most common type of testicular torsion in adolescents), testicular twisting may result from an abnormality of the tunica, in which the testis is abnormally positioned, or from a narrowing of the mesentery support. In *extravaginal torsion* (most common in neonates), loose attachment of the tunica vaginalis to the scrotal lining causes spermatic cord rotation above the testis. A sudden forceful contraction of the cremaster muscle may precipitate this condition.

Signs and symptoms

Testicular torsion typically produces excruciating pain in the affected testis or iliac fossa. Other features include nausea, vomiting, tachycardia, diaphoresis, and pallor.

Diagnosis

Physical examination reveals tense, tender swelling in the scrotum or inguinal canal, and hyperemia of the overlying skin. Systematic auscultation with a Doppler ultrasound stethoscope helps distinguish testicular torsion from strangulated hernia, undescended testes, or epididymitis.

Since torsion causes a loss of blood flow to the testes, the absence of pulsating sound from a painful testis confirms the diagnosis.

Treatment and additional considerations

Treatment consists of surgical repair by orchiopexy (fixation of a viable testis to

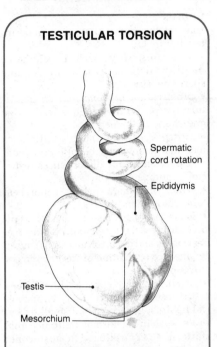

TESTICULAR TORSION

Spermatic cord rotation

Epididymis

Testis

Mesorchium

In extravaginal torsion, rotation of the spermatic cord above the testis causes strangulation and, eventually, infarction of the testis.

the scrotum) or, if the testis is not viable, orchiectomy (excision of the testis).

After surgery:
• the patient will need pain medication.
• an ice bag with a cover is usually applied to the patient's scrotum to reduce edema.
• the wound must be protected from contamination.

Aside from these considerations, the patient may perform as many normal daily activities as possible.

Male Infertility

Male infertility may be suspected whenever a couple fails to achieve pregnancy after about 1 year of regular unprotected intercourse. Approximately 40% to 50% of infertility problems in the United States are totally or partially attributed to the male. (See also, FEMALE INFERTILITY in Chapter 15.)

Causes

Some of the factors that cause male infertility include:

• *semen disorders,* such as volume or motility disturbances, or inadequate sperm density.

• *proliferation of abnormal or immature sperm,* with variations in the size and shape of the head.

• *systemic disease,* such as diabetes mellitus, neoplasms, hepatic and renal diseases, and viral disturbances, especially mumps orchitis.

• *genital infection,* such as gonorrhea, tuberculosis, and herpes.

• *disorders of the testes,* such as cryptorchidism, Sertoli-cell–only syndrome, varicocele, and ductal obstruction (caused by absence or ligation of vas deferens or infection).

• *genetic defects,* such as Klinefelter's (chromosomal pattern XXY; eunuchoidal habitus; gynecomastia; small testes) or Reifenstein's syndrome (chromosomal pattern 46XY; reduced testosterone; azoospermia; eunuchoidism; gynecomastia; hypospadias).

• *immunologic disorders,* such as autoimmune infertility or allergic orchitis.

• *endocrine imbalance* (rare) that disrupts pituitary gonadotropins, inhibiting spermatogenesis, testosterone production, or both; such imbalances occur in Kallmann's syndrome, panhypopituitarism, hypothyroidism, and congenital adrenal hyperplasia.

• *chemicals and drugs* which may inhibit gonadotropins or interfere with spermatogenesis, such as arsenic, methotrexate, medroxyprogesterone acetate, nitrofurantoin, monoamine oxidase inhibitors, and some antihypertensives.

• *sexual problems,* such as erectile dysfunction, ejaculatory incompetence or low libido.

Other factors may include age, occupation, and trauma to testes.

Signs and symptoms

The obvious indication of male infertility is, of course, failure to impregnate a fertile woman. Clinical features may include atrophied testes; empty scrotum; scrotal edema; varicocele or anteversion of the epididymis; inflamed seminal vesicles; beading or abnormal nodes on the spermatic cord and vas; penile nodes, warts, plaques, or hypospadias; and prostatic enlargement, nodules, swelling, or tenderness. In addition, male infertility is often apt to induce troublesome negative emotions in a couple—anger, hurt, disgust, guilt, and loss of self-esteem.

Diagnosis

Detailed patient history may reveal abnormal sexual development, delayed puberty, infertility in previous relationships, and a medical history of prolonged fever, mumps, impaired nutritional status, previous surgery, or trauma to genitalia. After a thorough patient history and physical examination, the most conclusive test for male infertility is semen analysis. Other laboratory tests include gonadotropin assay to determine integrity of pituitary gonadal axis, serum testosterone levels to determine end organ response to LH, urine 17-ketosteroid levels to measure testicular function, and testicular biopsy to help clarify unexplained oligospermia and azoospermia. Vasography and seminal vesiculography may be necessary.

Treatment

When anatomic dysfunctions or infections cause infertility, treatment consists of correcting the underlying problem. For patients with sexual dysfunctions, treatment includes education, counseling or therapy (on sexual techniques, coital frequency, and reproductive physiology), and proper nutrition with vitamin supplements. Decreased FSH levels may respond to vitamin B therapy; decreased LH levels, to chorionic gonadotropin therapy. Normal or elevated LH requires low dosages of testosterone. Decreased testosterone levels, decreased semen motility, and volume disturbances may respond to chorionic gonadotropin.

Patients with oligospermia who have a normal history and physical examination, normal hormonal assays, and no signs of systemic disease require emotional support and counseling, adequate nutrition, multivitamins, and selective therapeutic agents, such as clomiphene, chorionic gonadotropin, and low dosages of testosterone. Obvious alternatives to such treatment are adoption and artificial insemination.

Additional considerations
• The couple should be educated, as necessary, regarding reproductive and sexual functions, and about factors that may interfere with fertility, such as the use of lubricants and douches.
• The man with oligospermia must avoid habits such as wearing tight underwear or an athletic supporter, taking hot tub baths, or habitually riding a bicycle. These habits may interfere with normal spermatogenesis by elevating scrotal temperature. Cool scrotal temperatures are essential for adequate spermatogenesis.
• When possible, infertile couples should join group programs to share their feelings and concerns with other couples who have the same problem.
• To help prevent male infertility, all men should have regular physical examinations, protect their gonads during athletic activity, obtain prompt and correct treatment for venereal diseases, and undergo surgical correction for anatomic defects.

Precocious Puberty in Males

In precocious puberty, boys begin to mature sexually before age 10. It can occur as true precocious puberty, which is most common, with early maturation of the hypothalamic-pituitary-gonadal axis, development of secondary sex characteristics, gonadal development, and spermatogenesis; or as pseudoprecocious puberty, with development of secondary sex characteristics without gonadal development. Boys with true precocious puberty reportedly have fathered children at as young an age as 7 years.

In most boys with precocious puberty, sexual characteristics develop in essentially normal sequence; these children function normally when they reach adulthood.

Causes
True precocious puberty may be idiopathic (constitutional) or cerebral (neurogenic). In some patients, idiopathic precocity may be genetically transmitted as a dominant trait. Cerebral precocity results from pituitary or hypothalamic intracranial lesions that cause excessive secretion of gonadotropin.

Pseudoprecocious puberty may result from testicular tumors (hyperplasia, adenoma, or carcinoma) or from congenital adrenogenital syndrome. Testicular tumors create excessive testosterone levels; adrenogenital syndrome creates high levels of adrenocortical steroids.

Signs and symptoms
All boys with precocious puberty experience early bone development, causing initial growth spurt, early muscle development, and premature closure of the epiphyses, which results in stunted adult stature. Other features are adult hair pattern, penile growth, and bilateral enlarged testes. Symptoms of precocity due to cerebral lesions include nausea, vomiting, headache, visual disturbances, and internal hydrocephalus.

In pseudoprecocity caused by testicular tumors, adult hair patterns and acne develop. A discrepancy in testis size also occurs; the enlarged testis may be hard or may contain a palpable, isolated nodule. Adrenogenital syndrome produces adult skin tone, excessive hair (including beard), and deepened voice. A boy with this syndrome appears stocky and muscular; his penis, scrotal sac, and prostate are enlarged (but not the testes).

Diagnosis

Assessing the cause of precocious puberty requires a complete physical examination—including an examination of the skin, recording of physical measurements, and palpation of the testes to check for tumors. Detailed patient history can help evaluate recent growth pattern, behavior changes, family history of precocious puberty, or any hormonal ingestion.

In true precocity, laboratory results include the following:

• *Serum levels of luteinizing, follicle-stimulating, and adrenocorticotropic hormones* are elevated.
• *Plasma tests for testosterone* demonstrate elevated levels (equal to those of an adult male).
• *Evaluation of ejaculate* indicates true precocity by revealing presence of live spermatozoa.
• *Brain scan, skull X-rays, and EEG* can detect possible CNS tumors.
• *Skull and hand X-rays* reveal advanced bone age.

A child with an initial diagnosis of idiopathic precocious puberty should be reassessed regularly for possible tumors.

In pseudoprecocity, chromosomal karyotype analysis demonstrates abnormal pattern of autosomes and sex chromosomes. Elevated 24-hour urinary 17-ketosteroids and other steroid excretion levels also indicate pseudoprecocity.

Treatment

Boys with idiopathic precocious puberty generally require no medical treatment and, except for stunted growth, suffer no physical complications in adulthood. Supportive psychologic counseling is the most important therapy.

When precocious puberty is caused by tumors, the outlook is less encouraging. Brain tumors necessitate neurosurgery but commonly resist treatment and may prove fatal. Testicular tumors may be treated by removing the affected testis (orchiectomy). Malignant tumors additionally require chemotherapy and lymphatic radiation therapy, and have a poor prognosis.

Adrenogenital syndrome that causes precocious puberty may respond to lifelong therapy with maintenance doses of glucocorticoids (cortisol), to inhibit corticotropin production.

Additional considerations

• In most cases of precocious puberty, social and emotional development remain consistent with the child's chronologic age, not with his physical development. Parents must not place unrealistic demands on the child or expect him to act older than his age.
• The child needs reassurance that although his body is changing more rapidly than those of other boys, eventually they will experience the same changes. He should be helped to feel less self-conscious about his differences. One way is by suggesting clothing he can wear that de-emphasizes sexual development.
• The child with true precocity should receive sex education.
• The child and the parents need to be made aware of the medication's side effects (cushingoid symptoms).

Selected References

Barbach, Lonnie G. WOMEN DISCOVER ORGASM: A THERAPIST'S GUIDE TO A NEW TREATMENT APPROACH. New York: Macmillan Publishing Co., 1980.

Barnard, Martha U. HUMAN SEXUALITY FOR HEALTH PROFESSIONALS. Philadelphia: W.B. Saunders Co., 1978.

Budell, J. William. *Diagnosing Sexually Transmitted Diseases*, MEDICAL ASPECTS OF HUMAN SEXUALITY. 11:8:33, August 1977.

Dickinson, Robert L. ATLAS OF HUMAN SEX ANATOMY. Huntington, N.Y.: Robert E. Krieger

Publishing Co., 1969.

EDUCATION AND TREATMENT IN HUMAN SEXUALITY: THE TRAINING OF HEALTH PROFESSIONS. Albany, N.Y.: World Health Organization, 1975.

Fertel, N.S. *Vaginismus: A Review,* JOURNAL OF SEX AND MARITAL THERAPY. 3:2:113-132, 1977.

Furlow, W. *Surgical Management of Impotence Using the Inflatable Penile Prosthesis,* MAYO CLINIC PROCEEDINGS. 51:325-328, 1976.

Gagnon, John H. HUMAN SEXUALITIES. Glenview, Ill.: Scott, Foresman & Co., 1977.

Goldstein, Bernard. HUMAN SEXUALITY. New York: McGraw-Hill Book Co., 1976.

Green, Richard. HUMAN SEXUALITY, 2nd ed. Baltimore: Williams & Wilkins Co., 1979.

Hyde, Janet. UNDERSTANDING HUMAN SEXUALITY. New York: McGraw-Hill Book Co., 1979.

Kaplan, Helen S. THE NEW SEX THERAPY. New York: Brunner/Mazel, Inc., 1973.

Katchadourian, Herant A., and Donald T. Lunde. FUNDAMENTALS OF HUMAN SEXUALITY, 3rd ed. New York: Holt, Rinehart & Winston, Inc., 1980.

Kelly, Gary F. SEXUALITY—THE HUMAN PERSPECTIVE. Woodbury, N.Y.: Barron's Educational Series, Inc., 1979.

Kelman, Peter, and Burt Saxon. MODERN HUMAN SEXUALITY. Boston: Houghton Mifflin Co., 1976.

Kolodny, R., et al. TEXTBOOK OF HUMAN SEXUALITY FOR NURSES. Boston: Little, Brown & Co., 1979.

Levine, S. *Marital Sexual Dysfunction: Introductory Concepts,* ANNALS OF INTERNAL MEDICINE. 84:4:448-453.

Lopiccolo, J., and L. Lopiccolo, eds. HANDBOOK OF SEX THERAPY. New York: Plenum Publishing Corp., 1978.

McCary, James L. HUMAN SEXUALITY, 3rd ed. New York: D. Van Nostrand & Co., 1978.

Martin, Leonide. HEALTH CARE OF WOMEN. Philadelphia: J.B. Lippincott Co., 1978.

Masters, William H., and Virginia E. Johnson. HUMAN SEXUAL INADEQUACY. Boston: Little, Brown & Co., 1979.

Menning, B.E. *Resolve: A Support Group for Infertile Couples,* AMERICAN JOURNAL OF NURSING. 76:2:258-259, 1976.

Meyer, J.K., ed. CLINICAL MANAGEMENT OF SEXUAL DISORDERS. Baltimore: Williams & Wilkins Co., 1976.

Money, John, and Anke A. Ehrhardt. MAN AND WOMAN, BOY AND GIRL: DIFFERENTIATION AND DIMORPHISM OF GENDER IDENTITY FROM CONCEPTION TO MATURITY. Baltimore: Johns Hopkins University Press, 1973.

Munjack, D., and P. Kanna. *An Overview of Outcome in Frigidity: Treatment Effect and Effectiveness,* COMPREHENSIVE PSYCHIATRY. 17:3:401-413, 1976.

Nobel, Robert C. SEXUALLY TRANSMITTED DISEASES, GUIDE TO DIAGNOSIS AND THERAPY. New York: Medical Examination Publishing Co., 1977.

Schiavi, R.C., and D. White. *Androgens and Male Sexual Function,* JOURNAL OF SEX AND MARITAL THERAPY. 2:3, 1976.

SEX INFORMATION AND EDUCATION COUNCIL OF THE U.S. (SIECUS) REPORT. 9:1, September 1980.

Shane, J., et al. *The Infertile Couple,* CLINICAL SYMPOSIA. 28:5:2-40.

Smith, Donald R. GENERAL UROLOGY, 9th ed. Los Altos, Calif.: Lange Medical Pub., 1978.

Stangel, John J. FERTILITY AND CONCEPTION: AN ESSENTIAL GUIDE FOR CHILDLESS COUPLES. New York: New American Library, 1980.

Watts, R.J. *The Physiological Interrelationships Between Depression, Drugs, and Sexuality,* NURSING FORUM. 17:168-183, 1978.

Woods, Nancy Fugate. HUMAN SEXUALITY IN HEALTH AND ILLNESS, 2nd ed. St. Louis: C.V. Mosby Co., 1979.

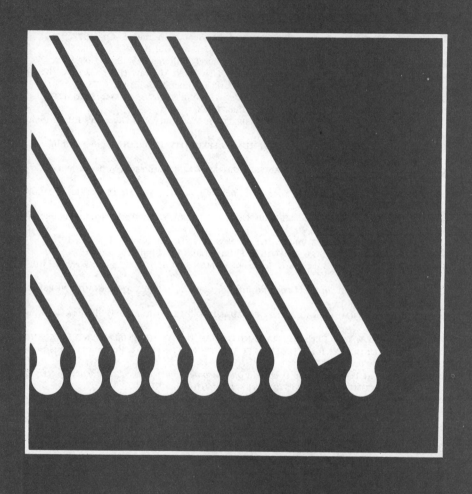

17 Hematologic Disorders

Hematologic Disorders

Introduction

Blood, one of the body's major fluid tissues, continuously circulates through the heart and blood vessels, carrying vital elements to every part of the body.

Blood basics

Blood performs several physiologically vital functions through its special components: the liquid portion (plasma), and the formed constituents (erythrocytes, leukocytes, thrombocytes) that are suspended in it. Erythrocytes (red blood cells [RBC]) carry oxygen to the tissues and remove carbon dioxide from them. Leukocytes (white blood cells [WBC]) participate in inflammatory and immune responses. Plasma (a clear straw-colored fluid) carries antibodies and nutrients to tissues and carries waste away; coagulation factors in plasma, with thrombocytes (platelets), control clotting.

Typically, the average person has 5 to 6 liters of circulating blood that constitute 5% to 7% of body weight (as much as 10% in premature newborns). Blood is three to five times more viscous than water, with an alkaline pH of 7.35 to 7.45, and is either bright red (arterial blood) or dark red (venous blood), depending on the degree of oxygen saturation and the hemoglobin level.

Formation and characteristics

The process of blood formation by hematopoiesis occurs primarily in the bone marrow, where primitive blood cells (stem cells) produce the precursors of erythrocytes (normoblasts), leukocytes, and thrombocytes. During embryonic development, blood cells are derived from mesenchyma, and form in the yolk sac. As the fetus matures, blood cells are produced in the liver, the spleen, and the thymus; by the fifth month of gestation, blood cells also begin to form in bone marrow. After birth, blood cells are usually produced only in the marrow.

Blood's function

The most important function of blood is to *transport oxygen* (bound to RBCs inside hemoglobin) from the lungs to the body tissues, and to *return carbon dioxide* from these tissues to the lungs. Blood also performs vital inflammatory and immunologic functions. It...

• produces and delivers antibodies (by way of WBCs) formed by plasma cells and lymphocytes
• transports granulocytes and monocytes to defend the body against pathogens by phagocytosis
• provides complement, a group of immunologically important protein substances in plasma.

Blood's other functions include control of hemostasis by platelets, plasma, and coagulation factors that repair tissue injuries and prevent or halt bleeding;

acid-base and fluid balance; regulation of body temperature by carrying off excess heat generated by the internal organs for dissipation through the skin; and transportation of nutrients and regulatory hormones to body tissues, and of metabolic wastes to the organs of excretion (kidneys, lungs, and skin).

Blood dysfunction

Because of the rapid reproduction of bone marrow cells, and the short life span and minimal storage in the bone marrow of circulating cells, bone marrow cells and their precursors are particularly vulnerable to physiologic changes that can affect cell production. Resulting blood disorders may be primary or secondary, quantitative or qualitative, or both; they may involve some or all blood components. Quantitative blood disorders result from increased or decreased cell production or cell destruction; qualitative blood disorders stem from intrinsic cell abnormalities or plasma component dysfunction. Specific causes of blood disorders include trauma, chronic disease, surgery, malnutrition, drugs, exposure to toxins and radiation, and genetic and congenital defects that disrupt production and function. For example, depressed bone marrow production or mechanical destruction of mature blood cells can reduce the number of RBCs, platelets, and granulocytes, resulting in pancytopenia (anemia, thrombocytopenia, granulocytopenia). Increased production of multiple bone

COAGULATION FACTORS		
FACTOR	**SYNONYM**	**LOCATION**
Factor I	Fibrinogen	Plasma
Factor II	Prothrombin	Plasma
Factor III	Tissue thromboplastin	Tissue cells
Factor IV	Calcium ion	Plasma
Factor V	Labile factor	Plasma
Factor VII	Stable factor	Plasma
Factor VIII	Antihemophilic globulin (AHG) or antihemophilic factor (AHF)	Plasma
Factor IX	Plasma thromboplastin component (PTC)	Plasma
Factor X	Stuart-Prower factor	Plasma
Factor XI	Plasma thromboplastin antecedent (PTA)	Plasma
Factor XII	Hageman factor	Plasma
Factor XIII	Fibrin stabilizing factor	Plasma

Adapted with permission from Ewald E. Selkurt, ed., BASIC PHYSIOLOGY FOR THE HEALTH SCIENCES (Boston: Little Brown & Co., 1975).

marrow components can follow myeloproliferative disorders.

Erythropoiesis

The tissues' demand for oxygen and the blood cells' ability to deliver it regulate RBC production. Consequently, hypoxia (or tissue anoxia) stimulates red cell production by triggering the formation and release of erythropoietin, a hormone (probably produced by the kidneys) that activates bone marrow to produce RBCs. Erythropoiesis may also be stimulated by androgens.

The actual formation of an erythrocyte begins with an uncommitted stem cell that may eventually develop into an RBC or a WBC. Such formation requires certain vitamins—B_{12} and folic acid—and minerals, such as copper, cobalt, and especially, iron, which is vital to hemoglobin's oxygen-carrying capacity. Iron is obtained from various foods, and is absorbed in the duodenum and upper jejunum, leaving any excess for temporary storage in reticuloendothelial cells, especially those in the liver. Iron excess is stored as ferritin and hemosiderin until it's released for use in the bone marrow to form new RBCs.

RBC disorders

RBC disorders include quantitative and qualitative abnormalities. Deficiency of RBCs (anemia) can follow any condition that destroys or inhibits the formation of these cells. Common factors leading to this deficiency include:
• drugs, toxins, ionizing radiation.
• congenital or acquired defects that cause bone marrow aplasia and suppress general hematopoiesis (aplastic anemia) or erythropoiesis.
• metabolic abnormalities (sideroblastic anemia).
• deficiencies of vitamins (vitamin B_{12} deficiency or pernicious anemia), iron or minerals (iron, folic acid, copper, and cobalt deficiency anemias) that cause inadequate RBC production.
• excessive chronic or acute blood loss (posthemorrhagic anemia).
• chronic illnesses, such as renal disease, malignancy, and chronic infections.
• intrinsically or extrinsically defective red cells (sickle cell anemia, hemolytic transfusion reaction).

Comparatively few conditions lead to excessive numbers of red cells:
• abnormal proliferation of all bone marrow elements (polycythemia vera)
• a single-element abnormality (for instance, an increase in RBCs that results from erythropoietin excess, which in turn results from hypoxemia or pulmonary disease)
• decreased plasma cell volume, which causes an apparent corresponding increase—relative, not absolute—in RBC concentration.

Function of white cells

WBCs, or leukocytes, protect the body against harmful bacteria and infection, and are classified as granular leukocytes (basophils, neutrophils, and eosinophils) or nongranular leukocytes (lymphocytes, monocytes, and plasma cells). Usually, WBCs are produced in bone marrow; however, lymphocytes and plasma cells are produced in lymphoid tissue as well. Although WBCs have a poorly defined tissue life span, they generally have a circulating half-life of less than 6 hours. However, some monocytes may survive for weeks or months.

Normally, WBCs number between 5,000 and 10,000/mm³, and comprise the following elements:
• *Neutrophils,* the predominant form of granulocyte, make up about 60% of white cells and help devour invading organisms by phagocytosis.
• *Eosinophils,* minor granulocytes, may defend against parasites and participate in allergic reactions.
• *Basophils,* minor granulocytes, may release heparin and histamine into the blood.
• *Monocytes,* along with neutrophils, help devour invading organisms by phagocytosis. They also help process antigens for lymphocytes and form macrophages in the tissues.
• *Lymphocytes* identify foreign organisms and may destroy them by antibody

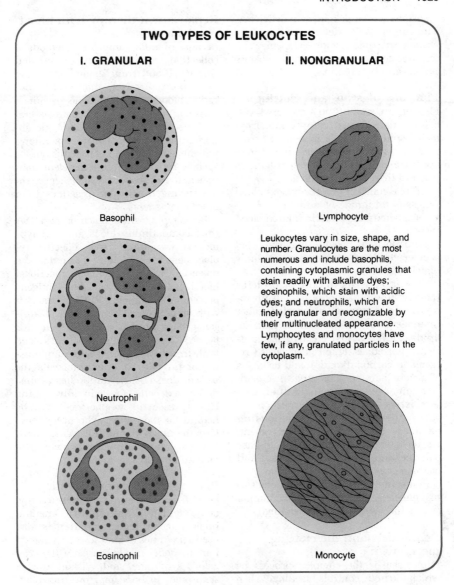

TWO TYPES OF LEUKOCYTES

I. GRANULAR

Basophil

Neutrophil

Eosinophil

II. NONGRANULAR

Lymphocyte

Leukocytes vary in size, shape, and number. Granulocytes are the most numerous and include basophils, containing cytoplasmic granules that stain readily with alkaline dyes; eosinophils, which stain with acidic dyes; and neutrophils, which are finely granular and recognizable by their multinucleated appearance. Lymphocytes and monocytes have few, if any, granulated particles in the cytoplasm.

Monocyte

formation or direct interaction.
• *Plasma cells* develop from lymphocytes and produce antibodies.

A temporary increase in production and release of mature WBCs (leukemic reaction) is a normal response to infection. However, an abnormal increase of immature WBC precursors and their accumulation in bone marrow or lymphoid tissue is characteristic of leuke-

mia. These nonfunctioning WBCs (blasts) provide no protection against infection, crowd out other vital components—RBCs, platelets, mature WBCs—and spill into the bloodstream, sometimes infiltrating organs and impairing organ functions.

Deficiencies of WBCs may reflect inadequate cell production, drug reactions, ionizing radiation, infiltrated bone marrow (leukemia), congenital defects, aplastic anemia, or folic acid deficiency. The major WBC deficiencies include granulocytopenia, lymphocytopenia, and less frequently, monocytopenia, eosinophilia, and basophilia.

Platelets, plasma, and clotting

Platelets are small (2 to 4 microns), colorless, disk-shaped cytoplasmic fragments split from cells in bone marrow megakaryocytes, and have a life span of approximately 10 days. These fragments perform three vital functions:
• initiate contraction of damaged blood vessels to minimize blood loss
• form hemostatic plugs in injured blood vessels
• with plasma, provide materials that accelerate blood coagulation—notably platelet factor 3.

Plasma consists mainly of proteins (chiefly albumin, globulin, and fibrinogen) held in aqueous suspension. Other components of plasma include glucose, lipids, amino acids, electrolytes, pigments, hormones, respiratory gases (oxygen and carbon dioxide), and products of metabolism, such as urea, uric acid, creatinine, and lactic acid. Its fluid characteristics—including osmotic pressure, viscosity, and suspension qualities—depend on its protein content. Plasma components regulate acid-base balance and immune responses, and mediate coagulation and nutrition.

In a complex process called hemostasis, platelets, plasma, and coagulation factors interact to control bleeding.

Hemostasis and the clotting mechanism

Hemostasis is the complex process by which the body controls bleeding. When a blood vessel ruptures, local vasoconstriction and platelet clumping (aggregation) at the site of the injury initially help prevent hemorrhage. However, formation of a more stable, secure clot requires initiation of the complex clotting mechanism known as the intrinsic cascade system. This mechanism is an interaction of platelets, plasma, and coagulation factors.

Replacement therapy with blood components

Because of today's improved methods of collection, component separation, and storage, blood transfusions are being used more effectively than ever. Separating blood into components permits a single unit of blood to benefit several patients with different hematologic abnormalities. Component therapy allows patients who need blood transfusions for specific replacement of a deficient component to receive this replacement without risking transfusion reactions from other components.

Blood typing, cross-matching, and HLA (histocompatibility locus antigen) typing are essential to safe, effective replacement therapy, and minimize the potential risk of transfusion reactions. Blood typing determines the antigens present in the patient's RBCs by reaction with standardized sera. (Critical antigen groups are those of ABO and Rh factor.) Cross-matching the patient's blood with transfusion blood before administration provides some assurance that the patient doesn't have antibodies against donor red cells. Occasionally, typing HLA (present in lymphocytes) may be helpful for the patient who needs long-term therapy with multiple transfusions. Usually, only family members can provide an appropriate match.

Bone marrow transplantation

One of the newest advances in treating acute leukemia and aplastic anemia, bone marrow transplantation is also used sometimes to treat severe combined immunodeficiency disease (SCID), Nezelof's syndrome, and Wiskott-Aldrich syndrome. In bone marrow transplantation, marrow from a twin or nontwin HLA identical donor (nearly always a sibling) is transfused into the recipient in an attempt to repopulate his bone marrow with normal cells. This procedure necessitates reverse isolation (preferably with laminar air flow) to protect the recipient from infection until the graft takes.

A hematologic disorder can affect

FOUR STAGES IN THE DEVELOPMENT OF NORMOBLASTS

In a four-stage process, primitive blood cells (stem cells) in the bone marrow differentiate into normoblasts—the precursors of erythrocytes. In each stage of normoblast development, the overall size of the normoblast decreases in proportion to a reduction in the size of its nucleus.

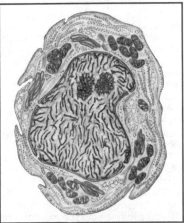

Stage I: Pronormoblast, which is usually irregular in shape, has a large nucleus that encompases about 80% of its cell area.

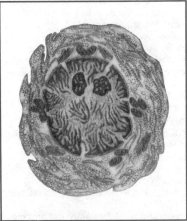

Stage II: Basophilic normoblast has a nucleus that occupies 75% of its cell area. During this stage, the normoblast becomes rounder.

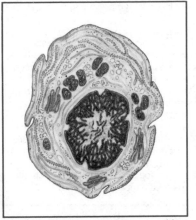

Stage III: Polychromatophilic normoblast has a nucleus that occupies only about 50% of its cell area. During this stage, large amounts of hemoglobin develop in the cytoplasm.

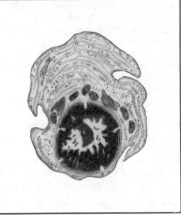

Stage IV: Orthochromatic normoblast, which is irregular in shape, has a nucleus that occupies only 25% of its cell area. During this stage, hemoglobin content continues to increase.

TESTS FOR BLOOD COMPOSITION, PRODUCTION, AND FUNCTION

Overall composition
- *Peripheral blood smear* shows maturity and morphologic characteristics of blood elements and determines qualitative abnormalities.
- *Complete blood count (CBC)* determines the actual number of blood elements in relation to volume and quantifies abnormalities.
- *Bone marrow aspiration* or *biopsy* allows evaluation of hematopoiesis by showing blood elements and precursors, and abnormal or malignant cells.

RBC function
- *Hematocrit (HCT)* (packed cell volume) measures the percentage of RBCs per fluid volume of whole blood.
- *Hemoglobin (Hb)* measures the amount (grams) of hemoglobin per 100 ml of blood, to determine oxygen-carrying capacity.
- *Reticulocyte count* allows assessment of RBC production by determining concentration of this early erythrocyte precursor.
- *Schilling test* determines absorption of vitamin B_{12} (necessary for erythropoiesis) by measuring excretion of radioactive B_{12} in the urine.
- *Mean corpuscular volume (MCV)* describes the red cell in terms of size.
- *Mean corpuscular hemoglobin (MCH)* determines average amount of hemoglobin per RBC.
- *Mean corpuscular hemoglobin concentration (MCHC)* establishes average hemoglobin concentration in 100 ml packed RBCs.
- *Serum bilirubin* measures liver function and extravascular RBC hemolysis.
- *Sugar-water test* assesses the susceptibility of RBCs to hemolyze with complement.
- *Direct Coombs' test* demonstrates the presence of IgG antibodies (such as antibodies to Rh factor) and/or complement on circulating RBCs.
- *Indirect Coombs' test*, a two-step test, detects the presence of IgG antibodies on RBCs in the serum.
- *Sideroblast test* detects stainable iron (available for hemoglobin synthesis) in normoblastic RBCs.

Hemostasis
- *Platelet count* determines number of platelets.
- *Prothrombin time (Quick's test, pro time, PT)* assists in evaluation of thrombin generation (extrinsic clotting mechanism).
- *Partial thromboplastin time (PTT)* aids evaluation of the adequacy of plasma-clotting factors (intrinsic clotting mechanism).
- *Thrombin time* detects abnormalities in thrombin fibrinogen reaction.
- *Activated partial thromboplastin time (APTT)* aids assessment of plasma-clotting factors (except factors VII and XIII) in the intrinsic clotting mechanism.

WBC function
- *WBC count, differential* establishes quantity and maturity of WBC elements (neutrophils [called polymorphonuclear granulocytes or bands], basophils, eosinophils, lymphocytes, monocytes).

Plasma
- *Erythrocyte sedimentation rate (ESR)* measures rate of RBCs settling from plasma and may reflect infection.
- *Electrophoresis of serum proteins* determines amount of various serum proteins (classified by mobility in response to an electrical field).
- *Immunoelectrophoresis of serum proteins* separates and classifies serum antibodies (immunoglobins) through specific antisera.
- *Fibrinogen (Factor I)* measures this coagulation factor in plasma.

nearly every aspect of the patient's life, perhaps resulting in life-threatening emergencies that require prompt medical treatment. With astute, sensitive care founded on a firm understanding of hematologic basics, the health care professional can help the patient survive such illnesses. In situations with poor prognoses, the health care professional can help the patient make the necessary adjustments to maintain an optimal quality of life.

ANEMIA

Copper Deficiency Anemia
(Hypocupremia)

Copper deficiency anemia is extremely rare in humans. Theoretically, copper deficiency impairs hemoglobin synthesis by inhibiting the absorption of iron in the gastrointestinal tract, the release of iron from body stores, and the utilization of iron by RBCs. Copper deficiency anemia is mild, hypochromic, and usually associated with iron deficiency anemia and other nutritional deficiencies. Copper deficiency may also impair normal development of bone, connective tissue, and the central nervous system.

Causes

Since an adult requires only 2 mg of copper daily, inadequate dietary copper intake is rare in adults. When copper deficiency anemia does occur in adults, it's usually secondary to:

• *disease states* associated with low protein levels (such as protein-calorie malnutrition and kwashiorkor).

• *substantial protein loss* (as in patients with nephrotic syndrome).

• *decreased gastrointestinal absorption* of copper (due to malabsorption syndromes, increased zinc intake, or resection of the stomach or small intestine).

• *total parenteral nutrition* (TPN) without a copper supplement.

• *Wilson's disease* (in which serum copper levels are low despite copper accumulation in the tissues).

Copper deficiency anemia may also occur in infants who are fed cow's milk that contains no dietary supplement, or who have malnutrition or malabsorption.

Signs and symptoms

Due to impaired hemoglobin synthesis, copper deficiency anemia characteristically leads to shortness of breath, pallor, fatigue, edema, poor wound healing, and anorexia. Prolonged copper deficiency may cause impaired mental development in infants and progressive mental deterioration in adults.

Diagnosis

Because it's a rare cause of anemia, copper deficiency is often overlooked. Leukopenia and severe neutropenia may be the first clues to this condition, which is confirmed by low serum copper levels (normal range in adults, 68 to 161 mcg/100 ml; in children, 45 to 110 mcg/100 ml). As in other anemias, hemoglobin is less than 10 g/100 ml, and RBC count may show microcytic hypochromia. Hypoalbuminemia, proteinuria, and glycosuria may also occur.

Treatment and additional considerations

Treatment of severe copper deficiency anemia necessitates I.V. replacement with copper sulfate, and supportive measures for associated symptoms. To prevent copper deficiency, patients should always receive a copper supplement during TPN and possibly after resection of the stomach or small intestine.

• Patients who are receiving TPN or who have had gastric or intestinal resections must be watched for signs of copper deficiency.

• New mothers who don't plan to breastfeed should not use powdered milk or unfortified cow's milk exclusively, without supplementing their infant's food with cereal and other copper-containing foods.

• The patient with copper deficiency

due to decreased dietary intake must eat a complete, balanced diet, including foods high in copper, such as oysters, shellfish, organ meats (especially brain, kidneys, and liver), nuts, dried legumes, raisins, and cocoa.

Pernicious Anemia
(Addison's anemia)

Pernicious anemia is a megaloblastic anemia characterized by decreased gastric production of hydrochloric acid and deficiency of intrinsic factor (IF), a substance normally secreted by the parietal cells of the gastric mucosa that is essential for vitamin B_{12} absorption. The resulting deficiency of vitamin B_{12} causes serious neurologic, gastric, and intestinal abnormalities. Untreated pernicious anemia may lead to permanent neurologic disability and death.

Pernicious anemia primarily affects persons of northern European ancestry; in the United States, it's most common in New England and the Great Lakes region, due to ethnic concentrations. It's rare in children, Blacks, and Asians. Onset is typically between ages 50 and 60; incidence rises with increasing age.

Causes

Familial incidence of pernicious anemia suggests a genetic predisposition. This disorder is significantly more common in patients with immunologically related diseases, such as thyroiditis, myxedema, and Graves' disease. These facts seem to support a widely held theory that an inherited autoimmune response causes gastric mucosal atrophy and, consequently, decreases hydrochloric acid and IF production. IF deficiency impairs vitamin B_{12} absorption; in turn, vitamin B_{12} deficiency inhibits the growth of all cells, especially the rapidly reproducing cells of the bone marrow and gastrointestinal tract. Since vitamin B_{12} is essential for RBC formation, this deficiency also leads to insufficient and deformed RBCs with poor oxygen-carrying capacity. Finally, vitamin B_{12} deficiency impairs myelin formation, which causes neurologic damage.

Signs and symptoms

Characteristically, pernicious anemia has an insidious onset but eventually causes an unmistakable triad of symptoms: weakness, sore tongue, and numbness and tingling in the extremities. The lips, gums, and tongue appear markedly bloodless. Hemolysis-induced hyperbilirubinemia may cause faintly jaundiced sclera and pale to bright yellow skin. In addition, the patient may become highly susceptible to infection, especially of the genitourinary tract.

Other systemic symptoms of pernicious anemia include the following:
• *Gastrointestinal:* Gastric mucosal atrophy and decreased hydrochloric acid production disturb digestion and lead to nausea, vomiting, anorexia, weight loss, flatulence, diarrhea, and constipation. Gingival bleeding and a sore, inflamed tongue may make eating painful and intensify anorexia.
• *Central nervous system:* Demyelination caused by vitamin B_{12} deficiency initially affects the peripheral nerves but gradually extends to the spinal cord. Consequently, the neurologic effects of pernicious anemia may include neuritis; weakness in extremities; peripheral numbness and paresthesias; disturbed position sense; lack of coordination; ataxia; impaired fine finger movement; positive Babinski's and Romberg's signs; light-headedness; altered vision (diplopia, blurred vision), taste, and hearing (tinnitus); optic muscle atrophy; loss of bowel and bladder control; and in males, impotence. Its effects on the nervous system may also produce irritability, poor

memory, headache, depression, and delirium. Although some of these symptoms are temporary, irreversible changes in the CNS may have occurred before treatment.

• *Cardiovascular:* Increasingly fragile cell membranes induce widespread destruction of RBCs, resulting in low hemoglobin levels. The impaired oxygen-carrying capacity of the blood secondary to lowered hemoglobin leads to weakness, fatigue, and light-headedness. Compensatory increased cardiac output results in palpitations, wide pulse pressure, dyspnea, orthopnea, tachycardia, premature beats, and eventually, congestive heart failure.

Diagnosis

A positive family history, typical ethnic heritage, and results of blood studies, bone marrow aspiration, gastric analysis, and the Schilling test establish the diagnosis. Laboratory screening must rule out other anemias with similar symptoms, such as folic acid deficiency anemia, since treatment differs. Diagnosis must also rule out vitamin B_{12} deficiency resulting from malabsorption due to gastrointestinal disorders, gastric surgery, radiation, or drug therapy.

Blood study results that suggest pernicious anemia include:

• decreased hemoglobin (4 to 5 g/100 ml) and decreased RBCs.

• increased mean corpuscular volume; because larger-than-normal RBCs *each* contain increased amounts of hemoglobin, mean corpuscular hemoglobin concentration is also increased.

• possible low WBC and platelet counts, and large, malformed platelets.

• serum vitamin B_{12} assay levels less than 0.1 mcg/ml.

Bone marrow aspiration reveals erythroid hyperplasia (crowded red bone marrow), with increased numbers of megaloblasts but few normally developing RBCs.

Gastric analysis shows absence of free hydrochloric acid after histamine or pentagastrin injection. Biopsy of gastric mucosa may be necessary.

The Schilling test is the definitive test for pernicious anemia. In this test, the patient receives a small (0.5 to 2 mcg) oral dose of radioactive vitamin B_{12} after fasting for 12 hours. A larger (1 mg) dose of nonradioactive vitamin B_{12} is given I.M. 2 hours later, as a parenteral flush, and the radioactivity of a 24-hour urine specimen is measured. About 7% of the radioactive B_{12} dose is excreted in the first 24 hours; persons with pernicious anemia excrete less than 3%. (Generally, vitamin B_{12} is absorbed, and excess amounts are excreted in the urine; in pernicious anemia, the vitamin remains unabsorbed and is passed in the stool.) When the Schilling test is repeated with IF added, the test shows normal excretion of vitamin B_{12}.

Treatment

Early parenteral vitamin B_{12} replacement can reverse pernicious anemia, minimize complications, and may prevent permanent neurologic damage. These injections rarely cause side effects or induce an allergic response. An initial high dose of parenteral vitamin B_{12} causes rapid RBC regeneration. Within 2 weeks, hemoglobin should rise to normal, and the patient's condition should markedly improve. Since rapid cell regeneration increases the patient's iron requirements, concomitant iron replacement is necessary at this time to prevent iron deficiency anemia. After the patient's condition improves, vitamin B_{12} doses can be decreased to maintenance levels and given monthly. Because such injections must be continued for life, patients should learn self-administration, if possible.

If anemia causes extreme fatigue, the patient may require bed rest until hemoglobin rises. If hemoglobin is dangerously low, he may need blood transfusions, digitalis, a diuretic, and a low-sodium diet for congestive heart failure. Most important is the replacement of vitamin B_{12} to control the condition that led to this failure. Appropriate antibiotics help combat accompanying infections.

Additional considerations

Supportive measures minimize the risk of complications and speed recovery. Patient and family teaching can promote compliance with lifelong vitamin B_{12} replacement.

• If the patient has severe anemia, activities, rest periods, and necessary diagnostic tests should be planned to conserve his energy. If the patient develops tachycardia, his activities are too strenuous.

• Accurate Schilling test results require that all urine over a 24-hour period is collected and that the specimens aren't contaminated with feces.

• The patient must guard against infections, and report signs of infection promptly, especially pulmonary and urinary tract infections, since his weakened condition may increase his susceptibility.

• The patient should eat a well-balanced diet, including foods high in vitamin B_{12} (meat, liver, fish, eggs, and milk). He should also eat between-meal snacks, and the family members should bring favorite foods from home.

• Since a sore mouth and tongue make eating painful, the dietitian should avoid giving the patient irritating foods. If these symptoms make talking difficult, a pad and pencil or some other aid will facilitate nonverbal communication. The patient should use diluted mouthwash or, with severe conditions, his mouth should be swabbed with tap water or warm saline solution.

• The patient with a sensory deficit must not use a heating pad, since it may cause burns.

• If the patient is incontinent, a regular bowel and bladder routine must be established. After the patient is discharged, a visiting health care professional should follow up on this schedule and make adjustments, as needed.

• If neurologic damage causes behavioral problems, the patient's mental and neurologic status must be assessed often. Tranquilizers may be ordered, as well as a jacket restraint for nighttime use.

• Vitamin B_{12} replacement isn't a permanent cure—these injections *must* be continued for life, even after symptoms subside.

• Patients who've had extensive gastric resections or who follow strict vegetarian diets can prevent pernicious anemia by taking vitamin B_{12} supplements regularly.

Folic Acid Deficiency Anemia

Folic acid deficiency anemia is a common, slowly progressive, megaloblastic anemia. It occurs most often in infants, adolescents, pregnant and lactating females, alcoholics, the elderly, and in persons with malignant or intestinal diseases.

Causes

Folic acid deficiency anemia follows insufficient intake of folic acid, which may result from:

• *poor diet* (common in alcoholics, elderly persons living alone, and infants, especially those with infections or diarrhea).

• *impaired absorption* (due to intestinal dysfunction, such as celiac disease, tropical sprue, regional jejunitis, or bowel resection).

• *excessive cooking*, which can destroy a high percentage of folic acids in foods.

• *limited storage capacity* in infants.

• *prolonged drug therapy* (anticonvulsants; estrogens, including estrogen-containing oral contraceptives).

• *increased folic acid requirement* during pregnancy; during rapid growth in infancy (common because of recent increase in survival of premature infants); during childhood and adolescence (because of general use of folate-poor cow's milk); and in patients with neoplastic diseases, and some skin diseases (chronic exfoliative dermatitis).

Signs and symptoms

Folic acid deficiency anemia gradually produces clinical features characteristic of other megaloblastic anemias, without the neurologic manifestations: progressive fatigue, shortness of breath, palpitations, weakness, glossitis, nausea, anorexia, headache, fainting, irritability, forgetfulness, pallor, and slight jaundice. Folic acid deficiency anemia does not cause neurologic impairment unless it's associated with vitamin B_{12} deficiency, as in pernicious anemia.

Diagnosis

Decreased serum folate (by assay using specific strains of *Lactobacillus casei*) confirms folic acid deficiency anemia. The Schilling test and a therapeutic trial of vitamin B_{12} injections distinguish between folic acid deficiency anemia and pernicious anemia. Significant blood findings include macrocytosis, decreased reticulocyte count, and abnormal platelets.

Treatment

Treatment consists primarily of folic acid supplements and elimination of contributing causes. Folic acid supplements may be given orally (usually 1 to 5 mg/day), or parenterally (to patients who are severely ill, have malabsorption, or are unable to take oral medication).

Additional considerations

When treating a patient with folic acid deficiency anemia, the health care professional should:
• teach the patient to meet daily folic acid requirements by including a food from each food group in every meal; explain that diet only reinforces folic acid supplementation and isn't therapeutic by itself; urge compliance with the prescribed course of therapy; advise the patient not to stop taking the supplements when he begins to feel better.

FOODS HIGH IN FOLIC ACID CONTENT

Folic acid (pteroylglutamic acid, folacin) is found in most body tissues, where it acts as a coenzyme in metabolic processes involving one carbon transfer. It is essential for formation and maturation of RBCs and for synthesis of DNA. Although its body stores are comparatively small (about 70 mg), this vitamin is plentiful in most well-balanced diets.

However, because it's water-soluble and heat-labile, it's easily destroyed by cooking. Also, approximately 20% of folic acid intake is excreted unabsorbed. Insufficient daily folic acid intake (< 50 mcg/day) usually induces folic acid deficiency within 4 months. Below is a list of foods high in folic acid content.

FOOD	mcg/100 g
Asparagus spears	109
Beef liver	294
Broccoli spears	54
Collards (cooked)	102
Mushrooms	24
Oatmeal	33
Peanut butter	57
Red beans	180
Wheat germ	305

• emphasize the importance of good oral hygiene if the patient has glossitis; suggest regular use of mild or diluted mouthwash and a soft toothbrush.
• watch fluid and electrolyte balance, particularly in the patient who has severe diarrhea and is receiving parenteral fluid replacement therapy.
• remember that anemia causes severe fatigue; schedule regular rest periods until the patient is able to resume normal activity.
• emphasize the importance of a well-balanced diet high in folic acid to prevent folic acid deficiency anemia; identify alcoholics with poor dietary habits, and try to arrange for appropriate counseling; tell mothers who are not breast-feeding to use commercially prepared formulas.

Acute Blood Loss Anemia

Acute blood loss anemia is a life-threatening condition that results from sudden loss of RBCs and consequent depletion of hemoglobin and iron stores. The primary concern with this disorder is a rapid decrease in total blood volume, which can be fatal.

Causes

Acute blood loss anemia usually develops after severe trauma, postoperative or postpartum hemorrhage, coagulation defects, invasive neoplasm, ruptured peptic ulcer, or arterial damage or erosion caused by ruptured aneurysm or varices.

Signs and symptoms

Acute blood loss anemia usually produces clinical features associated with hypoxia and hypovolemia. Common symptoms include fatigue, anorexia, pallor, and faintness. These effects may vary, depending on the rapidity, severity, and site of blood loss.

In acute hemorrhage, when the total volume of blood lost is between 20% and 30%, symptoms of vascular insufficiency appear: anxiety, restlessness, orthostatic hypotension, dyspnea, tachycardia, diaphoresis, headache, and cool, clammy skin. When the total volume of blood lost exceeds 30%, circulatory failure, shock, and coma may follow. When blood loss exceeds 40%, death is imminent, unless the patient receives immediate volume replacement.

Diagnosis

Laboratory findings reflect hypovolemia and anemia. Platelet count increases initially; coagulation times decrease. Reticulocyte count typically ranges from 0.5% to 2% of total normal erythrocyte count, peaks 4 to 7 days after blood loss (a persistent rise means continuing hemorrhage), then drops after iron stores are depleted. RBC count, hemoglobin, and hematocrit eventually decrease markedly but are unreliable signs of recent blood loss, because compensatory vasoconstriction and hemoconcentration temporarily maintain falsely normal levels. Unless bleeding is obvious, X-rays and other tests may be necessary to identify bleeding sites. Elevated BUN (more than 25 mg/dl), for example, may indicate hemorrhage into the gastrointestinal lumen.

Treatment

The goals of treatment are to control hemorrhage and restore blood volume to prevent or combat shock. Immediate infusion of I.V. fluids (noncolloid, electrolyte solutions, such as lactated Ringer's solution) and plasma expanders can increase circulating volume while donor blood is being typed and cross matched. If hemoglobin drops below 10 g/100 ml, infusion of packed or frozen-thawed RBCs can begin to restore blood volume. Whole blood transfusions should be used only to replace a dangerously depleted red cell mass that may lead to life-threatening tissue anoxia.

Additional considerations

When caring for a hemorrhaging patient, the hospital staff member should:
• assess vital signs frequently for early indications of hypovolemic shock (tachycardia, hypotension).
• maintain a calm environment and offer reassurance, since the patient with impending shock may experience severe apprehension; explain that this feeling is a temporary physiologic phenomenon.
• monitor parenteral infusions; carefully monitor central venous pressure (CVP) or pulmonary artery pressure to evaluate blood volume; watch closely for signs of circulatory overload (elevated CVP, onset of pulmonary rales, pulmonary edema) if the patient receives volume expanders or large volumes of whole

TRANSFUSIONS: BLOOD TYPE COMPATIBILITY

Precise blood typing and cross matching are essential—if the donor's blood is incompatible with the recipient's, the transfusion can be fatal. In most instances, determining the recipient's blood type and cross matching it with available donor blood take less than 1 hour.

The four blood groups are distinguished by their agglutinogen (antigen in RBCs) and their agglutinin (antibody in serum or plasma):

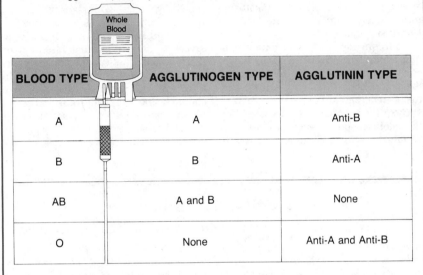

BLOOD TYPE	AGGLUTINOGEN TYPE	AGGLUTININ TYPE
A	A	Anti-B
B	B	Anti-A
AB	A and B	None
O	None	Anti-A and Anti-B

After determination of the recipient's blood type, it can be cross matched with a donor's. The following chart shows the groups that are compatible:

RECIPIENT		A	B	A B	O
COMPATIBLE DONOR	A	Yes	No	Yes	No
	B	No	Yes	Yes	No
	AB	No	No	Yes	No
	O	Yes	Yes	Yes	Yes

blood over a short time.
• double-check blood for transfusions (with another staff member) to make sure that the blood is for the right patient.
• watch carefully for signs of transfusion reaction (rash, hives, itching, fever, back pain, restlessness, shaking chills); take the patient's temperature before and after a transfusion; stop the transfusion immediately and notify the doctor if transfusion reaction occurs; assess vital signs frequently; substitute suitable volume expanders if the patient is in danger of shock; return the remaining blood to the blood bank, and record the transfusion reaction on the patient's chart.
• check for orthostatic hypotension (drop in systolic blood pressure of more than 15 mmHg, with a simultaneous rise in heart rate) when the patient sits up, before getting out of bed.
• administer oxygen, if needed, to relieve shortness of breath and ensure adequate oxygenation of vital organs.
• allow frequent rest periods, since the patient with anemia is easily fatigued.

Acute blood loss anemia can be prevented by watching for signs of bleeding in postoperative and postpartum patients, and in patients with histories of severe trauma, abnormal bleeding, or therapy with anticoagulants or drugs that irritate the gastrointestinal tract. In addition, all postoperative drainage should be monitored for frank and occult blood, and all patient histories checked on admission for use of anticoagulants or gastric irritants.

Hemochromatosis
(Bronze diabetes, Recklinghausen-Applebaum disease)

Hemochromatosis is a rare disorder characterized by iron overload in parenchymal cells, leading to cirrhosis (from iron deposits in the liver); diabetes (from iron deposits in the pancreas); cardiomegaly, with congestive heart failure and arrhythmias; and increased skin pigmentation. Prognosis depends on the extent of tissue damage at diagnosis. Hemochromatosis may be benign or fatal, depending on the amount and rapidity of parenchymal loading and the presence of hepatic disease from other causes. Death commonly results from hepatomas or myocardial damage.

Causes and incidence
Hemochromatosis may occur in several forms, with varying causes:
• *Erythropoietic:* This form of hemochromatosis is associated with hereditary sideroblastic anemia, β-thalassemia major, and other disorders characteristic of defective erythropoiesis.
• *Hepatic:* Such hemochromatosis seems directly related to hepatic disease that promotes excessive absorption of iron through abnormal mucosal regulation. Thus, it is often associated with alcoholism, malnutrition, viral hepatitis, and other disorders that impair iron utilization and absorption.
• *Idiopathic* (primary, familial, hereditary): Recent evidence suggests that hemochromatosis may be inherited as an autosomal dominant or recessive trait. Nearly half the relatives of patients with this disease also have a tendency toward increased iron absorption. Idiopathic hemochromatosis is about 10 times more common in males than in females, probably because females lose iron each month during menses. (In general, hemochromatosis rarely occurs before age 20; peak incidence is during the 40s.)

Rarely, the excessive ingestion of iron over many years (Bantu siderosis) results in hemochromatosis.

Increased iron absorption typical of hemochromatosis may result from an absence of pancreatic or gastric substances that normally regulate iron absorption. When plasma levels are normal, reticuloendothelial cells store most of the excess iron. When plasma levels are elevated, however, and transferrin levels rise above 60% saturation (compared with the normal 20% to 50%), some of the excess iron must be stored in parenchymal cells. In hemochromatosis, the slow accumulation of iron deposits in parenchymal cells causes tissue damage and typical clinical features.

Signs and symptoms
The course of hemochromatosis varies with dietary iron intake and ingestion of hepatotoxins, such as alcohol; it tends to be less severe in females. Characteristically, hemochromatosis produces the following cardinal signs:
• *diabetes* (most common sign), with subsequent weakness, lassitude, and weight loss. Diabetes results from fibrotic pancreatic changes and a reduction in the number of islets of Langerhans, with consequent diminished beta cell function.
• *cirrhotic hepatomegaly,* which may cause abdominal pain, spider angiomas, and rarely, ascites. Hemochromatosis is also associated with a rising incidence of hepatomas.
• *increased skin pigmentation* (usually bronze) from melanin accumulation (in 90% of patients). However, skin color may be metallic gray, caused by iron deposits in the skin itself.
• *cardiac dysfunction,* such as arrhythmias, cardiomyopathy, or progressive congestive heart failure.

Other common abnormalities in patients with hemochromatosis include testicular atrophy and loss of libido (possibly caused by depressed pituitary gonadotropin secretion), hypopituitarism, chondrocalcinosis (calcium deposits in cartilage), and arthritic joint pain from iron deposits in the synovial membrane.

Diagnosis
Diagnosis is based on observation of clinical features, and laboratory results that suggest iron excess:
• *serum or plasma iron concentration:* more than 225 to 325 mcg/100 ml
• *transferrin levels:* increased to 80% to 100% saturation
• *24-hour urine collection:* iron excretion 10 mg or more after administration of deferoxamine, an iron-chelating agent.

In patients with such abnormal findings, other appropriate tests may include liver biopsy and liver function studies, skin biopsy to test for iron deposits in the skin, glucose tolerance test to detect diabetes, EKG and chest X-ray to show cardiac involvement, and blood studies to check for anemia and for hypochromia and abnormally shaped RBCs, to rule out defective erythropoiesis as the cause of iron overload.

Treatment
Primary treatment is the removal of excess iron. Phlebotomy, the most effective way to remove excess iron, allows removal of at least 500 ml of blood weekly, until the serum iron level drops to less than 100 mcg/100 ml. Frequent phlebotomy may be necessary for 3 years or longer, depending on the patient's iron levels. Administration of deferoxamine mobilizes iron stores and promotes iron excretion but removes only about half as much iron as phlebotomy. Of course, associated conditions, such as diabetes, require appropriate treatment.

Additional considerations
Thorough patient teaching can improve patient compliance with treatment and can prevent complications. Sympathetic psychologic support can help the patient cope with the distorted body image that results from marked skin discoloration.

Supportive care includes:
• assessing skin color for characteristic changes (bronze, cyanotic, grayish).
• assisting during phlebotomy, and reassuring the patient during the procedure.
• administering deferoxamine by subcutaneous or I.M. injection, or by slow I.V. infusion with normal saline solution, as ordered; watching for signs of rapid infusion (flushing, urticaria, hypotension, or shock); explaining that deferoxamine may give urine a reddish tint.
• assessing dietary iron intake, and stressing compliance with treatment to

prevent life-threatening complications.
• advising alcoholics with this disorder that their risk of liver damage is greatly increased, and referring them to Alcoholics Anonymous or other supportive agencies.
• telling the patient's family they may have inherited hemochromatosis; teaching them how to recognize its effects, and encouraging screening to detect increased iron levels, so treatment can begin before tissue damage occurs; warning patients about the dangers of long-term self-medication with iron supplements.

Aplastic or Hypoplastic Anemias

Aplastic or hypoplastic anemias result from injury to or destruction of stem cells in bone marrow or the bone marrow matrix, causing pancytopenia (anemia, granulocytopenia, thrombocytopenia) and bone marrow hypoplasia. Although often used interchangeably with other terms for bone marrow failure, aplastic anemias properly refer to pancytopenia resulting from the decreased functional capacity of a hypoplastic, fatty bone marrow. These disorders generally produce fatal bleeding or infection, particularly when they're idiopathic or stem from chloramphenicol or from infectious hepatitis. Mortality for aplastic anemias with severe pancytopenia is 50% to 70%.

Causes and incidence
Aplastic anemias usually develop when damaged or destroyed stem cells inhibit RBC production. Less commonly, they develop when damaged bone marrow microvasculature creates an unfavorable environment for cell growth and maturation. Approximately half of such anemias result from drugs, toxic agents (such as benzene and chloramphenicol), or radiation. The rest may result from immunologic factors (suspected but unconfirmed) or severe disease, especially hepatitis.

Idiopathic anemias may be congenital. Two such forms of aplastic anemia have been identified: congenital hypoplastic anemia (anemia of Blackfan and Diamond) develops between ages 2 months and 3 months; Fanconi's syndrome, between birth and age 10. In Fanconi's syndrome, chromosomal abnormalities are usually associated with multiple congenital anomalies—such as dwarfism, and hypoplasia of the kidneys and spleen. In the absence of a consistent familial or genetic history of aplastic anemia, researchers suspect that these congenital abnormalities result from an induced change in the development of the fetus.

Signs and symptoms
Clinical features of aplastic anemias vary with the severity of pancytopenia but often develop insidiously. Anemic symptoms include progressive weakness and fatigue, shortness of breath, headache, pallor, and ultimately, tachycardia and congestive heart failure. Thrombocytopenia leads to ecchymosis, petechiae, and hemorrhage, especially from the mucous membranes (nose, gums, rectum, vagina) or into the retina or central nervous system. Neutropenia may lead to infection (fever, oral and rectal ulcers, sore throat), but without characteristic inflammation.

Diagnosis
Confirmation of aplastic anemia requires a series of laboratory tests:
• *RBCs* are usually normochromic and normocytic (although macrocytosis [larger than normal erythrocytes] and anisocytosis [excessive variation in erythrocyte size] may exist), with a total count of 1,000,000 or less. *Absolute reticulocyte count is very low.*
• *Serum iron* is elevated (unless bleeding occurs), but total iron-binding capacity is normal or slightly reduced.

BONE MARROW TRANSPLANTATION

In bone marrow transplantation, 500 to 700 ml of marrow are aspirated from the pelvic bones of a donor with HLA antigens compatible with the recipient. The donor is usually the recipient's twin or sibling. The donated marrow is filtered and then infused into the recipient in an attempt to repopulate his marrow with normal cells. This procedure has proven successful in treating severe aplastic anemia; it has resulted in long-term, healthy survivals for about half the patients who received such marrow transplantation. Transplantation may also be effective in treating acute leukemia and certain immunodeficiency diseases.

Because bone marrow transplantation carries serious risks, it requires reverse isolation, primary care and strict aseptic technique.

Before transplantation, the health care professional should:
• apply pressure dressings to the *donor's* aspiration sites after bone marrow aspiration is completed under local anesthetic; observe them for bleeding; relieve pain at these sites with analgesics and ice packs, as needed.
• admit the patient (recipient) to a reverse isolation unit with laminar air flow, if possible; obtain swabs for culture from each orifice; give the patient an antiseptic bath and shampoo; provide a sterile gown.
• assess the patient's understanding of bone marrow transplantation; correct any misconceptions, if necessary, and provide additional information; prepare the patient for a long stay in the hospital, but give encouragement by explaining that chances for recovery are good.
• give appropriate care if high-dose cyclophosphamide I.V. is given to suppress the immune system (usually given for 2 days, with I.V. fluids, furosemide, and urine alkalinization to force diuresis and prevent hemorrhagic cystitis). Care includes maintaining urine pH between 7 and 9; controlling nausea and vomiting with an antiemetic, such as prochlorperazine, as needed; giving allopurinol, as ordered, to prevent hyperuricemia resulting from tumor breakdown products; encouraging the patient to choose a wig or scarf before treatment begins, since alopecia is a common side effect.
• warn the patient that cataracts, gastrointestinal disturbances, and sterility are possible side effects of total bone irradiation, which is performed to induce total marrow aplasia; explain that radiation treatments and cyclophosphamide therapy are necessary to lower the body's resistance to the transplant.

During I.V. infusion of donated bone marrow, the professional should:
• monitor vital signs every 15 minutes for adverse reactions.
• watch for complications of marrow infusion, such as pulmonary embolus and volume overload.
• reassure the patient throughout the procedure.

After infusion is complete, the professional should:
• continue to monitor vital signs every 15 minutes for 2 to 4 hours after infusion, then every 4 hours; watch for fever and chills, which may be the only signs of infection (pus will not form at infection sites, because the patient doesn't have granulocytes); give prophylactic antibiotics, as ordered; avoid administering medications rectally or intramuscularly, to reduce the possibility of bleeding.
• administer methotrexate, as ordered, to prevent graft-versus-host (GVH) reaction, a potentially fatal complication of transplantation; watch for signs of GVH reaction, such as maculopapular rash, pancytopenia, jaundice, joint pain, and anasarca; remember that unchecked GVH reaction may cause massive, fatal hemorrhage.
• administer vitamins, and iron and folic acid supplements, as ordered. Blood products, such as platelets and packed RBCs, may also be indicated, depending on the results of daily blood studies.
• give good mouth care every 2 hours; use hydrogen peroxide and nystatin mouthwash, to prevent candidiasis and other mouth infections; provide meticulous skin care, paying special attention to pressure points and open sites, such as aspiration and I.V. sites.

Hemosiderin is present, and tissue iron storage is visible microscopically.

- *Platelet, neutrophil,* and *WBC counts* fall.
- *Coagulation tests* (bleeding time), reflecting decreased platelet count, are abnormal.
- Results of *bone marrow biopsies,* taken from several sites, may yield a "dry tap" or show severely hypocellular or aplastic marrow, with a varying amount of fat, fibrous tissue, or gelatinous replacement; absence of tagged iron (since the iron is deposited in the liver rather than in bone marrow) and megakaryocytes; and depression of erythroid elements.

Differential diagnosis must rule out paroxysmal nocturnal hemoglobinuria and other diseases in which pancytopenia is common.

Treatment

Effective treatment must eliminate any identifiable cause and provide vigorous supportive measures, such as packed red cell, platelet, and experimental HLA-matched leukocyte transfusions. Even after elimination of the cause, recovery can take months. Bone marrow transplantation is the treatment of choice for anemia due to severe aplasia and for patients who need constant RBC transfusions.

Reverse isolation is necessary to prevent infection in patients with low leukocyte counts. The infection itself may require specific antibiotics; however, these are not given prophylactically, because they tend to encourage resistant strains of organisms. Patients with low hemoglobin counts may need respiratory support with oxygen, in addition to blood transfusions.

Other appropriate forms of treatment include corticosteroids to stimulate erythroid production (successful in children, unsuccessful in adults), and marrow-stimulating agents, such as androgens (which are controversial).

Additional considerations

When treating a patient with aplastic anemia, the hospital staff member should:

- prevent hemorrhage if platelet count is low (less than 20,000/mm³) by avoiding I.M. injections, suggesting the use of an electric razor and a soft toothbrush, humidifying oxygen to prevent drying of mucous membranes (dry mucosa may bleed), and promoting regular bowel movements through the use of a stool softener and diet to prevent constipation (which may damage rectal mucosa and lead to bleeding); apply pressure to venipuncture sites until bleeding stops; detect bleeding problems early by routinely checking for blood in urine and stool, and assessing skin for petechiae.
- help prevent infection by washing hands thoroughly before entering the patient's room, by making sure the patient is receiving a nutritious diet (high in vitamins and proteins) to improve his resistance, and by encouraging meticulous mouth and perianal care.
- watch for life-threatening hemorrhage, infection, side effects of drug therapy, or blood transfusion reaction; make sure routine throat, urine, and blood cultures are done regularly and correctly to check for infection; teach the patient to recognize signs of infection, and tell him to report them immediately.
- schedule frequent rest periods if the patient has a low hemoglobin count, which causes fatigue, to compensate for inadequate oxygen exchange; administer oxygen therapy, as needed; check the patient's temperature before and after any blood transfusions to assess for a transfusion reaction; watch for other signs of transfusion reaction, such as rash, hives, itching, back pain, restlessness, and shaking chills.
- provide reassurance and emotional support to the patient and family by explaining the nature of this disease and its treatment, particularly if the patient has recurring acute episodes; explain the purpose of all prescribed drugs, and discuss possible side effects; tell the patient which side effects should be reported promptly; encourage the patient who doesn't require hospitalization to continue his normal life-style, with some restrictions (such as rest periods, as nec-

essary), until remission occurs.
- monitor blood studies carefully to prevent aplastic anemia in the patient receiving anemia-inducing drugs.
- support efforts to educate the public about the hazards of toxic agents; tell parents to keep toxic agents out of the reach of children; encourage persons who work with radiation to wear protective clothing and a radiation-detecting badge, and to observe plant safety precautions; tell persons who work with benzene (solvent) that 10 parts per million is the highest safe level, and that a delayed reaction to benzene may develop.

Sideroblastic Anemias

Sideroblastic anemias comprise a group of heterogenous disorders with a common defect—failure to use iron in hemoglobin synthesis, despite the availability of adequate iron stores. These anemias may be hereditary or acquired; the acquired form, in turn, can be primary or secondary. Hereditary sideroblastic anemia often responds to treatment with pyridoxine. Correction of the secondary acquired form depends on the causative disorder; the primary acquired (idiopathic) form, however, resists treatment and usually proves fatal within 10 years after onset of complications or a concomitant disease.

Causes and incidence
Hereditary sideroblastic anemia appears to be transmitted by X-linked inheritance, occurring mostly in young males; females are carriers and usually show no signs of this disorder.

The acquired form may be secondary to ingestion of or exposure to toxins, such as alcohol and lead, or to drugs, such as isoniazid and chloramphenicol. It can also occur as a complication of other diseases, such as rheumatoid arthritis, lupus erythematosus, multiple myeloma, tuberculosis, and severe infections.

The primary acquired form, in which the cause is unknown, is most common in the elderly, but occasionally develops in the young. It's often associated with thrombocytopenia or leukopenia.

In sideroblastic anemia, normoblasts (precursors of erythrocytes) fail to use iron to synthesize hemoglobin. As a result, iron deposits in the mitochondria of normoblasts, which are then termed ringed sideroblasts.

Signs and symptoms
Sideroblastic anemias usually produce nonspecific clinical effects, which may exist for several years before being identified. Such effects include anorexia, fatigue, weakness, dizziness, pale skin and mucous membranes, and occasionally, enlarged lymph nodes. Heart and liver failure may develop due to excessive

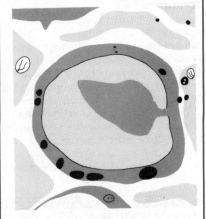

RINGED SIDEROBLAST

Electron microscopy shows large iron deposits in the mitochondria that surround the nucleus, forming the characteristic ringed sideroblast.

iron accumulation in these organs, causing dyspnea, exertional angina, slight jaundice, and hepatosplenomegaly. Hereditary sideroblastic anemia is associated with increased gastrointestinal absorption of iron, causing signs of hemosiderosis. Additional symptoms in secondary sideroblastic anemia depend upon the underlying cause.

Diagnosis

Ringed sideroblasts on microscopic examination of bone marrow aspirate, stained with Prussian blue or alizarin red dye, confirm this diagnosis. Microscopic examination of blood shows erythrocytes to be hypochromic or normochromic, and slightly macrocytic. Red cell precursors may be megaloblastic, with anisocytosis (abnormal variation in RBC size) and poikilocytosis (abnormal variation in RBC shape). Unlike iron deficiency anemia, sideroblastic anemia lowers hemoglobin, and raises serum iron and transferrin levels. In turn, faulty hemoglobin production raises urobilinogen and bilirubin levels. Platelets and leukocytes remain normal, but occasionally, thrombocytopenia or leukopenia occurs.

Treatment

Treatment of sideroblastic anemias depends on the underlying cause. The hereditary form usually responds to several weeks of treatment with high doses of pyridoxine (vitamin B_6). The acquired secondary form generally subsides after the causative drug or toxin is removed or the underlying condition is adequately treated. Folic acid supplements may also be beneficial when concomitant megaloblastic nuclear changes in RBC precursors are present. Elderly patients with

sideroblastic anemia—most commonly the primary acquired form—are less likely to improve quickly and are more likely to develop serious complications.

Carefully cross-matched transfusions (providing needed hemoglobin) or high doses of androgens are effective palliative measures for some patients with the primary acquired form of sideroblastic anemia. However, this form is essentially refractory to treatment, and usually leads to death from acute leukemia or from respiratory or cardiac complications.

Some patients with sideroblastic anemia may benefit from phlebotomy to prevent hemochromatosis. Phlebotomy steps up the rate of erythropoiesis and uses up excess iron stores; thus, it reduces serum and total-body iron levels.

Additional considerations

Health care and management are symptomatic and should emphasize patient teaching, including:

• administering medications, as ordered, and teaching the patient the importance of continuing prescribed therapy, even after he begins to feel better.

• providing frequent rest periods if the patient becomes easily fatigued.

• explaining the procedure thoroughly to help reduce anxiety if phlebotomy is scheduled; providing a high-protein diet, if phlebotomy must be repeated frequently, to help replace the protein lost during this procedure; encouraging the patient to follow a similar diet at home.

• always inquiring about the possibility of exposure to lead in the home (especially for children) or on the job.

• identifying and referring patients who abuse alcohol for appropriate therapy.

• supporting programs to educate the public about toxins, such as lead or alcohol, that can cause this disorder.

Thalassemia

Thalassemia, a hereditary group of hemolytic anemias, is characterized by defective synthesis in the polypeptide chains necessary for hemoglobin production. Conse-

quently, RBC synthesis is also impaired. Thalassemia is most common in persons of Mediterranean ancestry (especially Italian and Greek), but also occurs in Blacks and persons from southern China, Southeast Asia, and India.

β-Thalassemia is the most common form of this disorder, resulting from defective beta polypeptide chain synthesis. It occurs in three clinical forms: thalassemia major, intermedia, and minor. The severity of the resulting anemia depends on whether the patient is homozygous or heterozygous for the thalassemic trait. Prognosis for β-thalassemia varies. Patients with thalassemia major seldom survive to adulthood; children with thalassemia intermedia develop normally into adulthood, although puberty is usually delayed; persons with thalassemia minor can expect a normal life span.

Causes

Thalassemia major and *thalassemia intermedia* result from homozygous inheritance of the partially dominant autosomal gene responsible for this trait. *Thalassemia minor* results from heterozygous inheritance of the same gene. In all these disorders, total or partial deficiency of beta chain production impairs hemoglobin synthesis and results in continual production of fetal hemoglobin, even past the neonatal period.

Signs and symptoms

In thalassemia major (also known as Cooley's anemia, Mediterranean disease, and erythroblastic anemia), the infant is well at birth, but develops severe anemia, bone abnormalities, failure to thrive, and life-threatening complications. Often, the first signs are pallor, and yellow skin and scleras in infants aged 3 to 6 months. Later clinical features, in addition to severe anemia, include splenomegaly or hepatomegaly, with abdominal enlargement; frequent infections; bleeding tendencies (especially toward epistaxis); and anorexia.

Children with thalassemia major commonly have small bodies and large heads, and may also be mentally retarded. Infants may have mongoloid features, because bone marrow hyperactivity has thickened the bone at the base of the nose. As these children grow older, they become susceptible to pathologic fractures, as a result of expansion of the marrow cavities with thinning of the long bones. They are also subject to cardiac arrhythmias, heart failure, and other complications that result from iron deposits in the heart and in other tissues from repeated blood transfusions.

Thalassemia intermedia comprises moderate thalassemic disorders in homozygotes. Patients with this condition show some degree of anemia, jaundice, and splenomegaly, and possibly, signs of hemosiderosis due to increased intestinal absorption of iron.

Thalassemia minor may cause mild anemia but usually produces no symptoms and is often overlooked.

Diagnosis

A careful history, physical examination, laboratory tests, and X-rays help confirm this diagnosis.

In thalassemia major, laboratory results show lowered RBCs and hemoglobin and elevated reticulocytes, bilirubin,

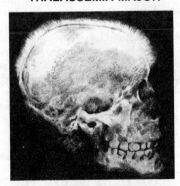

THALASSEMIA MAJOR

This X-ray shows a characteristic skull abnormality in thalassemia major: diploetic fibers extending from internal lamina.

and urinary and fecal urobilinogen. A low serum folate level indicates increased folate utilization by the hypertrophied bone marrow. A peripheral blood smear reveals target cells (extremely thin and fragile RBCs), pale nucleated RBCs, and marked anisocytosis.

X-rays of the skull and long bones show a thinning and widening of the marrow space in thalassemia major, because of overactive bone marrow. The bones of the skull and vertebrae may appear granular; long bones may show areas of osteoporosis. The phalanges may also be deformed (rectangular or biconvex). Hemoglobin electrophoresis demonstrates a significant rise in Hb F and a slight increase in Hb A_2. Diagnosis must rule out iron deficiency anemia, which also produces hypochromia and microcytic RBCs.

In thalassemia intermedia, laboratory results show hypochromia and microcytic RBCs, but the anemia is less severe than that in thalassemia major. In thalassemia minor, laboratory results show hypochromia (slightly lowered hemoglobin) and microcytic (notably small) RBCs. Hemoglobin electrophoresis shows a significant increase in Hb A_2 and a moderate rise in Hb F.

Treatment
Treatment of thalassemia major is essentially supportive. For example, infections require prompt treatment with appropriate antibiotics. Folic acid supplements help maintain folic acid levels in the face of increased requirements. Transfusions of packed RBCs raise hemoglobin levels but must be used judiciously to minimize iron overload. Splenectomy and bone marrow transplantation have been tried, but their effectiveness has not been confirmed.

Thalassemia intermedia and thalassemia minor generally don't require treatment.

Iron supplements are contraindicated in all forms of thalassemia.

Additional considerations
When treating a thalassemia patient, the health care professional should:
• watch for adverse reactions—shaking chills, fever, rash, itching, and hives—during and after RBC transfusions for thalassemia major.
• tell persons with thalassemia minor that their condition is benign.
• stress the importance of good nutrition, meticulous wound care, periodic dental checkups, and other measures to prevent infection.
• discuss with the parents of a young patient various options for healthy physical and creative outlets, after assessing the child's interests and activities. Such a child must avoid strenuous athletic activity because of increased oxygen demand and the tendency toward pathologic fractures, but he may participate in less stressful activities.
• teach parents to watch for signs of hepatitis and iron overload—always possible with frequent transfusions.
• refer parents for genetic counseling, since they may have questions about the vulnerability of future offspring; refer adult patients with thalassemia minor and thalassemia intermedia for genetic counseling—they need to recognize the risk of transmitting thalassemia major to their children if they marry another person with thalassemia. If such persons choose to marry and have children, all their children should be evaluated for thalassemia by age 1.

Anemia Secondary to Chronic Diseases

Certain chronic diseases depress bone marrow function and thereby induce secondary anemia. Such anemia is usually mild, although its severity varies with the underlying cause.

Causes

Chronic diseases most likely to induce secondary anemia are lung abscesses, tuberculosis, renal or hepatic failure, viral hepatitis, rheumatoid arthritis, rheumatic fever, bacterial endocarditis, osteomyelitis, and cancer. How chronic disease depresses bone marrow function is unknown.

Signs and symptoms

Secondary anemia usually develops about 1 to 2 months after onset of chronic disease. In many patients, the anemia is asymptomatic; the only clinical effects are those of the underlying disorder. In other patients, the features are clearly those of anemia. In mild anemia, such symptoms may include anorexia, listlessness, weight loss, and pallor. Such pallor results from a compensatory mechanism that shifts blood away from skin and peripheral tissues to increase blood flow to vital organs. If anemia is severe (rare), it may produce weakness, faintness, tachycardia, shortness of breath, and eventually, congestive heart failure.

Diagnosis

The most characteristic difference be-tween anemia secondary to chronic diseases and other anemias is that, in secondary anemia, serum iron levels drop despite adequate iron stores. Additional laboratory findings show RBCs that are normocytic and normochromic (sometimes hypochromic), normal or slightly raised reticulocyte count, shortened erythrocyte life span, and lowered total iron-binding capacity. Other laboratory values are consistent with the underlying disease.

Treatment and additional considerations

No standard form of therapy exists, other than treatment of the underlying cause. Therapy may include packed RBC transfusion (if anemia causes symptoms), but this is uncommon. Iron therapy is not beneficial; any drug therapy is specific to the underlying cause.

Health care is supportive and symptomatic. In addition, the health care professional should teach the patient about this disease so he knows his limitations, help him set realistic goals that take into account the fatigue that accompanies anemia, and urge regular medical checkups.

Iron Deficiency Anemia

Iron deficiency anemia is caused by an inadequate supply of iron for optimal formation of RBCs, resulting in smaller (microcytic) cells with less color on staining. Body stores of iron, including plasma iron, decrease, as does transferrin, which binds with and transports iron. Insufficient body stores of iron lead to a depleted RBC mass and, in turn, to a decreased hemoglobin concentration (hypochromia) and decreased oxygen-carrying capacity of the blood. A common disease worldwide, iron deficiency anemia affects 10% to 30% of the adult population of the United States.

Causes and incidence

Iron deficiency anemia results from:
• inadequate dietary intake of iron (less than 1 to 2 mg/day), as in prolonged unsupplemented breast- or bottle-feeding of infants, or during periods of stress, such as rapid growth in children and adolescents.

• iron malabsorption, as in chronic diarrhea, partial or total gastrectomy, and malabsorption syndromes, such as celiac disease.
• blood loss secondary to drug-induced gastrointestinal bleeding (from anticoagulants, aspirin, steroids), or due to heavy menses, hemorrhage from trauma,

gastrointestinal ulcers, malignancy, or varices.

• pregnancy, in which the mother's iron supply is diverted to the fetus for erythropoiesis.

• intravascular hemolysis-induced hemoglobinuria or paroxysmal nocturnal hemoglobinuria.

• mechanical erythrocyte trauma caused by a prosthetic heart valve.

Iron deficiency anemia occurs most commonly in premenopausal women, infants (particularly premature or low–birth-weight infants), children, and adolescents (especially girls).

Signs and symptoms

Because of the gradual progression of iron deficiency anemia, many patients are initially asymptomatic, except for symptoms of any underlying condition. They tend not to seek medical treatment until anemia is severe. At advanced stages, decreased hemoglobin and the consequent decrease in the blood's oxygen-carrying capacity cause the patient to develop dyspnea on exertion, fatigue, listlessness, pallor, inability to concentrate, irritability, headache, and a susceptibility to infection. Decreased oxygen perfusion causes the heart to compensate with increased cardiac output and tachycardia.

In patients with chronic iron deficiency anemia, nails become spoon-shaped and brittle, the corners of the mouth crack, the tongue turns smooth, and the patient complains of dysphagia. Associated neuromuscular effects include vasomotor disturbances, numbness and tingling of the extremities, and neuralgic pain.

Diagnosis

Blood studies (serum iron, total iron-binding capacity, ferritin levels) and stores in bone marrow may confirm iron deficiency anemia. However, the results of these tests can be misleading because of complicating factors, such as infection, pneumonia, blood transfusion, or iron supplements. Characteristic blood study results include:

• low hemoglobin levels (males, < 12g/100 ml; females, < 10g/100 ml)

• low hematocrit levels (males, < 47 ml/100 ml; females, < 42 ml/100 ml)

• low serum iron levels, with high binding capacity

• low serum ferritin levels

• low RBC count, with microcytic and hypochromic cells (in early stages, RBC count may be normal, except in infants and children)

• decreased mean corpuscular hemoglobin in severe anemia.

Bone marrow studies reveal depleted or absent iron stores (done by staining) and normoblastic hyperplasia.

Diagnosis must rule out other forms of anemia, such as those that result from thalassemia minor, malignancy, and chronic inflammatory, hepatic, and renal disease.

Prevention

The public health professional can play a vital role in the prevention of iron deficiency anemia by:

• teaching the basics of a nutritionally balanced diet—red meats, green vegetables, eggs, whole wheat, iron-fortified

---

ABSORPTION AND STORAGE OF IRON

Iron, which is essential to erythropoiesis, is abundant throughout the body. Two thirds of total body iron is found in hemoglobin; the other third, mostly in the reticuloendothelial system (liver, spleen, bone marrow), with small amounts in muscle, blood serum, and body cells.

Adequate dietary ingestion of iron and recirculation of iron released from disintegrating red cells maintain iron supplies. The duodenum and upper part of the small intestine absorb dietary iron. Such absorption depends on gastric acid content, the amount of reducing substances (ascorbic acid, for example) present in the alimentary canal, and dietary iron intake. If iron intake is deficient, the body gradually depletes its iron stores, causing decreased hemoglobin and, eventually, symptoms of iron deficiency anemia.

bread, and milk. (However, no food in itself contains enough iron to *treat* iron deficiency anemia; an average-sized person with anemia would have to eat at least 10 lb of steak daily to receive therapeutic amounts of iron.)

• emphasizing the need for high-risk individuals—such as premature infants, children under age 2, and pregnant women—to receive prophylactic oral iron, as ordered by a doctor. (Children under age 2 should also receive supplemental cereals and formulas high in iron.)

• assessing a family's dietary habits for iron intake and noting the influence of childhood eating patterns, cultural food preferences, and family income on adequate nutrition.

• encouraging the consumption of iron-rich foods and drinks, especially bread and milk, for families whose iron intake is deficient.

• carefully assessing a patient's drug history, since certain drugs, such as pancreatic enzymes and vitamin E, may interfere with iron metabolism and absorption, and since aspirin, steroids, and other drugs may cause gastrointestinal bleeding. (Patients who must take gastric irritants should be taught to take these medications with meals or milk.)

Treatment

The first priority of treatment is to determine the underlying cause of anemia. Once this is determined, iron replacement therapy can begin. Treatment of choice is an oral preparation of iron or a combination of iron and ascorbic acid (which enhances iron absorption). However, iron may have to be administered parenterally—if the patient is noncompliant to the oral preparation, if he needs more iron than he can take orally, if gastrointestinal malabsorption prevents iron absorption, or if a maximum rate of hemoglobin regeneration is desired.

Because total dose I.V. infusion is painless and requires fewer injections, it's usually preferred to I.M. administration. Pregnant patients and geriatric patients with severe anemia, for exam-

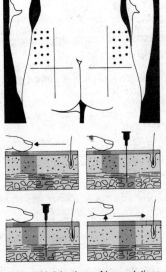

HOW TO INJECT IRON SOLUTIONS

For deep I.M. injections of iron solutions, the Z-track technique is used with a 19- to 20-gauge, 5- to 7.5-cm (2- to 3-in) needle to avoid subcutaneous irritation and discoloration from leaking medication. After drawing up the solution, a fresh needle is used to avoid tracking the solution through to subcutaneous tissue, and 0.5 cc of air is let into the syringe.

The skin, fat, and muscle at the injection site (in upper outer quadrant of buttocks only) is displaced firmly to one side. The needle is inserted after cleansing the area. The solution is slowly injected, followed by the 0.5 cc of air in the syringe. After waiting 10 seconds, the needle is pulled straight out, and tissues released.

Pressure is applied directly to the insertion site, but it is not massaged. The patient must avoid vigorous exercise for 15 to 30 minutes.

ple, should receive a total dose infusion of iron dextran in normal saline solution over 8 hours. To minimize the risk of an allergic reaction to iron, an I.V. test dose of 0.5 ml should be given first.

Additional considerations

When treating a patient for anemia, the health care professional should:

• monitor compliance with the prescribed iron supplement therapy; advise

SUPPORTIVE MANAGEMENT OF PATIENTS WITH ANEMIA

The anemic patient's nutritional needs can be met by:
• giving him small, frequent meals throughout the day if he is fatigued.
• serving soft, cool, bland foods if he has oral lesions.
• eliminating spicy foods, and including milk and dairy products in his diet if he has dyspepsia.
• having his family bring his favorite foods from home (unless his diet is restricted) and keeping him company during meals if he is anorexic and irritable.

Activities can be limited by:
• monitoring the patient's pulse rate during the specific activity to assess its effect. If his pulse accelerates rapidly and he develops hypotension with hypernoia, diaphoresis, light-headedness, palpitations, shortness of breath, or weakness, the activity is too strenuous.
• pacing his activities, and allowing for frequent rest periods.

The patient's susceptibility to infection can be decreased by:
• using strict aseptic technique.
• isolating the patient from infectious persons.
• instructing him to avoid crowds and other sources of infection; encouraging him to practice good hand-washing technique; stressing the importance of receiving necessary immunizations and prompt medical treatment for any sign of infection.

The patient can be prepared for diagnostic testing by:
• explaining erythropoiesis, the function of blood, and the purpose of diagnostic and therapeutic procedures.
• telling the patient how he can participate in diagnostic testing, and giving him an honest description of the pain or discomfort he will probably experience.
• scheduling all tests to avoid disrupting the patient's meals, sleep, and visiting hours.

Complications can be prevented by:
• observing for signs of bleeding that may exacerbate anemia; checking stool for occult bleeding; assessing for ecchymoses, gingival bleeding, and hematuria; monitoring vital signs.
• assisting with range-of-motion exercises and frequent turning, coughing, and deep breathing if the patient is confined to strict bed rest.
• giving washed RBCs, as ordered, in partial exchange if evidence of pump failure is present (blood transfusions are needed for severe anemia if hemoglobin is less than 5 g/100ml); carefully monitoring for signs of circulatory overload or transfusion reaction; watching for a change in pulse rate, blood pressure, or respirations, or onset of fever, chills, pruritus, or edema; stopping the transfusion and notifying the doctor if any of these signs develop.
• warning the patient to move about or change positions slowly to minimize dizziness induced by cerebral hypoxia.

---

the patient not to stop therapy even if he feels better, since replacement of iron stores takes time; check the patient's stool, which will be black if he's taking iron.
• advise the patient that milk or an antacid interferes with absorption; instruct the patient to drink iron in a liquid form through a straw to prevent staining the teeth.
• tell the patient to report any side effects of iron therapy, such as nausea, vomiting, diarrhea, or constipation, which may require a dosage adjustment.
• check the patient's history for allergies (the patient with other allergies may be allergic to iron, too).
• monitor the infusion rate carefully if the patient receives iron intravenously, and observe for an allergic reaction; stop the infusion and begin supportive treatment immediately if the patient shows signs of an adverse reaction; watch for dizziness and headache, and for thrombophlebitis around the I.V. site.
• use the Z-track injection method when administering iron I.M. to prevent skin discoloration, scarring, and irritating iron deposits in the skin.
• advise regular checkups, since an iron deficiency may recur.

Rare Hemolytic Anemias

CAUSES AND INCIDENCE	SYMPTOMS AND DIAGNOSIS	MANAGEMENT

INTRACORPUSCULAR ABNORMALITIES

G-6-PD deficiency
(glucose-6-phosphate dehydrogenase deficiency)

- Congenital sex-linked deficiency of this RBC enzyme, transmitted from mother to son, exaggerates susceptibility to hemolysis after ingestion of chemical oxidants (phenacetin, chloramphenicol, nitrofurantoin, sulfonamides, antimalarials, and in some Caucasians, fava beans).
- Severe infections for diabetic acidosis may also provoke hemolytic episodes.
- Common in persons of African or Mediterranean ancestry

- May be self-limiting (aging RBCs destroyed first)
- In severe cases, shortness of breath, fatigue, jaundice, dark urine, and possibly, hemoglobinuric renal failure (especially in Caucasians)
- Increased reticulocytes, hemoglobin, and serum bilirubin
- Decreased hematocrit
- Initially, Heinz bodies (particles of oxidized hemoglobin) present on RBCs

---

- Transfusions of whole blood or packed RBCs for rapid and severe hemolysis (as in favism)
- Exchange transfusion for infants with neonatal jaundice
- Osmotic diuresis for hemoglobinuria
- High-risk patients (and other family members) screened by direct blood assay and electrophoresis
- Patients given a list of oxidating agents to avoid

Hereditary spherocytosis

- Inherited autosomal dominant gene increases RBC membrane permeability and intracellular hypertonicity. Red cells become swollen, spherical, and rigid, and thus vulnerable to entrapment and destruction by spleen.

- Slight jaundice, anemia, splenomegaly, tendency to cholelithiasis (during infancy or delayed until adulthood)
- Small, spherical RBCs on peripheral blood smear

- Splenectomy corrects symptoms, but RBC defect persists In children, splenectomy is often delayed until age 3 or 4
- Patients or their parents told that this condition is inherited as a simple Mendelian dominant trait; it can be transmitted if only one parent carries the abnormal gene. This trait may skip generations

EXTRACORPUSCULAR ABNORMALITIES

Acquired hemolytic anemias

- Trauma (burns, snakebite)
- Underlying disease (infection, splenic disorders, systemic diseases [leukemias, lymphomas, lupus erythematosus])
- Medical and surgical procedures (incompatible blood transfusions, prosthetic heart valves)
- Others (heavy metal poisoning, autoimmunity resulting in antibodies against RBCs)

- With rapid hemolysis: chills, fever, jaundice, irritability, headache, abdominal pain, precordial spasm
- Nausea, vomiting, diarrhea, and eventually, decreased urinary output and shock

---

- Removal of underlying cause, when possible
- Blood transfusions for rapid hemolysis
- Intake and output, fluid and electrolytes, and vital signs monitored
- Adequate hydration and renal function maintained
- Patient warned to avoid hemolytic agent when applicable

Paroxysmal nocturnal hemoglobinuria (PNH)

- Acquired abnormality in RBC membrane increases susceptibility to lytic action of normal plasma components (magnesium, properdin, complement).
- Infection, immunization, or iron administration may provoke hemolytic episodes.
- May be associated with aplastic anemia or leukemia

- Nocturnal or early morning hemoglobinuria
- Yellow skin or mucous membranes
- Abdominal pain, headache, severe anemia, splenomegaly
- Tendency to venous thrombosis

- Transfusions of frozen or washed RBCs provide mature RBCs without adding components present in plasma, decreasing risk of increased hemolysis that accompanies transfusion of whole blood.
- Cautious use of heparin for venous thrombosis (may increase hemolysis)

POLYCYTHEMIAS

Polycythemia Vera
(Primary polycythemia, erythremia, polycythemia rubra vera, splenomegalic polycythemia, Vaquez-Osler disease)

Polycythemia vera is a chronic, myeloproliferative disorder characterized by increased RBC mass, leukocytosis, slight thrombocytosis, and increased hemoglobin concentration, with normal or decreased plasma volume. It usually occurs between ages 40 and 60, most commonly among males of Jewish ancestry; it rarely affects children or Blacks, and doesn't appear to be familial. Prognosis depends on age at diagnosis, treatment used, and complications. Mortality rate is high if polycythemia is untreated, or is associated with leukemia.

CLINICAL FEATURES OF POLYCYTHEMIA VERA

SYMPTOMS	CAUSE
Ear, Eye, Nose, and Throat • Visual disturbances (blurring, diplopia, scotoma, engorged veins of fundus and retina) and congestion of conjunctiva, retina, retinal veins, oral mucous membrane	• Hypervolemia and hyperviscosity
Central Nervous System • Headache or fullness in the head, lethargy, weakness, fatigue, syncope, tinnitus, paresthesia of digits, and impaired mentation	• Hypervolemia and hyperviscosity
Cardiovascular • Hypertension • Intermittent claudication, thrombosis and emboli, angina, thrombophlebitis • Hemorrhage	• Hypervolemia and hyperviscosity • Hypervolemia, thrombocytosis, and vascular disease • Engorgement of capillary beds
Skin • Pruritus (especially after hot bath) • Urticaria • Ruddy cyanosis • Night sweats • Ecchymosis	• Basophilia (secondary histamine release) • Altered histamine metabolism • Hypervolemia and hyperviscosity due to congested vessels, increased oxyhemoglobin, and reduced hemoglobin • Hypermetabolism • Hemorrhage
Gastrointestinal and hepatic • Epigastric distress • Early satiety and fullness • Peptic ulcer pain • Hepatosplenomegaly • Weight loss	• Hypervolemia and hyperviscosity • Hepatosplenomegaly • Gastric thrombosis and hemorrhage • Congestion, extramedullary hemopoiesis, and myeloid metaplasia • Hypermetabolism
Respiratory • Dyspnea	• Hypervolemia and hyperviscosity
Musculoskeletal • Joint symptoms	• Increased urate production secondary to nucleoprotein turnover

Causes

In polycythemia vera, uncontrolled and rapid cellular reproduction and maturation cause proliferation or hyperplasia of all bone marrow cells (panmyelosis). The cause of such uncontrolled cellular activity is unknown.

Signs and symptoms

Increased RBC mass results in hyperviscosity and inhibits blood flow to microcirculation. Subsequently, increased viscosity, diminished velocity, and thrombocytosis promote intravascular thrombosis. In its early stages, polycythemia vera usually produces no symptoms. (Increased hematocrit may be an incidental finding.) However, as altered circulation secondary to increased RBC mass produces hypervolemia and hypermetabolism, the patient may complain of a vague feeling of fullness in the head, headache, dizziness, and other symptoms, depending on the body system affected.

Paradoxically, hemorrhage is a complication of polycythemia vera. It may be due to defective platelet function or to hyperviscosity and the local effects from excess RBCs exerting pressure on distended venous and capillary walls.

Diagnosis

 Laboratory studies confirm polycythemia vera by showing increased RBC mass and normal arterial oxygen saturation in association with splenomegaly or two of the following:

- thrombocytosis
- leukocytosis
- elevated leukocyte alkaline phosphatase level
- elevated serum vitamin B_{12} or unbound B_{12}-binding capacity.

Another common finding is increased uric acid production, leading to hyperuricemia and hyperuricuria. Other laboratory results include increased blood histamine, decreased serum iron concentration, and decreased or normal urinary erythropoietin. Bone marrow biopsy reveals panmyelosis.

Treatment

Primary treatment controls hyperviscosity and hypervolemia by removing RBC mass and volume through phlebotomy, with fluid replacement. Later—or simultaneously (depending on the stage of the disease at diagnosis)—myelosuppressive agents such as radiophosphorus (^{32}P) inhibit cell proliferation. Phlebotomy immediately—but only temporarily—relieves symptoms (headache, vertigo, tinnitus) and lessens the risk of thrombosis or hemorrhage. However, after phlebotomy, a rebound effect may cause platelet and hematocrit counts to rise dramatically. Phlebotomy is repeated, depending on the results of regularly scheduled blood counts (ideally, every 2 to 4 weeks). Frequent phlebotomies cause iron deficiency anemia (250 mg iron is removed with each 500 ml whole blood), requiring iron replacement.

To control blood cell proliferation, ^{32}P can be given P.O. or I.V., as sodium phosphate, once every 12 weeks. The I.V. route is more effective because gastrointestinal absorption varies.

The therapeutic impact of ^{32}P may be delayed for 2 to 3 months. Repeated doses are usually given if hematocrit does not fall to 45%. Once absorbed, ^{32}P concentrates selectively in cells that actively participate in the mitotic cycle. Long-term therapy can induce remissions of 6 to 24 months and sometimes longer; however, ^{32}P has been linked to a rising incidence of leukemia.

Myelosuppressive chemotherapy with alkylating agents (chlorambucil, melphalan, busulfan, cyclophosphamide, uracil mustard) can also control blood cell proliferation. However, leukemia develops more commonly with chlorambucil than with ^{32}P. If needed, phlebotomy can supplement treatment with chemotherapy or ^{32}P.

Additional considerations

If the patient requires phlebotomy, the hospital staff member should:
- explain the procedure, and reassure the patient that it will relieve distressing symptoms; check blood pressure, pulse

rate, and respirations; make sure the patient is lying down comfortably to prevent vertigo and syncope; stay alert for tachycardia, clamminess, or complaints of vertigo and discontinue the procedure if these effects occur.

• check blood pressure and pulse rate immediately after phlebotomy; have the patient sit up for about 5 minutes before allowing him to walk to prevent vasovagal attack or orthostatic hypotension; administer 24 oz (720 ml) of juice or water.

The patient should watch for and report any symptoms of iron deficiency (pallor, weight loss, asthenia, glossitis).

During myelosuppressive chemotherapy, the staff member should:

• monitor CBC and platelet count before and during therapy; warn an outpatient with leukopenia that his resistance to infection is low; advise him to avoid crowds, and make sure he knows the symptoms of infection; follow hospital guidelines if leukopenia develops in a hospitalized patient who needs reverse isolation.

• tell the patient about possible side effects (nausea, vomiting, and susceptibility to infection) that may follow administration of an alkylating agent. Alopecia may follow the use of busulfan, cyclophosphamide, and uracil mustard. Sterile hemorrhagic cystitis may follow the use of cyclophosphamide (forcing fluids can prevent this side effect). Side effects must be watched for and reported. If nausea and vomiting occur, antiemetic therapy should be started and the patient's diet adjusted.

During treatment with ^{32}P, the staffer should:

• explain the procedure to relieve anxiety; tell the patient he may require repeated phlebotomies until ^{32}P takes effect; make sure there is a blood sample for CBC and platelet count before beginning treatment. (Note: The health care professional who administers ^{32}P should take radiation precautions to prevent contamination.)

• have the patient lie down during I.V. administration (to facilitate the procedure and prevent extravasation) and for 15 to 20 minutes afterward.

• keep the patient active and ambulatory to prevent thrombosis; prescribe a daily program of both active and passive range-of-motion exercises if bed rest is absolutely necessary.

• watch for complications, such as hypervolemia, thrombocytosis, and signs of an impending cerebrovascular accident (decreased sensation, numbness, transitory paralysis, fleeting blindness, headache, and epistaxis).

• regularly examine the patient closely for bleeding; tell him which are the most common bleeding sites (such as the nose, gingiva, and skin), so he can check for bleeding; advise him to report any abnormal bleeding promptly.

• give the patient additional fluids, administer allopurinol, as ordered, and alkalinize the urine to prevent uric acid calculi. These measures will compensate for increased uric acid production.

• suggest or provide small, frequent meals, followed by a rest period, if the patient has symptomatic splenomegaly, to prevent nausea and vomiting.

• report acute abdominal pain immediately. It may signal splenic infarction, renal calculi, or abdominal organ thrombosis.

Spurious Polycythemia

(Relative polycythemia, stress erythrocytosis, stress polycythemia, benign polycythemia, Gaisböck's syndrome, pseudopolycythemia)

Spurious polycythemia is characterized by increased hematocrit and normal or decreased RBC total mass; it results from decreasing plasma volume and subsequent hemoconcentration. This disease usually affects middle-aged persons and occurs more often in men than in women.

Causes
There are two possible causes of spurious polycythemia:
• *Dehydration:* Conditions that promote severe fluid loss decrease plasma levels and lead to hemoconcentration. Such conditions include persistent vomiting or diarrhea, burns, adrenocortical insufficiency, aggressive diuretic therapy, decreased fluid intake, diabetic acidosis, and renal disease.
• *Hemoconcentration due to stress:* Nervous stress decreases plasma levels and leads to hemoconcentration by some unknown mechanism (possibly by temporarily decreasing circulating plasma volume or vascular redistribution of erythrocytes). This form of erythrocytosis (chronically elevated hematocrit) is particularly common in the middle-aged man who is a chronic smoker and a type A personality (tense, hard-driving, anxious).

Other factors that may also predispose to spurious polycythemia include hypertension, thromboembolitic disease, elevated serum cholesterol and uric acid levels, and a familial tendency.

Signs and symptoms
The patient with spurious polycythemia usually has no specific symptoms; however, he may have many vague complaints, such as headaches, dizziness, and fatigue. Less commonly, he may develop diaphoresis, dyspnea, and claudication.

Typically, the patient has a ruddy appearance, a short neck, slight hypertension, and a tendency to hypoventilate when recumbent. He shows no associated hepatosplenomegaly but may have cardiac or pulmonary disease.

Diagnosis
Hemoglobin and hematocrit levels, and RBC count are elevated; RBC mass, arterial oxygen saturation, and bone marrow are normal. Plasma volume may be decreased or normal. Hypercholesterol-emia, hyperlipemia, or hyperuricemia may be present.

Spurious polycythemia is distinguishable from true polycythemia vera by its characteristic normal RBC mass, elevated hematocrit, and the absence of iron-deficiency anemia and leukocytosis.

Treatment
The principal goals of treatment are to correct dehydration and to prevent life-threatening thromboembolism. Rehydration with appropriate fluids and electrolytes is the primary therapy for spurious polycythemia secondary to dehydration. Therapy must also include appropriate measures to prevent continuing fluid loss.

Additional considerations
• During rehydration, intake and output must be carefully monitored to maintain fluid and electrolyte balance.
• Regular exercise and low-cholesterol diet can help prevent thromboemboli in predisposed patients. Antilipemics may also be necessary. Reduced calorie intake may be required for the obese patient.
• When appropriate, counseling about the patient's work habits and lack of relaxation should be suggested. If the patient is a smoker, he must understand how important it is that he stop smoking. If necessary, he should be referred to an antismoking program.
• The patient must get follow-up examinations every 3 to 4 months after leaving the hospital, to make sure the condition doesn't recur.
• Spurious polycythemia, all diagnostic measures, and therapy should be thoroughly explained. The hard-driving person predisposed to spurious polycythemia is likely to be more inquisitive and anxious than the average patient. His questions should be answered honestly, with care taken to reassure him that he can effectively control symptoms by complying with the prescribed treatment.

Secondary Polycythemia
(Reactive polycythemia)

Secondary polycythemia is a disorder characterized by excessive production of circulating RBCs due to hypoxia, tumor, or disease. It occurs in approximately 2 out of every 100,000 persons living at or near sea level; incidence rises among persons living at high altitudes.

Causes

Secondary polycythemia may result from increased production of erythropoietin. This hormone, which is possibly produced and secreted in the kidneys, stimulates bone marrow production of RBCs. This increased production may be an appropriate (compensatory) physiologic response to hypoxemia, which may result from:

• chronic obstructive pulmonary disease (COPD)
• hemoglobin abnormalities (such as carboxyhemoglobinemia)
• congestive heart failure (causing a decreased ventilation-perfusion ratio)
• right-to-left shunting of blood in the heart (as in transposition of the great vessels)
• central or peripheral alveolar hypoventilation (as in barbiturate intoxication or pickwickian syndrome)
• low oxygen content of air at high altitudes.

Increased production of erythropoietin may also be an inappropriate (pathologic) response to renal disease (such as Bartter's syndrome or pyelonephritis), to CNS disease (such as encephalitis and parkinsonism), or to disorders such as ovarian carcinoma, Cushing's syndrome, or adrenocortical carcinoma (in which ectopic foci of erythropoietin secretion occur). Rarely, secondary polycythemia results from a recessive genetic trait.

Signs and symptoms

In the hypoxic patient, suggestive physical findings include ruddy cyanotic skin, emphysema, and hypoxemia without hepatosplenomegaly or hypertension. Clubbing of the fingers may occur if the underlying disease is cardiovascular. When secondary polycythemia isn't caused by hypoxemia, it's usually an incidental finding during treatment for an underlying disease.

Diagnosis

Laboratory values for secondary polycythemia include increased RBC mass, urinary erythropoietin, and blood histamine, with decreased or normal arterial oxygen saturation. Bone marrow biopsies reveal hyperplasia confined to the erythroid series. Unlike polycythemia vera, secondary polycythemia isn't associated with leukocytosis.

Treatment

The goal of treatment is correction of the underlying disease or environmental condition. In severe secondary polycythemia where altitude is a contributing factor, relocation may be advisable. If secondary polycythemia has produced hazardous hyperviscosity or if the patient doesn't respond to treatment for the primary disease, reduction of blood volume by phlebotomy may be effective. Emergency phlebotomy is indicated for prevention of impending vascular occlusion or before emergency surgery. In the latter case, it's usually advisable to remove excess RBCs and reinfuse the patient's plasma. Because a patient with polycythemia risks hemorrhage during and after surgery, elective surgery should be avoided until polycythemia is controlled. Generally, secondary polycythemia disappears when the primary disease is corrected.

Additional considerations

Supportive care of the patient with secondary polycythemia includes:
• keeping the patient as active as possible to decrease the risk of thrombosis due to increased blood viscosity.
• reducing calorie and sodium intake to counteract the tendency to hypertension.
• checking blood pressure before and after a phlebotomy; giving the patient approximately 24 oz (720 ml) of water or juice to drink after the procedure; having him sit up for about 5 minutes before walking, to prevent syncope.
• emphasizing the importance of regular blood studies (every 2 to 3 months), even after the disease is controlled.
• teaching the patient and family about the underlying disorder; helping them understand its relationship to polycythemia and the measures needed to control both.

HEMORRHAGIC DISORDERS

Allergic Purpuras

(Henoch-Schönlein purpura, anaphylactoid purpura)

Allergic purpura, a nonthrombocytopenic purpura, is an acute or chronic vascular inflammation affecting the skin, joints, and gastrointestinal and genitourinary tracts, in association with allergy symptoms. When allergic purpura primarily affects the gastrointestinal tract, with accompanying joint pain, it is called Henoch-Schönlein syndrome or anaphylactoid purpura. However, the term allergic purpura applies to purpura associated with many other conditions, such as erythema nodosum. An acute attack of allergic purpura can last for several weeks and is potentially fatal (usually from renal failure); however, most patients do recover.

Fully developed, allergic purpura is persistent and debilitating, possibly leading to chronic glomerulonephritis (especially following a streptococcal infection). Allergic purpura affects males more often than females, and is most prevalent in children under age 7. Prognosis is more favorable for children than adults.

Causes

Although the causative agent may not be readily discernible, the most common identifiable cause of allergic purpura is probably an autoimmune reaction directed against vascular walls, triggered by a bacterial infection (particularly streptococcal infection). Other possible causes include allergic reactions to some antibiotics, analgesics, and vaccines; allergic reactions to insect bites; exposure to coal tar derivatives and other chemicals; and allergic reactions to some foods (wheat, eggs, milk, chocolate, etc.).

Signs and symptoms

Characteristic skin lesions of allergic purpura are purple, macular, ecchymotic, and of varying size, and are caused by vascular leakage into the skin and mucous membranes. The lesions usually appear in symmetric patterns on the arms and legs, and are accompanied by pruritus, paresthesia, and occasionally, angioneurotic edema. In children, skin lesions are generally urticarial and develop central red areas, which expand and become hemorrhagic. Scattered petechiae may appear on the legs, buttocks, and perineum.

Henoch-Schönlein syndrome commonly produces transient or severe colic, tenesmus and constipation, vomiting, and edema or hemorrhage of the mucous membranes of the bowel, resulting in gastrointestinal bleeding, occult blood in the stool, and possibly, intussusception. Such gastrointestinal abnormalities

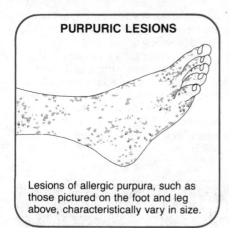

PURPURIC LESIONS

Lesions of allergic purpura, such as those pictured on the foot and leg above, characteristically vary in size.

may *precede* overt, cutaneous signs of purpura. Musculoskeletal symptoms, such as rheumatoid pains and periarticular effusions, mostly affect the legs and feet.

In about 25% to 50% of patients, allergic purpura is associated with genitourinary symptoms: nephritis; renal hemorrhages that may cause microscopic hematuria and disturb renal function; bleeding from the mucosal surfaces of the ureters, bladder, or urethra; and occasionally, glomerulonephritis. Other possible symptoms are moderate and irregular fever, headache, anorexia, and localized edema of the hands, feet, or scalp.

Diagnosis

Although no laboratory test clearly identifies allergic purpura, WBC count and ESR are elevated. Diagnosis therefore necessitates careful clinical observation, often during the second or third attack. Except for a positive tourniquet test, coagulation and platelet function tests are usually normal. Small bowel X-rays may reveal areas of transient edema; tests for

blood in the urine and stool are often positive. Increased BUN and creatinine may indicate renal involvement. Diagnosis must rule out other forms of non-thrombocytopenic purpura.

Treatment

Treatment is generally symptomatic; for example, severe allergic purpura may require steroids to relieve edema, and analgesics to relieve joint and abdominal pain. In some patients with chronic renal disease, immunosuppressive therapy with azathioprine may be helpful, along with identification of the provocative allergen. *Accurate allergy history is essential.*

Additional considerations

The health care professional caring for a patient with allergic purpura should:

• encourage maintenance of an elimination diet to help identify specific allergenic foods, so these foods can be eliminated from the patient's diet.

• monitor skin lesions, and abdominal and joint pain, providing analgesics, as needed.

• watch carefully for complications, such as gastrointestinal and genitourinary tract bleeding, edema, nausea, vomiting, headache, hypertension (with nephritis), increasing abdominal rigidity and tenderness, and absence of stool (with intussusception).

• perform or assist with passive or active range-of-motion exercises to prevent muscle atrophy in the bedridden patient.

• provide emotional support and reassurance, especially if the patient is temporarily disfigured by florid skin lesions.

• stress the need to *immediately* report *any* recurrence of symptoms after the acute stage, and to return for follow-up urinalysis.

Hereditary Hemorrhagic Telangiectasia
(Rendu-Osler-Weber disease)

Hereditary hemorrhagic telangiectasia is an inherited vascular disorder in which venules and capillaries dilate to form fragile masses of thin convoluted vessels (telangiectases), resulting in an abnormal tendency to hemorrhage. This disorder affects both sexes but may cause less severe bleeding in females.

Causes

Hereditary hemorrhagic telangiectasia is transmitted by autosomal dominant inheritance. It rarely skips generations. In its homozygous state, it may be lethal.

Signs and symptoms

Signs of hereditary hemorrhagic telangiectasia are present in childhood but increase in severity with age. Localized aggregations of dilated capillaries appear on the skin of the face, ears, scalp, hands, arms, and feet; under the nails; and on the mucous membranes of the nose, mouth, and stomach. These dilated capillaries cause frequent epistaxis, hemoptysis, and gastrointestinal bleeding, possibly leading to iron deficiency anemia. (In children, epistaxis is usually the first symptom.)

Characteristic telangiectases are violet, bleed spontaneously, may be flat or raised, blanch on pressure, and are nonpulsatile. They may be associated with sizable aneurysms in the hepatic or splenic arteries and the aorta. Visceral telangiectases are common in the liver, bladder, respiratory tract, and stomach. The type and distribution of these lesions are generally similar among family members.

Generalized capillary fragility, evidenced by spontaneous bleeding and spider hemangiomas of varying sizes, may exist without overt telangiectasia. Occasionally, vascular malformation may cause pulmonary arteriovenous fistulas; then, shunting of blood through the fistulas may lead to hypoxemia, recurring cerebral embolism, brain abscess, and clubbing of digits.

Diagnosis

Diagnosis rests on an established familial pattern of bleeding disorders and clinical evidence of telangiectasia and hemorrhage. Decreased hemoglobin and erythrocyte count, and bone marrow aspiration showing depleted iron stores confirm secondary iron deficiency ane-

mia. Other relevant laboratory tests show abnormal platelet function. However, coagulation tests are essentially irrelevant, because hemorrhage in telangiectasia results from vascular wall weakness.

Treatment

Supportive therapy includes blood transfusions and the administration of supplemental iron. Ancillary treatment includes applying pressure, vasoconstrictors, and thrombin to bleeding sites; excising bleeding sites (when accessible); and protecting the patient from trauma and unnecessary bleeding.

Parenteral administration of supplemental iron enhances absorption to maintain adequate iron stores and prevents gastric irritation. Administering antipyretics or antihistamines before blood transfusion, and using saline-washed cells, frozen blood, or other types of leukocyte-poor blood instead of whole blood transfusion, may prevent febrile transfusion reactions.

Additional considerations

• If the patient is receiving a blood transfusion, he will need a health care professional with him during the first 15 minutes to observe for possible adverse reactions. Afterward, he should be checked every 15

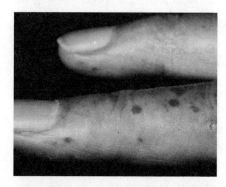

In hereditary hemorrhagic telangiectasia, localized aggregations of dilated capillaries may be flat or raised.

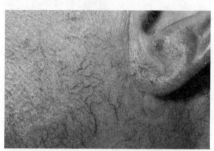

On the face shown above, spider hemangiomas reflect capillary fragility in hereditary hemorrhagic telangiectasia.

minutes for signs of febrile transfusion reaction (flushing, shaking chills, fever, headache, rash, tachycardia, hypertension), since such a patient is quite suscep-

tible to a reaction.

• The patient must be observed for indications of gastrointestinal bleeding, such as hematemesis and melena. He should also watch for and report such signs.

• If the patient requires an iron supplement, it is important to follow dosage instructions, and to take oral iron with meals to minimize gastric irritation or between meals to maximize absorption. The patient should be warned that iron turns stools dark green or black.

• The patient and family must be taught how to manage minor bleeding episodes, especially recurrent epistaxis, and to recognize major ones that necessitate emergency intervention.

• The patient can be referred for genetic counseling, as appropriate.

Thrombocytopenia

The most common cause of hemorrhagic disorders, thrombocytopenia is characterized by a deficient number of circulating platelets. Since platelets play a vital role in coagulation, this disease poses a serious threat to hemostasis. Prognosis is excellent in drug-induced thrombocytopenia if the offending drug is withdrawn; in such cases, recovery may be immediate. Otherwise, prognosis depends on response to treatment of the underlying cause.

Causes

Thrombocytopenia may be congenital or acquired. In either case, it usually results from decreased or defective production of platelets in the marrow (such as occurs in leukemia, aplastic anemia, or toxicity with certain drugs) or from increased destruction outside the marrow caused by an underlying disorder (such as cirrhosis of the liver, disseminated intravascular coagulation, or severe infection). Less commonly, it results from sequestration (hypersplenism, hypothermia) or platelet loss. Acquired thrombocytopenia may result from certain drugs, such as quinine, quinidine, sulfisoxazole, chlorothiazide, hydrochlorothiazide, phenylbutazone, oxyphenbutazone, rifampin, heparin, cyclophosphamide, and vinblastine sulfate.

An idiopathic form of thrombocytopenia commonly occurs in children.

Signs and symptoms

Thrombocytopenia typically produces a sudden onset of petechiae or ecchymoses in the skin, or bleeding into any mucous membrane (gastrointestinal, urinary, vaginal, or respiratory). As a result of such bleeding, the patient suffers malaise, fatigue, general weakness, and lethargy. In adults, large blood-filled bullae that are characteristic of thrombocytopenia appear in the mouth. In severe thrombocytopenia, hemorrhage may lead to tachycardia, shortness of breath, loss of consciousness, and death.

Diagnosis

Diagnosis necessitates a patient history (especially a drug history), physical examination, and laboratory tests. Coagulation tests show diminished platelet count (in adults, less than 200,000/ mm³), prolonged bleeding time, and normal prothrombin and partial thromboplastin times. If increased destruction of platelets is causing thrombocytopenia, bone marrow studies reveal a greater number of megakaryocytes (platelet precursors) and shortened platelet survival (several hours or days rather than the usual 7 to 10 days).

Treatment

Treatment varies with the underlying cause and may include corticosteroids to enhance vascular integrity. Removal of the offending agents in drug-induced thrombocytopenia or proper treatment of the underlying cause, when possible, is essential. Platelet transfusions are helpful only in treating complications of severe hemorrhage.

Additional considerations

When caring for the patient with thrombocytopenia, every possible precaution against bleeding must be taken. This includes:

• protecting the patient from trauma by keeping the side rails up, and padding them; promoting the use of an electric razor and a soft toothbrush, and avoiding all invasive procedures, such as venipuncture or urinary catheterization, if possible. When venipuncture is unavoidable, pressure should be exerted on the puncture site for at least 20 minutes or until the bleeding stops.

• monitoring platelet count daily.

• testing stool for guaiac and dipsticking urine and emesis for blood.

• watching for bleeding (petechiae, ecchymoses, surgical or gastrointestinal bleeding, menorrhagia).

• warning the patient to avoid aspirin in any form and other drugs that impair coagulation; teaching him how to recognize aspirin compounds listed on labels of over-the-counter remedies.

• advising the patient to avoid straining at stool or coughing, as both can lead to increased intracranial pressure, possibly causing cerebral hemorrhage in the patient with thrombocytopenia; providing a stool softener, if necessary.

• enforcing strict bed rest, if necessary, during periods of active bleeding.

• remembering when administering platelet concentrate that platelets are extremely fragile. They must be infused quickly, using the administration set recommended in the blood bank's trans-

---

CAUSES OF DECREASED CIRCULATING PLATELETS

Diminished or defective production

Congenital
• Wiskott-Aldrich syndrome
• Maternal ingestion of thiazides
• Neonatal rubella
• Thrombopoietin deficiency

Acquired
• Aplastic anemia
• Marrow infiltration (acute and chronic leukemias, tumor)
• Nutritional deficiency (B_{12}, folic acid)
• Myelosuppressive agents
• Drugs that directly influence platelet production (thiazides, alcohol, hormones)
• Radiation
• Viral infections (measles, dengue)

Increased peripheral destruction

Congenital
• Nonimmune (prematurity, erythroblastosis fetalis, infection)
• Immune (drug sensitivity, maternal ITP)

Acquired
• Nonimmune (infection, DIC, thrombotic thrombocytopenic purpura)
• Immune (drug-induced, especially with quinine and quinidine; posttransfusion purpura; acute and chronic ITP; sepsis; alcohol)

Sequestration
• Hypersplenism
• Hypothermia

Loss
• Hemorrhage
• Extracorporeal perfusion

Adapted with permission from William J. Williams et al., HEMATOLOGY (New York: McGraw-Hill Book Co., 1977).

fusion policy.
* monitoring for febrile reaction (flushing, chills, fever, headache, tachycardia, hypertension) during platelet transfusion. HLA-typed platelets may be ordered to prevent febrile reaction. If the patient has a history of minor reactions, he may benefit from acetaminophen and diphenhydramine before the transfusion.
* stressing the importance of avoiding the offending drug if thrombocytopenia is drug-induced.
* teaching the patient who must receive long-term steroid therapy to watch for and report cushingoid symptoms (acne, moon face, hirsutism, buffalo hump, hypertension, girdle obesity, thinning arms and legs, glycosuria, and edema); emphasizing that steroid doses must be discontinued gradually; monitoring fluid and electrolyte balance, and watching for infection, pathologic fractures, and mood changes.

Idiopathic Thrombocytopenic Purpura

Thrombocytopenia that results from immunologic platelet destruction is known as idiopathic thrombocytopenic purpura (ITP). This form of thrombocytopenia may be acute (postviral thrombocytopenia) or chronic (Werlhof's disease, purpura hemorrhagia, essential thrombocytopenia, autoimmune thrombocytopenia). Acute ITP usually affects children between ages 2 and 6; chronic ITP mainly affects adults under age 50, especially women between ages 20 and 40. Prognosis for acute ITP is excellent, with nearly four out of five patients recovering completely without specific treatment. Prognosis for chronic ITP is good; transient remissions lasting weeks or even years are common, especially among women.

Causes
ITP may be an autoimmune disorder, since antibodies that reduce the life span of platelets have been found in nearly all patients. The spleen probably helps to remove platelets modified by the antibody. Occasionally, ITP may be preceded by a viral infection, such as rubella or mumps. ITP may also be drug-induced or associated with lupus erythematosus or pregnancy.

Signs and symptoms
ITP produces clinical features that are common to all forms of thrombocytopenia: petechiae, ecchymoses, and mucosal bleeding from the mouth, nose, or gastrointestinal tract. Generally, hemorrhage is the only abnormal physical finding. Purpuric lesions may occur in vital organs, such as the brain, and may prove fatal. In acute ITP, which commonly occurs in children, onset is usually sudden and without warning, causing easy bruising, epistaxis, and bleeding gums. Onset of chronic ITP is insidious.

Diagnosis
Platelet count less than 20,000/mm³ and prolonged bleeding time suggest ITP. Platelet size and morphologic appearance may be abnormal; anemia may be

present if bleeding has occurred. As in thrombocytopenia, bone marrow studies show an abundance of megakaryocytes (platelet precursors) and a shortened circulating platelet survival time (several hours or days rather than the usual 7 to 10 days). Occasionally, platelet antibodies may be found in vitro, but this diagnosis is usually inferred from platelet survival data and the absence of an underlying disease.

Treatment

Corticosteroids, the initial treatment of choice for ITP, promote capillary integrity but are only temporarily effective in chronic ITP. Alternative treatments include immunosuppressive therapy (with vincristine sulfate, for example), plasmapheresis, and splenectomy in adults (85% successful). Before splenectomy, the patient may require blood, blood components, and vitamin K to correct anemia and coagulation defects. After splenectomy, he may need blood and component replacement, and platelet concentrate. Normally, however, platelets multiply spontaneously by themselves after splenectomy.

Additional considerations

Care for ITP is essentially the same as for thrombocytopenia, with emphasis on teaching the patient to observe for petechiae, ecchymoses, and other signs of recurrence, especially following acute ITP.

Patients who receive immunosuppressives for treatment must be monitored for signs of bone marrow depression, infection, mucositis, gastrointestinal tract ulceration, and severe diarrhea or vomiting. Immunosuppressives are frequently given before splenectomy.

Abnormal Platelet Function Disorders

Abnormal platelet function disorders are similar to thrombocytopenia but result from platelet dysfunction rather than platelet deficiency. They characteristically cause defects in platelet adhesion or procoagulation activity (ability to combine with plasma clotting factors to form a stable fibrin clot). Such disorders may also create defects in platelet aggregation and, occasionally, may produce abnormalities by preventing the release of adenosine diphosphate (defective platelet release reaction). Prognosis varies widely.

Causes

Abnormal platelet function disorders may be inherited (autosomal recessive) or acquired. Inherited disorders cause bone marrow production of platelets that are ineffective in the clotting mechanism. Acquired disorders result from the effects of drugs, such as aspirin; systemic diseases, such as uremia; or other hematologic disorders.

Signs and symptoms

Generally, the sudden appearance of petechiae or purpura, or excessive bruising and bleeding of the nose and gums are the first overt signs of platelet function disorders. More serious signs are external hemorrhage, internal hemorrhage into the muscles and visceral organs, or excessive bleeding during surgery.

Diagnosis

Prolonged bleeding time in a patient with both a normal platelet count and normal clotting factors suggests this diagnosis. Determination of the defective mechanism requires tests for platelet factor 3 (a component released by disintegrating platelets), and platelet retention and aggregation. Depending on the type of platelet dysfunction, some or all the test results may be abnormal.

Other typical laboratory findings are poor clot retraction and decreased pro-

PATIENT TEACHING AID

Precautions During Anticoagulation Therapy

Because your doctor has prescribed anticoagulant medication, you must be careful to prevent bleeding. Here are some helpful tips:

DO'S	DON'TS

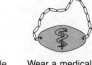
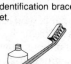

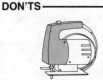

DO'S	**DON'TS**
Wear gloves while gardening. Wear a medical identification bracelet.	Don't self-medicate. Don't use power tools.
Use an electric shaver. Use a soft-bristled toothbrush.	Don't use alcohol excessively. Don't trim calluses and corns.

This patient teaching aid is intended for distribution to patients by doctors and nurses.
It should not be used without a doctor's approval.

thrombin conversion. Baseline testing includes CBC and differential, and appropriate tests to determine hemorrhage sites. In these disorders, plasma clotting factors, platelet counts, and prothrombin, activated partial thromboplastin, and thrombin times are usually normal.

Treatment

Platelet replacement is the only satisfactory treatment for inherited platelet dysfunction. However, acquired platelet function disorders respond to adequate treatment of the underlying disease or discontinuation of damaging drug therapy. Plasmapheresis effectively controls bleeding caused by a plasma element that's inhibiting platelet function. During this procedure, one or more units of whole blood are removed from the patient; the plasma is removed from the whole blood, and the remaining packed RBCs are reinfused.

Additional considerations

• An accurate patient history is needed, including onset of bleeding, use of drugs (especially aspirin), and bleeding disorders among family members.
• The patient must be watched closely for bleeding from skin, nose, gums, gastrointestinal tract, or an injury site.
• The patient must avoid unnecessary trauma. He should tell the dentist about this condition before undergoing oral surgery (following good oral hygiene may help him prevent such surgery). Staff members in the hospital must be alerted to the patient's hemorrhagic potential, especially during diagnostic tests that may cause trauma and bleeding.
• The patient undergoing plasmapheresis should be observed for hypovolemia, hypotension, tachycardia, vasoconstriction, and other signs of volume depletion.
• If platelet dysfunction is inherited, the patient and family will need help to understand and accept the nature of this disorder. They must be taught how to manage potential bleeding episodes, and must know that petechiae, ecchymoses, and bleeding from the nose, gums, and gastrointestinal tract signal abnormal bleed-

ing and should be reported immediately.
• The patient with a known coagulopathy or hepatic disease should avoid aspirin, aspirin compounds, and other agents that impair coagulation, because such drugs can precipitate severe bleeding episodes.
• The patient should wear a medical identification bracelet or carry a card identifying him as a potential bleeder.

Von Willebrand's Disease

Von Willebrand's disease is a hereditary bleeding disorder characterized by prolonged bleeding time, moderate deficiency of clotting Factor VIII$_{AHF}$ (antihemophilic factor), and impaired platelet function. This disease commonly causes bleeding from the skin or mucosal surfaces and, in females, excessive uterine bleeding. Bleeding may range from mild and asymptomatic to severe, potentially fatal hemorrhage. Prognosis, however, is usually good.

Causes and incidence
Unlike hemophilia, von Willebrand's disease is inherited as an autosomal dominant trait and occurs equally in males and females. One theory of pathophysiology holds that mild-to-moderate deficiency of Factor VIII and defective platelet adhesion prolong coagulation time. More specifically, this results from a deficiency of the von Willebrand factor (VWF), which appears to occupy the Factor VIII molecule and may be necessary for the production of Factor VIII and proper platelet function. Defective platelet function is characterized by:
• decreased agglutination and adhesion at the bleeding site.
• reduced platelet retention when filtered through a column of packed glass beads.
• diminished ristocetin-induced platelet aggregation.

Signs and symptoms
Von Willebrand's disease produces easy bruising, epistaxis, and bleeding from the gums. Severe forms of this disease may cause hemorrhage after laceration or surgery, menorrhagia, and gastrointestinal bleeding. Excessive postpartum bleeding is uncommon, because Factor VIII levels and bleeding time abnormalities become less pronounced during pregnancy. Massive soft-tissue hemorrhage and bleeding into joints rarely occur. Severity of bleeding may lessen with age, and bleeding episodes occur sporadically—a patient may bleed excessively after one dental extraction but not after another.

Diagnosis
Diagnosis is often difficult, because symptoms are mild, laboratory values are borderline, and Factor VIII levels fluctuate. However, a positive family history, typical bleeding patterns, and characteristic laboratory values can help establish diagnosis. Typical laboratory data include:
• prolonged bleeding time (more than 6 minutes)
• slightly prolonged partial thromboplastin time (more than 45 seconds)
• absent or reduced levels of Factor VIII-related antigens (VIII$_{AGN}$), and low Factor VIII activity level
• defective in vitro platelet aggregation (using the ristocetin coagulation factor assay test)
• normal platelet count and normal clot retraction.

Treatment
The aims of treatment are to shorten bleeding time by local measures and to replace Factor VIII (and, consequently, VWF) by infusion of cryoprecipitate or blood fractions that are rich in Factor VIII.

During bleeding episodes and before

even minor surgery, I.V. infusion of cryoprecipitate or fresh-frozen plasma (in quantities sufficient to raise Factor VIII levels to 50% of normal) generally shortens bleeding time.

Additional considerations

Care should include local measures to control bleeding, and patient teaching to prevent bleeding, unnecessary trauma, and complications.

• After surgery, bleeding time should be monitored for 24 to 48 hours, and the patient should be watched for signs of new bleeding.

• During a bleeding episode, the injured part must be immediately elevated and cold compresses and gentle pressure applied to the bleeding site.

• Parents of children with von Willebrand's disease should seek genetic counseling.

• The patient should consult his doctor after even minor trauma and before all surgery to determine if replacement of blood components is necessary.

• The patient should watch for signs of hepatitis within 6 weeks to 6 months after transfusion.

• The patient must avoid using aspirin and other drugs that impair platelet function.

• If the patient has a severe form of this disease, he should avoid contact sports.

Rare Inherited Factor Deficiencies

Normal blood clotting requires an adequate number of platelets and effective interaction among 12 coagulation factors. Deficiency of almost any one of these coagulation factors impairs normal blood clotting. Severe deficiency may cause massive and potentially fatal hemorrhage. Rare inherited deficiencies may occur in factors I, II, V, VII, X, XI, XII, and XIII. Deficiencies in Factor III (tissue thromboplastin) and Factor IV (calcium) are not inherited. Deficiencies in Factor VIII and Factor IX—which figure in hemophilia, von Willebrand's disease, and Christmas disease—can be inherited but are not considered rare. (There is no Factor VI.)

Rare inherited factor deficiencies affect both sexes. Factor XI deficiency (also called Rosenthal syndrome and hemophilia C) is most prevalent among persons of Jewish ancestry and may occur in association with Factor VIII deficiency.

Signs and symptoms

Most factor deficiencies cause easy or excessive bleeding, frequent epistaxis, prolonged bleeding after trauma, and in females, menorrhagia. Deficiencies in Factor V and Factor VII also have been associated with intracranial and gastrointestinal hemorrhages; Factor XIII deficiency, with intracranial hemorrhage alone. Factor XI deficiency is unique in that it causes delayed bleeding after trauma (such bleeding may occur 2 to 3 days after the trauma). Factor I (afibrinogenemia) and Factor XIII deficiencies are evident at birth, producing excessive umbilical cord bleeding. Factor XII deficiency has no discernible clinical effects.

Treatment and additional considerations

Treatment is generally supportive. It may include measures to control bleeding, such as application of gentle pressure or cold compresses, and elevation of the affected part, if possible. An acute bleeding episode usually necessitates administration of fresh or fresh-frozen plasma, or plasma fractions, depending on the factor deficiency. With Factor V or Factor XIII deficiency, transfusions may have to be continued for up to 2 weeks after the initial bleeding episode.

• The patient must be monitored for blood loss during an acute bleeding episode and after any surgical procedure.

• Transfusions of fresh or fresh-frozen

plasma, or any other blood components, should be given, as ordered.
• Patients with Factor V or Factor VII deficiency must be monitored for signs of gastrointestinal bleeding, and patients with Factor V, VII, or XIII deficiency must be watched for signs of CNS bleeding.

Disseminated Intravascular Coagulation
(Consumption coagulopathy, defibrination syndrome)

Disseminated intravascular coagulation (DIC) occurs as a complication of diseases and conditions that accelerate clotting, causing small blood vessel occlusion, organ necrosis, depletion of circulating clotting factors and platelets, and activation of the fibrinolytic system. This, in turn, can provoke severe hemorrhage. Clotting in the microcirculation usually affects the kidneys and extremities, but may occur in the brain, lungs, pituitary and adrenal glands, and gastrointestinal mucosa. Other conditions, such as vitamin K deficiency, hepatic disease, and anticoagulant therapy, may cause a similar hemorrhage. DIC is generally an acute condition but may be chronic in cancer patients. Prognosis depends on early detection and treatment, the severity of the hemorrhage, and treatment of the underlying disease or condition.

Causes

DIC may result from the following underlying disorders:
• *Infection:* gram-negative or gram-positive septicemia; viral, fungal, or rickettsial infection; protozoal infection (falciparum malaria)
• *Obstetric complications:* abruptio placentae, amniotic fluid embolism, toxemia, retained dead fetus
• *Neoplastic disease:* acute leukemia, metastatic carcinoma
• *Disorders that produce necrosis:* extensive burns and trauma, brain tissue destruction, transplant rejection, hepatic necrosis
• *Others:* heatstroke, hypovolemic shock, poisonous snakebite, cirrhosis, fat embolism, incompatible blood transfusion, cardiac arrest, surgery necessitating cardiopulmonary bypass, giant hemangioma, severe venous thrombosis, purpura fulminans.

It's not clear why such disorders lead to DIC; nor is it certain that they lead to it through a common mechanism. In many patients, the triggering mechanisms may be the entrance of foreign protein into the circulation, and vascular endothelial injury. Regardless of how DIC begins, the typical accelerated clotting results in generalized activation of prothrombin and a consequent excess of thrombin. Excess thrombin then converts fibrinogen to fibrin, abnormally increasing platelet aggregation and causing fibrin clots to form. This process consumes exorbitant amounts of coagulation factors (especially fibrinogen, prothrombin, platelets, and Factor V and Factor VIII), causing hypofibrinogenemia, hypoprothrombinemia, thrombocytopenia, and deficiencies in Factor V and Factor VIII. Circulating thrombin activates the fibrinolytic system, which lyses fibrin clots into fibrin degradation products. The hemorrhage that occurs may be due largely to the anticoagulant activity of the fibrin degradation products, as well as the depletion of plasma coagulation factors.

Signs and symptoms

The most significant clinical feature of DIC is abnormal bleeding, *without* an accompanying history of a serious hemorrhagic disorder. Principal signs of such bleeding include cutaneous oozing, petechiae, ecchymoses, and hematomas caused by bleeding into the skin. Bleeding from sites of surgical or invasive procedures (such as incisions or I.V. sites)

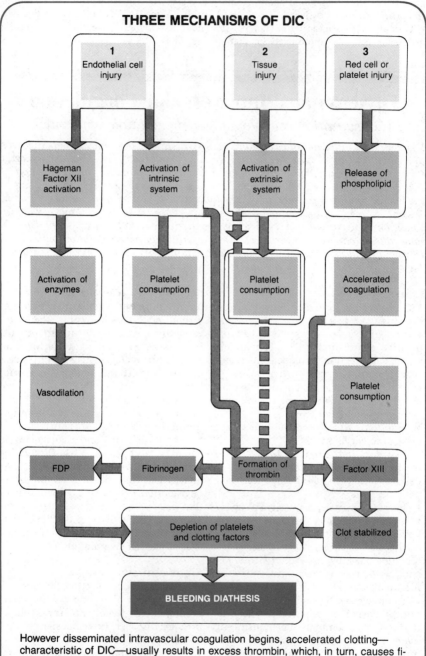

THREE MECHANISMS OF DIC

However disseminated intravascular coagulation begins, accelerated clotting—characteristic of DIC—usually results in excess thrombin, which, in turn, causes fibrinolysis with excess fibrin formation and fibrin degradation products (FDP), activation of fibrin-stabilizing factor (Factor XIII), consumption of platelet and clotting factors, and eventually, hemorrhage.

and from the gastrointestinal tract are equally significant signs, as are acrocyanosis and signs of acute tubular necrosis. Related symptoms and other possible effects include nausea, vomiting, dyspnea, convulsions, oliguria, coma, shock, failure of major organ systems, and severe muscle, back, and abdominal pain.

Diagnosis

Abnormal bleeding in the absence of a known hematologic disorder suggests DIC. Initial laboratory findings supporting a tentative diagnosis of DIC include:
• *prolonged prothrombin time:* > 15 seconds
• *prolonged partial thromboplastin time:* > 60 to 80 seconds
• *decreased fibrinogen levels:* < 150 mg%
• *decreased platelets:* < 100,000/mm³
• *increased fibrin degradation products:* often > 100 mcg/ml.

Other supportive data include positive fibrin monomers, diminished levels of factors V and VIII, fragmentation on RBCs, and decreased hemoglobin (< 10 g/100 ml). Assessment of renal status demonstrates reduction in urinary output (< 30 ml/hour), and elevated BUN (> 25 mg/100 ml) and serum creatinine (> 1.3 mg/100 ml).

Final confirmation of the diagnosis may be difficult, because many of these test results also occur in other disorders (primary fibrinolysis, for example). Additional diagnostic measures determine the underlying disorder.

Treatment

Successful management of DIC necessitates prompt recognition and adequate treatment of the underlying disorder. Treatment may be supportive (when the underlying disorder is self-limiting, for example) or highly specific. If the patient isn't actively bleeding, supportive care alone may reverse DIC. However, active bleeding may require heparin I.V. and administration of blood, fresh-frozen plasma, platelets, or packed RBCs to support hemostasis. Heparin's antithrombin activity neutralizes free-circulating thrombin, preventing proliferation of thrombin in the capillaries and further blood clotting.

Additional considerations

Health care must focus on early recognition of principal signs of abnormal bleeding, prompt treatment of the underlying disorders, and prevention of further bleeding. The hospital staff member should:
• avoid scrubbing bleeding areas to prevent clots from dislodging and causing fresh bleeding; use pressure, cold compresses, and topical hemostatic agents to control bleeding.
• protect the patient from injury; enforce complete bed rest during bleeding episodes; pad the side rails if the patient is very agitated.
• check all I.V. and venipuncture sites frequently for bleeding; apply pressure to injection sites for at least 10 minutes; alert other personnel to the patient's tendency to hemorrhage.
• monitor intake and output hourly in acute DIC, especially when administering blood products; watch for transfusion reactions and signs of fluid overload; weigh dressings and linen, and record drainage to measure the amount of blood lost; weigh the patient daily, particularly if there is renal involvement.
• watch for bleeding from the gastrointestinal and genitourinary tracts; measure the patient's abdominal girth at least every 4 hours if intra-abdominal bleeding is suspected, and monitor closely for signs of shock.
• monitor the results of serial blood studies (particularly hematocrit, hemoglobin, and coagulation times), which are usually performed every 6 hours.
• explain all diagnostic tests and procedures; allow time for questions.
• inform the family of the patient's progress; prepare them for his appearance (I.V.s, nasogastric tubes, bruises, dried blood); provide emotional support for the patient and family; enlist as needed the aid of a social worker and other members of the health care team in providing such support.

PLASMA CELL DYSCRASIAS

Macroglobulinemia
(Waldenström's macroglobulinemia)

Macroglobulinemia is a neoplastic disease of plasma and lymphoid cells that produces IgM antibodies. This disorder progresses slowly for many years, producing symptoms only late in its course. Eventually, it results in increased serum concentration of high–molecular-weight immunoglobulin (IgM) and leads to potentially fatal hyperviscosity, hemorrhage, thrombosis, hemolytic anemia, or infection. Patients with macroglobulinemia often have associated lymphomatous tumors that tend to cause rapid deterioration, even after treatment decreases IgM concentration. This disorder is most common in men over age 50 but can occur in women.

Causes

The cause of macroglobulinemia isn't known, but genetic predisposition is suspected. Some patients with this disorder have chromosomal abnormalities; their relatives may have similar immunoglobulin abnormalities.

More is known about the pathophysiology of macroglobulinemia. The high molecular weight and concentration of IgM produce highly viscous serum (hyperviscosity syndrome), which causes hemorrhagic diathesis, retinopathy with hemorrhage, and neurologic symptoms. Excessive serum IgM levels can interfere with platelet function and impair aggregation; they can also interact with or inhibit coagulation factors, causing hemolysis and agglutination of RBCs, which further exacerbate bleeding tendencies. Excess IgM is especially likely to induce agglutination of RBCs in low temperatures (Raynaud's phenomenon), resulting in vascular obstruction and hemolysis at the capillary level.

Signs and symptoms

Macroglobulinemia can be asymptomatic or can produce far-reaching clinical effects: hepatosplenomegaly, enlarged lymph nodes, ocular circulatory disturbances (retinal hemorrhage and sausagelike appearance of retinal veins), congestive heart failure, pallor and acrocyanosis in body parts exposed to cold, and diminished CNS circulation. The latter may produce acute cerebral dysfunction that resembles subarachnoid hemorrhage, with peripheral neuropathy, paresthesias, abnormal reflexes, confusion, obtundation, and coma. Anemia and platelet dysfunction may cause fatigue, weakness, weight loss, purpura, and bleeding (especially from the nose and the gastrointestinal tract).

Diagnosis

Patient history and physical examination revealing characteristic clinical features suggest macroglobulinemia. Increased relative serum viscosity (above 4) indicates the presence of high–molecular-weight immunoglobulins. Total serum protein and globulin levels are elevated; immunoelectrophoretic studies identify abnormal IgM levels as the cause of these high counts. Although a positive Sia water dilution test may suggest this disease, it isn't conclusively diagnostic, because the same result is possible in other conditions, especially rheumatoid arthritis.

Other blood studies show decreased hemoglobin levels, cryoglobulinemia (especially in patients with Raynaud's phenomenon), elevated ESR, increased leukocytes (more than 12,000/mm³), and prolonged bleeding and thrombin times. Bone marrow aspiration shows atypical plasma and lymphoid cells. In some patients, studies may also demonstrate Bence

Jones proteinuria and thrombocytopenia. Differential diagnosis must rule out chronic lymphocytic leukemia, lymphocytic lymphoma, and other plasma cell neoplasms.

Treatment
The patient who is asymptomatic requires no specific treatment but should be regularly monitored for developing clinical changes. Therapy depends on concurrent diseases and the extent of cellular infiltration in the bone marrow. Drug treatment often includes a 3-month course of alkylating agents, such as chlorambucil alone or combined with cyclophosphamide or melphalan. If serum viscosity is high and symptoms are severe, treatment consists of removing 4 to 6 units of plasma per day by plasmapheresis, possibly supplemented with prednisone and chlorambucil; it may also include blood transfusions for the patient with anemia, and splenectomy.

Additional considerations
Clinical care for patients with macroglobulinemia emphasizes measures to relieve symptoms such as epistaxis, reassurance and support during diagnostic and therapeutic procedures, and thorough patient teaching. The hospital staff member should:
• prepare the patient for side effects of chemotherapy (alopecia, gastrointestinal disturbances, and hemorrhagic cystitis); warn the patient receiving prednisone that his resistance to infection may be low, because this drug depresses the autoimmune system; tell him to prevent infection by avoiding crowds or infected persons.
• prepare the patient for plasmapheresis, if applicable. Because plasmapheresis necessitates the use of a dialysis-like machine, this procedure may be viewed as life-threatening. The purpose of plasmapheresis should be explained to the patient, and his vital signs should be monitored for changes.
• ensure correct patient-donor compatibility before administering blood transfusions (double-check to make sure you have the right blood for the right patient); observe for transfusion reaction, and discontinue treatment if it occurs; watch for hepatitis, a possible complication of blood transfusions.
• observe for complications, such as hemorrhage and thrombosis after splenectomy; monitor I.V. therapy, which should continue until bowel sounds return; ambulate the patient as soon as possible after surgery to prevent complications of venous stasis.
• support the patient with end-stage macroglobulinemia through the various stages of dying; keep the patient's family informed of his status and try to prepare them for his death.

Heavy Chain Diseases

Heavy chain diseases are extremely rare neoplasms of the lymphoplasmacytes. In these disorders, abnormal proliferation occurs among cells that produce immunoglobulins, causing incomplete heavy chains and no light chains. (Each immunoglobulin contains heavy and light chains as part of its molecular structure.) Five heavy chains exist, but only three—alpha (most common), gamma, and mu—have been related to lymphocytic disorders. Heavy chain diseases are usually progressively fatal, although complete remissions of the alpha type have occurred.

Causes and incidence
The cause of heavy chain disease is unknown. Only about 50 cases have been reported, mainly among elderly males.

Signs and symptoms
The alpha type of heavy chain disease causes gastrointestinal abnormalities, such as palpable abdominal mass, ab-

dominal pain, chronic diarrhea, severe malabsorption syndrome, marked weight loss, and steatorrhea. It's commonly associated with dehydration, electrolyte imbalance, and clubbing of the fingers.

The *gamma* type produces lymphadenopathy, anemia, malaise, fever, weakness, and hepatosplenomegaly. It may affect Waldeyer's tonsillar ring, producing palatal erythema and edema, with subsequent respiratory distress, and is generally associated with recurrent infections. A few patients with this form of heavy chain disease have developed plasma cell leukemia.

The *mu* type produces hepatosplenomegaly and symptoms of chronic lymphocytic leukemia, without enlarged peripheral lymph nodes.

Diagnosis
In both the alpha and gamma types, immunoelectrophoresis shows heavy chain protein fragments of IgA and IgG, respectively, in serum and sometimes in urine. This same procedure may reveal a greater number of kappa light chains in urine in the mu type. In all three types, serum electrophoresis may demonstrate hypogammaglobulinemia. In the gamma type, blood studies indicate mild-to-moderate anemia, leukopenia, hyperuricemia, thrombocytopenia, eosinophilia, and atypical lymphocytes or plasma cells. In the mu type, abnormal plasma cells appear in marrow aspirate.

Treatment and additional considerations
Treatment of heavy chain diseases is supportive and palliative, consisting chiefly of chemotherapy and radiation. In the mu type, the goal of treatment is to control the underlying disease.

• The patient should be taught how to relieve or minimize side effects of chemotherapy (nausea, stomatitis, alopecia, hemorrhagic cystitis) and radiation (dry throat, abdominal tenderness, skin erythema).

• Healthy skin and bowel function should be promoted. The patient will need an adequate diet, and should get plenty of rest. Changes in the patient's clinical status must be carefully recorded. The severely immunosuppressed patient should be isolated to prevent infection.

• The terminal patient and his family will need emotional support. The family should be kept informed of the patient's status, and may need help to accept and prepare for the patient's death.

MISCELLANEOUS DISORDERS

Granulocytopenia and Lymphocytopenia
(Agranulocytosis and lymphopenia)

Granulocytopenia is characterized by a marked reduction in the number of circulating granulocytes. Although this implies all the granulocytes (neutrophils, basophils, eosinophils) are reduced, granulocytopenia usually refers to decreased neutrophils. This disorder, which can occur at any age, is associated with infections and ulcerative lesions of the throat, gastrointestinal tract, other mucous membranes, and skin. Its severest form is known as agranulocytosis.

Lymphocytopenia, a rare disorder, is a deficiency of circulating lymphocytes (leukocytes produced mainly in lymph nodes).

In both granulocytopenia and lymphocytopenia, the total leukocyte count (WBC) may reach dangerously low levels, leaving the body unprotected against infection. Prognosis in both disorders depends on the underlying cause and whether it can be treated. Untreated, severe granulocytopenia can be fatal in 3 to 6 days.

Causes

Granulocytopenia may result from diminished production of granulocytes in bone marrow, increased peripheral destruction of granulocytes, or greater utilization of granulocytes. Diminished production of granulocytes in bone marrow generally stems from radiation or drug therapy; it's a common side effect of antimetabolites and alkylating agents, and may occur in the patient who is hypersensitive to antihistamines, phenothiazines, sulfonamides (and some sulfonamide derivatives, such as chlorothiazide), tranquilizers, and anticonvulsants. Drug-induced granulocytopenia usually develops slowly, and typically correlates with the dosage and duration of therapy. Production of granulocytes is also low in conditions such as aplastic anemia and bone marrow malignancies, and some hereditary disorders (infantile genetic agranulocytosis).

The growing loss of peripheral granulocytes is due to increased splenic sequestration, diseases that destroy peripheral blood cells (viral and bacterial infections), and drugs that act as haptens (carrying antigens that attack blood cells, and causing acute idiosyncratic or non–dose-related drug reactions). Infections such as infectious mononucleosis may result in granulocytopenia because of increased utilization of granulocytes.

Similarly, lymphocytopenia may result from decreased production, increased destruction, or loss of lymphocytes. For example, decreased production of lymphocytes may be secondary to a genetic or a thymic abnormality, or to immunodeficiency disorders, such as thymic dysplasia or ataxia-telangiectasia. Increased destruction of lymphocytes may be secondary to radiation or chemotherapy (alkylating agents). Loss of lymphocytes may follow postsurgical thoracic duct drainage, intestinal lymphangiectasia, or impaired intestinal lymphatic drainage (as in Whipple's disease).

A decline in the number of lymphocytes can also result from elevated plasma corticoid levels (due to stress, ACTH or

steroid treatment, or congestive heart failure). Associated conditions or diseases also include Hodgkin's disease, leukemia, aplastic anemia, sarcoidosis, myasthenia gravis, systemic lupus erythematosus, protein-calorie malnutrition, renal failure, terminal cancer, miliary tuberculosis, and in infants, severe combined immunodeficiency disorder (SCID).

Signs and symptoms

Patients with granulocytopenia typically experience slowly progressive fatigue and weakness, followed by the sudden onset of signs of overwhelming infection (fever, chills, tachycardia, anxiety, headache, and extreme prostration); ulcers in the mouth or colon; pharyngeal ulceration, possibly with associated necrosis; and septicemia, possibly leading to mild shock. If granulocytopenia is caused by an idiosyncratic drug reaction, signs of infection develop abruptly, without slowly progressive fatigue and weakness.

Patients with lymphocytopenia may exhibit enlarged lymph nodes, spleen, and tonsils, and signs of an associated disease.

Diagnosis

Diagnosis of granulocytopenia necessitates a thorough patient history to check for precipitating factors (recent drug or radiation therapy, or exposure). Physical examination for clinical effects of underlying disorders is also essential.

 Marked reduction in neutrophils (less than 500/mm³ leads to severe bacterial infections) and a WBC lower than 2,000/mm³, with few observable granulocytes on CBC, confirm granulocytopenia.

Examination of bone marrow generally shows a scarcity of granulocytic precursor cells beyond the most immature forms, but this finding may vary, depending on the cause.

A lymphocyte count less than 1,500/mm³ in adults or less than 3,000/mm³ in children indicates lymphocytopenia.

TRANSFUSION OF WBC CONCENTRATE

Content: WBCs, a few RBCs, some plasma

Indication: to increase the patient's white cell mass

Amount: 250 to 500 ml/unit

Administration: through a blood filter

Risks: hepatitis, febrile reaction from leukoagglutinins, and respiratory reactions.

Antipyretics and antihistamines will help prevent adverse reactions. Someone should stay with the patient during the transfusion, and he should be observed for flushing, shaking chills, fever, headache, rash, tachycardia, and hypertension. The transfusion must run slowly—at least 2 hours, and should not be stopped for hives or signs of a febrile reaction unless they are severe.

Symptoms of a respiratory reaction resemble those of pulmonary embolism: chest pain, dyspnea, and cyanosis. Such a reaction is generally due to the migration of white cells to the site of a pulmonary infection. If a respiratory reaction occurs, the transfusion should be halted and oxygen given; the reaction usually subsides within an hour.

Identifying the cause by clinical status, bone marrow and lymph node biopsies, or other appropriate tests helps establish the diagnosis.

Treatment

Effective management of granulocytopenia must include identification and elimination of the cause, if possible. Treatment must also control infection until the bone marrow can generate more leukocytes. This often means drug or radiation therapy must be discontinued and antibiotic treatment begun immediately, even while awaiting results of culture and sensitivity tests. Treatment may also include antifungal preparations and transfusion of WBC concentrate. Spontaneous restoration of leukocyte production in bone marrow generally occurs within 1 to 3 weeks.

Treatment of lymphocytopenia includes discontinuing or modifying the cause (such as alkylating drugs or thoracic drainage) and correctly managing any underlying disorders (such as Hodgkin's disease). For infants with SCID, therapy may include bone marrow transplantation.

Additional considerations

When treating a patient with either of these disorders, the hospital staff member should:

• monitor vital signs frequently; obtain cultures from blood, throat, urine, and sputum, as ordered; give antibiotics, as scheduled.

• explain the need for protective isolation (preferably with laminar air flow) to the patient and family; teach proper handwashing technique and how to correctly use gowns and masks; prevent patient contact with staff members or visitors with respiratory tract infections.

• maintain adequate nutrition and hydration, since malnutrition aggravates immunosuppression; make sure the patient with mouth ulcerations receives a high-calorie liquid diet; offer a straw to make drinking less painful.

• use warm saline water gargles and rinses, analgesics, and anesthetic lozenges, since good oral hygiene promotes patient comfort and facilitates the healing process.

• ensure adequate rest, which is essential to the mobilization of the body's defenses against infection; provide good skin and perineal care.

• monitor CBC and differential, blood culture results, serum electrolytes, intake and output, and daily weight.

• monitor the WBC of any patient receiving radiation or chemotherapy to help detect granulocytopenia and lymphocytopenia in the early, most treatable stages; take measures to avoid exposing a bone marrow-depressed patient to infection.

• advise the patient with known or suspected sensitivity to a drug that may lead to granulocytopenia or lymphocytopenia to alert medical personnel to this sensitivity in the future.

Hypersplenism

Hypersplenism is a syndrome marked by exaggerated splenic activity and possible splenomegaly. This disorder results in peripheral blood cell deficiency as the spleen traps and destroys peripheral blood cells.

Causes

Hypersplenism may be idiopathic (primary), or secondary to an extrasplenic disorder, such as chronic malaria, polycythemia vera, or rheumatoid arthritis. In hypersplenism, the spleen's normal filtering and phagocytic functions accelerate indiscriminately, automatically removing antibody-coated, aging, and abnormal cells, even though some cells may be functionally normal. The spleen may also temporarily sequester normal platelets and RBCs, withholding them from circulation. In this manner, the enlarged spleen may trap as much as 90% of the body's platelets and up to 45% of its RBC mass.

Signs and symptoms

Most patients with hypersplenism develop anemia, leukopenia, or thrombocytopenia, often with splenomegaly. They may contract bacterial infections frequently, bruise easily, hemorrhage spontaneously from the mucous membranes and gastrointestinal or genitourinary tract, and suffer ulcerations of the mouth, legs, and feet. They commonly develop fever, weakness, and palpitations. Patients with secondary hypersplenism may have other clinical abnormalities, depending on the underlying disease.

Diagnosis

Diagnosis requires evidence of abnormal splenic destruction or sequestration of RBCs or platelets, and splenomegaly.

 The most definitive test measures the accumulation of erythrocytes in the spleen and liver after I.V. infusion of chromium-labeled RBCs or platelets. A high spleen/liver ratio of radioactivity indicates splenic destruction

or sequestration. Complete blood count shows decreased hemoglobin (as low as 4 g/100 ml), WBC (less than 4,000/mm³), platelet count (less than 125,000), and reticulocyte count. Splenic biopsy, scan, and angiography may be useful; biopsy is hazardous, however, and should be avoided, if possible.

Treatment

Splenectomy is the treatment of choice if severe cytopenia (thrombocytopenia and granulocytopenia) occurs, but may be complicated by postoperative thromboembolic disease and infection. This procedure rarely cures the patient, especially if he has an underlying disease, but it does correct the effects of cytopenia. Occasionally, splenectomy may result in accelerated blood cell destruction in the bone marrow and liver. Secondary hypersplenism necessitates simultaneous treatment of the underlying disease.

CAUSES OF HYPERSPLENISM WITH SPLENOMEGALY

Infections: Subacute bacterial endocarditis, infectious mononucleosis, malaria, miliary tuberculosis
Connective tissue diseases: Rheumatoid arthritis, lupus erythematosus
Lympho- and myeloproliferative and hemolytic diseases: Lymphomas (Hodgkin's), leukemias (especially chronic lymphocytic and chronic myelocytic forms), polycythemia vera, hemolytic anemias (hereditary, chronic, acquired, acute)
Others: Metabolic disorders (Gaucher's, Niemann-Pick), splenic vein hypertension (cirrhosis, splenic and portal vein thrombosis, stenosis)

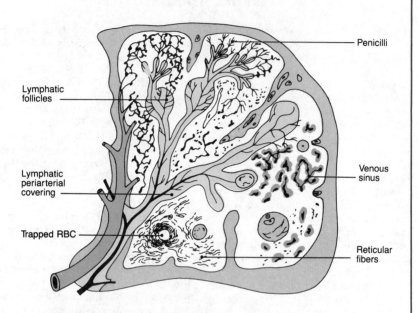

SPLENIC ENTRAPMENT OF BLOOD CELLS

Penicilli

Lymphatic follicles

Lymphatic periarterial covering

Trapped RBC

Venous sinus

Reticular fibers

In hypersplenism, a microscopic cross section of the spleen shows the location of reticular fibers which trap peripheral blood cells.

Additional considerations

If splenectomy is scheduled, preoperative transfusions of blood or blood products (fresh-frozen plasma, platelets) should be administered, as ordered, to replace deficient blood elements. Symptoms or complications of any underlying disorder should be treated also.

Postoperatively, the hospital staff member should: monitor vital signs; check for and immediately report any excessive drainage or apparent bleeding; watch for signs of infection, thromboembolic disease, and abdominal distention; keep the nasogastric tube patent and listen for bowel sounds; instruct the patient to perform deep breathing exercises; and encourage early ambulation to prevent respiratory complications and avoid venous stasis.

Selected References

Barker, Anne M., ed. *Clinical Implications of Laboratory Studies*, CRITICAL CARE QUARTERLY. 2:3, December 1979.

Beck, William S., ed. HEMATOLOGY, 2nd ed. Cambridge, Mass.: M.I.T. Press, 1977.

Berlin, N.I. *Diagnosis and Classifications of the Polycythemias*, SEMINARS IN HEMATOLOGY. 12:4:339-351.

BLOOD COMPONENT THERAPY. Washington, D.C.: American Association of Blood Banks, 1975.

Byrne, Judith. *Coagulation Studies: Part II, Tests of Plasma-clotting Factors*, NURSING77. 7:6:24-25, June 1977.

Byrne, Judith. *Hematological Studies: Part 2, A Review of the CBC: The Differential White Cell Count*, NURSING76. 6:11:15, November 1976.

Castle, W.B. *Myeloproliferative Disorders I: The Polycythemias*, HEMATOLOGY—HARVARD PATHOLOGY SERIES. 1:289-290.

Colvin, B.T. *Thalassemia*, NURSING MIRROR. 18-20, November 10, 1977.

Eichner. *Splenic Function: Too Much and Too Little*, AMERICAN JOURNAL OF MEDICINE. 66, 1979.

Erslev, Allan J., and Thomas G. Gabuzda. PATHOPHYSIOLOGY OF BLOOD, 2nd ed. Philadelphia: W.B. Saunders Co., 1979.

Frangione and Franklin. *Heavy Chain Diseases: Clinical Features and Molecular Significance of the Disordered Immunoglobulin Structure*, SEMINARS IN HEMATOLOGY. January 1973.

GENERAL PRINCIPLES OF BLOOD TRANSFUSION. Chicago: American Medical Association, 1977.

Hillman, R. *Blood-loss Anemia*, POSTGRADUATE MEDICINE. 64:88-94, October 1978.

Koss, L., and M. Eickholt. *Rapid Detection of Ringed Sideroblasts with Bromchlorophenol Blue*, AMERICAN JOURNAL OF CLINICAL PATHOLOGY. 70:738-740, November 1978.

Lee, et al. *Mu Chain Disease*, ANNALS OF INTERNAL MEDICINE. 75, 1971.

Lewis, Jessica, et al. BLEEDING DISORDERS. Garden City, N.Y.: Medical Examination Publishing Co., 1978.

Lichtman, Marshall A., ed. HEMATOLOGY FOR PRACTITIONERS. Boston: Little, Brown & Co., 1978.

Loeb, V. *Treatment of Polycythemia Vera*, CLINICS IN HEMATOLOGY. 4:2:441-456, June 1975.

Mengel, C., et al. *Anemia During Acute Infections: Role of Glucose-6-Phosphate Dehydrogenase*, ARCHIVES OF INTERNAL MEDICINE. 119:287-290.

New Light on von Willebrand's Disease, Congenital Hemorrhagic Disorder, JOURNAL OF THE AMERICAN MEDICAL ASSOCIATION. 238:15.

Reich, P. HEMATOLOGY: PHYSIOPATHOLOGIC BASIS FOR CLINICAL PRACTICE. Boston: Little, Brown & Co., 1978.

Ruddell, W.S., et al. *Pathogenesis of Gastric Cancer in Pernicious Anemia*, LANCET. 521-533, March 11, 1978.

Rutman, Roanne, et al. *Blood Therapy*, AMERICAN JOURNAL OF NURSING. 925-948, May 1979.

Stabbane, et al. *Mediterranean Lymphomas with Alpha Heavy Chain Monoclonal Gammopathy*, CANCER. 38, 1976.

Thomas, F., and S. Buckner. *Current Status of Bone Marrow Transplantation for Aplastic Anemia and Acute Leukemia*, BLOOD. 49:5, May 1977.

Thomas, Susan F. *Transfusing Granulocytes*, AMERICAN JOURNAL OF NURSING. 79:942-944, May 1979.

UCLA Bone Marrow Transplantation Group. *Bone Marrow Transplantation with Intensive Combination Chemotherapy/Radiation Therapy (SCARI) in Acute Leukemia*, ANNALS OF INTERNAL MEDICINE. 86:155-161, February 1977.

Vaz, D. *The Common Anemias: Nursing Approaches*, NURSING CLINICS OF NORTH AMERICA. 7:711-725, December 1972.

Wallner, S., et al. *The Anemia of Chronic Renal Failure and Chronic Diseases: In Vitro Studies of Erythropoiesis*, BLOOD. 47:4:561-569, April 1974.

Wasserman, L. *The Treatment of Polycythemia Vera*, SEMINARS IN HEMATOLOGY. 13:57-78, January 1976.

Weinreb, N., and C. Shih. *Spurious Polycythemia*, SEMINARS IN HEMATOLOGY. 12:397-407, October 1975.

Williams, William J., et al. HEMATOLOGY. New York: McGraw-Hill Book Co., 1977.

Wintrobe, Maxwell M., et al. CLINICAL HEMATOLOGY, 7th ed. Philadelphia: Lea & Febiger, 1974.

Zanjani, E.D. *Hematopoietic Factors in Polycythemia Vera*, SEMINARS IN HEMATOLOGY. 13:1, January 1976.

Zimmerman, S. *Bone Marrow Transplantation*, AMERICAN JOURNAL OF NURSING. 77:1311-1314, August 1977.

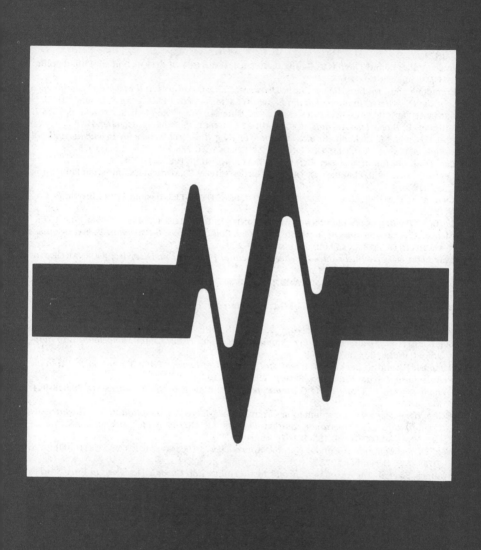

18 Cardiovascular Disorders

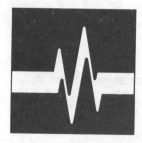

Cardiovascular Disorders

Introduction

The cardiovascular system begins its activity when the fetus is barely a month old and is the last to cease activity at the end of life. This system is so vital that its activity defines the presence of life.

Life-giving transport system

The heart, arteries, veins, and lymphatics form the cardiovascular network that serves as the body's transport system, bringing life-supporting oxygen and nutrients to cells, removing metabolic waste products, and carrying hormones from one part of the body to another. Often called the circulatory system, it may be divided into two branches: *pulmonary circulation,* in which blood picks up new oxygen and liberates the waste product carbon dioxide; and *systemic circulation* (includes coronary circulation), in which blood carries oxygen and nutrients to all active cells, while transporting waste products to the kidneys, liver, and skin for excretion. Circulation requires normal function of the heart, which propels blood through the system by continuous rhythmic contractions. Located behind the sternum, the heart is a muscular organ the size of a man's fist. It is composed of three layers: the *endocardium*—the smooth inner layer; the *myocardium*—the thick, muscular middle layer that contracts in rhythmic beats; and the *epicardium*—the thin, serous membrane that comprises the outer surface of the heart. Covering the entire heart is a sac-like membrane called the *pericardium.* It has two layers: a *visceral* layer that is in contact with the heart and a *parietal,* or outer, layer. To prevent irritation when the heart moves against this layer during contraction, fluid lubricates the parietal pericardium.

The heart has four chambers: two thin-walled chambers called *atria* and two thick-walled chambers called *ventricles.* The atria serve as reservoirs during ventricular contraction (systole) and as booster pumps during ventricular relaxation (diastole). The left ventricle propels blood through the systemic circulation. The right ventricle, which forces blood through the pulmonary circulation, is much thinner than the left, because it meets only one sixth the resistance of systemic circulation.

Heart valves

Two kinds of valves work inside the heart: *atrioventricular* and *semilunar.* The atrioventricular valve between the right atrium and ventricle has three leaflets, or cusps, and three papillary muscles; hence, it's called the tricuspid valve. The atrioventricular valve between the left atrium and ventricle consists of two cusps shaped like a miter and two papillary muscles, and is called the mitral valve. The tricuspid and mitral valves prevent blood backflow from the ventricles to the atria during ventricular contraction. The leaflets of both valves are attached to the papillary muscles of the ventricle by thin, fibrous bands called chordae tendineae; the leaflets separate and descend funnel-like into the ventricles during diastole, and are pushed upward and together during systole, to occlude the mitral and tricuspid orifices.

The two semilunar valves, so called because their cusps resemble half moons, prevent blood backflow from the aorta and pulmonary arteries into the ventricles when the chambers relax and fill with blood from the atria. These valves are named aortic and pulmonic for their respective arteries. However, the action of the valves is not entirely passive, since the papillary muscles contract during systole and prevent the leaflets from prolapse into the atria during ventricular contraction.

The cardiac cycle

Diastole is the phase of ventricular relaxation and filling. As diastole begins, ventricular pressure falls below arterial pressure, and the aortic and pulmonic valves close. As ventricular pressure continues to fall below atrial pressure, the mitral and tricuspid valves open, and blood flows rapidly into the ventricle. Atrial contraction then increases the volume of ventricular filling by pumping up to an additional 20% of blood into the

ventricle. When systole begins, the ventricular muscle contracts, raising ventricular pressure above atrial pressure and closing the mitral and tricuspid valves. When ventricular pressure finally becomes greater than that in the aorta and pulmonary artery, the aortic and pulmonic valves open, and the ventricles eject blood. Ventricular pressure continues to rise as blood is expelled from the heart. As systole ends, the ventricles relax and stop ejecting blood, and ventricular pressure falls, closing the pulmonic and aortic valves.

S_1 (the first heart sound) is heard as the ventricles contract and the atrioventricular valves close. S_1 is loudest at the apex of the heart, over the mitral area. S_2 (the second heart sound), which is normally rapid and sharp, occurs when the aortic and pulmonic valves close. S_2 is loudest at the base of the heart (second intercostal space on both sides of the sternum). Normally, the right heart valves close a fraction of a second later than the left valves, due to lower pressures in the right ventricle and pulmonary artery. Identifying these components during auscultation is usually difficult, except when inspiration coincides with the end of systole, causing slightly prolonged right ventricle ejection time, when the delayed closing of the pulmonic valve is heard as a split S_2.

Distention of the ventricles creates low-

PULSE POINTS

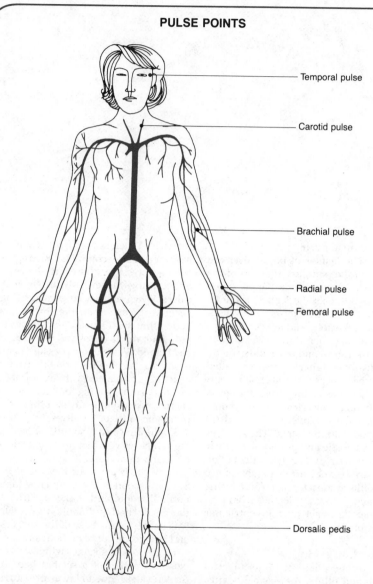

- Temporal pulse
- Carotid pulse
- Brachial pulse
- Radial pulse
- Femoral pulse
- Dorsalis pedis

Peripheral pulse rhythm should correspond exactly to the auscultatory heart rhythm. The character of the pulse may offer useful information. For example, pulsus alternans, a strong beat followed by a weak one, can mean myocardial weakness. A water-hammer (or Corrigan's) pulse, a forceful bounding pulse best felt in the carotid arteries or in the forearm, accompanies increased pulse pressure—often with capillary pulsations of the fingernails (Quincke's sign). This pulse usually indicates patent ductus or aortic regurgitation.

Pulsus biferiens, a double peripheral pulse for every apical beat, can signal aortic stenosis, hyperthyroidism, or some other disease. Pulsus bigeminus is a coupled rhythm; you feel its beat in pairs. Pulsus paradoxus is exaggerated waxing and waning of the arterial pressure (≥ 15 mmHg decrease in systolic blood pressure during inspiration).

frequency vibrations that can sometimes be heard as a third heart sound (S₃), often called a ventricular gallop. At the end of diastole, just before S₁, contraction of the atria forces blood into the already-filled ventricles, creating a rise in pressure and vibrations in the ventricles that can be heard as a fourth heart sound (S₄), dubbed an atrial gallop.

Cardiac conduction

The heart's conduction system is composed of specialized cells capable of generating and conducting rhythmic electrical impulses to stimulate heart contraction. Both the sympathetic and parasympathetic nervous systems influence the rate of electrical impulse generation. The sympathetic nervous system releases norepinephrine locally and increases heart rate; the parasympathetic system releases acetylcholine and slows heart rate. Normally, heart rate is faster in infants and slower in persons who exercise regularly. Body temperature, anxiety, and stress increase heart rate.

Adequate circulation or tissue perfusion depends on cardiac output and peripheral vascular resistance. Cardiac output is the quantity of blood pumped by the left ventricle into the aorta each minute; it is calculated by multiplying the stroke volume (the amount of blood the left ventricle ejects during systole) by heart rate (strokes per minute). Through an increase in either stroke volume or heart rate, cardiac output increases to meet cellular demand. Stroke volume depends on the volume of blood (or pressure exerted by the volume) in the ventricle at the end of diastole (preload), resistance to ejection (afterload), and the myocardium's contractile strength. Changes in preload, afterload, and contractile strength can alter the volume of blood ejected (stroke volume). In turn, the volume of blood ejected alters preload, afterload, and contractile strength.

Circulation and pulses

Blood circulates through three types of vessels: *arteries, veins,* and *capillaries.*

PULSE AMPLITUDE SCALE

To record your patient's pulse amplitude, use this standard scale:

  0: pulse not palpable.

  +1: pulse is thready, weak, difficult to find, may fade in and out, and disappears easily with pressure.

  +2: pulse is constant but not strong; light pressure must be applied or pulse will disappear.

  +3: pulse considered normal. Is easily palpable, does not disappear with pressure.

  +4: pulse is strong, bounding, and does not disappear with pressure.

The sturdy, pliable walls of the arteries distend and recoil to accommodate the volume of blood being sent out of the heart to the body. The major artery arching out of the left ventricle is the aorta. Its segments and subbranches ultimately divide into minute, thin-walled (one-celled) capillaries (so thin that oxygen and nutrients can diffuse out to cells). Capillaries then pass the blood to the veins, which return the blood to the heart. In the veins, valves prevent blood backflow.

Pulses can usually be felt wherever an artery runs close to the skin and over a bone or some other hard structure. The most easily found pulses are:
• *radial artery:* anterolateral aspect of the wrist
• *temporal artery:* in front of the ear, above and lateral to the eye
• *common carotid artery:* side of the neck
• *femoral artery:* groin.

The lymphatic system also plays a role in the cardiovascular network. Originating in tissue spaces, the lymphatic system drains fluid and other plasma components that build up in extravascular spaces and reroutes them back to the circulatory system as lymph, a fluid similar in composition to plasma. Lymphatics also extract bacteria and foreign bodies by reticular endothelial cells.

Cardiovascular assessment

To identify cardiovascular disorders,

PATTERNS OF CARDIAC PAIN

PERICARDITIS	ANGINA	MYOCARDIAL INFARCTION
ONSET AND DURATION: • Sudden onset; continuous pain lasting for days; residual soreness	*ONSET AND DURATION:* • Gradual or sudden onset; pain usually lasts less than 15 minutes and not more than 30 minutes (average: 3 minutes)	*ONSET AND DURATION:* • Sudden onset; pain ½ to 2 hours; residual soreness 1 to 3 days
LOCATION AND RADIATION: • Substernal pain to left of midline; radiation to back or subclavicular area	*LOCATION AND RADIATION:* • Substernal or anterior chest pain, not sharply localized; radiation to back, neck, arms, jaws, even upper abdomen or fingers	*LOCATION AND RADIATION:* • Substernal, midline, or anterior chest pain; radiation to jaws, neck, back, shoulders, or one or both arms
QUALITY AND INTENSITY: • Mild ache to severe pain, deep or superficial; "stabbing," "knife-like"	*QUALITY AND INTENSITY:* • Mild-to-moderate pressure; deep sensation; varied pattern of attacks; "tightness," "squeezing," "crushing"	*QUALITY AND INTENSITY:* • Persistent, severe pressure; deep sensation; "crushing," "squeezing," "heavy," "oppressive"
SIGNS AND SYMPTOMS: • Precordial friction rub; increased pain with movement, inspiration, laughing, coughing; decreased pain with sitting or leaning forward (sitting up pulls the heart away from the diaphragm)	*SIGNS AND SYMPTOMS:* • Dyspnea, diaphoresis, nausea, desire to void, belching, apprehension	*SIGNS AND SYMPTOMS:* • Nausea, vomiting, apprehension, dyspnea, diaphoresis, increased or decreased blood pressure; gallop heart sound, "sensation of impending doom"
PRECIPITATING FACTORS: • Myocardial infarction or upper respiratory tract infection; no relation to effort	*PRECIPITATING FACTORS:* • Exertion, stress, eating, cold or hot and humid weather	*PRECIPITATING FACTORS:* • Occurrence at rest or during physical exertion or emotional stress

assessment should include:
• examination for signs of underlying cardiovascular disorders, such as central cyanosis (disturbance in gas exchange), edema (congestive heart failure or valvular disease), and clubbing of the extremities (congenital cardiovascular disease).
• bilateral palpation of the peripheral pulses to evaluate their rate, equality, and quality on a scale from 0 (absent) to 4 + (bounding).
• inspection of the carotid arteries for equal appearance.
• palpation of the carotid arteries for thrills (fine vibrations due to irregular blood flow).
• auscultation of the carotid arteries for bruits (abnormal whooshing sounds).
• observation of pulsations in the jugular veins (more easily seen than felt).
• examination for jugular venous distention, a possible sign of right-sided heart failure, valvular stenosis, cardiac tamponade, or pulmonary embolism.
• bilateral blood pressure measurements, taken while the patient is lying, sitting, and standing.
• systematic auscultation of the anterior chest wall for each of the four heart sounds; in the aortic area (second intercostal space at the right sternal border), pulmonic area (second intercostal space at the left sternal border), tricuspid area (fifth intercostal space at the left sternal border), and mitral area (fifth intercostal space at the left midclavicular line). Each area is inspected for pulsations and palpated for thrills. Apical pulsation, or the point of maximum impulse (PMI), should be ⅜" to ¾" (1 to 2 cm) in diameter and positioned in the mitral area. Deviations may signal left ventricular hypertrophy, left-sided valvular disease, or right ventricular disease.

- auscultation for the vibrating sound of turbulent blood flow through a stenotic or incompetent valve indicating a murmur. A systolic murmur is heard between S_1 and S_2; a diastolic murmur, between S_2 and S_1. A continuous murmur begins during systole and continues into diastole.
- auscultation for the scratching or squeaking sound characteristic of a pericardial friction rub.

Special cardiovascular tests

After a thorough history, physical examination, and clinical observation, various tests provide diagnostic information.

Electrocardiography (EKG) is a primary tool for evaluating cardiac status. Through electrodes placed on the patient's limbs and over the precordium, an EKG measures electrical activity by recording currents transmitted by the heart. It can detect ischemia, conduction delay, chamber enlargement, and arrhythmias. In ambulatory electrocardiography (also known as Holter monitoring), a tape recording tracks as many as 100,000 cardiac cycles over a 12- or 24-hour period. This test is sometimes used to determine cardiac status after myocardial infarction, to assess the effectiveness of antiarrhythmic drugs, or to evaluate symptoms suggesting arrhythmia.

Chest X-rays may reveal cardiac enlargement and aortic dilation. For example, a heart larger than 50% of the thoracic diameter on a posteroanterior view is considered abnormally enlarged. Chest X-rays also assess pulmonary circulation. When pulmonary venous and arterial pressures rise, characteristic changes appear, such as dilation of the pulmonary venous shadows. When pulmonary venous pressure exceeds oncotic pressure of the blood, capillary fluid leaks into lung tissues, causing pulmonary edema. This fluid may settle in the alveoli, producing a butterfly pattern, or the lungs may appear cloudy or hazy; in the interlobular septa, sharp linear densities (Kerley's lines) may appear.

Exercise testing using a bicycle ergometer, treadmill, or short flight of stairs is a simple procedure to determine cardiac response to physical stress. This test measures blood pressure and EKG changes during an increasingly rigorous series of exercises. In addition to myocardial ischemia, it may cause abnormal blood pressure response or arrhythmias, which indicate failure of the circulatory system to adapt to exercise.

Cardiac catheterization evaluates chest pain, the need for coronary artery surgery, congenital heart defects, and valvular heart disease, and determines the extent of heart failure. Right heart catheterization involves threading a catheter through a vein (usually in the antecubital fossa) into the right heart, pulmonary artery, and its branches in the lungs to measure right atrial, right ventricular, pulmonary artery, and pulmonary capillary wedge pressures. A pulmonary arterial thermodilution catheter can measure cardiac output. Left heart catheterization entails inserting a catheter into an artery and threading it retrogradely through the aorta into the left ventricle. *Ventriculography* during left heart catheterization involves injecting radiopaque dye into the left ventricle to measure ejection fraction (portion of ventricular volume ejected per beat), and to disclose abnormal heart wall motion or mitral valve incompetence.

In *coronary arteriography*, radiopaque material injected into coronary arteries allows cineangiographic visualization of coronary arterial narrowing or occlusion.

Echocardiography uses echoes from pulsed high-frequency sound waves (ultrasound) to evaluate structures of the heart. In M-mode echocardiography, a small transducer placed on the chest wall in various positions and angles acts as both transmitter and receiver. It provides information about valve leaflets, sizes and dimensions of heart chambers, and thicknesses and motions of the septum and the ventricular walls. It can also show intracardiac masses (atrial tumors, for example), detect pericardial effusion, suggest idiopathic hyper-

EKG LEAD PLACEMENT

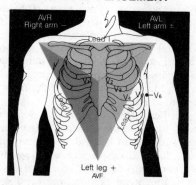

The twelve-lead EKG provides a three-dimensional view of cardiac activity through three sets of leads:
• Standard limb leads (I, II, III) record electrical activity from the heart to the extremities.
• Augmented leads (AVR, AVL, AVF) measure activity from the right and left shoulders and left leg.
• Precordial or chest leads (V_1 to V_6) show ventricular electrical activity.

trophic subaortic stenosis, and estimate cardiac output and ejection fraction. Echocardiography can also evaluate possible aortic dissection when it involves the ascending aorta. Two-dimensional echocardiography is a new, noninvasive technique that provides pictures of cardiac structures and their movements.

Phonocardiography graphically records the sounds of the cardiac cycle heard with a stethoscope. By simultaneously recording an EKG, this test can time heart sounds. It is used to measure ventricular function by calculating systolic time intervals.

In *gated blood pool scan*, a radioactive isotope remains in the intravascular compartment, allowing measurement of stroke volume, ventricular ejection fraction, and wall motion. *Myocardial imaging* uses radioactive agents (most often thallium 201) to detect abnormalities in coronary artery perfusion. These agents concentrate in normally perfused myocardium but not in ischemic areas. Non-

perfused areas, or "cold spots," may be permanent (scar tissue after myocardial infarction) or temporary (induced by transient ischemia). Thallium scanning with exercise tests identifies exercise-induced ischemia and evaluates abnormal findings on a stress EKG.

Acute infarct imaging documents muscle viability (not perfusion) through the use of technetium-labeled pyrophosphate. Unlike thallium, technetium accumulates only in irreversibly damaged myocardial tissue. Areas of necrosis appear as "hot spots" and can be detected only during acute infarction. This test determines the size and location of infarction but can produce false positive results.

Cardiac enzymes are cellular proteins released into the blood as a result of cell membrane injury. Their presence in the blood confirms acute myocardial infarction or severe cardiac trauma. All cardiac enzymes—creatine phosphokinase (CPK), lactic dehydrogenase (LDH), and serum glutamic-oxaloacetic transaminase (SGOT), for example—are also found in other cells. Fractionation of enzymes can determine the source of damaged cells. For example, three fractions of CPK are isolated, one of which (an isoenzyme called CPK-MB) is found only in cardiac cells. The presence of CPK-MB in the blood indicates injury to myocardial cells.

Arteriography consists of a fluoroscopic X-ray after arterial injection of contrast media. Similarly, *phlebography* defines the venous system after injection of contrast media into a vein. *Impedance plethysmography* evaluates the venous system to detect pressure changes (caused by changes in venous blood volume with deep breathing) transmitted to lower leg veins.

Managing cardiovascular disease

Cardiovascular disease poses a tremendous challenge, because proper diagnosis and treatment require a thorough understanding of cardiovascular anatomy, physiology, and pathophysiology. Because of their high anxiety levels, cardiac patients need support and reassurance, especially during stressful procedures such as cardiac catheterization, which may identify the need for open heart surgery. Cardiac rehabilitation programs are still experimental, developmental, and controversial in that the experts disagree about how much activity is safe and how to schedule its progression to normal. They agree, however, that the ideal rehabilitation program begins in the hospital and continues afterward, on an outpatient basis. Helping the patient resume a satisfying lifestyle requires careful planning and comprehensive teaching. Hospitals and community organizations across the United States and Canada are initiating formal cardiac rehabilitation programs that emphasize the recognition, prevention, and treatment of cardiovascular disease. The patient and his family should be informed about such programs in their area.

CONGENITAL ACYANOTIC DEFECTS

Ventricular Septal Defect

In ventricular septal defect (VSD), the most common congenital heart disorder, an opening in the septum between the ventricles allows blood to shunt between the left and right ventricles. VSD accounts for up to 30% of all congenital heart defects. Prognosis is good for small defects that close spontaneously or are correctable surgically, but poor for extremely large, untreated, or irreparable defects, which are sometimes fatal by age 1, usually from secondary complications.

Causes
In infants with VSD, the ventricular septum fails to close completely by the eighth week of gestation, as it would normally. VSD occurs in some infants with fetal alcohol syndrome, but a causal relationship has not been established. Although most children with congenital heart defects are otherwise normal, in some, VSD coexists with additional birth defects, especially Down's syndrome and other autosomal trisomies, renal anomalies, and such cardiac defects as patent ductus arteriosus and coarctation of the aorta. VSDs are usually located in the membranous or muscular portion of the ventricular septum, and vary in size. Some muscular defects are small and close spontaneously; in some membranous defects, the entire septum is absent, creating a single ventricle.

VSD isn't readily apparent at birth because right and left ventricular pressures are approximately equal, so blood doesn't shunt through the defect. As the pulmonary vasculature gradually relaxes, between 4 and 8 weeks after birth, right ventricular pressure decreases, allowing blood to shunt from the left to the right ventricle.

Signs and symptoms
Clinical features of VSD vary with the size of the defect, the effect of the shunting on the pulmonary vasculature, and the infant's age. In a small VSD, shunting is minimal, and pulmonary artery pressure and heart size remain normal. Such defects may eventually close spontaneously without ever causing symptoms.

Large VSD shunts cause left atrial, and right and left ventricular hypertrophy, due to increasing pulmonary resistance and right ventricular pressure. Eventually, biventricular congestive heart failure and cyanosis (from reversal of shunt direction) occur. Resulting cardiac hypertrophy may make the anterior chest wall prominent. A large VSD also increases the risk of pneumonia.

Infants with large VSDs are thin, small for their age, and gain weight slowly. They may develop congestive heart failure, with dusky skin; liver, heart, and spleen enlargement because of systemic venous congestion; diaphoresis; feeding difficulties; rapid, grunting respirations; and increased heart rate. They may also develop severe pulmonary hypertension, with right-to-left shunt (Eisenmenger's complex), causing cyanosis and clubbing of the nailbeds. The typical murmur associated with a VSD is harsh, and its frequency varies from one beat to the next. In the newborn, a moderately loud early systolic murmur may be heard along the lower left sternal border. About the second or third day after birth, the murmur may become louder and longer, then shorten again in 3 to 6 weeks. In infants, the murmur may be loudest near the base of the heart and may suggest pulmonary stenosis. A small VSD may produce a functional murmur or a characteristic loud, harsh systolic murmur. Moderate-sized and large VSDs produce audible murmurs (at least a grade 3 pansystolic), loudest at the fourth intercostal space, usually accompanied by a thrill. Palpation reveals displacement of the point of maximal impulse to the left. When pulmonary hypertension or mitral stenosis is present, a diastolic murmur may be audible on auscultation, the systolic murmur becomes quieter, and S_2 is accentuated.

Diagnosis

Diagnostic tests include the following:
• *Chest X-ray* is normal in small defects; in large VSDs, it shows left atrial and left ventricular enlargement, and prominent pulmonary vascular markings.
• *EKG* is normal in children with small VSDs; in large VSDs, it shows left and right ventricular hypertrophy, suggesting pulmonary hypertension.
• *Echocardiography* may detect a large VSD and its location in the septum, determine the size of a left-to-right shunt, and suggest pulmonary hypertension, but is more useful in identifying associated lesions and complications.

 • *Cardiac catheterization* determines the size of the VSD and calculates the degree of shunting through a comparison of blood oxygen saturation in each ventricle. Catheterization also determines the extent of pulmonary hypertension and can rule out associated defects.

Treatment

Large defects usually require early surgical correction, before irreversible pulmonary vascular disease develops. Surgery consists of simple suture closure or insertion of a patch graft, using cardiopulmonary bypass. If the child has other defects and will benefit from delaying surgery, pulmonary artery banding normalizes pressures and flow distal to the band and prevents pulmonary vascular disease, allowing postponement of surgical correction. (Pulmonary artery banding is necessary only when the child has severe symptoms or other complications.) A rare complication of VSD repair is complete heart block from interference with the bundle of His during surgery. (Heart block may necessitate temporary or permanent pacemaker implantation.)

Before surgery, treatment consists of:
• bed rest, oxygen, digoxin, sodium restriction, and diuretics to prevent congestive heart failure.
• careful monitoring by physical examination, X-ray, and EKG for severe pulmonary hypertension, which, if it develops, indicates an imminent need for surgery.
• measures to prevent infection (prophylactic antibiotics, for example, to prevent infective endocarditis).

Postoperative treatment may include nitroprusside to dilate peripheral blood vessels and lessen left ventricular workload while increasing cardiac output; catecholamines by continuous I.V. infusion to maintain blood pressure and cardiac output; diuretics to increase urinary output; analgesics; mechanical ventilation; and possibly, a temporary pacemaker.

Additional considerations

Although the parents of an infant or child with VSD often suspect something is wrong with their child before diagnosis, they may need psychologic support to accept this serious cardiac disorder. Because surgery often is delayed or uncertain, parents must reduce the risk of complications until the child is ready for surgery or until the defect closes. For example, parents should:

• watch for signs of congestive heart failure, such as poor feeding, sweating, heavy breathing, and fatigue.

• watch for signs of digoxin toxicity (anorexa, nausea, vomiting) if the child is taking this medication. Parents should be reminded to keep medication out of the reach of children.

• recognize and report early signs of infection, and avoid exposing their child to crowds or persons with infections.

After surgery to correct VSD, the child's parents still need support. They'll probably feel reassured if they can participate in the child's care as much as possible.

Caring for the child after surgery includes careful monitoring of the child's vital signs, and fluid intake and output. An overbed warmer may be used to maintain his body temperature. In addition, the child's care includes:

• giving catecholamines, nitroprusside, diuretics, and analgesics.

• obtaining central venous pressure, arterial blood pressure, and left atrial or pulmonary artery pressure readings.

• assessing heart rate and rhythm for signs of conduction block.

• checking oxygenation, especially if the child requires mechanical ventilation.

• frequent suctioning, to ensure a patent airway and to prevent atelectasis and pneumonia.

• monitoring pacemaker effectiveness (if appropriate). Signs of pacemaker failure include bradycardia and hypotension.

Atrial Septal Defect

In an atrial septal defect (ASD), an opening between the left and right atria allows shunting of blood between the chambers. Ostium secundum defect (most common) occurs in the region of the fossa ovalis and, occasionally, extends inferiorly, close to the vena cava; sinus venosus defect occurs in the superior-posterior portion of the atrial septum, sometimes extending into the vena cava, and is almost always associated with abnormal drainage of pulmonary veins into the right atrium; ostium primum, a defect of the primitive septum, occurs in the inferior portion of the septum primum and is usually associated with atrioventricular valve abnormalities (cleft mitral valve) and conduction defects. ASD accounts for about 10% of congenital heart defects and appears almost twice as often in females as in males, with a strong familial tendency. Although ASD is usually a benign defect during infancy, delayed development of symptoms and complications makes it one of the most common congenital heart defects diagnosed in adults. Prognosis is excellent in asymptomatic persons, but poor in those with cyanosis and severe, untreated defects.

Causes

The cause of ASD is unknown. In this condition, blood shunts from left to right because left atrial pressure normally is slightly higher than right atrial pressure; this pressure difference is sufficient to force large amounts of blood through a defect. The left-to-right shunt results in right heart volume overload, affecting the right atrium, right ventricle, and pulmonary arteries. Eventually, the right atrium enlarges, and the right ventricle dilates to accommodate the increased blood volume. If obstructive pulmonary vascular disease develops as a consequence of the shunt (rare in children), pulmonary artery pressure rises, resulting in right ventricular hypertrophy and decreased pulmonary vascular compliance. In some patients, decreased right ventricular compliance causes reversal of the direction of the shunt, which results in unoxygenated blood entering the systemic circulation, causing cyanosis.

Signs and symptoms

ASD often goes undetected in preschoolers; such children may complain about feeling tired only after extreme exertion and may have frequent respiratory tract infections but otherwise appear normal and healthy. However, they may show growth retardation if they have large shunts. Children with ASD rarely develop congestive heart failure, pulmonary hypertension, infective endocarditis, or other complications. However, as adults, they usually manifest pronounced symptoms, such as fatigability and dyspnea on exertion, frequently to the point of severe limitation of activity (especially after age 40).

In children, auscultation reveals an early to midsystolic murmur, superficial in quality, heard at the second or third intercostal space. In patients with large shunts—as a result of increased tricuspid valve flow—a low-pitched diastolic murmur is heard at the lower left sternal border, which becomes more pronounced on inspiration. Although the murmur's intensity is a rough indicator of the size of the left-to-right shunt, its low pitch sometimes makes it difficult to hear. An early to midsystolic click at the apex may indicate impending mitral valve prolapse. Occasionally, a late systolic apical murmur of mitral insufficiency can be heard.

In older patients with large uncorrected defects and obstructive pulmonary vascular disease, auscultation reveals right ventricular hypertrophy, with an accentuated S_2 and fixed wide splitting due to delayed closure of the pulmonic valve. A pulmonary ejection click and an audible S_4 may also be pres-

ent. Clubbing of the fingers, and cyanosis become evident; syncope and hemoptysis may occur with severe pulmonary vascular disease.

Diagnosis

A history of increasing fatigue and characteristic physical features suggest ASD. The following findings support this diagnosis:

• *Chest X-ray* shows an enlarged right atrium and right ventricle, and a prominent pulmonary artery.

• *EKG* may be normal but often shows prolonged P-R interval, varying degrees of right bundle branch block, right ventricular hypertrophy, atrial fibrillation (particularly in severe cases after the third decade of life), and in ostium primum, left axis deviation.

• *Echocardiography* measures the extent of right ventricular enlargement and may locate the defect. (Other causes of right ventricular enlargement—for example, tricuspid insufficiency—must be ruled out.)

 • *Cardiac catheterization* confirms ASD by demonstrating that right atrial blood is more oxygenated than superior vena cava blood—indicating a left-to-right shunt—and determines the degree of shunting and pulmonary vascular disease.

Treatment and additional considerations

Since ASD seldom produces complications in infants and toddlers, surgical repair can be delayed until they reach preschool or early school age. If the defect is large, immediate and temporary surgical closure with sutures or a patch graft may be necessary. For a small ASD, insertion of an umbrella-like patch using a cardiac catheter is an alternative to open heart surgery.

The parents and child need an explanation of cardiac catheterization, as well as pre-test and post-test procedures. Drawings and a tour of the catheterization lab will help both parents and child understand the explanation.

If surgery is scheduled, parents and child may be shown the ICU and introduced to the staff. The ICU staff can explain how tubes, dressings, and monitoring equipment are used during postoperative care.

After surgery, the ICU staff will closely monitor the child's vital signs, central venous and intra-arterial pressures, and fluid intake and output. They'll also watch for atrial arrhythmias, since surgical correction of ASD is only about 50% successful in eliminating these arrhythmias.

Coarctation of the Aorta

Coarctation is a narrowing of the aorta, usually just below the left subclavian artery, near the site where the ligamentum arteriosum (the remnant of the ductus arteriosus, a fetal blood vessel) joins the pulmonary artery to the aorta. Coarctation is often classified as preductal (occurring above the ligamentum arteriosum) or postductal (occurring below). Both types are associated with other congenital heart anomalies, most commonly tubular hypoplasia of the aortic arch and patent ductus arteriosus. Ventricular septal defect and transposition of the great vessels often accompany preductal coarctation; bicuspid aortic valve and aortic stenosis often accompany postductal coarctation. Generally, prognosis for coarctation of the aorta depends on the severity of associated congenital anomalies; prognosis for isolated coarctation is good if corrective surgery is performed before this condition induces degenerative changes.

Causes and incidence

Coarctation of the aorta may develop as a result of spasm and constriction of the smooth muscle in the ductus arteriosus as it closes. Possibly, this contractile tissue extends into the aortic wall, causing narrowing. The obstructive process causes hypertension in the aortic branches above the constriction (arteries that supply the arms and brain) and diminished pressure in the vessels below the constriction.

Hypertension increases the pressure load on the left ventricle and causes dilation of the proximal aorta and ventricular hypertrophy. Untreated, this condition may lead to left heart failure and, rarely, to cerebral hemorrhage and aortic rupture. If ventricular septal defect accompanies coarctation, blood shunts left to right, straining the right heart. This leads to pulmonary hypertension and, eventually, right heart hypertrophy and failure.

Coarctation of the aorta accounts for about 7% of all congenital heart defects in children and is twice as common in males as in females. When it occurs in females, it's often associated with Turner's syndrome, an absence or defect of the second sex chromosome, causing ovarian dysgenesis.

Signs and symptoms

Clinical features vary with age. During the first year of life, when aortic coarctation often causes congestive heart failure, the infant displays dyspnea, pulmonary edema, tachypnea, pallor, failure to thrive, cardiomegaly, and hepatomegaly. Coarctation causes cyanosis if it's associated with transposition of the great vessels; it causes peripheral cyanosis in the terminal stages of severe untreated coarctation.

If coarctation is asymptomatic in infancy, it usually remains so throughout adolescence, as collateral circulation develops to bypass the narrowed segment. After adolescence, this defect produces dyspnea, claudication, headaches, epistaxis, weak or absent femoral pulses, and hypertension in the upper extremities despite collateral circulation. Fre-

COARCTATION OF THE AORTA

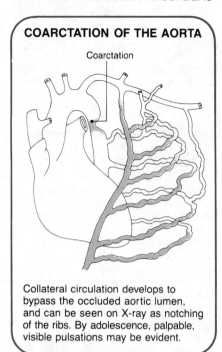

Coarctation

Collateral circulation develops to bypass the occluded aortic lumen, and can be seen on X-ray as notching of the ribs. By adolescence, palpable, visible pulsations may be evident.

quently, it causes resting systolic hypertension and wide pulse pressure; high diastolic pressure readings are the same in both the arms and legs. Coarctation may also produce a visible aortic pulsation in the suprasternal notch; a soft systolic ejection murmur along the left sternal border, and an S_4, caused by left ventricular failure.

Diagnosis

The cardinal signs of coarctation of the aorta are resting systolic hypertension and wide pulse pressure (high systolic readings when measured in the arms; normal or depressed readings when measured in the legs). The following tests support this diagnosis:

• *Chest X-ray* may demonstrate left ventricular hypertrophy, congestive heart failure, a wide descending aorta, and notching of the undersurfaces of the ribs, due to extensive collateral circulation.

• *EKG* may eventually reveal left ventricular hypertrophy.

• *Echocardiography* may show increased left ventricular muscle thickness and, possibly, aortic valve abnormalities and the site of the coarctation.

• *Cardiac catheterization* and *aortography* are indicated in the presence of other cardiac abnormalities. Cardiac catheterization evaluates collateral circulation, and measures pressure in the right and left ventricles and in the ascending and descending aortas (on both sides of the obstruction); aortography may locate the site and extent of coarctation.

Treatment

Surgical resection with end-to-end anastomosis of the aorta or insertion of a prosthetic graft is the treatment of choice. Such surgery is usually necessary during infancy if associated anomalies are present. However, careful medical management with digitalis, fluid restriction, and antihypertensive therapy generally permits postponement of surgery in a symptomatic child with a single defect until the child is between ages 3 and 6. Ideally, surgical repair for an asymptomatic child is deferred until ages 8 to 12.

Additional considerations

Coarctation in an infant may require rapid digitalization. If so, he'll be observed closely for signs of digitalis toxicity (anorexia, nausea, vomiting).

Medical care also includes:

• monitoring vital signs.

• carefully balancing fluid intake and output, especially if the infant is receiving diuretics with fluid restriction.

• regulating environmental temperature, using an overbed warmer, if necessary.

After corrective surgery, the infant's blood pressure is monitored continuously with an arterial line. In addition, postoperative care includes:

• taking regular pressure-cuff blood pressure readings in each extremity (except the extremity with the aterial line in place).

• monitoring blood glucose levels to detect possible hypoglycemia.

• administering nitroprusside or trimethaphan by continuous I.V. infusion, if the infant develops hypertension.

• promoting adequate respiratory function by turning the infant and encouraging coughing and deep breathing.

• monitoring chest tubes for patency.

• providing pain relief.

• encouraging a gradual increase in activity.

The parents of an infant or child with coarctation of the aorta need emotional support. In addition, they need an explanation of the disorder and its treatment. To care for the child at home, they need to know drug dosages and side effects. If an older child is asymptomatic but requires antihypertensives, the need for compliance should be stressed. If the child's scheduled for corrective surgery, he should be told what to expect during his hospitalization.

Patent Ductus Arteriosus

The ductus arteriosus is a fetal blood vessel that connects the pulmonary artery to the descending aorta. In patent ductus arteriosus (PDA), the lumen of the ductus remains open after birth. This creates a left-to-right shunt of blood from the aorta to the pulmonary artery and results in recirculation of arterial blood through the lungs. Initially, PDA may produce no clinical effects, but in time, it can precipitate pulmonary vascular disease, causing symptoms to appear by age 40. Prognosis is good if the shunt is small or surgical repair is effective. Otherwise, PDA may advance to intractable congestive heart failure, which may be fatal.

Causes and incidence

PDA affects twice as many females as males and is the most common congenital heart disease found in adults. Normally, the ductus closes within days to weeks after birth. Failure to close is most prevalent in premature infants, probably as a result of abnormalities in oxygenation (with normal lung function) or the relaxant action of ductal prostaglandin E, which prevents ductus spasm and contracture necessary for closure. PDA often accompanies rubella syndrome and may be associated with other congenital defects, such as coarctation of the aorta, ventricular septal defect, and pulmonary and aortic stenoses.

In PDA, the relative resistances in the pulmonary and systemic vasculature, and the size of the ductus determine the amount of left-to-right shunting. The left atrium and left ventricle must accommodate the increased pulmonary venous return, in turn increasing left heart filling pressure and workload, and possibly causing left heart failure. In the final stages of untreated PDA, severe obstructive pulmonary vascular disease may develop and cause the shunt to reverse (right to left); unoxygenated blood thus enters the systemic circulation, resulting in cyanosis.

Signs and symptoms

In infants, especially those who are premature, a large PDA usually produces respiratory distress, with signs of congestive heart failure due to the tremendous volume of blood shunted to the lungs through a patent ductus and the increasing left heart workload. Other characteristic features may include heightened susceptibility to respiratory tract infections, slow motor development, and failure to thrive. In adults with undetected PDA, pulmonary vascular disease may develop, and by age 40, they may display fatigability, and dyspnea on exertion. About 10% of these persons also develop infective endocarditis.

Auscultation reveals the classic machinery murmur (Gibson murmur): a continuous murmur (during systole and diastole) best heard at the base of the heart, at the second left intercostal space under the left clavicle in 85% of children with PDA. This murmur may also obscure S_2. However, with a right-to-left shunt, such a murmur may be absent. Auscultation of infants and children with large PDAs may detect a middiastolic rumble heard at the apex, a systolic ejection sound, or S_3. Palpation may reveal a thrill at the left sternal border and a prominent left ventricular impulse. Peripheral arterial pulses are bounding (Corrigan's pulse); pulse pressure is widened, due to an elevation in systolic blood pressure and primarily to a drop in diastolic pressure.

Diagnosis

• *Chest X-ray* shows increased pulmonary vascular markings, normal heart size, and if the shunt is large, an enlarged left atrium, left ventricle, aorta, and pulmonary artery.
• *EKG* may indicate left ventricular hypertrophy and, in pulmonary vascular disease, biventricular hypertrophy.
• *Echocardiography* reveals an enlarged left atrium and left ventricle, or right ventricular hypertrophy from pulmonary vascular disease; it also detects PDA.
• *Cardiac catheterization* shows pulmonary arterial oxygen content higher than right ventricular content because of the influx of aortic blood, suggesting diagnosis. Increased pulmonary artery pressure indicates a large shunt or, if it exceeds systemic arterial pressure, severe pulmonary vascular disease. Catheterization allows calculation of blood volume crossing the ductus and can rule out associated cardiac defects.

Treatment

Asymptomatic infants with PDA require no immediate treatment. Those with congestive heart failure require fluid restriction, diuretics, and digitalis to minimize or control symptoms. If these measures can't control congestive heart failure, surgery is necessary to ligate the ductus. If symptoms are mild, surgical correction is usually delayed until pre-school age. Before surgery, children with PDA require antibiotics to protect against infective endocarditis.

Other forms of therapy include cardiac catheterization to deposit a plug in the ductus to stop shunting, or administration of indomethacin (a prostaglandin inhibitor that appears promising in treating premature infants) to induce ductus spasm and closure.

Additional considerations

Every premature infant should be watched carefully for signs of PDA, especially respiratory distress resulting from congestive heart failure (which may develop rapidly in an infant). Frequent assessments of vital signs, electrolyte levels, fluid intake and output, and EKG readout strips are essential.

In addition, the infant's response to diuretics, digitalis, and other drugs must be monitored closely. For example, he must be watched for signs of digitalis toxicity (anorexia, nausea, vomiting, cardiac arrhythmias). And if he receives indomethacin for ductus closure, he must be watched for side effects such as diarrhea, jaundice, bleeding, or renal dysfunction.

The infant's family should be informed about the disorder and its treatment, and given emotional support, especially when surgery's scheduled. If the patient's an older child, he should be given the explanation, too. He may be less apprehensive about surgery if he meets the ICU staff beforehand. They can show him I.V. and monitoring equipment, and explain postoperative procedures.

Following surgery, the child's vital signs, fluid intake and output, and arterial and venous pressures should be monitored regularly. Pain relief is provided as needed.

After discharge, the child's activity restrictions are governed by his own tolerance and energy levels. Parents should be advised against overprotecting the child as his tolerance for physical activity increases.

Parents should also understand the need for regular medical follow-up examinations for their child. In addition, they must remember to inform any doctor who treats their child in the future about the child's medical history—even if he is treating the child for an unrelated medical problem.

CONGENITAL CYANOTIC DEFECTS

Tetralogy of Fallot

Tetralogy of Fallot is a complex of four congenital heart defects: ventricular septal defect (VSD), right ventricular outflow tract obstruction (pulmonary stenosis), right ventricular hypertrophy, and dextroposition of the aorta, with overriding of the VSD. Blood shunts right to left through the VSD, permitting unoxygenated blood to mix with oxygenated blood, resulting in cyanosis. Tetralogy of Fallot sometimes coexists with other congenital heart defects, such as patent ductus arteriosus or atrial septal defect. It accounts for about 10% of all congenital heart diseases, and occurs equally in boys and girls. Before surgical advances made correction possible, approximately one third of these children died in infancy.

Causes
The cause of tetralogy of Fallot is unknown, but it may result from embryologic hypoplasia of the outflow tract of the right ventricle, and has been associated with fetal alcohol syndrome and the ingestion of thalidomide during pregnancy.

Signs and symptoms
The degree of pulmonary stenosis, interacting with the size of the VSD, determines the clinical and hemodynamic effects of this complex defect. The VSD usually lies in the outflow tract of the right ventricle and is generally large enough to permit equalization of right and left ventricular pressures. However, systemic vascular resistance to pulmonary stenosis affects the direction and magnitude of shunt flow across the VSD. Severe obstruction of right ventricular outflow produces a right-to-left shunt, causing decreased systemic arterial oxygen saturation, cyanosis, reduced pulmonary blood flow, and hypoplasia of the entire pulmonary vasculature. Milder forms of pulmonary stenosis result in a left-to-right shunt, causing increased right ventricular pressure and, eventually, right ventricular hypertrophy.

Generally, the hallmark of the disorder is cyanosis, which usually becomes evident within several months after birth, but may be present at birth if the infant has severe pulmonary stenosis. Between ages 2 months and 2 years, children with tetralogy of Fallot may experience cyanotic, or "blue," spells. Such spells are caused by increased right-to-left shunting, possibly caused by spasm of the right ventricular outflow tract, increased systemic venous return, or decreased systemic arterial resistance.

Exercise, crying, straining, infection, or fever can precipitate blue spells. Blue spells are characterized by dyspnea; deep, sighing respirations; bradycardia; fainting; seizures; and loss of consciousness. Older children may also develop other signs of poor oxygenation, such as clubbing of fingers and toes, diminished exercise tolerance, increasing dyspnea on exertion, growth retardation, and eating difficulties. These children habitually squat when they feel short of breath; this decreases venous return of unoxygenated blood from the legs and increases systemic arterial resistance.

Children with tetralogy of Fallot also risk developing cerebral abscesses, pulmonary thrombosis, venous thrombosis or cerebral embolism, and infective endocarditis.

In females with tetralogy of Fallot who live to childbearing age, incidence of spontaneous abortion, premature births, and low birth weight rises.

Diagnosis

In a patient with tetralogy of Fallot, auscultation detects a loud systolic heart murmur (best heard along the left sternal border), which may diminish or obscure the pulmonic component of S_2. A prominent ejection click is heard immediately after S_1. However, in severe pulmonary stenosis, the continuous murmur of a patent ductus obscures the systolic murmur. Palpation may reveal a cardiac thrill at the left sternal border.

The results of special tests also support the diagnosis:

• *Chest X-ray* may demonstrate decreased pulmonary vascular marking, depending on the severity of the pulmonary obstruction, and a boot-shaped cardiac silhouette.

• *EKG* shows right ventricular hypertrophy, right axis deviation, and possibly, right atrial hypertrophy.

• *Echocardiography* identifies septal overriding of the aorta, further substantiates both the VSD and pulmonary stenosis, and depicts an enlarged right atrium and right ventricle.

 • *Cardiac catheterization* confirms diagnosis by detecting pulmonary stenosis and the VSD, visualizing the overriding aorta, and ruling out other cyanotic heart defects. This test also detects decreased oxygen saturation of aortic blood.

• Laboratory findings reveal diminished arterial oxygen saturation; polycythemia (hematocrit may be more than 60%), if the cyanosis is severe and long-standing, predisposing to thrombosis.

Treatment

Effective management of tetralogy of Fallot necessitates prevention and treatment of complications, measures to relieve cyanosis, and palliative or corrective surgery. During cyanotic spells, the knee-chest position and administration of oxygen and morphine improve oxygenation. Propranolol (a beta-adrenergic blocking agent) may relieve spasm of the right ventricular outflow tract and improve oxygen saturation.

Palliative surgery is performed on infants with severe complications, such as potentially fatal hypoxic spells. The goal of surgery is to enhance blood flow to the lungs to reduce hypoxia; this may be accomplished by joining the subclavian artery to the pulmonary artery (Blalock-Taussig procedure), by joining the descending aorta to the pulmonary artery (Potts-Smith-Gibson), or by joining the ascending aorta to the right pulmonary artery (Waterston). Supportive measures include prophylactic antibiotics to prevent infective endocarditis or cerebral abscess administered before, during, and after bowel, bladder or any other surgery, or dental extractions. Treatment may also include phlebotomy in children with polycythemia.

Complete corrective surgery to relieve pulmonary stenosis and close the VSD, directing left ventricular outflow to the aorta, requires cardiopulmonary bypass with hypothermia to decrease oxygen utilization during surgery, especially in young children. This is usually accomplished by age 2.

Additional considerations

Although a child with tetralogy of Fallot will be small for his age, he can engage in normal physical activity. Parents, who may become overprotective, need to be reassured that a child will know when to rest and limit his own activity.

The child's parents must learn to recognize the signs of serious hypoxic spells (dramatically increased cyanosis; deep, sighing respirations; loss of consciousness). If the child suffers a hypoxic spell, his parents should place him in a knee-chest position and seek medical advice at once. Emergency treatment may be necessary.

To prevent infective endocarditis and other infections, parents should keep

NORMAL HEART

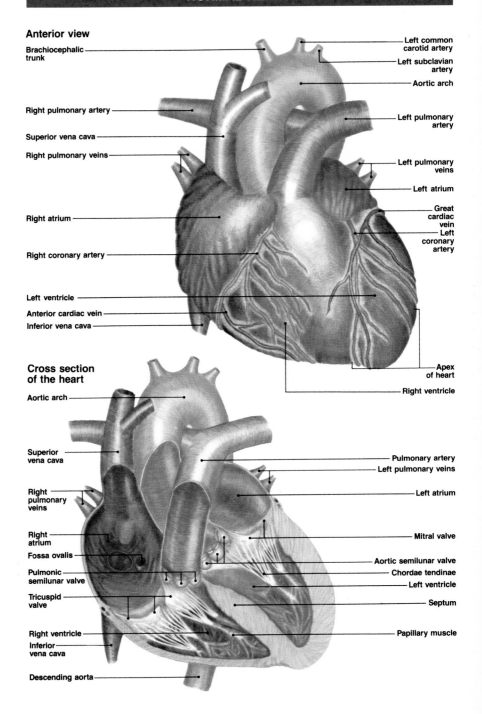

Anterior view

Brachiocephalic trunk

Right pulmonary artery

Superior vena cava

Right pulmonary veins

Right atrium

Right coronary artery

Left ventricle

Anterior cardiac vein

Inferior vena cava

Left common carotid artery

Left subclavian artery

Aortic arch

Left pulmonary artery

Left pulmonary veins

Left atrium

Great cardiac vein

Left coronary artery

Apex of heart

Right ventricle

Cross section of the heart

Aortic arch

Superior vena cava

Right pulmonary veins

Right atrium

Fossa ovalis

Pulmonic semilunar valve

Tricuspid valve

Right ventricle

Inferior vena cava

Descending aorta

Pulmonary artery

Left pulmonary veins

Left atrium

Mitral valve

Aortic semilunar valve

Chordae tendinae

Left ventricle

Septum

Papillary muscle

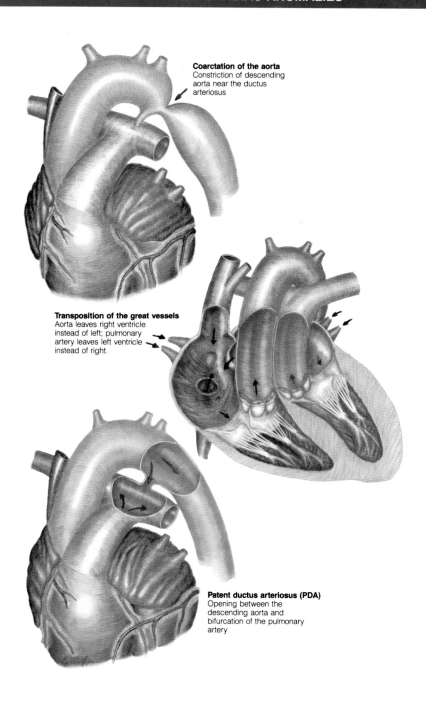

Coarctation of the aorta
Constriction of descending aorta near the ductus arteriosus

Transposition of the great vessels
Aorta leaves right ventricle instead of left; pulmonary artery leaves left ventricle instead of right.

Patent ductus arteriosus (PDA)
Opening between the descending aorta and bifurcation of the pulmonary artery

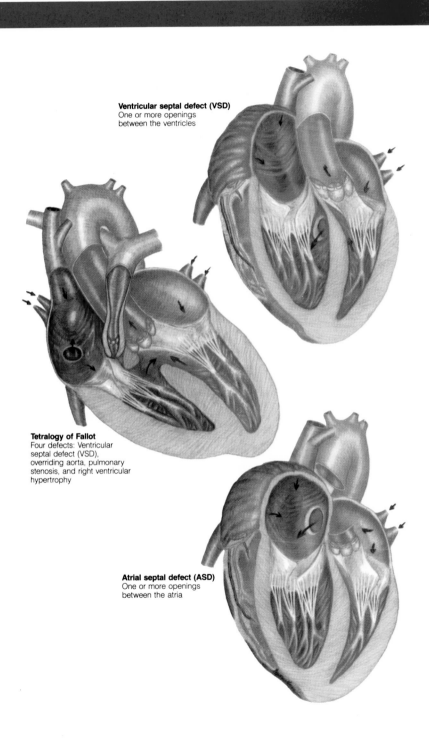

Ventricular septal defect (VSD)
One or more openings
between the ventricles

Tetralogy of Fallot
Four defects: Ventricular
septal defect (VSD),
overriding aorta, pulmonary
stenosis, and right ventricular
hypertrophy

Atrial septal defect (ASD)
One or more openings
between the atria

MAJOR BLOOD VESSELS

Arteries

Veins

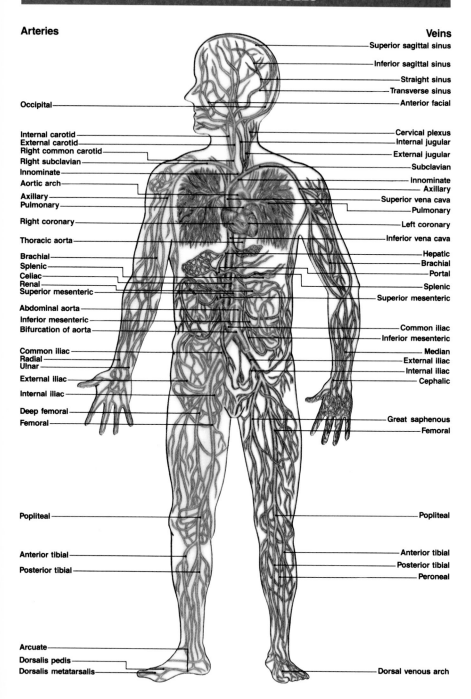

Occipital

Internal carotid
External carotid
Right common carotid
Right subclavian
Innominate
Aortic arch
Axillary
Pulmonary

Right coronary

Thoracic aorta

Brachial
Splenic
Celiac
Renal
Superior mesenteric

Abdominal aorta
Inferior mesenteric
Bifurcation of aorta

Common iliac
Radial
Ulnar

External iliac

Internal iliac

Deep femoral
Femoral

Popliteal

Anterior tibial

Posterior tibial

Arcuate
Dorsalis pedis
Dorsalis metatarsalis

Superior sagittal sinus
Inferior sagittal sinus
Straight sinus
Transverse sinus
Anterior facial

Cervical plexus
Internal jugular
External jugular
Subclavian
Innominate
Axillary
Superior vena cava
Pulmonary
Left coronary
Inferior vena cava
Hepatic
Brachial
Portal
Splenic
Superior mesenteric

Common iliac
Inferior mesenteric
Median
External iliac
Internal iliac
Cephalic

Great saphenous
Femoral

Popliteal

Anterior tibial
Posterior tibial
Peroneal

Dorsal venous arch

their child away from persons with infections, and encourage him to brush his teeth regularly. Immediate treatment is needed for ear, nose, or throat infections, and dental caries. If antibiotics are prescribed following medical or dental treatment, completion of the prescribed regimen is essential.

If the child requires medical attention, even for an unrelated problem, parents should immediately inform the doctor of the child's history of tetralogy of Fallot. The doctor must take this serious heart defect into consideration before treating the child.

Whenever the child's hospitalized, the hospital staff also must be alerted to the child's condition. Because of the right-to-left shunt through the VSD, I.V. lines should be treated with special care, like arterial lines. A clot dislodged from a catheter tip into a vein can cross the VSD and cause cerebral embolism. A cerebral embolism also can result if air enters a venous line.

If the child undergoes palliative surgery, such as the Blalock-Taussig procedure, his arterial blood gas values will be closely monitored in the ICU. However, the arm on the operative side won't be used for measuring blood pressure, inserting I.V. lines, or drawing blood samples. Blood perfusion in this arm diminishes greatly until collateral circulation develops. A warning against using this arm for such procedures should appear on the child's chart and at his bedside.

After corrective surgery, the child must be watched for right bundle branch block, or other disturbances of atrioventricular conduction, and ventricular ectopic beats. If atrioventricular block develops, with a low heart rate, a temporary external pacemaker may be needed.

If blood pressure or cardiac output isn't adequate, catecholamines may be given by continuous I.V. infusion. Nitroprusside (to decrease left ventricular workload) may also be given.

Other possible postoperative complications include bleeding, right-sided heart failure, and respiratory failure.

Postoperative care includes:

• direct monitoring of left atrial pressure.

• frequent checking of vital signs, arterial blood gas values, and color.

• monitoring of central venous and pulmonary artery pressures with a pulmonary artery catheter.

• regular suctioning to prevent atelectasis and pneumonia.

• administering medications (such as catecholamines or nitroprusside), as ordered.

After discharge, the child may still need prophylactic antibiotics, digoxin, diuretics, and other drugs. For example, prophylactic antibiotics to prevent infective endocarditis may still be required. Parents must know how and when to give these drugs, and should understand the importance of complying with the prescribed regimen.

Parents must watch for signs of digitalis toxicity (anorexia, nausea, vomiting), and report them to the doctor at once. In addition, they should be cautioned against becoming overprotective as the child's tolerance for physical activity increases.

Transposition of the Great Vessels
(Transposition of the great arteries)

In this congenital heart defect, the arteries are reversed: the aorta arises from the right ventricle and the pulmonary artery from the left ventricle, producing two noncommunicating circulatory systems (pulmonary and systemic). Transposition accounts for up to 5% of all congenital heart defects and often coexists with other congenital heart defects. It affects males two to three times more often than females.

Causes

Transposition of the great vessels results from faulty embryonic development, but the cause of such development is unknown.

In transposition, oxygenated blood returning to the left side of the heart is carried back to the lungs by a transposed pulmonary artery; unoxygenated blood returning to the right side of the heart is carried to the systemic circulation by a transposed aorta.

Communication between the pulmonary and systemic circulations is necessary for survival. In infants with isolated transposition, blood mixes only at the patent foramen ovale (an opening in the atrial septum) and at the patent ductus arteriosus, resulting in slight mixing of unoxygenated systemic blood and oxygenated pulmonary blood. In infants with concurrent cardiac defects such as atrial septal defect (ASD) or ventricular septal defect (VSD), greater mixing of systemic and pulmonary blood occurs.

Signs and symptoms

Within the first few hours after birth, neonates with transposition of the great vessels, but without associated heart defects, generally show cyanosis, tachypnea, and dyspnea, which worsen with crying. After several days or weeks, such infants usually develop signs of congestive heart failure (gallop rhythm, tachycardia, dyspnea, hepatomegaly) and cardiomegaly (from increased workload). S_2 is louder than normal, because the anteriorly transposed aorta is directly behind the sternum; often, however, no murmur can be heard during the first few days of life. Associated defects (ASD or VSD) that allow arterial and venous blood to mix may minimize cyanosis but may also cause other complications (especially severe congestive heart failure).

As infants with this defect grow older, cyanosis is their most prominent abnormality. However, they also develop diminished exercise tolerance, fatigability, coughing, clubbing of fingers, and murmurs if ASD, VSD, patent ductus arteriosus, or pulmonary stenosis is present.

Diagnosis

• *Chest X-rays* are normal in the first days of life. Within days to weeks, right atrial and right ventricular enlargement characteristically cause the heart to appear oblong (resembling an egg on its side). X-rays also show increased pulmonary vascular markings, except when pulmonary stenosis accompanies transposition.

• *EKG* reveals right axis deviation and right ventricular hypertrophy.

• *Echocardiography* demonstrates the reversed position of the aorta and pulmonary artery, and records echoes from both semilunar valves simultaneously, due to the displacement of the aortic valve.

• *Cardiac catheterization* reveals decreased oxygen saturation in left ventricular blood and aortic blood; increased right atrial, right ventricular, and pulmonary artery oxygen saturation; and right ventricular systolic pressure equal to systemic pressure (with a large VSD).

• *Dye injection* reveals the transposed vessels, and *aortography* detects a patent ductus arteriosus, if present.

• *Arterial blood gas measurements* indicate hypoxia and secondary metabolic acidosis.

Treatment

Until the infant can tolerate corrective surgery, emergency atrial balloon septostomy (Rashkind procedure) creates an ASD if there is none, thereby improving oxygenation by allowing the pulmonary and systemic circulations to mix. Atrial balloon septostomy requires passage of a balloon-tipped catheter through the foramen ovale, and subsequent inflation and withdrawal across the atrial septum. This procedure, performed during cardiac catheterization, alleviates hypoxia and some symptoms of congestive heart failure. Afterward, digoxin and diuretics can lessen congestive heart failure until the infant is ready to withstand corrective surgery

SURGICAL REPAIR OF TRANSPOSITION OF THE GREAT VESSELS *(Mustard Procedure)*

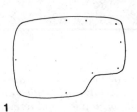
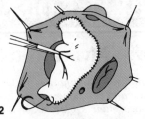
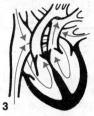

1   **2**   **3**

A Dacron patch (fig. 1) is sutured in the excised atrial septum (fig. 2) to divert pulmonary venous return to the tricuspid valve, and systemic venous return to the mitral valve (fig. 3).

(usually between ages 3 months and 3 years). The Mustard procedure, the most common corrective technique, replaces the atrial septum with a Dacron or pericardial partition that allows systemic venous blood to be channeled to the pulmonary artery—which carries the blood to the lungs for oxygenation—and oxygenated blood returning to the heart to be channeled through the pulmonary veins into the aorta. The Senny procedure accomplishes the same result, using the atrial septum to create partitions to redirect blood flow. The patient with a coexisting VSD requires patch closure of this additional defect. Surgery also corrects other heart defects, such as pulmonary stenosis.

Additional considerations

If the child's scheduled for cardiac catheterization and the Rashkind procedure, parents need an explanation of both procedures. For example, they should understand that the Rashkind procedure improves the child's chances for survival until he is old enough to tolerate more extensive corrective surgery.

Before and after the procedures, the child's vital signs, arterial blood gases, urinary output, and central venous pressure will be monitored closely for any sign of congestive heart failure. In addition, he'll receive digoxin and I.V. fluids.

To care for the child at home, parents must learn to recognize signs of congestive heart failure and digoxin toxicity (anorexia, nausea, vomiting). Any such signs should be reported immediately. Regular checkups are essential for monitoring the child's cardiovascular status.

When the child's scheduled for corrective surgery, both the parents and the child should receive an explanation of the operation and postoperative care. The child may be introduced to the ICU staff and shown the tubes, catheters, dressings, and monitoring equipment he'll see after surgery.

Preoperatively, his arterial blood gases, acid-base balance, fluid intake and output, and vital signs will be watched closely. Postoperatively, the child's care includes:
• monitoring blood pressure, skin color, heart rate, urinary output, central venous and left atrial pressures, cardiac output, and level of consciousness.
• measuring arterial blood gases to evaluate adequacy of mechanical ventilation.
• watching for signs of supraventricular conduction blocks, atrioventricular blocks, impaired sinoatrial function, and arrhythmias.

Parents need emotional support to help them accept their child's condition. Although they should protect him from exposure to infection, they shouldn't become overprotective. The child will know his own limits and should be encouraged to assume new activity levels.

ACQUIRED INFLAMMATORY HEART DISEASE

Myocarditis

Myocarditis is focal or diffuse inflammation of the cardiac muscle (myocardium). It may be acute or chronic and can occur at any age. Frequently, myocarditis fails to produce specific cardiovascular symptoms or EKG abnormalities, and recovery is usually spontaneous, without residual defects. Occasionally, myocarditis is complicated by congestive heart failure and, rarely, leads to cardiomyopathy.

Causes
Myocarditis results from:
• *viral infections* (most common cause in the United States): Coxsackievirus A and B strains and, possibly, poliomyelitis, influenza, rubeola, rubella, and adeno- and echoviruses
• *bacterial infections:* diphtheria, tuberculosis, typhoid fever, tetanus, and staphylococcal, pneumococcal, and gonococcal infections
• *hypersensitive immune reactions:* acute rheumatic fever and postcardiotomy syndrome
• *radiation therapy:* large doses of radiation to the chest in treating lung or breast cancer
• *chemical poisons:* such as chronic alcoholism
• *parasitic infections:* especially South American trypanosomiasis (Chagas' disease) in infants and immunosuppressed adults; also, toxoplasmosis
• *helminthic infections:* such as trichinosis.

Signs and symptoms
Myocarditis usually causes nonspecific symptoms—such as fatigue, dyspnea, palpitations, and fever—that reflect the accompanying systemic infection. Occasionally, it may produce mild, continuous pressure or soreness in the chest (unlike the recurring, stress-related pain of angina pectoris). Although myocarditis is generally uncomplicated and self-limiting, it may induce myofibril degeneration that results in right and left heart failure, with cardiomegaly, neck vein distention, dyspnea, resting or exertional tachycardia disproportionate to the degree of fever, and supraventricular and ventricular arrhythmias. Sometimes myocarditis recurs, or produces cardiomyopathy, arrhythmias, thromboembolism, and chronic valvulitis, when it results from rheumatic fever.

Diagnosis
Patient history commonly reveals recent febrile upper respiratory tract infection, viral pharyngitis, or tonsillitis. Physical examination shows supraventricular and ventricular arrhythmias, S_3 and S_4 gallops, a faint S_1, possibly a murmur of mitral regurgitation (from papillary muscle dysfunction), and if pericarditis is present, a pericardial friction rub.

Laboratory tests can't unequivocally confirm myocarditis, but the following findings support this diagnosis:
• cardiac enzymes: elevated creatine phosphokinase (CPK), CPK isoenzyme (CPK_2), SGOT, and lactic dehydrogenase
• increased WBC and ESR
• elevated antibody titers (such as antistreptolysin O [ASO titer] in rheumatic fever).

EKG changes are the most reliable diagnostic aid, and typically show diffuse ST segment and T wave abnormalities as in pericarditis, conduction defects (prolonged P-R interval), and other supraventricular ectopic arrhythmias.

Stool and throat cultures may identify bacteria or isolate the virus.

Treatment

Treatment includes antibiotics for bacterial infection, modified bed rest to decrease heart workload, and careful management of complications. Congestive heart failure requires restriction of activity to minimize myocardial oxygen consumption, supplemental oxygen therapy, sodium restriction, diuretics to decrease fluid retention, and digitalis to increase myocardial contractility. However, digitalis necessitates cautious administration, since some patients with myocarditis may show a paradoxical sensitivity to even small doses. Arrhythmias necessitate prompt but cautious administration of antiarrhythmics, such as quinidine or procainamide, since these drugs depress myocardial contractility. Thromboembolism requires anticoagulation therapy. Because corticosteroids may aggravate the underlying infection by suppressing systemic defense mechanisms, they are used mainly to combat life-threatening complications, such as intractable heart failure.

Additional considerations

Health care for a patient suffering from myocarditis includes:
• regularly assessing cardiovascular status.
• watching for signs of congestive heart failure (rales, dyspnea, hypotension, tachycardia, increased central venous pressure, neck vein distention, edema, weight gain, or decreased urinary output).
• checking for changes in cardiac rhythm or conduction.
• observing for signs of digitalis toxicity (anorexia, nausea, vomiting, blurred vision, cardiac arrhythmias).
• treating electrolyte imbalance (may promote digitalis toxicity), or hypoxia.

Bed rest is important to recovery. The patient should be helped with bathing and provided with a bedside commode, since using a commode stresses the heart less than using a bedpan. During recovery, the patient can gradually resume normal activities, but he should avoid competitive sports.

Endocarditis

(Infective endocarditis, bacterial endocarditis)

Endocarditis is an infection of the endocardium, heart valves, or cardiac prosthesis, resulting from bacterial (or, in intravenous drug abusers, fungal) invasion. This invasion produces vegetative growths on the heart valves, endocardial lining of a heart chamber, or the endothelium of a blood vessel that may embolize to the spleen, kidneys, central nervous system, and lungs. Untreated endocarditis is usually fatal, but with proper treatment, 70% of patients recover. Prognosis is worst when endocarditis causes severe valvular damage, leading to insufficiency and congestive heart failure, or when it involves a prosthetic valve.

Causes

Acute infective endocarditis usually results from bacteremia that follows septic thrombophlebitis, open heart surgery involving prosthetic valves, or skin, bone, and pulmonary infections. The most common causative organisms are group A nonhemolytic streptococcus (rheumatic endocarditis), pneumococcus, staphylococcus, and rarely, gonococcus. This form of endocarditis also occurs in intravenous drug abusers, possibly from *Staphylococcus aureus*, pseudomonas, *Candida*, or usually harmless skin saprophytes.

Subacute infective endocarditis typically occurs in persons with acquired valvular or congenital cardiac lesions. It can also follow dental, genitourinary, gynecologic, and gastrointestinal procedures. The most common infecting organisms are *Streptococcus viridans*, which normally inhabits the upper respiratory tract, and *Streptococcus faecalis* (enterococcus), generally found in gastrointestinal and perineal flora.

Preexisting rheumatic endocardial lesions are a common predisposing factor in bacterial endocarditis. Rheumatic endocarditis commonly affects the mitral valve; less frequently, the aortic or tricuspid valve; and rarely, the pulmonic valve.

In infective endocarditis, fibrin and platelets aggregate on the valve tissue and engulf circulating bacteria or fungi that flourish and produce friable verrucous vegetations. Such vegetations may cover the valve surfaces, causing ulceration and necrosis; they may also extend to the chordae tendineae, leading to their rupture and subsequent valvular insufficiency. Sometimes vegetations form on the endocardium, usually in areas altered by rheumatic, congenital, or syphilitic heart disease, although they may also form on normal surfaces.

Signs and symptoms

Early clinical features of endocarditis are nonspecific, and include weakness, fatigue, weight loss, anorexia, arthralgia, night sweats, and in 90% of patients, an intermittent fever that may recur for weeks. Endocarditis often causes a loud, regurgitant murmur typical of the underlying rheumatic or congenital heart disease. A suddenly changing murmur or the discovery of a new murmur in the presence of fever is a classic physical sign of endocarditis.

In about 30% of patients with subacute endocarditis, embolization from vegetating lesions or diseased valve tissue may produce typical features of splenic, renal, cerebral, or pulmonary infarction, or peripheral vascular occlusion:

• *splenic infarction:* pain in the upper left quadrant, radiating to the left shoulder; abdominal rigidity

• *renal infarction:* hematuria, pyuria, flank pain, decreased urinary output

• *cerebral infarction:* hemiparesis, aphasia, or other neurologic deficits

• *pulmonary infarction* (most common in right-sided endocarditis, which often occurs among intravenous drug abusers and after cardiac surgery): cough, pleuritic pain, pleural friction rub, dyspnea, and hemoptysis

• *peripheral vascular occlusion:* numbness and tingling in an arm, leg, finger, or toe, or signs of impending peripheral gangrene.

Other symptoms include petechiae of the skin (especially common on the upper anterior trunk) and the buccal, pharyngeal, or conjunctival mucosa, and splinter hemorrhages under the nails. Rarely, endocarditis produces Osler's nodes (tender, raised, subcutaneous lesions on the fingers or toes), Roth's spots (hemorrhagic areas with white centers on the retina), and Janeway lesions (purplish macules on the palms or soles).

Diagnosis

 Three or more blood cultures during a 24- to 48-hour period identify the causative organism in up to 90% of patients. The remaining 10% may have negative blood cultures, possibly suggesting fungal infection. Other abnormal but nonspecific laboratory results include:

• elevated WBC

• abnormal histocytes (macrophages)

• elevated ESR

• normocytic, normochromic anemia

PROSTHETIC VALVE ENDOCARDITIS

Increasing use of prosthetic heart valve implants has given rise to prosthetic valve endocarditis, an infection of the artificial valve along the suture line. This disorder can be either acute or subacute. Signs and symptoms usually are similar to those of other forms of endocarditis, although sometimes the only symptoms are fever and murmur from valve dysfunction. Treatment consists of antibiotic therapy and often, surgery to replace the infected prosthetic valve.

(in subacute bacterial endocarditis)
• rheumatoid factor, in about half of all patients with endocarditis.

Echocardiography may identify valvular damage; EKG may show atrial fibrillation and other arrhythmias that accompany valvular disease.

Treatment

The goal of treatment is to eradicate the infecting organism. Therapy should start promptly and continue over several weeks. Antibiotic selection is based on sensitivity studies of the infecting organism—or the probable organism, if blood cultures are negative. I.V. antibiotic therapy usually lasts about 4 weeks.

Supportive treatment includes bed rest, aspirin for fever and aches, and sufficient fluid intake. Severe valvular damage, especially aortic regurgitation or infection of cardiac prosthesis, may require corrective surgery if refractory heart failure develops.

Additional considerations

To avoid a possible allergic reaction, the patient's allergy history must be determined before antibiotic treatment begins. The prescribed antibiotics must be in a stable form and compatible with other medications given, and should be administered on a regular schedule to maintain consistent antibiotic levels in the blood.

During treatment of a patient with endocarditis, various complications may arise. These include:
• infiltration or inflammation at the venipuncture site, possible complications of long-term I.V. therapy. Regular site rotation may prevent these complications.
• embolization, which may cause peripheral vascular occlusion, or splenic, renal, cerebral, or pulmonary infarction. Embolization may occur within the first 3 months after treatment begins. Signs of embolization include hematuria, pleuritic chest pain, upper left quadrant pain, and paresis.
• renal emboli or drug toxicity. Both complications can be identified by closely

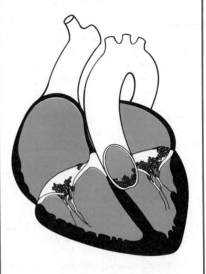

DEGENERATIVE CHANGES OF ENDOCARDITIS

Typical vegetations on the endocardium produced by fibrin and platelet deposits on infection sites

monitoring renal status (BUN, creatinine, and urinary output).
• congestive heart failure. Signs include dyspnea, tachypnea, tachycardia, rales, neck vein distention, edema, and weight gain.

The patient and his family should be taught about the disease and the need for prolonged treatment. They should watch closely for fever, anorexia, and other signs of relapse, which may occur about 2 weeks after treatment stops. During recovery, the patient should gradually increase physical activity, but he must be careful to avoid excessive exertion.

A susceptible patient needs prophylatic antibiotics before, during and after dental work, childbirth, and genitourinary, gastrointestinal, or gynecologic procedures. He should be taught the symptoms of endocarditis, and should notify his doctor at once if he detects any of them.

Pericarditis

Pericarditis is an inflammation of the pericardium, the fibroserous sac that envelops, supports, and protects the heart. It occurs in both acute and chronic forms. Acute pericarditis can be fibrinous or effusive, with purulent serous or hemorrhagic exudate; chronic constrictive pericarditis is characterized by dense fibrous pericardial thickening. Prognosis depends on the underlying cause but is generally good in acute pericarditis, unless constriction occurs.

Causes

Common causes of this disease include:
• bacterial, fungal, or viral infection (infectious pericarditis)
• neoplasms (primary, or metastases from lungs, breasts, or other organs)
• high-dose radiation to the chest
• uremia
• hypersensitivity or autoimmune disease, such as rheumatic fever (most common cause of pericarditis in children), systemic lupus erythematosus, and rheumatoid arthritis
• postcardiac injury, such as myocardial infarction (which later causes an autoimmune reaction [Dressler's syndrome] in the pericardium), trauma, or surgery that leaves the pericardium intact but causes blood to leak into the pericardial cavity
• drugs, such as hydralazine or procainamide
• idiopathic factors (most common in acute pericarditis).

Less common causes include aortic aneurysm with pericardial leakage, and myxedema with cholesterol deposits in the pericardium.

Signs and symptoms

Acute pericarditis typically produces a sharp and often sudden pain that usually starts over the sternum and radiates to the neck, shoulders, back, and arms. However, unlike the pain of myocardial infarction, pericardial pain is often pleuritic, increasing with deep inspiration and decreasing when the patient sits up and leans forward, pulling the heart away from the diaphragmatic pleurae of the lungs.

Pericardial effusion, the major complication of acute pericarditis, may produce effects of heart failure—such as dyspnea, orthopnea, and tachycardia—ill-defined substernal chest pain, and a feeling of fullness in the chest. If the fluid accumulates rapidly, cardiac tamponade may occur, resulting in pallor, clammy skin, hypotension, pulsus paradoxus (a decrease in blood pressure ≥ 15 mmHg during slow inspiration), neck vein distention, and eventually, cardiovascular collapse and death.

Chronic constrictive pericarditis causes a gradual increase in systemic venous pressure and produces symptoms similar to those of chronic right heart failure (fluid retention, ascites, hepatomegaly).

Diagnosis

Since pericarditis often coexists with other conditions, diagnosis of acute pericarditis depends on typical clinical features and elimination of other possible causes. A classic symptom, the pericardial friction rub, is a grating sound heard as the heart moves. It can usually be auscultated best during forced expiration, while the patient leans forward or is on his hands and knees in bed. It may have up to three components, corresponding to the timing of atrial systole, ventricular systole, and the rapid-filling phase of ventricular diastole. Occasionally, this friction rub is heard only briefly or not at all. Nevertheless, its presence, together with other characteristic features, is diagnostic of acute pericarditis. In addition, if acute pericarditis has caused very large pericardial effusions, physical examination reveals increased cardiac dullness and diminished or absent apical impulse and distant heart sounds.

In patients with chronic pericarditis, acute inflammation or effusions do not occur—only restricted cardiac filling.

Laboratory results reflect inflammation and may identify its cause:

• normal or elevated WBC, especially in infectious pericarditis

• elevated ESR

• slightly elevated cardiac enzymes with associated myocarditis

• culture of pericardial fluid obtained by open surgical drainage or cardiocentesis (sometimes identifies a causative organism in bacterial or fungal pericarditis)

• EKG shows the following changes in acute pericarditis: elevation of ST segments in the standard limb leads and most precordial leads without significant changes in QRS morphology that occur with myocardial infarction; atrial ectopic rhythms, such as atrial fibrillation; and in pericardial effusion, diminished QRS voltage.

Other laboratory data include BUN to check for uremia, antistreptolysin O titers to detect rheumatic fever, and a purified protein derivative skin test to check for tuberculosis. In pericardial effusion, echocardiography is diagnostic when it shows an echofree space between the ventricular wall and the pericardium.

Treatment

The goal of treatment is to relieve symptoms and manage underlying systemic disease. In acute idiopathic pericarditis, postmyocardial infarction pericarditis, and post-thoracotomy pericarditis, treatment consists of bed rest as long as fever and pain persist, and nonsteroidal drugs, such as aspirin and indomethacin, to relieve pain and reduce inflammation. If these drugs fail to relieve symptoms, corticosteroids may be used. Although corticosteroids produce rapid and effective relief, they must be used cautiously because symptomatic episodes may recur when therapy is discontinued.

Infectious pericarditis that results from disease of the left pleural space, mediastinal abscesses, or septicemia requires antibiotics, surgical drainage, or both. If cardiac tamponade develops, the doctor may perform emergency pericardiocentesis. Signs of cardiac tamponade include pulsus paradoxus, neck vein distention, dyspnea, and shock.

Recurrent pericarditis may necessitate partial pericardectomy (surgical removal of part of the pericardium), creating a "window" that allows fluid to drain into the pleural space. In constrictive pericarditis, total pericardectomy to permit adequate filling and contraction of the heart may be necessary. Treatment must also include management of rheumatic fever, uremia, tuberculosis, and other underlying disorders.

Additional considerations

A patient with pericarditis needs complete bed rest. In addition, health care includes:

• assessing pain in relation to respiration and body position, to distinguish pericardial pain from possible myocardial ischemic pain.

• placing the patient in an upright position, to relieve dyspnea and pain.

• providing analgesics and oxygen.

• reassuring the acute pericarditis patient that his condition is temporary and treatable.

• monitoring for signs of cardiac compression or cardiac tamponade, possible complications of pericardial effusion. Signs include decreased blood pressure, increased central venous pressure, and pulsus paradoxus. Since cardiac tamponade must be treated immediately, a pericardiocentesis set must be readily available whenever pericardial effusion is suspected.

• explaining diagnostic procedures and treatment to the patient. If surgery is necessary, he should learn deep breathing and coughing exercises beforehand. (Postoperative care is similar to that given following cardiothoracic surgery.)

Rheumatic Fever and Rheumatic Heart Disease

Acute rheumatic fever is a systemic inflammatory disease of childhood, often recurrent, that follows a Group A beta-hemolytic streptococcal infection. Rheumatic heart disease refers to the cardiac manifestations of rheumatic fever, and includes pancarditis (myocarditis, pericarditis, and endocarditis) during the early acute phase and chronic valvular disease later. Long-term antibiotic therapy can minimize recurrence of rheumatic fever, reducing the risk of permanent cardiac damage and eventual valvular deformity. However, severe pancarditis occasionally produces fatal congestive heart failure during the acute phase. Of the patients who survive this complication, about 20% die within 10 years.

Causes and incidence

Rheumatic fever appears to be a hypersensitivity reaction to a Group A beta-hemolytic streptococcal infection, in which antibodies manufactured to combat streptococci react and produce characteristic lesions at specific tissue sites, especially in the heart and joints. Since very few persons (0.3%) with streptococcal infections ever contract rheumatic fever, altered host resistance must be involved in its development or recurrence. Although rheumatic fever tends to be familial, this may merely reflect contributing environmental factors. For example, in lower socioeconomic groups, incidence is highest in children between ages 5 and 15, probably as a result of malnutrition and crowded living conditions. This disease strikes most often during cool, damp weather in the winter and early spring. In the United States, it's most common in the northern states.

Signs and symptoms

In 95% of patients, rheumatic fever characteristically follows a streptococcal infection that appeared a few days to 6 weeks earlier. A temperature of at least 100.4° F. (38° C.) occurs, and most patients complain of migratory joint pain or *polyarthritis*. Swelling, redness, and signs of effusion usually accompany such pain, which most commonly affects the knees, ankles, elbows, or hips. In 5% of patients (generally those with carditis), rheumatic fever causes skin lesions such as *erythema marginatum*, a nonpruritic, macular, transient rash that gives rise to red lesions with blanched centers. Rheumatic fever may also produce firm, movable, nontender, *subcutaneous nodules* about 3 mm to 2 cm in diameter, usually near tendons or bony prominences of joints (especially the elbows, knuckles, wrists, and knees) and less often on the scalp and backs of the hands. These nodules persist for a few days to several weeks and, like erythema marginatum, often accompany carditis.

Later, rheumatic fever may cause transient *chorea*, which develops up to 6 months after the original streptococcal infection. Mild chorea may produce hyperirritability, a deterioration in handwriting, or inability to concentrate. Severe chorea causes purposeless, nonrepetitive, involuntary muscle spasms; poor muscle coordination; and weakness. Chorea always resolves without residual neurologic damage.

The most destructive effect of rheumatic fever is *carditis*, which develops in up to 50% of patients and may affect the endocardium, myocardium, pericardium, or the heart valves. Pericarditis causes a pericardial friction rub and, occasionally, pain and effusion. Myocarditis produces characteristic lesions called Aschoff's bodies (in the acute stages), and cellular swelling and fragmentation of interstitial collagen, leading to formation of a progressively fibrotic nodule and interstitial scars. Endocarditis causes valve leaflet swelling, erosion along the lines of leaflet closure, and blood, platelet, and fibrin deposits, which form beadlike vegetations. Endocarditis affects the mitral valve most often in females; the aortic, most often in males. In both females and males, endocarditis affects the tricuspid valves occasionally and the pulmonic only rarely.

Severe rheumatic carditis may cause congestive heart failure, with dyspnea, upper right quadrant pain, tachycardia, tachypnea, a hacking nonproductive cough, edema, and significant mitral and aortic murmurs. The most common of such murmurs include:

• a systolic murmur of mitral regurgitation (high-pitched, blowing, holosystolic, loudest at apex, possibly radiating to the anterior axillary line).
• a midsystolic murmur due to stiffening and swelling of the mitral leaflet
• occasionally, a diastolic murmur of aortic regurgitation (low-pitched, rumbling, and almost inaudible). Valvular disease may eventually result in chronic valvular stenosis and insufficiency, including mitral stenosis and regurgitation, and aortic regurgitation. In children, mitral insufficiency remains the major sequela of rheumatic heart disease.

Diagnosis
Diagnosis depends on recognition of one or more of the classic symptoms (carditis, polyarthritis, chorea, erythema marginatum, or subcutaneous nodules) and a detailed patient history. Laboratory data support the diagnosis:
• *WBC* and *ESR* may be elevated (especially during the acute phase); blood studies show slight anemia, due to suppressed erythropoiesis during inflammation.
• *C-reactive protein* is positive (especially during acute phase).
• *Cardiac enzymes* may be increased in severe carditis.
• *Antistreptolysin O titer* is elevated in 95% of patients within 2 months of onset.
• *EKG* changes are not diagnostic; however, 20% of patients show a prolonged P-R interval.

• *Chest X-rays* show normal heart size (except with myocarditis, congestive heart failure, or pericardial effusion).
• *Echocardiography* helps identify valvular damage.
• *Cardiac catheterization* evaluates valvular damage and left ventricular function in severe cardiac dysfunction.

Treatment
Effective management eradicates the streptococcal infection, relieves symptoms, and prevents recurrence, reducing the chance of permanent cardiac damage. During the acute phase, treatment includes penicillin or (for patients with penicillin hypersensitivity) erythromycin. Salicylates, such as aspirin, relieve fever and minimize joint swelling and pain; if carditis is present or salicylates fail to relieve pain and inflammation, corticosteroids may be used. Supportive treatment requires strict bed rest for about 5 weeks during the acute phase with active carditis, followed by a progressive increase in physical activity, depending on clinical and laboratory findings and the response to treatment.

After the acute phase subsides, a monthly I.M. injection of penicillin G benzathine, or daily doses of oral sulfadiazine or penicillin G may be used to prevent recurrence. Such preventive treatment usually continues for at least 5 years or until age 25. Congestive heart failure necessitates continued bed rest and diuretics. Severe mitral or aortic valvular dysfunction causing persistent congestive heart failure requires corrective valvular surgery, including commissurotomy (separation of the adherent, thickened leaflets of the mitral valve), valvuloplasty (repair of valve), or valve replacement (with prosthetic valve). Corrective valvular surgery is rarely necessary before late adolescence or early adulthood.

Additional considerations
Because rheumatic fever and rheumatic heart disease require prolonged treatment, the health care plan should include comprehensive patient teaching to pro-

mote compliance with the prescribed therapy.

• Before being given penicillin, the patient or (if the patient's a child) his parents must be questioned if they ever had a hypersensitive reaction to it. Even if the patient has never had a reaction to penicillin, such a reaction is still possible. If the patient develops a rash, fever, chills, or other signs of allergy *at any time* during penicillin therapy the drug should be stopped and the doctor called immediately.

• The patient and his family should also watch for and report early signs of congestive heart failure, such as dyspnea and a hacking, nonproductive cough.

• Bed rest, which is very important during the acute phase of the disease, may be promoted by appropriate, physically undemanding diversions. After the acute phase, the family and friends should spend as much time as possible with the patient to minimize boredom. Parents should secure tutorial services to help the child keep up with schoolwork during the long convalescence.

• Parents may need help overcoming any guilt feelings they may have about their child's illness. They should not be distressed by their failure to seek treatment for streptococcal infection, since this illness often seems no worse than a cold. Instead they need to vent their frustrations during the long, tedious recovery. If the child has severe carditis, they will need help preparing for permanent changes in the child's life-style.

• The patient and family should be taught about this disease and its treatment. Parents must watch for and immediately report signs of recurrent streptococcal infection—sudden sore throat, diffuse throat redness and oropharyngeal exudate, swollen and tender cervical lymph glands, pain on swallowing, temperature of 101° to 104° F. (38.3° to 40° C.), headache, and nausea. They should try to keep their child away from persons with respiratory tract infections.

• Good dental hygiene to prevent gingival infection is important. The patient and his family must understand the need to comply with prolonged antibiotic therapy and follow-up care, and the need for additional antibiotics during dental surgery. They may want or need a visiting nurse to oversee home care.

VALVULAR HEART DISEASE

Valvular Heart Disease

In valvular heart disease, one or more valves malfunction, producing regurgitation (a backflow of blood through the valves due to incompetent closure) or stenosis (an incomplete opening of the valves). Either one of these conditions can lead to heart failure.

Valvular heart disease occurs in varying forms:

• *Mitral insufficiency:* Blood from the left ventricle flows back into the left atrium during systole, causing the atrium to enlarge to accommodate the backflow. The ventricle also dilates to accommodate the increased volume of blood from the atrium and to compensate for diminishing cardiac output. Ventricular hypertrophy and increased end-diastolic pressure result in increased pulmonary artery pressure, eventually leading to right ventricular failure.

• *Mitral stenosis:* Narrowing of the valve by valvular abnormalities, fibrosis, or calcification obstructs blood flow from the left atrium to the left ventricle. Consequently, left atrial pressure rises and the chamber dilates. Greater resistance

FORMS OF VALVULAR HEART DISEASE

CAUSES AND INCIDENCE	CLINICAL FEATURES	DIAGNOSTIC MEASURES
Mitral stenosis		
• Results from rheumatic fever (most common cause) • Most common in females • May be associated with other congenital anomalies, such as tetralogy of Fallot	• Dyspnea on exertion, paroxysmal nocturnal dyspnea, orthopnea, weakness, fatigue, palpitations • Peripheral edema, jugular venous distention, ascites, hepatomegaly (right ventricular failure in severe pulmonary hypertension) • Rales, cardiac arrhythmias (atrial fibrillation), signs of systemic emboli • Auscultation reveals a loud S_1 or opening snap, and a diastolic murmur at the apex.	• Cardiac catheterization demonstrates diastolic pressure gradient across valve: elevated left atrial, pulmonary capillary wedge (PCWP > 15) with severe pulmonary hypertension, and pulmonary arterial pressures; elevated right heart pressure; decreased cardiac output. Valve size may be < 1.0 cm² in severe disease. Angiography may reveal abnormal contraction of the left ventricle. May not be indicated in patients with isolated mitral stenosis with mild symptoms • X-ray: left atrial and ventricular enlargement, enlarged pulmonary arteries, mitral valve calcification • Echocardiography: thickened mitral valve leaflets, left atrial enlargement • Electrocardiography: left atrial hypertrophy, atrial fibrillation, right ventricular hypertrophy, right axis deviation
Mitral insufficiency		
• Results from rheumatic fever, idiopathic hypertrophic subaortic stenosis (IHSS), mitral valve prolapse, myocardial infarction, severe left ventricular failure, ruptured chordae tendineae • Associated with other congenital anomalies, such as transposition of the great vessels • Rare in children without other congenital anomalies	• Orthopnea, dyspnea, fatigue, angina, palpitations • Peripheral edema, jugular venous distention, hepatomegaly (right ventricular failure) • Tachycardia, rales, pulmonary edema • Auscultation reveals a holosystolic murmur at apex, possible split S_2, and an S_3.	• Cardiac catheterization: mitral regurgitation, with increased left ventricular end-diastolic volume and pressure; increased atrial and pulmonary capillary wedge pressures; and decreased cardiac output • X-ray: left atrial and ventricular enlargement, pulmonary venous congestion • Echocardiography: abnormal valve leaflet motion, left atrial enlargement • Electrocardiography: may show left atrial and ventricular hypertrophy, sinus tachycardia, atrial fibrillation.

FORMS OF VALVULAR HEART DISEASE (continued)

CAUSES AND INCIDENCE	CLINICAL FEATURES	DIAGNOSTIC MEASURES
Tricuspid insufficiency		
• Results from right ventricular failure, rheumatic fever, and rarely, trauma and endocarditis • Associated with congenital disorders	• Dyspnea and fatigue • May lead to peripheral edema, jugular venous distention, hepatomegaly, and ascites (right ventricular failure) • Auscultation reveals possible S$_3$ and systolic murmur at lower left sternal border that increases with inspiration	• Right heart catheterization: high atrial pressure, tricuspid regurgitation, decreased or normal cardiac output, other valvular abnormalities (if present) • X-ray: right atrial dilation, right ventricular enlargement • Echocardiography: shows systolic prolapse of tricuspid value, right atrial enlargement • Electrocardiography: right atrial or right ventricular hypertrophy, atrial fibrillation
Tricuspid stenosis		
• Results from rheumatic fever • May be congenital • Associated with mitral or aortic valve disease • Most common in women	• May be symptomatic with dyspnea, fatigue, syncope • Possibly peripheral edema, jugular venous distention, hepatomegaly, and ascites (right ventricular failure) • Auscultation reveals diastolic murmur at lower left sternal border that increases with inspiration	• Cardiac catheterization: increased pressure gradient across valve, increased right atrial pressure, decreased cardiac output • X-ray: right atrial enlargement • Echocardiography: leaflet abnormality, right atrial enlargement • Electrocardiography: right atrial hypertrophy, right or left ventricular hypertrophy, atrial fibrillation
Pulmonic stenosis		
• Results from congenital stenosis of valve cusp or rheumatic heart disease (infrequent) • Associated with other congenital heart defects, such as tetralogy of Fallot	• Asymptomatic or symptomatic with dyspnea on exertion, fatigue, chest pain, syncope • May lead to peripheral edema, jugular venous distention, hepatomegaly (right ventricular failure) • Auscultation reveals a systolic murmur at the left sternal border, a split S$_2$ with a delayed or absent pulmonic component	• Cardiac catheterization: increased right ventricular pressure, decreased pulmonary artery pressure, abnormal valve orifice • Electrocardiography: may show right ventricular hypertrophy, right axis deviation, right atrial hypertrophy, atrial fibrillation

FORMS OF VALVULAR HEART DISEASE (continued)

CAUSES AND INCIDENCE	CLINICAL FEATURES	DIAGNOSTIC MEASURES
Pulmonic insufficiency • May be congenital or may result from pulmonary hypertension	• Dyspnea, weakness, fatigue, chest pain • Peripheral edema, jugular venous distention, hepatomegaly (right ventricular failure) • Auscultation reveals diastolic murmur in pulmonic area.	• Cardiac catheterization: pulmonary regurgitation, increased right ventricular pressure, associated cardiac defects • X-ray: right ventricular and pulmonary arterial enlargement • Electrocardiography: right ventricular or right atrial enlargement
Aortic insufficiency • Results from rheumatic fever, syphilis, hypertension, endocarditis, or may be idiopathic • Associated with Marfan's syndrome • Most common in males	• Dyspnea, cough, fatigue, palpitations, angina, syncope • Pulmonary venous congestion, congestive heart failure, pulmonary edema (left ventricular failure), "pulsating" nailbeds (Quincke's sign) • Rapidly rising and collapsing pulses (pulsus biferiens), cardiac arrhythmias, wide pulse pressure in severe regurgitation • Auscultation may reveal an S_3 and a diastolic blowing murmur at left sternal border. • Palpation and visualization of apical impulse in chronic disease	• Cardiac catheterization: reduction in arterial diastolic pressures, aortic regurgitation, other valvular abnormalities, and increased left ventricular end-diastolic pressure • X-ray: left ventricular enlargement, pulmonary venous congestion • Echocardiography: left ventricular enlargement, alterations in mitral valve movement (indirect indication of aortic valve disease), and mitral thickening • Electrocardiography: sinus tachycardia, left ventricular hypertrophy, left atrial hypertrophy in severe disease
Aortic stenosis • Results from congenital aortic bicuspid valve (associated with coarctation of the aorta), congenital stenosis of valve cusps, rheumatic fever, or atherosclerosis in the aged • Most common in males	• Dyspnea on exertion, paroxysmal nocturnal dyspnea, fatigue, syncope, angina, palpitations • Pulmonary venous congestion, congestive heart failure, pulmonary edema (left ventricular failure) • Diminished carotid pulses, decreased cardiac output, cardiac arrhythmias; may have pulsus alternans • Auscultation reveals systolic murmur heard at base or in carotids and, possibly, an S_4.	• Cardiac catheterization: pressure gradient across valve (indicating obstruction), increased left ventricular end-diastolic pressures • X-ray: valvular calcification, left ventricular enlargement, pulmonary venous congestion • Echocardiography: thickened aortic valve and left ventricular wall, possibly coexistent with mitral valve stenosis • Electrocardiography: left ventricular hypertrophy

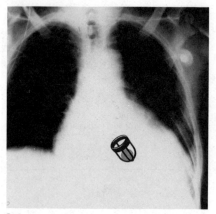

Severe valvular heart disease may require surgical insertion of a prosthetic mitral valve, such as the Starr Edwards valve illustrated in the X-ray above.

to blood flow causes pulmonary hypertension, right ventricular hypertrophy, and eventually, right ventricular failure.

• *Aortic insufficiency:* Blood flows back into the left ventricle during diastole, causing a fluid overload in the ventricle, which, in turn, dilates and, ultimately, hypertrophies. The excess volume causes a fluid overload in the left atrium and, finally, in the pulmonary system. Left ventricular failure and pulmonary edema eventually result.

• *Aortic stenosis:* Increased left ventricular pressure attempts to overcome the resistance of the narrowed valvular opening. The added workload causes a greater demand for oxygen, while diminished cardiac output causes poor coronary artery perfusion, ischemia of the left ventricle, and eventually, left ventricular failure.

• *Pulmonic insufficiency:* Blood that entered the pulmonary artery flows back into the right ventricle during diastole, causing a fluid overload in the ventricle, ventricular hypertrophy, and finally, right ventricular failure.

• *Pulmonic stenosis:* Obstructed right ventricular outflow causes right ventricular hypertrophy in an attempt to overcome resistance to the narrow valvular opening. Right ventricular failure ultimately results.

• *Tricuspid insufficiency:* Blood flows back into the right atrium during systole, decreasing blood flow to the left side of the heart. Cardiac output also lessens. Fluid overload in the right side of the heart can eventually lead to right ventricular failure.

• *Tricuspid stenosis:* Obstructed blood flow from the right atrium to the right ventricle causes the right atrium to dilate and hypertrophy. This increases pressure in the vena cava and eventually leads to right ventricular failure.

Treatment and additional considerations

Treatment of valvular heart disease depends on the nature and severity of associated symptoms. For example, heart failure requires digoxin, diuretics, a sodium-restricted diet, and in acute cases, oxygen. Atrial fibrillation requires digoxin or electrical conversion, and if pulmonary edema occurs, oxygen and I.V. administration of diuretics.

If the patient has severe symptoms that can't be managed medically, open heart surgery using cardiopulmonary bypass for valve replacement is indicated. Other appropriate measures include anticoagulant therapy to prevent thrombus formation around diseased or replaced valves, and prophylactic antibiotics before and after surgery or dental care.

Other care includes:

• watching closely for signs of heart failure or pulmonary edema, and side effects of drug therapy.

• teaching the patient about diet restrictions, medications, symptoms that should be reported, and the importance of consistent follow-up care.

• watching for hypotension, arrhythmias, and thrombus formation if the patient undergoes surgery; monitoring vital signs, arterial blood gases, intake and output, daily weights, blood chemistries, chest X-rays, and pulmonary artery catheter readings.

DEGENERATIVE CARDIOVASCULAR DISORDERS

Hypertension

Hypertension, an intermittent or sustained elevation in diastolic or systolic blood pressure, occurs as two major types: essential (idiopathic) hypertension, the most common, and secondary hypertension, which results from renal disease or another identifiable cause. Malignant hypertension is a severe, fulminant form of hypertension common to both types. Hypertension is a major cause of cerebrovascular accident, cardiac disease, and renal failure. Prognosis is good if this disorder is detected early and treatment begins before complications develop. Severely elevated blood pressure (hypertensive crisis) may be fatal.

Causes and incidence

Hypertension affects 15% to 20% of adults in the United States. If untreated, this disorder carries a high mortality. Risk factors for essential hypertension include family history, race (most common in Blacks), stress, obesity, a high dietary intake of saturated fats or sodium, use of tobacco or oral contraceptives, sedentary life-style, and aging.

Secondary hypertension may result from renal vascular disease; pheochromocytoma; primary hyperaldosteronism; Cushing's syndrome; dysfunctions of the thyroid, pituitary, or parathyroid glands; and neurologic disorders.

Cardiac output and peripheral vascular resistance determine blood pressure. Increased blood volume, increased cardiac rate, or arteriolar vasoconstriction that increases peripheral resistance causes blood pressure to rise, but the relationship of these mechanisms to sustained hypertension is unclear. Increased blood pressure may also result from the breakdown or inappropriate response of mechanisms that intrinsically regulate it.

• Renin-angiotensin system is a neural mechanism that utilizes renin, a renal enzyme, to form angiotensin, a substance that directly produces vasoconstriction or indirectly stimulates the adrenal cortex to produce aldosterone, which in turn increases sodium reabsorption. Thus, hypertonic stimulated release of antidiuretic hormone from the pituitary gland follows, in turn increasing water reabsorption, plasma volume, cardiac output, and blood pressure.

• Changes in renal arterial pressure stimulate autoregulation of the blood pressure by the kidneys. A decrease in pressure, for example, causes a decline in glomerular filtration rate and an increased tubular reabsorption of water, which, in turn, increases blood volume, cardiac output, and ultimately, blood pressure.

• Baroreceptors (pressure receptors) in the aortic arch, carotid sinus, and other large central arteries stimulate the vasomotor center to increase sympathetic stimulation of the heart by increasing epinephrine and norepinephrine levels. This, in turn, increases cardiac output by strengthening the contractile force, increasing the heart rate and augmenting peripheral resistance by vasoconstriction. Stress can also stimulate the sympathetic nervous system to increase cardiac output and peripheral vascular resistance.

Signs and symptoms

Hypertension usually does not produce clinical effects until vascular changes in the heart, brain, or kidneys occur. Severely elevated blood pressure damages the intima of small vessels, resulting in

HYPERTENSIVE CRISIS

Hypertensive crisis is an acute, life-threatening rise in blood pressure (diastolic usually over 120 mmHg). It may develop in hypertensive patients after abrupt discontinuation of anti-hypertensive medication; increased salt consumption; increased production of renin, epinephrine, and norepinephrine; and added stress. This emergency requires immediate and vigorous treatment to lower blood pressure and thereby prevent cerebrovascular accident, left heart failure, and pulmonary edema.

Hypertensive crisis produces severe and widespread symptoms, including headache, drowsiness, mental clouding, vomiting, focal neurologic signs (such as paresthesias), and if pulmonary edema is present, shortness of breath and hemoptysis. Treatment to rapidly lower blood pressure and thereby prevent hypertensive encephalopathy may include vasodilators, such as I.V. nitroprusside, hydralazine, or dia-zoxide; a potent diuretic, such as furosemide; and a sympathetic blocker, such as methyldopa, trimethaphan, or phentolamine.

In the early stages of antihypertensive I.V. therapy, blood pressure and heart rate must be monitored frequently (as often as every 1 to 3 minutes with some drugs) for a precipitous drop, indicating hypersensitivity to the prescribed medications. Blood pressure level must be maintained.

The patient should be kept calm; if he's excited, a sedative may be necessary. Intake and output should be recorded accurately, and the reasons for fluid restriction explained. The patient must be watched closely for hypotension, and until blood pressure is stable at a desirable level, checked for signs of heart failure, such as tachycardia, tachypnea, dyspnea, pulmonary rales, S_3 or S_4 gallops, neck vein distention, cyanosis, and edema.

cation of the damaged vessels:
- brain: cerebrovascular accident
- retina: blindness
- heart: myocardial infarction
- kidneys: proteinuria, edema, and eventually, renal failure.

Hypertension also increases the heart's workload, leading to left ventricular hypertrophy and, eventually, to left ventricular failure, congestive heart failure, and pulmonary edema.

Diagnosis

 Serial blood pressure measurements on a sphygmomanometer of more than 140/90 in persons under age 50, or 150/95 in persons over age 50 confirm hypertension. During physical examination, auscultation may reveal bruits over the abdominal aorta and the carotid, renal, and femoral arteries; ophthalmoscopy reveals arteriovenous nicking and, in hypertensive encephalopathy, papilledema. Patient history and the following additional tests may show predisposing factors and help identify an underlying cause, such as renal disease:
- *Urinalysis:* Protein, RBCs, and WBCs may indicate glomerulonephritis.
- *Intravenous pyelography:* Renal atrophy indicates chronic renal disease; one kidney more than 5/8" (1.5 cm) shorter than the other suggests unilateral renal disease.
- *Serum potassium:* Levels less than 3.5 mEq/liter may indicate adrenal dysfunction (primary hyperaldosteronism).
- *BUN and creatinine:* BUN normal or elevated to more than 20 mg/100 ml, and creatinine normal or elevated to more than 1.5 mg/100 ml suggest renal disease.

Other tests help detect cardiovascular damage and other complications:
- *EKG* may show left ventricular hypertrophy or ischemia.
- *Chest X-ray* may show cardiomegaly.

Treatment

Although essential hypertension has no cure, drugs and modifications in diet and life-style can control it. Drug therapy

fibrin accumulation in the vessels, development of local edema, and possibly, intravascular clotting. Symptoms produced by this process depend on the lo-

usually begins with a diuretic alone and sympathetic blockers or vasodilators added, as needed. Life-style and dietary changes may include weight loss, relaxation techniques, regular exercise, and restriction of sodium and saturated fat intake.

Treatment of secondary hypertension includes correction of the underlying cause, in addition to controlling hypertensive effects.

Additional considerations

• To encourage compliance with antihypertensive therapy, a daily routine for taking medication can be established. The patient must be warned that uncontrolled hypertension may cause stroke and heart attack. He should report drug side effects and avoid over-the-counter cold and sinus medications, since these contain potentially harmful vasoconstrictors.

• A change in dietary habits should be encouraged. The obese patient will need help in planning a reducing diet; he should avoid foods high in sodium (pickles, potato chips, canned soups, cold cuts) and eliminate table salt.

• The patient may need help to examine and modify his life-style (such as eliminating sources of stress and exercising regularly, as appropriate).

If a patient is hospitalized with hypertension, the hospital staff member should:

• find out if he was taking his prescribed medication; ask why if he wasn't; refer the patient to an appropriate social service agency if he can't afford the medication; tell the patient and family to keep a record of drugs used in the past, noting especially which ones were or were not effective; suggest recording this information on a card so the patient can show it to his doctor.

When routine blood pressure screening reveals elevated pressure, the staffer should:

• make sure the cuff size is appropriate for the circumference of the patient's upper arm.

• take the pressure in both arms in lying, sitting, and standing positions.

• ask the patient if he smoked, drank a beverage containing caffeine, or was emotionally upset before the test.

• advise the patient to return for blood pressure testing at frequent and regular intervals if his blood pressure is borderline.

Measures that will help identify hypertension and prevent untreated hypertension include: participating in education programs dealing with hypertension and ways to reduce risk factors; encouraging participation in blood pressure screening programs; routinely screening all patients, especially those at risk (Blacks, and persons with family histories of hypertension, stroke, or heart attack).

Coronary Artery Disease

The dominant effect of coronary artery disease is the loss of oxygen and nutrients to myocardial tissue because of diminished coronary blood flow. This disease is near-epidemic in the Western world. Coronary artery disease occurs more often in men than in women, in Caucasians, and in the middle-aged and the elderly. In the past, this disorder rarely affected women who were premenopausal, but that is no longer the case, perhaps because many women now take oral contraceptives, smoke cigarettes, and are employed in stressful jobs that used to be held exclusively by men.

Causes

Atherosclerosis is the usual cause of coronary artery disease. In this form of arteriosclerosis, fatty, fibrous plaques narrow the lumen of the coronary arteries, reduce the volume of blood that can flow through them, and lead to myocardial ischemia. Plaque formation also predisposes to thrombosis, which can provoke myocardial infarction.

Atherosclerosis usually develops in high-flow, high-pressure arteries, such as those in the heart, brain, kidneys, and in the aorta, especially at bifurcation points. It has been linked to many risk factors: family history, hypertension, obesity, smoking, diabetes mellitus, stress, sedentary life-style, and high serum cholesterol and/or triglyceride levels.

Uncommon causes of reduced coronary artery blood flow include dissecting aneurysms, infectious vasculitis, syphilis, and congenital defects in the coronary vascular system. Coronary artery spasms may also impede blood flow.

Signs and symptoms

The classic symptom of coronary artery disease is angina, the direct result of inadequate flow of oxygen to the myocardium. It's usually described as a burning, squeezing, or crushing tightness in the substernal or precordial chest that radiates to the left arm, neck, jaw, or shoulder blade. Typically, the patient clenches his fist over his chest or rubs his left arm when describing the pain, which is often accompanied by nausea, vomiting, fainting, sweating, and cool extremities. Anginal episodes most often follow physical exertion but may also follow emotional excitement or exposure to cold.

Angina has three major forms: *stable* (pain is predictable in frequency and duration, and can be relieved with nitrates and rest), *unstable* (pain increases in frequency and duration, and is more easily induced), or *decubitus* (anginal pain recurs even at rest). Severe and prolonged anginal pain generally suggests myocardial infarction, with potentially fatal arrhythmias and mechanical failure.

Diagnosis

• Patient history—including the frequency and duration of angina, and the presence of associated risk factors—is crucial in evaluating coronary artery disease. Additional diagnostic measures include the following:

• *EKG during angina* shows ischemia and, possibly, arrhythmias, such as premature ventricular contraction. EKG is apt to be normal when the patient is painfree. Arrhythmias may occur without infarction, secondary to ischemia.

• *Treadmill or bicycle exercise test* may provoke chest pain and EKG signs of myocardial ischemia in response to physical exertion.

• *Coronary angiography* reveals coronary artery stenosis or obstruction, collateral circulation, and the condition of the coronary arteries beyond the narrowing.

• *Myocardial perfusion imaging* with thallium 201 detects ischemic areas of the myocardium, which are visualized as "cold spots."

Treatment

The goal of treatment in patients with angina is to either reduce myocardial oxygen demand or increase oxygen supply. Therapy consists primarily of nitrates, such as nitroglycerin (given sublingually or P.O., or applied topically in ointment form), isosorbide dinitrate (sublingually or P.O.), or propranolol (P.O.). Obstructive lesions may necessitate coronary artery bypass surgery using vein grafts. Angioplasty, an experimental procedure, may be performed during cardiac catheterization to compress fatty deposits and relieve occlusion in patients with no calcification and partial occlusion. This procedure carries a certain risk, but its morbidity is lower than that for surgery.

Because coronary artery disease is so widespread, prevention is of incalculable importance. Dietary restrictions aimed at reducing intake of calories (in obesity) and of salt, fats, and cholesterol serve to minimize the risk, especially when supplemented with regular exercise. Abstention from smoking and reduction of stress are also beneficial. Other preventive actions include control of hypertension (with sympathetic blocking agents, such as methyldopa and propranolol, or diuretics, such as hydrochlorothiazide); control of elevated serum cholesterol or triglyceride levels (with antilipemics, such as clofibrate, sitosterols, and niacin); and measures to minimize platelet aggregation and the danger of blood clots (with aspirin or sulfinpyrazone, which may be prescribed after myocardial infarction; however, their effectiveness is still unproven).

Additional considerations

When caring for a patient with coronary artery disease, the hospital staff member should:

• monitor blood pressure and heart rate during anginal episodes; take an EKG during anginal episodes and before administering nitroglycerin or other nitrates; record duration of pain, amount of medication required to relieve it, and accompanying symptoms.

• keep nitroglycerin available for immediate use; instruct the patient to call whenever he feels chest pain; place the call bell within easy reach.

• explain cardiac catheterization to the patient before the procedure; make sure he knows why it is necessary, understands the risks involved, and realizes that its results may indicate a need for surgery.

• review the expected course of treatment with the patient and family after catheterization; monitor the catheter site (usually the groin or the antecubital fossa) for bleeding; check for distal pulses; make sure the patient drinks plenty of fluids to counter the diuretic effect of the dye; assess potassium levels.

• explain any surgical procedure to the patient and family, and answer their questions; take them on a tour of the ICU, and introduce them to the ICU staff.

• provide meticulous I.V., pulmonary artery catheter, and endotracheal tube care after surgery; monitor blood pressure, intake and output, breath sounds, and EKG, watching for signs of ischemia and arrhythmias; observe for and record chest pain; give vigorous chest physiotherapy.

• before discharge, emphasize the importance of following the prescribed medication regimen (antihypertensives, nitrates, antilipemics, for example), exercise program, and dietary restrictions; encourage moderate but regular exercise; refer the patient to a self-help program if he cannot stop smoking.

Myocardial Infarction
(Heart attack)

In myocardial infarction (MI), reduced blood flow through one of the coronary arteries results in myocardial ischemia and necrosis. In cardiovascular disease, the leading cause of death in the United States and Western Europe, death usually results from the cardiac damage or complications of MI. Mortality is high when treatment is delayed, and almost half of sudden deaths due to an MI occur before hospitalization, within 1 hour of the onset of symptoms. Prognosis improves if vigorous treatment begins immediately.

Causes and incidence

Predisposing factors to coronary artery disease and, in turn, MI include:

• positive family history
• hypertension
• smoking
• elevated serum triglyceride and cholesterol levels

• diabetes mellitus
• obesity, or excessive intake of saturated fats, carbohydrates, and/or salt
• sedentary life-style
• aging
• stress or a Type A personality (aggressive, ambitious, competitive attitude, addiction to work, chronic

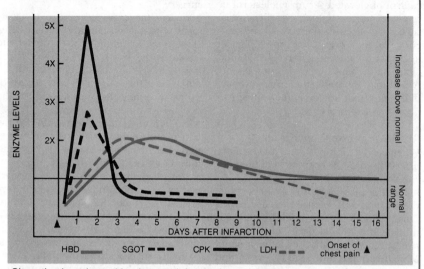

HOW SERUM ENZYME LEVELS CHANGE IN MYOCARDIAL INFARCTION

Since they're released by damaged tissue, determinations of serum enzymes—catalytic proteins that vary in concentration in specific organs—are essential to identify the compromised organ and assess the extent of its damage. The following most significant serum enzymes help diagnose myocardial infarction:
• serum glutamic-oxaloacetic transaminase (SGOT): in heart muscle and liver and, less extensively, in skeletal muscle, kidneys, and RBCs
• lactic dehydrogenase (LDH): in heart, brain, kidneys, liver, skeletal muscle, and erythrocytes; classified as five subtypes, of which LDH_1 and LDH_2 are the most important in myocardial infarction
• hydroxybutyrate dehydrogenase (HBD): an indirect measurement of LDH_1 and LDH_2
• creatine phosphokinase (CPK): in the heart, skeletal muscle, and brain.

impatience).

Males are more susceptible to MI than females, although incidence is rising among females, especially those who smoke and take oral contraceptives.

The site of the MI depends on the vessels involved. Occlusion of the circumflex branch of the left coronary artery causes a lateral wall infarction; occlusion of the anterior descending branch of the left coronary artery, an anterior wall infarction. True posterior wall infarctions generally result from occlusion of the right coronary artery or one of its branches. In transmural MI, tissue damage extends through all myocardial layers; in subendocardial MI, only to the innermost layer.

Signs and symptoms

The cardinal symptom of MI is persistent, crushing substernal pain that may radiate to the left arm, jaw, neck, or shoulder blades. Such pain is often described as "heavy," "squeezing," or "crushing," and may persist for 12 hours or more. However, in some MI patients—particularly the elderly or diabetics—pain may not occur at all; in others, it may be mild and confused with indigestion. In patients with coronary artery disease, angina of increasing frequency, severity, or duration (especially when not precipitated by exertion, a heavy meal, or cold and wind) may signal an impending infarction.

Other clinical effects include a feeling

of impending doom, fatigue, nausea, vomiting, and shortness of breath. The patient may experience catecholamine responses, such as coolness in extremities, perspiration, anxiety, and restlessness. Fever is unusual at the onset of an MI, but a low-grade temperature elevation may develop during the next few days. Blood pressure may vary among MI patients; hypo- or hypertension may be present.

The most common postmyocardial infarction complications include recurrent or persistent chest pain, arrhythmias, left ventricular failure (resulting in congestive heart failure or acute pulmonary edema), and cardiogenic shock. Unusual but potentially lethal complications that may develop soon after infarction include thromboembolism; papillary muscle dysfunction or rupture, causing mitral regurgitation; rupture of ventricular septum, causing ventricular septal defect; rupture of the myocardium; and ventricular aneurysm. Within 2 weeks to several months after infarction, Dressler's syndrome may develop, characterized by pericarditis, pericardial friction rub, chest pain, fever, and possibly, pleurisy or pneumonitis, and leukocytosis.

Diagnosis

 A history of coronary artery disease, persistent chest pain, changes in EKG, and elevated serum enzyme levels over a 72-hour period usually confirm MI. Auscultation may reveal diminished heart sounds, gallops, and in papillary dysfunction, the apical systolic murmur of mitral regurgitation over the mitral valve area.

When clinical features are equivocal, it's essential to assume MI until special tests rule it out. Diagnostic laboratory results include the following:
• *serial 12-lead EKG:* EKG abnormalities may be absent or inconclusive during the first few hours following an MI. When present, characteristic abnormalities show serial ST-T changes in subendocardial MI and Q waves representing transmural MI.

• *serial serum enzymes:* elevated creatine phosphokinase (CPK)—especially elevated CPK-MB isoenzyme, the cardiac muscle fraction of CPK—lactic dehydrogenase (LDH) isoenzymes—especially LDH$_1$, and LDH$_2$—SGOT, and alpha hydroxybutyric dehydrogenase
• *elevated ESR and WBC*
• *serial chest X-rays:* normal in MI, but with development of congestive heart failure show cardiomegaly, pulmonary vascular congestion, or bilateral pleural effusion.

Scans using I.V. technetium 99 can identify acutely damaged muscle by picking up radioactive nucleotide, which appears as a "hot spot" on the film. They are useful in localizing a recent MI.

Treatment

The goals of treatment are to relieve chest pain, to stabilize heart rhythm, and to reduce cardiac workload. Arrhythmias, the predominant problem during the first 48 hours after the infarction, may require antiarrhythmics, possibly a pacemaker, and rarely, electrocardioversion.

Other therapy includes:
• lidocaine for ventricular arrhythmias or, if lidocaine is ineffective, other drugs, such as procainamide, quinidine, bretylium, or disopyramide.
• atropine I.V. or a temporary pacemaker to treat heart block.
• nitroglycerin or isosorbide dinitrate to relieve pain by redistributing blood to ischemic area of myocardium, increasing cardiac output, and reducing myocardial workload.
• morphine or meperidine I.V. for pain and sedation.
• complete bed rest to decrease cardiac workload.
• oxygen administration (by face mask or nasal cannula) at a modest flow rate for 24 to 48 hours; a lower concentration is necessary if the patient has chronic obstructive pulmonary disease.
• pulmonary artery catheterization to detect left ventricular failure and to monitor response to treatment.
• drugs that increase contractility or

COMPLICATIONS OF MYOCARDIAL INFARCTION

COMPLICATION	DIAGNOSIS	TREATMENT
Arrhythmias	• In inferior wall MI, EKG shows bradycardia and junctional rhythms or AV block; in anterior wall MI, tachycardia or heart block; in all MIs, premature ventricular contractions, ventricular tachycardia, or ventricular fibrillation.	• Antiarrhythmics, cardioversion, and pacemaker
Congestive heart failure	• In left heart failure, chest X-rays show venous congestion and cardiomegaly. • Catheterization shows increased pulmonary artery, pulmonary capillary wedge, left ventricular end-diastolic pressures and central venous pressure.	• Diuretics, vasodilators, inotropics, cardiac glycosides
Cardiogenic shock	• Catheterization shows decreased cardiac output, and increased pulmonary artery and pulmonary capillary wedge pressures. • Other signs include hypotension, tachycardia, decreased level of consciousness, decreased urinary output, and neck vein distention, and cool, pale, moist skin.	• I.V. fluids, vasodilators, cardiotonics, cardiac glycosides, intra-aortic ballon pump (IABP), and beta-adrenergic stimulants
Mitral regurgitation	• Auscultation reveals rales and apical holosystolic murmur. • Catheterization shows increased pulmonary artery and pulmonary capillary wedge pressures. • Dyspnea is prominent.	• Nitroglycerin, nitroprusside, IABP, and surgical replacement of the mitral valve and concomitant myocardial revascularization
Ventricular septal rupture	• In left-to-right shunt, auscultation reveals a harsh holosystolic murmur and thrill. • Catheterization shows increased pulmonary artery and pulmonary capillary wedge pressures. • Confirmation by increased oxygen saturation of right ventricle and pulmonary artery.	• Surgical correction (may be postponed several weeks), IABP, nitroglycerin, or nitroprusside
Pericarditis	• Auscultation reveals a friction rub. • Chest pain is relieved by sitting up.	• Aspirin or other analgesics
Ventricular aneurysm	• Chest X-ray may show cardiomegaly. • EKG may show arrhythmias and persistent ST segment elevation. • Left ventriculography shows altered left ventricular motion (akinesis) or parodoxical motion (dyskinesis). • Complications include congestive heart failure, arrhythmias, and systemic embolization.	• Cardioversion, antiarrhythmics, vasodilators, anticoagulants, cardiotonic glycosides (digitalis), and diuretics. If conservative treatment fails to control complications, surgical resection is necessary
Dressler's syndrome	• Auscultation reveals a friction rub. • Chest X-rays may show pleural effusion.	Anti-inflammatory agents, such as aspirin or corticosteroids

blood pressure, or an intra-aortic balloon pump for cardiogenic shock.

Additional considerations

Health care is directed toward detecting complications, preventing further myocardial damage, and promoting comfort, rest, and emotional well-being. Most patients with MI receive treatment in the CCU, under constant observation for complications.

When treating an MI patient, the hospital staff member should:

• monitor and record EKG, blood pressure, temperature, and heart and breath sounds on admission to the CCU.

• assess pain, and administer morphine or meperidine I.V., as ordered; always record the severity and duration of pain; avoid giving I.M. injections, since they elevate CPK levels and render this test unreliable for MI, unless CPK isoenzymes are available (absorption of I.M. injections from the muscle is unpredictable due to low cardiac output and diminished peripheral perfusion).

• frequently monitor EKG to detect rate changes or arrhythmias; place rhythm strips in the patient's chart periodically, for evaluation.

• obtain EKG, blood pressure, and pulmonary artery catheter measurements to determine changes during episodes of chest pain.

• watch for signs of fluid retention (rales, cough, tachypnea, edema), which may indicate impending heart failure; monitor daily weight, intake and output, respirations, serum enzymes, and blood pressure; listen for adventitious breath sounds (patients on bed rest frequently have atelectatic rales, which may disappear after coughing) and for S_3 or S_4 gallops.

• plan patient care to maximize uninterrupted rest.

• ask the dietary department to provide a clear liquid diet until nausea subsides (a low-cholesterol, low-sodium diet, without caffeine-containing beverages, may be ordered).

• provide a stool softener to prevent straining at stool, which causes vagal stimulation and may slow heart rate; allow the patient to use a bedside commode, and provide as much privacy as possible.

• assist with range-of-motion exercises; turn the patient often if he is completely immobilized by a severe MI; use antiembolism stockings to help prevent venostasis and thrombophlebitis.

• provide emotional support, and help reduce stress and anxiety; administer tranquilizers, as needed; explain procedures and answer questions—an explanation of the CCU environment and routine can lessen the patient's anxiety; involve the patient and his family as much as possible in his care, to prevent dependence.

Preparing the MI patient for discharge includes:

• thoroughly explaining dosages and therapy to promote compliance with drug regimen and other treatment measures; warning about drug side effects, and advising the patient to watch for and report signs of toxicity (anorexia, nausea, vomiting, and yellow vision, for example, if the patient is receiving digitalis).

• reviewing dietary restrictions; providing a list of foods the patient should avoid if he must follow a low-sodium or low-fat and low-cholesterol diet; having the dietitian speak to the patient and family, if needed.

• counseling the patient about resuming sexual activity.

• advising the patient about appropriate responses to new or recurrent symptoms.

• advising the patient to report to the doctor typical or atypical chest pain. Postinfarction syndrome may develop, producing chest pain that must be differentiated from recurrent MI, pulmonary infarct, or congestive heart failure.

• explaining the purpose and use of a Holter monitor, if necessary.

• stressing the need to stop smoking; referring the patient to a self-help group, if necessary.

Congestive Heart Failure

Congestive heart failure (CHF) is a syndrome characterized by myocardial dysfunction that leads to impaired pump performance (diminished cardiac output) or to frank heart failure and abnormal circulatory congestion. Congestion of systemic venous circulation may result in peripheral edema or hepatomegaly; congestion of pulmonary circulation may cause pulmonary edema, an acute life-threatening emergency. Pump failure usually occurs in a damaged left ventricle (left heart failure) but may happen in the right ventricle (right heart failure) primarily, or secondary to left heart failure. Sometimes, left and right heart failures develop simultaneously. Although CHF may be acute (as a direct result of myocardial infarction), it's generally a chronic disorder associated with retention of salt and water by the kidneys. Advances in diagnostic and therapeutic techniques have greatly improved the outlook for patients with CHF, but prognosis still depends on the underlying cause and its response to treatment.

Causes

CHF may result from a primary abnormality of the heart muscle—such as an infarction—inadequate myocardial perfusion due to coronary artery disease, or cardiomyopathy. Other causes include:

• mechanical disturbances in ventricular filling during diastole when there's too little blood for the ventricle to pump, as in mitral stenosis secondary to rheumatic heart disease or constrictive pericarditis and atrial fibrillation.

• systolic hemodynamic disturbances, such as excessive cardiac workload due to volume overloading or pressure overload, that limit the heart's pumping ability. These disturbances can result from mitral or aortic regurgitation, which causes volume overloading, and aortic stenosis or systemic hypertension, which results in increased resistance to ventricular emptying.

Reduced cardiac output triggers three compensatory mechanisms: *ventricular dilation, hypertrophy,* and *increased sympathetic activity.* These mechanisms improve cardiac output at the expense of increased ventricular work. In *cardiac dilation,* an increase in end-diastolic ventricular volume (preload) causes increased stroke work and stroke volume during contraction, stretching cardiac muscle fibers beyond optimum limits and producing pulmonary congestion and pulmonary hypertension, which, in turn, lead to right ventricular failure.

In *ventricular hypertrophy,* an increase in muscle mass or diameter of the left ventricle allows the heart to pump against increased resistance (impedance) to the outflow of blood. An increase in ventricular diastolic pressure necessary to fill the enlarged ventricle may compromise diastolic coronary blood flow, limiting the oxygen supply to the ventricle, causing ischemia and impaired muscle contractility.

Increased sympathetic activity occurs as a response to decreased cardiac output and blood pressure by enhancing peripheral vascular resistance, contractility, heart rate, and venous return. Signs of increased sympathetic activity, such as cool extremities and clamminess, may indicate impending heart failure. Increased sympathetic activity also restricts blood flow to the kidneys, which respond by reducing the glomerular filtration rate and increasing tubular reabsorption of salt and water, in turn expanding the circulating blood volume. This renal mechanism, if unchecked, can aggravate congestion and produce overt edema.

Chronic CHF may worsen as a result of respiratory tract infections, pulmonary embolism, added emotional stress, increased salt or water intake, or failure to comply with prescribed therapy.

Signs and symptoms

Left heart failure produces fatigue, dyspnea (exertional, paroxysmal nocturnal); right heart failure causes engorgement of veins (when the patient is upright, neck veins may appear distended, feel rigid, and show exaggerated pulsations), and hepatomegaly. Many patients complain of a slight but persistent cold and dry cough combined with wheezing, which may be confused with an allergic reaction.

Later symptoms include tachypnea, palpitations, dependent edema, unexplained steady weight gain, nausea, chest tightness, slowed mental response, anorexia, hypotension, diaphoresis, narrow pulse pressure, pallor, and oliguria. Auscultation reveals a gallop rhythm (S_3) and rales on inspiration; the liver may be palpable and slightly tender.

In later stages of congestive heart failure, dullness develops over the lung bases, as well as hemoptysis and cyanosis, marked hepatomegaly, pitting ankle edema, and in bedridden patients, edema over the sacrum.

Complications include pulmonary edema; venostasis, with predisposition to thromboembolism (especially with prolonged bed rest); cerebral insufficiency; and renal insufficiency, with severe electrolyte imbalance.

Diagnosis

• *EKG* reflects heart strain or enlargement, or ischemia. It may also reveal atrial enlargement, tachycardia, and extrasystoles suggesting CHF.
• *Chest X-ray* shows increased pulmonary vascular markings, interstitial edema, or pleural effusion and cardiomegaly.
• *Pulmonary artery monitoring* demonstrates elevated pulmonary artery and capillary wedge pressures, which reflect left ventricular end-diastolic pressure in left heart failure, and elevated right atrial pressure or central venous pressure in right heart failure.

MANAGING PULMONARY EDEMA

INITIAL STAGE

SYMPTOMS
• Persistent cough
• Slight dyspnea/orthopnea
• Exercise intolerance
• Restlessness and anxiety
• Crepitant rales at lung bases
• Diastolic gallop

CLINICAL RESPONSIBILITIES
• checking color and amount of expectoration.
• positioning patient for comfort.
• auscultating chest for rales and S_3.
• medicate, as ordered.
• monitoring apical and radial pulses.
• assisting patient with all needs, to conserve strength.
• providing emotional support (through all stages) for patient and family.

ACUTE STAGE

SYMPTOMS
• Acute shortness of breath
• Respirations—rapid, noisy (audible wheeze, rales)
• Cough—more intense and productive of frothy, blood-tinged sputum
• Cyanosis—cold, clammy skin
• Tachycardia—arrhythmias
• Hypotension

CLINICAL RESPONSIBILITIES
• giving oxygen (preferably by high-concentration mask or IPPB).
• inserting I.V., if not already done.
• aspirating nasopharynx, as needed.
• applying rotating tourniquets.
• giving digitalis, morphine, and potent diuretics (e.g., furosemide), as ordered.
• inserting Foley catheter.
• calculating intake and output accurately.
• drawing blood to measure arterial blood gases.
• attaching cardiac monitor leads, and observing EKG.
• preparing for phlebotomy, if necessary.
• keeping resuscitation equipment available.

ADVANCED STAGE

SYMPTOMS
• Decreased level of consciousness
• Ventricular arrhythmias; shock
• Diminished breath sounds

CLINICAL RESPONSIBILITIES
• being prepared for cardioversion.
• assisting with intubation and mechanical ventilation, and resuscitating, if necessary.

Treatment

The aim of therapy is to improve pump function by reversing the compensatory mechanisms producing the clinical effects. CHF can be controlled quickly by treatment consisting of:
• diuresis to reduce total blood volume and circulatory congestion
• prolonged bed rest
• digitalis to strengthen myocardial contractility
• vasodilators to increase cardiac output by reducing the impedance to ventricular outflow (afterload)
• antiembolism stockings to prevent venostasis and possible thromboembolism.

Pulmonary edema requires morphine, as a venodilator, to diminish blood return to the heart; supplemental oxygen; and possibly, rotating tourniquets or phlebotomy for immediate decongestion by abruptly limiting venous return.

After recovery, the patient usually must continue taking digitalis and diuretics and must remain under medical supervision. If the patient with valve dysfunction has recurrent acute CHF, surgical replacement may be necessary.

Additional considerations

During the acute phase, the hospital staff member should:
• weigh the patient daily and check for peripheral edema; carefully monitor I.V. intake and urinary output (especially in the patient receiving diuretics), vital signs (for increased respiratory rate, heart rate, and narrowing pulse pressure), and mental status; auscultate the heart for abnormal sounds (S_3 gallop) and the lungs for rales or rhonchi; report changes immediately.
• frequently monitor BUN, creatinine, and serum potassium, sodium, chloride, and magnesium levels.
• when using rotating tourniquets, check radial and pedal pulses often to ensure the tourniquets aren't too tight; remove *one* tourniquet at a time at the completion of tourniquet therapy to prevent a sudden upsurge in circulating volume.
• check vital signs often during phlebotomy; make sure the patient has an I.V. line in place since fluid replacement may be necessary.
• prevent deep-vein thrombosis due to vascular congestion by assisting with range-of-motion exercises, enforcing bed rest, applying antiembolism stockings, and watching for calf pain and tenderness.

To prepare the patient for discharge, the staff member should:
• advise the patient to avoid foods high in sodium, such as canned or commercially prepared foods and dairy products, to curb fluid overload.
• tell the patient that potassium lost through diuretics must be replaced by taking a prescribed potassium supplement and eating high-potassium foods, such as bananas, apricots, and orange juice.
• emphasize the importance of taking digitalis exactly as prescribed, and instruct the patient to watch for signs of toxicity (anorexia, nausea, vomiting, yellow vision, cardiac arrhythmias).

The patient should notify the doctor if his pulse is unusually irregular or less than 60 beats per minute, or if he experiences dizziness, blurred vision, shortness of breath, a persistent dry cough, palpitations, increased fatigue, paroxysmal nocturnal dyspnea, swollen ankles, or decreased urinary output; or if he gains 3 to 5 lb (1.35 to 2.25 kg) in a week.

Congestive Cardiomyopathy

Congestive cardiomyopathy results from extensively damaged myocardial muscle fibers. This disorder interferes with myocardial metabolism and grossly dilates the ventricles without proportional compensatory hypertrophy, causing the heart to take on a globular shape and to contract poorly during systole. Congestive cardiomyopathy leads to intractable congestive heart failure, arrhythmias, and emboli. Since this disease is usually not diagnosed until it's in the advanced stages, prognosis is generally poor.

Causes

The cause of most cardiomyopathies is unknown. Occasionally, congestive cardiomyopathies are not primary myocardial diseases but rather result from myocardial destruction by toxic, infectious, or metabolic agents, such as certain viruses, endocrine and electrolyte disorders, and nutritional deficiencies. Other causes include muscle disorders (myasthenia gravis, progressive muscular dystrophy, myotonic dystrophy), infiltrative disorders (hemochromatosis, amyloidosis), and sarcoidosis.

Cardiomyopathy is a possible complication of alcoholism. In such cases, cardiomyopathy may improve somewhat with abstinence from alcohol but recurs when the patient resumes drinking. How viruses may induce cardiomyopathy is still unclear, but investigation is focused on a possible link between viral myocarditis and subsequent congestive cardiomyopathy, especially after infection with coxsackievirus B, poliovirus, and influenza virus.

Metabolic cardiomyopathies are related to endocrine and electrolyte disorders and nutritional deficiencies. Thus, congestive cardiomyopathy may develop in patients with hyperthyroidism, pheochromocytoma, beriberi (thiamine deficiency), and kwashiorkor (protein deficiency). Cardiomyopathy may also result from rheumatic fever, especially among children with myocarditis.

Ante- or postpartal cardiomyopathy may develop during the last trimester or within months after delivery. Its cause is unknown, but it occurs most frequently in multiparous women over age 30, particularly those with malnutrition or preeclampsia. In these patients, cardiomegaly and congestive heart failure may reverse with treatment, allowing a subsequent normal pregnancy. If cardiomegaly persists despite treatment, prognosis is extremely poor.

Signs and symptoms

In congestive cardiomyopathy, the heart ejects blood less efficiently than normal. Consequently, a large volume of blood remains in the left ventricle after systole, causing signs of congestive heart failure—both left-sided (shortness of breath, orthopnea, dyspnea on exertion, paroxysmal nocturnal dyspnea, fatigue, and an irritating dry cough at night) and right-sided (edema, liver engorgement, and jugular venous distention). Congestive cardiomyopathy also produces peripheral cyanosis, and sinus tachycardia or atrial fibrillation in some patients, secondary to low cardiac output. Auscultation reveals diffuse apical impulses, pansystolic murmur (mitral and tricuspid regurgitation secondary to cardiomegaly and weak papillary muscles), and S_3 and S_4 gallop rhythms.

Diagnosis

No single test confirms congestive cardiomyopathy. Diagnosis requires elimination of other possible causes of congestive heart failure and arrhythmias.

• *EKG* and *angiography* rule out ischemic heart disease; the EKG may also show biventricular hypertrophy, sinus tachycardia, atrial enlargement, and in 20% of patients, atrial fibrillation.

• *Chest X-ray* demonstrates cardiomegaly—usually affecting all heart chambers—pulmonary congestion, or pleural effusion.

Treatment

In congestive cardiomyopathy, the goal of treatment is to correct the underlying cause and to improve the heart's pumping ability with digitalis, diuretics, oxygen, and a restricted-sodium diet. Therapy may also include prolonged bed rest, selective use of steroids, and possibly, pericardiotomy, which is still investigational. Vasodilators reduce preload

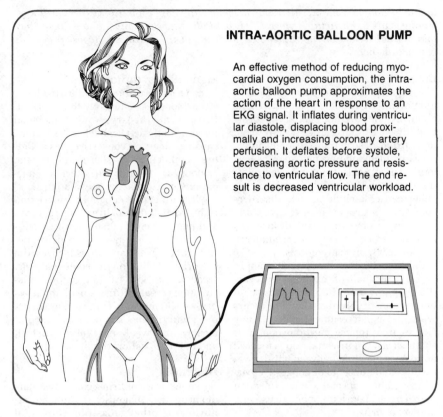

INTRA-AORTIC BALLOON PUMP

An effective method of reducing myocardial oxygen consumption, the intra-aortic balloon pump approximates the action of the heart in response to an EKG signal. It inflates during ventricular diastole, displacing blood proximally and increasing coronary artery perfusion. It deflates before systole, decreasing aortic pressure and resistance to ventricular flow. The end result is decreased ventricular workload.

and afterload, thereby decreasing congestion and increasing cardiac output. Acute heart failure necessitates vasodilation with nitroprusside I.V. or, more recently, nitroglycerin I.V. Although not yet approved for use in the United States, Salbutamol I.V. shows promise in improving cardiac status. Long-term treatment may include phenoxybenzamine, prazosin, hydralazine, isosorbide dinitrate, and if the patient is on prolonged bed rest, anticoagulants.

Additional considerations

• Daily care for the patient with acute failure includes monitoring for signs of progressive failure (decreased arterial pulses, increased neck vein distention) and compromised renal perfusion (oliguria, increased BUN and creatinine, and electrolyte imbalances). The patient should be weighed daily.

• If the patient is receiving vasodilators, blood pressure and heart rate must be checked frequently.
• If the patient becomes hypotensive, the infusion must be stopped and he should be placed in a supine position with legs elevated to increase venous return to the heart and to ensure cerebral blood flow.
• If the patient is receiving diuretics, he should be monitored for signs of resolving congestion (decreased rales and dyspnea) or too vigorous diuresis. He must be watched for signs of hypokalemia, especially if therapy includes digitalis.
• If hospitalization becomes prolonged, the patient should try to spend occasional weekends away from the hospital. Visiting hours should be flexible. Therapeutic restrictions and uncertain prognosis usually cause profound anxiety and depression, so he will need support and encouragment to express his feelings.

Before discharge, the patient should be taught about his illness and its treatment to help ensure continued compliance with therapy. He will have to restrict his sodium intake, watch for weight gain, and take digitalis as prescribed and watch for its toxic effects (anorexia, nausea, vomiting, yellow vision).

Idiopathic Hypertrophic Subaortic Stenosis

Idiopathic hypertrophic subaortic stenosis (IHSS) is a primary disease of cardiac muscle characterized by left ventricular hypertrophy and thickening of the ventricular septum, without concomitant dilation of the cavity. In IHSS cardiac output may be low, normal, or high, depending on whether stenosis is obstructive or nonobstructive. If cardiac output is normal or high, IHSS may go undetected for years; but low cardiac output may lead to potentially fatal congestive heart failure. The course of IHSS varies; some patients demonstrate progressive deterioration, while others remain stable for several years.

Causes

Despite being designated as idiopathic, in almost all cases, IHSS is inherited as a non–sex-linked autosomal dominant trait. Most patients with IHSS have obstructive disease, resulting from the combined effects of ventricular septum hypertrophy and the movement of the anterior mitral valve leaflet into the outflow tract during systole. Eventually, left ventricular dysfunction, due to rigidity and decreased compliance, causes pump failure.

Signs and symptoms

Generally, clinical features of IHSS don't appear until the disease is well advanced, when atrial dilation and, possibly, atrial fibrillation abruptly reduce blood flow to the left ventricle. Reduced inflow and subsequent low output may produce angina pectoris, arrhythmias, dyspnea, syncope, congestive heart failure, and sudden death. Auscultation reveals a medium-pitched systolic ejection murmur along the left sternal border and at the apex; palpation reveals a peripheral pulse with a characteristic double impulse (pulsus biferiens) and, with atrial fibrillation, an irregular pulse.

Diagnosis

Diagnosis of IHSS depends on typical clinical findings and the following test results:

• *Echocardiography* (most useful) shows increased thickness of the interventricular septum and abnormal motion of the anterior mitral leaflet during systole, occluding left ventricular outflow in obstructive IHSS.
• *Cardiac catheterization* reveals elevated left ventricular end-diastolic pressure and, possibly, mitral insufficiency.
• *EKG* usually demonstrates left ventricular hypertrophy, ST segment and T wave abnormalities, deep waves (due to hypertrophy, not infarction), left anterior hemiblock, ventricular arrhythmias, and possibly, atrial fibrillation.
• *Phonocardiography* confirms an early systolic murmur.

Treatment

The goals of treatment of IHSS are to relax the ventricle and to relieve outflow tract obstruction. Propranolol, a beta-adrenergic blocking agent, slows heart rate and increases ventricular filling by relaxing the obstructing muscle, thereby reducing angina, syncope, dyspnea, and arrhythmias. However, propranolol may aggravate symptoms of cardiac decompensation. Atrial fibrillation necessitates digitalis or cardioversion to treat the arrhythmia, and because of the high risk of systemic embolism, anticoagulant therapy until fibrillation subsides. Since vasodilators, such as nitroglycerin, reduce venous return by permitting pooling of blood in the periphery, decreasing ventricular volume and chamber size, and may cause further obstruction, they're contraindicated in patients with IHSS. Also contraindicated are sympathetic stimulators, such as isoproterenol, which enhance cardiac contractility and myocardial demands for oxygen, intensifying the obstruction.

If drug therapy fails, surgery is indicated. Ventricular myotomy (resection of the hypertrophied septum) alone or combined with mitral valve replacement may ease outflow tract obstruction and relieve symptoms. However, ventricular myotomy may cause complications, such as complete heart block and ventricular septal defect, and is still considered experimental.

Additional considerations

• Because syncope or sudden death may follow well-tolerated exercise, such patients must avoid strenuous physical activity, such as running.
• Medication should be administered, as ordered, but nitroglycerin should *not* be used for chest pain because it can worsen obstruction. The patient should not stop taking propranolol abruptly, since doing so may cause rebound effects, resulting in myocardial infarction or sudden death. The patient's tolerance for increased dosage of propranolol can be determined by taking his pulse to check for bradycardia, and having him stand and walk around slowly to check for orthostatic hypotension.
• The patient may need psychologic support. If he is hospitalized for a prolonged time, a hospital staff member should be flexible with visiting hours, and encourage occasional weekends away from the hospital, if possible. The patient should seek psychosocial counseling to help him and his family accept the restricted life-style imposed by this chronic disease and cope with the poor prognosis.
• If the patient is a child, his parents should arrange for him to continue his studies in the hospital.
• Since sudden cardiac arrest is possible, the patient's family should learn cardiopulmonary resuscitation.

Restrictive Cardiomyopathy

Restrictive cardiomyopathy, a disorder of the myocardial musculature, is characterized by restricted ventricular filling (the result of left ventricular hypertrophy), and endocardial fibrosis and thickening. Severe restrictive cardiomyopathy is irreversible.

Causes

An extremely rare disorder, primary restrictive cardiomyopathy is of unknown etiology. However, restrictive cardiomyopathy syndrome, a manifestation of amyloidosis, results from infiltration of amyloid into the intracellular spaces in the myocardium, endocardium, and subendocardium.

In both forms of restrictive cardiomyopathy, the myocardium becomes rigid, with poor distention during diastole, inhibiting complete ventricular filling, and fails to contract completely during systole, resulting in low cardiac output.

Signs and symptoms

Because it lowers cardiac output and leads to congestive heart failure, restrictive cardiomyopathy produces fatigue, dyspnea, orthopnea, chest pain, generalized edema, liver engorgement, peripheral cyanosis, and pallor.

Diagnosis

• In advanced stages of this disease, *chest X-ray* shows massive cardiomegaly affecting all four chambers of the heart.

• *Echocardiography* rules out constrictive pericarditis as the cause of restricted filling by detecting increased left ventricular muscle mass and differences in end-diastolic pressures between the ventricles.

• *EKG* may show low-voltage complexes or hypertrophy.

• *Arterial pulsation* reveals blunt carotid upstroke with small volume.

• *Cardiac catheterization* demonstrates increased left ventricular end-diastolic pressure and rules out constrictive pericarditis as the cause of restricted filling.

Treatment

Although no therapy currently exists for restricted ventricular filling, digitalis, diuretics, and a restricted sodium diet are beneficial by easing the symptoms of congestive heart failure. Oral vasodilators—such as isosorbide dinitrate, prazosin, and hydralazine—may control intractable congestive heart failure. Anticoagulant therapy may be necessary to prevent thrombophlebitis in the patient restricted to prolonged bed rest.

Additional considerations

• In the acute phase, heart rate and rhythm, blood pressure, urinary output, and pulmonary artery pressure readings must be monitored to help guide treatment.

• The patient will need psychologic support, and should have appropriate diversionary activities if restricted to prolonged bed rest. Since the poor prognosis for severe restrictive cardiomyopathy usually causes profound anxiety and depression, he will need support, understanding, and encouragement; also, psychosocial counseling to help him cope with his restricted life-style. The hospital staff member should be flexible with visiting hours whenever possible.

• Before discharge, the patient must know how to watch for signs of digoxin toxicity (anorexia, nausea, vomiting, yellow vision) and should report them. He must also record and report weight gain, and if sodium restriction is ordered, should avoid canned vegetables, pickles, smoked meats, and excessive use of table salt.

CARDIAC COMPLICATIONS

Hypovolemic Shock
(Hypovolemic shock syndrome)

In hypovolemic shock, reduced intravascular blood volume causes circulatory dysfunction and inadequate tissue perfusion. Without sufficient blood or fluid replacement, hypovolemic shock syndrome may lead to irreversible cerebral and renal damage, cardiac arrest, and ultimately, death. Hypovolemic shock syndrome necessitates early recognition of signs and symptoms, and prompt, aggressive treatment to improve prognosis.

Causes

Hypovolemic shock usually results from acute blood loss—about one fifth of total volume. Such massive blood loss may result from gastrointestinal bleeding, internal hemorrhage (hemothorax, hemoperitoneum), or external hemorrhage (accidental or surgical trauma), or from any condition that reduces circulating intravascular plasma volume or other body fluids, such as in severe burns. Other underlying causes of hypovolemic shock include intestinal obstruction, peritonitis, acute pancreatitis, ascites and dehydration from excessive perspiration, severe diarrhea or protracted vomiting, diabetes insipidus, diuresis, or inadequate fluid intake.

USING MEDICAL ANTI-SHOCK TROUSERS EFFECTIVELY

Medical Anti-shock Trousers (MAST) counteracts bleeding and hypovolemia by slowing or stopping arterial bleeding; by forcing any available blood from the lower body to the heart, brain, and other vital organs; and by preventing return of the available circulating blood volume to the lower extremities.

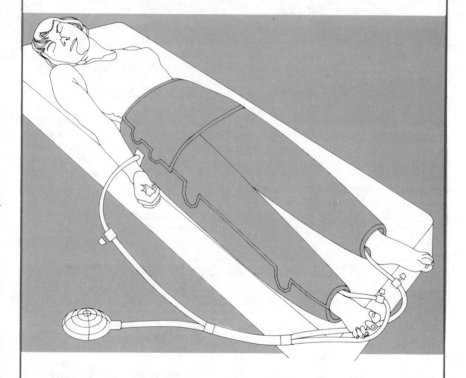

CLINICAL CONSIDERATIONS
• MAST must not be applied if positions or wounds show or suggest major intrathoracic or intracranial vascular injury; or if the patient has open extremity bleeding, pulmonary edema, or trauma above the level of MAST application.
• While the patient is wearing MAST, his vital signs must be monitored, especially blood pressure, apical and radial pulse rates, and respirations. Extremities should be checked for pedal pulses, color, warmth, and numbness; MAST must not be too constricting.
• MAST should only be taken off the patient when a doctor is present, when fluids are available for transfusion, and when anesthesia and surgical teams are available.
• MAST must be cleaned with warm soap and water, not with solvents or by autoclaving. Then, it should be air dried, prior to being stored for future use.

Signs and symptoms

Hypovolemic shock produces a syndrome of hypotension, with narrowing pulse pressure; decreased sensorium; tachycardia; rapid, shallow respirations; reduced urinary output (less than 25 ml/hour); and cold, pale, clammy skin. Metabolic acidosis with an accumulation of lactic acid develops as a result of tissue anoxia, as cellular metabolism shifts from aerobic to anaerobic pathways. Disseminated intravascular coagulation (DIC) is a possible complication of hypovolemic shock.

Diagnosis

No single symptom or diagnostic test establishes the diagnosis or severity of shock. Laboratory findings include:
• elevated potassium, serum lactate, and BUN levels.
• increased urine specific gravity (more than 1.020) and urine osmolality.
• decreased blood pH and PO_2, and increased PCO_2.

In addition, gastroscopy, aspiration of gastric contents through a nasogastric tube, and X-rays identify internal bleeding sites; coagulation studies may detect coagulopathy from DIC.

Treatment

Emergency treatment measures consist of prompt, adequate blood and fluid replacement to restore intravascular volume and raise blood pressure. Saline solution, then possibly plasma proteins (albumin), other plasma expanders, or lactated Ringer's solution, may produce volume expansion until whole blood can be matched. Application of Medical Anti-shock Trousers (MAST) may be helpful. Treatment may also include oxygen administration, identification of bleeding site, control of bleeding by direct measures (such as pressure and elevation of an extremity), and possibly, surgery.

Additional considerations

Management of hypovolemic shock necessitates prompt, aggressive supportive measures, and careful assessment and monitoring of vital signs. This includes:
• checking for a patent airway and adequate circulation; starting cardiopulmonary resuscitation if blood pressure and heart rate are absent.
• placing the patient flat in bed, with his legs elevated about 30° to increase blood flow by promoting venous return to the heart.
• recording blood pressure, pulse rate,

PATHOPHYSIOLOGY OF HYPOVOLEMIC SHOCK

Normally, the body compensates for a loss of blood or fluid by constricting arteriolar beds, increasing heart rate and contractile force, and redistributing fluids. These compensation mechanisms are effective enough to maintain stable vital signs, even after a 10% blood loss. But by the time blood or fluid loss reaches 15% to 25%, these mechanisms fail to maintain cardiac output, and blood pressure drops.

Baroreceptors (pressure-sensitive stretch receptors) in the aorta and carotid bodies trigger sympathetic nerve fibers. As a result, the adrenals release norepinephrine and epinephrine, causing vasoconstriction, which sharply reduces the blood flow to peripheral muscle and some of the vital organs (kidneys, liver, and lungs). Some cells, therefore, no longer receive oxygen, and cellular metabolism shifts from aerobic to anaerobic pathways, producing an accumulation of lactic acid, which is not metabolized to yield needed energy. Impaired renal or hepatic function causes this acid to accumulate and results in metabolic acidosis.

To compensate for metabolic acidosis, the patient hyperventilates to exhale more CO_2 and, in doing so, induces respiratory alkalosis. Since he may be unable to maintain the physical exertion required for hyperventilation, he may eventually need respiratory support, either oxygen by mask or mechanical ventilation.

Eventually, the compensatory mechanisms that serve to maintain acid-base balance fail, and cellular function is severely impaired, leading to cell death and subsequent organ failure.

INVASIVE MONITORING IN HYPOVOLEMIC SHOCK

KIND OF MONITORING	TEST RESULTS	SIGNIFICANCE
Intra-arterial pressure monitoring (for systemic arterial pressure)	• Hypotension (< 90 mmHg auscultatory systolic blood pressure) • Central blood pressure may be 10 to 20 mmHg higher than brachial reading	• Impaired ventricular ejection or alterations in vascular compliance or resistance
Central venous pressure ([CVP]—a good guide for I.V. fluid monitoring because of definitive response [increase or decrease] to fluid loading)	• Decreased central venous pressure (< 8 cm H_2O) • Reading may not reflect an accurate right ventricular filling pressure and does not reflect left heart function	• Inadequate intravascular volume to produce a right ventricular filling pressure necessary for ventricular ejection
Pulmonary artery pressure The flow-directed, balloon-tipped, pulmonary artery thermodilution catheter is a quadruple-lumen catheter inserted through the right heart into the pulmonary artery to measure cardiac output, as well as right atrial, pulmonary artery, or pulmonary capillary wedge pressure (a reliable indicator of left heart function and fluid overload)	• Decreased right atrial, pulmonary artery, and pulmonary capillary wedge pressures (PCWP < 12 mmHg) • Reading reflects an accurate mean left atrial pressure • Decreased cardiac output (with thermodilution catheter)	• Inadequate intravascular volume to produce a left ventricular filling pressure necessary for ventricular ejection

peripheral pulses, respirations, and other vital signs every 15 minutes, and EKG continuously. Systolic blood pressure less than 80 mmHg usually results in inadequate coronary artery blood flow, cardiac ischemia, arrhythmias, and further complications of low cardiac output. When blood pressure drops below 80 mmHg, the oxygen flow rate must be increased, and the doctor notified immediately. A progressive drop in blood pressure, accompanied by a thready pulse, generally signals inadequate cardiac output from reduced intravascular volume. The doctor should be notified, and the infusion rate increased.
• starting I.V.s with normal saline or lactated Ringer's solution, using a large-bore catheter (14G), which allows easier administration of later blood transfusions. (I.V.s should *not* be started in the legs of a patient in shock who has suffered abdominal trauma, since infused fluid may escape through the ruptured vessel into the abdomen.)
• inserting a Foley catheter, if needed, to measure hourly urinary output. If output is less than 30 ml/hour in adults, the fluid infusion rate can be increased, but the patient must be watched for signs of fluid overload, such as an increase in pulmonary capillary wedge pressure (PCWP). The doctor should be notified if urinary output does not improve. An osmotic diuretic, such as mannitol, may be ordered to increase renal blood flow and urinary output. The proper amount of fluid can be determined by checking blood pressure, urinary output, central venous pressure (CVP), or PCWP. (To increase accuracy, CVP should be measured at the level of the right atrium, using the same reference point on the chest each time.)

• drawing an arterial blood sample to measure blood gas levels; administering oxygen to ensure adequate oxygenation of tissues; adjusting the oxygen flow rate to a higher or lower level, as blood gas measurements indicate.

• drawing venous blood for CBC, electrolytes, type and cross match, and coagulation studies.

• assessing skin color and temperature during therapy, and noting any changes.

Cold, clammy skin may be a sign of continuing peripheral vascular constriction, indicating progressive shock.

• watching for signs of impending coagulopathy (petechiae, bruising, bleeding or oozing from gums or venipuncture sites).

• explaining all procedures and their purpose; providing emotional support to the patient and family throughout these emergency measures.

Cardiogenic Shock

Sometimes called pump failure, cardiogenic shock is a condition of diminished cardiac output that severely impairs tissue perfusion. It reflects severe left ventricular failure, and occurs as a serious complication in nearly 15% of all patients hospitalized with acute myocardial infarction. Cardiogenic shock typically affects patients whose area of infarction exceeds 40% of muscle mass; in such patients, the fatality rate may exceed 85%. Most patients with cardiogenic shock die within 24 hours of onset. Prognosis for those who survive is extremely poor.

Causes

Cardiogenic shock can result from any condition that causes significant left ventricular dysfunction with reduced cardiac output, such as myocardial infarction (most common), myocardial ischemia, papillary muscle dysfunction, or end-stage cardiomyopathy. Regardless of the underlying cause, left ventricular dysfunction sets into motion a series of compensatory mechanisms that attempt to increase cardiac output and, in turn, maintain vital organ function.

As cardiac output falls in left ventricular dysfunction, aortic and carotid baroreceptors initiate sympathetic nervous responses, which increase heart rate, left ventricular filling pressure, and peripheral resistance to flow, to enhance venous return to the heart. These compensatory responses initially stabilize the patient but later cause deterioration with rising oxygen demands of the already compromised myocardium. These events comprise a vicious circle of low cardiac output, sympathetic compensation, myocardial ischemia, and even lower cardiac output.

Signs and symptoms

Cardiogenic shock produces signs of poor tissue perfusion: cold, pale, clammy skin; a drop in systolic blood pressure to 30 mmHg below baseline, or a sustained reading below 80 mmHg not attributable to medication; tachycardia; rapid, shallow respirations; oliguria (less than 20 ml urine/hour); restlessness, and mental confusion and obtundation; narrowing pulse pressure; and cyanosis. Although many of these clinical features also occur in congestive heart failure and other shock syndromes, they are usually more profound in cardiogenic shock.

Diagnosis

Auscultation detects gallop rhythm, faint heart sounds, and possibly, if the shock results from rupture of the ventricular septum or papillary muscles, a holosystolic murmur. Other abnormal clinical findings include:

• *pulmonary artery pressure monitoring:* increased pulmonary artery pressure (PAP), and increased pulmonary capillary wedge pressure (PCWP), reflecting a rise in left ventricular end-diastolic pressure (preload) and increased resistance to left ventricular emptying (afterload) due to ineffective pumping. Thermodilution technique measures decreased cardiac index (less than 2.2 liters/minute).

• *invasive arterial pressure monitoring:* hypotension due to impaired ventricular ejection

• *arterial blood gases:* may show metabolic acidosis and hypoxia

• *EKG:* possible evidence of acute myocardial infarction, ischemia, or ventricular aneurysm

• *enzyme levels:* elevated creatine phosphokinase (CPK), lactic dehydrogenase (LDH), SGOT, and SGPT, which point to myocardial infarction or ischemia, and suggest congestive heart failure or shock. CPK and LDH isoenzyme determinations may confirm acute myocardial infarction.

Additional tests determine other conditions that can lead to pump dysfunction and failure, such as cardiac dysrhythmias, cardiac tamponade, papillary muscle infarct or rupture, ventricular septal rupture, pulmonary emboli, venous pooling (associated with venodilators and continuous intermittent positive pressure breathing), and hypovolemia.

Treatment

The aim of treatment is to enhance cardiovascular status by increasing cardiac output, improving myocardial perfusion, and decreasing cardiac workload with combinations of various cardiovascular drugs and mechanical-assist techniques. Drug therapy may include dopamine I.V., a vasopressor that increases cardiac output, blood pressure, and renal blood flow; levarterenol (norepinephrine), when a more potent vasoconstrictor is necessary; and nitroprusside I.V., a vasodilator that may be used with a vasopressor to further improve cardiac output by decreasing peripheral vascular resistance (afterload) and reducing left ventricular enddiastolic pressure (preload). The intraaortic balloon pump (IABP) is a mechanical-assist device that attempts to improve coronary artery perfusion and decrease cardiac workload. The inflatable balloon pump is surgically inserted through the femoral artery into the descending thoracic aorta. The balloon inflates during diastole to increase coronary artery perfusion pressure and deflates before systole (before the aortic valve opens) to reduce resistance to ejection (afterload) and therefore lessen cardiac workload. Improved ventricular ejection, which significantly improves cardiac output, and a subsequent vasodilation in the peripheral vasculature lead to lower preload volume.

Additional considerations

• At the first sign of cardiogenic shock, blood pressure and heart rate must be immediately checked. If the patient is hypotensive or has difficulty breathing, he must be checked for a patent I.V. line and a patent airway, and be given oxygen to promote adequate oxygenation of tissues. A doctor should be notified.

• Arterial blood gases should be monitored to measure oxygenation and detect acidosis from poor tissue perfusion. Oxygen flow can be increased as indicated by blood gas measurements. CBC and electrolytes should be checked.

• After diagnosis, cardiac rhythm must be monitored continuously. Skin color and temperature, and other vital signs should be assessed often. The patient must be watched for a drop in systolic blood pressure to less than 80 mmHg (usually results in inadequate coronary artery blood flow, which may produce cardiac ischemia or cardiac arrhythmias, and further compromise cardiac output). Hypotension must be reported.

• A Foley catheter may be inserted to measure urinary output. The doctor should be notified if output drops below 30 ml/hour. The patient may need an osmotic diuretic, such as mannitol, to increase renal tubular flow and prevent acute tubular necrosis.

• PAP and PCWP should be monitored with a pulmonary artery catheter, and, if equipment is available, cardiac output should also be checked. A high PCWP indicates congestive heart failure and must be reported immediately.

• When a patient is on the IABP, repositioning him often and performing passive range-of-motion exercises will prevent skin breakdown. However, the patient's "ballooned" leg should not be flexed at the hip, since this may displace or fracture the catheter. Pedal pulses, and skin temperature and color must be assessed to make sure circulation to the leg is adequate. The dressing on the insertion site should be frequently checked for bleeding, and changed, if needed. The site should also be checked for he-matoma or signs of infection, and any drainage cultured.

• After the patient has become hemodynamically stable, the frequency of balloon inflation is gradually reduced to wean him from the IABP. During weaning, he must be carefully watched for monitor changes, chest pain, and other signs of recurring cardiac ischemia and shock.

• Since the patient and family may be anxious about the ICU, IABP, and other tubes and devices, they may need psychologic support and reassurance. To ease emotional stress, care should allow frequent rest periods and provide as much privacy as possible.

Ventricular Aneurysm

Ventricular aneurysm is an outpouching, almost always of the left ventricle, that produces ventricular wall dysfunction in about 20% of patients after myocardial infarction (MI). Ventricular aneurysm may develop within weeks after MI or may be delayed for years. Untreated ventricular aneurysm can lead to arrhythmias, systemic embolization, or congestive heart failure, and is potentially fatal. Resection improves prognosis in congestive heart failure or refractory patients who have developed ventricular arrhythmias.

Causes

When MI destroys a large muscular section of the left ventricle, necrosis reduces the ventricular wall to a thin sheath of fibrous tissue. Under intracardiac pressure, this thin layer stretches and forms a separate noncontractile sac (aneurysm). Abnormal muscular wall movement accompanies ventricular aneurysm and includes akinesia (lack of movement), dyskinesia (paradoxical movement), asynergia (decreased and inadequate movement), and asynchrony (uncoordinated movement). During systolic ejection, the abnormal muscular wall movements associated with the aneurysm cause the remaining normally functioning myocardial fibers to increase the force of contraction in order to maintain stroke volume and cardiac output. At the same time, a portion of the stroke volume is lost to passive distention of the noncontractile sac.

Signs and symptoms

Ventricular aneurysm may cause arrhythmias—such as premature ventricular contractions or ventricular tachycardia—palpitations, signs of cardiac dysfunction (weakness on exertion, fatigue, angina), and occasionally, a visible or palpable systolic precordial bulge. This condition may also lead to left ventricular dysfunction, with chronic congestive heart failure (dyspnea, fatigue, edema, rales, gallop rhythm, neck vein distention); pulmonary edema; systemic embolization; and with left ventricular failure, pulsus alternans. Ventricular aneurysms enlarge but rarely rupture.

Diagnosis

Persistent ventricular arrhythmias, onset of heart failure, or systemic embolization in a patient with left ventricular failure and a history of MI strongly suggests ventricular aneurysm. Indicative tests

include the following:
- *Left ventriculography* reveals left ventricular enlargement, with an area of akinesia or dyskinesia (during cineangiography) and diminished cardiac function.
- *EKG* may show persistent ST-T wave elevations after infarction.
- *Chest X-ray* may demonstrate an abnormal bulge distorting the heart's contour if the aneurysm is large; the X-ray may be normal if the aneurysm is small.
- *Noninvasive nuclear cardiology scan* may indicate the site of infarction and suggest the area of aneurysm.

Treatment

Depending on the size of the aneurysm, and the complications, treatment may necessitate only routine medical examination to follow the patient's condition, or aggressive measures for intractable ventricular arrhythmias, congestive heart failure, and emboli.

Emergency treatment of ventricular arrhythmia includes antiarrhythmics I.V. or electrocardioversion. Preventive treatment continues with oral antiarrhythmics, such as procainamide, quinidine, or disopyramide.

Emergency treatment for congestive heart failure with pulmonary edema includes oxygen, digitalis I.V., furosemide I.V., morphine sulfate I.V., and when necessary, nitroprusside I.V. and intubation. Maintenance therapy may include nitrates, prazosin, and hydralazine P.O. Systemic embolization requires anticoagulation therapy or embolectomy. Refractory ventricular tachycardia, heart failure, recurrent arterial embolization, and persistent angina with coronary artery occlusion may necessitate surgery, of which the most effective procedure is aneurysmectomy, with myocardial revascularization.

Additional considerations

- If ventricular tachycardia occurs, blood pressure and heart rate should be monitored. If cardiac arrest develops, cardiopulmonary resuscitation (CPR) must be started and assistance, resuscitative equipment, and medication obtained.
- In a patient with congestive heart failure, the following require close monitoring: vital signs, heart sounds, intake and output, fluid and electrolyte balances, and BUN and creatinine levels. Because of the threat of systemic embolization, peripheral pulses and the color and temperature of extremities should be frequently checked. The patient must be watched for sudden changes in sensorium that indicate cerebral embolization and for any signs that suggest renal failure or progressive myocardial infarction.
- If arrhythmias necessitate cardioversion, a sufficient amount of conducting jelly should be used to prevent chest burns. If the patient is conscious, diazepam I.V. should be given, as ordered, before cardioversion. Cardioversion treatment—a lifesaving method using brief electroshock to the heart—should be explained. If the patient is receiving antiarrhythmics, appropriate laboratory tests must be checked. For instance, if he takes procainamide, antinuclear antibodies must be checked because this drug may induce lupus erythematosus syndrome.

If the patient is scheduled to undergo resection, the hospital staff member should:
- explain before surgery what's included in expected postoperative care in the ICU (including use of endotracheal tube, ventilator, hemodynamic monitoring, chest tubes, and drainage bottle).
- monitor vital signs, intake and output, heart sounds, and pulmonary artery catheter after surgery; watch for signs of infection, such as fever and excessive drainage from incision.

To prepare the patient for discharge, the staffer should:
- teach the patient how to take his pulse (observing for irregularity and rate changes); urge him to follow his medication regimen strictly (even if he has to set an alarm to take medication during the night) and to watch for side effects.
- refer the family to a community-based CPR training program since arrhythmias can cause sudden death.

Cardiac Tamponade

In cardiac tamponade, a rapid, unchecked rise in intrapericardial pressure impairs diastolic filling of the heart. The rise in pressure usually results from blood or fluid accumulation in the pericardial sac. If fluid accumulates rapidly, this condition is commonly fatal and necessitates emergency lifesaving measures. Slow accumulation and rise in pressure, as in pericardial effusion associated with malignancies, may not produce immediate symptoms, since the fibrous wall of the pericardial sac can gradually stretch to accommodate as much as 1 to 2 liters of fluid.

Causes

Increased intrapericardial pressure and consequent cardiac tamponade may result from:
• effusion (in malignancy, bacterial infections, tuberculosis, and rarely, acute rheumatic fever).
• hemorrhage from trauma (such as gunshot or stab wounds of the chest, and perforation by catheter during cardiac or central venous catheterization, or postcardiac surgery).
• hemorrhage from nontraumatic causes (such as rupture of the heart or great vessels, or anticoagulant therapy in a patient with pericarditis).

Signs and symptoms

Cardiac tamponade classically produces increased venous pressure with neck vein distention, reduced arterial blood pressure, muffled heart sounds on auscultation, and pulsus paradoxus (an abnormal inspiratory drop in systemic blood pressure greater than 15 mmHg). These classic symptoms represent failure of physiologic compensatory mechanisms to override the effects of rapidly rising pericardial pressure, which limits diastolic filling of the ventricles and reduces stroke volume to a critically low level. Generally, ventricular end-systolic volume is not changed significantly, since the contractile force of the ventricles remains intact even in severe tamponade. The increasing pericardial pressure is transmitted equally across the heart cavities, producing a proportionate rise in intracardiac pressure, especially both atrial pressures and end-diastolic ventricular pressures. Cardiac tamponade may also produce dyspnea, tachycardia, narrow pulse pressure, restlessness, and hepatomegaly.

Diagnosis

Diagnosis usually relies on classic clinical features. Laboratory results may include the following:
• *Chest X-ray* shows slightly widened mediastinum and cardiomegaly.
• *EKG* is rarely diagnostic of tamponade but is useful to rule out other cardiac disorders. It may reveal changes produced by acute pericarditis.
• *Pulmonary artery catheterization* detects increased right atrial pressure, right ventricular diastolic pressure, and central venous pressure.
• *Echocardiography* records pericardial effusion.

Treatment

The goal of treatment is to relieve intrapericardial pressure and cardiac compression by removing accumulated blood or fluid. Pericardiocentesis (needle aspiration of the pericardial cavity) or surgical creation of an opening dramatically improves systemic arterial pressure and cardiac output with aspiration of as little as 25 ml of fluid. Such treatment necessitates continuous hemodynamic and EKG monitoring in the ICU. Trial volume loading with temporary I.V. normal saline solution with albumin, and perhaps an inotropic drug, such as isoproterenol, is necessary in the hypotensive patient to maintain cardiac output. Although this drug normally improves myocardial function, it may further compromise an ischemic myocardium after myocardial infarction.

Depending on the cause of tamponade, additional treatment may include:
• *in traumatic injury:* blood transfusion or a thoracotomy to drain reaccumulating fluid or to repair bleeding sites
• *in heparin-induced tamponade:* the heparin antagonist protamine sulfate
• *in warfarin-induced tamponade:* vitamin K.

Additional considerations
If the patient is to undergo pericardiocentesis, the hospital staff member should:
• explain the procedure to the patient; keep a pericardial aspiration needle attached to a 50 ml syringe by a three-way stopcock, an EKG machine, and an emergency cart with a defibrillator at the bedside; make sure the equipment is turned on and ready for immediate use; position the patient at a 45° to 60° angle to facilitate correct needle insertion; connect the precordial EKG lead to the hub of the aspiration needle with an alligator clamp and connecting wire, and assist with fluid aspiration (when the needle touches the myocardium, there will be an ST segment elevation or premature ventricular contractions).

• monitor blood pressure and central venous pressure (CVP) during and after pericardiocentesis; infuse I.V. solutions, as ordered, to maintain blood pressure; watch for a decrease in CVP and a concomitant rise in blood pressure, which indicate relief of cardiac compression.
• watch for complications of pericardiocentesis, such as ventricular fibrillation, vagovagal arrest, or coronary artery or cardiac chamber puncture; closely monitor EKG changes, blood pressure, pulse rate, level of consciousness, and urinary output.

If the patient is scheduled for thoracotomy, the hospital staff member should:
• explain the procedure to the patient; tell him what to expect postoperatively (chest tubes, drainage bottles, and administration of oxygen); teach him how to turn, deep breathe, and cough.
• give antibiotics, protamine sulfate, or vitamin K, as ordered.
• postoperatively, monitor critical parameters, such as vital signs and arterial blood gases, and assess the patient's heart and breath sounds; give pain medication, as ordered; maintain the chest drainage system, and be alert for complications, such as hemorrhage, cardiac arrhythmias, and pulmonary or renal dysfunction.

Cardiac Arrest

Cardiac arrest is the sudden cessation of the heart's pumping function. Untreated, it's rapidly fatal; a delay in treatment of only 3 to 5 minutes may produce irreversible brain damage. In the United States, cardiac arrest accounts for more than 350,000 deaths a year—most occurring outside the hospital. However, prompt, aggressive treatment and early entry into the emergency medical services system may prevent many of these deaths.

Causes
Cardiac arrest may result from circulatory collapse caused by a dissociation between mechanical and electrical heart functions (electromechanical dissociation). Although its mechanism is not fully understood, electromechanical dissociation may result from failure in the

calcium transport system, and is associated with severe myocardial ischemia and necrosis.

Other causes of cardiac arrest include:
• *ventricular fibrillation,* resulting from myocardial infarction, heart failure, anesthetics, electrical shock, electrolyte disturbances (hyper- or hypokalemia,

acidosis), ventricular irritation (from cardiac pacing wires, cardiac catheterization), or acute hemorrhage.

• *ventricular standstill* or *asystole,* from hypoxia, acidosis and/or hypercapnia, vagal stimulation, and hyperkalemia.

Signs and symptoms
Cardiac arrest doesn't usually occur without premonitory clues. For example, cardiac arrest is apt to quickly follow loss of peripheral blood pressure, changes in EKG patterns, respiratory failure, or sudden tachycardia or bradycardia. Typically, imminent cardiac arrest produces bradycardia and hypotension, followed by seizure, loss of consciousness, cessation of respiration, and absence of peripheral pulses or heart sounds. Pupillary dilation, a sign of inadequate cerebral perfusion, occurs secondary to cardiac arrest.

Diagnosis

Absence of central pulses (carotid or femoral) and respiration, and loss of consciousness confirm cardiac arrest. Treatment must begin immediately to restore vital functions and prevent cerebral damage and death secondary to anoxia. Later, EKG can detect recurrent arrhythmias that may have provoked cardiac arrest, or enzyme studies can confirm myocardial infarction.

Treatment
Treatment attempts to restore an effective heart rhythm that can sustain cardiac output through basic and advanced life support techniques.

Basic life support (BLS) is emergency first aid treatment for both respiratory and cardiac arrests. It establishes an adequate airway, ventilation through artificial means, and circulatory assistance through external (closed) cardiac massage. BLS, properly administered, continues until the patient recovers, can be transported to receive more advanced life support, or is pronounced dead by a doctor.

Management of cardiac arrest then proceeds to advanced life support (ALS), which provides adjunctive treatment by trained personnel to maintain effective ventilation and circulation. ALS includes cardiac monitoring—especially for dysrhythmias—I.V. therapy, defibrillation, and postresuscitative care.

Additional considerations
• All health care personnel should be

SOME ESSENTIAL DRUGS FOR TREATMENT OF CARDIAC ARREST	
DRUG	**ACTION**
Sodium bicarbonate	Neutralizes acidosis from lactic acid and carbon dioxide retention
Epinephrine	Increases heart rate and arterial blood pressure
Atropine	Treats severe bradycardia (accompanied by hypotension)
Lidocaine	Treats arrhythmias of ventricular origin
Calcium chloride	In electromechanical dissociation or ventricular standstill, restores effective cardiac contractions
Isoproterenol	Increases cardiac output; achieves immediate control of bradycardia refractory to atropine

trained in cardiopulmonary resuscitation (CPR), and should know their hospital's procedure for managing cardiac arrest—its method for alerting a cardiac arrest team, and the location and use of emergency equipment and drugs.

• Early signs of cardiac arrest, such as hypotension and bradycardia, are important in high-risk patients, especially those with ischemic heart disease.

• Respiratory status should be assessed frequently by drawing arterial blood gas samples, and adjusting oxygen concentrations accordingly. Mechanical ventilation may be necessary.

During recovery from cardiac arrest:

• I.V. lines must be kept patent to ensure rapid administration of drugs. For patients with ventricular arrhythmias, I.V. lidocaine should be kept at bedside for bolus administration.

• Metabolic abnormalities should be monitored by frequent arterial blood gas samples. Conditions that may precipitate a second arrest include arrhythmias, hypoxia, acidosis, and hypokalemia. The patient should be watched for these.

• Renal status should be monitored by measuring hourly urinary output and specific gravity, and daily electrolytes, BUN, or creatinine levels. An osmotic diuretic may be ordered to increase urinary output and reverse acute renal failure.

• Cardiac status is assessed by checking level of consciousness, skin color and temperature, and peripheral pulses, and monitoring pulmonary artery catheter readings, cardiac output using thermodilution technique, and direct arterial blood pressure.

• Neurologic status is determined by checking for signs of cerebral edema and other CNS complications (elevated temperature, wide pulse pressure, diminished responsiveness, or seizure activity).

• Complications of CPR include rib or sternal fractures, cardiac tamponade, and pneumothorax.

• If CPR fails, the family should be given psychologic support.

Cardiac Arrhythmias

In cardiac arrhythmias, abnormal electrical conduction or automaticity changes heart rate and rhythm. Arrhythmias vary in severity, from those that are mild, asymptomatic, and require no treatment (such as sinus arrhythmia, in which heart rate increases and decreases with respiration) to catastrophic ventricular fibrillation, which necessitates immediate resuscitation. Arrhythmias are generally classified according to their origin (ventricular or supraventricular). Their effect on cardiac output and blood pressure, partially influenced by the site of origin, determines their clinical significance.

Causes

Arrhythmias may be congenital, or may result from myocardial anoxia, infarction, hypertrophy of muscle fiber from hypertension or valvular heart disease, toxic doses of cardioactive drugs (such as digoxin), or degeneration of conductive tissue necessary to maintain normal heart rhythm (sick sinus syndrome).

Additional considerations

When caring for a patient with cardiac arrhythmia, the hospital staff member should:

• assess an unmonitored patient for rhythm disturbances; watch for signs of hypoperfusion (changes in level of consciousness, hypotension, diminished urinary output, poor peripheral perfusion) if the patient's pulse is abnormally rapid, slow, or irregular.

• document any arrhythmias in a monitored patient, and assess for possible causes and effects.

• rapidly assess the level of consciousness, respirations, and pulse, when life-

CARDIAC ARRHYTHMIAS

Normal sinus rhythm (NSR) in adults

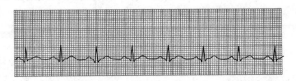

- Ventricular and atrial rates of 60 to 100 beats per minute (BPM)
- QRS complexes and P waves regular and uniform
- P-R interval 0.12 to 0.2 seconds
- QRS duration < 0.12 seconds
- Identical atrial and ventricular rates, with constant P-R interval

---

Sinus arrhythmia

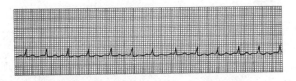

CAUSES	DESCRIPTION	TREATMENT
• Usually a normal variation of NSR; associated with sinus bradycardia	• Slight irregularity of heartbeat, usually corresponding to respiratory cycle • P-R interval increases with inspiration and decreases with expiration	• None

---

Sinus tachycardia

CAUSES	DESCRIPTION	TREATMENT
• Normal physiologic response to fever, exercise, anxiety, pain, dehydration; may also accompany shock, left ventricular failure, cardiac tamponade, anemia, hyperthyroidism, hypovolemia, pulmonary embolus • May result from treatment with vagolytic and sympathetic stimulating drugs	• Rate > 100 BPM; rarely, > 160 BPM • Every QRS wave follows a P wave	• Underlying cause is corrected

CARDIAC ARRHYTHMIAS (continued)

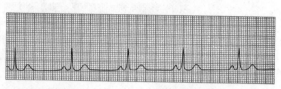

Sinus bradycardia

CAUSES

- Increased intracranial pressure; increased vagal tone due to bowel straining, vomiting, intubation, mechanical ventilation; sick sinus syndrome or hypothyroidism
- Treatment with beta-blockers and sympatholytic drugs
- May be normal in athletes

DESCRIPTION

- Rate- 60 BPM
- A QRS complex follows each P wave

TREATMENT

- For signs of low cardiac output, dizziness, weakness, altered level of consciousness, or low blood pressure, at least 0.4 mg atropine every 5 minutes
- Temporary ventricular pacemaker or isoproterenol, if atropine fails

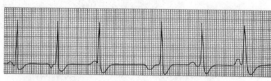

Sinoatrial arrest or block (sinus arrest)

CAUSES

- Vagal stimulation, digitalis or quinidine toxicity
- Often a sign of sick sinus syndrome

DESCRIPTION

- NSR interrupted by unexpectedly prolonged P-P interval, often terminated by a junctional escape beat, or return to NSR
- QRS complexes uniform but irregular

TREATMENT

- A pacemaker for repeated episodes

Wandering atrial pacemaker

CAUSES

- Seen in rheumatic pancarditis as a result of inflammation involving the SA node, digitalis toxicity, sick sinus syndrome

DESCRIPTION

- Rate varies
- QRS complexes uniform in shape but irregular in rhythm
- P waves irregular with changing configuration, indicating they're not all from sinus node or single atrial focus
- P-R interval varies from short to normal

TREATMENT

- If patient is taking digitalis, it is discontinued
- No other treatment

CARDIAC ARRHYTHMIAS (continued)

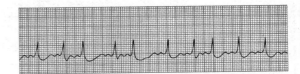

Premature atrial contraction (PAC)

CAUSES

- Congestive heart failure, ischemic heart disease, acute respiratory failure, or COPD
- May result from treatment with digitalis, aminophylline, or adrenergic drugs; or from anxiety, excessive caffeine ingestion
- Occasional PAC may be normal

DESCRIPTION

- Premature, occasionally abnormal-looking P waves
- QRS complexes follow, except in very early or blocked PACs
- P wave often buried in the preceding T wave or can often be identified in the preceding T wave

TREATMENT

- If more than six times per minute or frequency is increasing, digitalis, quinidine, or propranolol is given; after revascularization surgery, propranolol
- Known causes, such as caffeine or drugs, are eliminated

Paroxysmal atrial tachycardia (PAT) or paroxysmal supraventricular tachycardia

CAUSES

- Intrinsic abnormality of AV conduction system
- Congenital accessory atrial conduction pathway
- Physical or psychologic stress, hypoxia, hypokalemia, caffeine, marijuana, stimulants, digitalis toxicity

DESCRIPTION

- Heart rate > 140 BPM; rarely exceeds 250 BPM
- P waves regular but aberrant; difficult to differentiate from preceding T wave
- Onset and termination of arrhythmia occur suddenly
- May cause palpitations and light-headedness

TREATMENT

- Vagal maneuvers, sympathetic blockers (propranolol, digitalis [when not caused by digitalis toxicity], quinidine), or calcium blockers to alter AV node conduction
- Elective cardioversion, if patient is symptomatic and unresponsive to drugs

---

Atrial flutter

CAUSES

- Heart failure, valvular heart disease, pulmonary embolism, digitalis toxicity, postoperative revascularization

DESCRIPTION

- Ventricular rate depends on degree of AV block (usually 60 to 100 BPM)
- Atrial rate 240 to 400 BPM and regular
- QRS complexes uniform in shape, but often irregular in rate
- P waves may have sawtooth configuration

TREATMENT

- Digitalis (unless arrhythmia is due to digitalis toxicity), propranolol, or quinidine
- May require synchronized cardioversion, atrial pacemaker, or vagal stimulation

CARDIAC ARRHYTHMIAS (continued)

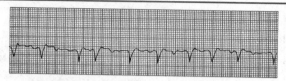

Atrial fibrillation

CAUSES

• Congestive heart failure, COPD, hyperthyroidism, sepsis, pulmonary embolus, mitral stenosis, digitalis toxicity (rarely), atrial irritation, postcoronary bypass or valve replacement surgery

DESCRIPTION

• Atrial rate > 400 BPM
• Ventricular rate varies
• QRS complexes uniform in shape, but at irregular intervals
• P-R interval indiscernible
• No P waves, or P waves appear as erratic, irregular baseline F waves
• Irregular QRS rate

TREATMENT

• Digitalis and quinidine to slow ventricular rate, and quinidine to convert rhythm to NSR; diuretics, such as furosemide, for congestive heart failure
• May require elective cardioversion for rapid rate

Nodal rhythm
(AV junctional rhythm)

CAUSES

• Digitalis toxicity, inferior wall myocardial infarction or ischemia, hypoxia, vagal stimulation
• Acute rheumatic fever
• Valve surgery

DESCRIPTION

• Ventricular rate usually 40 to 60 BPM (60 to 100 BPM is accelerated junctional rhythm)
• P waves may precede, be hidden within (absent), or follow QRS; if visible, they're altered
• QRS duration is normal, except in aberrant conduction.
• Patient may be asymptomatic unless ventricular rate is very slow

TREATMENT

• Symptomatic
• Atropine, with slow rate
• If patient is taking digitalis, it is discontinued

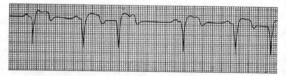

Premature nodal contractions (PNC) or junctional premature beats

CAUSES

• Myocardial infarction or ischemia, digitalis toxicity, excessive caffeine ingestion

DESCRIPTION

• Underlying rhythm is sinus or atrial
• QRS complexes of uniform shape but irregular rate
• P waves irregular, with premature beat; may precede, be hidden within, or follow QRS

TREATMENT

• Underlying cause is corrected
• Quinidine or disopyramide, as ordered
• If patient is taking digitalis, it is discontinued

CARDIAC ARRHYTHMIAS (continued)

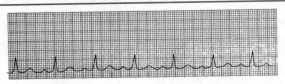

First-degree AV block

CAUSES

• Inferior myocardial ischemia or infarction, hypothyroidism, digitalis toxicity, potassium imbalance

DESCRIPTION

• P-R interval prolonged > 0.2 seconds
• QRS complex normal

TREATMENT

• If patient is taking digitalis, it is discontinued
• Underlying cause is corrected. Otherwise, patient is watched for increasing block

---

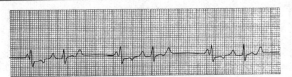

Second-degree AV block
Mobitz Type I (Wenckebach)

CAUSES

• *Mobitz Type I:* Inferior wall myocardial infarction, digitalis toxicity, vagal stimulation

DESCRIPTION

• *Mobitz Type I:* P-R interval becomes progressively longer with each cycle until QRS disappears (dropped beat). After a dropped beat, P-R interval is shorter. Ventricular rate is irregular; atrial rhythm, regular

TREATMENT

• *Mobitz Type I:* atropine if patient is symptomatic
• Digitalis is discontinued
• *Mobitz Type II:* temporary pacemaker, sometimes followed by permanent pacemaker
• Atropine, for slow rate
• If patient is taking digitalis, it is discontinued

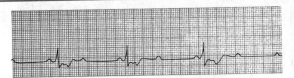

Second-degree AV block
Mobitz Type II

CAUSES

• *Mobitz Type II:* Degenerative disease of conduction system, ischemia of AV node in anterior myocardial infarction, digitalis toxicity, anteroseptal infarction

DESCRIPTION

• *Mobitz Type II:* P-R interval is constant, with QRS complex dropped at regular intervals
• Ventricular rhythm may be irregular, with varying degree of block
• Atrial rate regular

TREATMENT

• *Mobitz Type II:* temporary pacemaker, sometimes followed by permanent pacemaker
• Atropine, for slow rate
• If patient is taking digitalis, it is discontinued

CARDIAC ARRHYTHMIAS (continued)

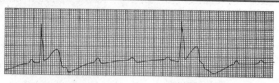

Third-degree AV block (complete heart block)

CAUSES
- Ischemic heart disease or infarction; postsurgical complications of mitral valve replacement; digitalis toxicity; hypoxia sometimes causing syncope due to decreased cerebral blood flow, as in Stokes-Adams syndrome

DESCRIPTION
- Atrial rate regular; ventricular rate, slow and regular
- No relationship between P waves and QRS complexes
- No constant P-R interval
- QRS interval normal (nodal pacemaker); wide and bizarre (ventricular pacemaker)

TREATMENT
- Usually requires temporary pacemaker, followed by permanent pacemaker
- Epinephrine or isoproterenol

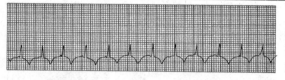

Nodal tachycardia (junctional tachycardia)

CAUSES
- Digitalis toxicity, myocarditis, cardiomyopathy, myocardial ischemia or infarct

DESCRIPTION
- Onset of rhythm often sudden, occurring in bursts
- Ventricular rate > 100 BPM
- Other characteristics same as junctional rhythm

TREATMENT
- Vagal stimulation
- Propranolol, quinidine, digitalis (if cause is not digitalis toxicity)
- Elective cardioversion

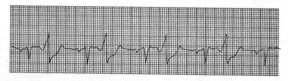

Premature ventricular contraction (PVC)

CAUSES
- Heart failure; old or acute myocardial infarction or contusion with trauma; myocardial irritation by ventricular catheter, such as a pacemaker; hypoxia, as in anemia and acute respiratory failure; drug toxicity (digitalis, aminophylline, tricyclic antidepressants, beta-adrenergics [isoproterenol or dopamine]); electrolyte imbalances (especially hypokalemia); psychologic stress

DESCRIPTION
- Beat occurs prematurely, usually followed by a complete compensatory pause after PVC; irregular pulse
- QRS complex wide and distorted
- Can occur singly, in pairs, or in threes; and can alternate with normal beats
- Focus can be from one or more sites
- PVCs are most ominous when clustered, multifocal, with R wave on T pattern

TREATMENT
- Lidocaine I.V. bolus and drip infusion; procainamide I.V. If induced by digitalis toxicity, this drug is stopped; if induced by hypokalemia, potassium chloride I.V. is given

CARDIAC ARRHYTHMIAS (continued)

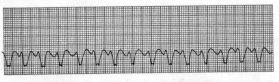

Ventricular tachycardia (VT)

CAUSES
- Myocardial ischemia, infarction, or aneurysm; ventricular catheters; digitalis or quinidine toxicity; hypokalemia; hypercalcemia; anxiety

DESCRIPTION
- Ventricular rate 140 to 220 BPM; may be regular
- QRS complexes are wide, bizarre, and independent of P waves
- No visible P waves
- Can produce chest pain, anxiety, palpitations, dyspnea, shock, coma, and death

TREATMENT
- CPR (if cardiac arrest occurs), followed by lidocaine I.V. (bolus and drip infusion); if level of consciousness is decreased, synchronized cardioversion is used
- For recurrent episodes, bretylium tosylate is used

Ventricular fibrillation

CAUSES
- Myocardial ischemia or infarction, untreated ventricular tachycardia, electrolyte imbalances (hypokalemia and alkalosis, hyperkalemia and hypercalcemia), digitalis or quinidine toxicity, electric shock, hypothermia

DESCRIPTION
- Ventricular rhythm rapid and chaotic
- QRS complexes are wide and irregular; no visible P waves
- Loss of consciousness, with no peripheral pulses, blood pressure, or respirations; possible seizures; and sudden death

TREATMENT
- CPR
- Asynchronized countershock (400 watts/second). If rhythm doesn't return, patient is shocked again
- Drugs, such as lidocaine or bretylium tosylate I.V. (for recurrent episodes)

Ventricular standstill (asystole)

CAUSES
- Acute respiratory failure, myocardial ischemia or infarction, ruptured ventricular aneurysm, aortic valve disease, or hyperkalemia

DESCRIPTION
- Primary ventricular standstill—regular P waves, no QRS complexes
- Secondary ventricular standstill—QRS complexes wide and slurred, occurring at irregular intervals; agonal heart rhythm
- Loss of consciousness, with no peripheral pulses, blood pressure, or respirations

TREATMENT
- CPR
- Endotracheal intubation, pacemaker should be available
- Epinephrine, calcium gluconate, and sodium bicarbonate
- Cardiac monitoring

HOLTER MONITORING

Tape-recorded ambulatory electrocardiography (Holter monitoring) permits monitoring of all cardiac cycles over a prescribed period (usually 24 hours). This type of monitoring has proven useful for patients recuperating from myocardial infarctions, receiving antiarrhythmic drugs, or using pacemakers. It can record rate, rhythm, and conduction abnormalities, as well as cardiac responses to typical environmental stimuli, and is especially useful in diagnosing arrhythmias. Holter monitoring has many advantages:

• With minimal equipment, the doctor can hook up a patient to one or more EKG leads. (Equipment includes the monitor, its carrying case, a belt, skin electrodes, alcohol swabs, a blank cassette tape, a patient diary, and a test analysis report.)

• Leads are recorded on a tape in a portable cassette recorder that the patient can wear easily. After the recorder is connected to a cardiac monitor for test readings, the electrodes are attached to the patient, and he goes through a typical day, with the Holter monitor in place. He is encouraged to engage in activities that usually precipitate symptoms, and is instructed to keep a diary of the exact times of symptoms and activities, and of any medication he takes, so the impact of these factors can be correlated with EKG patterns.

• With a high-speed computer scanner, the doctor can review 24 hours of tape in minutes to detect important rhythm changes. He can also correlate

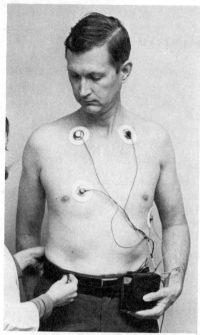

The Holter monitor should be strapped around the patient's waist to create a secure but comfortable fit. If the belt is too loose, the monitor's weight will pull on the electrodes.

the patient's symptoms, such as lightheadedness, with the documented arrhythmias.

• The Holter monitor can capture a sporadic rhythm disturbance that an office or stress-test EKG might miss.

---

threatening arrhythmias develop, and initiate cardiopulmonary resuscitation, as indicated.

• evaluate for altered cardiac output resulting from arrhythmias; consider potentially progressive or ominous arrhythmias in determining the course of action; administer medications, and prepare to assist with medical procedures (for example, cardioversion or pacemaker insertion).

• monitor for predisposing factors—such

as fluid and electrolyte imbalance—and signs of drug toxicity, especially with digoxin; report signs of suspected drug toxicity immediately and withhold the next dose.

• provide adequate oxygen and reduce heart workload to prevent arrhythmias in a postoperative cardiac patient, while carefully maintaining metabolic, neurologic, respiratory, and hemodynamic status.

- install a fresh battery before each insertion to avoid temporary pacemaker malfunction; carefully secure the external catheter wires and the pacemaker box; assess the threshold daily; watch closely for premature contractions, a sign of myocardial irritation.
- restrict the patient's activity after pacemaker insertion, as ordered, to avert permanent malfunction; monitor the pulse rate regularly, and watch for signs of decreased cardiac output.
- warn the patient about environmental hazards, as indicated by the pacemaker manufacturer, which may include microwave ovens, electrical appliances, some ham radios, and radar. Since many contemporary pacemakers are enclosed in metal containers, these hazards may not present a problem; however, in doubtful situations, 24-hour Holter monitoring may be helpful.
- tell the patient to report light-headedness or syncope, and stress the importance of regular checkups.

NORMAL CARDIAC CONDUCTION

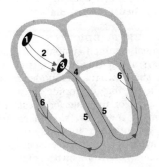

Each electrical impulse travels from the SA node (1) through the internodal tracts (2), producing atrial contraction. The impulse slows momentarily as it passes through the AV junction (3) to the bundle of His (4). Then, it descends the left and right bundle branches (5) and reaches Purkinje's fibers (6), stimulating ventricular contraction.

VASCULAR DISORDERS

Thoracic Aneurysm

Thoracic aneurysm is an abnormal widening of the ascending, transverse, or descending portion of the aorta. The aneurysm may be dissecting, a hemorrhagic separation in the aortic wall, usually within the medial layer; saccular, an outpouching of the arterial wall, with a narrow neck; or fusiform, a spindle-shaped enlargement encompassing the entire aortic circumference. Some aneurysms progress to serious and, eventually, lethal complications, such as rupture of untreated thoracic dissecting aneurysm into the pericardium, with resulting tamponade.

Causes and incidence

Commonly, a thoracic aneurysm results from atherosclerosis, which weakens the aortic wall and gradually distends the lumen at the weakened area. The initiating factor in dissecting aneurysm (in about 60% of patients) is an intimal tear in the ascending aorta. Other causes include:

- infection (mycotic aneurysms) of the aortic arch and descending segments.
- congenital disorders, such as coarctation of the aorta, and Marfan's syndrome (often associated with dissecting aneurysm).
- trauma, usually of the descending thoracic aorta, as a result of an automobile accident that damages the aorta by shearing it transversely (acceleration-deceleration injuries).
- syphilis, usually of the ascending aorta (now uncommon because of effective

antibiotic therapy).
• hypertension (in dissecting aneurysm).

Thoracic aneurysms are most common in men between ages 50 and 70; dissecting aneurysms, in Blacks.

Signs and symptoms

The most common symptom of thoracic aneurysm is pain. In dissecting aneurysm, such pain may be sudden in onset, with a tearing or ripping sensation in the thorax or the anterior chest. It may extend to the neck, shoulders, lower back, or abdomen but rarely to the jaw and arms, which distinguishes dissecting aneurysm from myocardial infarction.

Accompanying signs include syncope, pallor, sweating, shortness of breath, increased pulse rate, cyanosis, leg weakness or transient paralysis, diastolic murmur (caused by aortic regurgitation), and abrupt loss of radial and femoral pulses or wide variations in pulses or blood pressure between arms and legs. Paradoxically, although the patient appears to be in shock, systolic blood pressure is often normal or significantly elevated.

Clinical effects caused by thoracic aneurysms (saccular or fusiform) vary according to the size and location of the aneurysm, and the compression, distortion, or erosion of surrounding structures, such as the lungs, trachea, larynx and recurrent laryngeal nerve, esophagus, and spinal nerves.

Characteristic associated symptoms may include a substernal ache in the shoulders, lower back, or abdomen; marked respiratory distress (dyspnea, brassy cough, wheezing); hoarseness or loss of voice; dysphagia (rare); and possibly, paresthesias or neuralgia. Such aneurysms can occasionally rupture.

Diagnosis

Diagnosis relies on patient history, clinical features, and appropriate tests. In an asymptomatic patient, diagnosis often occurs accidentally, through posteroanterior and oblique chest X-rays showing widening of the aorta (most obvious when compared with a previous chest X-ray). Other tests help confirm aneurysm:
• *Aortography,* the most definitive test, shows the lumen of the aneurysm, its size and location, and the false lumen in dissecting aneurysm.
• *EKG* is not diagnostic but helps differentiate between thoracic aneurysm and myocardial infarction.
• *Echocardiography* may help identify dissecting aneurysm of the aortic root.
• *Hemoglobin* may be normal or decreased, due to frank bleeding or blood loss into the hematoma from a slow-leaking aneurysm.

Treatment

Dissecting aneurysm is an extreme emergency that requires prompt surgery and stabilizing measures: antihypertensives, such as nitroprusside; negative inotropic agents that decrease the force of contractility, such as propranolol; oxygen therapy for respiratory distress; narcotics for pain; I.V. fluids; and if necessary, whole blood transfusions.

Surgery is comparable to open heart surgery, and consists of resecting the aneurysm, restoring normal blood flow through a Dacron or Teflon graft replacement, and with aortic valve insufficiency, aortic valve replacement.

Postoperative measures include careful monitoring and continuous assessment in the ICU, antibiotics to prevent infection, endotracheal and chest tubes for respiratory management, EKG monitoring for cardiac management, and pulmonary artery catheterization for hemodynamic management.

Additional considerations

The hospital staff member should:
• carefully monitor blood pressure, pulmonary capillary wedge pressure, and central venous pressure; assess pain, respirations, and carotid, radial, and femoral pulses.
• make sure laboratory tests include CBC with differential count, electrolyte determinations, type and cross match for whole blood, arterial blood gas deter-

TYPES OF AORTIC ANEURYSMS

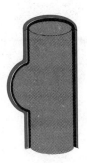 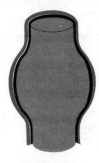 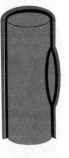 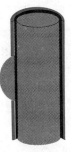

- *Saccular*—unilateral pouchlike bulge with a narrow neck

- *Fusiform*—a spindle-shaped bulge encompassing the entire diameter of the vessel

- *Dissecting*—a hemorrhagic separation of the medial layer of the vessel wall, which creates a false lumen

- *False aneurysm*—pulsating hematoma resulting from trauma and often mistaken for an abdominal aneurysm

minations, and urinalysis.
- insert a Foley catheter; administer 5% dextrose in water or lactated Ringer's solution, and antibiotics, as ordered. carefully monitor nitroprusside I.V. and use a separate I.V. line for infusion; adjust the dose by slowly increasing the infusion rate; check blood pressure every 5 minutes until it stabilizes; give whole blood transfusion with suspected bleeding from aneurysm.
- explain diagnostic tests; explain the procedure if surgery is scheduled as well as expected postoperative care (I.V.s, endotracheal and drainage tubes, cardiac monitoring, ventilation).

After repair of thoracic aneurysm, the staffer should:
- carefully assess level of consciousness; monitor vital signs, pulmonary artery and capillary wedge and central venous pressures, pulse rate, urinary output, and pain.
- check respiratory function; carefully observe and record type and amount of chest tube drainage, and frequently assess heart and lung sounds.

- monitor I.V. therapy.
- give medications, as ordered.
- watch for signs of infection, especially fever, and excessive drainage on dressing.
- assist with range-of-motion exercises of legs to prevent thromboembolic phenomenon (due to venostasis during prolonged bed rest).
- encourage and assist the patient in turning, coughing, and deep breathing after stabilization of vital signs and respiration; provide intermittent positive pressure breathing, if necessary, to promote lung expansion; help the patient walk as soon as he's able.
- ensure compliance with antihypertensive therapy by explaining before discharge the need for such drugs and the expected side effects; teach the patient how to monitor his blood pressure; refer him to community agencies for continued support and assistance, as needed.
- offer the patient and family psychologic support throughout hospitalization; answer all questions honestly, and provide reassurance.

Abdominal Aneurysm

Abdominal aneurysm, an abnormal dilation in the arterial wall, generally occurs in the aorta between the renal arteries and iliac branches. Such aneurysms are four times more common in men than in women and are most prevalent in Caucasians aged 50 to 80. Over 50% of all persons with untreated abdominal aneurysms die, primarily from aneurysmal rupture, within 2 years of diagnosis; over 85%, within 5 years.

Causes

About 95% of abdominal aortic aneurysms result from arteriosclerosis; the rest, from cystic medial necrosis, trauma, syphilis, and other infections. These aneurysms develop slowly. First, a focal weakness in the muscular layer of the aorta (tunica media), due to degenerative changes, allows the inner layer (tunica intima) and outer layer (tunica adventitia) to stretch outward. Blood pressure within the aorta progressively weakens the vessel walls and enlarges the aneurysm.

Signs and symptoms

Although abdominal aneurysms usually don't manifest symptoms, most are evident (unless the patient is obese) as a pulsating mass in the periumbilical area, accompanied by a systolic bruit over the aorta. Some tenderness may be present on deep palpation. A large aneurysm may produce symptoms that mimic renal calculi, lumbar disk disease, and duodenal compression. Abdominal aneurysms rarely cause diminished peripheral pulses or claudication, unless embolization occurs.

Lumbar pain that radiates to the flank and groin from pressure on lumbar nerves may signify enlargement and imminent rupture. If the aneurysm ruptures into the peritoneal cavity, it causes severe, persistent abdominal and back pain, mimicking renal or ureteral colic. Signs of hemorrhage—such as weakness, sweating, tachycardia, and hypotension—may be subtle, since rupture into the retroperitoneal space produces a tamponade effect that prevents continued hemorrhage. Patients with such rupture may remain stable for hours before shock and death occur, although 20% die immediately.

Diagnosis

Since an abdominal aneurysm rarely produces symptoms, it's often detected accidentally as the result of an X-ray or a routine physical examination. Several tests can confirm suspected abdominal aneurysm:

• *Serial ultrasound* (sonography) is accurate and allows determination of aneurysm size, shape, and location.

• *Anteroposterior and lateral X-rays* of the abdomen can detect aortic calcification, which outlines the mass, at least 75% of the time.

• *Aortography* shows the condition of vessels proximal and distal to the aneurysm and the extent of the aneurysm but may underestimate aneurysm diameter, because it visualizes only the flow channel and not the surrounding clot.

Treatment

Usually, abdominal aneurysm requires resection of the aneurysm and replacement of the damaged aortic section with a Dacron graft. If the aneurysm is small and asymptomatic, surgery may be delayed; however, small aneurysms may also rupture. Regular physical examination and ultrasound checks are necessary to detect enlargement, which may forewarn rupture. Large aneurysms or those that produce symptoms involve a significant risk of rupture and necessitate immediate repair. In patients with poor distal runoff, external grafting may be done.

COMMON FUSIFORM ABDOMINAL ANEURYSMS

During surgery, a Dacron crimp prosthesis replaces or encloses weakened area.

BEFORE SURGERY

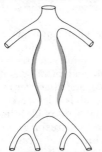

Aneurysm below renal arteries and above bifurcation

AFTER SURGERY

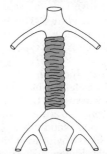

The prosthesis extends distal to the renal arteries to above the aortic bifurcation.

BEFORE SURGERY

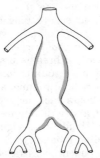

Aneurysm below renal arteries involving the iliac branches

AFTER SURGERY

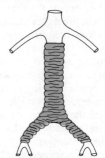

The prosthesis extends to the common femorals.

BEFORE SURGERY

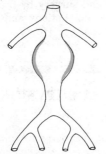

Small aneurysm in a patient with poor distal runoff (poor risk)

AFTER SURGERY

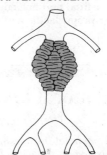

The external prosthesis encircles the aneurysm and is held in place with sutures.

Additional considerations

Abdominal aneurysm requires meticulous care, psychologic support, and comprehensive patient teaching. Following diagnosis, if rupture is not imminent, elective surgery allows time for additional preoperative tests to evaluate the patient's clinical status. The hospital staff member should:
• monitor vital signs, and type and cross match blood.
• obtain kidney function tests (BUN, creatinine, electrolytes), blood samples (CBC with differential), EKG and cardiac evaluation, baseline pulmonary function tests, and blood gases.
• be alert for signs of rupture which may be immediately fatal; watch closely for any signs of acute blood loss (decreasing blood pressure, increasing pulse and respiratory rate, cool, clammy skin, restlessness, and decreased sensorium).

If rupture does occur, the first priority is to get the patient to surgery immediately! Medical Anti-shock Trousers may be used while transporting to surgery. Surgery allows direct compression of the aorta to control hemorrhage. Large amounts of blood may be needed during the resuscitative period to replace blood loss. In such a patient, renal failure due to ischemia is a major postoperative complication, possibly requiring hemodialysis.

Before elective surgery, the staffer should:
• weigh the patient, insert a Foley catheter, an I.V., and assist with insertion of arterial line and pulmonary artery catheter to monitor fluid and hemodynamic balance; give prophylactic antibiotics, as ordered.
• explain the surgical procedure, and the expected postoperative care in the ICU for patients undergoing complex abdominal surgery (I.V.s, endotracheal and nasogastric intubation, mechanical ventilation).

After surgery, in the ICU, the staffer should:
• monitor vital signs, intake and hourly output, neurologic status (level of consciousness, pupil size, sensation in arms and legs), and blood gases, assess the depth, rate, and character of respirations and lung sounds at least every hour.
• watch for signs of bleeding (increased pulse rate and respirations, hypotension), which may occur retroperitoneally from the graft site; check abdominal dressings for excessive bleeding or drainage; be alert for temperature elevations and other signs of infection. After nasogastric intubation for intestinal decompression, the tube should be irrigated frequently to ensure patency, and the amount and type of drainage recorded.
• suction the endotracheal tube often. If the patient can breathe unassisted, and has good lung sounds and adequate blood gases, tidal volume, and vital capacity 24 hours after surgery, he will be extubated and will require oxygen by mask. He should be weighed daily to evaluate fluid balance.
• help the patient walk as soon as possible (generally the second day after surgery).
• provide psychologic support for the patient and family; help ease their fears about the ICU, the threat of impending rupture, and surgery by providing appropriate explanations and answering all questions.

Femoral and Popliteal Aneurysms
(Peripheral arterial aneurysms)

Femoral and popliteal aneurysms are the end result of progressive atherosclerotic changes occurring in the walls (medial layer) of these major peripheral arteries. These aneurysmal formations may be fusiform *(spindle-shaped) or* saccular *(pouch-like), with fusiform occurring three times more frequently. They may be singular or multiple segmental lesions, often affecting both legs, and may accompany other*

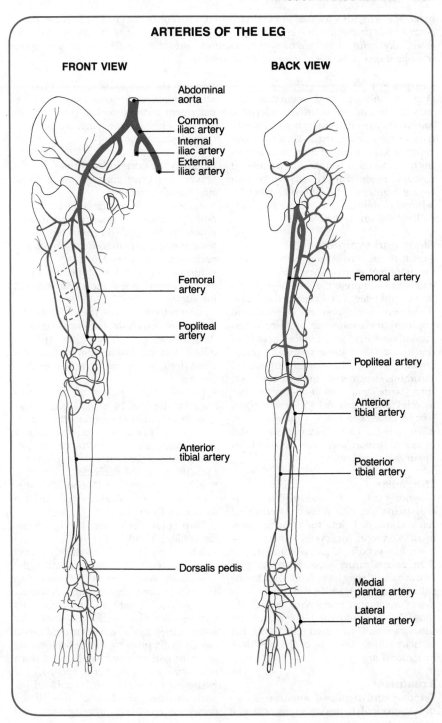

ARTERIES OF THE LEG

FRONT VIEW

BACK VIEW

Abdominal aorta

Common iliac artery

Internal iliac artery

External iliac artery

Femoral artery

Popliteal artery

Anterior tibial artery

Dorsalis pedis

Femoral artery

Popliteal artery

Anterior tibial artery

Posterior tibial artery

Medial plantar artery

Lateral plantar artery

arterial aneurysms located in the abdominal aorta or iliac arteries. This condition occurs most frequently in men over age 50. The clinical course is usually progressive, eventually ending in thrombosis, embolization, and gangrene. Elective surgery before complications arise greatly improves prognosis.

Causes

Femoral and popliteal aneurysms are usually secondary to atherosclerosis. Rarely, they result from congenital weakness in the arterial wall. They may also result from trauma (blunt or penetrating), bacterial infection, or peripheral vascular reconstructive surgery (which causes "suture line" aneurysms, whereby a blood clot forms a second lumen, also called false aneurysms).

Signs and symptoms

Popliteal aneurysms may cause pain in the popliteal space when they're large enough to compress the medial popliteal nerve, and edema and venous distention if the vein is compressed. Femoral and popliteal aneurysms can produce symptoms of severe ischemia in the leg or foot, due to acute thrombosis within the aneurysmal sac, embolization of mural thrombus fragments, and rarely, rupture. Acute symptoms of aneurysm after arterial occlusion include severe pain, loss of pulse and color, coldness in the affected leg or foot, and gangrene. Distal petechial hemorrhages may develop from aneurysmal emboli.

Diagnosis

Diagnosis is usually confirmed by bilateral palpation that reveals a pulsating mass above or below the inguinal ligament in femoral aneurysm. When thrombosis has occurred, palpation detects a firm, nonpulsating mass. Arteriography or ultrasound may be indicated in doubtful situations. Arteriography may also detect associated aneurysms, especially those in the abdominal aorta and the iliac arteries. Ultrasound may be helpful in determining the size of the popliteal or femoral artery.

Treatment

Femoral and popliteal aneurysms require surgical bypass and reconstruction of the artery, usually with an autogenous saphenous vein graft replacement. Arterial occlusion that causes severe ischemia and gangrene may require leg amputation.

Additional considerations

Before corrective surgery, the hospital staff member should:
• assess and record circulatory status, noting location and quality of peripheral pulses in the affected arm or leg.
• administer prophylactic antibiotics or anticoagulants, as ordered.
• discuss expected postoperative procedures, and review the explanation of the surgery.

After arterial surgery, the staffer should:
• monitor carefully for early signs of thrombosis or graft occlusion (loss of pulse, decreased skin temperature and sensation, severe pain) and infection (fever).
• palpate distal pulses at least every hour for the first 24 hours, then as frequently as ordered; correlate these findings with preoperative circulatory assessment; mark the sites on the patient's skin where pulses are palpable, to facilitate repeated checks.
• help the patient walk soon after surgery, to prevent venostasis and possible thrombus formation.

To prepare the patient for discharge, the staffer should:
• tell the patient to immediately report any recurrence of symptoms, since the saphenous vein graft replacement can fail or another aneurysm may develop.
• explain to the patient with popliteal artery resection that swelling may persist for some time; make sure antiembolism stockings fit properly, if applicable, and teach the patient how to apply them; warn against wearing constrictive apparel.
• suggest measures to prevent bleeding, such as using an electric razor, if the patient is receiving anticoagulants; tell

the patient to report any signs of bleeding immediately (bleeding gums, tarry stools, easy bruising); explain the importance of follow-up blood studies to monitor anticoagulant therapy; warn him to avoid trauma, tobacco, and aspirin.

Aortic Arch Syndrome

(Takayasu's disease, pulseless disease, brachiocephalic arteritis, panaortitis, primary arteritis of the aortic arch, obliterative aortic disease, aortitis syndrome)

Aortic arch syndrome is progressive obliteration of the aorta and its branches, eventually causing bilateral loss of pulse in the arms, loss of carotid pulse, and tissue ischemia, especially of the nervous system. This rare disease occurs preponderantly in Oriental women aged 18 to 40 but may be seen in women of other races. It's usually fatal within 2 to 5 years after diagnosis, as a result of heart failure, hypertension, or neurologic complications.

Causes

Aortic arch syndrome may be an autoimmune response, since laboratory results in persons with this disorder show elevated alpha and gamma globulins, and positive complement fixation. This disease produces a nonspecific inflammation of the arterial wall (primarily the adventitia and media) and, later, scarring and thickening of the intima, which leads to thrombus formation and occlusion of the aortic arch branches.

Signs and symptoms

Early in its course, aortic arch syndrome produces nonspecific systemic symptoms similar to those of collagen vascular disease, including malaise, pallor, nausea, night sweats, arthralgias, anorexia, and weight loss. However, as the disease progresses, variable symptoms of cardiovascular dysfunction develop secondary to extensive involvement of arch vessels:
• *brachiocephalic (innominate) artery* (most common site): local pain in the neck, shoulders, and chest; bruits; and loss of radial and carotid pulses
• *carotid arteries:* diplopia, blurred vision, transient blindness, focal neurologic deficits, fainting, syncope, and dizziness due to cerebral ischemia
• *subclavian arteries:* paresthesias, and intermittent claudication, loss of pulses, and decreased blood pressure in the arms. The extent of symptoms depends on the degree of involvement and the development of collateral circulation.

Occasionally, aortic arch syndrome may affect the coronary arteries, generally secondary to aortic thickening, producing narrowing of the coronary arteries. This condition may lead to myocardial ischemia and infarction.

Diagnosis

While typical clinical findings suggest aortic arch syndrome, diagnosis requires aortography of the aortic arch to identify the affected vessels and the extent of damage. Supportive laboratory results include the following:
• elevated WBC and ESR
• decreased hemoglobin
• positive LE cell preparation and complement fixation
• serum protein electrophoresis demonstrating increased alpha and gamma globulins.

In addition, chest X-rays may reveal cardiomegaly, rib-notching from collateral circulation, and calcification of damaged blood vessels.

Treatment

Treatment of aortic arch syndrome includes surgical repair, with bypass grafting or thromboendarterectomy for symptomatic relief. However, the long-term outlook is poor because of the progressive nature of the disease and the number of damaged arteries. Anticoagulant and corticosteroid (prednisone) therapy improves prognosis if it begins before irreversible organ damage has occurred. Decreasing ESR reflects the effectiveness of corticosteroid therapy.

Additional considerations

Patients with aortic arch syndrome require supportive pre- and postoperative care, patient teaching, and psychologic support to help them cope with this inevitably fatal disease.

The health care professional should:
• explain necessary diagnostic procedures, such as X-rays and aortography.
• preoperatively, provide an explanation of the surgical procedure and postoperative care, such as intensive care monitoring; I.V. therapy; and coughing, deep breathing, and leg exercises to prevent thrombus formation.
• postoperatively, be alert for signs of arterial occlusion or thrombosis; monitor vital signs, and intake and output, and observe for signs of infection (chills, fever, excessive or foul-smelling wound drainage).
• before long-term corticosteroid and anticoagulant therapy, explain its purpose, expected results, proper dosage, and drug side effects; warn against stopping corticosteroids abruptly; warn the patient to avoid aspirin and aspirin-containing compounds, to use a safety razor, and to avoid trauma, to prevent bleeding from anticoagulant therapy; stress the need for serial blood studies (prothrombin times) throughout therapy.
• assess neurologic functions carefully; if the patient has suffered a stroke due to occluded carotid arteries, refer the patient to an appropriate community agency for continued rehabilitation after discharge, if necessary.
• provide psychologic support and encouragement for the patient and family; refer the patient for psychiatric or social services, if necessary.

Thrombophlebitis

An acute condition characterized by inflammation and thrombus formation, thrombophlebitis may occur in deep (inter- or intramuscular) or superficial (subcutaneous) veins. Deep-vein thrombophlebitis affects small veins, such as the soleal venous sinuses, or large veins, such as the vena cava, and the femoral, iliac, subclavian veins. This disorder is frequently progressive, leading to pulmonary embolism, a potentially lethal complication. Superficial thrombophlebitis is usually self-limiting and rarely leads to pulmonary embolism. Thrombophlebitis often begins with localized inflammation alone (phlebitis); but such inflammation rapidly provokes thrombus formation. Rarely, venous thrombosis develops without associated inflammation of the vein (phlebothrombosis).

Causes

A thrombus occurs when an alteration in the epithelial lining causes platelet aggregation and consequent fibrin entrapment of RBCs, WBCs, and additional platelets. Thrombus formation is more rapid in areas where blood flow is slower, due to greater contact between platelet and thrombin accumulation. The rapidly expanding thrombus initiates a chemical inflammatory process in the vessel epithelium, which leads to fibrosis. The enlarging clot may occlude the vessel lumen partially or totally, or it may detach and embolize, to lodge elsewhere in the systemic circulation.

Deep-vein thrombophlebitis may be idiopathic, but it usually results from endothelial damage, accelerated blood clotting, and reduced blood flow. Predisposing factors are prolonged bed rest, trauma, surgery, childbirth, and use of oral contraceptives, such as estrogens.

Causes of superficial thrombophlebitis include trauma, infection, I.V. drug abuse, and chemical irritation, due to the extensive use of the I.V. route for medications and diagnostic tests.

Signs and symptoms

In both types of thrombophlebitis, clinical features vary with the site and length of the affected vein. Although deep-vein thrombophlebitis may occur asymptomatically, it may also produce severe pain, fever, chills, malaise, and possibly, swelling and cyanosis of the affected arm or leg. Superficial thrombophlebitis produces visible and palpable signs, such as heat, pain, swelling, rubor, tenderness, and induration along the length of the affected vein. Extensive vein involvement may cause lymphadenitis.

Diagnosis

Some patients may display signs of inflammation and, possibly, a positive Homans' sign (pain on dorsiflexion of the foot) during physical examination; others are asymptomatic. Consequently, essential laboratory tests include:

• *Doppler ultrasonography:* to identify reduced blood flow to a specific area and any obstruction to venous flow, particularly in iliofemoral deep-vein thrombophlebitis.

• *plethysmography:* to show decreased circulation distal to affected area; more sensitive than ultrasound in detecting deep-vein thrombophlebitis.

• *phlebography* (usually confirms diagnosis): to show filling defects and diverted blood flow. This test is limited, since it fails to show the deep venous system.

Diagnosis must rule out arterial occlusive disease, lymphangitis, cellulitis, and myositis.

Diagnosis of superficial thrombophlebitis is based on physical examination (redness and warmth over affected area, palpable vein, and pain during palpation or compression).

CHRONIC VENOUS INSUFFICIENCY

Chronic venous insufficiency results from the valvular destruction of deep-vein thrombophlebitis, usually in the iliac and femoral veins, and occasionally, the saphenous veins. It's often accompanied by incompetence of the communicating veins at the ankle, causing increased venous pressure and fluid migration into the interstitial tissue. Clinical effects include chronic swelling of the affected leg from edema, leading to tissue fibrosis, and induration; skin discoloration from extravasation of blood in subcutaneous tissue; and stasis ulcers around the ankle.

Treatment of small ulcers includes bed rest, elevation of the legs, warm soaks, and antimicrobial therapy for infection. Treatment to counteract increased venous pressure, the result of reflux from the deep venous system to surface veins, may include compression dressings, such as a sponge rubber pressure dressing or a zinc gelatin boot (Unna's boot). This therapy begins after massive swelling subsides with leg elevation and bed rest.

Large stasis ulcers unresponsive to conservative treatment may require excision and skin grafting. Health care includes daily inspection to assess healing. Other care is the same as for varicose veins.

Treatment

The goals of treatment are to control thrombus development, prevent complications, and relieve pain. Symptomatic measures include bed rest, with elevation of the affected arm or leg; warm, moist soaks to the affected area; and analgesics, as ordered. After the acute episode of deep-vein thrombophlebitis subsides, the patient may begin to walk while wearing antiembolism stockings.

Treatment may also include anticoagulants (initially, heparin; later, warfarin) to prolong clotting time. Full anticoagulant dose must be discontinued during the operative period, due to the risk of hemorrhage. Postoperatively, prophylactic doses may reduce the risk of

VARICOSE VEINS

Varicose veins are dilated, tortuous veins, usually affecting the subcutaneous leg veins—the saphenous veins and their branches. They can result from congenital weakness of the valves or venous wall; from diseases of the venous system, such as deep-vein thrombophlebitis; or from conditions that produce prolonged venostasis, such as pregnancy, or from occupations that necessitate standing for an extended period of time.

Varicose veins may be asymptomatic or produce mild to severe leg symptoms, including a feeling of heaviness; cramps at night; diffuse, dull aching after prolonged standing or walking; aching during menses; fatigability; palpable nodules; and with deep-vein incompetency, orthostatic edema and stasis pigmentation of the calves and ankles.

In mild to moderate varicose veins, antiembolism stockings or elastic bandages counteract pedal and ankle swelling by supporting the veins and improving circulation. An exercise program, such as walking, promotes muscular contraction and forces blood through the veins, thereby minimizing venous pooling. Severe varicose veins may necessitate stripping and ligation, or as an alternative to surgery, injection of a sclerosing agent into small affected vein segments.

Measures to promote comfort and minimize worsening of varicosities include:
• discouraging the patient from wearing constrictive clothing.
• advising the patient to elevate his legs whenever possible and to avoid prolonged standing or sitting.

Care after stripping and ligation, or injection of a sclerosing agent includes:
• administering analgesics to relieve pain.
• elevating the affected leg.
• frequently checking circulation in toes (color and temperature), and observing elastic bandages for bleeding; rewrapping bandages at least once every 8 hours, wrapping from toe to thigh, with the leg elevated.
• watching for signs of complications, such as sensory loss in the leg (which could indicate saphenous nerve damage), calf pain (thrombophlebitis), and fever (infection).

---

pulmonary embolism. Rarely, deep-vein thrombophlebitis may cause complete venous occlusion, which necessitates venous interruption through simple ligation to vein plication, or clipping.

Therapy for severe superficial thrombophlebitis may include an anti-inflammatory, such as phenylbutazone, and antiembolism stockings.

Additional considerations
Patient teaching, identification of high-risk patients, and measures to prevent venostasis can prevent deep-vein thrombophlebitis; close monitoring of anticoagulant therapy can prevent serious complications, such as internal hemorrhage.

Bed rest, as ordered, must be enforced, and the affected arm or leg should be elevated. If pillows are used for leg elevation, they should be placed so they support the entire length of the affected extremity to prevent compression of the popliteal space.

Warm soaks will increase circulation to the affected area and will relieve pain and inflammation. Analgesics may be ordered to relieve pain.

The circumference of the affected arm or leg must be measured and recorded and this measurement compared to the normal one. Marking the skin over the measured area will ensure accuracy and consistency of serial measurements.

Heparin I.V. should be administered, as ordered, with an infusion monitor or pump to control the flow rate, if necessary.

Partial thromboplastin time must be measured regularly for the patient on heparin therapy, and prothrombin time for the patient on warfarin (therapeutic anticoagulation values for both are one and a half to two times control values). Signs of bleeding are dark, tarry stools, coffee-ground vomitus, and ecchymoses. The patient should use an electric razor and avoid medications containing aspirin.

Signs of pulmonary emboli include rales, dyspnea, hemoptysis, and hypotension.

Preparing the patient for discharge includes:

• emphasizing the importance of follow-up blood studies to monitor anticoagulant therapy.

• teaching the patient or his family how to give subcutaneous injections if he is being discharged on heparin therapy; arranging for a visiting nurse if he re-

quires further assistance.

• telling the patient to avoid prolonged sitting or standing to help prevent recurrence.

• teaching the patient how to properly use antiembolism stockings.

• preventing thrombophlebitis in high-risk patients by performing range-of-motion exercises while the patient is on bed rest, using intermittent pneumatic calf massage during lengthy surgical or diagnostic procedures, applying antiembolism stockings postoperatively, and encouraging early ambulation.

Polyarteritis

(Polyarteritis nodosa, periarteritis nodosa, necrotizing angiitis)

Polyarteritis is a relatively rare disorder that produces widespread segmental inflammation and necrosis in the small and medium arteries. This disorder can cause arterial damage throughout the body. Although prognosis depends on the severity and location of the lesions, and varies from complete remission to death (usually from renal failure, myocardial infarction, or gastrointestinal bleeding), the outlook is generally poor. Polyarteritis is most prevalent in men aged 30 to 50.

Causes

Although the cause of polyarteritis is unknown, some evidence supports the theory that this disorder is immunologically mediated. Initially, polyarteritis produces focal lesions in the medial arterial layer. These lesions may eventually extend into the adventitial and the intimal layers as well, and may produce palpable beadlike projections along the course of the artery. The inflammatory lesions are randomly distributed throughout the vessel and may not affect its entire circumference. Arterial wall changes may precipitate fibrosis and eventual weakening, resulting in arterial occlusion, thrombosis, infarction, or aneurysm.

Signs and symptoms

Clinical features of polyarteritis may vary widely, as does its course, which may be acute, chronic, or intermittent. Early symptoms of polyarteritis are nonspecific, and usually include fever, leu-

kocytosis, general weakness, weight loss, and anorexia. Other symptoms depend on the organ or system affected and the severity of the lesions:

• *kidneys:* proteinuria, microscopic hematuria, hypertension

• *gastrointestinal tract:* abdominal pain, nausea, vomiting, diarrhea, anorexia, bleeding

• *musculoskeletal system:* arthralgia, myalgia, muscle weakness

• *cardiovascular system:* chest pain, cardiac arrhythmias, pericarditis, congestive heart failure

• *liver:* hepatic failure (ascites, hepatomegaly, jaundice, coma)

• *peripheral nervous system:* sensory and motor deficits, headache, possible seizures.

Diagnosis

Since no single test confirms polyarteritis, diagnosis relies on a combination of patient history, clinical features, lesion biopsy, and arteriography. Diagnosis must rule out other types of vasculitis.

Treatment
Treatment is usually symptomatic, through long-term use of corticosteroids, usually prednisone. Unfortunately, relapses are common after discontinuing therapy. Immunosuppressive drugs, such as azathioprine, are investigational. Depending on complications, treatment may include fluid management, antihypertensive therapy, digitalis, and antibiotics. (Caution: Sulfonamides or penicillins may exacerbate polyarteritis.)

Additional considerations
When treating a patient with polyarteritis, the health care professional should:
• monitor intake and output, and vital signs, particularly blood pressure; watch for signs of infection, and remember that corticosteroids may mask infection; be alert for signs of cutaneous involvement (tender, subcutaneous nodules) and possible pulmonary involvement (pleuritis, with or without effusion).
• position the patient with arthralgia or myalgia comfortably; assist with range-of-motion exercises if he's bedridden.
• teach the patient and family about the nature of the disease; instruct the patient to avoid drugs that could exacerbate his condition (sulfonamides, penicillins, iodides, diuretics, anticonvulsants); stress the importance of moderately restricting sodium intake to minimize side effects of corticosteroid therapy.
• provide emotional support to help the patient and family cope with polyarteritis and the side effects of corticosteroid therapy (moon face, buffalo hump, hirsutism, purplish striae); encourage them to share their feelings, and help them set realistic expectations.

Raynaud's Disease

Raynaud's disease is one of several primary arteriospastic disorders characterized by episodic vasospasm in the small peripheral arteries and arterioles, precipitated by exposure to cold or stress. This condition occurs bilaterally and usually affects the hands or, less often, the feet. Raynaud's disease is most prevalent in females, particularly between puberty and age 40. It is a benign condition, requiring no specific treatment and with no serious sequelae.

Raynaud's phenomenon, however, a condition often associated with several connective tissue disorders—such as scleroderma, systemic lupus erythematosus, or polymyositis—has a progressive course, leading to ischemia, gangrene, and amputation. Distinction between the two disorders is difficult, because some patients who experience mild symptoms of Raynaud's disease for several years may later develop overt connective tissue disease—especially scleroderma.

Causes
Although the cause of Raynaud's disease is unknown, several theories have been proposed to account for the reduced digital blood flow: intrinsic vascular wall hyperactivity to cold, increased vasomotor tone due to sympathetic stimulation, and antigen-antibody immune response (the most probable theory, since abnormal immunologic test results accompany Raynaud's phenomenon).

Signs and symptoms
After exposure to cold or stress, the skin on the fingers typically blanches, then becomes cyanotic before changing to red, and from cold to normal temperature. Numbness and tingling may also occur. These symptoms are relieved by warmth.

In long-standing disease, trophic changes, such as sclerodactyly, ulcerations, or chronic paronychia, may result.

Although it's extremely uncommon (developing in only 1% of persons with this disease), minimal cutaneous gangrene necessitates amputation of one or more phalanges.

Diagnosis

Clinical criteria that establish Raynaud's disease include skin color changes induced by cold or stress; bilateral involvement; absence of gangrene or, if present, minimal cutaneous gangrene; normal arterial pulses; and patient history of clinical symptoms of longer than 2 years' duration. Diagnosis must also rule out secondary disease processes, such as chronic arterial occlusive or connective tissue disease.

Treatment

Initially, treatment consists of avoidance of cold, mechanical, or chemical injury; cessation of smoking; and reassurance that symptoms are benign. Since drug side effects, especially from vasodilators, may be more bothersome than the disease itself, drug therapy is reserved for unusually severe symptoms. Such therapy may include phenoxybenzamine or reserpine. Sympathectomy may be helpful when conservative modalities fail to prevent ischemic ulcers, and becomes necessary in less than 25% of patients.

Additional considerations

• The patient should try to avoid exposure to the cold. She should always wear mittens or gloves in cold weather, or when handling cold items—such as frozen foods—or defrosting the refrigerator or freezer.
• The patient must avoid stressful situations, when possible, and stop smoking (nicotine is a vasoconstrictor).
• The patient should inspect the skin frequently and seek immediate care for signs of skin breakdown or infection.
• The patient must understand the use and side effects of any therapeutic drugs.
• The patient will need psychologic support and reassurance to allay her fear of amputation and disfigurement.

Buerger's Disease
(Thromboangiitis obliterans)

Buerger's disease—an inflammatory, nonatheromatous occlusive condition—causes segmental lesions and subsequent thrombus formation in the small and medium arteries (and sometimes the veins), resulting in decreased blood flow to the feet and legs. This disorder may produce ulceration and, eventually, gangrene.

Causes

Although the cause of Buerger's disease is unknown, a definite link exists to smoking, suggesting a hypersensitivity reaction to nicotine. Incidence is highest among men of Jewish ancestry, aged 20 to 40, who smoke heavily.

Signs and symptoms

Buerger's disease typically produces intermittent claudication of the instep, which is aggravated by exercise and relieved by rest. During exposure to low temperature, the feet initially become cold, cyanotic, and numb; later, they redden, become hot, and tingle. Occasionally, Buerger's disease also affects the hands, possibly resulting in painful fingertip ulcerations. Other symptoms include impaired peripheral pulses, migratory superficial thrombophlebitis, and in later stages, ulceration, muscle atrophy, and gangrene.

Diagnosis

Patient history and physical examination strongly suggest Buerger's disease. Supportive tests include Doppler ultrasonography and plethysmography to show diminished circulation in the peripheral vessels, and arteriography to locate lesions and rule out atherosclerosis.

Treatment and additional considerations

The primary goals of treatment are to relieve symptoms and prevent complications. Such therapy may include an exercise program that uses gravity to fill and drain the blood vessels, or, in severe disease, a lumbar sympathectomy to increase blood supply to the skin. Amputation may be necessary for nonhealing ulcers, intractable pain, or gangrene.

• To enhance the effectiveness of treatment, the patient must discontinue smoking permanently.

• The patient should try to avoid precipitating factors, such as emotional stress, exposure to extreme temperatures, and trauma.

• Proper foot care is important, especially wearing well-fitting shoes and cotton or wool socks; inspecting the feet daily for cuts, abrasions, and signs of skin breakdown; and seeking medical attention immediately after any trauma.

• If the patient has ulcers and gangrene, bed rest must be enforced and a bed cradle should be used to prevent pressure from bed linens. The feet should be protected with soft padding, such as cotton batting, washed gently with a mild soap and tepid water, rinsed thoroughly, and patted dry with a soft towel.

• The patient will need psychologic support. If necessary, he should be referred for psychologic counseling to help him cope with restrictions imposed by this chronic disease. If he has undergone amputation, he should be referred for assistance and equipment.

Arterial Occlusive Disease

Arterial occlusive disease is the obstruction or narrowing of the lumen of the aorta and its major branches, causing an interruption of blood flow, usually to the legs and feet. This disorder may affect the carotid, vertebral, innominate, subclavian, mesenteric, and celiac arteries. Occlusions may be acute or chronic, and often cause severe ischemia, skin ulceration, and gangrene. Arterial occlusive disease is more common in males than in females. Prognosis depends on the location of the occlusion, the development of collateral circulation to counteract reduced blood flow, and in acute disease, the time elapsed between occlusion and its removal.

Causes

Arterial occlusive disease is a frequent complication of atherosclerosis. The occlusive mechanism may be endogenous, due to emboli or thrombosis, or exogenous, due to trauma or fracture. Predisposing factors include smoking; aging; conditions such as hypertension, hyperlipemia, and diabetes; and family history of vascular disorders, myocardial infarction, or cerebrovascular accident.

Diagnosis

Diagnosis of arterial occlusive disease is usually indicated by patient history and physical examination. Diagnostic tests include the following:

• *Arteriography* demonstrates the type (thrombus or embolus), location, and degree of obstruction, and collateral circulation; this procedure is particularly useful in chronic disease or for evaluating candidates for reconstructive surgery.

• *Doppler ultrasonography* and *plethysmography* are noninvasive tests that, in acute disease, show decreased blood flow distal to the occlusion.

• *Ophthalmodynamometry* helps determine degree of obstruction in the internal carotid artery by comparing ophthalmic artery to brachial artery pressure on the affected side. More than 20% difference suggests insufficiency.

• *EEG* and *CAT scan* may be necessary to rule out brain lesions.

Treatment
Generally, treatment depends on the cause, location, and size of the obstruction. In mild chronic disease, treatment usually consists of supportive measures and drug therapy with vasodilators, such as pa-paverine, or in carotid artery occlusion, antiplatelet therapy with dipyridamole and aspirin.

Acute disease usually necessitates surgery to restore circulation to the affected area. Appropriate surgery may include:
• *embolectomy:* balloon-tipped Fogarty catheter used to remove thrombotic material from artery; used mainly for mes-

ARTERIAL OCCLUSIVE DISEASE

SITE OF OCCLUSION	SIGNS AND SYMPTOMS
Carotid arterial system • Internal carotids • External carotids	Neurologic dysfunction: transient ischemic attacks (TIAs) due to reduced cerbral circulation produce unilateral sensory or motor dysfunction (transient monocular blindness, hemiparesis), possible aphasia or dysarthria, confusion, decreased mentation, and headache. These recurrent clinical features usually last 5 to 10 minutes but may persist up to 24 hours, and may herald a stroke. Absent or decreased pulsation with an auscultatory bruit over the affected vessels
Vertebrobasilar system • Vertebral arteries • Basilar arteries	Neurologic dysfunction: TIAs of brain stem and cerebellum produce binocular visual disturbances, vertigo, dysarthria, and "drop attacks" (falling down without loss of consciousness). Less common than carotid TIA
Innominate • Brachiocephalic artery	Neurologic dysfunction: signs and symptoms of vertebrobasilar occlusion. Indications of ischemia (claudication) of right arm; possible bruit over right side of neck
Subclavian artery	Subclavian steal syndrome (characterized by the backflow of blood from the brain through the vertebral artery on the same side as the occlusion, into the subclavian artery distal to the occlusion); clinical effects of vertebrobasilar occlusion and exercise-induced arm claudication. Possible gangrene, usually limited to the digits
Mesenteric artery • Superior (most commonly affected) • Celiac axis • Inferior	Bowel ischemia, infarct necrosis, and gangrene; sudden, acute abdominal pain; nausea and vomiting; diarrhea; leukocytosis; and shock due to massive intraluminal fluid and plasma loss
Aortic bifurcation (saddle block occlusion) a medical emergency associated with cardiac embolization	Sensory and motor deficits (muscle weakness, numbness, paresthesias, paralysis), and signs of ischemia (sudden pain; cold, pale legs with decreased or absent peripheral pulses) in both legs
Iliac artery (Leriche's syndrome)	Intermittent claudication of lower back, buttocks, and thighs, relieved by rest; absent or reduced femoral or distal pulses; possible bruit over femoral arteries
Femoral and popliteal artery (associated with aneurysm formation)	Intermittent claudication of calves on exertion, ischemic pain in feet, pretrophic pain (heralds necrosis and ulceration), leg pallor and coolness, blanching of feet on elevation, gangrene

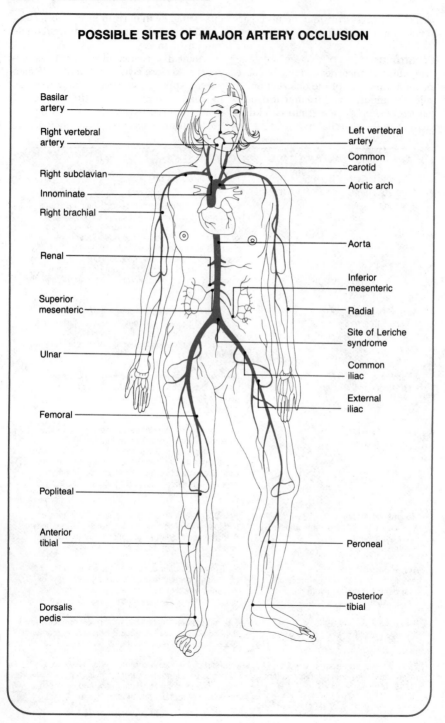

POSSIBLE SITES OF MAJOR ARTERY OCCLUSION

enteric, femoral, or popliteal occlusion
- *thromboendarterectomy:* opening of the artery and removal of the obstructing thrombus (atherosclerotic plaque) and the medial layer of the arterial wall; usually performed after angiography; often used with autogenous vein or Dacron bypass surgery (femoral-popliteal or aortofemoral)
- *patch grafting:* removal of the thrombosed segment and replacement with an autogenous vein or Dacron graft
- *bypass graft:* diversion of blood flow through an anastomosed autogenous or woven Dacron graft to bypass the thrombosed arterial segment
- *lumbar sympathectomy:* may be an adjunct to reconstructive surgery.

Amputation becomes necessary with failure of arterial reconstructive surgery, gangrene, uncontrollable infection, or intractable pain.

Other therapy includes heparin to prevent emboli in patients with embolic occlusion, and bowel resection after restoration of blood flow in patients with occlusion of the mesenteric artery.

Additional considerations

Comprehensive patient teaching, such as proper foot care, is needed. All diagnostic tests and procedures should be explained. The patient should stop smoking and follow the prescribed medical regimen.

Preoperatively, during an acute episode, the hospital staff member should:
- assess circulatory status by checking for the most distal pulses and inspecting skin color and temperature.
- provide pain relief.
- administer heparin by continuous I.V. drip, as ordered; use an infusion monitor or pump to ensure proper flow rate.
- wrap the affected foot in soft cotton batting, and reposition it frequently to prevent pressure on any one area; strictly avoid elevating or applying heat to the affected leg.
- watch for signs of fluid and electrolyte imbalance, and monitor intake and output for signs of renal failure (urine output less than 30 ml/hour); check for signs

of cerebrovascular accident (numbness in an arm or leg, and intermittent blindness) if the patient has carotid, innominate, vertebral, or subclavian artery occlusion.

Postoperatively, the staffer should:
- monitor vital signs; continuously assess circulatory function by inspecting skin color and temperature and by checking for distal pulses; compare earlier assessments and observations in charting; watch for signs of hemorrhage (tachycardia, hypotension), and check dressing for excessive bleeding.
- assess neurologic status frequently in carotid, innominate, vertebral, or subclavian artery occlusion for changes in level of consciousness or muscle strength, and pupil size.
- connect nasogastric tube to low intermittent suction in mesenteric artery occlusion; monitor intake and output (low urine output may indicate damage to renal arteries during surgery); check bowel sounds for return of peristalsis. Increasing abdominal distention and tenderness may indicate extension of bowel ischemia with resulting gangrene, necessitating further excision, or may indicate peritonitis.
- check distal pulses for adequate circulation in saddle block occlusion; watch for signs of renal failure and mesenteric artery occlusion (severe abdominal pain), and for cardiac arrhythmias, which may precipitate embolus formation.
- monitor urine output in iliac artery occlusion for signs of renal failure from decreased perfusion to the kidneys, as a result of surgery; provide meticulous catheter care.
- assist with early ambulation in both femoral and popliteal artery occlusions, but don't allow the patient to sit for an extended period.
- check stump carefully for drainage after amputation; note and record its color and amount of drainage, if it occurs, and the time; elevate the stump, as ordered, and administer adequate analgesic medication; explain phantom limb pain phenomenon, which is common, to the patient.

- tell the patient before discharge to watch for signs of recurrence (pain, pallor, numbness, paralysis, absence of pulse) due to graft occlusion or occlusion at another site; warn against constrictive clothing, and prolonged bending or sitting.

MISCELLANEOUS DISORDERS

Benign Cardiac Tumors

Benign cardiac tumors can arise from the endocardium, myocardium, and pericardium, and constitute 75% of all primary lesions found in the heart. Myxomas and rhabdomyomas are the two most common benign tumors, with myxomas accounting for at least half of these. Rarer benign tumors include fibromas, lipomas, teratomas, angiomas, and hamartomas. Although histologically benign, these tumors can be fatal, and often produce cardiac dysfunction, such as pericardial effusion and tamponade, potentially lethal arrhythmias, refractory heart failure, and sudden death. Clinical course for this rare disorder varies with tumor type and location. With early recognition of signs and symptoms, removal of benign cardiac tumors by open heart surgery can greatly improve prognosis.

Causes and incidence

Myxomas may develop from mural thrombi or may be of neoplastic origin (true tumor). As single or multiple lesions, myxomas arise from the endocardium and occupy the left atrium three times more often than the right; however, they may be bilateral. Myxomas are most prevalent in women between ages 30 and 60. *Angiomas* and *lipomas* may be intracavitary, occurring in the atria.

Rhabdomyomas may result from congenital tissue malformation, or from a localized disorder of glycogen metabolism resulting from an enzyme defect. They may not be true tumors and, when multiple, coexist with tuberous sclerosis of the brain. Rhabdomyomas usually arise from the myocardium and may extend inward—protruding into the left ventricle—or outward—onto the epicardium. These tumors account for 35% of nonproliferative tumors in children under age 3, most of whom die within the first year of life. Rarer myocardial tumors may include *fibromas, hamartomas,* and *mesotheliomas. Teratomas* and other rare benign cardiac tumors, including angiomas, derive from abnormal embryonic development. Teratomas usually arise from the pericardium, as do rarer benign cardiac tumors, including *leiomyomas* and *neurofibromas.*

Some benign tumors are common to all three cardiac layers.

Signs and symptoms

Overt clinical effects develop only after tumor growth impairs heart function. Benign tumors may produce symptoms that simulate familiar cardiac disorders. For this reason, these tumors have been dubbed the great imitators of cardiovascular disease.

The hallmark of benign intracavitary tumors is disruption of cardiac filling and emptying. Symptoms of left atrial myxoma are due to mitral valve obstruction by the tumor, mimicking mitral stenosis. Clinical effects include syncope (especially with change in position) and shocklike syndrome, resulting from a reduction in cardiac output; pulmonary venous congestion; signs of occlusive vascular disease, resulting from embolization; and possibly, seizures or coma. A murmur of mitral regurgitation may also occur. Right atrial myxoma produces symptoms resulting from rapid and unrelenting right heart failure (fatigue, peripheral edema, hepatomegaly, neck vein distention) with fever, weight loss, and murmur. Right atrial myxomas mimic constrictive pericarditis, tricuspid stenosis, and other cardiac disorders. Cyanosis and neck vein distention may result from superior vena cava obstruction.

Typical signs of right ventricular myxomas include syncope, fever of unknown origin, and murmurs of pulmonary and tricuspid valve obstruction. Rhabdomyomas may obstruct the right ventricular outflow tract, simulating pulmonary stenosis. Left ventricular tumors, such as fibromas arising from the aortic valve, may produce signs of left heart failure, mimicking aortic stenosis or hypertrophic subaortic stenosis; such tumors cause hemodynamic alterations upon changes in body position. Teratomas and other pericardial tumors mimic acute pericarditis, and cause precordial pain, friction rub, and signs of pericardial effusion and tamponade. Myocardial tumors may involve the heart wall, valves, or conduction system. Although these tumors rarely cause obstructive disorders, they may cause arrhythmias and sudden death.

Diagnosis
A patient history and physical examination showing characteristic clinical findings suggest benign cardiac tumors. However, laboratory tests must rule out other cardiac disorders that produce similar symptoms.
• *Chest X-ray* may reveal an abnormal cardiac silhouette, widening of the mediastinum, and intracavitary tumor calcification, but it cannot distinguish between pericardial effusion and pericardial tumors.
• *EKG* often shows axis deviation or ventricular hypertrophy in ventricular myxomas; in other endocardial myxomas, it may show arrhythmias and conduction disturbances, such as bundle branch block, abnormal P waves, and ST segment changes.
• *Abnormal laboratory results* in myxomas include increased serum enzymes

(lactic dehydrogenase and SGOT), ESR, and alkaline phosphatase; leukocytosis; hyperglobulinemia; and occasionally, increased hemoglobin in right atrial myxoma (polycythemia).
• *Cardiac catheterization*, the most reliable diagnostic tool, shows filling defects, compression, pressure changes in cardiac chambers, or displacement of the major blood vessels and mediastinal structures. However, it cannot distinguish between benign and malignant tumors or large thrombi. This procedure risks dislodgment of tumor fragments, resulting in embolism.
• *Echocardiography* can identify atrial tumors that occupy the mitral or tricuspid valve leaflets, and differentiates left atrial myxomas from mitral stenosis.

Treatment
Depending on tumor size and location, open heart surgery using complete cardiopulmonary bypass can remove many benign cardiac tumors; subsequent valve replacement or septal repair with a Dacron graft may be necessary. Before surgery and for symptomatic relief of pericardial tumors, pericardiocentesis can remove fluid accumulation. Symptomatic treatment for inoperable tumors includes pacemaker for heart block, and digitalis, diuretics, and vasodilators for congestive heart failure.

Additional considerations
Benign cardiac tumors necessitate intensive care monitoring before and after surgery. Preoperatively, the hospital staff member should:
• auscultate for friction rubs and murmurs; note EKG changes and report and treat arrhythmias; watch for symptoms of decreased cardiac output (syncope, shock), of left heart failure (dyspnea, cyanosis, rales in chest), and of right heart failure (fatigue, peripheral edema, hepatomegaly); assess for signs of cardiac tamponade in patients with pericardial tumors; watch for signs of pulmonary and systemic embolization.
• explain all diagnostic procedures carefully; tell the patient what to expect

after surgery (endotracheal and chest tubes, ventilator, cardiac monitor, Foley catheter, and venous and pulmonary arterial lines).
• instruct the patient to avoid positions that further obstruct cardiac blood flow, causing dizziness and reduced cardiac output.

Postoperatively, the staffer should:
• monitor vital signs, level of consciousness, respiratory status, intake and output, and hemodynamic pressures; record any chest tube drainage, and suction the endotracheal tube frequently; watch for, report, and treat arrhythmias.
• have the patient turn, cough, and breathe deeply at regular intervals when vital signs stabilize; give medications (antibiotics, digitalis preparations, diuretics), as ordered.
• provide emotional support, especially for parents of infants with rhabdomyomas—many of these infants die soon after birth. Since the word tumor conjures visions of cancer, the benign nature of these lesions should be emphasized.

Athletic Heart Syndrome

Athletic heart syndrome comprises a series of related cardiac changes that develop as an anatomic and physiologic response to strenuous exercise. Such changes, which do not necessarily impair heart function, include biventricular hypertrophy, intermittent systolic ejection murmur, S₃ gallop, arrhythmias, ST-T wave abnormalities, decreased heart rate, and increased stroke volume, left ventricular stroke work, and cardiac output. Because of the large number of persons currently participating in physical fitness, the incidence of athletic heart syndrome is rising.

Causes
Athletic heart syndrome is probably an adaptive physiologic response to maintain optimal cardiac performance during physical endurance training. To compensate for the sustained hemodynamic burden produced by exercise, left ventricular internal dimension (measured by left ventricular end-diastolic volumes) and cardiac wall thickness increase, enhancing contractility, improving cardiac output, and delivering more oxygen during maximum workloads.

Signs and symptoms
This syndrome usually doesn't produce symptoms, although it may cause chest pounding or an irregular heartbeat after strenuous activity.

Diagnosis
Athletic heart syndrome is often detected during a routine physical examination or hospitalization for an athletic injury, with the following findings:
• *History* reveals endurance training.

• *Chest X-ray* shows enlarged right and left ventricles and, occasionally, an enlarged left atrium and aortic root.
• *Echocardiography* demonstrates increased cardiac mass, including ventricular hypertrophy and, possibly, an enlarged left atrium.
• *Chest auscultation* may reveal a slow heart rate with intermittent systolic ejection murmur along the left sternal border, S₃ gallop over the mitral area (can be a normal finding in youth), and hyperdynamic ventricular impulse at point of maximum impulse.
• *EKG* (resting and during exercise) may show sinus bradycardia (as low as 40 beats per minute), increased QRS and T amplitude in both standard and precordial leads, elevated ST segment in precordial leads (V_2 to V_5), appearance of U wave due to abnormal repolarization or left ventricular hypertrophy, and arrhythmias.

Isolated findings—bradycardia, for example—may indicate primary organic heart disease or may be a normal finding.

Treatment and additional considerations

Athletic heart syndrome doesn't necessitate treatment, but underlying cardiac disease may require the athlete to discontinue training.
• The patient should understand the purpose of diagnostic procedures, and should be told that while there is no evidence that strenuous exercise causes heart damage or increases the risk of early death from cardiac disease, the long-term effects of athletic heart syndrome are still unknown and are being studied.
• The patient should know that future risk of heart disease is closely linked to a family history of cardiovascular disorders. To minimize future risk, he should have regular checkups with resting and exercise EKGs.
• An extensive medical evaluation of the patient may be necessary to distinguish normal variations from disease states.

Coronary Artery Spasm

In coronary artery spasm, a spontaneous sustained contraction of one or more coronary arteries causes ischemia and dysfunction of the heart muscle supplied by these arteries. This disorder also causes Prinzmetal's angina and even myocardial infarction in patients with unoccluded coronary arteries.

Causes

The direct cause of coronary artery spasm is unknown, but possible contributing factors include:
• intimal hemorrhage into the medial layer of the blood vessel, causing irritation and subsequent spasm; spasm may worsen with an arteriosclerotic obstruction.
• hyperventilation, decreasing hydrogen ions (with normal or increased calcium ion levels), causing vasoconstriction; hydrogen ions normally act as a calcium antagonist.
• elevated catecholamine levels, which produce an overall rise in sympathetic tone (alpha-adrenergic stimulation) in the coronary arteries and increase the risk of spasms.

Signs and symptoms

The primary clinical feature of coronary artery spasm is angina (oppressive substernal discomfort, radiating to the jaw and the ulnar aspect of the left arm). But, unlike classic angina, this pain commonly occurs spontaneously and is unrelated to physical exertion or emotional stress; it's also more severe, usually lasts longer, and may be cyclic, frequently recurring every day at the same time. Such painful ischemic attacks may change heart rate, lower blood pressure, and occasionally, cause fainting due to diminished cardiac output. If the spasm occurs in the left coronary artery, the mitral valve may prolapse during the ischemic attack and produce a loud systolic murmur and, possibly, pulmonary edema, with dyspnea, rales, and hemoptysis.

Diagnosis

Coronary arteriography confirms coronary artery spasm by showing uninduced spontaneous spasm in a patient with a history of spontaneous anginal attacks, or an ergonovine-induced spasm in a patient with unoccluded coronary arteries or an artery with an occlusion of less than 50%.

During pain, EKG shows ST elevation, with an upright or inverted T wave, reflecting myocardial ischemia; the EKG returns to normal when the pain subsides. Serial EKGs also are often normal during painfree periods. Ambulatory EKG using a Holter monitor helps detect ST changes during cyclic chest pain and may reveal serious arrhythmias.

Treatment

Drug therapy reduces coronary artery spasm. Nitrates—such as nitroglycerin (I.V. or sublingual), isosorbide dinitrate P.O., or nitroglycerin ointment—relieve chest pain by decreasing myocardial oxygen requirements and perhaps redistributing myocardial blood flow. The effectiveness of diltiazem and nifedipine (calcium antagonists that decrease vascular resistance) and of phenoxybenzamine and phentolamine (alpha adrenergic blockers) in reducing chest pain is under investigation.

Additional considerations

• Before cardiac catheterization and angiography, the procedure should be explained to the patient. He must understand that the procedure is invasive, and may reproduce coronary artery spasm and chest pain under controlled conditions, but such pain will be treated immediately with nitroglycerin.

• After cardiac catheterization and angiography, blood pressure and pulse rate should be checked frequently. The patient must be watched for signs of bleeding or infection at the catheter entry site (the arm or groin).

• The patient has to drink plenty of liquids to replace fluid lost through dye-induced diuresis. He should rest in bed for about 6 hours, then gradually resume normal activity.

• Blood pressure and pulse rate should be monitored throughout nifedipine therapy. A drop in blood pressure and a reflex increase in pulse rate are expected, but severe hypotension or tachycardia must be reported. The patient should report dizziness, undue fatigue, gastrointestinal distress, and abnormal sweating.

• The use of sublingual nitroglycerin for chest pain should be explained and reinforced. The patient must carry nitroglycerin tablets at all times, in a tightly closed, dark bottle with no cotton. He should keep the medication away from heat and sunlight, throw away old tablets every 3 months and replace them with new ones, and take the tablet while sitting. He may experience flushing or dizziness soon after taking the medication but should not be alarmed by it. Whenever the patient's chest pain doesn't subside in 10 minutes, or after 3 tablets of nitroglycerin, he should go immediately to the nearest emergency room.

• The patient receiving oral isosorbide dinitrate instead of nitroglycerin should take tablets on an empty stomach. If nitroglycerin ointment is ordered, the patient must be shown how to apply it.

• Because coronary artery spasm is sometimes associated with atherosclerotic disease, the patient should know the risk factors associated with this disease. He should stop smoking (since this may provoke spasm), avoid overeating, especially foods high in cholesterol (eggs, red meats), use alcohol sparingly (less than 1 oz [30 ml] per day); and maintain a proper balance of exercise and rest. He must realize the importance of reporting changes in the character of chest pain. If the patient is hypertensive, then his compliance with antihypertensive therapy is critical.

Selected References

Adams, Nancy R., ed. *Hemodynamic Monitoring*, CRITICAL CARE QUARTERLY. 2:2, September 1979.

Adelman, A.G., et al. *Current Concepts of Primary Cardiomyopathies*, CARDIOVASCULAR MEDICINE. 5:495-507, 1977.

Andreoli, Kathleen G. COMPREHENSIVE CARDIAC CARE: A TEXT FOR NURSES AND OTHER HEALTH PROFESSIONALS, 3rd ed. St. Louis: C.V. Mosby Co., 1975.

Argenta, Louis, et al. *A Comparison of the Hemodynamic Effects of Inotropic Agents*, ANNALS OF THORACIC SURGERY. 22:1:51-57, July 1976.

Bergan, John J., and J.S. Yao, eds. VENOUS PROBLEMS. Chicago: Year Book Medical Pubs., 1978.

Buda, A. J. *Coronary Artery Spasm and Mitral Valve Prolapse,* AMERICAN HEART JOURNAL. 95:4:457-462, 1978.

Budassi, Susan A., ed. *Cardiopulmonary Resuscitation,* CRITICAL CARE QUARTERLY. 1:1, May 1978.

Chewning, Betty. STAFF MANUAL FOR TEACHING PATIENTS ABOUT HYPERTENSION. Chicago: American Hospital Assn., 1979.

DeBakey, Michael E., and George P. Noon. *Aneurysms of the Thoracic Aorta,* MODERN CONCEPTS OF CARDIOVASCULAR DISEASE. 44:10, October 1975.

Elenbaas, Robert M., ed. *Pharmacologic Management of Shock,* CRITICAL CARE QUARTERLY. 2:4, March 1980.

Firmin, R., et al. *A Case of Rhabdomyosarcoma of the Right Ventricle,* BRITISH HEART JOURNAL. 40:1426-1428, 1978.

Graham, S., and A. Sellers. *Atrial Myxoma with Multiple Myeloma,* ARCHIVES OF INTERNAL MEDICINE. 139:116-117, 1979.

Hancock, E.W. *Management of Pericardial Disease,* MODERN CONCEPTS OF CARDIOVASCULAR DISEASE. January 1979.

Hathaway, Rebecca G. *Hemodynamic Monitoring in Shock,* JOURNAL OF EMERGENCY NURSING. 3:37-42, 1977.

Hathaway, Rebecca G. *The Swan-Ganz Catheter: A Review,* NURSING CLINICS OF NORTH AMERICA. 13:389-407, 1978.

Helfant, R.H. *Coronary Artery Spasm and Provocative Testing in Ischemic Heart Disease,* AMERICAN JOURNAL OF CARDIOLOGY. 41:787-789, 1978.

Hurst, J. Willis, and R. Bruce Logue, eds. THE HEART, 3rd ed. New York: McGraw-Hill Book Co., 1974.

Johnson, Sarah, and Rolf Gunnar. *Treatment of Shock in Myocardial Infarction,* JOURNAL OF THE AMERICAN MEDICAL ASSOCIATION. 237:19:2106-2108, May 9, 1977.

Kaplan, Norman M. CLINICAL HYPERTENSION, 2nd ed. Baltimore: Williams & Wilkins Co., 1978.

Krovetz, J., et al. HANDBOOK OF PEDIATRIC CARDIOLOGY, 2nd ed. Baltimore: University Park Press, 1979.

Lester, Robert, and Gallen Wagner. *Acute Myocardial Infarction,* MEDICAL CLINICS OF NORTH AMERICA. 63:1, January 1979.

Levy, Robert I., et al., eds. NUTRITION, LIPIDS, AND CORONARY HEART DISEASE. New York: Raven Press, 1979.

Masiri, A., et al. *Coronary Vasospasm as a Possible Cause of Myocardial Infarction,* NEW ENGLAND JOURNAL OF MEDICINE. 299:23:1271-1277, 1978.

Massie, Barrie, and Chatterjee Kanu. *Vasodilator Therapy of Pump Failure Complicating Acute Myocardial Infarction,* MEDICAL CLINICS OF NORTH AMERICA. 63:1:25-52, January 1979.

Morgan, Beverly L., ed. *Symposium on Pediatric Cardiology,* PEDIATRIC CLINICS OF NORTH AMERICA. 25:4, November 1978.

Moser, Marvin, et al. *Report of the Joint National Committee on the Detection, Evaluation, and Treatment of High Blood Pressure,* JOURNAL OF THE AMERICAN MEDICAL ASSOCIATION. 237:3:255-261, January 17, 1977.

Mullen, D.C. *Abdominal Aortic Aneurysm,* HOSPITAL MEDICINE. 12:60-61, August 1976.

Nagger, C.Z. *Ultrasound in Medical Diagnosis: Neurologic and Abdominal Applications,* HEART AND LUNG. 6:829-837, September-October 1977.

Rutherford, Robert B., ed. VASCULAR SURGERY. Philadelphia: W.B. Saunders Co., 1977.

Sacksteder, Sara, et al. *Common Congenital Cardiac Defects,* AMERICAN JOURNAL OF NURSING. 266-272, February 1978.

Small, Donald. *Cellular Mechanisms for Lipid Deposition in Athero-Sclerosis, Part I,* NEW ENGLAND JOURNAL OF MEDICINE. 297:16:873-877, October 20, 1977.

Tanner, Gloria. *Heart Failure in the MI Patient,* AMERICAN JOURNAL OF NURSING. 77:2:230-234, February 1977.

Tyler, M.L. *Basic Cardiopulmonary Resuscitation,* NURSING CLINICS OF NORTH AMERICA. 13:499-512, 1978.

Wheat, Myron, J. *Acute Dissecting Aneurysms of the Aorta,* PRIMARY CARDIOLOGY. July-August 1978.

Wilson, R.F., and J.A. Wilson. *Pathophysiology, Diagnosis and Treatment of Shock,* JOURNAL OF EMERGENCY NURSING. 3:11-25, 1977.

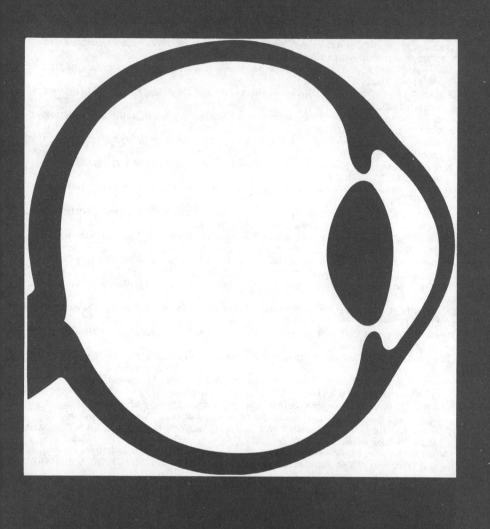

19 Eye Disorders

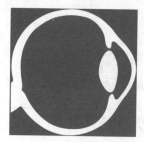

Eye Disorders

Introduction

Vision, the most complex sense, has recently been the focus of some of the greatest medical and surgical innovations. Disorders that affect the eye generally lead to vision loss or impairment; therefore, routine ophthalmic examinations and early treatment of these disorders are essential.

Review of anatomy

The visual system consists mainly of the bony orbit, which houses the eye; the contents of the orbit, including the eyeball, optic nerves, extraocular muscles, cranial nerves, blood vessels, orbital fat, and lacrimal system; and the eyelids, which protect and cover the eye.

The *orbit* (or socket) encloses the eye in a protective recess in the skull. It consists of seven bones—frontal, sphenoid, zygomatic, maxilla, palatine, ethmoid, and lacrimal. These bones form a cone, the apex of which points toward the brain; the base of the cone forms the orbital rim. The periorbita covers the bones of the orbit.

Extraocular muscles hold the eyes in place and control their coordinated movement. Each muscle has a primary action; four have secondary actions:

• *superior rectus:* primary, rotates the eye upward; secondary, rotates the eye inward

• *inferior rectus:* primary, rotates the eye downward; secondary, rotates the eye inward

• *lateral rectus:* primary, turns the eye outward (laterally)

• *medial rectus:* primary, turns the eye inward (medially)

• *superior oblique:* primary, turns the eye downward; secondary, turns the eye downward and inward

• *inferior oblique:* primary, turns the eye upward; secondary, turns the eye upward and outward

The actions of these muscles are mutually antagonistic: as one contracts, its opposing muscle relaxes.

Ocular layers

The eye has three structural layers: the sclera and cornea, the uveal tract, and the retina.

The *sclera* is the dense, white, fibrous outer protective coat of the eye. It meets the cornea at the limbus (corneoscleral junction) anteriorly, and the dural sheath of the optic nerve posteriorly. The lamina cribrosa is a sievelike structure composed of a few strands of scleral tissue that passes over the optic disk. The sclera is covered by the episclera, a thin layer of fine elastic tissue.

The *cornea* is the transparent, avascular, curved layer of the eye that is continuous with the sclera. The cornea consists of five layers: the epithelium, which contains sensory nerves; Bowman's membrane, the basement membrane for the epithelial cells; the stroma, or supporting tissue (90% of the corneal structure); Descemet's membrane, containing many elastic fibers; and the endothelium, a single layer of cells that acts as a pump to maintain proper hydration of the cornea. Aqueous humor bathes the surface of the cornea, maintaining intraocular pressure by volume and rate of outflow. The cornea's sole function is to refract light rays.

The middle layer of the eye, the *uveal tract,* is pigmented and vascular. It consists of the iris and the ciliary body in the anterior portion, and the choroid in the posterior portion. In the center of the iris is the pupil. The sphincter and dilator muscles control the amount of light

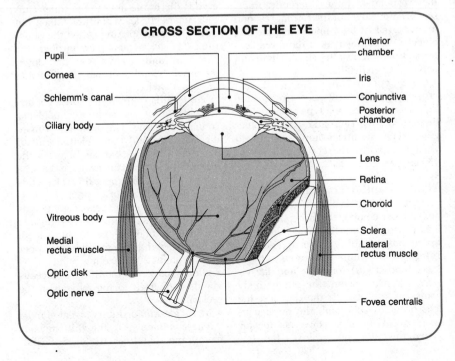

CROSS SECTION OF THE EYE

Pupil
Cornea
Schlemm's canal
Ciliary body
Vitreous body
Medial rectus muscle
Optic disk
Optic nerve

Anterior chamber
Iris
Conjunctiva
Posterior chamber
Lens
Retina
Choroid
Sclera
Lateral rectus muscle
Fovea centralis

that enters the eye through the pupil, while the pupil itself allows aqueous humor to flow from the posterior chamber into the anterior chamber.

The anterior iris joins the posterior corneal surface at an angle, where many small collecting channels form the trabecular meshwork. Aqueous humor drains through these channels into an encircling venous system called the canal of Schlemm.

The *ciliary body,* which extends from the root of the iris to the ora serrata, produces aqueous humor and controls lens accommodation through its action on the zonules of Zinn. The *choroid,* the largest part of the uveal tract, is made up of blood vessels and is bound by Bruch's membrane.

The *retina,* the most essential structure, receives the light rays from all other parts of the eye. The retina extends from the ora serrata to the optic nerve; the retinal pigment epithelium (RPE) adheres lightly to the choroid. Located next to the RPE are rods and cones. Although both rods and cones are light receptors, they respond to light differently. Rods, scattered throughout the retina, respond to low levels of light and detect moving objects; cones, located in the fovea centralis, function best in brighter light and perceive finer details.

Three types of cones contain different visual pigments and react to specific light wavelengths: one type reacts to red light, one to green, and one to blue-violet. The eye mixes these colors into various shades; the cones can detect 150 shades.

The lens and accommodation

The *lens* of the eye is biconvex, avascular, and almost completely transparent; the lens capsule is a semipermeable membrane that can admit water and electrolytes. The lens changes shape (accommodation) for near and far vision. For near vision, the ciliary body contracts and relaxes the zonules, the lens becomes spherical, the pupil constricts, and the eyes converge; for far vision, the ciliary body relaxes, the zon-

ules tighten, the lens becomes flatter, the eyes straighten, and the pupils dilate. The lens refines the refraction necessary to focus a clear image on the retina.

The *vitreous body,* which is 99% water and a small amount of insoluble protein, composes two thirds of the volume of the eye. This gelatinous body gives the eye its shape and contributes to the refraction of light rays. The vitreous is firmly attached to part of the ciliary body and to a small section of the retina; it contacts but doesn't adhere to the lens, zonules, retina, and optic nerve head.

Lacrimal network and eyelids

The lacrimal apparatus consists of the lacrimal gland, upper and lower canaliculi, lacrimal sac, and nasolacrimal duct. The gland, located in a shallow fossa beneath the superior temporal orbital rim, secretes tears, which keep the cornea and conjunctiva moist. These tears flow through 8 to 12 excretory ducts, and contain lysozyme, an enzyme that protects the conjunctiva from bacterial invasion. With every blink, the eyelids direct the flow to the inner canthus, where the tears pool and then drain through a tiny opening called the punctum. The tears then pass through the canaliculi and lacrimal sac, and down the nasolacrimal duct, which opens into the nasal cavity.

The eyelids (palpebrae) consist of tarsal plates that are composed of dense connective tissue. The orbital septum—the fascia behind the orbicularis oculi muscle—acts as a barrier between the lids and the orbit. The levator palpebrae muscle elevates the upper lid. The eyelids contain three types of glands:

• *meibomian glands:* sebaceous glands in the tarsal plates that secrete an oily substance to lubricate the tear film; about 25 of these glands are found in the upper lid and about 20 in the lower lid

• *glands of Zeis:* modified sebaceous glands connected to the follicles of the eyelashes

• *Moll's glands:* ordinary sweat glands.

The *conjunctiva* is the thin mucous membrane that lines the eyelids (palpebral conjunctiva), folds over at the fornix, and covers the surface of the eyeball (bulbar conjunctiva). The ophthalmic and lacrimal arteries supply blood to the lids. The space between the open lids is the palpebral fissure; the juncture of the upper and lower lids is the canthus. The junction near the nose is called the nasal, medial, or inner canthus; the junction on the temporal side, the lateral or external canthus.

Depth perception

In normal binocular vision, a perceived image is projected onto the two foveae. Impulses then travel along the optic pathways to the occipital cortex, which perceives a single image. However, the cortex receives two images—each from a slightly different angle—giving the images perspective and providing depth perception.

Vision testing

Several tests assess visual acuity and identify visual defects:

• *Ishihara's test* determines color blindness by using a series of plates composed of a colored background, with a letter, number, or pattern of a contrasting color located in the center of each plate. The patient with deficient color perception can't perceive the differences in color or, consequently, the designs formed by the color contrasts.

• The *Snellen chart* or other eye charts evaluate visual acuity. Such charts use progressively smaller letters or symbols to determine central vision on a numerical scale. A person with normal acuity should be able to read the letters or recognize the symbols on the 20-foot line of the eye chart at a distance of 20 feet.

• *Ophthalmoscopy,* direct ophthalmoscopy or binocular indirect ophthalmoscopy, allows examination of the interior of the eye after the pupil has been dilated with a mydriatic.

• *Refraction tests* may be performed with or without cycloplegics. In cycloplegic refraction, eyedrops weaken the accommodative power of the ciliary muscle, which facilitates the use of an

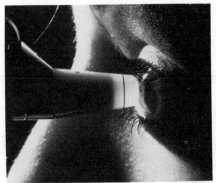

Applanation tonometry determines intraocular pressure by measuring the force required to flatten a small area of the central cornea.

ophthalmoscope. A retinoscope directs a beam of light into the pupil; the light's shadow is neutralized by placing the appropriate lens in front of the eye.

• *Maddox rod test* assesses muscle dysfunction; it's especially useful to disclose and measure heterophoria (the tendency of the eyes to deviate).

• *Duction test* checks eye movement in all directions of gaze. While one eye is covered, the other eye follows a moving light. This test detects any weakness of rotation due to muscle paralysis or structural dysfunction.

• The *test for convergence* locates the breaking point of fusion. For this test, the examiner holds a small object in front of the patient's nose and slowly brings it closer to the patient. Normally, the patient can maintain convergence until the object reaches the bridge of the nose. The point at which the eyes "break" is termed the near point of convergence and is given a number.

• The *cover-uncover test* assesses muscle deviation. The patient stares at a small, fixed object—first, from a distance of 20′ (6 m); then, from 12″ (30 cm). The examiner covers the patient's eyes one at a time, noting any movement of the uncovered eye, the direction of any deviation, and the rate at which the eyes recover normal binocular vision when latent heterophoria is present. A corollary test, the alternate-cover test, also tests for deviation.

• *Slit-lamp examination* allows a well-illuminated microscopic examination of the eyelids and the anterior segment of the eyeball.

• *Visual field* tests the function of the retina, the optic nerve, and the optic pathways when both central and peripheral visual fields are examined.

• *Schiøtz tonometry* and *applanation tonometry* measure intraocular pressure. After instilling a local anesthetic in the patient's eye, the examiner places the Schiøtz tonometer lightly on the corneal surface and measures the indentation of the cornea produced by a given weight. Applanation tonometry gauges the force required to flatten, rather than indent, a small area of central cornea.

• *Gonioscopy* allows for direct visualization of the anterior chamber angle through use of a goniolens; a slit lamp is used as the light source and microscope.

• *Ophthalmodynamometry* measures the relative central retinal artery pressures and indirectly assesses carotid artery flow on each side.

• *Fluorescein angiography* evaluates the anatomic and physiologic states of the blood vessels in the choroid and the retina after I.V. injection of fluorescein dye; the results are viewed through an ophthalmoscope or are recorded by photographs of the fundus.

EYELIDS AND LACRIMAL DUCTS

Blepharitis

A common inflammation, especially in children, blepharitis produces a red-rimmed appearance of the margins of the eyelids. It's frequently chronic and often bilateral, and can affect both upper and lower lids. It usually occurs as seborrheic (nonulcerative) blepharitis, characterized by greasy scales; or as staphylococcal (ulcerative) blepharitis, characterized by dry scales, with tiny ulcerated areas along the lid margins. Both types may coexist. Blepharitis tends to recur and become chronic. It can be controlled if treatment begins before onset of ocular involvement.

Causes and incidence
Seborrheic blepharitis generally results from seborrhea of the scalp, eyebrows, and ears; ulcerative blepharitis, from *Staphylococcus aureus* infection. (Persons with this infection may also be apt to develop chalazions and styes.) Blepharitis may also result from pediculosis (from *Phthirus pubis* or *Pediculus humanus* var. *capitis*) of the brows and lashes, which irritates the lid margins.

Signs and symptoms
Clinical features of blepharitis include itching, burning, foreign-body sensation, and sticky, crusted eyelids on waking. This constant irritation results in unconscious rubbing of the eyes (causing reddened rims) or continual blinking. Other signs include greasy scales in seborrheic blepharitis; flaky scales on lashes, loss of lashes, ulcerated areas on lid margins in ulcerative blepharitis; and nits on lashes in pediculosis.

Diagnosis
Diagnosis depends on patient history and characteristic symptoms. In ulcerative blepharitis, culture of ulcerated lid margin shows *S. aureus*. In pediculosis, examination of the lashes reveals nits.

Treatment
Early treatment is essential to prevent recurrence or complications. Treatment depends on the type of blepharitis:

• *seborrheic blepharitis:* daily shampooing (using a mild shampoo on a damp applicator stick or a washcloth) to remove scales from the lid margins; also, frequent shampooing of the scalp and eyebrows
• *ulcerative blepharitis:* sulfonamide eye ointment or an appropriate antibiotic
• *blepharitis resulting from pediculosis:* removal of nits (with forceps), or application of ophthalmic physostigmine ointment as an insecticide (this may cause pupil constriction and, possibly, headache, conjunctival irritation, and blurred vision from the film of ointment on the cornea).

Additional considerations

• The patient should remove scales from the lid margins daily, with an applicator stick or clean washcloth.
• The patient should apply warm compresses by: running warm water into a clean bowl; immersing a clean cloth in the water and wringing it out; placing it against the closed eyelid, but being careful not to burn the skin; holding the compress in place until it cools; and continuing this procedure for 15 minutes.
• If blepharitis results from pediculosis, the patient's family and other contacts should be checked and local health authorities notified.

Exophthalmos
(Proptosis)

Exophthalmos is the unilateral or bilateral bulging or protrusion of the eyeballs, or their apparent forward displacement (as with lid retraction). Prognosis depends on the underlying cause.

Causes

Exophthalmos usually results from thyroid disorders, such as Graves' disease (thyrotoxicosis), in which forward displacement of the eyeballs and lid retraction occur. Unilateral exophthalmos most commonly results from trauma (such as fracture of the ethmoid bone, which allows air from the sinus to enter the orbit, displacing the soft tissue and the eyeball). Exophthalmos may also stem from hemorrhage, varicosities, thrombosis, aneurysms, and edema, which similarly displace the eyeballs.

Other systemic and ocular causes include the following:
• *diseases:* leukemia and lymphoma
• *infection:* orbital cellulitis, panophthalmitis, and infection of the lacrimal gland or orbital tissues
• *tumors:* especially in children—rhabdomyosarcomas, gliomas of the optic nerve, dermoid cysts, teratomas, metastatic neuroblastomas, and African lymphoma; in adults—lacrimal gland tumors, mucoceles, meningiomas, and

metastatic carcinomas
• *parasitic cysts:* in surrounding tissue
• *paralysis of extraocular muscles:* relaxation of eyeball retractors, congenital macrophthalmia, and high myopia.

Signs and symptoms

The obvious effect is a bulging eyeball. A common feature is diplopia, if edema disrupts the visual axis. A rim of the sclera may be visible around the limbus, and the patient may blink infrequently. Other symptoms depend on the cause: Pain may accompany traumatic exophthalmos; a tumor may produce conjunctival hyperemia or chemosis; retraction of the upper lid predisposes to exposure keratitis. If exophthalmos is associated with cavernous sinus thrombosis, the patient may exhibit paresis of the muscles supplied by cranial nerves III, IV, and VI; limited ocular movement; and a septic-type (high) fever.

Diagnosis

Exophthalmos is obvious on physical

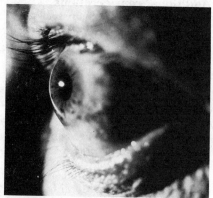

This photo of exophthalmos shows characteristic forward protrusion of the eye from the orbit.

examination; exophthalmometer readings confirm diagnosis by showing the degree of anterior projection and asymmetry between the eyes (normal bar readings range from 12 to 20 mm). Other diagnostic measures identify the cause:
• *X-rays* show orbital fracture, or bony erosion by an orbital tumor.
• *CAT scan* detects pathology (lesions in the optic nerve, orbit, or ocular muscle) in the area within the orbit that is, relatively, radiologically blind.
• *Culture* of discharge from cellulitis or panophthalmitis determines the infecting organism; sensitivity testing indicates appropriate antibiotic therapy.
• *Biopsy* of orbital tissue may be necessary if initial treatment fails.

Treatment
The goal of treatment is to correct the underlying cause. For example, eye trauma may require cold compresses for the first 24 hours, followed by warm compresses, and prophylactic antibiotic

therapy. After edema subsides, surgery may be necessary. Eye infection requires treatment with broad-spectrum antibiotics during the 24 hours preceding positive identification of the organism, followed by specific antibiotics. A patient with exophthalmos resulting from an orbital tumor may initially benefit from antibiotic or corticosteroid therapy. Eventually, however, surgical exploration of the orbit and, depending on the tumor, excision of the tumor, enucleation, or exenteration are necessary.

Treatment of Graves' disease may include antithyroid drug therapy, or partial or total thyroidectomy to control hyperthyroidism; initial high doses of systemic corticosteroids, such as prednisone, for optic neuropathy; guanethidine (10%) eyedrops to temporarily correct lid retraction and improve appearance; and if lid retraction is severe, application of protective lubricants.

Surgery may include lateral tarsorrhaphy (suturing the lateral sections of the eyelids together) to correct lid retraction, or Krönlein's operation (removal of the superior and lateral orbital walls) to decompress the orbit. Such decompression is necessary if vision is threatened.

Additional considerations
• If medication (steroids, antibiotics) is ordered, the patient's response to therapy should be carefully documented.
• Cold and warm compresses should be applied for fractures or other trauma.
• The patient will need appropriate postoperative care.
• Tests and procedures must be thoroughly explained.
• Emotional support should be given, especially to the patient with sudden onset of exophthalmos.

Ptosis

Ptosis (drooping of the upper eyelid) may be congenital or acquired, unilateral or bilateral, constant or intermittent. Severe ptosis usually responds well to treatment; slight ptosis may require no treatment at all.

Causes and incidence

Congenital ptosis is transmitted as an autosomal dominant trait or results from a congenital anomaly in which the levator muscles of the eyelids fail to develop. This condition is usually bilateral.

Acquired ptosis may result from any of the following:

• *age* (senile ptosis), which causes loss of tone in the levator muscles, usually producing bilateral ptosis

• *mechanical factors* that make the eyelid heavy, such as swelling caused by a foreign body on the palpebral surface of the eyelid or by edema, inflammation produced by a tumor or pseudotumor, or an extra fatty fold

• *myogenic factors*, such as muscular dystrophy or myasthenia gravis (in which the defect seems to be in humoral transmission at the myoneural junction)

• *neurogenic (paralytic) factors* from interference in innervation of the eyelid by the oculomotor nerve (cranial nerve III), most commonly due to trauma, diabetes, or carotid aneurysm

• *nutritional factors*, especially Wernicke's syndrome, due to severe chronic alcoholism, hyperemesis gravidarum, and other malnutrition-producing states.

Signs and symptoms

An infant with congenital ptosis has a smooth, flat upper eyelid, without the tarsal fold normally caused by the pull of the levator muscle; associated weakness of the superior rectus muscle is not uncommon.

The child with unilateral ptosis that covers the pupil can develop an amblyopic eye from disuse or lack of eye stimulation. In bilateral ptosis, the child may elevate his brow in an attempt to compensate, wrinkling his forehead in an effort to raise the upper lid. Also, the child may tilt his head backward to see.

In myasthenia gravis, ptosis results from fatigue and characteristically appears in the evening, but is relieved by rest. Oculomotor nerve damage produces a fixed, dilated pupil; divergent strabismus; and slight depression of the eyeball.

Diagnosis

 A physical examination that consists of measuring palpebral fissure widths, range of lid movement, and relation of lid margin to upper border of the cornea confirms ptosis. Diagnosis also includes tests to determine the underlying cause:

• *glucose tolerance test:* diabetes

• *edrophonium test:* myasthenia gravis (in acquired ptosis with no history of trauma)

• *ophthalmologic examination:* foreign bodies

• *patient history:* Wernicke's syndrome

• *cerebral arteriography:* aneurysm.

Treatment

Slight ptosis that doesn't produce deformity or loss of vision requires no treatment. Severe ptosis that interferes with vision or is cosmetically undesirable usually necessitates resection of the weak levator muscles. Surgery to correct congenital ptosis is usually performed at age 3 or 4, but it may be done earlier if ptosis is unilateral, since the totally occluded pupil may cause an amblyopic eye. If surgery is undesirable, special glasses with an attached suspended crutch on the frames may elevate the eyelid.

Effective treatment of ptosis also requires treatment of the underlying cause. For example, in patients with myasthenia gravis, neostigmine may be prescribed to increase the effect of acetylcholine and aid transmission of nerve impulses to muscles.

Additional considerations

The hospital staff member should:

• report any bleeding immediately; watch for blood on the pressure patch or head bandage after surgery to correct ptosis. (This bandage is worn for 24 hours after surgery, to prevent swelling.)

• emphasize to the patient and family the importance of preventing accidental trauma to the surgical site until healing is complete (6 weeks). Damage to the suture line can precipitate recurrence of ptosis.

Orbital Cellulitis

Orbital cellulitis is an acute infection of the orbital tissues and eyelids that doesn't involve the eyeball. With treatment, prognosis is good; if cellulitis is not treated, infection may spread to the cavernous sinus or the meninges.

Causes and incidence

Orbital cellulitis is usually secondary to streptococcal, staphylococcal, or pneumococcal infection of nearby structures. These organisms then invade the orbit, frequently by direct extension through the sinuses (especially the ethmoidal sinus), the bloodstream, or the lymphatic ducts. Primary orbital cellulitis results from orbital trauma that permits entry of bacteria, such as an insect bite. It's most common in young children.

Signs and symptoms

Orbital cellulitis generally produces unilateral eyelid edema, hyperemia of the orbital tissues, reddened eyelids, and matted lashes. Although the eyeball is initially unaffected, proptosis may develop later (because of edematous tissues within the bony confines of the orbit). Other indications include extreme orbital pain, impaired eye movement, chemosis, and purulent discharge from indurated areas. The severity of associated systemic symptoms (chills, fever, and malaise that may progress to marked debility) varies according to the cause.

Complications include posterior extension, causing cavernous sinus thrombosis, meningitis, or brain abscess, and, rarely, atrophy and subsequent loss of vision secondary to optic neuritis.

Diagnosis

Typical clinical features establish diagnosis. Wound culture and sensitivity testing determine the causative organism and specific antibiotic therapy. Other supportive tests include:
• *WBC* (elevated from infection of the orbital tissues) and *ophthalmologic examination* (to rule out cavernous sinus thrombosis).

Treatment

Prompt treatment is necessary to prevent complications. Primary treatment consists of appropriate antibiotic therapy, depending on the results of culture and sensitivity tests. Systemic antibiotics (I.V., P.O.), as well as eyedrops or ointment, will be ordered. Supportive therapy consists of fluids; warm, moist compresses; and bed rest. If antibiotic therapy fails, incision and drainage may be necessary.

Additional considerations

• Vital signs must be monitored, and fluid and electrolyte balance maintained.
• Compresses should be applied every 3 to 4 hours to localize inflammation and relieve discomfort, and the patient should be taught how to apply these compresses. Pain medication, as ordered, can be given after assessing pain level.
• Before discharge, the patient must understand the importance of completing prescribed antibiotic therapy. To prevent orbital cellulitis, he should maintain good general hygiene, and carefully cleanse abrasions and cuts that occur near the orbit. Early treatment of orbital cellulitis will prevent infection from spreading.

Dacryocystitis

Dacryocystitis is a common infection of the lacrimal sac. In adults, it results from an obstruction (dacryostenosis) of the nasolacrimal duct (most often in women over age 40) or from trauma; in infants, it results from congenital atresia of the nasolacrimal duct. Dacryocystitis can be acute or chronic and is usually unilateral.

Causes

The most common infecting organism in acute dacryocystitis is *Staphylococcus aureus* or, occasionally, beta-hemolytic streptococcus. In chronic dacryocystitis, *Streptococcus pneumoniae* and, sometimes, a fungus—such as *Candida albicans*—are the causative organisms.

In infants, atresia of the nasolacrimal ducts results from failure of canalization; or, in the first few weeks of life, from blockage when the membrane that separates the lower part of the nasolacrimal duct and the inferior nasal meatus fails to open spontaneously before tear secretion. It may also result from obstruction of the duct by gross abnormalities of the nasal bones.

Signs and symptoms

The hallmark of both acute and chronic forms of dacryocystitis is constant tearing. Other symptoms of acute dacryocystitis include inflammation and tenderness over the nasolacrimal sac; pressure over this area may produce purulent discharge from the punctum. In the chronic form, a mucoid discharge may be expressed from the tear sac.

Diagnosis

Clinical features and a physical examination suggest dacryocystitis. Culture of the discharged material demonstrates *S. aureus* and, occasionally, beta-hemolytic streptococcus in acute dacryocystitis; *S. pneumoniae* or *C. albicans* in the chronic form. WBC may be elevated in the acute form; in the chronic form, it's generally normal. An X-ray

after injection of a radiopaque medium (dacryocystography) locates the atresia.

Treatment

Treatment of acute dacryocystitis consists of application of warm compresses, and topical and systemic antibiotic therapy. Chronic dacryocystitis may eventually require dacryocystorhinostomy.

Therapy for nasolacrimal duct obstruction in an infant consists of careful massage of the area over the lacrimal sac 4 times a day for 2 to 3 months. If this fails to open the duct, dilation of the punctum and probing of the duct are necessary. Postoperative management requires a pressure patch over the area of the eye, and nasal packing.

Additional considerations

• The patient's history should be checked for possible allergy to antibiotics before administration. He must understand the importance of complying precisely with prescribed antibiotic therapy.

• After surgery, the adult patient should lie on the operative side, with his arm behind him and his head tilted forward on a pillow, to facilitate drainage of blood. This position keeps the sinuses on the opposite side free of secretions and aids breathing.

• Blood loss can be monitored by counting dressings used to collect the blood.

• Ice compresses should be applied postoperatively. After the patch and packing are removed (24 to 48 hours after surgery), a small adhesive bandage should be placed over the suture line to protect it.

Chalazion

A chalazion is a granulomatous inflammation of a meibomian gland in the upper or lower eyelid. This common eye disorder is characterized by localized swelling, and usually develops slowly over several weeks. A chalazion may become large enough to press on the eyeball, producing astigmatism; a large chalazion seldom subsides spontaneously. It's generally benign and chronic, and can occur at any age; in some patients, it's apt to recur.

Causes

Obstruction of the meibomian (sebaceous) gland duct causes a chalazion.

Signs and symptoms

A chalazion occurs as a painless, hard lump that usually *points toward* the conjunctival side of the eyelid. Eversion of the lid reveals a red or red-yellow elevated area on the conjunctival surface.

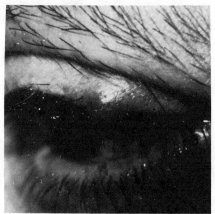

Chalazion, a nontender granulomatous inflammation of a meibomian gland on the upper eyelid.

Diagnosis

Diagnosis requires visual examination and palpation of the eyelid, revealing a small bump or nodule. Persistently recurrent chalazions, especially in an adult, necessitate biopsy, to rule out meibomian cancer.

Treatment and additional considerations

Initially, treatment of a chalazion consists of application of warm compresses to open the lumen of the gland and, occasionally, instillation of sulfonamide eyedrops. If such therapy fails, or if the chalazion presses on the eyeball or causes a severe cosmetic problem, incision and curettage under local anesthetic may be necessary. After such surgery, a pressure eyepatch applied for 8 to 24 hours controls bleeding and swelling. After removal of the patch, treatment again consists of warm compresses applied for 10 to 15 minutes, 2 to 4 times daily, and antimicrobial eyedrops or ointment to prevent secondary infection.

Care includes:
- teaching proper lid hygiene to the patient disposed to chalazions (water and mild baby shampoo applied with a cotton applicator).
- instructing the patient how to properly apply *warm* compresses, such as taking special care to avoid burning the skin, always using a clean cloth, and discarding used compresses; telling the patient to apply warm compresses at the first sign of lid irritation, to increase the blood supply and keep the lumen open.

Stye
(Hordeolum)

A localized, purulent staphylococcal infection, a stye can occur externally (in the lumen of the smaller glands of Zeis or in the sweat glands of Moll) or internally (in the larger meibomian gland). A stye can occur at any age. Generally, this infection responds well to treatment but tends to recur; an untreated stye can lead to cellulitis of the eyelid.

Signs and symptoms

Typically, a stye produces redness, swelling, and pain. An abscess frequently forms at the lid margin, with an eyelash pointing outward from its center.

Diagnosis

Visual examination generally confirms this infection. Culture of purulent material from the abscess usually reveals a staphylococcal organism.

Treatment

Treatment consists of warm compresses applied for 10 to 15 minutes, 4 times a day for 3 to 4 days, to facilitate drainage of the abscess, to relieve pain and inflammation, and to promote suppuration. Drug therapy includes a topical sulfonamide or antibiotic eyedrops or ointment, and occasionally, a systemic antibiotic. If conservative treatment fails, incision and drainage may be necessary.

Additional considerations

• The patient should use a clean cloth for each application of warm compresses, and should dispose of it or launder it separately to prevent spreading this infection to family members. For the

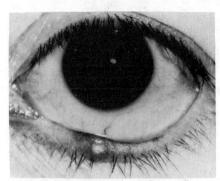

A stye is a localized red, swollen, and tender abscess of the lid glands.

same reason, the patient should avoid sharing towels and washcloths, and should follow good general hygiene.

• The patient must not squeeze the stye; this spreads the infection and may cause cellulitis.

• The patient or family members must be taught the proper technique for instilling eyedrops or ointments into the cul-de-sac of the lower eyelid.

CONJUNCTIVA

Inclusion Conjunctivitis
(Inclusion blennorrhea)

A fairly common disease, inclusion conjunctivitis is an acute ocular inflammation resulting from infection by Chlamydia oculogenitalis. *Although inclusion conjunctivitis occasionally becomes chronic, prognosis is generally good.*

Causes

C. oculogenitalis (an organism of the psittacosis-lymphogranuloma venereum-trachoma group that may be a large, atypical virus) usually infects the urethra in males and the cervix in females, and is transmitted during sexual activity. Since contaminated cervical secretions infect the eyes of the neonate during birth, inclusion conjunctivitis is an important cause of ophthalmia neonatorum. Transmission of *C. oculogenitalis* can also occur through the water in im-

properly chlorinated swimming pools. Rarely, inclusion conjunctivitis results from autoinfection, when an infected person transfers the virus from his genitourinary tract to his own eyes.

Signs and symptoms

Inclusion conjunctivitis develops 5 to 10 days after contamination (it takes longer to develop than gonococcal ophthalmia). In a newborn, the lower eyelids redden, and a thick, purulent discharge develops. In children and adults, follicles appear inside the lower eyelids; such follicles don't form in infants because the lymphoid tissue is not yet well developed. Children and adults also develop preauricular lymphadenopathy and, as a complication, otitis media. Inclusion conjunctivitis may persist for weeks or months, possibly with superficial corneal involvement. In newborns, pseudomembranes may form, which can lead to conjunctival scarring.

Diagnosis

Clinical features and a history of recent swimming in pools suggest inclusion conjunctivitis.

Examination of Giemsa-stained conjunctival scraping reveals cytoplasmic inclusion bodies in conjunctival epithelial cells, many polymorphonuclear leukocytes, and a negative culture for bacteria.

Treatment

Treatment consists of eyedrops of 1% tetracycline in oil, erythromycin ophthalmic ointment or sulfonamide eyedrops 5 or 6 times daily for 2 weeks for infants, and oral tetracycline or erythromycin for 3 weeks for adults. In severe inclusion conjunctivitis, adults may require concomitant systemic sulfonamide therapy.

Additional considerations

• The patient's eyes must be kept as clean as possible. The eyes should be cleaned from the inner to the outer canthus. Warm soaks can be applied, as needed, and the amount and color of drainage should be recorded.

• If the patient's eyes are sensitive to light, the room should be kept dark. He may need appropriate diversionary activities.

• Further spread of inclusion conjunctivitis can be prevented by: washing hands thoroughly before and after administering eye medications; suggesting genital examination of the mother of an infected newborn or of any adult with inclusion conjunctivitis; obtaining a history of recent sexual contacts, so they can be examined for inclusion conjunctivitis.

Conjunctivitis

Conjunctivitis is characterized by hyperemia of the conjunctiva due to infection, allergy, or chemical reactions. This disorder usually occurs as benign, self-limiting pinkeye; it may also be chronic, possibly indicating degenerative changes or damage from repeated acute attacks. In the Western hemisphere, conjunctivitis is probably the most common eye disorder.

Causes

The most common causative organisms are the following:

• *bacterial: Staphylococcus aureus, Streptococcus pneumoniae, Neisseria gonorrhoeae, Neisseria meningitidis*

• *chlamydial: Chlamydia trachomatis; Chlamydia oculogenitalis* (inclusion conjunctivitis)

• *viral:* adenovirus types 3, 7, and 8; herpes simplex virus, Type 1.

Other causes include allergic reactions to pollen, grass, topical medications, air pollutants, smoke, or unknown seasonal allergens (vernal conjunctivitis); occupational irritants (acids and alkalies); rickettsial diseases (Rocky Mountain spotted fever); parasitic diseases caused by *Phthirus pubis, Schistosoma haematobium*; and rarely, fungal infections.

Vernal conjunctivitis (also called seasonal or warm-weather conjunctivitis) results from allergy to an unidentified allergen. This form of conjunctivitis is bilateral; it usually begins before puberty and persists for about 10 years. It is sometimes associated with other signs of allergy commonly related to grass or pollen sensitivity.

An idiopathic form of conjunctivitis may be associated with certain systemic diseases, such as erythema multiforme, chronic follicular conjunctivitis (orphan's conjunctivitis), and thyroid disease. Conjunctivitis may be secondary to pneumococcal dacryocystitis or canaliculitis due to candidal infection.

Signs and symptoms

Conjunctivitis commonly produces hyperemia of the conjunctiva, sometimes accompanied by discharge, tearing, pain, and with corneal involvement, photophobia. It generally doesn't affect vision. Conjunctivitis usually begins in one eye and rapidly spreads to the other by contamination of towels, washcloths, or the patient's own hand.

Acute bacterial conjunctivitis (pinkeye) usually lasts only 2 weeks. The patient typically complains of itching, burning, and the sensation of a foreign body in his eye. His eyelids show a crust of sticky, mucopurulent discharge. If the disorder is due to *N. gonorrhoeae,* however, the patient exhibits a profuse, purulent discharge.

Viral conjunctivitis produces copious tearing with minimal exudate, and enlargement of the preauricular lymph node. Some viruses follow a chronic course and produce severe disabling disease, while others last 2 to 3 weeks.

Diagnosis

Physical examination reveals injection of the conjunctival vessels. In children, possible systemic symptoms include sore throat or fever. Monocytes are predominant in stained smears of conjunctival scrapings if the disorder is caused by a virus; polymorphonuclear cells (neutrophils), if due to bacteria; and eosinophils, if allergy-related. Culture and sensitivity tests identify the causative bacterial organism and indicate appropriate antibiotic therapy.

Treatment

Treatment of conjunctivitis varies with

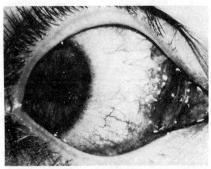

Allergy, infection, or physical or chemical trauma can cause an inflammation of the conjunctiva, which produces redness, pain, swelling, lacrimation, and possible discharge.

the cause. Bacterial conjunctivitis requires topical application of the appropriate antibiotic or sulfonamide. Although viral conjunctivitis resists treatment, a sulfonamide or broad-spectrum antibiotic eyedrops may prevent secondary infection. Herpes simplex infection generally responds to treatment with idoxuridine or vidarabine ointment, but the infection may persist for 2 to 3 weeks. Treatment of vernal (allergic) conjunctivitis includes administration of vasoconstrictor eyedrops, such as epinephrine; cold compresses to relieve itching; and occasionally, oral antihistamines.

Instillation of 1% silver nitrate into the eyes of newborns prevents gonococcal conjunctivitis.

Additional considerations

Health care includes:
• teaching proper handwashing technique, since some forms of conjunctivitis are highly contagious; stressing the risk of spreading infection to family members by sharing washcloths, towels, and pillows; warning against rubbing the infected eye, which can spread the infection to the other eye and to other persons.
• applying warm compresses and therapeutic ointment or drops, as ordered; avoiding irrigating the eye, as this will spread infection; having the patient wash his hands before he uses the medication, and telling him to use clean washcloths

or towels frequently so he doesn't infect his other eye.
• teaching the patient to instill eyedrops and ointments correctly—without the bottle tip touching his eye or lashes.

• stressing the importance of safety glasses for the patient who works near chemical irritants.
• notifying public health authorities if cultures show *N. gonorrhoeae.*

Trachoma

The most common cause of blindness in underdeveloped areas of the world, trachoma is a chronic form of keratoconjunctivitis. This infection is usually confined to the eye but can also localize in the urethra. Although trachoma itself is self-limiting, it causes permanent damage to the cornea and conjunctiva; severe trachoma may lead to blindness, especially if a secondary bacterial infection develops. Early diagnosis and treatment (before trachoma results in scar formation) ensure recovery but without immunity to reinfection. Trachoma is prevalent in Africa, Latin America, and Asia, particularly in children; in the United States, it is prevalent among the American Indians of the Southwest.

Causes
Trachoma results from infection by *Chlamydia trachomatis,* an organism of the psittacosis-lymphogranuloma venereum-trachoma group. These organisms, whose characteristics place them between true viruses and rickettsiae, display some bacterial properties; they are transmitted from eye to eye by flies and gnats in endemic areas. Trachoma is spread by close contact between family members or among schoolchildren. Other prediposing factors include poverty, and poor hygiene due to lack of water, especially in desert areas.

Signs and symptoms
Trachoma begins with a mild infection resembling bacterial conjunctivitis (visible conjunctival follicles, red and edematous eyelids, pain, photophobia, tearing, and exudation). After about 1 month, if the infection is untreated, conjunctival follicles enlarge into inflamed papillae that later become yellow or gray. At this stage, small blood vessels invade the cornea under the upper lid (superior pannus). Eventually, severe scarring and contraction of the eyelids cause entropion; the eyelids turn inward and the lashes rub against the cornea, producing

corneal scarring and visual distortion. Severe conjunctival scarring may obstruct the lacrimal ducts and cause dry eyes.

Diagnosis
Follicular conjunctivitis with corneal infiltration, and pannus or conjunctival scarring suggest trachoma, especially in endemic areas, when these symptoms persist longer than 3 weeks.

 Microscopic examination of a Giemsa-stained conjunctival scraping confirms diagnosis by showing cytoplasmic inclusion bodies, some polymorphonuclear reaction, plasma cells, Leber's cells (large macrophages containing phagocytosed debris), and follicle cells.

Treatment and additional considerations
Primary treatment of trachoma consists of 3 to 4 weeks of topical or systemic antibiotic therapy with tetracycline, erythromycin, or sulfonamides. (Tetracycline is contraindicated in pregnant females because it may adversely affect epiphyseal development in the fetus, and in children under age 7, in whom it may cause permanent discoloration of teeth.)

Severe entropion necessitates surgery.

• The patient must understand the importance of handwashing and making the best use of available water supplies to maintain good personal hygiene. To prevent trachoma, patients should avoid allowing flies or gnats to settle around the eyes.

• No definitive preventive measure exists (available vaccines offer temporary and partial protection, at best). Patients must comply with the prescribed drug therapy.

• If eyedrops are ordered, the patient or family members must be taught how to instill them correctly.

CORNEA

Keratoconus

Keratoconus is a rare, degenerative eye disorder typified by thinning and anterior protrusion of the cornea. It predominantly affects females (70%), is usually bilateral, and begins during puberty. With treatment, prognosis is generally good.

Causes
Keratoconus is probably transmitted as an autosomal recessive trait. It's commonly associated with Down's and Marfan's syndromes, and atopic dermatitis; less commonly, with retinitis pigmentosa, vernal catarrh (allergic conjunctivitis due to spring pollens), and aniridia (congenital absence of the iris).

Signs and symptoms
Generally, the first symptom of keratoconus is blurred vision, possibly accompanied by acute hydrops of the cornea, in which central corneal edema impairs vision. Another feature is cone-shaped corneas, which produce indentations in the lower eyelids when the patient looks down (Munson's sign).

Diagnosis
Visual examination with only a flashlight reveals ruptures (similar to stretch marks) in Descemet's membrane (a clear, elastic membrane, one of the five corneal layers).

Distorted corneal reflection on examination with a Placido's disk (used to measure the amount and character of corneal astigmatism), and abnormal keratometer readings (used to measure corneal curves) confirm keratoconus. The fundus of the eye isn't clearly visible, due to corneal distortion. Retinoscopy reveals an irregular shadow.

Treatment and additional considerations
In the early stages of the disorder, hard contact lenses, or spectacle lenses with high astigmatic correction rectify the corneal astigmatism and improve visual acuity. Cornea transplantation (penetrating keratoplasty) is necessary in patients with acute hydrops that has left a central scar after healing, or in patients with corneal thinning that threatens perforation. Such surgery is effective in 90% of patients. Preoperatively, the hospital staff member should:

• instill eyedrops to protect the lens by induced miosis.

• make sure the patient understands that strict bed rest may be necessary for 24 hours after surgery.

After cornea transplantation, the staffer should:

• tell the patient not to bend over or perform activities that may cause stress or increase intraocular pressure; place the call button within easy reach, and help with personal care, as needed.

• administer analgesics for pain, as or-

dered; report persistent pain immediately, since it may indicate hemorrhage, infection, or ineffectiveness of the prescribed pain medication.
• encourage gradual return to normal activity; instruct the patient to return after discharge for regular checkups.

Efforts to promote postmortem donations of healthy corneas to an eye bank should be supported. Persons who are interested in making such donations should be taught how to do so.

Keratitis

Keratitis, inflammation of the cornea, may be acute or chronic, superficial or deep. Superficial keratitis is fairly common and may develop at any age. Prognosis is good, with treatment. Untreated, recurrent keratitis may lead to blindness.

Causes
Keratitis usually results from infection by herpes simplex type 1 virus (such as dendriform keratitis). It may also result from exposure, due to the patient's inability to close his eyelids, or from congenital syphilis (interstitial keratitis). Less commonly, it stems from bacterial and fungal infections.

Signs and symptoms
Usually unilateral, keratitis produces opacities of the cornea, mild irritation, tearing, and photophobia. If the infection is in the center of the cornea, it may produce blurred vision. When keratitis results from exposure, it usually affects the lower portion of the cornea.

Diagnosis

Slit-lamp examination confirms keratitis. If keratitis is due to herpes simplex virus, staining the eye with a fluorescein strip produces one or more small branchlike (dendritic) lesions; touching the cornea with cotton reveals reduced corneal sensation. Vision testing may show slightly decreased acuity. Patient history may reveal a recent infection of the upper respiratory tract accompanied by cold sores (also caused by herpes simplex type 1 virus).

Treatment
Treatment of acute keratitis due to herpes simplex virus consists of idoxuridine eyedrops and ointment, or vidarabine ointment; and of recurrent herpetic keratitis, trifluridine. A broad-spectrum antibiotic may prevent secondary bacterial infection. Chronic dendriform keratitis may respond more quickly to vidarabine. Long-term topical therapy may be necessary. (Corticosteroid therapy is contraindicated in dendriform keratitis or any other viral or fungal disease of the cornea; such therapy may exacerbate the infection and predispose to corneal perforation.) When keratitis results from fungal infection, treatment consists of natamycin.

Keratitis due to exposure requires application of moisturizing ointment to the exposed cornea, and a plastic bubble eyeshield or eyepatch. In patients with severe corneal scarring, treatment may include keratoplasty (cornea transplantation).

Additional considerations
Patients predisposed to cold sores should be checked for keratitis. They should know that stress, trauma, fever, colds, and overexposure to the sun may trigger flare-ups.

The patient should be told that the ointment may temporarily blur his vision.

The exposed corneas of unconscious patients with half-opened eyes can be protected by cleaning the eyes daily, applying moisturizing ointment, or covering the eyes with a plastic bubble eyeshield.

Corneal Abrasion

A corneal abrasion is a scratch on the surface epithelium of the cornea, often caused by a foreign body. An abrasion, or foreign body in the eye is the most common eye injury. With treatment, prognosis is usually good.

Causes

A corneal abrasion usually results from a foreign body, such as a cinder or a piece of dust, dirt, or grit, that becomes embedded under the eyelid. Even if the foreign body is washed out by tears, it may still injure the cornea. Small pieces of metal that get in the eyes of workers who don't wear protective glasses quickly form a rust ring on the cornea and cause corneal abrasion. Such abrasions also commonly occur in the eyes of persons who fall asleep wearing hard contact lenses.

A corneal scratch produced by a fingernail, a piece of paper, or other organic substance may cause a persistent lesion. The epithelium doesn't always heal properly, and a recurrent corneal erosion may develop, with delayed effects more severe than the original injury.

Signs and symptoms

Typically, corneal abrasions produce redness, increased tearing, a sensation of "something in the eye," and because the cornea is richly endowed with nerve endings from the trigeminal nerve (cranial nerve V), pain disproportionate to the size of the injury. A corneal abrasion may affect visual acuity, depending on the size and location of the injury.

Diagnosis

History of eye trauma or prolonged wearing of contact lenses, and typical symptoms suggest corneal abrasion.

Staining the cornea with fluorescein stain confirms the diagnosis: The injured area appears green when examined with a flashlight. Slit-lamp examination discloses the depth of the abrasion.

Examining the eye with a flashlight may reveal a foreign body on the cornea; the eyelid must be everted to check for a foreign body embedded under the lid.

Before beginning treatment, a test to determine visual acuity provides a medical baseline and a legal safeguard.

Treatment and additional considerations

Treatment of a deeply embedded foreign body consists of removal with a foreign body spud, using a topical anesthetic. A rust ring on the cornea can be removed with an ophthalmic burr, after applying a topical anesthetic. When only partial removal is possible, re-epithelialization lifts the ring to the surface again, and allows complete removal the following day.

Treatment also includes instillation of broad-spectrum antibiotic eyedrops in the affected eye every 3 to 4 hours. Initial application of a pressure patch prevents further irritation when the patient blinks.

• Before beginning treatment, the patient's visual acuity in the affected eye should be checked.

• If a foreign body is visible, the eye is irrigated with normal saline solution.

• The patient should be reassured that the corneal epithelium usually heals in 24 to 48 hours.

• The patient must follow the antibiotic eyedrop therapy ordered, since an untreated corneal infection can lead to ulceration and permanent loss of vision. The patient should be taught the proper way to instill eye medications.

• Safety glasses are absolutely necessary to protect workers' eyes from flying fragments. Persons wearing contact lenses should follow instructions for wearing and caring for them, to prevent trauma.

way to instill eye medications.
• Safety glasses are absolutely necessary to protect workers' eyes from flying frag-

ments. Persons wearing contact lenses should follow instructions for wearing and caring for them, to prevent trauma.

Corneal Ulcers

A major cause of blindness worldwide, ulcers produce corneal scarring or perforation. They occur in the central or marginal areas of the cornea, vary in shape and size, and may be singular or multiple. Marginal ulcers are the most common form. Prompt treatment (within hours of onset) can prevent visual impairment.

Causes

Corneal ulcers generally result from bacterial, viral, or fungal infections. Common bacterial sources include *Staphylococcus aureus, Pseudomonas aeruginosa, Streptococcus viridans, Streptococcus (Diplococcus) pneumoniae,* and *Moraxella liquefaciens;* viral sources, herpes simplex type 1, variola, vaccinia, and varicella-zoster viruses; common fungal sources, *Candida, Fusarium,* and *Cephalosporium.*

Other causes include trauma, exposure, reactions to bacterial infections, toxins, and allergens. Tuberculoprotein causes a classic phlyctenular keratoconjunctivitis; vitamin A deficiency results in xerophthalmia; and fifth cranial nerve lesions, neurotropic ulcers.

Signs and symptoms

Typically, corneal ulceration begins with pain (aggravated by blinking), followed by increased tearing. Eventually, central corneal ulceration produces pronounced visual blurring. The eye may appear injected, from congestion in the conjunctival blood vessels. Purulent discharge is possible with a bacterial ulcer.

Diagnosis

Patient history—possibly indicating trauma—and examination, using a flashlight, that reveals irregular corneal surface suggest corneal ulcer. Exudate may be present on the cornea, and a hypopyon (accumulation of white cells or pus in the anterior chamber) may produce cloudiness or color change.

Fluorescein dye, instilled in the conjunctival sac, stains the outline of the ulcer and confirms the diagnosis.

Culture and sensitivity testing of corneal scraping may identify the causative bacteria or fungus, and indicate appropriate antibiotic or antifungal therapy.

Treatment and additional considerations

Generally, treatment consists of systemic and topical broad-spectrum antibiotics until culture results identify the causative organism. The goals of treatment are to eliminate the underlying cause of the ulcer and to relieve pain:
• *infection by P. aeruginosa:* polymyxin B and gentamicin, administered topically and by subconjunctival injection, or carbenicillin and tobramycin I.V. Since this type of corneal ulcer spreads so rapidly, it can cause corneal perforation and loss of the eye within 48 hours. Immediate treatment and isolation of hospitalized patients are required. *Note:* Treatment of a corneal ulcer due to bacterial infection should *never* include an eyepatch, since patching creates the dark, warm, moist environment ideal for bacterial growth.
• *herpes simplex type 1 virus:* hourly topical application of idoxuridine or vidarabine. Corneal ulcers resulting from a viral infection often recur, in which case, trifluridine becomes the treatment of choice.
• *varicella-zoster virus:* topical sulfon-

amide ointment applied three to four times daily to prevent secondary infection. These lesions are unilateral, following the pathway of the fifth cranial nerve, and are quite painful, requiring analgesics. Associated anterior uveitis requires cycloplegic eyedrops. The patient should be observed for signs of secondary glaucoma (increased intraocular pressure, transient vision loss, and halos around lights).

• *fungi:* topical instillation of natamycin for *Fusarium, Cephalosporium,* and *Candida.*

• *hypersensitivity reactions:* topical corticosteroids, such as dexamethasone and hydrocortisone.

• *hypovitaminosis A:* correction of dietary deficiency or gastrointestinal malabsorption of vitamin A.

• *neurotropic ulcers or exposure keratitis:* frequent instillation of artificial tears or lubricating ointments and use of a plastic bubble eyeshield.

Prompt treatment is essential for all forms of corneal ulcer, to prevent complications and permanent visual impairment.

UVEAL TRACT, RETINA, AND LENS

Uveitis

Uveitis is inflammation of the uveal tract. It occurs as anterior uveitis, which affects the iris (iritis), or both the iris and the ciliary body (iridocyclitis); as posterior uveitis, which affects the choroid (choroiditis), or both the choroid and the retina (chorioretinitis); or as panuveitis, which affects the entire uveal tract. Untreated anterior uveitis progresses to posterior uveitis, causing scarring, cataracts, and glaucoma. With immediate treatment, anterior uveitis usually subsides after a few days to several weeks; however, recurrence is likely. Posterior uveitis generally produces some residual visual loss and marked blurring of vision.

Causes

Anterior uveitis occurs in two forms, although clinical distinction is not always possible. The granulomatous form follows microbial infection resulting from debilitating disease (tuberculosis, histoplasmosis, toxoplasmosis); the nongranulomatous form, from an improperly healed corneal abrasion, particularly when the abrasion results from a sharp object, rheumatoid arthritis, sarcoidosis, or idiopathic causes.

Posterior uveitis is always granulomatous, and results from debilitating disease or as a complication of unresolved iritis.

Signs and symptoms

Anterior uveitis produces moderate to severe eye pain, severe injection, photophobia, and a small, nonreactive pupil from iris spasm that inhibits eye accommodation.

Onset of symptoms in posterior uveitis is insidious. The patient may complain of floating spots, pain (less severe than in iritis), and photophobia (less severe than in anterior uveitis). Posterior synechiae (adhesions of the iris to the lens) or scar formation causes distortion of the shape of the pupil, cataract, glaucoma, retinal detachment, and anterior uveitis. Posterior uveitis also causes gradual blurring of vision, and injection.

Diagnosis

In both anterior and posterior uveitises, a slit-lamp examination shows keratitic precipitates (round, pale deposits on the corneal endothelium) and Koeppe nodules in the iris, especially if the underlying disorder is sarcoidosis. In posterior

GRANULOMATOUS AND NONGRANULOMATOUS UVEITIS

FACTOR	GRANULOMATOUS	NONGRANULOMATOUS
Location	• Any part of uveal tract, but usually the posterior part	• Anterior portion: iris, ciliary body
Onset	• Insidious	• Acute
Pain	• None or slight	• Marked
Photophobia	• Slight	• Marked
Course	• Chronic	• Acute
Prognosis	• Fair to poor	• Good
Recurrence	• Occasional	• Common

Adapted with permission from Lillian S. Brunner and Doris S. Suddarth, TEXTBOOK OF MEDICAL-SURGICAL NURSING (Philadelphia: J.B. Lippincott Co., 1980).

uveitis, a large inflamed area is also visible with the slit lamp. In both forms, skin tests for tuberculosis and histoplasmosis, and chest X-rays assist in determining the cause.

Treatment

Vigorous and prompt management of both anterior and posterior uveitises is required to prevent complications. Treatment of the underlying cause is essential. In addition, pupil dilation with mydriatics, such as scopolamine, rests the eye and prevents the formation of posterior synechiae. In anterior uveitis, treatment also includes corticosteroid drops to reduce inflammation and promote healing. In posterior uveitis, therapy includes systemic corticosteroids (prednisone), diuretics (such as acetazolamide) to reduce intraocular pressure, epinephrine eyedrops to reduce tearing and photophobia, and possibly, subconjunctival or retrobulbar injections of steroids.

Additional considerations

Care of the patient with uveitis includes:
• encouraging bed rest during the acute phase of posterior uveitis.
• before discharge, teaching the patient the proper method of instilling eyedrops to prevent scarring, which can cause cataracts or glaucoma.
• suggesting the use of dark glasses to ease the discomfort of photophobia.
• instructing the patient to watch for and report side effects of systemic corticosteroid therapy (edema, muscle weakness).
• stressing the importance of follow-up care because of the strong likelihood of recurrence; telling the patient to immediately seek treatment at first signs of iritis.

Retinal Detachment

In retinal detachment, the sensory portion of the retina separates from the pigment epithelium of the choroid. Retinal detachment is usually unilateral and most commonly affects males. New surgical techniques allow reattachment in more than 90% of patients. However, prognosis for good visual acuity is uncertain after prolonged detachment of the macula.

Causes

Any retinal tear or hole allows the liquid vitreous to seep between the retina and choroid, pushing the retina off the choroid. In adults, retinal detachment usually results from degenerative changes of aging, which cause a spontaneous retinal hole as the vitreous framework shrinks and pulls away from the retina. Predisposing factors include myopia, cataracts, surgery, and trauma. Retinal detachment may also follow retinopathy from systemic diseases—such as severe hypertension, chronic glomerulonephritis, periarteritis nodosa, and diabetes mellitus—and vascular disturbances in the retina and choroid, such as retinal vein occlusion or choroidal carcinoma.

In children, retinal detachment usually results from trauma or high myopia; less frequently, from choroidal or retinal tumors, inflammation, or vascular diseases. Idiopathic detachments are uncommon in children; most cases appear to be hereditary.

Signs and symptoms

Initially, the patient may complain of floating spots and recurrent flashes of light. However, as detachment progresses, he experiences gradual, painless vision loss.

Diagnosis

Diagnosis depends on ophthalmoscopy after full pupil dilation.

Such examination shows the usually pink retina as gray and opaque, with an indefinite margin. In severe detachment, examination reveals folds in the retina and a ballooning out of the area. Indirect ophthalmoscopy is also used to search the retina for additional tears.

Treatment

Treatment depends on the location and severity of the detachment but usually includes restriction of eye movements through bed rest, sedation, an eyepatch, and proper head positioning, so the tear or hole is in a dependent position in relation to the rest of the eye. Retinal detachment rarely heals spontaneously;

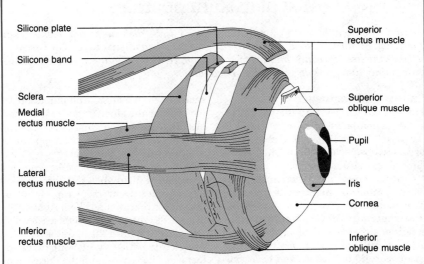

SURGICAL CORRECTION OF RETINAL DETACHMENT

Silicone plate
Silicone band
Sclera
Medial rectus muscle
Lateral rectus muscle
Inferior rectus muscle

Superior rectus muscle
Superior oblique muscle
Pupil
Iris
Cornea
Inferior oblique muscle

In scleral buckling, cryotherapy (cold therapy), photocoagulation (laser therapy), or diathermy (heat therapy) creates a sterile inflammatory reaction that causes retinal readherence. The surgeon then implants a silicone plate at the site of reattachment beneath the dissected scleral flaps. When the flaps are sutured together, the pressure exerted on the plate indents (buckles) the eyeball and gently pushes the choroid closer to the retinal hole.

surgery, consisting of scleral buckling, is necessary to seal the retina in place as it heals.

Additional considerations
• The patient will need emotional support, since he may be understandably distraught because of his loss of vision. A relaxing atmosphere, and a call bell within easy reach, will help him stay calm and relaxed.
• To prepare the patient for surgery, his face should be washed with a surgical soap preparation, and his eyelashes cut off to minimize the risk of infection. The patient is given antibiotics and mydriatic eyedrops (adults get scopolamine, and children a combination of cyclopentolate and phenylephrine).
• Postoperatively, patient positioning is important. Generally the head of the bed is elevated about 30°. The patient should not bend over, strain, or rub his eyes, but he is allowed to move his head in any direction. He should try to ambulate as soon as possible. If bed rest is prolonged, he should be encouraged to do leg exercises to prevent thrombophlebitis.
• The eye should be gently cleansed with warm compresses. Then topical ophthalmic medication should be instilled. The patient usually will need mydriatic drops to keep the pupil dilated and to reduce inflammation.
• The patient must be carefully observed for possible complications, such as hemorrhagic choroidal detachment or retinal redetachment. The patient and family should be taught how to instill eyedrops and ointments, and must understand the importance of follow-up examinations. The patient should use dark glasses in bright light because of the dilated pupil.

Vascular Retinopathies

Vascular retinopathies are noninflammatory retinal disorders that result from interference with the blood supply to the eyes. The four distinct types of vascular retinopathy are central retinal artery occlusion, central retinal vein occlusion, diabetic retinopathy, and hypertensive retinopathy.

Causes and incidence
The retinal arteries feed the capillaries and thus maintain blood circulation in the retina. When one of these vessels becomes obstructed, diminished blood flow causes visual deficits.

Central retinal artery occlusion may be idiopathic, or may result from embolism, atherosclerosis, infection (syphilis, rheumatic fever, hepatitis), or conditions that retard blood flow, such as temporal arteritis, massive hemorrhage, carotid occlusion, and heart failure. This disorder is rare, usually occurs unilaterally, and most commonly affects the elderly.

Causes of *central retinal vein occlusion* include external compression of the retinal vein, trauma, diabetes, phlebitis, thrombosis, granulomatous diseases, generalized infection, inflammation of the orbit or the sinuses, gastrointestinal bleeding, glaucoma, and atherosclerosis. This form of vascular retinopathy is most prevalent in the elderly.

Diabetic retinopathy results from juvenile or adult diabetes. Microcirculatory changes occur more rapidly when diabetes is poorly controlled. About 75% of patients with juvenile diabetes develop retinopathy within 20 years of onset of diabetes. In patients with adult diabetes, incidence increases with the duration of diabetes. For example, 80% of patients who have had diabetes for 20 to 25 years develop retinopathy. This condition is a leading cause of acquired adult blindness.

Hypertensive retinopathy results from prolonged hypertensive disease, produc-

DIAGNOSTIC TESTS FOR VASCULAR RETINOPATHIES

CENTRAL RETINAL ARTERY OCCLUSION	CENTRAL RETINAL VEIN OCCLUSION	DIABETIC RETINOPATHY	HYPERTENSIVE RETINOPATHY
• **Ophthalmoscopy (direct or indirect):** shows emptying of retinal arterioles during transient attack. • **Slit-lamp examination:** within 2 hours of onset, shows clumps or segmentation in artery; later, milky white retina around disk due to swelling and necrosis of ganglion cells caused by reduced blood supply; also shows cherry-red spot in macula that subsides after several weeks. • **Ophthalmodynamometry:** approximately measures the relative pressures in the central retinal arteries and indirectly assesses internal carotid artery obstruction. • **Ultrasonography:** reveals condition of blood vessels. • **Physical examination:** reveals underlying cause.	• **Slit-lamp examination:** shows retinal hemorrhage, retinal vein engorgement, white patches among hemorrhages, edema around the disk. • **Ultrasonography:** confirms or rules out occlusion of blood vessels. • **Physical examination:** reveals underlying cause.	• **Slit-lamp examination:** shows thickening of retinal capillary walls. • **Indirect ophthalmoscopy:** shows retinal changes such as microaneurysms (earliest change), retinal hemorrhages and edema, venous dilation and twisting, exudates, vitreous hemorrhage, proliferation of fibrin into vitreous due to retinal holes, growth of new blood vessels, and microinfarcts of nerve fiber layer. • **Fluorescein angiography:** shows leakage of fluorescein from dilated vessels, and differentiates between microaneurysms and true hemorrhages. • **History:** diabetes	• **Ophthalmoscopy (direct or indirect):** in early stages, shows hard, shiny deposits, tiny hemorrhages, and elevated arterial blood pressure; in late stages, cotton wool patches, exudates, retinal edema, papilledema due to ischemia and capillary insufficiency, hemorrhages, and microaneurysms. • **History:** hypertension

ing retinal vasospasm, and consequent damage and narrowing of the arteriolar lumen.

Signs and symptoms

Central retinal artery occlusion produces sudden, painless, unilateral loss of vision (partial or complete). It may follow amaurosis partialis fugax, or transient episodes of unilateral loss of vision lasting from a few seconds to minutes, probably due to vasospasm. This condition causes permanent blindness unless treatment begins within hours of onset.

Central retinal vein occlusion causes reduced visual acuity, allowing perception of only hand movement and light. This condition is painless, except when caused by glaucoma. Prognosis is poor—

5% to 20% of patients with this type of vascular retinopathy develop secondary glaucoma within 3 to 4 months following occlusion.

Diabetic retinopathy typically produces an edematous retina, which scatters light, causing glare; visual acuity decreases in later stages. If this disorder occurs in a simple form, prognosis is good when treated promptly; in a malignant (proliferative) form, prognosis is poor (50% of patients become blind within 5 years).

Symptoms of hypertensive retinopathy depend on location of retinopathy. For example, mild visual disturbances, such as blurred vision, result from retinopathy located near the fovea centralis. Prognosis varies with the severity of the disorder. Severe, prolonged disease pro-

VASCULAR RETINOPATHIES

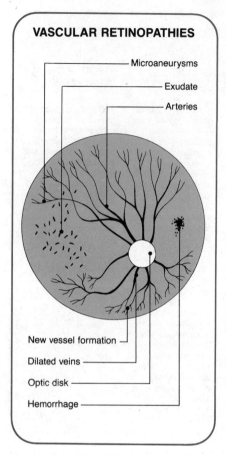

- Microaneurysms
- Exudate
- Arteries
- New vessel formation
- Dilated veins
- Optic disk
- Hemorrhage

oxygen, 5% carbon dioxide by face mask to improve circulation; global massage to move the embolus; anticoagulants (such as heparin or warfarin); and anterior chamber tap or acetazolamide to reduce intraocular pressure. Hospitalization and testing are necessary to determine the cause and to prevent occlusion in the other eye.

Therapy for central retinal vein occlusion includes anticoagulants to prevent additional thrombi, and management of underlying causes. If therapy is unsuccessful, enucleation may be necessary.

Treatment of diabetic retinopathy consists of sealing retinal holes and areas of new vessel leakage with an argon laser (photocoagulation), although degenerative changes are difficult to treat. Hypertensive retinopathy necessitates antihypertensive therapy. In all types of vascular retinopathy, vitrectomy may partially restore sight following vitreous hemorrhage.

Additional considerations
- *Immediate* treatment is necessary when a patient complains of sudden, unilateral loss of vision. Blindness may be permanent if treatment is delayed.
- A baseline blood pressure reading should be obtained before inhalation treatment with oxygen and carbon dioxide is begun. Blood pressure must be monitored carefully during treatment, since such a patient is commonly hypertensive. If blood pressure rises markedly, therapy must be stopped immediately.
- Drug therapy may include anticoagulants to prevent embolism and acetazolamide to reduce intraocular pressure.
- The patient must follow the prescribed treatment carefully to prevent the disorder from developing bilaterally or causing further visual impairment.

duces blindness; mild, prolonged disease, visual defects.

Diagnosis
Appropriate diagnostic tests depend on the type of vascular retinopathy.

Treatment
In central retinal artery occlusion, treatment must begin within several hours of onset, and includes inhalation of 95%

Cataract

A common cause of vision loss, a cataract is a gradually developing opacity of the lens or lens capsule of the eye. Cataracts commonly occur bilaterally, with each progressing independently. Two possible exceptions are traumatic cataracts, which are usually unilateral, and congenital cataracts, which may remain stationary. progress. Cataracts are most prevalent in persons over age 70, as part of aging. Prognosis is generally good; surgery improves vision in 95% of affected persons.

Causes

Cataracts have various causes:
- *Senile cataracts* develop in the elderly, probably because of changes in the chemical state of lens proteins.
- *Congenital cataracts* occur in newborns as genetic defects or due to maternal rubella during the first trimester.
- *Traumatic cataracts* develop after a foreign body injures the lens with sufficient force to allow aqueous or vitreous humor to enter the lens capsule.
- *Complicated cataracts* occur secondary to uveitis, glaucoma, retinitis pigmentosa, or detached retina.
- *Toxic cataracts* result from drug or chemical toxicity with ergot, dinitrophenol, naphthalene, and phenothiazines, or from galactose in patients with galactosemia.

Signs and symptoms

Typically, a patient with a cataract experiences painless, gradual blurring and loss of vision. As the cataract progresses, the normally black pupil turns milky white. Some patients see halos around lights and blinding glare from headlights when they drive at night; others complain of poor reading vision, and of an unpleasant glare and poor vision in bright sunlight. Patients with central opacities can see better in dim light than in bright light.

Diagnosis

On examination, shining a penlight on the pupil reveals the white area behind the pupil (unnoticeable until the cataract is advanced) and suggests a cataract.

 Ophthalmoscopy or slit-lamp examination confirms the diagnosis by revealing a dark area or shadow in the normally homogenous red reflex.

Treatment

Treatment consists of surgical extraction of the defective lens and postoperative correction of visual deficits. Surgical procedures for such extraction include the following:
- *Intracapsular cataract extraction*, the most common procedure, removes the entire lens with the capsule intact by cryoextraction (the moist lens sticks to a extremely cold metal probe for easy and safe removal with gentle traction).
- *Extracapsular cataract extraction* removes the cortex and lens, and retains the posterior lens capsule; this procedure is often used for children and young adults.
- *Phacoemulsion* fragments the lens with ultrasonic vibrations and aspirates the pieces; occasionally, this procedure is performed on patients under age 30.
- *Discission* ruptures the lens capsule, allowing the aqueous humor access to the lens, to be slowly digested.

Possible complications of surgery include wound rupture from loosening of sutures, hyphema, prolapse of the iris into the anterior chamber, loss of vitreous, adhesions, infection, pupillary block glaucoma, and retinal detachment.

Postoperatively, visual deficits can be corrected by various methods. Initially, the patient receives temporary cataract spectacle lenses that are usually made of dark glass to prevent glare. About 3 months after surgery, he receives permanent lenses, which affect central vision only; the patient must turn his head for peripheral vision. However, after unilateral cataract extraction, the patient generally complains of diplopia, since he doesn't have normal binocular vision.

Another effective postoperative procedure consists of fitting the patient with contact lenses 1 month after surgery; these lenses eliminate the distortion often produced by glasses. In addition to decreasing magnification, they restore both central and peripheral vision. Instead of prescribing glasses or contact lenses, some surgeons implant an intraocular lens directly behind the cornea during cataract surgery.

Additional considerations

After surgery to extract a cataract, the hospital staff member should:
• maintain 30° elevation of the head of the bed; warn the patient to avoid activities that increase intraocular pressure (bending, straining, or lying flat).
• urge the patient to protect the eye from accidental injury by wearing a Fox shield (a metal shield with perforations) or glasses during the day, and a Fox shield at night.
• administer mydriatic drops, as ordered, to dilate the pupil and keep it at rest, antibiotic ointment or drops to prevent infection, and steroids to reduce inflammation.
• watch for complications, such as prolapse of the iris, a sudden sharp pain in the eye, or hyphema, and report them immediately.
• teach correct instillation of eyedrops before discharge (usually 1 to 5 days after uncomplicated surgery), and instruct the patient to notify the doctor immediately if he experiences sharp eye pain; caution him about activity restrictions, and advise him that it takes several weeks to adjust to wearing cataract spectacle lenses.

Retinitis Pigmentosa

Retinitis pigmentosa is a genetically induced, progressive destruction of the retinal rods, resulting in atrophy of the pigment epithelium and eventual blindness. Incidence ranges from 1 in 2,000 to 1 in 7,000 live births. Retinitis pigmentosa often accompanies other hereditary disorders in several distinct syndromes; the most common is Laurence-Moon-Biedl syndrome, typified by visual destruction from retinitis pigmentosa, obesity, mental retardation, polydactyly, and hypogenitalism.

Causes

About 80% of children with retinitis pigmentosa inherit it as an autosomal recessive trait. Onset occurs before age 20, initially affecting night and peripheral vision, and progresses inevitably—sometimes rapidly—to blindness before age 50. Retinitis pigmentosa can also be transmitted as an X-linked trait, producing the least common but most severe form of the disease, usually causing blindness before age 40.

Typically, in all forms of retinitis pigmentosa, the retinal rods slowly deteriorate; subsequently, the rest of the retina and pigment epithelium atrophy. Clumps of pigment resembling bone corpuscles aggregate in the equatorial region of the retina, and ultimately involve the macular and peripheral regions. In advanced stages, the retinal arterioles narrow, and the disk appears pale and waxy.

Signs and symptoms

Generally, night blindness occurs while the patient is in his teens. As the disease progresses, his visual field gradually constricts, causing tunnel or "gun-barrel" vision and, possibly, other ocular disorders, such as cataracts, choroidal sclerosis, macular degeneration, glaucoma, keratoconus, or scotomata (blind spots). Eventually, blindness follows invasion of the macula.

Diagnosis

A detailed family history may imply predisposition to retinitis pigmentosa. In a patient whose history suggests this condition, the following tests help confirm diagnosis.
• *Electroretinography* shows a retinal response time slower than normal or absent.
• *Visual field testing* (using a tangent screen) detects ring scotomata.

• *Fluorescein angiography* visualizes white dots (areas of dyspigmentation) in the epithelium.
• *Ophthalmoscopy* may initially show normal fundi but later reveals characteristic black pigmentary disturbance.

Treatment
Although extensive research continues, no cure exists for retinitis pigmentosa.

Additional considerations
• The patient and family should be taught about the various aspects of retinitis pigmentosa. They should know that it's a hereditary disease, and should seek genetic counseling for young adults who risk transmitting it to their children.
• The patient should wear dark glasses in bright sunlight, and should know that he might not be able to drive a car at night. (Special new glasses can help patients with retinitis pigmentosa see at night but are experimental and expensive.)
• The patient should be referred to a social service agency or to the National Retinitis Pigmentosa Foundation for information and for counseling to prepare him for eventual blindness. He should consider learning braille.
• Since the prospect of blindness is frightening, the patient will need emotional support and guidance.

MISCELLANEOUS

Optic Atrophy

Optic atrophy, or degeneration of the optic nerve, can develop spontaneously (primary) or follow inflammation or edema of the nerve head (secondary). Some forms of this condition may subside without treatment, but degeneration of the optic nerve is irreversible.

Causes
Optic atrophy usually results from CNS disorders, such as:
• pressure against the optic nerve, resulting from aneurysms or from intraorbital or intracranial tumors (descending optic atrophy)
• optic neuritis, in multiple sclerosis, retrobulbar neuritis, and tabes.

Other causes include retinitis pigmentosa; chronic papilledema and papillitis; congential syphilis; glaucoma; central retinal artery or vein occlusion that interrupts the blood supply to the optic nerve, causing degeneration of ganglion cells (ascending optic atrophy); trauma; and ingestion of toxins, such as methanol and quinine.

Symptoms and diagnosis
Optic atrophy produces painless loss of either visual field or visual acuity, or both. Loss of vision may be abrupt or gradual, depending on the cause.

Slit-lamp examination and ophthalmoscopy confirm the diagnosis. Slit-lamp examination reveals pallor of the optic disk, and a nonreactive pupil that dilates instead of constricting when exposed to light. Ophthalmoscopy shows pallor of the nerve head from loss of microvascular circulation in the disk and deposit of fibrous or glial tissue. Visual field testing may show a scotoma.

Treatment and additional considerations
Generally, treatment of optic atrophy consists of correcting the underlying cause to prevent further vision loss. Steroids are given to decrease inflammation and swelling. In patients with multiple sclerosis and resulting optic neuritis, optic atrophy of-

ten subsides spontaneously.

During diagnostic procedures and treatment the patient will need symptomatic health care. The patient who is visually compromised will need help performing daily activities.

Understanding all procedures will help the patient minimize his anxiety. He will need emotional support to help him deal with his loss of vision.

Extraocular Motor Nerve Palsies
(Ophthalmoplegia)

Extraocular motor nerve palsies are dysfunctions of the third, fourth, and sixth cranial nerves. The oculomotor (third cranial) nerve innervates the inferior, medial, and superior rectus muscles; the inferior oblique extraocular muscles; the pupilloconstrictor muscles; and the levator palpebrae muscles. The trochlear (fourth cranial) nerve innervates the superior oblique muscles; the abducens (sixth cranial) nerve innervates the lateral rectus muscles. Complete dysfunction of the third cranial nerve is called total oculomotor ophthalmoplegia and may be associated with other CNS abnormalities.

Causes

The most common causes of extraocular motor nerve palsies are diabetic neuropathy, and pressure from an aneurysm or brain tumor. Other causes vary, depending on the particular cranial nerve involved:

• *Third nerve palsy* (acute ophthalmoplegia) also results from brain stem ischemia or other cerebrovascular disorders, poisoning (lead, carbon monoxide, botulism), alcohol abuse, infections (measles, encephalitis), trauma to the extraocular muscles, myasthenia gravis, or tumors in the cavernous sinus area.

• *Fourth nerve (trochlear) palsy* also results from closed-head trauma (blowout fracture) or sinus surgery.

• *Sixth nerve (abducens) palsy* also results from increased intracranial pressure, brain abscess, meningitis, arterial brain occlusion, infections of the petrous bone (rare), lateral sinus thrombosis, myasthenia gravis, and thyrotropic exophthalmos.

Signs and symptoms

The most characteristic clinical effect of extraocular motor nerve palsies is diplopia of recent onset, which varies in different visual fields, depending on the muscles affected.

Typically, the patient with third nerve palsy exhibits ptosis, exotropia (eye looks outward), pupil dilation, and unresponsiveness to light; the eye is unable to move and cannot accommodate.

The patient with fourth nerve palsy displays diplopia and an inability to rotate the eye downward or upward. Such a patient develops ocular torticollis (wryneck) from repeatedly tilting his head to one side to compensate for vertical diplopia.

Sixth nerve palsy causes one eye to turn; the eye cannot abduct beyond the midline. To compensate for diplopia, the patient turns his head to one side and develops torticollis.

Diagnosis

Diagnosis necessitates a complete neuroophthalmologic examination and a thorough patient history. Differential diagnosis of third, fourth, or sixth nerve palsy depends on the specific motor defect exhibited by the patient. For all extraocular motor nerve palsies, skull X-rays and CAT scans rule out tumors. The patient is also evaluated for an aneurysm or diabetes. If sixth nerve palsy results from infection, culture and sensitivity tests identify the causative organism and determine specific antibiotic therapy.

Treatment and additional considerations

Identification of the underlying cause is essential, since treatment varies accordingly. Neurosurgery is necessary if the cause is a brain tumor or an aneurysm. For infection, massive doses of antibiotics I.V. may be appropriate. Otherwise, treatment and health care vary according to symptoms.

Nystagmus

Nystagmus is recurring, involuntary eyeball movement. Such movement may be horizontal, vertical, rotating, or mixed; it produces blurred vision and difficulty in focusing. Nystagmus is classified according to eye movement characteristics and may be jerking or pendular. Prognosis varies with the underlying cause.

Causes

Although nystagmus may be congenital, it is usually an acquired disorder. *Jerking nystagmus*, the most common type, results from excessive stimulation of the vestibular apparatus in the inner ear or from lesions of the brain stem or cerebellum. This disorder occurs in acute labyrinthitis, Ménière's disease, multiple sclerosis, vascular lesions (especially in patients with hypertension), and any inflammation of the brain (such as encephalitis). Jerking nystagmus may also result from drug and alcohol toxicity, and congenital neurologic disorders.

Pendular nystagmus results from improper transmission of visual impulses to the brain in the presence of corneal opacification, high astigmatism, congenital cataract or congenital anomalies of the optic disk, or bilateral macular lesions. Other causes include optic atrophy and albinism.

Signs and symptoms

In jerking nystagmus, the eyeballs oscillate faster in one direction than in the other; in pendular nystagmus, horizontal movements are approximately equal in both directions. If nystagmus results from a localized lesion, it may be unilateral; if from systemic disease, it's usually bilateral.

Diagnosis

The opticokinetic drum test is useful in diagnosing the underlying cause of nystagmus. In this test, the patient looks at a rapidly rotating, vertically striped drum—first at the stripes themselves, then quickly in the direction from which the stripes are coming, producing a normal jerking movement of the eyeballs. The absence of such a response suggests a CNS disturbance (such as a brain stem lesion).

Injecting warm or cold water into the external ear canal (caloric stimulation) also can precipitate nystagmus in an unaffected person. In patients with labyrinthine disorders, the response is abnormal (hypo- or hyperactive) or absent.

Positional testing involves quickly changing the patient's position from supine to upright, and turning his head from side to side, precipitating nystagmus. The direction of the nystagmus response aids diagnosis.

Treatment and additional considerations

The goal of treatment of nystagmus is to correct the underlying cause, if possible. Unfortunately, the underlying cause often has no known cure (for example, brain stem lesions or multiple sclerosis). Eyeglasses can correct visual disturbances, such as high astigmatism. The patient can help himself see by positioning his head in a certain way; if he can't focus with both eyes, he can turn his head and use only one eye.

A clear, thorough explanation of all testing procedures will help minimize the patient's anxiety.

The patient with nystagmus of rapid onset will need emotional support, since the disorder may be caused by a brain stem lesion or some other severe neurologic disturbance.

Strabismus

(Cross-eye, squint, heterotropia, walleye)

Strabismus is a condition of eye deviation due to the absence of normal, parallel, or coordinated eye movement. It may be concomitant, in which the degree of deviation doesn't vary with the direction of gaze; inconcomitant, in which the degree of deviation varies with the direction of gaze; obvious (tropia); or latent (phoria), apparent in children when they cry or are angry. Possible deviations include esotropia (eyes deviate inward), exotropia (eyes deviate outward), and vertical strabismus, such as hypertropia (one eye higher than the other) or hypotropia (one eye lower than the other). Prognosis varies according to the cause and severity of the condition, and the timing of treatment. For example, disorders of muscle imbalance are largely correctable (by orthoptic training or surgery) if treatment begins in early childhood. If treatment is delayed, some residual defect may persist. Strabismus affects about 2% of the population.

Causes

The most common cause of strabismus in children (about half of all cases) is amblyopia (lazy eye). This condition results from the suppression of vision in one eye due to unilateral myopia, or from double vision due to deviations such as esotropia or hypertropia. Esotropia may result from muscle imbalance (basic esotropia) or farsightedness (accommodative esotropia) or both. In accommodative esotropia, the child's attempt to compensate for the farsightedness af-

fects the convergent reflex, and the eyes cross. Misalignment of the eyes leads to suppression of one of the eyes, causing amblyopia, if it develops before age 5.

Strabismus frequently accompanies severe CNS disturbances, such as Down's syndrome, cerebral palsy, or mental retardation.

Signs and symptoms

Deviation of visual alignment and absence of coordinated eye movement are obvious at examination.

In addition, strabismus causes diplopia and the inability to see objects clearly.

Diagnosis

Generally, obvious deviation and uncoordinated eye movement establish this diagnosis. Ophthalmologic tests help ascertain the cause:

• *Visual acuity test* evaluates the degree of visual defect.

• *Retinoscopy* determines refractive error; usually done with eyes dilated.

• *Maddox rods test* assesses specific muscle involvement.

• *Convergence test* shows distance at which convergence is sustained.

• *Duction test* reveals limitation of eye

Note the medial deviation of the patient's left eye in this photo of esotropia.

movement.
• *Cover-uncover test* demonstrates eye deviation and the rate of recovery to original alignment.
• *Alternate-cover test* shows intermittent or latent deviation.
• *Neurologic examination* determines whether condition is muscular or neurologic in origin, and should be performed on all patients with strabismus.

Treatment
Initial treatment is generally conservative, and includes patching the normal eye and prescribing therapeutic eye exercises to force the affected eye to work (especially in amblyopia); corrective glasses may keep the eye straight and counteract farsightedness (especially in accommodative esotropia). Surgery is often necessary for cosmetic and psychologic reasons to correct strabismus due to basic esotropia, or residual accommodative esotropia after correction with glasses. The earlier this surgery is performed, the better the chance for correction. Surgical correction includes recession (moving the muscle posteriorly from its original insertion) or resection (shortening the muscle). Possible complications of surgery include over- or undercorrection, slipped muscle, and perforation of the globe. Postoperative therapy may include patching the affected eye, topical antibiotics, eye exercises, and glasses. It may be necessary to repeat surgery.

Additional considerations
• Postoperatively, a young child may require elbow restraints to prevent him from rubbing his eyes.
• Antibiotic ointment and antiemetics may be ordered.
• After surgery, the child should be checked carefully to see that the eye appears to move in all visual fields. If it doesn't, the muscle may have slipped. The surgeon must be notified immediately, so the child can be returned to the operating room for muscle repair.
• If the child must wear an eyepatch postoperatively, his parents should know that he'll lose depth perception and should be careful while playing or performing everyday activities, such as descending stairs.
• Parents should seek early treatment for their child to prevent vision loss from strabismus. If surgery is recommended, they should know that more than one operation may be necessary.

Glaucoma

The most preventable cause of blindness, glaucoma is abnormally increased intraocular pressure, which may produce severe and permanent vision defects. It occurs in several forms: chronic open-angle (most common), and acute or chronic closed-angle. Glaucoma affects 2% of the U.S. population over age 40—women more often than men—and accounts for 15% of all cases of blindness in the United States. Occasionally, glaucoma may be due to a congenital defect, inherited as an autosomal recessive trait. In all forms of glaucoma, prognosis is usually good with early diagnosis and treatment.

Causes and incidence
Chronic open-angle glaucoma results from overproduction of aqueous humor or obstruction to its outflow through the trabecular network, the canal of Schlemm, or aqueous veins. This form of glaucoma is frequently familial in origin, and affects 90% of all patients with glaucoma.

Acute closed-angle (narrow-angle) glaucoma results from obstruction to the outflow of aqueous humor due to anatomically narrow angles between the anterior iris and the posterior corneal surface, shallow anterior chambers, a

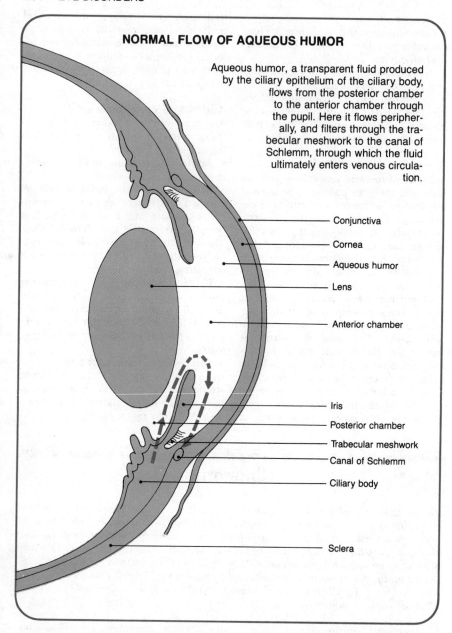

NORMAL FLOW OF AQUEOUS HUMOR

Aqueous humor, a transparent fluid produced by the ciliary epithelium of the ciliary body, flows from the posterior chamber to the anterior chamber through the pupil. Here it flows peripherally, and filters through the trabecular meshwork to the canal of Schlemm, through which the fluid ultimately enters venous circulation.

- Conjunctiva
- Cornea
- Aqueous humor
- Lens
- Anterior chamber
- Iris
- Posterior chamber
- Trabecular meshwork
- Canal of Schlemm
- Ciliary body
- Sclera

thickened iris that causes angle closure on pupil dilation, or a bulging iris that presses on the trabeculae, closing the angle (peripheral anterior synechiae).

Chronic closed-angle glaucoma follows an untreated attack of acute closed-angle glaucoma, or mild, recurring, acute attacks that produce increasing adhesions in the trabeculae.

Signs and symptoms
Chronic open-angle glaucoma is usually

bilateral, with insidious onset and a slowly progressive course. Symptoms appear late in the disease and include mild aching in the eyes, loss of peripheral vision, seeing halos around lights, and reduced visual acuity (especially at night) that is uncorrectable with glasses.

Acute closed-angle glaucoma typically has a rapid onset, constituting an ophthalmic emergency. Symptoms may include unilateral inflammation and pain, pressure over the eye, moderate pupil dilation that is nonreactive to light, a cloudy cornea, blurring and decreased visual acuity, photophobia, and seeing halos around lights. Increased intraocular pressure may induce nausea and vomiting, which may cause glaucoma to be misinterpreted as gastrointestinal distress. Unless treated promptly, this acute form of glaucoma produces blindness in 3 to 5 days.

Chronic closed-angle glaucoma has a gradual onset. It usually produces no symptoms, although blurred vision or seeing halos around lights is possible. If untreated, this type of glaucoma progresses to absolute glaucoma, the final stage of this disease, producing pain and blindness. Enucleation may be necessary to relieve extreme pain.

Diagnosis

Schiøtz or applanation tonometry confirms glaucoma by detecting increased intraocular pressure. Gonioscopy enables differentiation between chronic open-angle glaucoma, and acute or chronic closed-angle glaucoma by determining the angle of the anterior chamber of the eye. The angle is normal in chronic open-angle glaucoma. However, in older patients, partial closure of the angle may also occur, so that two forms of glaucoma may coexist.

Other relevant diagnostic measures include the following:

• *Ophthalmoscopy and slit-lamp examination:* Cupping and atrophy of the optic disk are visible in chronic open-angle glaucoma and late in chronic closed-angle glaucoma; a pale disk appears in acute closed-angle glaucoma.

• *Fingertip tension:* On gentle palpation of closed eyelids, one eye feels harder than the other in acute closed-angle glaucoma.

• *Perimetry or visual field tests:* The extent of chronic open-angle or chronic closed-angle deterioration is evaluated by determining peripheral vision loss.

Treatment

For chronic open-angle glaucoma, treatment initially decreases aqueous humor production through beta-blockers, such as timolol (contraindicated for asthmatics or patients with bradycardia); epinephrine to lower intraocular pressure; or diuretics, such as acetazolamide. Drug treatment also includes miotic eyedrops, such as pilocarpine, to facilitate the outflow of aqueous humor. Patients who are unresponsive to drug therapy may require a surgical filtering procedure that creates an opening for aqueous outflow.

Acute closed-angle glaucoma is an ocular emergency requiring immediate treatment to lower the high intraocular pressure. If pressure doesn't decrease

---

BLINDNESS

Blindness affects 28 million people worldwide. In the United States, blindness is legally defined as optimal visual acuity of 20/200 or less in the better eye after best correction, or a visual field not exceeding 20° in the better eye.

According to the World Health Organization, the most common causes of preventable blindness worldwide are trachoma, onchocerciasis (roundworm infection transmitted by a blackfly and other species of *Simulium*), and xerophthalmia (dryness of conjunctiva and cornea from vitamin A deficiency).

In the United States, the most common causes of acquired blindness are glaucoma, senile macular degeneration, and diabetic retinopathy. However, incidence of blindness from glaucoma is decreasing due to early detection and treatment. Rarer causes of acquired blindness include herpes simplex keratitis, cataracts, and retinal detachment.

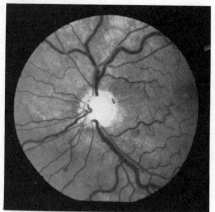

Ophthalmoscopy and slit-lamp examination show cupping of the optic disk characteristic of chronic glaucoma.

with drug therapy, peripheral iridectomy must be performed promptly to save the patient's vision. Iridectomy relieves pressure by excising part of the iris to reestablish aqueous humor outflow. A prophylactic iridectomy is performed a few days later on the opposite eye to prevent an acute episode of glaucoma in the normal eye. Preoperative drug therapy lowers intraocular pressure with acetazolamide, mannitol (20%), pilocarpine (constricts the pupil, forcing the iris away from the trabeculae, allowing fluid to escape), and oral glycerin (50%) to force fluid from the eye by making the blood hypertonic. Severe pain may necessitate narcotic analgesics.

In the patient with chronic closedangle glaucoma, pilocarpine drops terminate an acute attack or prevent one until peripheral iridectomy is performed. Surgery is bilateral to prevent onset of glaucoma in the normal eye. In chronic closed-angle glaucoma, a surgical filtering procedure may be effective.

Additional considerations
• The patient must understand the importance of meticulous compliance with prescribed drug therapy to prevent disk changes, loss of vision, and the need for surgery.
• The patient with acute closed-angle glaucoma should be given medications, as ordered, and should be prepared physically and psychologically for surgery.
• Postoperative care after peripheral iridectomy includes cycloplegic eyedrops to relax the ciliary muscle and to decrease inflammation, thus preventing adhesions. *Note:* Cycloplegics must be used only in the affected eye. The use of these drops in the normal eye may precipitate an attack of acute closed-angle glaucoma in this eye, threatening the patient's residual vision.
• Ambulation should be encouraged immediately after surgery.
• Following surgical filtering, postoperative care includes dilation and topical steroids to rest the pupil.
• The importance of glaucoma screening for early detection and prevention must be stressed. All persons over age 30, especially those with family histories of glaucoma, should have an annual tonometric examination.

Selected References

Adler, F. H. TEXTBOOK OF OPHTHALMOLOGY. Philadelphia: W.B. Saunders Co., 1968.

Bedford, M.A. COLOR ATLAS OF OPHTHALMOLOGICAL DIAGNOSES. Chicago: Year Book Medical Pubs., 1971.

Boyd-Monk, Heather. *Examining the External Eye, Part 1,* NURSING80. 10:5:58-62, May 1980.

Boyd-Monk, Heather. *Helping the Corneal Transplant Patient to See Again,* NURSING78. 8:2:47-52, February 1978.

Boyd-Monk, Heather. *Screening For Glaucoma,* NURSING79. 9:8:42-45, August 1979.

Cogan, David G. NEUROLOGY OF THE OCULAR MUSCLES, 2nd ed. Springfield, Ill.: Charles C. Thomas Pub., 1978.

Conn, Howard F., and Rex B. Conn, Jr. CURRENT DIAGNOSIS. Philadelphia: W.B. Saunders Co., 1980.

Gray, Henry. ANATOMY OF THE HUMAN BODY. Philadelphia: Lea & Febiger, 1973.

Harley, Robinson D., ed. PEDIATRIC OPHTHALMOLOGY. Philadelphia: W.B. Saunders Co., 1975.

Havener, William H. SYNOPSIS OF OPHTHALMOLOGY, 5th ed. St. Louis: C.V. Mosby Co., 1979.

Luckman, J., and K.C. Sorensen. MECIAL/SURGICAL NURSING, 2nd ed. Philadelphia: W.B. Saunders Co., 1980.

MacFaden, J.S. *Caring for the Patient with a Primary Retinal Detachment*, AMERICAN JOURNAL OF NURSING. 80:5:920-921, May 1980.

Moses, Robert A. ADLER'S PHYSIOLOGY OF THE EYE: CLINICAL APPLICATION, 6th ed. St. Louis: C.V. Mosby Co., 1975.

Newell, Frank W. OPHTHALMOLOGY—PRINCIPLES AND CONCEPTS. St. Louis: C.V. Mosby Co., 1974.

Paton, David. *Glaucomas: Diagnosis and Treatment*, CLINICAL SYMPOSIA. Summit, N.J.: Ciba Pharmaceutical Co. 28:2, 1976.

Perrin, Elizabeth D. *Laser Therapy for Diabetic Retinopathy*, AMERICAN JOURNAL OF NURSING. 80:4:664-665, April 1980.

Reinecke, Robert D., ed. STRABISMUS. New York: Grune & Stratton, 1978.

Saunders, William H., et al. NURSING CARE IN EYE, EAR, NOSE AND THROAT DISORDERS. St. Louis: C.V. Mosby Co., 1979.

Scheie, Harold G., and Daniel M. Alert. TEXTBOOK OF OPHTHALMOLOGY, 9th ed. Philadelphia: W.B. Saunders Co., 1977.

Vaughan, Daniel, and Taylor Asbury. GENERAL OPHTHALMOLOGY, 8th ed. Los Altos, Calif.: Lange Medical Publications, 1977.

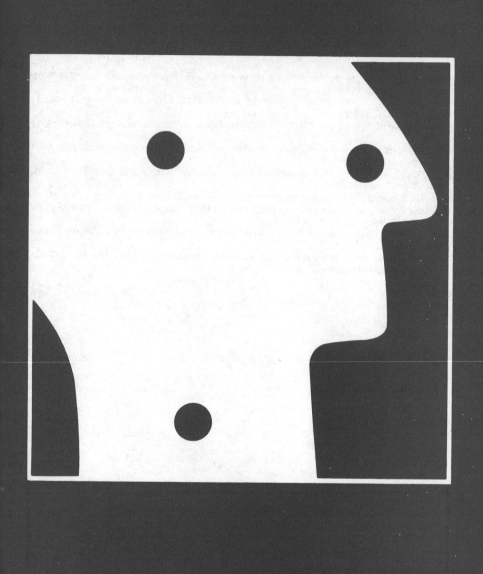

20 Ear, Nose, and Throat Disorders

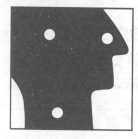

Ear, Nose, and Throat Disorders

Introduction

Most ear, nose, and throat disorders rarely prove fatal (except for those resulting from neoplasm) but may cause serious social, cosmetic, and communication problems. Untreated hearing loss or deafness can drastically impair ability to interact with society; ear disorders may also impair equilibrium. Nasal disorders can cause disturbing changes in facial features and interfere with breathing and tasting. Diseases arising in the throat may threaten airway patency and interfere with speech. Despite their relatively minor standing in the spectrum of human disease, these disorders can cause considerable discomfort and pain, and require thorough assessment and prompt treatment.

The ear

Hearing begins when sound waves reach the tympanic membrane, which then vibrates the ossicles in the middle ear cavity. The stapes transmits these vibrations to the perilymphatic fluid in the inner ear by vibrating against the oval window. The vibrations then pass across the cochlea's fluid receptor cells, in the basilar membrane, stimulating movement of the hair cells of the organ of Corti and initiating auditory nerve impulses to the brain.

The inner ear structures also maintain the body's equilibrium and balance through the fluid in the semicircular canals. This fluid is set in motion by body movement and stimulates nerve cells that line the canals. These cells, in turn, transmit impulses to the brain by way of the vestibular branch of the acoustic nerve.

Although the ear can respond to sounds that vibrate at frequencies from 20 to 20,000 hertz (Hz), the range of normal speech is from 250 to 4,000 Hz, with 70% falling between 500 and 2,000 Hz. The ratio between sound intensities, the decibel (db), is the lowest volume at which any given sound can be heard. A faint whisper registers 10 to 15 db; average conversation, 50 to 60 db; a shout, 85 to 90 db. Hearing damage may follow exposure to sounds louder than 90 db.

Assessment

After a patient history of ear disease is obtained, the auricle and surrounding tissue is inspected for deformities, lumps, and skin lesions. The patient is asked if he has ear pain. If inflammation is present, the ear is checked for tenderness by moving the auricle and pressing on the tragus and the mastoid process. The ear canal is examined for excessive cerumen, discharge, or foreign bodies.

The patient is asked if he's had episodes of vertigo or blurred vision. He is tested for vertigo by having him stand on one foot and close his eyes, or having him walk a straight line with his eyes closed. He is then asked if he always falls to the same side and if the room seems to be spinning.

Audiometric testing

Audiometric testing evaluates hearing and determines the type and extent of hearing loss. The simplest but least reliable method for judging hearing acuity consists of covering one of the patient's ears, standing 18″ to 24″ (45 to 60 cm) from the uncovered ear, and whispering a short phrase or series of numbers. (The patient's vision is blocked to prevent lip reading.) The patient is then asked to repeat the phrase or series of numbers. To test hearing at both high and low frequencies, the test can be repeated in a normal speaking voice. (As an alternative, a ticking watch can be held to the patient's ear.)

If a hearing loss is identified, further testing is necessary to determine if the loss is conductive or sensorineural. A conductive loss can result from faulty bone conduction (inability of the eighth cranial nerve to respond to sound waves traveling through the skull) or faulty air conduction (impaired transmission of sound through ear structures to the auditory nerve and, ultimately, the brain).

The following tests assess bone and air conduction:

• *Rinne test:* The base of a lightly vibrating tuning fork is placed on the mastoid process until it's no longer heard (bone conduction [BC]). Then the fork

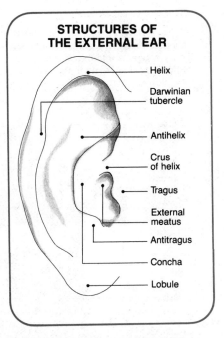

STRUCTURES OF THE EXTERNAL EAR

- Helix
- Darwinian tubercle
- Antihelix
- Crus of helix
- Tragus
- External meatus
- Antitragus
- Concha
- Lobule

is moved to the front of the meatus, where the patient should continue to hear the vibrations (air conduction [AC]). Normal AC time is about twice as long as BC time, but precise time measurement is difficult.

• *Weber test* (used for testing unilateral hearing loss): The handle of a lightly vibrating tuning fork is placed on the midline of the forehead. Normally, the patient should hear sounds equally in both ears. With conductive hearing loss, sound lateralizes (localizes) to the ear with the poorest hearing; with sensorineural loss, to the normal ear.

After identification of the hearing loss as conductive, sensorineural, or mixed, further audiometric testing determines the extent of hearing loss. These tests include pure tone audiometry, speech audiometry, impedance audiometry, and tympanometry.

• *Pure tone audiometry* produces a series of pure tones of calibrated loudness (db) at different frequencies (400 to 3,000 Hz). Speech threshold represents the loudness at which a person with nor-

mal hearing can perceive the tone. Both air and bone conduction are measured for each ear, and the results are plotted on a graph. If hearing is normal, the line is plotted at zero db.

• *Speech audiometry* uses the same technique as pure tone audiometry, but speech, instead of pure tones, is transmitted through the headset. (A person with normal hearing can hear and correctly repeat 95% to 100% of transmitted words.)

• *Impedance audiometry* detects middle ear pathology, precisely determining the degree of tympanic membrane and middle ear mobility. One end of the impedance audiometer, a probe with

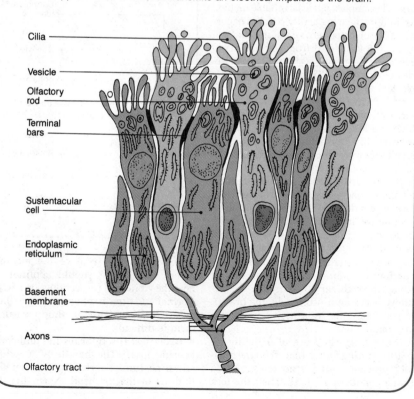

SENSE OF SMELL

Although the exact mechanism of olfactory perception is unknown, the most likely theory suggests that the sticky mucus covering the olfactory cells traps airborne odorous molecules. As the molecules fit into appropriate receptors on the cell surface, the opposite end of the cell transmits an electrical impulse to the brain.

Cilia

Vesicle

Olfactory rod

Terminal bars

Sustentacular cell

Endoplasmic reticulum

Basement membrane

Axons

Olfactory tract

three small tubes, is inserted into the external canal; the other end is attached to an oscillator. One tube delivers a low tone of variable intensity, the second contains a microphone, and the third, an air pump. A mobile tympanic membrane reflects minimal sound waves and produces a low-voltage curve on the graph. When the tympanic membrane shows decreased mobility, it reflects maximal sound waves and produces a high-voltage curve.

• *Tympanometry,* using the impedance audiometer, measures tympanic membrane compliance to air pressure variations in the external canal and determines the degree of negative pressure in the middle ear.

The nose

As air travels to the superior turbinate, it touches sensory hairs (cilia) in the mucosal surface, which then add, retain, or remove moisture and particles in the air to ensure the safe delivery of humid, bacteria-free air to the pharynx and lungs. In addition, when air touches mucosal cilia, stimulation of the first cranial nerve sends nerve impulses to the olfactory area of the frontal cortex, providing the sense of smell.

Assessment

The external nose should be checked for redness, edema, lumps, tumors, or poor alignment. Marked septal cartilage depression may be symptomatic of saddle deformity due to destruction of the septum from trauma or congenital syphilis; extreme lateral deviation, from injury; and thin, narrow nostrils, from chronically enlarged adenoids. Reddened nostrils may indicate frequent noseblowing as a result of acute allergies or infectious rhinitis. Dilated and engorged blood vessels may suggest chronic alcoholism or constant exposure to the elements. A bulbous, discolored nose may be a sign of chronic rosacea.

With a nasal speculum and adequate lighting, nasal mucosa should be checked for pallor and edema (allergic rhinitis) or redness and inflammation (viral rhin-

itis), dried mucous plugs (which may obstruct air exchange), furuncles, and polyps. Also, the patient should be examined for abnormal appearance of capillaries, a deviated or perforated septum, nasal discharge (color, consistency, odor) and blood. Profuse, thin, watery discharge may indicate allergy or cold; excessive, thin, purulent discharge may indicate cold or chronic sinus infection.

Sinus inflammation can be checked by applying pressure to the nostrils, orbital rims, and cheeks. Pain after pressure above the upper orbital rims indicates frontal sinus irritation; after pressure to the cheeks, maxillary sinus irritation. To check for sinusitis, equal pressure is applied bilaterally. Greater discomfort over one area suggests sinusitis.

The throat

Parts of the throat include the pharynx, epiglottis, and larynx. The pharynx is the passageway for food and air to the larynx and esophagus. The epiglottis diverts material away from the glottis during swallowing. The larynx produces sounds by vibrating expired air through the vocal cords. Changes in vocal cord length and air pressure affect pitch and voice intensity. The larynx also stimulates the vital cough reflex when a foreign body touches its sensitive mucosa.

Assessment

The mouth and throat are inspected using a bright light and a tongue blade. The patient is checked for inflammation or white patches, and any irregularities on the tongue or throat. Vital signs and respiratory status are assessed. The health care professional must be careful not to compromise the patient's airway. Respiratory distress (dyspnea, tachycardia, tachypnea, inspiratory stridor, increasing restlessness) and changes in skin color, such as circumoral or nail-bed cyanosis, must be watched for and reported immediately. The main diagnostic test used in throat assessment is a culture, usually taken by swab, to identify the infecting organism when exudate is present.

EXTERNAL EAR

Otitis Externa
(External otitis, swimmer's ear)

Otitis externa, inflammation of the skin of the external ear canal and auricle, may be acute or chronic. It is most common in the summer. With treatment, acute otitis externa usually subsides within 7 days—although it may become chronic—and tends to recur.

Causes and incidence
Otitis externa usually results from bacteria, such as pseudomonas, *Proteus vulgaris,* streptococci, and *Staphylococcus aureus,* and sometimes, fungi, such as *Aspergillus niger* and *Candida albicans* (fungal otitis externa is most common in the Tropics). Occasionally, chronic otitis externa results from dermatologic conditions, such as seborrhea or psoriasis. Predisposing factors include:
• swimming in contaminated water; cerumen creates a culture medium for the waterborne organism.
• cleaning the ear canal with a cotton swab, bobby pin, finger, or other foreign objects; this irritates the ear canal and possibly introduces the infecting microorganism.
• exposure to dust, hair care products, or other irritants, which causes the patient to scratch his ear, excoriating the auricle and canal.
• regular use of earphones, earplugs, or earmuffs, which trap moisture in the ear canal, creating a culture medium for infection.
• chronic drainage from a perforated tympanic membrane.

Signs and symptoms
Acute otitis externa characteristically produces moderate to severe pain that is exacerbated by manipulation of the auricle or tragus, clenching the teeth, opening the mouth, or chewing. Its other clinical effects may include fever, foulsmelling aural discharge, regional cellulitis, and partial hearing loss.

Fungal otitis externa may be asymptomatic, although *A. niger* produces a black or gray, blotting-paper–like growth in the ear canal. In chronic otitis externa, pruritus replaces pain, which may lead to scaling and skin thickening. Aural discharge may also occur.

Diagnosis

Physical examination confirms otitis externa. In acute otitis externa, otoscopy reveals a swollen external ear canal (sometimes to the point of complete closure), periauricular lymphadenopathy (tender nodes in front of the tragus, behind the ear, or in the upper neck), and occasionally, regional cellulitis.

In fungal otitis externa, removal of characteristic growth shows thick, red epithelium. Culture and sensitivity tests identify the causative organism and determine appropriate antibiotic treatment. Pain on palpation of the tragus or auricle distinguishes acute otitis externa from otitis media.

In chronic otitis externa, physical examination shows thick red epithelium in the ear canal. Severe chronic otitis externa may reflect underlying diabetes mellitus, hypothyroidism, or nephritis.

Treatment
To relieve the pain of acute otitis externa, treatment includes heat therapy to the periauricular region (heat lamp; hot, wet compresses; heating pad), aspirin or acetaminophen, and codeine. Instil-

DIFFERENTIAL DIAGNOSIS OF ACUTE
OTITIS EXTERNA AND ACUTE OTITIS MEDIA

ACUTE OTITIS EXTERNA
(PREVALENT IN SUMMER)

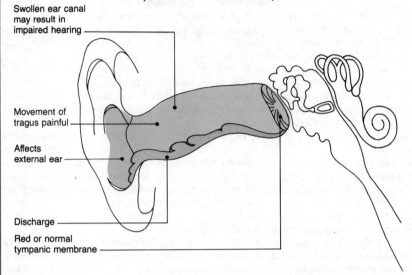

Swollen ear canal
may result in
impaired hearing

Movement of
tragus painful

Affects
external ear

Discharge

Red or normal
tympanic membrane

ACUTE OTITIS MEDIA
(PREVALENT IN WINTER)

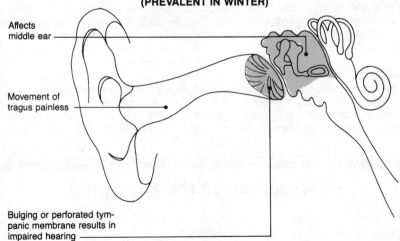

Affects
middle ear

Movement of
tragus painless

Bulging or perforated tympanic membrane results in
impaired hearing

lation of antibiotic eardrops (with or without hydrocortisone) follows cleansing of the ear and removal of debris. If fever persists or regional cellulitis develops, a systemic antibiotic is necessary.

As with other forms of this disorder, fungal otitis externa necessitates careful cleansing of the ear. Application of a keratolytic or 2% salicylic acid in cream containing nystatin may help treat otitis externa resulting from candidal organisms. Instillation of slightly acidic eardrops creates an unfavorable environment in the ear canal for most fungi, as well as pseudomonas. No specific treatment exists for otitis externa caused by A. niger, except repeated cleansing of the ear canal with baby oil.

In chronic otitis externa, primary treatment consists of cleansing the ear and removing debris. Supplemental therapy includes instillation of antibiotic eardrops or application of antibiotic ointment or cream (neomycin, bacitracin, or polymyxin, possibly combined with hydrocortisone). Another ointment contains phenol, salicylic acid, precipitated sulfur, and petrolatum, and produces exfoliative and antipruritic effects.

For mild chronic otitis externa, treatment may include instilling antibiotic eardrops once or twice weekly and wearing specially fitted earplugs (molded to the patient's ear) while showering, shampooing, or swimming.

Additional considerations

If the patient has acute otitis externa, the health care professional should:
• monitor vital signs, particularly temperature; watch for and record the type and amount of aural drainage.
• remove debris and gently cleanse the ear canal with mild Burow's solution (aluminum acetate); place a wisp of cotton soaked with solution into the ear, and apply a saturated compress directly to the auricle; dry the ear gently but thoroughly afterward. (In severe otitis externa, such cleansing may be delayed until after initial treatment with antibiotic eardrops.)
• pull the pinna upward and backward to straighten the canal to instill eardrops in an adult; insert a wisp of cotton moistened with eardrops into the ear to ensure that the drops reach the epithelium.
• cleanse the ear thoroughly if the patient has chronic otitis externa; use wet soaks intermittently on oozing or infected skin; cleanse the ear canal well if the patient has a chronic fungal infection, then apply an exfoliative ointment.

To prevent otitis externa, the professional should:
• advise the patient to use lamb's wool earplugs coated with petrolatum to keep water out of the ears when showering or shampooing.
• tell the patient to wear earplugs or to keep his head above water when swimming; to instill two or three drops of 3% boric acid solution in 70% alcohol before and after swimming to toughen the skin of the external ear canal.
• warn against cleaning the ears with cotton swabs, bobby pins, or foreign objects.
• urge prompt treatment of otitis media to prevent perforation of the tympanic membrane (otitis media may also lead to the more benign otitis externa).

Obstructions of the Ear Canal

Obstructions of the ear canal can interfere with auditory function and lead to infection, inflammation, or conductive hearing loss.

Causes and incidence

Common causes of ear obstructions include impacted cerumen, due to a narrow ear canal; excessive secretion of cerumen; or a foreign body, including insects. Children's ears may be obstructed by a variety of objects, such as toys, beans, peas, pebbles, beads, erasers, or paper.

Signs and symptoms
Obstructions may be painful, especially if a foreign body is deep in the canal. The degree of hearing loss depends on the degree of obstruction. An insect in the ear causes a distressing buzzing sound or sensation of movement.

Diagnosis
 Diagnosis requires a history of ear pain or hearing loss, and physical examination to confirm obstruction. Parents may discover foreign objects in children's ears if the objects aren't inserted too deeply in the canal.

Treatment
The aim of treatment is removal of the obstruction; specific treatment depends on the cause.

Impacted cerumen can be removed by gently scraping the ear canal with a cerumen spoon or by irrigating the canal using an ear syringe or an aerated water jet (such as Water Pik), on low setting, and a solution of equal parts of hydrogen peroxide and warm water. A gentle stream is directed toward the upper wall of the canal, to prevent excessive pressure on the tympanic membrane. The irrigating fluid and cerumen are collected in a small basin held below the patient's ear.

Irrigation is contraindicated in patients with suspected perforation of the tympanic membrane, and should be stopped immediately if it causes pain, nausea, or dizziness. Extremely hard or firmly impacted cerumen may necessitate preliminary softening by instillation of warm glycerin, a few drops of mineral oil, or a ceruminolytic, such as carbamide peroxide, before irrigation.

An insect in the ear can be quickly killed by instillation of 70% alcohol solution or a few drops of mineral oil into the ear canal; it can then be removed with a cerumen spoon, or forceps.

Paper or vegetables may be difficult to remove. Wet paper must be allowed to dry before extraction with forceps. Vegetables require preliminary irrigation with 70% alcohol solution (water may cause vegetables to swell within the ear) or can be removed with forceps or an ear hook. The patient with a large or firmly embedded object often requires referral to an otolaryngologist for extraction of the object under a general anesthetic.

Additional considerations
The health care professional should:
- instill eardrops or irrigate the canal.
- refer the patient to an otolaryngologist, as needed.
- tell patients, especially children, not to insert foreign objects in their ears.

To prevent obstruction in patients with hard cerumen, one or two drops of mineral, olive, or baby oil should be instilled in the ears at night, followed by one or two drops of hydrogen peroxide in the morning, and cleansing of the external meatus *only* with soft cotton. This should be done once a week.

Benign Tumors of the Ear Canal

Benign tumors may develop anywhere in the ear canal. Common types include keloids, osteomas, and sebaceous cysts; their causes vary. These tumors rarely become malignant, and with proper treatment, prognosis is excellent.

Signs and symptoms
A benign ear tumor is usually asymptomatic, unless it becomes infected, in which case pain, fever, or inflammation may result. (Pain is often a sign of malignancy.) If the tumor grows large enough

CAUSES AND CHARACTERISTICS OF BENIGN EAR TUMORS

TUMOR	CAUSES AND INCIDENCE	CHARACTERISTICS
Keloid	• Surgery or trauma, such as ear-piercing • Most common in Blacks	• Hypertrophy and fibrosis of scar tissue • Commonly recurs
Osteoma	• Idiopathic growth • Predisposing factor, swimming in cold water • Three times more common in males than in females • Seldom occurs before adolescence	• Bony outgrowth from wall of external auditory meatus • Usually bilateral and multiple (exostoses)
Sebaceous cyst	• Obstruction of a sebaceous gland	• Painless mass filled with oily, fatty, glandular secretions • May occur on external ear (especially postauricular area) and outer one third of external auditory canal

to obstruct the ear canal by itself or through accumulated cerumen and debris, it may cause hearing loss and the sensation of pressure.

Diagnosis

 Clinical features and patient history suggest a benign tumor of the ear canal; otoscopy confirms it. To rule out malignancy, the doctor may perform a biopsy.

Treatment

Generally, a benign tumor requires surgical excision if it obstructs the ear canal, is cosmetically undesirable, or becomes malignant.

Treatment of a keloid may include radiation in the early stages and, for patients predisposed to recurrence, surgery, followed by a single dose of radiation and a long-acting steroid (usually an injection of hydrocortisone acetate). Excision must be complete, but even this may not prevent recurrence.

Surgical excision of an osteoma is particularly difficult because of the osteoma's proximity to the facial nerves. Treatment, therefore, consists of shaving the osteoma with a mechanical burr or drill.

A sebaceous cyst requires preliminary treatment with antibiotics, to reduce inflammation. To prevent recurrence, excision must include the sac or capsule of the cyst.

Additional considerations

Since treatment of benign ear tumors generally doesn't require hospitalization, health care focuses on providing patient teaching and giving emotional support.

• All diagnostic procedures and treatment must be thoroughly explained to the patient and his family.

• After surgery, the patient should be taught good aural hygiene—the ear should be kept clean and dry. The patient must not insert anything in his ear or allow water to get in it.

• The patient should be taught how to recognize signs of infection (pain, fever, redness, swelling). He should report any such signs immediately.

MIDDLE EAR

Otitis Media

Otitis media, inflammation of the middle ear, may be suppurative or secretory, acute or chronic. Acute otitis media is common in children; its incidence rises during the winter months, paralleling the seasonal rise in nonbacterial respiratory tract infections. With prompt treatment, prognosis for acute otitis media is excellent; however, prolonged accumulation of fluid within the middle ear cavity causes chronic otitis media, with possible perforation of the tympanic membrane. Chronic suppurative otitis media may lead to scarring, adhesions, and severe structural or functional ear damage; chronic secretory otitis media, with its persistent inflammation and pressure, may cause conductive hearing loss.

Causes

Otitis media results from disruption of eustachian tube patency. In the suppurative form, respiratory tract infection, allergic reaction, or positional changes (such as holding an infant supine during feeding) allow nasopharyngeal flora to reflux through the eustachian tube and colonize the middle ear. Suppurative otitis media usually results from bacterial infection with pneumococcus, *Hemophilus influenzae* (the most common cause in children under age 6), beta-hemolytic streptococci, staphylococci, and gram-negative bacteria (most common cause in neonates, particularly among premature infants). Predisposing factors include the normally wider, shorter, more horizontal eustachian tubes and increased lymphoid tissue in children, and anatomic anomalies, such as cleft palate. Chronic suppurative otitis media results from inadequate treatment of acute otitis episodes or from infection by resistant strains of bacteria.

Secretory otitis media results from obstruction of the eustachian tube. This causes a buildup of negative pressure in the middle ear that promotes transudation of sterile serous fluid from blood vessels in the membrane of the middle ear. Such effusion may be secondary to eustachian tube dysfunction from viral infection, or allergy. It may also follow barotrauma (pressure injury caused by inability to equalize pressures between the environment and the middle ear), such as that during rapid aircraft descent in a person with an upper respiratory tract infection or during rapid underwater ascent in scuba diving (barotitis media). Chronic secretory otitis media follows persistent eustachian tube dysfunction from mechanical obstruction (adenoidal tissue overgrowth, tumors), edema (allergic rhinitis, chronic sinus infection), or inadequate treatment of acute suppurative otitis media.

Signs and symptoms

Clinical features of acute suppurative otitis media include severe, deep, throbbing pain (from pressure behind the tympanic membrane); signs of upper respiratory tract infection (sneezing, coughing); mild to very high fever; hearing loss (usually mild and conductive); dizziness; nausea; and vomiting. Other possible effects include bulging of the tympanic membrane, with concomitant erythema, and purulent drainage in the ear canal from tympanic membrane rupture. However, many patients are asymptomatic.

Acute secretory otitis media produces severe conductive hearing loss—which varies from 15 to 35 db, depending on the thickness and amount of fluid in the middle ear cavity—and, possibly, a sensation of fullness in the ear and popping, crackling, or clicking sounds on swallowing or with jaw movement. Accumulation of fluid may also cause the patient to hear an echo when he speaks and to experience a vague feeling of top heaviness. However, acute secretory otitis media is frequently asymptomatic.

Chronic otitis media usually begins in childhood and persists into adulthood. Its cumulative effects include thickening and scarring of the tympanic membrane; decreased or absent tympanic membrane mobility; cholesteatoma (a cystlike mass in the middle ear); and with chronic suppurative otitis media, painless purulent discharge. Associated conductive hearing loss varies with the size and type of tympanic membrane perforation and ossicular destruction. Complications may include abscesses (brain, subperiosteal, and epidural), sigmoid sinus or jugular vein thrombosis, septicemia, meningitis, suppurative labyrinthitis, facial paralysis, and otitis externa.

Diagnosis

In acute suppurative otitis media, otoscopy reveals obscured or distorted bony landmarks of the tympanic membrane. Pneumatoscopy can show decreased tympanic membrane mobility, but this procedure is painful and therefore contraindicated with an obviously bulging, erythematous tympanic membrane. The pain pattern is diagnostically significant: in acute suppurative otitis media, for example, pulling the auricle *doesn't* exacerbate the pain.

In acute secretory otitis media, otoscopy demonstrates tympanic membrane retraction, which causes the bony landmarks to appear more prominent. This examination also detects clear or amber fluid behind the tympanic membrane, possibly with a meniscus and bubbles. If hemorrhage into the middle ear has occurred, as in barotrauma, the tympanic membrane appears blue-black.

In chronic otitis media, patient history discloses recurrent or unresolved otitis media. Otoscopy shows thickening and sometimes scarring, and decreased mobility of the tympanic membrane; pneumatoscopy, decreased or absent tympanic

membrane movement. History of recent air travel or scuba diving suggests barotitis media.

Treatment

In acute suppurative otitis media, antibiotic therapy includes ampicillin (for children under age 6), penicillin (for persons over age 6), or erythromycin and sulfisoxazole (for those allergic to penicillin). Aspirin or acetaminophen controls pain and fever; oral or local nasal decongestants improve eustachian tube patency. Severe, painful bulging of the tympanic membrane necessitates myringotomy. Broad-spectrum antibiotics (sulfisoxazole, co-trimoxazole) can help prevent acute suppurative otitis media in high-risk patients, such as children with recurring episodes of otitis. However, in patients with recurring otitis, antibiotics must be used sparingly and with discretion, to prevent development of resistant strains of bacteria.

In acute secretory otitis media, inflation of the eustachian tube by performing Valsalva's maneuver several times a day may be the only treatment required. Otherwise, nasopharyngeal decongestant therapy is needed for at least 2 weeks and, sometimes, indefinitely, with periodic evaluation. If decongestant therapy fails, myringotomy and aspiration of middle ear fluid are necessary, followed by insertion of a polyethylene tube into the tympanic membrane, for immediate and prolonged equalization of pressure. The tube falls out spontaneously after 9 to 12 months. Concomitant treatment of the underlying cause (such as elimination of allergens, or adenoidectomy for hypertrophied adenoids) is also essential.

Treatment of chronic otitis media includes antibiotics for exacerbations of acute otitis media, elimination of eustachian tube obstruction, treatment of otitis externa (when present), myringoplasty (tympanic membrane graft) and tympanoplasty to reconstruct middle ear structures when thickening and scarring are present, and possibly, mastoidectomy. Cholesteatoma requires excision.

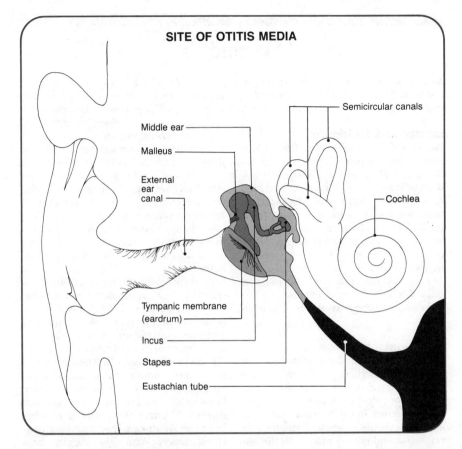

SITE OF OTITIS MEDIA

Semicircular canals

Middle ear

Malleus

External ear canal

Cochlea

Tympanic membrane (eardrum)

Incus

Stapes

Eustachian tube

Additional considerations

When treating a patient with otitis media, the health care professional should:
• explain all diagnostic tests and procedures; maintain drainage flow after myringotomy; never place cotton or plugs deep in the ear canal; use sterile cotton placed loosely in the external ear to absorb drainage; change the cotton whenever it gets damp to prevent infection, and wash hands before and after giving ear care; watch for and report headache, fever, severe pain, or disorientation.
• reinforce dressings after tympanoplasty, and observe for excessive bleeding from the ear canal; administer analgesics, as needed; warn the patient against blowing his nose or getting the ear wet when bathing.
• encourage the patient to complete the prescribed course of antibiotic treatment; teach correct use of nasopharyngeal decongestants.
• suggest application of heat to the ear to relieve pain.
• advise the patient with acute secretory otitis media to watch for and report signs of secondary infection, such as pain and fever.
• encourage early treatment for upper respiratory tract infections.
• instruct parents not to feed their infant in a supine position or put him to bed with a bottle.
• instruct the patient to perform Valsalva's maneuver several times daily to promote eustachian tube patency.
• advise against forceful noseblowing, since this can drive infected secretions into the middle ear.

Mastoiditis

Mastoiditis is a bacterial infection and inflammation of the air cells of the mastoid antrum. Although prognosis is good with early treatment, possible complications include meningitis, facial paralysis, brain abscess, and suppurative labyrinthitis.

Causes and incidence

Bacteria that cause mastoiditis include pneumococcus (usually in children under age 6), *Hemophilus influenzae*, beta-hemolytic streptococci, staphylococci, and gram-negative organisms. Mastoiditis is usually a complication of chronic otitis media and, less frequently, of acute otitis media. An accumulation of pus under pressure in the middle ear cavity results in necrosis of adjacent tissue and extension of the infection into the mastoid cells. Chronic systemic diseases or immunosuppression may also lead to mastoiditis.

Signs and symptoms

Primary clinical features include a dull ache and tenderness in the area of the mastoid process, low-grade fever, and a thick, purulent discharge that gradually becomes more profuse, possibly leading to otitis externa. Postauricular erythema and edema may push the auricle out from the head; pressure within the edematous mastoid antrum may produce swelling and obstruction of the external ear canal, causing conductive hearing loss.

Diagnosis

X-rays of the mastoid area reveal hazy mastoid air cells; the bony walls between the cells appear decalcified. Examination shows a dull, thickened, and edematous tympanic membrane, if the membrane isn't concealed by obstruction. During examination, the external ear canal is cleaned; persistent oozing into the canal indicates perforation of the tympanic membrane.

Treatment

Treatment of mastoiditis consists of intense parenteral antibiotic therapy. If bone damage is minimal, myringotomy drains purulent fluid and provides a specimen of discharge for culture and sensitivity testing. Recurrent or persistent infection, or signs of intracranial complications necessitate simple mastoidectomy. This procedure involves removal of the diseased bone and cleansing of the affected area, after which a drain is inserted.

A chronically inflamed mastoid requires radical mastoidectomy (excision of the posterior wall of the ear canal, remnants of the tympanic membrane, and the malleus and incus [although these bones are usually destroyed by infection before surgery]). The stapes and facial nerve remain intact. Radical mastoidectomy, which is seldom necessary because of antibiotic therapy, does not drastically affect the patient's hearing because significant hearing loss precedes surgery. With either surgical procedure, the patient continues oral antibiotic therapy for several weeks after surgery and hospital discharge.

Additional considerations

Health care of a patient with mastoiditis includes:

• giving pain medication, as needed, after simple mastoidectomy; checking wound drainage, and reinforcing dressings (the surgeon usually changes the dressing daily and removes the drain in 72 hours); checking the patient's hearing, and watching for signs of complications, especially infection (either localized or extending to the brain); facial nerve paralysis, with unilateral facial drooping; bleeding; and vertigo, especially when the patient stands.

• packing the wound with petrolatum

gauze or gauze treated with an antibiotic ointment after radical mastoidectomy; giving pain medication before the packing is removed, on the fourth or fifth postoperative day.
• keeping the side rails up, and assisting the patient with ambulation; giving antiemetics, as ordered and as needed. The patient may feel dizzy and nauseated for several days afterward because of stimulation to the inner ear during surgery.
• teaching the patient and family how to change the dressing, and telling them to avoid getting it wet; urging compliance with prescribed antibiotic treatment, and promoting regular follow-up care.

Otosclerosis

The most common cause of conductive deafness, otosclerosis is the slow formation of spongy bone in the otic capsule, particularly at the oval window. It occurs in at least 10% of Caucasians, and is twice as prevalent in females as in males, usually between ages 15 and 30. With surgery, prognosis is good.

Causes
Otosclerosis appears to result from a genetic factor transmitted as an autosomal dominant trait; many patients with this disorder report family histories of hearing loss (excluding presbycusis). Pregnancy may trigger onset of this condition.

Signs and symptoms
Spongy bone in the otic capsule immobilizes the footplate of the normally mobile stapes, disrupting the conduction of vibrations from the tympanic membrane to the cochlea. This causes slowly progressive unilateral hearing loss, which may advance to bilateral deafness. Other symptoms include tinnitus (low and medium pitch) and paracusis of Willis (hearing conversation better in a noisy environment than in a quiet one).

Diagnosis
 Early diagnosis is based on a Rinne test that shows bone conduction lasting longer than air conduction (normally, the reverse is true). As otosclerosis progresses, bone conduction also deteriorates. Audiometric testing reveals hearing loss ranging from 60 db, in early stages, to total loss, as the disease advances. Weber's test detects sound lateralizing to the more affected ear. Physical examination reveals a normal tympanic membrane.

Treatment
Generally, treatment consists of stapedectomy (removal of the stapes) and insertion of a prosthesis, to restore partial or total hearing. This procedure is performed on only one ear at a time, beginning with the ear that has suffered greater damage. Postoperatively, treatment includes hospitalization for 2 to 3 days and antibiotics to prevent infection. If stapedectomy is not possible, a hearing aid (air conduction aid with molded ear insert receiver) enables the patient to hear conversation in normal surroundings, although this therapy isn't as effective as stapedectomy.

Additional considerations
• During the first 24 hours following surgery, the patient must lie flat, with his head turned so that the affected ear faces upward (to maintain the position of the graft). Enforced bed rest is necessary for 48 hours. Since the patient may be dizzy, the bed side rails should be kept up, and walking tried slowly. Pain and vertigo may be relieved with repositioning or prescribed medication.
• The patient should avoid loud noises and sudden pressure changes (such as those that occur while diving or flying)

until healing is complete (usually 6 months). Also, he must not blow his nose for at least 1 week to prevent contaminated air and bacteria from entering the eustachian tube.
• The patient must protect his ears against cold, avoid activities that provoke dizziness, such as straining, bending, or heavy lifting, and if possible, avoid contact with anyone who has an upper respiratory tract infection. The patient and family should be taught how to change the external ear dressing (eye or gauze pad) and care for the incision. Completing the prescribed antibiotic regimen and returning for scheduled follow-up care will help detect changes before they become permanent.

Infectious Myringitis

Acute infectious myringitis is characterized by inflammation, hemorrhage, and effusion of fluid into the tissue at the end of the external ear canal and the tympanic membrane. This self-limiting disorder (resolving spontaneously within 3 days to 2 weeks) often follows acute otitis media or upper respiratory tract infection and frequently occurs epidemically in children.

Chronic granular myringitis, a rare inflammation of the squamous layer of the tympanic membrane, causes gradual hearing loss. Without specific treatment, this condition can lead to stenosis of the ear canal, as granulation extends from the tympanic membrane to the external ear.

Causes

Acute infectious myringitis usually follows viral infection, but may also result from infection with bacteria, (pneumococcus, *Hemophilus influenzae*, beta-hemolytic streptococci, staphylococci) or any other organism that may cause acute otitis media. Myringitis is a rare sequela of atypical pneumonia caused by *Mycoplasma pneumoniae*. The cause of chronic granular myringitis is unknown.

Signs and symptoms

Acute infectious myringitis begins with severe ear pain, commonly accompanied by tenderness over the mastoid process. Small, reddened, inflamed blebs form in the canal, on the tympanic membrane, and with bacterial invasion, in the middle ear. Fever and hearing loss are rare unless fluid accumulates in the middle ear or a large bleb totally obstructs the external auditory meatus. Spontaneous rupture of these blebs may cause bloody discharge. Chronic granular myringitis produces pruritus, purulent discharge, and gradual hearing loss.

Diagnosis

Diagnosis of acute infectious myringitis is based on physical examination showing characteristic blebs, and typical patient history. Culture and sensitivity testing of exudate identify any secondary infection present. In chronic granular myringitis, physical examination may reveal granulation extending from the tympanic membrane to the external ear.

Treatment and additional considerations

Hospitalization is usually not required for the patient with acute infectious myringitis. Treatment consists of measures to relieve pain: analgesics, such as aspirin or acetaminophen, and application of heat to the external ear are usually sufficient, but severe pain may necessitate use of codeine. Systemic or topical antibiotics prevent or treat secondary infection. Incision of blebs and evacuation of serum and blood may relieve pressure and help drain exudate but do not speed recovery.

Treatment of chronic granular myringitis consists of systemic antibiotics or local anti-inflammatory antibiotic combination eardrops, and surgical excision and cautery. If stenosis is present, surgical reconstruction is necessary.

The patient must understand the importance of completing prescribed antibiotic therapy. He should be taught how to instill topical antibiotics (eardrops) and, when appropriate, the necessity for the incision of blebs should be explained to him. Early treatment of acute otitis media will help prevent infectious myringitis.

INNER EAR

Ménière's Disease

(Endolymphatic hydrops)

Ménière's disease, a labyrinthine dysfunction, produces severe vertigo, sensorineural hearing loss, and tinnitus. It usually affects adults, men slightly more often than women, between ages 30 and 60. After multiple attacks over several years, this disorder leads to residual tinnitus and hearing loss.

Causes
Overproduction or decreased absorption of endolymph results in endolymphatic hydrops or endolymphatic hypertension, with consequent degeneration of the vestibular and cochlear hair cells. This condition may stem from autonomic nervous system dysfunction that produces a temporary constriction of blood vessels supplying the inner ear. In some women, premenstrual edema may precipitate attacks of Ménière's disease.

Signs and symptoms
Ménière's disease produces three characteristic effects: severe vertigo, tinnitus, and sensorineural hearing loss. Fullness or blocked feeling in the ear is also quite common. Violent paroxysmal attacks last from 10 minutes to several hours. During an acute attack, associated symptoms include severe nausea, vomiting, sweating, giddiness, and nystagmus (direction varies). Also, vertigo may cause loss of balance and falling to the affected side. To lessen these symptoms, the patient may instinctively assume a characteristic posture—lying on the unaffected ear and looking in the direction of the affected ear. Initially, the patient may be asymptomatic between attacks, except for residual tinnitus that worsens during an attack. Such attacks may occur several times a year, or remissions may last as long as several years. Eventually, these attacks become less frequent, as hearing loss progresses (usually unilateral), and they may cease when hearing loss is total.

Diagnosis
Presence of all three typical symptoms suggests Ménière's disease. Caloric testing supports diagnosis by precipitating a severe attack. During this test, instillation of 0.2 ml of ice water into each ear, while the patient lies with his head elevated 30°, usually provokes an acute attack in the patient with Ménière's disease; normally, it causes only dizziness in a person who is not affected with the disorder. Electronystagmography, and X-rays of the internal meatus may be necessary for differential diagnosis.

Treatment
Treatment with atropine may stop an attack in 20 to 30 minutes. Epinephrine or diphenhydramine may be necessary in a severe attack; dimenhydrinate, meclizine, diphenhydramine, or promethazine may be effective in a milder attack.

Long-term management includes use of a diuretic or vasodilator, and restricted sodium intake. Prophylactic antihistamines or mild sedatives (phenobarbital, diazepam) may also be helpful. If Ménière's disease persists after more than 2 years of treatment or produces incapacitating vertigo, surgical destruction of the affected labyrinth may be necessary. This procedure permanently relieves symptoms but at the expense of irreversible hearing loss.

Additional considerations

To minimize dizziness during an attack of Ménière's disease, the patient should avoid reading, and exposure to glaring lights. To prevent falls, the bed side rails must be kept up, and the patient should not get out of bed or walk without assistance. Because such attacks are apt to begin quite rapidly, the patient must avoid sudden position changes and any tasks that vertigo makes hazardous.

Health care of a patient with Ménière's disease includes:

• recording fluid intake and output and characteristics of emesis if the patient is vomiting before surgery; administering antiemetics, as ordered, and giving small amounts of fluid frequently.

• explaining diagnostic tests, and offering reassurance and emotional support.

• carefully recording fluid intake and output postoperatively; telling the patient to expect dizziness and nausea for 1 to 2 days after surgery; giving prophylactic antibiotics and antiemetics, as ordered.

Labyrinthitis

Labyrinthitis, an inflammation of the labyrinth of the inner ear, frequently incapacitates the patient by producing severe vertigo that lasts for 3 to 5 days; symptoms gradually subside over a 3- to 6-week period. This disorder is rare, although viral labyrinthitis is often associated with upper respiratory tract infections.

Causes

Labyrinthitis results from the same organisms that cause acute febrile diseases, such as pneumonia, influenza, and especially, chronic otitis media. In chronic otitis media, cholesteatoma formation erodes the bone of the labyrinth, allowing bacteria to enter from the middle ear. Other causes include toxic drug ingestion, excessive use of alcohol, allergy, and severe fatigue.

Signs and symptoms

Since the inner ear controls both hearing and balance, this infection typically produces severe vertigo (with any movement of the head) and progressive sensorineural hearing loss. Vertigo begins gradually but peaks within 48 hours, causing loss of balance and falling in the direction of the affected ear. Other clinical features include spontaneous nystagmus, with jerking movements of the eyes toward the unaffected ear, nausea, vomiting, and giddiness; with cholesteatoma, signs of middle ear disease; and with severe bacterial infection, purulent drainage. To minimize giddiness and nystagmus, the patient may assume a characteristic posture—lying on the unaffected ear and looking in the direction of the affected ear.

Diagnosis

Typical clinical picture and history of upper respiratory tract infection suggest labyrinthitis. Diagnostic measures include culture and sensitivity testing, if purulent drainage is present, and occasionally, audiometric testing. When an infectious etiology can't be found, testing must be done to rule out a brain lesion or Ménière's disease.

Treatment

Symptomatic treatment includes bed rest,

with the head immobilized between pillows; meclizine P.O. to control vertigo; and massive doses of antibiotics to combat diffuse purulent labyrinthitis. Oral fluids can prevent dehydration from vomiting; for severe nausea and vomiting, I.V. fluids may be necessary.

When conservative management fails, treatment necessitates surgical excision of the cholesteatoma and drainage of the infected areas of the middle and inner ear. Prevention is possible by early and vigorous treatment of predisposing conditions, such as otitis media and any local or systemic infection.

Additional considerations

During hospitalization, the bedside rails must be kept up to prevent falls. If vomiting is severe, antiemetics and I.V. fluids may be required. Accurate intake and output records are necessary to prevent fluid or electrolyte imbalance.

The patient should be reassured that recovery is certain but may take as long as 6 weeks. He should limit activities that vertigo may make hazardous, such as climbing a ladder or driving a car.

Hearing Loss

Hearing loss results from a mechanical or nervous impediment to the transmission of sound waves. The major forms of hearing loss are classified as conductive loss (interrupted passage of sound from the external ear to the junction of the stapes and oval window); sensorineural loss (impaired cochlea or acoustic [eighth cranial] nerve dysfunction, causing failure of transmission of sound impulses within the inner ear or brain); or mixed (combined dysfunction of conduction and sensorineural transmission). Hearing loss may be partial or total and is calculated from the American Medical Association formula: hearing is 1.5% impaired for every decibel that the pure tone average exceeds 25 db.

Causes and incidence

Congenital hearing loss may be transmitted as a dominant, autosomal dominant, autosomal recessive, or sex-linked recessive trait. Hearing loss in neonates may also result from trauma, toxicity, or infection during pregnancy or delivery. Predisposing factors include a family history of hearing loss or known hereditary disorders (otosclerosis, for example), maternal exposure to rubella or syphilis during pregnancy, use of ototoxic drugs during pregnancy, prolonged fetal anoxia during delivery, and congenital abnormalities of the ears, nose, or throat. Premature or low–birth-weight infants are most likely to have structural or functional hearing impairments; those with serum bilirubin levels greater than 20 mg/100 ml also risk hearing impairment from the toxic effect of high serum bilirubin levels on the brain. In addition, trauma during delivery may cause intracranial hemorrhage and damage the cochlea or acoustic nerve.

Sudden deafness refers to sudden hearing loss in a person with no prior hearing impairment. This condition is considered a medical emergency, because prompt treatment may restore full hearing. Its causes and predisposing factors may include:

• acute infections, especially mumps (most common cause of unilateral sensorineural hearing loss in children), and other bacterial and viral infections, such as rubella, rubeola, influenza, herpes zoster, and infectious mononucleosis; and mycoplasma infections.

• metabolic disorders (diabetes mellitus, hypothyroidism, hyperlipoproteinemia).

• vascular disorders, such as hypertension, arteriosclerosis.

• head trauma or brain tumors.

• ototoxic drugs (tobramycin, streptomycin, quinine, gentamicin, furosemide, ethacrynic acid).

• neurologic disorders (multiple sclerosis, neurosyphilis).

• blood dyscrasias (leukemia and hypercoagulation).

Noise-induced hearing loss, which may be transient or permanent, may follow prolonged exposure to loud noise (85 to 90 db) or brief exposure to extremely loud noise (greater than 90 db). Such hearing loss is common in workers subjected to constant industrial noise and in military personnel, hunters, and rock musicians.

Presbycusis, an otologic effect of aging, results from a loss of hair cells in the organ of Corti. This disorder causes sensorineural hearing loss, usually of high-frequency tones.

Signs and symptoms
Although congenital hearing loss may produce no obvious signs of hearing impairment at birth, deficient response to auditory stimuli generally becomes apparent within 2 to 3 days. As the child grows older, hearing loss impairs speech development.

Sudden deafness may be conductive, sensorineural, or mixed, depending on etiology. Associated clinical features depend on the underlying cause.

Noise-induced hearing loss causes sensorineural damage, the extent of which depends on the duration and intensity of the noise. Initially, the patient loses perception of certain frequencies (around 4,000 Hz) but, with continued exposure, eventually loses perception of all frequencies.

Presbycusis usually produces tinnitus and the inability to understand the spoken word.

Diagnosis

Patient, family, and occupational histories and a complete audiologic examination usually provide ample evidence of hearing loss and suggest possible causes or predisposing factors. The Weber, the Rinne, and specialized audiologic tests differentiate between conductive and sensorineural hearing loss.

Treatment
After identifying the underlying cause, therapy for congenital hearing loss refractory to surgery consists of developing the patient's ability to communicate through sign language, speech reading, or other effective means. Measures to prevent congenital hearing loss include aggressively immunizing children against rubella, to reduce the risk of maternal exposure during pregnancy; educating pregnant women about the dangers of exposure to drugs, chemicals, or infection; and careful monitoring during labor and delivery to prevent fetal anoxia.

Treatment of sudden deafness requires prompt identification of the underlying cause. Prevention necessitates educating patients and health-care professionals about the many causes of sudden deafness and the ways to recognize and treat them.

In persons with noise-induced hearing loss, overnight rest usually restores normal hearing in those who have been exposed to noise levels greater than 90 db for several hours; but not in those who have been exposed to such noise repeatedly. As hearing deteriorates, treatment must include speech and hearing rehabilitation, since hearing aids are rarely helpful. Prevention of noise-induced hearing loss requires public recognition of the dangers of noise exposure and insistence on the use, as mandated by law, of protective devices, such as earplugs, during occupational exposure to noise.

Presbycusis usually requires the use of a hearing aid.

Additional considerations
When caring for a patient with hearing loss, the hospital staff member should:

• stand in a well-lit area directly in front of the patient with hearing loss who can read lips, and speak to him slowly and distinctly; approach the patient within his visual range, and elicit his attention

by raising your arm or waving—touching him may be unnecessarily startling.
• make other staff members and hospital personnel aware of the patient's handicap and his established method of communication; carefully explain all diagnostic tests and hospital procedures in a way the patient understands.
• make sure the patient with a hearing loss is in an area where he can observe unit activities and persons approaching, since such a patient depends totally on visual clues.
• speak slowly and distinctly in a low tone when addressing an older patient—avoid shouting.

• provide emotional support and encouragement to the patient learning to use a hearing aid; teach him how the aid works and how to maintain it.
• refer children with suspected hearing loss to an audiologist or otolaryngologist for further evaluation.
• help prevent hearing loss by watching for signs of hearing impairment in patients receiving ototoxic drugs, emphasizing the danger of excessive exposure to noise, stressing to pregnant women the danger of exposure to drugs, chemicals, and infection (especially rubella), and encouraging the use of protective devices in a noisy environment.

Motion Sickness

Motion sickness is characterized by loss of equilibrium, associated with nausea and vomiting that result from irregular or rhythmic movements or from the sensation of motion. Removal of the stimulus restores normal equilibrium.

Causes and incidence
Motion sickness may result from excessive stimulation of the labyrinthine receptors of the inner ear by certain motions, such as those experienced in a car, boat, plane, or swing. The disorder may also be caused by confusion in the cerebellum from conflicting sensory input; visual stimulus (a moving horizon) conflicts with labyrinthine perception. Predisposing factors include tension or fear, offensive odors, or sights and sounds associated with a previous attack. Motion sickness from cars, elevators, trains, and swings is most common in children; from boats and airplanes, in adults. Persons who suffer from one kind of motion sickness are not necessarily susceptible to other types.

Signs and symptoms
Typically, motion sickness induces nausea, vomiting, headache, dizziness, fatigue, diaphoresis, and occasionally, difficulty in breathing, leading to a sensation of suffocation. These symptoms usually subside when the precipitating stimulus is removed, but they may persist for several hours or days.

Treatment and additional considerations
The best way to treat the disorder is to stop the motion that's causing it. If this is impossible, as on an ocean voyage, the patient will benefit from lying down, closing his eyes, and attempting to sleep. Antiemetics, such as dimenhydrinate, cyclizine, and meclizine, may prevent or relieve motion sickness.

The patient should avoid exposure to precipitating motion whenever possible. The traveler can minimize motion sickness by sitting where motion is least apparent (near the wing section in an aircraft, in the center of a boat, or in the front seat of an automobile). He should attempt to keep his head still, and keep his eyes closed or focused on a distant and stationary object. An elevated car seat may help prevent motion sickness in a child, by allowing him to see out the front window.

The patient should avoid eating or

drinking for at least 4 hours before traveling, and take an antiemetic 30 to 60 minutes before traveling. The patient with prostate enlargement or glaucoma should consult a doctor or pharmacist before taking antiemetics, because such medications can exacerbate these disorders.

NOSE

Epistaxis
(Nosebleed)

Epistaxis may be either a primary disorder or secondary to another condition. Such bleeding in children generally originates in the anterior nasal septum and tends to be mild. In adults, such bleeding is most likely to originate in the posterior septum and can be severe. Epistaxis is twice as common in children as in adults.

Causes
Epistaxis usually follows trauma from external or internal causes: a blow to the nose, nosepicking, or insertion of a foreign body. Less commonly, it follows polyps; acute or chronic infections, such as sinusitis or rhinitis, which cause congestion and eventual bleeding of the capillary blood vessels; or inhalation of chemicals that irritate the nasal mucosa.

Predisposing factors include anticoagulant therapy; hypertension; chronic use of aspirin; high altitudes and dry climates; sclerotic vessel disease; Hodgkin's disease; scurvy; vitamin K deficiency; rheumatic fever; and blood dyscrasias, such as hemophilia, purpura, leukemia, and some anemias.

Signs and symptoms
Blood oozing from the nostrils usually originates in the anterior nose and is bright red. Blood from the back of the throat originates in the posterior area and may be dark or bright red (often mistaken for hemoptysis due to expectoration). Epistaxis is generally unilateral, except when due to dyscrasia or severe trauma. In severe epistaxis, blood may seep behind the nasal septum; it may also appear in the middle ear and in the corners of the eyes.

Associated clinical effects depend on the severity of bleeding. Moderate blood loss may produce light-headedness, dizziness, and slight respiratory difficulty; severe hemorrhage causes a drop in blood pressure, rapid and bounding pulse, dyspnea, pallor, and other indications of progressive shock. Bleeding is considered severe if it persists longer than 10 minutes after pressure is applied and may cause blood loss as great as 1 liter/hour in adults.

Diagnosis
 Although simple observation confirms epistaxis, inspection with a bright light and nasal speculum is necessary to locate the site of bleeding.

Relevant laboratory values include:
• gradual reduction in hemoglobin and hematocrit (often inaccurate immediately following epistaxis, due to hemoconcentration).
• decreased platelet count in a patient with blood dyscrasia.
• prothrombin time and partial thromboplastin time showing a coagulation time twice the control, due to a bleeding disorder or anticoagulant therapy.

Diagnosis must rule out underlying systemic causes of epistaxis, especially disseminated intravascular coagulation and rheumatic fever. Bruises or concomitant bleeding elsewhere probably indicates a hematologic disorder.

INSERTION OF AN ANTERIOR-POSTERIOR NASAL PACK

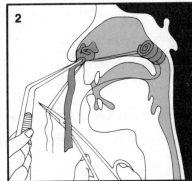

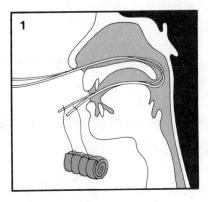

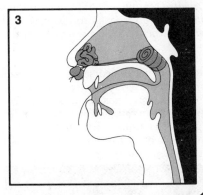

The first step in the insertion of an anterior-posterior nasal pack is the insertion of catheters in the nostrils. After drawing the catheters through the mouth, a suture from the pack is tied to each (fig. 1), which positions the pack in place as the catheters are drawn back through the nostrils. While the sutures are held tightly, packing is inserted into the anterior nose (fig. 2). The sutures are then secured around a dental roll; the middle suture extends from the mouth (fig. 3) and is tied to the cheek.

Treatment

For anterior bleeding, treatment consists of application of a cotton ball saturated with epinephrine to the bleeding site, external pressure, followed by cauterization with electrocautery or silver nitrate stick. If these measures don't control the bleeding, petrolatum gauze nasal packing may be needed.

For posterior bleeding, therapy includes gauze packing inserted through the nose, or postnasal packing inserted through the mouth, depending on the bleeding site. (Gauze packing generally remains in place for 24 to 48 hours; postnasal packing, 48 to 72 hours.) Antibiotics may be appropriate if packing must remain in place for longer than 24 hours. If local measures fail to control bleeding, additional treatment may include supplemental vitamin K or C, and for severe bleeding, blood transfusions and surgical ligation of a bleeding artery. Carbazochrome may help control epistaxis by correcting abnormal capillary permeability.

Additional considerations

Epistaxis can be controlled by:
• elevating the patient's head.
• compressing the soft portion of the nostrils against the septum continuously for 5 to 10 minutes; applying an ice collar or cold, wet compresses to the nose; notifying the doctor if bleeding continues after 10 minutes of pressure.

• monitoring vital signs and skin color, and recording blood loss.
• instructing patient to breathe through the mouth; telling him not to swallow blood, to talk, or to blow his nose.
• keeping vasoconstrictors, such as phenylephrine, handy.
• reassuring the patient and family that epistaxis usually *looks* worse than it is.

To prevent recurrence of epistaxis, the health care professional should:

• instruct the patient not to pick his nose or insert foreign objects in it; emphasize the need for follow-up examinations and periodic blood studies after an episode of epistaxis; advise prompt treatment of nasal infection or irritation, to prevent recurring nose trauma.
• suggest humidifiers for persons who live in dry climates or at high elevations, or whose homes are heated with circulating hot air.

Septal Perforation and Deviation

Perforated septum, a hole in the nasal septum between the two air passages, usually occurs in the anterior cartilaginous septum but may occur in the bony septum. Deviated septum, a shift from the midline, is common in most adults. This condition may be severe enough to obstruct the passage of air through the nostrils. With surgical correction, prognosis for either perforated or deviated septum is good.

Causes and incidence

Generally, perforated septum is caused by traumatic irritation, most commonly from excessive nosepicking; less frequently, from repeated cauterization for epistaxis or from penetrating septal injury. It may also result from perichon-

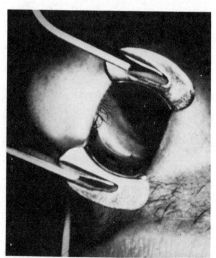

In the photograph above, the nasal septum shows obvious perforation of the cartilage between the two air passages.

dritis, an infection that gradually erodes the perichondrial layer and cartilage, finally forming an ulcer that perforates the septum. Other causes of septal perforation include syphilis, tuberculosis, untreated septal hematoma, inhalation of irritating chemicals, snorting cocaine, chronic nasal infections, nasal carcinoma, granuloma, and chronic sinusitis.

Deviated septum commonly develops during normal growth, as the septum shifts from one side to the other. Consequently, few adults have perfectly straight septa. Nasal trauma resulting from a fall, a blow to the nose, or surgery further exaggerates the deviation. Congenital deviated septum is rare.

Signs and symptoms

A small septal perforation is usually asymptomatic but may produce a whistle on inspiration. A large perforation causes rhinitis, epistaxis, nasal crusting, and watery discharge.

In deviated septum, the patient develops an apparently crooked nose, as the midline deflects to one side. The predominant symptom of severe deflection, however, is nasal obstruction. Other manifestations include a sensation of fullness in the face, shortness of breath, nasal discharge, recurring epistaxis, infection, sinusitis, and headache.

Diagnosis

Although clinical features suggest septal perforation or deviation, confirmation requires inspection of the nasal mucosa with bright light and a nasal speculum.

Treatment

Symptomatic treatment of perforated septum includes decongestants to reduce nasal congestion by local vasoconstriction, local application of lanolin or petrolatum to prevent ulceration and crusting, and antibiotics to combat infection. Surgery may be necessary to graft part of the perichondrial layer over the perforation. Also, a plastic or Silastic "button" prosthesis may be used to close the perforation.

Symptomatic treatment of deviated septum usually includes analgesics to relieve headache; decongestants to minimize secretions; and as necessary, vasoconstrictors, nasal packing, or cautery to control hemorrhage. Manipulation of the nasal septum at birth can correct congenital deviated septum.

Corrective surgical procedures include:
- *reconstruction of the nasal septum by submucous resection* to reposition the nasal septal cartilage and relieve nasal obstruction.
- *rhinoplasty* to correct nasal structure deformity by intranasal incisions.
- *septoplasty* to relieve nasal obstruction and enhance cosmetic appearance.

Additional considerations

- In the patient with perforated septum, a cotton applicator should be used to apply petrolatum to the nasal mucosa. This will minimize crusting and ulceration.
- The patient with perforation or severe deviation must avoid blowing his nose. To relieve nasal congestion, saline nosedrops can be instilled and a humidifier should be used.

- To treat epistaxis, the head of the bed should be elevated, and the patient instructed to expectorate any blood into an emesis basin. The outer portion of the nose should be compressed against the septum for 10 to 15 minutes, and ice packs applied.
- If corrective surgery is scheduled, the patient can expect postoperative facial edema, periorbital bruising, and nasal packing, which remains in place for 12 to 24 hours. The patient must breathe through his mouth. After surgery for deviated septum, the patient may also have a splint on his nose.
- To reduce or prevent edema and promote drainage, the patient can be placed in semi-Fowler's position. A cool-mist vaporizer will liquefy secretions and facilitate normal breathing. To lessen facial edema and pain, crushed ice in a rubber glove or a small ice bag can be applied intermittently over the eyes and nose for 24 hours.
- Because the patient is breathing through his mouth, he will need frequent and meticulous mouth care.
- The mustache dressing or drip pad should be changed, as needed, and the color, consistency, and amount of drainage recorded. While nasal packing is in place, slight, bright red drainage, with clots may appear. After packing is removed, the patient must be watched for purulent discharge, an indication of infection.
- Signs of excessive swallowing, hematoma, or a falling or flapping septum (depressed, or soft and unstable septum) must be watched for and reported. Intranasal examination is necessary to detect hematoma formation. Any of these complications requires surgical correction.
- Sedatives and analgesics, as ordered, should be administered. Because of its anticoagulant properties, aspirin is contraindicated after surgery for septal deviation or perforation.
- Noseblowing may cause bruising and swelling even after nasal packing is removed. After surgery, the patient must limit physical activity for 2 or 3 days, and if he's a smoker, he must stop smoking for at least 2 days.

Sinusitis

Sinusitis, inflammation of the paranasal sinuses, may be acute, subacute, chronic, allergic, or hyperplastic. Acute sinusitis usually results from the common cold and lingers in subacute form in only about 10% of patients. Chronic sinusitis follows persistent bacterial infection; allergic sinusitis accompanies allergic rhinitis; hyperplastic sinusitis is a combination of purulent acute sinusitis and allergic sinusitis or rhinitis. Prognosis is good for all types.

Causes and incidence
Sinusitis usually results from bacterial infection (pneumococci, *Hemophilus influenzae*, anaerobes) or, less frequently, from viral infection. Bacterial invasion generally occurs when a cold spreads to the sinuses. Excessive noseblowing during an acute infection forces infected material into the sinuses.

Predisposing factors include any condition that interferes with drainage and ventilation of the sinuses, such as chronic nasal edema, viscous mucus, or nasal polyps. Bacterial invasion may also result from swimming in contaminated water or from a sudden change in temperature.

Signs and symptoms
The primary indication of *acute sinusitis* is nasal congestion, followed by a gradual buildup of pressure in the affected sinus. For 24 to 48 hours after onset, nasal discharge may be blood-tinged, later becoming purulent. Associated symptoms include malaise, sore throat, headache, and low-grade fever (temperature of 99° to 99.5° F. [37.2° to 37.5° C.]).

Characteristic pain depends on the affected sinus: maxillary sinusitis causes pain over the cheeks and upper teeth; ethmoid sinusitis, pain over the eyes; frontal sinusitis, pain over the eyebrows; and sphenoid sinusitis (rare), pain behind the eyes.

Purulent nasal drainage that continues longer than 3 weeks after an acute infection subsides suggests *subacute sinusitis*. Other clinical features of the subacute form include a stuffy nose,

vague facial discomfort, fatigue, and a nonproductive cough.

The effects of *chronic sinusitis* are similar to those of acute sinusitis, but the chronic form causes continuous mucopurulent discharge.

The effects of *allergic sinusitis* are the same as those of allergic rhinitis—prominent symptoms are sneezing, frontal headache, watery nasal discharge, and a stuffy, burning, itchy nose.

In *hyperplastic sinusitis,* bacterial growth on diseased tissue causes pronounced tissue edema; thickening of the mucosal lining and the development of mucosal polyps produce chronic stuffiness of the nose, and headaches.

Diagnosis
The following measures are useful in diagnosing sinusitis:
• *Sinus X-rays* reveal cloudiness in the affected sinus, air-fluid levels, or thickened mucosal lining.
• *Antral puncture* provides a specimen for culture and sensitivity identification of the infecting organism.
• *Transillumination* allows inspection of the sinus cavities by passing a light through them; purulent drainage prevents passage of light.
• *Nasal examination* reveals inflammation and pus.

Treatment
Analgesics (meperidine or codeine) are the primary treatment for acute sinusitis. Other appropriate measures include vasoconstrictors, such as epinephrine or phenylephrine, to decrease nasal secretions. Steam inhalation also promotes

vasoconstriction, in addition to encouraging drainage.

Antibiotics are necessary to combat persistent infection. Penicillin is usually the antibiotic of choice, but therapy varies according to the results of culture and sensitivity testing. Local applications of heat may help to relieve pain and congestion.

In subacute sinusitis, antibiotic therapy replaces analgesics as the primary treatment. As in acute sinusitis, vasoconstrictors may lessen nasal secretions. After the acute infection subsides, sinus irrigations (needle puncture followed by saline wash) may be helpful, occasionally followed by corticosteroids to decrease inflammation.

Treatment of allergic sinusitis must include treatment of allergic rhinitis—administration of antihistamines, identification of allergens by skin testing, and desensitization by immunotherapy. Severe allergic symptoms may require treatment with corticosteroids and epinephrine.

In both chronic sinusitis and hyperplastic sinusitis, nasal irrigation may relieve pain and congestion. If irrigation fails to relieve symptoms, one or more sinuses may require surgery.

Additional considerations

When caring for a patient with sinusitis, the health care professional should:
• enforce bed rest, and encourage the patient to drink plenty of fluids, to promote drainage; not elevate the head of the bed more than 30°.
• apply warm compresses continuously, or 4 times daily for 2-hour intervals, to relieve pain and promote drainage; give analgesics and antihistamines, as needed.
• watch for and report complications, such as vomiting, chills, fever, edema of the forehead or eyelids, blurred or double vision, and personality changes.
• place the patient in semi-Fowler's position to prevent edema and promote drainage; apply ice compresses or a rubber glove filled with ice chips over the nose, and iced saline gauze over the eyes to relieve edema and pain, and minimize

---

SURGERY FOR CHRONIC AND HYPERPLASTIC SINUSITIS

For maxillary sinusitis:
• *Nasal window procedure* creates an opening in the sinus, allowing secretions and pus to drain through the nose.
• *Caldwell-Luc procedure* removes diseased mucosa in the maxillary sinus through an incision under the upper lip.

For chronic ethmoid sinusitis:
• *Ethmoidectomy* removes all infected tissue through an external or intranasal incision into the ethmoidal sinus.

For sphenoid sinusitis:
• *External ethmoidectomy* removes infected ethmoidal sinus tissue through a crescent-shaped incision, beginning under the inner eyebrow and extending along the side of the nose.

For chronic frontal sinusitis:
• *Fronto-ethmoidectomy* removes infected frontal sinus tissue through an extended external ethmoidectomy.
• *Osteoplastic flap* drains the sinuses through an incision across the skull, behind the hairline.

---

bleeding; continue these measures for 24 hours.
• tell the patient who requires surgery what to expect postoperatively, such as having nasal packing in place for 12 to 24 hours following surgery, having to breathe through his mouth, and not being able to blow his nose. After surgery, he must be monitored for excessive drainage or bleeding and watched for complications.
• frequently change the mustache dressing or drip pad, and record the consistency, amount, and color of drainage (expect scant, bright red, and clotty drainage).
• provide meticulous mouth care, because the patient will be breathing through his mouth.
• tell the patient that even after the packing is removed, noseblowing may cause bleeding and swelling. If the patient is a smoker, he must not smoke for at least 2 to 3 days following surgery.

Nasal Polyps

Benign and edematous growths, nasal polyps are usually multiple, mobile, and bilateral. Nasal polyps may become large and numerous enough to cause nasal distention and enlargement of the bony framework, possibly occluding the airway. They are more common in adults than in children and tend to recur.

Causes

Nasal polyps are usually produced by the continuous pressure resulting from a chronic allergy that causes prolonged mucous membrane edema in the nose and sinuses. Other predisposing factors include chronic sinusitis, chronic rhinitis, and recurrent nasal infections.

Signs and symptoms

Nasal obstruction is the primary indication of nasal polyps. Such obstruction causes anosmia, a sensation of fullness in the face, nasal discharge, and shortness of breath. Associated clinical features are usually symptomatic of allergic rhinitis.

Diagnosis

Diagnosis of nasal polyps is aided by the following tests:

• *X-rays of sinuses and nasal passages* reveal soft tissue shadows over the affected areas.

• *Examination with a nasal speculum* shows a dry, red surface, with clear or gray growths. Large growths may resemble tumors.

Nasal polyps occurring in children require further testing to rule out cystic fibrosis.

Treatment

Generally, treatment consists of cortisone (either systemically or by direct injection into the polyps) to temporarily reduce the polyp. Treatment of the underlying cause may include antihistamines and corticosteroids to control allergy, and antibiotic therapy if infection is present. Local application of an astringent shrinks hypertrophied tissue. However, medical management alone is rarely effective.

Consequently, the treatment of choice is polypectomy (intranasal removal of the nasal polyp with a wire snare), usually performed under a local anesthetic. Continued recurrence may require surgical opening of the ethmoidal and the maxillary sinuses, and evacuation of diseased tissue.

Additional considerations

Antihistamines should be given, as ordered, for the patient with allergies. He can be prepared for scheduled surgery by telling him what to expect postoperatively, such as nasal packing for 1 to 2 days after surgery.

After surgery care includes:

• monitoring for excessive bleeding or other drainage, and promoting patient comfort.

• elevating the head of the bed to facilitate breathing, reduce swelling, and promote adequate drainage; changing the mustache dressing or drip pad, as needed, and recording the consistency, amount, and color of nasal drainage.

• intermittently applying ice compresses over the nostrils to lessen swelling, prevent bleeding, and relieve pain.

• elevating the head of the bed, monitoring vital signs, and advising the patient not to swallow blood if nasal bleeding occurs (most likely after packing is removed); compressing the outside of the nose against the septum for 10 to 15 minutes; notifying the doctor immediately if bleeding persists.

To prevent nasal polyps, patients with allergies should avoid exposure to allergens and take antihistamines at the first sign of an allergic reaction. They should also avoid overuse of nosedrops and sprays.

Nasal Papillomas

A papilloma is a benign epithelial tissue overgrowth within the intranasal mucosa. Inverted papillomas grow into the underlying tissue, usually at the junction of the antrum and the ethmoidal sinus; they generally occur singly but sometimes are associated with a squamous cell malignancy. Exophytic papillomas, which also tend to occur singly, arise from epithelial tissue, commonly on the surface of the nasal septum. Both types of papillomas are most prevalent in males. Recurrence is likely, even after surgical excision.

Causes
A papilloma may arise as a benign precursor of a neoplasm or as a response to tissue injury or viral infection, but its cause is unknown.

Signs and symptoms
Both inverted and exophytic papillomas typically produce symptoms related to unilateral nasal obstruction—stuffiness, postnasal drip, headache, shortness of breath, dyspnea, and rarely, severe respiratory distress, nasal drainage, and infection. Epistaxis is most likely to occur with exophytic papillomas.

Diagnosis

On examination of the nasal mucosa, inverted papillomas usually appear large, bulky, highly vascular, and edematous; color varies from dark red to gray; consistency, from firm to friable. Exophytic papillomas are commonly raised, firm, and rubbery; pink to gray; and securely attached by a broad or pedunculated base to the mucous membrane. Histologic examination of excised tissue confirms the diagnosis.

Treatment
The most effective treatment is wide surgical excision or diathermy, with careful inspection of adjacent tissues and sinuses to rule out extension. Since an exophytic papilloma is pedunculated, a suture tied around the growth may cause it to atrophy and fall off; this process takes 1 or 2 days and produces minimal bleeding. Aspirin or acetaminophen, and decongestants may relieve symptoms.

Additional considerations
• If bleeding occurs, the head of the bed should be raised, and the patient should expectorate blood into an emesis basin. The sides of the nose should be compressed against the septum for 10 to 15 minutes, and if necessary, ice packs applied to the area. If bleeding doesn't stop, the doctor must be notified.
• Checking for airway obstruction can be done by placing a hand under the patient's nostrils, and watching for signs of mild shortness of breath.
• If surgery is scheduled, the patient should be told what to expect postoperatively: that his nostrils will probably be packed and that he'll have to breathe through his mouth. He must not blow his nose. (Packing is usually removed 12 to 24 hours after surgery.)

Postoperatively care includes:
• monitoring vital signs and respiratory status; administering analgesics and facilitating breathing with a cool-mist vaporizer; providing good mouth care.
• frequently changing the mustache dressing or drip pad to ensure proper absorption of drainage; recording type and amount of drainage. While the nasal packing is in place, scant, usually bright red, clotted drainage is probable; the amount of drainage often increases for a few hours after the packing is removed.

Because papillomas tend to recur, the patient should seek medical attention at the first sign of nasal discomfort, discharge, or congestion that doesn't subside with conservative treatment.

THROAT

Pharyngitis

The most common throat disorder, pharyngitis is an acute or chronic inflammation of the pharynx. It is widespread among adults who live or work in dusty or very dry environments, use their voices excessively, habitually use tobacco or alcohol, or suffer from chronic sinusitis, persistent coughs, or allergies.

Causes
Pharyngitis is caused by a virus (90% of patients) or bacteria (most often streptococcus, especially in children). Acute pharyngitis may precede the common cold or other communicable diseases; chronic pharyngitis is often an extension of nasopharyngeal obstruction or inflammation.

Signs and symptoms
Pharyngitis typically produces a sore throat and slight difficulty in swallowing. Oddly, swallowing saliva is usually more painful than swallowing food. Pharyngitis may also cause the sensation of a lump in the throat, as well as a constant, aggravating urge to swallow. Associated features may include mild fever, headache, and muscle and joint pain (especially in bacterial pharyngitis). Uncomplicated pharyngitis usually subsides in 3 to 10 days.

Diagnosis
Physical examination of the pharynx reveals generalized redness and inflammation of the posterior wall, and red, edematous mucous membranes studded with white or yellow follicles. Exudate is usually confined to the lymphoid areas of the throat, sparing the tonsillar pillars. Throat culture may identify bacterial organisms, if they are the cause of the inflammation.

Treatment
Treatment of acute viral pharyngitis is usually symptomatic, and consists mainly of rest, warm saline gargles, throat lozenges containing a mild anesthetic, plenty of fluids, and analgesics, as needed. If the patient can't swallow fluids, hospitalization may be required, for I.V. hydration.

Bacterial pharyngitis necessitates rigorous treatment with penicillin—or another broad-spectrum antibiotic, if the patient is allergic to penicillin—since streptococcus is the chief infecting organism. Antibiotic therapy should continue for 48 hours after visible signs of infection have disappeared, or for at least 7 to 10 days.

Chronic pharyngitis requires the same supportive measures as acute pharyngitis but with greater emphasis on eliminating the underlying cause, such as an allergen. Preventive measures include adequate humidification and avoiding excessive exposure to air conditioning. In addition, the patient should be urged to stop smoking.

Additional considerations
Health care includes:
• administering analgesics and warm saline gargles, as ordered and as appropriate; encouraging the patient to drink plenty of fluids (up to 2,500 ml/day); monitoring intake and output scrupulously, and watching for signs of dehydration (cracked lips, dry mucous membranes, low urinary output); providing meticulous mouth care to prevent dry lips and oral pyoderma, and maintaining a restful environment.
• obtaining throat cultures, and administering antibiotics, as ordered; emphasizing the importance of completing the full course of antibiotic therapy if the patient has acute bacterial pharyngitis;

teaching the patient with chronic pharyngitis how to minimize sources of throat irritation in the environment, such as using a bedside humidifier; referring the patient to a self-help group to stop smoking, if appropriate.

Tonsillitis

Tonsillitis, or inflammation of the tonsils, can be acute or chronic. The uncomplicated acute form usually lasts 4 to 6 days and commonly affects children between ages 5 and 10. The presence of proven chronic tonsillitis justifies tonsillectomy, the only effective treatment. Tonsils tend to hypertrophy during childhood and atrophy after puberty.

Causes
Tonsillitis generally results from infection with beta-hemolytic streptococci but can result from other bacteria or viruses.

Signs and symptoms
Acute tonsillitis commonly begins with a mild to severe sore throat. A very young child, unable to complain about a sore throat, may stop eating. Tonsillitis may also produce dysphagia, fever, swelling and tenderness of the lymph glands in the submandibular area, muscle and joint pain, chills, malaise, headache, and pain (frequently referred to the ears). Excess secretions may elicit the complaint of a constant urge to swallow; the back of the throat may feel constricted. Such discomfort usually subsides after 72 hours.

Chronic tonsillitis produces a recurrent sore throat and purulent drainage in the tonsillar crypts. Frequent attacks of acute tonsillitis may also occur. Complications include obstruction from tonsillar hypertrophy and peritonsillar abscess.

Diagnosis
Diagnostic confirmation requires a thorough throat examination that reveals:
• generalized inflammation of the pharyngeal wall.
• swollen tonsils that project from between the pillars of the fauces and exude white or yellow follicles.
• purulent drainage when pressure is applied to the tonsillar pillars.
• possible edematous and inflamed uvula.

Culture may determine the infecting organism and indicate appropriate antibiotic therapy. Leukocytosis is also usually present. Differential diagnosis rules out infectious mononucleosis and diphtheria.

Treatment
Treatment of acute tonsillitis requires rest, adequate fluid intake, administration of aspirin or acetaminophen, and for bacterial infection, antibiotics. When the causative organism is Group A beta-hemolytic streptococcus, penicillin is the drug of choice (erythromycin or another broad-spectrum antibiotic may be given if the patient is allergic to penicillin). To prevent complications, antibiotic therapy should continue for 10 days. Chronic tonsillitis or the development of complications (obstructions from tonsillar hypertrophy, peritonsillar abscess) may require a tonsillectomy, but only after the patient has been free of tonsillar or respiratory tract infections for 3 to 4 weeks.

Additional considerations
• Despite dysphagia, the patient must drink plenty of fluids, especially if he has a fever. A child can be offered ice cream and flavored drinks and ices. Gargling may soothe the throat, unless it exacerbates pain. The patient and parents must understand the importance of completing the prescribed antibiotic

treatment.

• Before tonsillectomy, the adult patient should know that a local anesthetic prevents pain but allows a sensation of pressure during surgery. The patient can expect considerable throat discomfort and some bleeding postoperatively.

• For the pediatric patient, the explanation of the surgery should be simple and nonthreatening. The child can be shown the operating and recovery rooms, and have the hospital routine briefly explained to him. A parent should stay with the child, if allowed.

• Postoperatively, a patent airway should be maintained. To prevent aspiration, the patient can be placed on his side. Vital signs must be monitored, and the patient checked for bleeding. Excessive bleeding, increased pulse rate or dropping blood pressure must be reported immediately. After the patient is fully alert and the gag reflex has returned, he can drink water. Later, he should drink nonirritating fluids, walk, and take frequent deep breaths to prevent pulmonary complications. He should be given pain medication, a needed.

• Before discharge, the patient or parents will need written instructions on home care. They can expect a white scab to form in the throat between 5 and 10 days postoperatively. They should report bleeding, ear discomfort, or a fever that lasts longer than 3 days.

Adenoid Hyperplasia
(Adenoid hypertrophy)

A fairly common childhood condition, adenoid hyperplasia is enlargement of the lymphoid tissue of the nasopharynx. Although adenoidal tissue is usually small at birth (¾" to 1¼" [2 to 3 cm]), it grows rapidly until age 3 and reaches maximal size by age 5; normally, it then begins to slowly atrophy. In adenoid hyperplasia, however, this tissue continues to grow.

Causes
Although the cause of adenoid hyperplasia is unknown, contributing factors may include heredity, repeated infection, chronic nasal congestion, persistent allergy, insufficient aeration, and inefficient nasal breathing. Inflammation due to repeated infection enhances the risk of respiratory obstruction.

Signs and symptoms
Typically, adenoid hyperplasia produces symptoms of respiratory obstruction, especially mouth breathing, snoring at night, and frequent, prolonged head colds. Persistent mouth breathing during the formative years produces distinctive changes in facial features (adenoid facies)—typically, the face becomes slightly elongated, the mouth always open, the palate highly arched, the upper lip shortened, and the eyes take on a vacant expression.

Occasionally, the child is incapable of mouth breathing, snores loudly at night, and may eventually show effects of nocturnal respiratory insufficiency, such as intercostal retractions and nasal flaring; this may lead to pulmonary hypertension and cor pulmonale. Adenoid hyperplasia can also obstruct the eustachian tube and predispose to otitis media, which in turn can lead to fluctuating conductive hearing loss (reversible with treatment). Stasis of nasal secretions from adenoidal inflammation can lead to sinusitis.

Diagnosis
 Nasopharyngoscopy or rhinoscopy confirms adenoid hyperplasia by visualizing abnormal tissue mass. In nasopharyngoscopy, a small flexible scope with fiberoptic lighting is inserted through the nostrils to visualize the adenoids; in rhinoscopy, light is re-

flected on a hand mirror for the same purpose. Lateral pharyngeal X-rays show obliteration of the nasopharyngeal air column.

Treatment
Adenoidectomy is the treatment of choice of adenoid hyperplasia, and is commonly recommended for the patient with prolonged mouth breathing, nasal speech, adenoid facies, recurrent otitis media, constant nasopharyngitis, and nocturnal respiratory distress. This procedure usually eliminates recurrent nasal infections and ear complications, and reverses any secondary hearing loss.

Additional considerations
Since adenoid hyperplasia occurs exclusively in children, the health care plan should focus on sympathetic preoperative care and diligent postoperative monitoring.

Before surgery, the health care professional should:
- arrange for the patient and parents to tour relevant areas of the hospital; describe the hospital routine in a nonthreatening manner.
- explain adenoidectomy to the child, using illustrations, if necessary, and detail the recovery process; reassure him that he'll probably need to be hospitalized only two nights (the nights before and after surgery); encourage one parent to stay with the child if hospital protocol allows and participate in his care.

After surgery, the professional should:
- maintain a patent airway; position the child on his side, with head down, to prevent aspiration of draining secretions; frequently check the throat for bleeding, especially during the first postoperative night; be alert for vomiting of old, partially digested blood ("coffee ground"); closely monitor vital signs, and report excessive bleeding, rise in pulse rate, drop in blood pressure, tachypnea, and restlessness.
- offer cracked ice or water, if no bleeding occurs, when the patient is awake.
- tell the parents that their child may temporarily have a nasal voice.

Velopharyngeal Insufficiency

Velopharyngeal insufficiency results from failure of the velopharyngeal sphincter to close properly during speech, giving the voice a hypernasal quality and permitting nasal emission (air escape during pronunciation of particular consonants). This disorder commonly occurs in persons who undergo surgery for cleft palate and those with submucous cleft palates. Middle ear disease and hearing loss frequently accompany this disorder.

Causes
Velopharyngeal insufficiency can result from an inherited palate abnormality (short palate, pharyngomegaly, submucous cleft palate), or it can be an acquired disorder from tonsillectomy, adenoidectomy, or palatal paresis.

Signs and symptoms
Generally, this condition causes unintelligible speech, marked by hypernasality, nasal emission, poor consonant definition, and a weak voice. The person's efforts to correct this problem result in speech maladjustments characteristic of cleft palate. In addition, he experiences dysphagia. If velopharyngeal insufficiency is severe, he may regurgitate liquids and solid food through the nose.

Diagnosis
Fiberoptic nasopharyngoscopy, which permits monitoring of velopharyngeal patency during speech, suggests this diagnosis. Another helpful diagnostic procedure is ultrasound scanning, which shows air-tissue overlap, reflecting the degree of velopharyngeal sphincter in-

competence (an opening greater than 20 mm² results in unintelligible speech).

Treatment
Treatment consists of corrective surgery, usually at age 6 or 7. The preferred surgical method is the *pharyngeal flap procedure,* which diverts a tissue flap from the pharynx to the soft palate. Other appropriate surgical procedures include:
• *palatal push-back,* which separates the hard and soft palates to allow insertion of an obturator, thus lengthening the soft palate.
• *pharyngoplasty,* which rotates pharyngeal flaps to lengthen the soft palate and narrow the pharynx.
• *augmentation pharyngoplasty,* which narrows the velopharyngeal opening by enlarging the pharyngeal wall with a retropharyngeal implant (injected Teflon or Silastic). The disadvantages of this procedure include infection, and implant displacement.
• *velopharyngeal sphincter reconstruction,* which uses free muscle implantation to reconstruct the sphincter.

Surgery eliminates hypernasality and nasal emission, but speech maladjustments persist and usually necessitate speech therapy, depending on the patient's age. Immediate postoperative therapy includes antibiotics and a clear, liquid diet for the first 3 days, followed by a soft diet for 2 weeks.

Additional considerations
Postoperatively, the health care professional should:
• maintain a patent airway (edema of the nasopharynx may obstruct the airway); position the patient on his side, and suction the dependent side of his mouth; be careful not to insert the suction catheter into the pharynx.
• control postoperative agitation, which may provoke pharyngeal bleeding, with sedation, as ordered.
• administer high-humidity oxygen, as ordered.
• monitor vital signs frequently, and report any changes immediately; observe for bleeding from the mouth or nose; check intake and output, and watch for signs of dehydration, particularly if the patient has dysphagia; give reassurance that such difficulty will subside as swelling diminishes.
• advise the patient that speech therapy, if ordered, requires time and effort on his part, but with persistence and practice, his speech will improve; emphasize before discharge the importance of completing the prescribed antibiotic therapy.

Throat Abscesses

Throat abscesses may be peritonsillar (quinsy) or retropharyngeal. Peritonsillar abscess forms in the connective tissue space between the tonsil capsule and constrictor muscle of the pharynx. Retropharyngeal abscess, or abscess of the potential space, forms between the posterior pharyngeal wall and prevertebral fascia. With treatment, the prognosis for both types of abscesses is good.

Causes and incidence
Peritonsillar abscess is a complication of acute tonsillitis, usually after streptococcal or staphylococcal infection. It occurs more often in adolescents and young adults than in children.

Acute retropharyngeal abscess results from infection in the retropharyngeal lymph glands, which may follow an upper respiratory tract bacterial infection. Because these lymph glands, present at birth, begin to atrophy after age 2, acute retropharyngeal abscess most commonly affects infants and children under age 2.

Chronic retropharyngeal abscess results from tuberculosis of the cervical spine (Pott's disease) and may occur at any age.

Signs and symptoms

Key symptoms of peritonsillar abscess include severe throat pain, occasional ear pain on the same side as the abscess, and tenderness of the submandibular gland. Dysphagia causes drooling. Trismus may occur as a result of edema and infection spreading from the peritonsillar space to the pterygoid muscles. Other effects include fever, chills, malaise, rancid breath, nausea, muffled speech, dehydration, cervical adenopathy, and localized or systemic sepsis.

Clinical features of retropharyngeal abscess include pain, dysphagia, fever, and when the abscess is located in the upper pharynx, nasal obstruction; with a low-positioned abscess, dyspnea, progressive inspiratory stridor (from laryngeal obstruction), neck hyperextension, and in children, drooling and muffled crying. A grossly enlarged abscess may press on the larynx, producing edema, or may erode into major blood vessels, causing sudden death from asphyxia or aspiration.

Diagnosis

Diagnosis of peritonsillar abscess begins with a patient history of staphylococcal or streptococcal infection. Examination of the throat shows swelling of the soft palate on the abscessed side, with displacement of the uvula to the opposite side; red, edematous mucous membranes; and tonsil displacement toward the midline. Culture may reveal streptococcal or staphylococcal infection.

Diagnosis of retropharyngeal abscess is based on patient history of nasopharyngitis or pharyngitis, and physical examination revealing a soft, red bulging of the posterior pharyngeal wall. X-rays show the larynx pushed forward, and a widened space between the posterior pharyngeal wall and vertebrae. Culture and sensitivity tests isolate the causative organism and determine the appropriate antibiotic.

Treatment

For early-stage peritonsillar abscess, large doses of penicillin or another broad-spectrum antibiotic are necessary. For late-stage abscess, with cellulitis of the tonsillar space, primary treatment is usually incision and drainage under a local anesthetic, followed by antibiotic therapy for 7 to 10 days. Tonsillectomy, scheduled no sooner than 1 month after healing, prevents recurrence but is recommended only after several episodes.

In acute retropharyngeal abscess, the primary treatment is incision and drainage through the pharyngeal wall. In chronic retropharyngeal abscess, drainage is performed through an external incision behind the sternomastoid muscle. During incision and drainage, strong, continuous mouth suction is necessary to prevent aspiration of pus. Postoperative drug therapy includes antibiotics (usually penicillin) and analgesics.

Additional considerations

Before and during incision and drainage, care includes:
• being alert for signs of respiratory obstruction (inspiratory stridor, dyspnea, increasing restlessness, or cyanosis); keeping emergency airway equipment nearby.
• explaining drainage procedure to the patient or his parents (since the procedure is generally done under a local anesthetic, the patient may be apprehensive).
• assisting with incision and drainage; placing the patient in a semirecumbent or sitting position to allow easy expectoration and suction of pus and blood.

After incision and drainage, care includes:
• giving antibiotics, analgesics, and antipyretics; stressing the importance of completing prescribed antibiotic therapy.
• monitoring vital signs, and reporting any significant changes or bleeding; assessing pain and treating accordingly.
• ensuring adequate hydration with I.V. therapy if the patient is unable to swallow; monitoring fluid intake and output, and watching for dehydration.
• providing meticulous mouth care; applying petrolatum to the patient's lips; promoting healing with warm saline gargles or throat irrigations for 24 to 36 hours after incision and drainage.

Vocal Cord Paralysis

Vocal cord paralysis results from disease of or injury to the superior or, most often, the recurrent laryngeal nerve.

Causes

Vocal cord paralysis commonly results from the accidental severing of the recurrent laryngeal nerve or of one of its extralaryngeal branches, during thyroidectomy. Other causes include pressure from an aortic aneurysm or from an enlarged atrium (in patients with mitral stenosis), bronchial or esophageal carcinoma, hypertrophy of the thyroid gland, trauma (such as neck injuries), and neuritis due to infections or metallic poisoning.

Vocal cord paralysis can also result from hysteria and, rarely, CNS lesions.

Signs and symptoms

Indications of vocal cord paralysis depend on whether the paralysis is unilateral or bilateral, and on the position of the cord or cords when paralyzed. Unilateral paralysis, the most common form, may cause vocal weakness and hoarseness; bilateral paralysis produces vocal weakness, and incapacitating airway obstruction if the cords become paralyzed in the adducted position.

Diagnosis

Patient history and characteristic features suggest vocal cord paralysis.

 Visualization by indirect laryngoscopy shows one or both cords fixed in an adducted or partially abducted position, and confirms the diagnosis.

Treatment

Treatment of unilateral paralysis consists of injection of Teflon into the paralyzed cord, under direct laryngoscopy. This procedure enlarges the cord and brings it closer to the other cord, which usually strengthens the voice and protects the airway from aspiration. Bilateral cord paralysis in an adducted position generally necessitates tracheotomy to restore a patent airway.

Alternative therapy for adults includes arytenoidectomy to open the glottis, and lateral fixation of the arytenoid cartilage through an external neck incision. Excision or fixation of the arytenoid improves airway patency but produces residual voice impairment.

Treatment of hysterical aphonia may include psychotherapy and, for some patients, hypnosis.

Additional considerations

If the patient chooses direct laryngoscopy and Teflon injection, he must understand the procedures thoroughly. He should know that these measures will improve his voice but won't restore it to normal.

Many patients with bilateral cord paralysis prefer to keep a tracheostomy instead of having an arytenoidectomy; their voices are generally better with a tracheostomy alone than after corrective surgery.

If the patient is scheduled to undergo a tracheotomy, the hospital staff member should:

• explain the procedure thoroughly, and offer reassurance. Since the procedure is performed under a local anesthetic, the patient may be apprehensive.

• teach the patient how to suction, clean, and change the tracheostomy tube.

• reassure the patient that he can still speak by covering the lumen of the tracheostomy tube with his finger or a tracheostomy plug.

If the patient elects to have an arytenoidectomy, he should understand its consequences, and be aware that the tracheostomy will remain in place until the edema has subsided and the airway is patent.

Vocal Cord Nodules and Polyps

Vocal cord nodules result from hypertrophy of fibrous tissue and form at the point where the cords come together forcibly. Vocal cord polyps are chronic, subepithelial, edematous masses. Both nodules and polyps have good prognoses, unless continued voice abuse causes recurrence, with subsequent scarring and permanent hoarseness.

Causes and incidence

Vocal cord nodules and polyps usually result from voice abuse, especially in the presence of infection. Consequently, they're most common in teachers, singers, and sports fans, and in energetic children (ages 8 to 12) who continually shout while playing. Polyps are common in adults who smoke, live in dry climates, or have allergies.

Signs and symptoms

Nodules and polyps inhibit the approximation of vocal cords and produce painless hoarseness. The voice may also develop a breathy or husky quality.

Diagnosis

Persistent hoarseness suggests vocal cord nodules and polyps; visualization by indirect laryngoscopy confirms it. In the patient with vocal cord nodules, laryngoscopy initially shows small red nodes; later, white solid nodes on one or both cords. In the patient with polyps, laryngoscopy reveals unilateral or, occasionally, bilateral, sessile or pedunculated polyps of varying size, anywhere on the vocal cords.

Treatment

Conservative management of small vocal cord nodules and polyps includes humidification, speech therapy (voice rest, training to reduce the intensity and duration of voice production), and treatment of any underlying allergies.

When conservative treatment fails to relieve hoarseness, nodules or polyps require removal under direct laryngoscopy. Microlaryngoscopy may be done for small lesions, to avoid injuring the

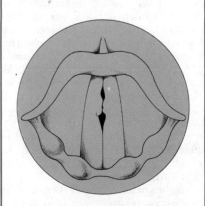

VOCAL CORD NODULES

Posterior two thirds

Open glottis

Anterior one third

The most common site of vocal cord nodules is the point of maximal vibration and impact (junction of the anterior one third and the posterior two thirds of the vocal cord).

Vocal cord nodules affect the voice by inhibiting proper closure of the vocal cords during phonation.

vocal cord surface. If nodules or polyps are bilateral, excision may be performed in two stages: one cord is allowed to heal before excision of polyps on the other cord. Two-stage excision prevents laryngeal web, which occurs when epithelial tissue is removed from adjacent cord surfaces, and these surfaces grow together. For children, treatment consists of speech therapy. If possible, surgery should be delayed until the child is old enough to benefit from voice training, or until he can understand the need to abstain from voice abuse.

Additional considerations

When caring for a patient with vocal cord nodules or polyps, the health care professional should:

• stress the importance postoperatively of resting the voice for 10 days to 2 weeks while the vocal cords heal; provide an alternative means of communication— Magic Slate, pad and pencil, or alphabet board; place a sign over the bed to remind visitors that the patient shouldn't talk; mark the intercom so other hospital personnel are aware the patient can't answer; minimize the need to speak by trying to anticipate the patient's needs.
• encourage the smoker to stop smoking entirely or, at the very least, to refrain from smoking during recovery from surgery.
• utilize a vaporizer to increase humidity and decrease throat irritation.
• make sure the patient receives speech therapy after healing, if necessary, since continued voice abuse causes recurrence.

Laryngitis

A common disorder, laryngitis is acute or chronic inflammation of the vocal cords. Acute laryngitis may occur as an isolated infection or as part of a generalized bacterial or viral upper respiratory tract infection. Repeated attacks of acute laryngitis cause inflammatory changes associated with chronic laryngitis.

Causes and incidence

Acute laryngitis usually results from infection or excessive use of the voice, an occupational hazard in certain vocations (teaching, public speaking, singing, for example). It may also result from leisuretime activities (such as cheering at a sports event), inhalation of smoke or fumes, or aspiration of caustic chemicals. Causes of chronic laryngitis include chronic upper respiratory tract disorders (sinusitis, bronchitis, nasal polyps, allergy), mouth breathing, smoking, constant exposure to dust or other irritants, and alcohol abuse.

Signs and symptoms

Acute laryngitis typically begins with hoarseness, ranging from mild to complete loss of voice. Associated clinical features include pain (especially when swallowing or speaking), dry cough, fever, laryngeal edema, and malaise. In chronic laryngitis, persistent hoarseness is usually the only symptom.

Diagnosis

 Indirect laryngoscopy confirms diagnosis by revealing red, inflamed, and occasionally, hemorrhagic vocal cords, with rounded rather than sharp edges, and exudate. Bilateral swelling may be present, which restricts movement but doesn't cause paralysis.

Treatment

Primary treatment consists of resting the voice. For viral infection, symptomatic care includes analgesics and throat lozenges for pain relief. Bacterial infection requires antibiotic therapy. Severe, acute laryngitis may necessitate hospitalization. Occasionally, when laryngeal edema results in airway obstruction, tracheotomy may be necessary. In chronic laryngitis, effective treatment must eliminate the underlying cause.

Additional considerations
• The hospitalized patient must be given an explanation of why he should not talk. A sign can be placed over his bed to remind others of this restriction. He should be given a Magic Slate or a pad and pencil for communication. The intercom panel must be marked so other hospital personnel are aware the patient can't answer. Trying to anticipate the patient's needs will minimize his need to talk.

• The patient can maintain adequate humidification by using a vaporizer or humidifier during the winter; by avoiding air conditioning during the summer (because it dehumidifies); by using medicated throat lozenges; and by not smoking. He should complete prescribed antibiotics.

• A detailed patient history will help determine the cause of chronic laryngitis. The patient will need encouragement to modify predisposing habits.

Juvenile Angiofibroma

An uncommon disorder, juvenile angiofibroma is a highly vascular, nasopharyngeal tumor made up of masses of fibrous tissue that contain many thin-walled blood vessels. These tumors are found primarily in adolescent males, and are extremely rare in females. Incidence is higher in Egypt, India, Southeast Asia, and Kenya than in the United States and Europe. Prognosis is good with treatment.

Causes
Although its cause is unknown, juvenile angiofibroma has been identified as a type of hemangioma. This tumor grows on one side of the posterior nares, and may completely fill the nasopharynx, nose, paranasal sinuses, and possibly, the orbit. More often sessile than polypoid, juvenile angiofibroma is nonencapsulated and invades surrounding tissue.

Signs and symptoms
Juvenile angiofibroma produces unilateral or bilateral nasal obstruction and severe recurrent epistaxis, usually between ages 7 and 21. Recurrent epistaxic episodes eventually cause secondary anemia. Associated effects include purulent rhinorrhea, facial deformity, and nasal speech. Serous otitis media and hearing loss may result from eustachian tube obstruction.

Diagnosis
Physical examination with a nasopharyngeal mirror or nasal speculum permits visualization of the tumor, which appears as a blue mass in the nose or nasopharynx. X-rays show a bowing of the posterior wall of the maxillary sinus. Angiography determines the size and

JUVENILE ANGIOFIBROMA

This tumor affects the posterior nares, producing nasal obstruction and recurrent epistaxis.

location of the tumor and also shows the source of vascularization. Biopsy of the tumor is contraindicated because of the danger of hemorrhage.

Treatment
Several surgical methods, ranging from avulsion to cryosurgical techniques, comprise the treatment of choice. Surgical excision is preferred after embolization with Teflon or absorbable gelatin sponge, to decrease vascularization. Whichever surgical method is used, this tumor must be removed in its entirety and not in pieces. Preoperative hormonal therapy may decrease the tumor's size and vascularity. Blood transfusions may be necessary during avulsion. Radiation therapy produces only a temporary regression in an angiofibroma but is the treatment of choice if the tumor has expanded into the cranium or orbit. Because the tumor is multilobular and locally invasive, symptomatic recurrences are common (about 30% of patients) during the first year after treatment, but are uncommon after 2 years.

Additional considerations
When caring for a patient with juvenile angiofibroma, the hospital staff member should:
- explain all diagnostic and surgical procedures; provide emotional support—severe epistaxis frightens many persons to the point of panic; check hemoglobin and hematocrit for anemia.
- report excessive bleeding after surgery immediately; make sure an adequate supply of typed and cross-matched blood is available for transfusion.
- monitor for any change in vital signs; provide good oral hygiene; use a bedside vaporizer to raise humidity.
- during blood transfusion, watch for transfusion reactions, such as fever, chills, or a rash; discontinue the blood transfusion if any of these reactions occur and notify the doctor immediately.
- teach the family how to apply pressure over the affected area; instruct them to seek immediate attention if bleeding occurs after discharge; stress the importance of providing adequate humidification at home to keep nasal mucosa moist.

Contact Ulcers

Contact ulcers are erosions on the laryngeal mucosa that cause gradual tissue necrosis. They appear on laryngeal mucosa over the arytenoid cartilage, where the vocal cords come together forcibly. Contact ulcers are relatively common in the United States, particularly in middle-aged, urban, professional men. Contact ulcers respond well to rest or excision, but recurrence is common.

Causes
Contact ulcers most commonly result from vocal strain, especially during laryngitis. Other causes include laryngeal trauma from endotracheal intubation, and emotional stress.

Signs and symptoms
Typical indications of contact ulcers are hoarseness of varying intensity and mild dysphagia. Other symptoms may include laryngeal tenderness during external palpation, and granulation from prolonged ulceration.

Diagnosis
 Indirect laryngoscopy permits visualization of the ulcer and granulation tissue, confirming the diagnosis. Biopsy under direct laryngoscopy is necessary to rule out neoplasm.

Treatment and additional considerations
Supportive measures include prolonged and absolute voice rest, adequate humidification, and aerosol therapy. Drug therapy may include antibiotics and

tranquilizers. Psychotherapy may help prevent recurrence. Laryngoscopic removal of excessive granulomatous tissue is necessary after confirmation.

Health care of the patient with contact ulcers includes:

• explaining laryngoscopy fully to the patient; giving preoperative sedation.

• allowing the patient nothing by mouth after laryngoscopy until the effect of the anesthetic wears off (usually 2 hours).

• supplying a Magic Slate or a pencil and pad to help the patient communicate while resting his voice; placing a sign over the bed to remind visitors that the patient must not speak.

• providing emotional support, since many patients are distressed by enforced silence.

Selected References

Ausband, John R., ed. EAR, NOSE AND THROAT DISORDERS: A PRACTITIONERS GUIDE. Garden City, N.Y.: Medical Examination Publishing Co., 1974.

Batsakis, John G. TUMORS OF THE HEAD AND NECK: CLINICAL AND PATHOLOGICAL CONSIDERATIONS, 2nd ed. Baltimore: Williams & Wilkins Co., 1979.

Bluestone, Charles, and Paul Shurin. *Middle Ear Disease in Children,* PEDIATRIC CLINICS OF NORTH AMERICA. 21:2:379-400, May 1974.

Bruch, William. *Otitis Media,* PEDIATRIC NURSING. 5:1:9-12, January/February 1979.

DeWeese, David D., and William H. Saunders. TEXTBOOK OF OTOLARYNGOLOGY, 5th ed. St. Louis: C.V. Mosby Co., 1977.

Downs, Marion, *Auditory Screening,* OTOLARYNGOLOGIC CLINICS OF NORTH AMERICA. 11:3:611-629, October 1978.

Eliachar, Isaac. *Audiologic Manifestations in Otitis Media,* OTOLARYNGOLOGIC CLINICS OF NORTH AMERICA. 11:3:769-776, October 1978.

Hall, Ian Simson, and Bernard H. Colman. DISEASES OF THE NOSE, THROAT AND EAR. New York: Churchill Livingstone Inc., 1976.

Havener, William H., et al. NURSING CARE IN EYE, EAR, NOSE AND THROAT DISORDERS. St. Louis: C.V. Mosby Co., 1975.

Heffer, Allan, *Hearing Loss Due to Noise Exposure,* OTOLARYNGOLOGIC CLINICS OF NORTH AMERICA. 11:3:723-740, October 1978.

Lee, K.J. DIFFERENTIAL DIAGNOSIS IN OTOLARYNGOLOGY. New York: Arco Publishing Co., 1978.

Mechner, E. *Examination of the Ear,* AMERICAN JOURNAL OF NURSING. 75:3:1-24, March 1975.

Mortimer, Edward. *Suppurative Otitis Media: A Pediatric View,* OTOLARYNGOLOGIC CLINICS OF NORTH AMERICA. 9:3:679-687, October 1976.

Paparella, Michael M., and Donald A. Shunrick. OTOLARYNGOLOGY, Vols. 1, 2, and 3. Philadelphia: W.B. Saunders Co., 1973.

Paparella, Michael, et al. *Hearing Loss—A Common Medical Responsibility Symposium,* POSTGRADUATE MEDICINE. 62:4:93-143, October 1977.

Saunders, William H., et al. NURSING CARE IN EYE, EAR, NOSE AND THROAT DISORDERS, 4th ed. St. Louis: C.V. Mosby Co., 1979.

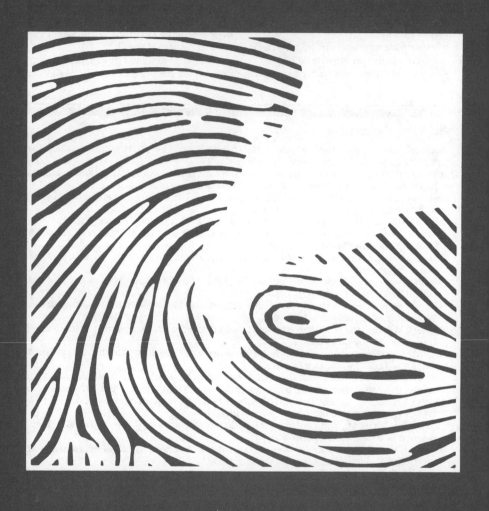

21 Skin Disorders

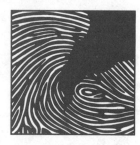

Skin Disorders

Introduction

Skin is man's front-line protective barrier between internal structures and the external environment. It's tough, resilient, and virtually impermeable to aqueous solutions, bacteria, or toxic compounds. It also performs many vital functions. Skin protects against trauma, regulates body temperature, serves as an organ of excretion and sensation, and synthesizes vitamin D in the presence of ultraviolet light. Skin varies in thickness and other qualities from one part of the body to another, which often accounts for the distribution of skin diseases.

Skin has three primary layers: *epidermis*, *dermis*, and *subcutaneous tissue*. The epidermis—the outermost layer—as its primary function, produces keratin. This layer is generally thin but is thicker in areas subject to constant pressure or friction, such as the soles and palms. Epidermis contains two sublayers: the *stratum corneum*, an outer, horny layer of keratin that protects the body against harmful environmental substances and restricts water loss; and the *cellular stratum*, where keratin cells are synthesized. The *basement membrane* lies beneath the cellular stratum and joins the epidermis to the dermis.

The cellular stratum, the deepest layer of the epidermis, consists of the *basal layer*, where mitosis takes place; the *stratum spinosum*, where cells begin to flatten, and fibrils—precursors of kera-

tin—start to appear; and the *stratum granulosum*, made up of cells containing deeply staining granules of keratohyalin, which are generally thought to become the keratin that forms the stratum corneum. A skin cell moves from the basal layer of the cellular stratum to the stratum corneum in about 14 days. After another 14 days, normal wear and tear on the skin cause it to slough off. The epidermis also contains melanocytes, which produce the melanin that gives the skin its color, and a yellow pigment called carotene.

The *dermis*, the second primary layer of the skin, consists of three fibrous proteins, fibroblasts, and an intervening ground substance. The proteins are collagen, which strengthens the skin to prevent it from tearing; elastin to give it resilience; and reticulin, which helps make up the basement membrane. The ground substance contains primarily jellylike mucopolysaccharides; this substance makes the skin soft and compressible. Two distinct layers comprise the dermis: the papillary dermis (top layer) and the reticular dermis (bottom layer).

Subcutaneous tissue, the third primary layer of the skin, consists mainly of fat (containing mostly triglycerides), which provides heat, insulation, shock absorption, and a reserve of calories. Both sensory and motor nerves (autonomic fibers) are found in the dermis and the subcutaneous tissue.

Appendages: Nails, glands, and hair

Nails are epidermal cells converted to hard keratin. The bed on which the nail rests is highly vascular, making the nail appear pink; the whitish, crescent-shaped area extending beyond the proximal nail fold, called the lunula—most visible in the thumbnail—marks the end of the matrix, the site of mitosis and of nail growth.

Sebaceous glands, found everywhere on the body except the palms and soles, serve as appendages of the dermis. These glands generally excrete sebum into hair follicles, but in some cases, they empty directly onto the skin surface. Sebum is an oily substance that helps keep the skin and hair from drying out and prevents water and heat loss. Sebaceous glands abound on the scalp, forehead, cheeks, chin, back, and genitalia, and may be stimulated by sex hormones—primarily testosterone.

Appendages found in the dermis and the subcutaneous tissue include *eccrine* and *apocrine glands,* and *hair.* Eccrine sweat glands open directly onto the skin and regulate body temperature. Innervated by sympathetic nerves, these sweat glands are distributed throughout the body, except for the lips, ears, and parts of the genitalia. They secrete a solution made up mostly of water and sodium chloride; the prime stimulus for eccrine gland secretion is heat. Other stimuli include muscular exertion and emotional stress.

Apocrine sweat glands appear chiefly in the axillae and genitalia; they are responsible for producing body odor and are stimulated by emotional stress. The sweat produced is sterile but undergoes bacterial decomposition on the skin surface. These glands become functional after puberty. (Ceruminous glands, located in the external ear canal, appear to be modified sweat glands and secrete a waxy substance known as cerumen.)

Hair grows on most of the body, except for the palms, the soles, and parts of the genitalia. An individual hair consists of a shaft (a column of keratinized cells), a root (embedded in the dermis), the hair follicle (the root and its covering), and the hair papilla (a loop of capillaries at the base of the follicle). Mitosis at the base of the follicle causes the hair to grow, while the papilla provides nourishment for mitosis. Small bundles of involuntary muscles known as arrectores pilorum cling to hair follicles. When these muscles contract, usually during moments of fear or shock, the hairs stand on end, and the person is said to have goose bumps or gooseflesh. Melanin in the outer layer of the hair shaft gives the

PRIMARY SKIN LESIONS

MACULE
(flat, circumscribed area with change in normal skin)

VESICLE
(serous fluid-filled lesion)

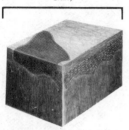

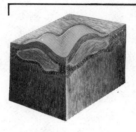

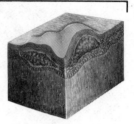

Patch (usually > 1 cm)—flat area of skin with change in color

Bulla (> 1 cm)—larger circumscribed area containing free serous fluid

Pustule (size varies)—lesion containing purulent fluid

PAPULE
(solid, elevated mass)

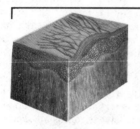

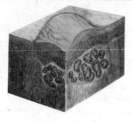

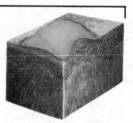

Plaque—formed by confluence of papules

Nodule or tumor (usually > 1 cm)—palpable, solid, and round

Wheal—circumscribed area of edema, usually transient

hair its distinctive color, which is directly related to the number of melanocytes (melanin-producing cells) in the hair bulb.

Vascular influence

Skin contains a vast arteriovenous network, extending from subcutaneous tissue to the dermis. These blood vessels provide oxygen and nutrients to sensory nerves (which control touch, temperature, and pain), motor nerves (which control the activities of sweat glands, the arterioles, and smooth muscles of the skin), and skin appendages. Blood flow also influences skin coloring, since the amount of oxygen carried to capillaries in the dermis can produce transient changes in color. For example, decreased oxygen supply can turn the skin pale or bluish; increased oxygen can turn it pink or ruddy.

Assessing skin disorders

Assessment begins with a thorough patient history to determine whether a skin disorder is an acute flare-up, recurrent problem, or chronic condition. The patient should be asked how long he's had the disorder; how a typical flare-up or attack begins; whether or not it itches; and what medications—systemic or topical—have been used to treat it. Also, if any family members, friends, or contacts have the same disorder, and if the patient lives or works in an environment that could cause the condition.

Examination of a patient with a skin disorder includes: being sure to look everywhere—mucous membranes, hair, scalp, axillae, groin, palms, soles, nails; noting moisture, temperature, texture, thickness, mobility, edema, turgor, and any irregularities in skin color; looking for skin lesions; recording the color, size, and location of any lesion; trying to determine which is the primary lesion—the one that appeared first and always starts in normal skin. The patient might be able to point it out.

If more than one lesion is in evidence, the pattern of distribution should be noted. Lesions can be localized (isolated), regional, general, or universal (total), involving the entire skin, hair, and nails. Also, whether the lesions are unilateral or bilateral, symmetric or asymmetric should be observed, and the arrangement of the lesions (clustered or linear configuration, for example) noted.

Diagnostic aids

After simple observation, and examination of the affected area of the skin with a dermatoscope, for morphologic detail, the following clinical diagnostic techniques may help to identify skin disorders:
• *Diascopy,* in which a lesion is covered with a microscopic slide or piece of clear plastic, helps determine whether dilated capillaries or extravasated blood is causing the redness of a lesion.
• *Sidelighting* shows minor elevations or depressions in lesions; it also helps determine the configuration and degree of

SECONDARY CHANGES IN PRIMARY SKIN LESIONS

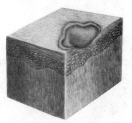

Erosion—circumscribed, partial loss of epidermis

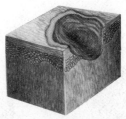

Ulcer—irregularly sized and shaped excavations penetrating into dermis

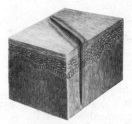

Fissure—linear ulcer

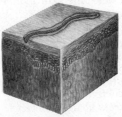

Excoriation—abrasion or scratch mark (linear break produced manually)

SECONDARY CHANGES IN PRIMARY SKIN LESIONS

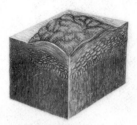

Crust—variously colored masses of exudate from skin

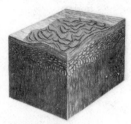

Scale—loose fragments of keratin in stratum corneum

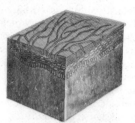

Lichenification—thick and roughened skin, exaggerated skin lines

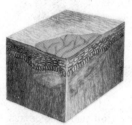

Atrophy—thin skin without normal markings

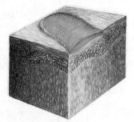

Scar—permanent fibrous tissue at site of healed injury

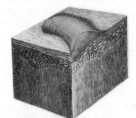

Keloid—hypertrophied scar

eruption.

• *Subdued lighting* highlights the difference between normal skin and circumscribed lesions that are hypo- or hyperpigmented.

• *Microscopic immunofluorescence* identifies immunoglobulins and elastic tissue in detecting skin manifestations of immunologically mediated disease.

• *Potassium hydroxide preparations* permit examination for mycelia in fungal infections.

• *Gram's stains and exudate cultures* help identify the organism responsible for an underlying infection.

• *Patch tests* identify contact sensitivity (usually with dermatitis).

• *Biopsy* determines histology of cells, and may be diagnostic, confirmatory, or inconclusive, depending on the disease.

Special considerations

When assessing a skin disorder, the health care professional should keep in mind its distressing social and psychologic implications. Unlike internal disorders, such as cardiac disease or diabetes mellitus, a skin condition is usually obvious and disfiguring. Understandably, the psychologic implications are most acute when skin disorders affect the face—especially during adolescence, an emotionally turbulent time of life. But such disorders can also create tremendous psychologic problems for adults. A skin disease often interferes with a person's ability to work because the condition affects the hands or because it distresses the patient to such an extent that he can't function.

For these reasons, the professional

should be empathetic and accepting. Above all, he must not be afraid to touch such a patient; most skin disorders are not contagious. Touching the patient naturally and without hesitation helps show acceptance of the dermatologic condition. Such acceptance is no less important than teaching the patient about the disease, and carrying out prescribed treatment.

BACTERIAL INFECTION

Impetigo
(Impetigo contagiosa)

A contagious, superficial skin infection, impetigo occurs in nonbullous and bullous forms. This vesiculopustular eruptive disorder spreads most easily among infants, young children, and the elderly. Predisposing factors such as poor hygiene, anemia, malnutrition, and a warm climate favor outbreaks of this infection, most of which occur during the late summer and early fall. Impetigo can complicate chickenpox, eczema, or other skin conditions marked by open lesions.

Causes
Beta-hemolytic streptococcus usually produces nonbullous impetigo; coagulase-positive *Staphylococcus aureus* generally causes bullous impetigo.

Signs and symptoms
Streptococcal impetigo typically begins with a small red macule that turns into a vesicle, becoming pustular in a matter of hours. When the vesicle breaks, a characteristic thick yellow crust forms from the exudate. Autoinoculation may cause satellite lesions to appear. Other clinical features include pruritus, burning, and regional lymphadenopathy.

A rare but serious complication of streptococcal impetigo is glomerulonephritis. Infants and very young children may develop aural impetigo or otitis externa, but the lesions usually clear without treatment in 2 to 3 weeks, unless an underlying disorder, such as eczema, is present.

In *staphylococcal impetigo*, a thin-walled vesicle opens, and a thin, clear crust forms from the exudate. As in the streptococcal form, the lesion consists of a central clearing, circumscribed by an outer rim—much like a ringworm lesion—and commonly appears on the face or other exposed areas. Both forms usually produce painless itching, and may appear simultaneously and be clinically indistinguishable.

Diagnosis

Characteristic lesions suggest impetigo; microscopic visualization of the causative organism in a Gram's stain of vesicle fluid usually confirms *S. aureus* infection and justifies anti-

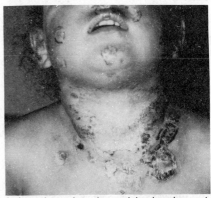
In impetigo, when the vesicles break, crust forms from the exudate. This infection is especially contagious among young children.

ECTHYMA

Ecthyma is a superficial skin infection that usually causes scarring. It generally results from infection by beta-hemolytic streptococcus. Ecthyma differs from impetigo in that its characteristic ulcer results from deeper penetration of the skin by the infecting organism (involving the lower epidermis and dermis), and the overlying crust tends to be piled high (1 to 3 cm). These lesions often occur on the posterior aspects of the thighs and buttocks. Autoinoculation can transmit ecthyma to other parts of the body, especially to sites that have been scratched open. (Ecthyma often results from the scratching of chigger bites.) Therapy is basically the same as for impetigo, beginning with removal of the crust, but response may be slower. Widespread ulcers may require parenteral antibiotics.

antibiotics (usually penicillin, or erythromycin for patients who are allergic to penicillin), which also help prevent glomerulonephritis. Therapy also includes removal of the exudate by washing the lesions two to three times a day with soap and water, or for stubborn crusts, warm soaks or compresses of normal saline or a diluted soap solution before application of topical antibiotics (usually polymyxin B and bacitracin). Topical antibiotics are less effective than systemic antibiotics.

Additional considerations

• The patient should be told not to scratch, since this exacerbates impetigo. Parents should cut a child's fingernails. The patient should be checked for penicillin allergy before any medication is given. The patient must continue prescribed medications even after lesions have healed.

• The patient or family should be taught how to care for impetiginous lesions. Frequent bathing using a bactericidal soap will help prevent further spread of this highly contagious infection. The patient must not share towels, washcloths, or bed linens with family members. He must understand the importance of following proper handwashing technique.

• All family members should be checked for impetigo. If this infection is present in a schoolchild, his school should be notified.

biotic therapy. Culture and sensitivity testing of fluid or denuded skin may indicate the most appropriate antibiotic, but therapy should not be delayed for laboratory results, which can take 3 days. WBC may be elevated in the presence of infection.

Treatment

Generally, treatment consists of systemic

Folliculitis, Furunculosis, and Carbunculosis

Folliculitis is a bacterial infection of the hair follicle that causes the formation of a pustule. The infection can be superficial (follicular impetigo or Bockhart's impetigo) or deep (sycosis barbae). Folliculitis may also lead to the development of furuncles (furunculosis), commonly known as boils, or carbuncles (carbunculosis). Prognosis depends on the severity of the infection and on the patient's physical condition and ability to resist infection.

Causes

The most common cause of folliculitis, furunculosis, or carbunculosis is coagulase-positive *Staphylococcus aureus*. For furunculosis, predisposing fac-

tors include an infected wound elsewhere on the body, poor personal hygiene, debilitation, diabetes, exposure to chemicals (cutting oils), and management of skin lesions with tar or with occlusive therapy, using steroids. Furunculosis generally follows folliculitis exacerbated by irritation, pressure, friction, or perspiration. Carbunculosis follows persistent S. *aureus* infection and furunculosis.

Signs and symptoms

Pustules of folliculitis usually appear on the scalp, arms, and legs in children; on the face of bearded men (sycosis barbae); and on the eyelids (styes). Deep folliculitis may be painful.

Folliculitis may progress to the hard, painful nodules of furunculosis, which commonly develop on the neck, face, axillae, and buttocks. For several days these nodules enlarge, and then rupture, discharging pus and necrotic material. After the nodules rupture, pain subsides, but erythema and edema may persist for days or weeks.

Carbunculosis is marked by extremely painful, deep abscesses that drain through multiple openings onto the skin surface, usually around several hair follicles. Fever and malaise may accompany these lesions.

Diagnosis

The obvious skin lesion confirms follicu-

FORMS OF BACTERIAL SKIN INFECTION

Degree of hair follicle involvement in bacterial skin infection ranges from superficial erythema and pustule of a single follicle to deep abscesses (carbuncles) involving several follicles.

Superficial folliculitis (*erythema and pustule in a single follicle*)

Carbuncle (*deep follicular abscesses of several follicles with several draining points*)

Furuncle (*red, tender nodule surrounding a follicle with one draining point*)

Deep folliculitis (*extensive follicular involvement*)

litis, furunculosis, or carbunculosis. Wound culture shows *S. aureus*. In carbunculosis, patient history reveals preexistent furunculosis. CBC may show elevated WBC (leukocytosis).

Treatment

Treatment of folliculitis consists of cleansing the infected area thoroughly with soap and water; applying hot, wet compresses to promote vasodilation and drainage of infected material from the lesions; topical antibiotics, such as bacitracin and polymyxin B; and in recurrent infection, systemic antibiotics.

Furunculosis may also require incision and drainage of ripe lesions after application of hot, wet compresses, and topical antibiotics after drainage. Treatment of carbunculosis requires systemic antibiotics.

Additional considerations

Health care for a patient with folliculitis, furunculosis, or carbunculosis is basically supportive, and emphasizes patient teaching of scrupulous personal and family hygiene, dietary modifications (reduced intake of sugars and fats), and precautions to prevent spreading infection. These include:

• cautioning the patient never to squeeze a boil, since this may cause it to rupture into the surrounding area.

• urging the patient not to share his towel and washcloth, to avoid spreading bacteria to family members; telling him that these items should be boiled in hot water before being reused, that he should change his clothes and bedsheets daily, and that these also should be washed in hot water; encouraging the patient to change dressings frequently and to discard them promptly in paper bags.

• advising the patient with recurrent furunculosis to have a physical examination, since an underlying disease, such as diabetes, may be present.

Erythrasma

A superficial, bacterial skin infection, erythrasma commonly affects the skin folds, especially of the groin, axillae, and toe webs; rarely, it is generalized. This condition is usually chronic but may be intermittent, with recurring periods of exacerbation.

Causes and incidence

The bacterium *Corynebacterium minutissimum* causes erythrasma by colonization of the skin rather than by invasion. It affects persons of all ages and both sexes equally, with one exception: the genitocrural form is slightly more common in males than in females. Predisposing factors include heat and humidity, diabetes, obesity, poor personal hygiene, and debilitation. This infection is not known to be contagious.

Signs and symptoms

The most common form of erythrasma is found in the toe webs, and produces scaling, fissuring, and maceration.

In both the toe-web and genitocrural forms, plaques are pink but may turn brown; in the genitocrural form, plaques are circumscribed, scaly, and pruritic.

Diagnosis

 The characteristic coral glow of infected areas during a Wood's light examination in a darkened room confirms diagnosis. A false negative reaction to this test is possible if the patient has bathed during the previous 48 hours. Gram's stains of the scales rule out fungal infection, psoriasis, seborrheic dermatitis, or intertrigo, all of which mimic erythrasma.

Treatment and additional considerations

Treatment consists of administering keratolytics, such as salicylic acid; washing with antibacterial soap; and applying topical antibiotics. Resistant infection may necessitate systemic antibiotics; erythromycin in particular appears to be effective against erythrasma. Clearing usually occurs in 2 to 3 weeks.

The use of keratolytics should be explained to the patient, and he should be advised to dry the skin thoroughly after bathing with an antibacterial soap, since moisture promotes bacterial growth.

If the patient is receiving systemic antibiotics, he must understand the importance of taking them exactly as prescribed, and the need for follow-up.

Staphylococcal Scalded Skin Syndrome

A severe skin disorder, staphylococcal scalded skin syndrome (SSSS) is marked by epidermal erythema, peeling, and necrosis that give the skin a scalded appearance. SSSS is most prevalent in infants aged 1 to 3 months but may develop in children; it's uncommon in adults. This disease follows a consistent pattern of progression, and most patients recover fully. Mortality is 2% to 3%, with death usually resulting from complications of fluid and electrolyte loss, sepsis, and involvement of other body systems.

Causes

The causative organism in SSSS is Group 2 *Staphylococcus aureus*, primarily phage type 71. Predisposing factors may include impaired immunity and renal insufficiency—present to some extent in the normal neonate, due to immature development of these systems.

Signs and symptoms

SSSS can often be traced to a prodromal upper respiratory tract infection, possibly with concomitant purulent conjunctivitis. Cutaneous changes progress through three stages:

• *Erythema:* Erythema becomes visible, usually around the mouth and other orifices, and may spread in widening circles over the entire body surface. The skin becomes tender; Nikolsky's sign (sloughing of the skin when friction is applied) may appear.

• *Exfoliation* (24 to 48 hours later): In the more common, localized form of this disease, superficial erosions and minimal crusting occur, generally around body orifices, and may spread to exposed areas of the skin. In the more severe forms of this disease, large, flaccid bullae erupt and may spread to cover extensive areas of the body. These bullae

eventually rupture, revealing sections of denuded skin.

• *Desquamation:* In this final stage, affected areas dry up, and powdery scales form. Normal skin replaces these scales in 5 to 7 days.

Diagnosis

Diagnosis requires careful observation of the three-stage progression of this disease. Results of exfoliative cytology and biopsy aid in differential diagnosis, ruling out erythema multiforme and drug-induced toxic epidermal necrolysis, both of which are similar to SSSS. Isolation of Group 2 *S. aureus* on cultures of skin lesions confirms the diagnosis. However, skin lesions sometimes appear sterile.

Treatment and additional considerations

Treatment includes systemic antibiotics—usually penicillinase-resistant penicillin—to prevent secondary infections, and replacement measures to maintain fluid and electrolyte balance.

• The neonate may require special care, including placement in a warming infant incubator to maintain body temperature and provide isolation.

• Intake and output must be carefully

monitored to assess fluid and electrolyte balance. In severe cases, I.V. fluid replacement may be necessary.
• Vital signs should be checked often, watching especially for a sudden rise in temperature, indicating sepsis, which requires prompt, aggressive treatment.
• Skin integrity must be maintained. Using strict aseptic technique can help preclude secondary infection, especially during the exfoliative stage, because of open lesions. Affected areas should be left uncovered or loosely covered to prevent friction and sloughing of the skin. Cotton placed between severely affected fingers and toes will help prevent webbing.
• During the recovery period the patient should be given warm baths and soaks, and exfoliated areas should be debrided.
• Parents should be reassured that complications are rare and residual scars are unlikely.

FUNGAL INFECTION

Tinea Versicolor
(Pityriasis versicolor)

A chronic, superficial, fungal infection, tinea versicolor may produce a multicolored rash, commonly on the upper trunk. This condition, primarily a cosmetic defect, usually affects young persons, especially during warm weather, and is most prevalent in tropical countries. Recurrence is common.

Causes
The agent that causes tinea versicolor is *Pityrosporon orbiculare (Microsporum furfur)*. Whether this condition is infectious or merely a proliferation of normal skin fungi is uncertain.

Signs and symptoms
Tinea versicolor typically produces raised

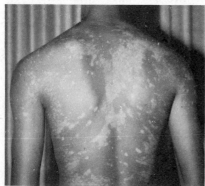

In dark-skinned patients, tinea versicolor causes hypopigmented areas (white patches) that fail to tan.

or macular, round or oval, slightly scaly lesions on the upper trunk, which may extend to the lower abdomen, neck, arms, and rarely, the face. These lesions are usually tawny but may range from hypopigmented (white) patches in dark-skinned patients to hyperpigmented (brown) patches in fair-skinned patients. Some areas don't tan when exposed to sunlight, causing the cosmetic defect for which most persons seek medical help. Inflammation, burning, and itching are possible but usually absent.

Diagnosis
 Visualization of lesions during Wood's light examination strongly suggests tinea versicolor; microscopic examination of skin scrapings prepared in potassium hydroxide solution confirms it by showing hyphae and clusters of yeast.

Treatment and additional considerations
The most effective treatment is selenium

sulfide suspension applied twice weekly for 4 weeks. Also effective are 20% sodium thiosulfate, 15% sodium hyposulfite, and 2% micropulverized sulfur plus 2% salicylic acid solutions, applied twice daily to affected areas for several months; however, these solutions may be unacceptable because of unpleasant odor.

The patient should apply selenium sulfide suspension full strength at bedtime, no more often than twice weekly for 4 weeks (daily use may prove irritating, especially in skin folds). He should bathe and dry completely before applying the suspension and wash it off first thing in the morning.

The patient must know that his fungal infection is cured even though depigmented spots may persist after treatment; gradual exposure to the sun or ultraviolet light can restore normal color.

Since recurrence of tinea versicolor is common, the patient should watch for new areas of discoloration.

Dermatophytosis
(Ringworm)

Dermatophytosis may affect the scalp (tinea capitis), body (tinea corporis), nails (tinea unguium), feet (tinea pedis), groin (tinea cruris), and bearded skin (tinea barbae). Tinea infections are quite prevalent in the United States, and are usually more common in males than in females. With effective treatment, the cure rate is very high, although about 20% of infected persons develop chronic conditions.

Causes

Tinea infections (except for tinea versicolor) result from dermatophytes (fungi) of the genera *Trichophyton, Microsporum,* and *Epidermophyton.*

Transmission can occur directly (through contact with infected lesions) or indirectly (through contact with contaminated articles, such as shoes, towels, or shower stalls).

Signs and symptoms

Lesions vary in appearance and duration. *Tinea capitis,* which mainly affects children, is characterized by small, spreading papules on the scalp, causing patchy hair loss with scaling. These papules may progress to inflamed, pus-filled lesions (kerions).

Tinea corporis produces flat lesions on the skin at any site except the scalp, bearded skin, or feet. These lesions may be dry and scaly or moist and crusty; as they enlarge, their centers heal, causing the classic ring-shaped appearance. In *tinea unguium* (onychomycosis), infection typically starts at the tip of one or more toenails (fingernail infection is less common) and produces gradual thickening, discoloration, and crumbling of the nail, with accumulation of subungual debris. Eventually, the nail may be destroyed completely.

Tinea pedis causes scaling and blisters between the toes. Severe infection may result in inflammation, with severe itching and pain on walking. A dry, squamous inflammation may affect the entire sole. *Tinea cruris* (jock itch) produces red, raised, sharply defined, itchy lesions in the groin that may extend to the buttocks, inner thighs, and the external genitalia. Warm weather and tight clothing encourage fungus growth. *Tinea barbae* is an uncommon infection that affects the facial area of men where there is beard.

Diagnosis

 Microscopic examination of lesion scrapings prepared in potassium hydroxide solution usually confirms tinea infection. Other diagnostic procedures include Wood's light examination for some types of tinea capitis, and culture of the infecting organism;

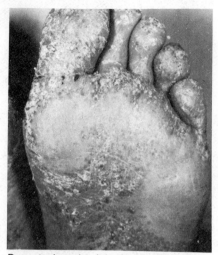

Dermatophytosis of the feet (tinea pedis) is popularly called athlete's foot. This infection causes macerated, scaling lesions, which may spread from the interdigital spaces to the sole. Diagnosis must rule out other possible causes of signs and symptoms; for example, eczema, psoriasis, contact dermatitis, and maceration by tight, ill-fitting shoes.

however, culturing may delay treatment.

Treatment

Tinea infections usually respond to treatment with griseofulvin P.O., which is especially effective in tinea infections of the skin, hair, and nails; tinea pedis requires concomitant use of a topical agent. (Griseofulvin is contraindicated in the patient with porphyria; it may also necessitate an increase in dosage during anticoagulant [warfarin] therapy.) Topical application of antifungals, such as clotrimazole, miconazole, haloprogin, or tolnaftate for localized infections, is also effective. Supportive measures include open wet dressings, removal of scabs and scales, and application of keratolytics, such as salicylic acid, to soften and remove hyperkeratotic lesions of the heels or soles.

Additional considerations

Management of tinea infections requires careful application of topical agents, ob-servation for sensitivity reactions (marked irritation), and patient teaching.

• For tinea capitis, care includes: keeping topical medications away from the patient's eyes; discontinuing medications if condition worsens; using good handwashing technique, and teaching the patient to do the same; advising the patient to wash his towels, bedclothes, and combs frequently in hot water, and to avoid sharing them to prevent spread of infection to others; suggesting that family members be checked for tinea capitis.

• For tinea corporis, care includes: using abdominal pads between skin folds for the patient with excessive abdominal girth and changing pads frequently; checking daily for excoriated, newly denuded areas of skin; applying open wet dressings two or three times daily to decrease inflammation and help remove scales.

• For tinea unguium, care includes: keeping the patient's nails short and straight; gently removing debris under the nails with an emery board; preparing the patient for prolonged therapy and possible side effects of griseofulvin, such as headache, nausea, vomiting, and photosensitivity.

• For tinea pedis, care includes: encouraging the patient to expose feet to air when possible, to wear sandals or leather shoes, and cotton socks (especially with hyperhidrosis), and to wash his feet twice daily. After drying them thoroughly, he should evenly apply an antifungal powder, to absorb perspiration and prevent excoriation. In severe infection, the patient may need to disinfect his socks in boiling water.

• For tinea cruris, care includes: instructing the patient to dry the affected area thoroughly after bathing and to evenly apply antifungal powder; advising him to wear loose-fitting clothing, which should be changed frequently and laundered in hot water; suggesting sitz baths to relieve itching.

• For tinea barbae, care includes: suggesting the patient let his beard grow (whiskers may be trimmed with scissors, not a razor). If he must shave, he should use an electric razor instead of a blade.

PARASITIC INFESTATIONS

Scabies

An age-old skin infection, scabies results from infestation with Sarcoptes scabiei *var.* hominis *(commonly known as the itch mite), which provokes a sensitivity reaction. Scabies occurs worldwide and is predisposed by overcrowding and poor hygiene—conditions that can make it endemic.*

Causes

Mites can live their entire life cycles in the skin of humans, causing chronic infection. The female mite burrows into the skin to lay her eggs, from which larvae emerge to copulate and then reburrow under the skin. Transmission occurs through skin contact or venereally. The adult mite can survive without a human host for only 2 or 3 days.

Signs and symptoms

Typically, scabies causes itching, which intensifies at night. Characteristic lesions are usually excoriated, and may appear as erythematous nodules. These threadlike lesions are approximately ⅜″ long and generally occur between fingers, on flexor surfaces of the wrists, on elbows, in axillary folds, at the waistline, on nipples in females, and on genitalia in males. In infants, the burrows (lesions) may appear on the head and neck. Intense scratching can lead to severe excoriation and secondary bacterial infection. Itching may become generalized secondary to sensitization.

Diagnosis

 Visual examination of the contents of the scabietic burrow may reveal the itch mite. If not, a drop of mineral oil placed over the burrow, followed by superficial scraping and examination of expressed material under a low-power microscope, may reveal ova, or mite feces. However, excoriation or inflammation of the burrow often makes such identification difficult. If scabies is strongly suspected but positive identification of the mite is impossible, skin clearing with a therapeutic trial of a pediculicide confirms the diagnosis.

Treatment

Generally, treatment consists of bathing with soap and water, followed by application of a pediculicide. Gamma benzene hexachloride cream should be applied and left on for 24 hours. Because this cream is not ovicidal, this application must be repeated in 1 week. Another pediculicide, crotamiton cream, may be applied twice in 48 hours. Persistent pruritus is usually due to mite sensitization or contact dermatitis, which may develop from repeated use of pediculicides, rather than from continued infection. An antipruritic emollient or topical steroid is often prescribed to reduce itching. Intralesional steroids may resolve erythematous nodules. Approx-

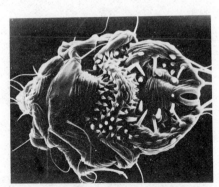

Sarcoptes scabiei—the itch mite—has a hard shell and measures a microscopic 0.1 mm.

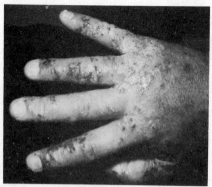

This photo of scabies lesions shows erythematous nodules with excoriation. These lesions are usually highly pruritic.

imately 10% of a pediculicide is absorbed systemically; therefore, a 6% to 10% solution of sulfur, which is less toxic, applied for 3 consecutive days, is an alternative therapy for infants and pregnant females. Widespread bacterial infections require systemic antibiotics.

Additional considerations
• The patient should apply gamma benzene hexachloride cream from the neck down, making sure to cover his entire body. (He may need assistance to reach all body areas.) Afterward, the patient must wait about 15 minutes before dressing and must avoid bathing for 24 hours. All contaminated clothing and linens must be washed or dry-cleaned.
• Family members and other close personal contacts of the patient must be checked for possible symptoms.
• If a hospitalized patient has scabies, transmission to other patients can be prevented by: practicing good handwashing technique or wearing gloves when touching the patient; observing wound and skin precautions for 24 hours after treatment with a pediculicide; gas autoclaving blood pressure cuffs before using them on other patients; isolating linens until the patient is noninfectious, and thoroughly disinfecting the patient's room after discharge.

Cutaneous Larva Migrans
(Creeping eruption)

Cutaneous larva migrans is a skin reaction to infestation by nematodes (hookworms or roundworms) that usually infect dogs and cats. It most often affects persons who come in contact with infected soil or sand, such as children and farmers. Eruptions clear completely with treatment.

Causes
Under favorable conditions—warmth, moisture, sandy soil—hookworm or roundworm ova present in feces of affected animals (such as dogs and cats) hatch into larvae, which can then burrow into human skin on contact. After penetrating its host, the larva becomes trapped under the skin, unable to reach the intestines to complete its normal life cycle. The parasite begins to move around, producing the peculiar, tunnel-like lesions that are alternately meandering and linear, reflecting the nematode's persistent and unsuccessful attempts to escape its host.

Signs and symptoms
A transient rash or, possibly, a small vesicle appears at the point of penetration, usually on an exposed area that has come in contact with the ground, such as the feet, legs, or buttocks. As the parasite migrates, it etches a noticeable thin, raised, red line on the skin, which may become vesicular and encrusted. Pruritus quickly develops, often with crusting and secondary infection following excoriation. The larva's apparently random path can cover from 1 mm to 1 cm a day. Penetration of more than one larva may involve a much larger area of the skin, marking it with many tracks.

Diagnosis

Characteristic migratory lesions strongly suggest cutaneous larva migrans. Patient history usually reveals contact with warm, moist soil within the past several months.

Treatment and additional considerations

Thiabendazole, applied locally in a 2% solution with dimethyl sulfoxide, is the treatment of choice. Severe infections may require administration of 50 mg/kg thiabendazole P.O. for 2 or 3 days. The patient must be told that side effects of systemic thiabendazole include nausea, vomiting, abdominal pain, and dizziness.

Prevention requires patient teaching about the existence of these parasites, sanitation of beaches and sandboxes, and proper pet care.

Patient and family should be reassured that larva migrans lesions usually clear 1 to 2 weeks after treatment. The im-

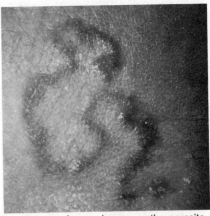

In cutaneous larva migrans, as the parasite migrates, it etches a noticeable red line on the skin. These lesions are thin, raised, and alternately meandering and linear.

portance of adhering to the treatment regimen should be stressed.

Pediculosis

Pediculosis is caused by parasitic forms of lice: Pediculus humanus *var.* capitis *causes pediculosis capitis (head lice);* Pediculus humanus *var.* corporis *causes pediculosis corporis (body lice); and* Phthirus pubis *causes pediculosis pubis (crab lice). These lice feed on human blood and lay their eggs (nits) in body hairs or clothing fibers. After the nits hatch, the lice must feed within 24 hours or die; they mature in about 2 to 3 weeks. When a louse bites, it injects a toxin into the skin that produces mild irritation and a purpuric spot. Repeated bites cause sensitization to the toxin, leading to more serious inflammation. Treatment can effectively eliminate lice.*

Causes and incidence

P. humanus var. *capitis* (most common species) feeds on the scalp and, rarely, in the eyebrows, eyelashes, and beard. This form of pediculosis is caused by overcrowded conditions and poor personal hygiene, and commonly affects children, especially girls. It spreads through shared clothing, hats, combs, and hairbrushes.

P. humanus var. *corporis* lives in the seams of clothing, next to the skin, leaving only to feed on blood. Common causes include prolonged wearing of the same

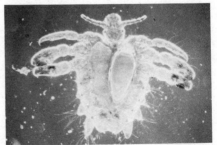

Phthirus pubis (pubic or "crab" louse) is slightly translucent; its first set of legs is shorter than its second and third.

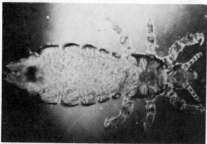

Pediculus humanus var. *corporis* (body louse) has a long abdomen, and all its legs are approximately the same length.

clothing (which might occur in cold climates), overcrowding, and poor personal hygiene. It spreads through shared clothing and bedsheets.

P. pubis is primarily found in pubic hairs, but this species may extend to the eyebrows, eyelashes, and axillary or body hair. Pediculosis pubis is transmitted through sexual intercourse or by contact with clothes, bedsheets, or towels harboring lice.

Signs and symptoms
Clinical features of pediculosis capitis include itching; excoriation (with severe itching); matted, foul-smelling, lusterless hair (in severe cases); occipital and cervical lymphadenopathy; and a rash on the trunk, probably due to sensitization. Adult lice migrate from the scalp and deposit oval, gray-white nits on hair shafts.

Pediculosis corporis initially produces small red papules (usually on the shoul-

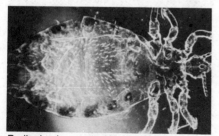

Pediculus humanus var. *capitis* (head louse) is similar in appearance to *P. humanus* var. *corporis*.

ders, trunk, or buttocks), which change to urticaria from scratching. Later, rashes or wheals (probably a sensitivity reaction) may develop. Untreated pediculosis corporis may lead to dry, discolored, thickly encrusted, scaly skin, with bacterial infection and scarring. In severe cases, headache, fever, and malaise may accompany the cutaneous symptoms.

Pediculosis pubis causes skin irritation from scratching, which is usually more obvious than the bites. Small gray-blue spots (maculae caeruleae) may appear on the thighs or upper body.

Diagnosis
Pediculosis is visible on physical examination:
• *in pediculosis capitis:* oval, grayish nits that can't be shaken loose like dandruff (the closer the nits are to the end of the hair shaft, the longer the infection has been present, since the ova are laid close to the scalp).
• *in pediculosis corporis:* characteristic skin lesions; nits found on clothing.
• *in pediculosis pubis:* nits stuck to pubic hairs, which feel grainy to the touch.

Treatment
For pediculosis capitis, treatment consists of gamma benzene hexachloride (GBH) cream rubbed into the scalp at night, then rinsed out in the morning with GBH shampoo (this treatment should be repeated the following night). A fine-tooth comb dipped in vinegar removes nits from hair; washing hair with ordinary shampoo removes crustations.

Pediculosis corporis requires bathing with soap and water to remove lice from the body; in severe infestation, treatment with GBH may be necessary. Lice may be removed from clothes by washing, ironing, or dry-cleaning. Storing clothes for more than 30 days, or placing them in dry heat of 140° F. (77.7° C.) kills lice. If clothes can't be washed or changed, application of 10% DDT or 10% GBH powder is effective.

Treatment of pediculosis pubis includes application of GBH ointment, cream, or lotion (which is then left on for 24 hours), or shampooing the affected area with GBH shampoo. Treatment should be repeated in 1 week. Clothes and bedsheets must be laundered to prevent reinfestation.

Additional considerations
• Patients need to know how to use the creams, ointments, powders, and shampoos that eliminate lice. To prevent self-infestation, the health care professional should avoid prolonged contact with the patient's hair, clothing, and bedsheets.
• The patient with pediculosis pubis should be asked for a history of recent sexual contacts, so that the contacts can be examined and treated.
• To prevent the spread of pediculosis to other hospitalized persons, all high-risk patients should be examined on admission, especially the elderly who depend on others for care, those admitted from nursing homes, or persons living in crowded conditions.

FOLLICULAR & GLANDULAR DISORDERS

Acne Vulgaris

An inflammatory disease of the sebaceous follicles, acne vulgaris primarily affects adolescents, although lesions can appear as early as age 8. Although acne strikes boys more often and more severely, it usually occurs in girls at an earlier age and tends to affect them for a longer period, sometimes into adulthood. Prognosis is good with treatment.

Causes
The cause of acne is unknown, but theories regarding dietary influences (including the nearly universally held "chocolate causes acne" theory) appear to be groundless. Research now centers on hormonal dysfunction and oversecretion of sebum as possible primary causes.

Predisposing factors include the use of oral contraceptives (many females experience an acne flare-up during their first few menstrual cycles on oral contraceptives or after they stop using them); certain medications, including corticosteroids, adrenocorticotropic hormone, androgens, iodides, bromides, trimethadione, phenytoin, isoniazid, lithium, and halothane; cobalt irradiation; or hyperalimentation therapy. Other predisposing factors are exposure to heavy oils, greases, or tars; trauma or rubbing from tight clothing; cosmetics; emotional stress; or unfavorable climate.

More is known about the pathogenesis of acne. Androgens stimulate sebaceous gland growth, and production of sebum, which is secreted into dilated hair follicles that contain bacteria. The bacteria, usually *Propionibacterium acnes* and *Staphylococcus epidermidis*—which are normal flora on the skin—secrete lipase. This enzyme interacts with sebum to produce free fatty acids, which provoke inflammation. Concurrently, the hair follicles produce increased amounts of keratin, which joins with the sebum to form a plug in the dilated follicle.

Signs and symptoms
The acne plug may appear as a closed comedo, or whitehead (if it doesn't protrude from the follicle but is covered by the epidermis), or as an open comedo, or blackhead (if it does protrude and isn't covered by the epidermis). The black coloration is caused by the melanin or pigment produced by the follicle, not by dirt. Eventually, an enlarged plug can rupture or leak, spreading its contents into the dermis. This results in inflammation and the subsequent characteristic acne pustules, papules, or in severe

forms, acne cysts or abscesses. Chronic, recurring lesions produce distinctive acne scars.

Diagnosis

The appearance of characteristic lesions, especially in an adolescent, confirms the presence of acne. Patient history may indicate a predisposing cause, such as oral contraceptives.

Treatment

Common therapy for severe acne includes benzoyl peroxide, a powerful antibacterial, alone or in combination with tretinoin, a keratolytic (retinoic acid or topical vitamin A); both agents may irritate the skin. Topical antibiotics, such as tetracycline, erythromycin, and clindamycin, may prove helpful.

Systemic therapy consists primarily of antibiotics, usually tetracycline, to decrease bacterial growth until the patient is in remission; then a lower dosage is used for long-term maintenance. Tetracycline is contraindicated during pregnancy because it discolors the teeth of the fetus. Alternate drugs are erythromycin and minocycline (systemic clindamycin should not be used because of the risk of pseudomembranous enterocolitis). Exacerbation of pustules or abscesses during antibiotic therapy requires a culture to identify a possible secondary bacterial infection.

Females with particularly stubborn acne may benefit from the administration of estrogens to inhibit androgen activity. However, this is usually a last resort, since improvement rarely occurs before 2 to 4 months and exacerbations may follow its discontinuation.

Other treatments include intralesional corticosteroid injections (into cysts or abscesses), exposure to ultraviolet light (but never when a photosensitizing agent, such as tretinoin, is being used), cryotherapy, or surgery. Although there's no evidence that certain foods cause acne, the patient may want to eliminate from his diet foods he associates with flareups, for psychologic reasons.

Additional considerations

• Special attention should be paid to the patient's drug history, since certain medications, such as oral contraceptives, may cause an acne flare-up.

• An attempt should be made to identify predisposing factors, such as emotional stress, which may be eliminated or modified.

• The causes of acne must be explained to the patient and family. They should understand that the prescribed treatment is more likely to improve acne than a strict diet and fanatic scrubbing with soap and water. In fact, overzealous washing can worsen the lesions. Written instructions regarding treatment can be given to them.

• The patient receiving tretinoin should apply it at least 30 minutes after washing his face and at least 1 hour before bedtime. He must avoid using this medication around the eyes or lips. After treatments, the patient should closely observe his skin, which should look pink and dry. If it appears red or starts to peel, the preparation may have to be weakened or applied less often. The patient must avoid exposure to sunlight or use a sunscreening agent, since tretinoin is photosensitizing. If the prescribed regimen includes tretinoin and benzoyl peroxide, one preparation should be used in the morning and the other at night. Applying the two agents together may cause skin irritation.

• The patient should take tetracycline on an empty stomach, and should not take it along with antacids or milk since it interacts with metallic ions in dairy products and antacids.

• The patient should know that acne takes a long time to clear—even years for complete resolution. He should continue local skin care even after acne clears. The side effects of all medications should be explained and included in any written instructions.

• Special attention must be paid to the patient's perception of his physical appearance. Adolescents are especially traumatized by acne in today's appearance-conscious culture.

Hirsutism

A distressing disorder usually found in women and children, hirsutism is the excessive growth of body hair, typically in an adult male distribution pattern. This condition commonly occurs spontaneously but may also develop as a secondary disorder of various underlying diseases. It must always be distinguished from hypertrichosis. Prognosis varies with the cause and the effectiveness of treatment.

Causes

Idiopathic hirsutism probably stems from a hereditary trait, since the patient usually has a family history of the disorder. Causes of secondary hirsutism include endocrine abnormalities related to pituitary dysfunction (acromegaly, precocious puberty), adrenal dysfunction (Cushing's disease, congenital adrenal hyperplasia, or Cushing's syndrome), and ovarian lesions (such as polycystic ovary syndrome); and iatrogenic factors (such as corticosteroid therapy or the use of testosterone).

Signs and symptoms

Hirsutism typically produces enlarged hair follicles, as well as enlargement and hyperpigmentation of the hairs themselves. Excessive growth of facial hair is the most common complaint and the one for which most patients seek medical help. The pattern of hirsutism varies widely, depending on the patient's race and age. An elderly woman, for example, commonly shows increased hair growth on the chin and upper lip. In secondary hirsutism, signs of masculinization may appear—deepening of the voice, increased muscle mass and size of genitalia, menstrual irregularity, and decreased breast size.

Diagnosis

Family history of hirsutism, absence of menstrual abnormalities or signs of masculinization, and a normal pelvic examination strongly suggest idiopathic hirsutism. Diagnostic measures for secondary hirsutism depend on associated symptoms that suggest an underlying disorder.

Treatment

At the patient's request (primarily for cosmetic purposes), treatment of idiopathic hirsutism consists of eliminating excess hair by any of several methods: scissors and shaving, depilatory creams, or removal of the entire hair shaft with tweezers or wax. Bleaching with hydrogen peroxide may also be satisfactory. Electrolysis, a slow and expensive process, can destroy hair bulbs permanently, but this procedure works best when only a few hairs need to be re-

HYPERTRICHOSIS

Hypertrichosis is a localized or generalized condition in males and females that is marked by excessive hair growth. Localized hypertrichosis usually results from local trauma, chemical irritation, or hormonal stimulation; pigmented nevi (Becker's nevus, for example) may also contain hairs. Generalized hypertrichosis results from neurologic or psychiatric disorders, such as encephalitis, multiple sclerosis, concussion, anorexia nervosa, or schizophrenia; contributing factors include juvenile hypothyroidism, porphyria cutanea tarda, and the use of drugs such as phenytoin.

Hypertrichosis lanuginosa is a generalized proliferation of fine, lanugo-type hair (sometimes called down, or woolly hair). Such hair may be present at birth but generally disappears shortly thereafter. This condition may become chronic, with persistent lanugo-type hair growing over the entire body, or may develop suddenly later in life; it is very rare and usually results from malignancy.

moved. (A history of keloid formation contraindicates this procedure.)

Treatment of secondary hirsutism depends on the underlying disorder.

Additional considerations

Care for patients with idiopathic hirsutism focuses on emotional support and patient teaching; appropriate care for patients with secondary hirsutism depends on the treatment of the underlying disease. Care by a health care professional includes:

• providing emotional support by being sensitive to the patient's feelings about her appearance.

• watching for signs of contact dermatitis in patients being treated with depilatory creams, especially the elderly; watching for infection of hair follicles after hair removal with tweezers or wax.

• suggesting the patient consult a cosmetologist about makeup or bleaching agents to disguise excess facial hair

---

Alopecia

Alopecia, or hair loss, usually occurs on the scalp; hair loss elsewhere on the body is less common and less conspicuous. In the nonscarring form of this disorder (noncicatricial alopecia), the hair follicle can generally regrow hair. But scarring alopecia usually destroys the hair follicle, making hair loss irreversible.

Causes and incidence

The most common form of nonscarring alopecia is male-pattern alopecia, which appears to be related to androgen levels and to aging. Genetic predisposition commonly influences time of onset, degree of baldness, speed with which it spreads, and pattern of hair loss. Male-pattern alopecia may also occur in women, but it's rarely severe.

Other forms of nonscarring alopecia include:

• *physiologic alopecia* (usually temporary): sudden hair loss in infants, loss of straight hairline in adolescents, and diffuse hair loss after childbirth

• *alopecia areata* (idiopathic form): generally reversible and self-limiting; occurs most frequently in young and middle-aged adults of both sexes

• *trichotillomania*: compulsive pulling out of one's own hair; most common in children.

Predisposing factors of nonscarring alopecia also include radiation, many types of drug therapies and drug reactions, bacterial and fungal infections, psoriasis, seborrhea, and endocrine disorders, such as thyroid, parathyroid, and pituitary dysfunctions.

Scarring alopecia causes irreversible hair loss. It may result from physical or chemical trauma, or chronic tension on a hair shaft, such as braiding or rolling the hair. Diseases that produce alopecia include destructive skin tumors, granulomas, lupus erythematosus, scleroderma, follicular lichen planus, and severe bacterial or viral infections, such as folliculitis or herpes simplex.

Signs and symptoms

In male-pattern alopecia, hair loss is gradual, and usually affects the thinner, shorter, and less pigmented hairs of the frontal and parietal portions of the scalp. In women, hair loss is generally more diffuse; completely bald areas are uncommon but may occur.

Alopecia areata affects small patches of the scalp but may also occur as alopecia totalis, which involves the entire scalp, or as alopecia universalis, which involves the entire body. Although mild erythema may occur initially, affected areas of scalp or skin appear normal. "Exclamation point" hairs (loose hairs with dark, rough, brushlike tips on narrow, less pigmented shafts) occur at the periphery of new patches. Regrowth initially appears as fine, white, downy hair, which is gradually replaced by normal hair.

In trichotillomania, patchy, incomplete areas of hair loss with many broken hairs appear primarily on the scalp but may occur on other areas as well, such as the eyebrows.

Diagnosis

 Physical examination is usually sufficient to confirm alopecia. In trichotillomania, an occlusive dressing can establish diagnosis by allowing new hair to grow, revealing that the hair is being pulled out. Diagnosis must also identify any underlying disorder that might be causing alopecia.

Treatment

No treatment reverses male-pattern alopecia, although hair follicles can be surgically redistributed by autografting.

In alopecia areata, treatment is often unnecessary, as spontaneous regrowth is common. Intralesional corticosteroid injections are beneficial for small patches and may produce regrowth in 4 to 6 weeks. In trichotillomania, an occlusive dressing encourages normal hair growth, simply by calling attention to the problem (and to the possible need for

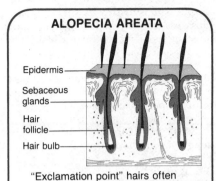

ALOPECIA AREATA

Epidermis

Sebaceous glands

Hair follicle

Hair bulb

"Exclamation point" hairs often border new patches of alopecia areata. Not seen in any other type of alopecia, these hairs indicate the patch is expanding.

psychiatric counseling). Treatment of other types of alopecia varies according to the underlying cause.

Additional considerations

A woman with male-pattern alopecia will need reassurance that it doesn't lead to total baldness, and that wearing a wig won't cause greater hair loss.

The erratic, recurrent nature of alopecia areata should be explained to the patient. He may need reassurance that complete regrowth is possible. Interim use of a wig can be suggested.

Rosacea

A chronic skin eruption, rosacea produces flushing and dilation of the small blood vessels in the face, especially the nose and cheeks. Papules and pustules may also occur, but without the characteristic comedones of acne vulgaris. Rosacea is most common in Caucasian women between ages 30 and 50. When it occurs in men, however, it's usually more severe and often associated with rhinophyma, which is characterized by dilated follicles and thickened, bulbous skin on the nose. Ocular involvement may result in blepharitis, conjunctivitis, uveitis, or keratitis. Rosacea usually spreads slowly and rarely subsides spontaneously.

Causes

Although the cause of rosacea is unknown, stress, infection, vitamin deficiency, and endocrine abnormalities can aggravate this condition. Anything that produces flushing—for example, hot beverages, such as tea or coffee; tobacco; alcohol; spicy foods; physical activity; sunlight; and extreme heat or cold—can also aggravate rosacea.

Signs and symptoms

Rosacea generally begins with periodic flushing across the central oval of the face, accompanied later by telangiectasias, papules, pustules, and nodules. Rhinophyma is commonly associated with severe rosacea but may occur alone. Rhinophyma usually appears first on the lower half of the nose, and produces red, thickened skin and follicular enlargement. Related ocular lesions are uncommon.

Diagnosis

 Typical vascular and acneiform lesions—without the comedones characteristically associated with acne vulgaris—and rhinophyma in severe cases confirm rosacea.

Treatment and additional considerations

Treatment of the acneiform component of rosacea consists of tetracycline P.O. in gradually decreasing doses as symptoms subside. Topical application of hydrocortisone ointment reduces erythema and inflammation. Other treatment may include electrolysis to destroy large, dilated blood vessels, and removal of excess tissue in patients with rhinophyma. Care also includes:
• instructing the patient to avoid hot beverages, alcohol, and other possible causes of flushing.
• assessing the effect of rosacea on body image. Since it's always apparent on the face, support and reassurance are essential.

DISORDERS OF PIGMENTATION

Vitiligo

Marked by stark-white skin patches that may cause a serious cosmetic problem, vitiligo results from the destruction and loss of pigment cells. This condition affects about 1% of the U.S. population, usually persons between ages 10 and 30, with peak incidence around age 20. It shows no racial preference, but the distinctive patches are most prominent in Blacks. Vitiligo doesn't favor one sex; however, women tend to seek treatment more often than men. Repigmentation therapy, which is widely used in treating vitiligo, may necessitate several summers of exposure to sunlight; the effects of this treatment may not be permanent.

Causes

Although the cause of vitiligo is unknown, inheritance seems a definite etiologic factor, since about 30% of patients with vitiligo have family members with the same condition. Other theories implicate enzymatic self-destructing mechanisms, autoimmune mechanisms, and abnormal neurogenic stimuli.

Some link exists between vitiligo and several other disorders that it often accompanies—thyroid dysfunction, pernicious anemia, Addison's disease, aseptic meningitis, diabetes mellitus, photophobia, hearing defects, alopecia areata, and halo nevi.

The most frequently reported precipitating factor is a stressful physical or psychologic event—severe sunburn, surgery, pregnancy, loss of job, bereavement, or some other source of distress. Chemical agents, such as phenols and catechols, may also cause this condition.

Signs and symptoms

Vitiligo produces depigmented or stark-white patches on the skin; on fair-skinned Caucasians, these are almost imperceptible. Lesions are usually bilaterally symmetric with sharp borders, which, occasionally, are raised and hyperpigmented. These unique patches generally appear over bony prominences, around orifices (eyes, mouth), within body folds, and at sites of trauma. The hair within these lesions may also turn white. Since hair follicles and certain parts of the eyes also contain pigment cells, vitiligo may be associated with premature graying of the hair and ocular pigmentary changes.

Diagnosis

Diagnosis requires accurate history of onset and of associated illnesses, family history, and clinical observation of characteristic lesions. Other skin disorders, such as tinea versicolor or piebaldism, must be ruled out.

 In fair-skinned patients, Wood's light examination in a darkened room detects vitiliginous patches; depigmented skin reflects the light, while pigmented skin absorbs it. Skin biopsy for electron microscopy reveals an absence of pigment cells. If autoimmune or endocrine disturbances are suspected, other laboratory studies (thyroid indexes, for example) are appropriate.

Treatment

Repigmentation therapy combines systemic and topical psoralen compounds (8-methoxypsoralen and trioxsalen) with exposure to sunlight or artificial ultraviolet light, wavelength A (UVA). New pigment rises from hair follicles and appears on the skin as small freckles, which gradually enlarge and coalesce. Consequently, parts of the body containing few hair follicles (such as the fingertips) may prove refractory to this therapy.

Since psoralens and UVA affect the entire skin surface, systemic therapy enhances the contrast between normal and vitiliginous skin. Therefore, white, vitiliginous areas are accented by normal skin, which tans darker than usual (application of a sunscreen to normal skin may minimize the contrast and prevent sunburn).

Depigmentation therapy is suggested for vitiligo affecting over 50% of body

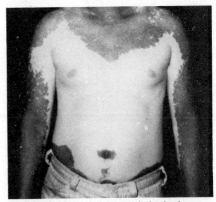

This photo shows characteristic depigmented skin patches in vitiligo. These patches are usually bilaterally symmetric, with distinct borders.

surface. A cream containing 20% monobenzone ether of hydroquinone permanently destroys pigment cells in unaffected areas of the skin and produces a uniform skin tone. This medication is applied initially to a small area of normal skin once daily to test for unfavorable reactions (contact dermatitis, for example). In the absence of adverse effects, the patient begins applying the cream twice daily to those areas he wishes to depigment first. *Note:* Depigmentation is permanent and results in extreme sensitivity to sunlight.

Commercial cosmetics may also help cover or de-emphasize vitiliginous skin. Some patients prefer dyes because these remain on the skin for several days, although the results are not always satisfactory. Complete avoidance of exposure to sunlight through the use of screening agents and protective clothing may minimize vitiliginous lesions in Caucasians. However, this restriction is often impractical.

Additional considerations

• The patient needs to use psoralen medications (topically or systemically) three or four times weekly. He should know the best time for exposure to sunlight is between 11 a.m. and 2 p.m. (*Note:* Systemic psoralens should be taken 2 hours before exposure to sun; topical solutions should be applied 30 to 60 minutes before exposure.) Patients with vitiligo must use a sunscreen (SPF 8-10) to protect both affected and normal skin during exposure, and should wear sunglasses after taking the medication. If periorbital areas require exposure, the patient should keep his eyes closed during treatment.

• The patient receiving depigmentation therapy should wear protective clothing and use a sunscreen. He will need a thorough explanation of the therapy, and should be given plenty of time to decide whether to undergo this treatment. He must understand that the results of depigmentation are permanent, and that chronic photosensitivity may severely restrict his life-style.

• The patient should not buy any commercial cosmetics or dyes without trying them first, since some products may not be suitable.

• Repigmentation therapy for the child with vitiligo should be modified to avoid unnecessary restrictions. Parents may give the initial dose of psoralen medication at 1 p.m. and then let the child go out to play as usual. After this, medication should be given 30 minutes earlier each day of treatment, provided the child's skin doesn't turn more than slightly pink from exposure. If marked erythema develops, parents must discontinue treatment and notify the doctor. Eventually, the child should be able to take the medication at 9:30 a.m. and play outdoors the rest of the day without side effects. Parents should dress the child in clothing that permits maximum exposure of vitiliginous areas to the sun.

• Patients undergoing repigmentation therapy should be reminded that exposure to sunlight also darkens normal skin. After being exposed to UVA for the prescribed amount of time, the patient must apply a sunscreen if he plans to be exposed to sunlight also. If sunburn occurs, the patient should discontinue therapy temporarily and apply open wet dressings (using thin sheeting) to affected areas for 15 to 20 minutes, 4 or 5 times daily or as necessary for comfort. After application of wet dressings, the skin must be allowed to air-dry. A soothing, lubricating cream or lotion can be applied while the skin is still slightly moist.

• Patient teaching should be reinforced with written instructions.

• The patient will need sensitivity to comfort his emotional needs. This disfiguring condition may cause a great deal of distress for the patient. Since the course of vitiligo is unpredictable, promotion of unrealistic hope for a total cure must be avoided.

Melasma

(Chloasma, mask of pregnancy)

A patchy, hypermelanotic skin disorder, melasma poses a serious cosmetic problem. Although it tends to occur equally in all races, the light-brown color characteristic of melasma is most evident in dark-skinned Caucasians. Melasma affects females more often than males; it may be chronic but is never life-threatening.

Causes

The cause of melasma is unknown. Histologically, hyperpigmentation results from increased melanin production, although the number of melanocytes remains normal. Melasma appears to be related to the increased hormonal levels associated with pregnancy, ovarian carcinoma, and the use of oral contraceptives. Progestational agents, phenytoin, and mephenytoin may also contribute to this disorder. Exposure to sunlight stimulates melasma, but this disorder may develop without any apparent predisposing factor. There are no associated endocrine disorders with this form.

Signs and symptoms

Melasma produces large, brown, irregular patches, symmetrically distributed on the forehead, cheeks, and sides of the nose. Less commonly, it may occur on the neck, upper lip, and temples.

Diagnosis

Observation of characteristic dark patches on the face usually confirms melasma. Patient history may reveal predisposing factors.

Treatment and additional considerations

Treatment consists primarily of application of bleaching agents containing 2% to 4% hydroquinone, to inhibit melanin synthesis. This medication is applied twice daily, with results usually evident within 8 weeks. Adjunctive measures include avoidance of sunlight, use of sunblockers to screen harmful ultraviolet rays, and discontinuation of oral contraceptives.

• The patient should be taught to avoid sunlight by using sunblockers and wearing a wide-brimmed hat or visor when outdoors. She should be aware that although bleaching agents may achieve the desired cosmetic effect, periodic treatments may be necessary to maintain it. Opaque cosmetics may help mask areas of deep pigmentation.

• The patient will need reassurance that melasma is treatable. Serial photographs will help show the patient that the patches on her face are improving with treatment.

Berlock Dermatitis

(Berloque dermatitis)

Berlock dermatitis is a unique skin reaction to psoralen-type photosensitizers. A fairly common but noncontagious condition, it usually affects women and children. Prognosis is good.

Causes

Berlock dermatitis may result from use of oil of bergamot, which contains photosensitizing psoralen, and exposure to ultraviolet light. Oil of bergamot, an extract from the peel of a small orange grown in southern France and Italy, is commonly a component of perfumes, colognes, and pomades. Psoralen photosensitizers (specifically furocoumarins, such as 5- and 8-methoxypsoralen) may also occur in clover, cockleburs, buttercups, meadow grass, limes, figs, dill, parsley, celery, and carrot greens.

Signs and symptoms

Berlock dermatitis produces an acute erythematous, vesicular, sunburnlike reaction. The affected area becomes hyperpigmented, with darker pigmentation around the border. Lesions erupt around the neck in a highly irregular pattern, corresponding to areas where the applied perfume or cologne came in contact with the neck. Sometimes these lesions appear pendantlike (*berloque* means pendant in French).

Diagnosis

Characteristic skin eruptions, and patient history of recent exposure to psoralens and other causative agents suggest berlock dermatitis.

Treatment and additional considerations

Therapy must identify and eliminate the cause. Topical steroids may relieve discomfort. The patient must avoid prolonged exposure to sunlight or ultraviolet light. He should be given reassurance that hyperpigmented areas will disappear within several months after treatment begins.

INFLAMMATORY REACTION

Dermatitis

Dermatitis, inflammation of the skin, occurs in several forms: atopic (discussed here), contact, chronic, seborrheic, nummular, exfoliative, and stasis dermatitises (discussed below). Atopic dermatitis (atopic or infantile eczema, neurodermatitis constitutionalis, Besnier's prurigo) is a chronic inflammatory response often associated with other atopic diseases, such as bronchial asthma, allergic rhinitis, and chronic urticaria. It usually develops in infants and toddlers between ages 1 month and 1 year, commonly in those with strong family histories of atopic disease. These children often acquire other atopic disorders as they grow older. Typically, this form of dermatitis subsides spontaneously by age 3 and stays in remission until prepuberty (ages 10 to 12), when it often flares up again.

Causes and incidence

Atopic dermatitis is the cutaneous manifestation of a delayed, cell-mediated allergic response (not a T cell disease, but related to IgE), resulting from the same allergens (pollen, wool, silk, fur, ointment, detergent, or perfume) that provoke other atopic diseases. Such allergens also include certain foods, particularly wheat, milk, and eggs. Atopic dermatitis tends to flare up in response to extremes in temperature and humidity. Other causes of flare-ups are sweating and psychologic stress.

In approximately 70% of patients with atopic dermatitis, positive skin tests and

DERMATITIS AND ECZEMA

TYPE	CAUSES	SIGNS AND SYMPTOMS
Seborrheic dermatitis 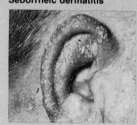	• Unknown; stress, and neurologic conditions may be predisposing factors	• Eruptions in areas with many sebaceous glands (usually scalp, face, and trunk) and in skin folds • Itching, redness, and inflammation of affected areas; lesions may appear greasy; fissures may occur • Indistinct, occasionally yellowish, scaly patches from excess stratum corneum (dandruff may be a mild seborrheic dermatitis)
Nummular dermatitis 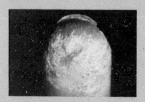	• Possibly precipitated by stress; or dryness, irritants, or scratching	• Round, nummular (coin-shaped) lesions, usually on arms and legs, with distinct borders of crusts and scales • Possible oozing and severe itching • Summertime remissions common, with wintertime recurrence

carefully controlled food elimination diets identify at least one allergen but rarely determine the primary cause.

An important secondary cause of atopic dermatitis is irritation, which seems to change the epidermal structure, allowing IgE activity to increase. Consequently, chronic skin irritation usually continues even after exposure to the allergen has ended or after the irritation has been systemically controlled.

Signs and symptoms

Atopic skin lesions generally begin as erythematous areas on excessively dry skin. In children, such lesions typically appear on the forehead, cheeks, and extensor surfaces of the arms and legs; in adults, at flexion points (antecubital fossa, popliteal area, and neck). During flareups, pruritus and scratching cause edema, vesiculation (sometimes vesicles are pus-filled), and scaling. Eventually, chronic atopic lesions lead to multiple areas of dry, scaly skin, with white dermatographia, blanching, and lichenification.

Common secondary conditions associated with atopic dermatitis include viral, fungal, or bacterial infections, and ocular disorders. Because of intense pruritus, the upper eyelid is commonly hyperpigmented and swollen, producing a double fold under the lower lid (Morgan's, Dennie's, or Mongolian fold). Atopic cataracts usually develop between ages 20 and 40. Kaposi's varicelliform eruption, a potentially fatal generalized viral infection, may develop if the patient with atopic dermatitis comes in contact with a person who has herpes simplex.

Diagnosis

Positive family history of allergy and chronic inflammation suggest atopic dermatitis. Typical distribution of skin lesions rules out other inflammatory skin lesions, such as diaper rash (lesions confined to the diapered area), seborrheic dermatitis (no pigmentation changes, or lichenification occurs in chronic lesions), and chronic contact dermatitis (lesions affect hands and forearms, sparing antecubital and popliteal areas). Serum IgE levels are elevated.

DIAGNOSIS	TREATMENT AND INTERVENTION
• Patient history and physical findings, especially distribution of lesions in sebaceous gland areas, confirm seborrheic dermatitis. • Diagnosis must rule out psoriasis.	• Removal of scales with frequent washing and shampooing with selenium sulfide suspension (most effective), zinc pyrithione, or tar and salicylic acid shampoo • Application of fluorinated steroids to nonhairy areas
• Physical findings and patient history confirm nummular dermatitis; a middle-aged or older patient may have a history of atopic dermatitis. • Diagnosis must rule out fungal infections, atopic or contact dermatitis, and psoriasis.	• Elimination of known irritants • Measures to relieve dry skin: increased humidification; limited frequency of baths and use of bland soap and bath oils; and application of emollients • Application of wet dressings in acute phase • Topical steroids (occlusive dressing or intralesional injections) for persistent lesions • Tar preparations and antihistamines to control itching • Antibiotics for secondary infection • Other intervention similar to atopic dermatitis

DERMATITIS AND ECZEMA (continued)

TYPE	CAUSES	SIGNS AND SYMPTOMS
Contact dermatitis 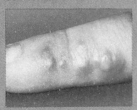	• Mild irritants: chronic exposure to detergents or solvents • Strong irritants: damage on contact with acids or alkalis • Allergens: sensitization after repeated exposure	• Mild irritants and allergens: erythema, and small vesicles that ooze, scale, and itch • Strong irritants: blisters and ulcerations • Classic allergic response: clearly defined lesions, with straight lines following points of contact • Severe allergic reaction: marked edema of affected areas
Chronic dermatitis 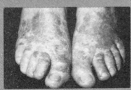	• Usually unknown but may result from progressive contact dermatitis • Secondary factors: trauma, infections, redistribution of normal flora, photosensitivity, and food sensitivity, which may perpetuate this condition	• Thick, lichenified, single or multiple lesions on any part of the body (often on the hands) • Inflammation and scaling • Recurrence follows long remissions.
Localized neurodermatitis (lichen simplex chronicus, essential pruritus) 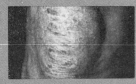	• Chronic scratching or rubbing of a primary lesion or insect bite, or other skin irritation	• Intense, sometimes continual scratching • Thick, sharp-bordered, possibly dry, scaly lesions, with raised papules • Usually affects easily reached areas, such as ankles, lower legs, anogenital area, back of neck, and ears
Exfoliative dermatitis 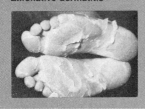	• Usually, preexisting skin lesions progress to exfoliative stage, such as in contact dermatitis, drug reaction, lymphoma, or leukemia.	• Generalized dermatitis, with acute loss of stratum corneum, and erythema and scaling • Sensation of tight skin • Hair loss • Possible fever, sensitivity to cold, shivering, gynecomastia, and lymphadenopathy
Stasis dermatitis 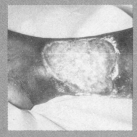	• Secondary to peripheral vascular diseases affecting legs, such as recurrent thrombophlebitis and resultant chronic venous insufficiency	• Varicosities and edema common, but obvious vascular insufficiency not always present • Usually affects the lower leg, just above internal malleolus, or sites of trauma or irritation • Early signs: dusky red deposits of hemosiderin in skin, with itching and dimpling of subcutaneous tissue. Later signs: edema, redness, and scaling of large area of legs • Fissures, crusts, and ulcers may develop

DIAGNOSIS	TREATMENT AND INTERVENTION
• Patient history • Patch testing to identify allergens • Shape and distribution of lesions suggest contact dermatitis.	• Elimination of known allergens and decreased exposure to irritants; wearing protective clothing, such as gloves; and washing immediately after contact with irritants or allergens • Topical anti-inflammatory agents (including steroids), systemic steroids for edema and bullae, antihistamines, and local applications of Burow's solution (for blisters) • Sensitization to topical medications may occur. • Other intervention similar to atopic dermatitis
• No characteristic pattern or course; diagnosis relies on detailed patient history and physical findings.	• Same as for contact dermatitis • Antibiotics for secondary infection • Avoidance of excessive washing and drying of hands, and of accumulation of soaps and detergents under rings • Use of emollients with topical steroids
• Physical findings confirm diagnosis.	• Lesions disappear about 2 weeks after scratching stops. • Fixed dressing or Unna's boot, to cover affected area • Steroids under occlusion or by intralesional injection • Antihistamines and open wet dressings • Emollients • Inform patient about underlying cause.
• Diagnosis requires identification of the underlying cause.	• Hospitalization, with protective isolation and hygienic measures to prevent secondary bacterial infection • Open wet dressings, with colloidal baths • Bland lotions over topical steroids • Maintenance of constant environmental temperature to prevent chilling or overheating • Careful monitoring of renal and cardiac status • Systemic antibiotics and steroids • Other intervention similar to atopic dermatitis
• Diagnosis requires positive history of venous insufficiency and physical findings, such as varicosities.	• Measures to prevent venous stasis: avoidance of prolonged sitting or standing, use of support stockings, and weight reduction in obesity • Corrective surgery for underlying cause • After ulcer develops, encourage rest periods, with legs elevated; open wet dressings; Unna's boot (zinc gelatin dressing provides continuous pressure to affected areas); antibiotics for secondary infection after wound culture.

Treatment and additional considerations

Effective treatment of atopic dermatitis lesions consists of eliminating allergens and avoiding irritants, extreme temperature changes, and other precipitating factors; local and systemic measures are used to relieve itching and inflammation. Topical application of a corticosteroid cream, especially after bathing, often alleviates inflammation. However, systemic corticosteroid therapy, because of its many side effects, should be used only during exacerbations. Weak tar preparations and ultraviolet B light therapy are used to increase the thickness of the stratum corneum. Antibiotics should be used for secondary infection if a bacterial agent has been cultured.

When treating a patient with atopic dermatitis, the health care professional should:

• warn that drowsiness is possible with the use of antihistamines to relieve daytime itching; suggest methods for inducing natural sleep, if nocturnal itching interferes with sleep.

• complement medical treatment by helping the patient set up an individual schedule and plan for daily skin care; instruct the patient to limit bathing, according to the severity of the lesions; tell the patient to bathe with a special nonfatty soap and tepid water, but to avoid using any soap when lesions are acutely inflamed; advise the patient to shampoo frequently and apply corticosteroid cream afterward, to keep his fingernails short to limit excoriation and secondary infections caused by scratching, and to lubricate his skin after a tub bath.

• apply occlusive dressings (such as plastic film) intermittently to help clear lichenified skin, and secure the dressings with nonallergenic tape.

• inform the patient that irritants, such as detergents and wool clothing, and emotional stress exacerbate atopic dermatitis.

• be careful not to show any anxiety or revulsion when touching the lesions during treatment; help the patient accept his altered body image, and encourage him to verbalize his feelings; remember that coping with disfigurement is extremely difficult, especially for children and adolescents; arrange for counseling, if necessary, to relieve emotional distress and help the patient deal with the disease more effectively.

MISCELLANEOUS DISORDERS

Toxic Epidermal Necrolysis
(Scalded skin syndrome)

Toxic epidermal necrolysis (TEN) is a rare, severe skin disorder that causes epidermal erythema, superficial necrosis, and skin erosions. The skin appears to be scalded; hence the term scalded skin syndrome. Mortality is high (30%), especially among the debilitated and the elderly. Reepithelialization is slow, and residual scarring is common. TEN primarily affects adults.

Causes

The immediate cause of this disease is still obscure, but it may be a reaction to a toxin, an allergen, or both. TEN usually results from a drug reaction—most commonly to butazones, sulfonamides, penicillins, barbiturates, and hydantoins, but may be linked to other drugs as well. TEN may reflect an immune response or may be related to overwhelming physiologic stress, (coexisting sepsis, neoplastic diseases, and drug treatment). Airborne toxins, such as carbon monoxide, have also been linked to TEN.

Signs and symptoms

Early symptoms of TEN include inflammation of the mucous membranes, a burning sensation in the conjunctivae, malaise, fever, and generalized skin tenderness. After such prodromal symptoms, TEN erupts in three phases:
- diffuse, erythematous rash
- vesiculation and blistering
- large-scale epidermal necrolysis and desquamation.

Large, flaccid bullae that rupture easily expose extensive areas of denuded skin, permitting loss of tissue fluids and electrolytes, and widespread systemic involvement. Systemic complications may include bronchopneumonia, pulmonary edema, gastrointestinal and esophageal hemorrhage, shock, renal failure, sepsis, and disseminated intravascular coagulation; these conditions markedly increase the mortality.

Diagnosis

 Diagnosis is based on clinical status at the peak stage of disease. Nikolsky's sign (skin sloughs off with slight friction) is present in erythematous areas. Culture and Gram's stain of lesions determine whether infection is present. Supportive findings include leukocytosis, elevated transaminase (SGOT and SGPT) levels, albuminuria, and fluid and electrolyte imbalances.

Exfoliative cytology and biopsy aid in ruling out erythema multiforme and exfoliative dermatitis.

Treatment and additional considerations

Treatment consists of high-dose systemic corticosteroids and maintenance of fluid and electrolyte balance with I.V. fluid replacement. Frequent determinations of hemoglobin and hematocrit, electrolytes, serum proteins, and blood gases are necessary.

Health care includes:
- monitoring vital signs, central venous pressure, and urinary output; watching for signs of renal failure (decreased urinary output) and bleeding; reporting temperature elevations immediately, and obtaining blood cultures and sensitivity tests promptly, as ordered, to detect and treat septic infection.
- preventing secondary infection—protective isolation and prophylactic antibiotic therapy may be necessary.
- maintaining skin integrity as much as possible. The patient should not wear clothing and should be covered loosely to prevent friction and sloughing of skin. A turning frame is helpful.
- administering analgesics, as needed; applying cool, sterile compresses to relieve discomfort.
- providing frequent eye care to remove exudate, since ocular lesions are common.
- providing emotional support for the patient and family.

Warts

(Verrucae)

Warts are common, benign, viral infections of the skin and adjacent mucous membranes. Although their incidence is highest in children and young adults, warts may occur at any age. Prognosis varies: some warts disappear readily with treatment; others necessitate more vigorous and prolonged treatment.

Causes

Warts are caused by infection with the human papillomavirus, a group of ether-resistant, DNA-containing papovaviruses. Mode of transmission is probably through direct contact, but autoinoculation is possible.

Signs and symptoms

Clinical manifestations depend on the

REMOVING WARTS BY ELECTROSURGERY

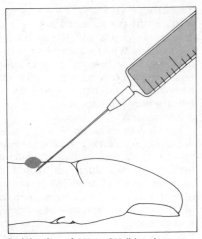

1. Injection of 1% to 2% lidocaine under and around the wart, avoiding wart itself

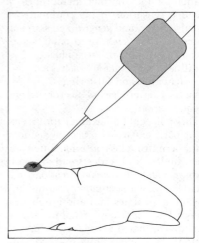

2. Desiccation of the wart

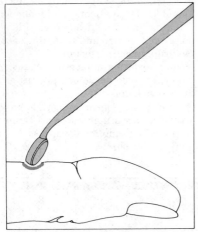

3. Removal of the wart tissue with a curette and small, curved scissors

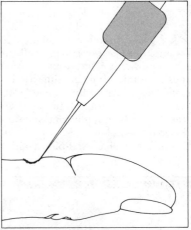

4. Light desiccation of the area to control bleeding and prevent recurrence

type of wart and its location:
• *common* (verruca vulgaris): rough, elevated, rounded surface; appears most frequently on extremities, particularly hands and fingers; most prevalent in children and young adults
• *filiform:* single, thin, threadlike pro-jection; commonly occurs around the face and neck
• *periungual:* rough, irregularly shaped, elevated surface; occurs around edges of finger- and toenails. When severe, the wart may extend under the nail and lift it off the nailbed, causing pain.

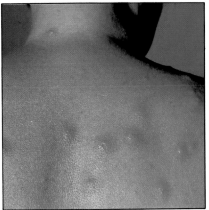

An allergic reaction to tetanus toxin may cause raised, red, itchy wheals.

These circumscribed, reddish skin lesions indicate a barbiturate reaction.

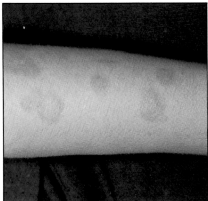

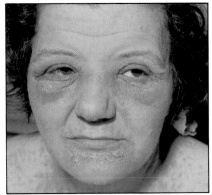

Spread over the patient's head, neck and shoulders, this generalized maculopapular rash is a common reaction to penicillin and other drugs in the penicillin family.

This raised, morbilliform (measles-like) rash, caused by ampicillin reaction, is another possible reaction to drugs in the penicillin family.

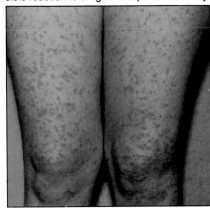

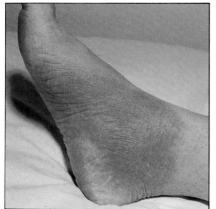

An aspirin reaction may cause a limited erythematous rash, like the one appearing on this patient's ankle.

In a sensitive patient, a sulfa drug may cause the painful, bulbous reaction shown here.

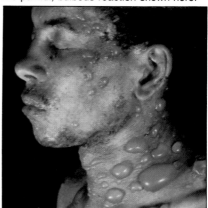

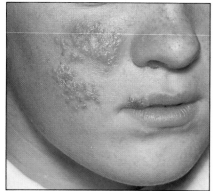

Herpes simplex causes recurrent, painful fever blisters (vesicles) on the mouth and face.

Urticaria (hives) are itchy, dermal wheals which may be caused by reaction to drugs, foods, environment, or climate changes.

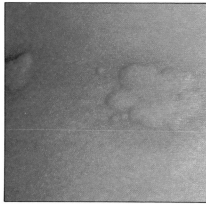

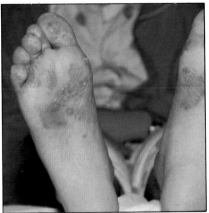

Nummular eczema, shown here, is characterized by patchy, scaly lesions.

Nummular eczema tends to occur symmetrically on the extremities.

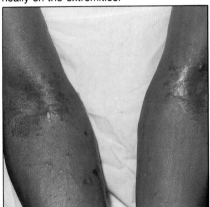

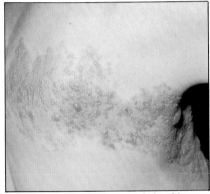

These vesicles are characteristic of herpes zoster (shingles). Typically, they erupt along a peripheral nerve in the torso, as shown here.

After about 10 days, herpes zoster lesions begin to dry and form scabs.

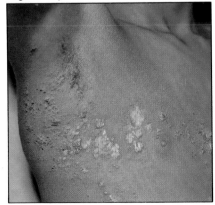

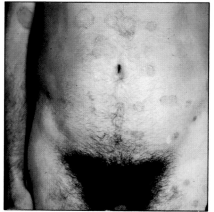

Tinea (ringworm) corporis, a fungus infection, causes flat, round lesions on the body.

Tinea capitis is ringworm of the scalp. It causes small, spreading papules, as shown here, and commonly affects children.

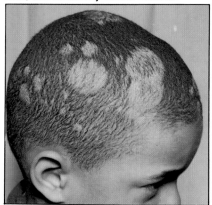

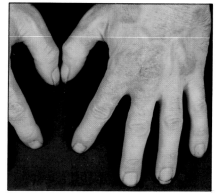

Contact dermatitis occurs after skin contact with an irritating substance. This patient's contact dermatitis has been complicated by a hemolytic *streptococcus* infection.

Basal cell carcinoma, which usually appears on the face, is most prevalent among fair-skinned Caucasians over age 40. In later stages, it may produce a rodent ulcer, like the one shown here.

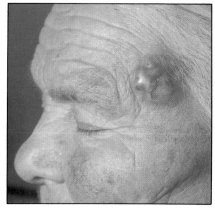

• *flat:* multiple groupings of up to several hundred slightly raised lesions with smooth, flat, or slightly rounded tops; .common on the face, neck, chest, knees, dorsa of hands, wrists, and flexor surfaces of the forearms; usually occur in children but can affect adults. Distribution is often linear, because these warts can spread from scratching or shaving.

• *plantar:* slightly elevated or flat; occurs singly or in large clusters (mosaic warts), primarily at pressure points of the feet

• *digitate:* fingerlike, horny projection arising from a pea-shaped base; occurs on scalp or near hairline

• *condyloma acuminatum* (moist wart): usually small, pink to red, moist, and soft; may occur singly or in large cauliflowerlike clusters on the penis, scrotum, vulva, and anus. Although this type of wart may be transmitted through sexual contact, it's not always venereal in origin.

Diagnosis

Visual examination usually confirms diagnosis. Plantar warts can be differentiated from corns and calluses by certain distinguishing features. Plantar warts obliterate natural lines of the skin, may contain red or black capillary dots that are easily discernible if the surface of the wart is shaved down with a scapel, and are painful on application of pressure. Both plantar warts and corns have a soft, pulpy core surrounded by a thick callous ring; plantar warts and calluses are flush with the skin surface.

Recurrent anal warts require sigmoidoscopy to rule out internal involvement, which may necessitate surgery.

Treatment and additional considerations

Treatment of warts varies according to location, size, number, pain level (present and projected), history of therapy, the patient's age, and compliance with treatment. Most persons eventually develop an immune response that causes warts to dis-

appear spontaneously and require no treatment.

Treatment may include:

• *Electrodesiccation and curettage:* High-frequency electric current destroys the wart, and is followed by surgical removal of dead tissue at the base and application of an antibiotic ointment (such as polysporin), covered with a bandage, for 48 hours. This method is effective for common, filiform, and occasionally, plantar warts.

• *Cryotherapy:* Liquid nitrogen or solid carbon dioxide kills the wart; the resulting dried blister is removed several days later. If initial treatment isn't successful, it can be repeated at 2- to 4-week intervals. This method is useful for either periungual warts or for common warts on the face, extremities, penis, vagina, or anus.

• *Acid therapy* (primary or adjunctive): The patient applies plaster patches impregnated with acid (such as 40% salicylic acid plasters), or acid drops (such as 5% to 16.7% salicylic and lactic acid in flexible collodion) every 12 to 24 hours for 2 to 4 weeks. This method is not recommended for areas where perspiration is heavy or that are likely to get wet, or for exposed body parts where patches are cosmetically undesirable.

• *25% podophyllum in compound with tincture of benzoin (for venereal warts):* For protection, adjacent unaffected skin is covered with dimethicone or petrolatum before each treatment. The solution is then applied on moist warts. The patient must lie still while it dries, leave it on for 4 hours, and then wash it off with soap and water. Treatment may be repeated every 3 to 4 days and, in some cases, the compound must be left on a maximum of 24 hours, depending on the patient's tolerance. Triamcinolone cream 0.1% should be applied to relieve any post-treatment inflammation.

Antiviral drugs for treating warts are under investigation; suggestion and hypnosis are occasionally successful, especially with children. Perseverance with prescribed therapy is essential. The patient's sexual partner may also require treatment.

Psoriasis

Psoriasis is a chronic, recurrent disease marked by epidermal proliferation. Its lesions, which appear as erythematous papules and plaques covered with silvery scales, vary widely in severity and distribution. It affects about 2% of the population in the United States, and incidence is higher among Caucasians than other races. Although this disorder is most common in adults, it may strike at any age, including infancy. Psoriasis is characterized by recurring remissions and exacerbations. Flare-ups are often related to specific systemic and environmental factors but may be unpredictable; they can usually be controlled with therapy.

Causes

The tendency to develop psoriasis is genetically determined. Researchers have discovered significantly higher than normal incidence of certain histocompatibility antigens (HLA) in patients with psoriasis, suggesting a possible autoimmune deficiency. Onset of disease is also influenced by environmental factors. Trauma can trigger the isomorphic effect, or Koebner's phenomenon, in which lesions develop at sites of injury. Infections, especially those resulting from beta-hemolytic streptococcus, may cause a flare of guttate (drop-shaped) lesions. Other contributing factors include pregnancy, endocrine changes, climatic conditions (cold weather tends to exacerbate psoriasis), and emotional stress.

Generally, a skin cell takes 14 days to move from the basal layer to the stratum corneum, where after 14 days of normal wear and tear, it's sloughed off. The life cycle of a normal skin cell is 28 days, compared to only 4 days for a psoriatic skin cell. This markedly shortened cycle doesn't allow time for the cell to mature. Consequently, the stratum corneum becomes thick and flaky, producing the cardinal manifestations of psoriasis.

Signs and symptoms

The most common complaint of the patient with psoriasis is itching and, occasionally, pain from dry, cracked, encrusted lesions. Psoriatic lesions are erythematous and usually form well-defined plaques, sometimes covering large areas of the body. Such lesions most commonly appear on the scalp, chest, elbows, knees, back, and buttocks. The plaques consist of characteristic silver scales that either flake off easily or can thicken, covering the lesion. Removal of psoriatic scales frequently produces fine bleeding points (Auspitz sign). Occasionally, small guttate lesions appear, either alone or with plaques; these lesions are typically thin and erythematous, with few scales.

Widespread shedding of scales is common in exfoliative or erythrodermic psoriasis and may also develop in chronic psoriasis.

Rarely, psoriasis becomes pustular, taking one of two forms. In localized

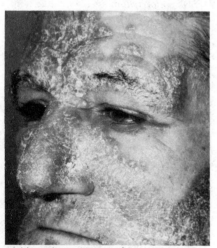

In this patient with psoriasis, plaques consisting of silver scales cover a large area of the face.

pustular psoriasis (Barber), pustules appear on the palms and soles, and remain sterile until opened. In generalized pustular psoriasis (Von Zumbusch), which often occurs with fever, leukocytosis, and malaise, groups of pustules coalesce to form lakes of pus on the skin. These pustules also remain sterile until opened and commonly involve the tongue and oral mucosa.

In approximately 30% of patients, psoriasis spreads to the fingernails (more often than the toenails), producing small indentations or pits, and yellow or brown discoloration. In severe cases, the accumulation of thick crumbly debris under the nail causes the nail to separate from the nailbed.

Many patients with psoriasis develop arthritic symptoms, usually in one or more joints of the fingers or toes, or sometimes in the sacroiliac joints, which may progress to spondylitis. Such patients may complain of morning stiffness. Joint symptoms show no consistent linkage to the course of the cutaneous manifestations of psoriasis; they demonstrate remissions and exacerbations similar to those of rheumatoid arthritis.

Diagnosis
Diagnosis depends on patient history, appearance of the lesions, and if needed, the results of skin biopsy. Typically, serum uric acid level is elevated, due to accelerated nucleic acid degradation, but indications of gout are absent. HLA antigens 13 and 17 may be present.

Treatment
Treatment depends on the type of psoriasis, the extent of the disease and the patient's response to it, and what effect the disease has on the patient's life-style. Unfortunately, no permanent cure exists, and all methods of treatment are merely palliative.

Removal of psoriatic scales necessitates application of occlusive ointment bases, such as petrolatum, salicylic acid preparations, or preparations containing urea. These medications soften the scales, which can then be removed in an oatmeal bath.

Methods to retard rapid cell production include exposure to ultraviolet light (wavelength B [UVB] or natural sunlight) to the point of minimal erythema. Tar preparations or crude coal tar itself may be applied to affected areas about 15 minutes before exposure, or may be left on overnight and wiped off the next morning. As treatment continues, exposure time to ultraviolet light can be increased gradually.

Steroid creams are useful to control psoriasis. A potent fluorinated steroid works well, except on the face and intertriginous areas. These creams require application three or four times a day, preferably after washing or bathing to facilitate absorption, and possibly with occlusive dressings—plastic wrap, plastic gloves or booties, or a vinyl exercise suit—especially overnight. Small, stubborn plaques that resist local treatment may require intralesional steroid injections. Anthralin, combined with a paste mixture, may be used for well-defined plaques but must not be applied to unaffected areas, because this synthetic compound may cause an allergic reaction; it also stains the skin. This medication is often used concurrently with steroids; anthralin is applied at night and steroids during the day.

In a patient with severe chronic psoriasis, the Goeckerman regimen—which combines tar baths and UVB treatments—may help achieve remission and clear the skin in 3 to 5 weeks. The Ingram technique is a variation of this treatment, using anthralin instead of tar. An experimental program called PUVA combines administration of methoxsalen with exposure to ultraviolet light, wavelength A (UVA). As a last resort, a cytotoxin, usually methotrexate, may be useful for severe and refractory psoriasis.

Low-dosage antihistamines (to minimize side effects), oatmeal baths, emollients (perhaps mixed with phenol and menthol), and open wet dressings may help relieve pruritus. Aspirin and local heat application help alleviate the pain of psoriatic arthritis; severe cases may require nonsteroidal anti-inflammatory drugs, such as indomethacin.

Therapy for psoriasis of the scalp often consists of a tar shampoo, followed by application of a steroid lotion while the hair is still wet. No effective treatment exists for psoriasis of the nails. The nails usually improve as skin lesions improve.

Additional considerations

The proper care plan should include patient teaching, careful monitoring for side effects of therapy, and sympathetic support.

• The patient must understand his prescribed therapy, and should be given written instructions to avoid confusion. He must know the correct way to apply prescribed creams and lotions. A steroid cream, for example, is applied in a thin film and rubbed into the skin until the cream disappears. Steroid creams are usually covered with an occlusive dressing and left on overnight. Anthralin is applied with a downward motion to avoid rubbing it into the follicles. Gloves are worn, since anthralin stains the skin. After application, the patient may dust himself with powder to prevent anthralin from rubbing off on his clothes. The patient must never put an occlusive dressing over anthralin. He can use mineral oil, then soap and water, to remove anthralin. The patient must avoid scrubbing his skin vigorously, to prevent Koebner's phenomenon. If a medication has been applied to the scales to soften them, the patient should use a soft brush to remove them.

• The patient must be watched for side effects, especially allergic reactions to anthralin, atrophy and acne from steroids, and burning, itching, nausea, and squamous cell epitheliomas from PUVA. The patient on methotrexate should be tested weekly for RBC, WBC, and platelet counts, since cytotoxins may cause hepatic or bone marrow toxicity. Liver biopsy may be done to assess the effects of methotrexate.

• The patient receiving PUVA therapy must stay out of the sun on the day of treatment, and should protect his eyes with special sunglasses that screen UVA for 24 hours after treatment. He must also wear goggles during exposure to ultraviolet light.

• Psoriasis can cause psychologic problems. The patient should know that psoriasis is not contagious, and although exacerbations and remissions occur, they're controllable with treatment. However, he must also understand there is no cure. Since stressful situations tend to exacerbate psoriasis, the patient must learn to cope with these situations. The relationship between psoriasis and arthritis should be explained, along with the fact that psoriasis causes no other systemic disturbances. All patients should be referred to the National Psoriasis Foundation, which provides information and directs patients to local chapters.

Lichen Planus

A benign but pruritic skin eruption, lichen planus usually produces scaling, purple papules, marked by white lines or spots. Such eruptions occur most often in middle-aged persons and are uncommon in the young or elderly. Lichen planus, a relatively rare disorder, is found in all geographic areas, with equal distribution among races. In most patients, it resolves spontaneously in 6 to 18 months; in a few, chronic lichen planus may persist for several years.

Causes

The cause of lichen planus is unknown, but possible causes may include a virus, an immunologic defect, or psychogenic factors, such as fatigue or severe emotional stress. Eruptions similar to lichen planus have been induced by certain chemicals and drugs.

Signs and symptoms

Lichen planus may develop suddenly or insidiously. Initial lesions commonly appear on the arms or legs, and evolve into the generalized eruption of flat, glistening, purple papules, marked with white lines or spots (Wickham's striae). These lesions may be linear, due to scratching, or coalesce into plaques. Lesions often affect the mucous membranes (especially the buccal mucosa), male genitalia, and less often, the nails. Mild-to-severe pruritus is common.

Diagnosis

 Although characteristic skin lesions frequently establish the diagnosis of lichen planus, confirmation may necessitate skin biopsy.

Treatment

Treatment is essentially symptomatic.

The goal of therapy is to relieve itching with topical fluorinated steroids, with occlusive dressings; intralesional injections of steroids; oatmeal baths; and antihistamines. Vitamin A in the form of retinoic acid may shrink lesions but is not generally recommended. Systemic corticosteroids, given in early acute stages, may shorten the duration of the disease. If a drug is suspected as the cause, it should be discontinued. Treatment of lichen planus associated with emotional stress may require counseling to identify stressors and teach more effective coping mechanisms.

Additional considerations

Medications should be given, as ordered, and the patient informed of possible side effects, especially drowsiness produced by antihistamines.

The patient may need emotional support. He should be reassured that lichen planus, although annoying and unsightly, is usually a benign, self-limiting condition.

Corns and Calluses

Usually located on areas of repeated trauma (most often the feet), corns and calluses are acquired skin conditions marked by hyperkeratosis of the stratum corneum. Prognosis is good with proper foot care.

Causes and incidence

A corn is a hyperkeratotic area that usually results from external pressure, such as that from ill-fitting shoes, or less commonly, from internal pressure, such as that caused by a protruding underlying bone (due to arthritis, for example). A callus is an area of thickened skin, generally found on the foot or hand, produced by external pressure or friction. Persons whose activities produce repeated trauma (for example, manual laborers or guitarists) commonly develop calluses.

The severity of a corn or callus depends on the degree and duration of trauma.

Signs and symptoms

Both corns and calluses cause pain through pressure on underlying tissue by localized thickened skin. Corns contain a central keratinous core, are smaller and more clearly defined than calluses, and are usually more painful. The pain they cause may be dull and constant or sharp when pressure is applied. "Soft" corns are caused by the pressure of a bony prominence. They appear as whitish thickenings and are commonly found between the toes, most often in the fourth interdigital web. "Hard" corns are sharply delineated and conical, and appear most frequently over the dorsolateral aspect of the fifth toe.

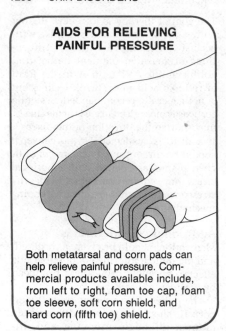

AIDS FOR RELIEVING PAINFUL PRESSURE

Both metatarsal and corn pads can help relieve painful pressure. Commercial products available include, from left to right, foam toe cap, foam toe sleeve, soft corn shield, and hard corn (fifth toe) shield.

Calluses have indefinite borders and may be quite large. They usually produce dull pain on pressure, rather than constant pain. Although calluses commonly appear over plantar warts, they're distinguished from these warts by normal skin markings.

Diagnosis
Diagnosis depends on careful physical examination of the affected area and on patient history revealing chronic trauma.

Treatment
Surgical debridement may be performed to remove the nucleus of a corn, usually under a local anesthetic. In intermittent debridement, keratolytics—usually 40% salicylic acid plasters—are applied to affected areas. Injections of corticosteroids beneath the corn may be necessary to relieve pain. However, the simplest and best treatment is essentially preventive—avoidance of trauma. Corns and calluses disappear after the source of trauma has been removed. Metatarsal pads may redistribute the weight-bearing areas of the foot; corn pads may prevent painful pressure.

Patients with persistent corns or calluses require referral to a podiatrist or dermatologist; those with corns or calluses caused by a bony malformation, as in arthritis, require orthopedic consultation.

Additional considerations
The patient must know how to apply salicylic acid plasters. The plaster should be large enough to cover the affected area. The sticky side is placed down on the foot, then the plaster is covered with adhesive tape. Plasters are usually taken off after an overnight application but may be left in place for as long as 7 days. After removing the plaster, the patient should soak the area in water and abrade the soft, macerated skin with a towel or pumice stone. He should then reapply the plaster, and repeat the entire procedure until all the hyperkeratotic skin has been removed. The patient must avoid removing corns or calluses with a sharp instrument, such as a razor blade or knife.

The patient should wear properly fitted shoes. Metatarsal or corn pads can be used to relieve pressure. He may need to be referred to a podiatrist, dermatologist, or orthopedist.

The patient should be assured that corns or calluses can be corrected with proper care.

Pityriasis Rosea

An acute, self-limiting, inflammatory skin disease, pityriasis rosea produces a "herald" patch—which usually goes undetected—followed by a generalized eruption of papulosquamous lesions. Although this noncontagious disorder may develop at any age, it's most apt to occur in adolescents and young adults. Incidence rises in the spring and fall.

Causes
The cause of pityriasis rosea is unknown, but the brief course of the disease and the virtual absence of recurrence suggest a viral agent or an autoimmune disorder.

Signs and symptoms
Pityriasis typically begins with an erythematous "herald" patch, which may appear anywhere on the body. Although this slightly raised, oval lesion is about 2 to 6 cm in diameter, approximately 25% of patients don't notice it. A few days to several weeks later, yellow-tan or erythematous patches with scaly edges (about 0.5 to 1 cm in diameter) erupt on the trunk and extremities—and sometimes on the face, hands, and feet in adolescents. Eruption continues for 7 to 10 days, and the patches persist for 2 to 6 weeks. Occasionally, these patches are macular, vesicular, or urticarial. A characteristic of this disease is the arrangement of lesions along body cleavage lines, producing a pattern similar to that of a pine tree. Accompanying pruritus is usually mild but may be severe.

Diagnosis
Characteristic skin lesions support the diagnosis. Differential diagnosis must also rule out secondary syphilis (through serologic testing), dermatophytosis, and drug reaction.

Treatment and additional considerations
Treatment focuses on relief of pruritus, with emollients, oatmeal baths, antihistamines, and occasionally, exposure to ultraviolet light or sunlight. Topical steroids in a hydrophilic cream base may be beneficial. Rarely, if inflammation is severe, systemic corticosteroids may be required.
- The patient should be reassured that pityriasis rosea is noncontagious, that spontaneous remission usually occurs in 2 to 6 weeks, and that lesions generally don't recur.
- The patient must avoid scratching. He should be told that hot baths may intensify itching. The use of antipruritics should be encouraged.

Hyperhidrosis

Hyperhidrosis is the excessive secretion of sweat from the eccrine glands. It usually occurs in the axillae (typically after puberty) and on the palms and soles (often starting during infancy or childhood).

Causes
Genetic factors may contribute to the development of hyperhidrosis, and in susceptible individuals, emotional stress appears to be the most prominent cause. Increased CNS impulses may provoke excessive release of acetylcholine, producing a heightened sweat response. Exercise and a hot climate can cause profuse sweating in these patients. Certain drugs, such as antipyretics, emetics, meperidine, and anticholinesterase, have been known to increase sweating.

In addition, hyperhidrosis often occurs as a clinical manifestation of an underlying disorder. Infections and chronic diseases, such as tuberculosis, malaria, or lymphoma, may cause excessive nighttime sweating. A person with diabetes often demonstrates hyperhidrosis during a hypoglycemic crisis. Other predisposing conditions include pheochromocytomas; cardiovascular disorders, such as shock or heart failure; CNS disturbances (most often lesions of the hypothalamus); withdrawal from drugs or alcohol; menopause; and Graves' disease.

Signs and symptoms
Axillary hyperhidrosis frequently produces such extreme sweating that patients often ruin their clothes in 1 day and develop contact dermatitis from clothing dyes; similarly, hyperhidrosis of the soles can easily damage a pair of shoes. Profuse sweating from both the soles and palms hinders the patient's ability to work and interact socially. Patients with this condition often report increased emotional strain.

Diagnosis
Clinical observations and patient history confirm hyperhidrosis.

Treatment
Treatment of choice is application of 20% aluminum chloride in absolute ethanol. Formaldehyde may also be used but may lead to allergic contact sensitization. Glutaraldehyde produces less contact sensitivity than formaldehyde but stains the skin; it's used more often on the feet than on the hands, as a soak or applied directly several times a week and then weekly, as needed. Therapy sometimes includes anticholinergics, except in patients with glaucoma or prostatic hypertrophy. Severe hyperhidrosis unresponsive to conservative therapy may require local axillary removal of sweat glands or, as a last resort, a cervicothoracic or lumbar sympathectomy.

Additional considerations
The patient will need support and reassurance, since hyperhidrosis may be socially embarrassing. Nightly, he should apply aluminum chloride in absolute ethanol to dry axillae, soles, or palms. The area should be covered with plastic wrap for 6 to 8 hours, and then washed with soap and water. This procedure should be repeated for several consecutive nights, until profuse daytime sweating subsides. Frequency of treatments can then be reduced. The patient with hyperhidrosis of the soles should wear leather sandals and white or colorfast cotton socks whenever possible to keep his feet cool. (The dye in colored socks can irritate his skin.)

Pemphigus

Pemphigus is a rare, chronic, blistering disease that causes superficial and deep lesions. In pemphigus foliaceus and its variant forms—pemphigus erythematosus and fogo selvagem—the characteristic bullous lesions are superficial; in both pemphigus vulgaris, the most common form of this disease, and pemphigus vegetans, a rare variant, the lesions extend deeper in the epidermis. The mortality of pemphigus vulgaris is high, even with treatment.

Causes and incidence
The cause of pemphigus is unknown, but an autoimmune reaction may contribute to its development.

Pemphigus foliaceus primarily affects the elderly and, occasionally, children, and is slightly more common in persons of Jewish ancestry than in other ethnic groups.

Pemphigus vulgaris often strikes the debilitated and is most prevalent in persons of Jewish or Mediterranean descent. This form may occur at any age but is most likely to appear between ages 40 and 50.

Signs and symptoms
Pemphigus foliaceus usually develops slowly. It may begin with bullous lesions, commonly on the head and trunk. As these lesions spread to other parts of the body, they become moist, scaly, and malodorous. Nikolsky's sign is present— the outer layer of skin can easily be

rubbed off by sliding a finger over it. Denudation of the lesions results in extensive areas of erythematous skin, with large, loose scales and crusts. Pruritus and burning are usual. Oral lesions are uncommon.

Pemphigus vulgaris can have an acute onset and progress rapidly, or it can be chronic. This form of the disease commonly starts in a specific location, favoring the same parts of the body as pemphigus foliaceus, and becomes increasingly generalized; it usually involves the mucous membranes. Initial involvement of the oral mucosa (in 50%) heralds a more fulminating course. The bullae may be tender or painful and are usually flaccid, varying in size from small to large and leaving sizable areas of denuded skin when they rupture. The exudate may be clear, bloody, or purulent. Nikolsky's sign is again present, but pruritus is less common than in pemphigus foliaceus.

Diagnosis
Characteristic clinical features, patient history, and histopathologic and immunofluorescence studies confirm pemphigus.

Treatment
Treatment of choice is administration of corticosteroids, supplemented with immunosuppressives. Acutely ill patients require high doses of corticosteroids, usually prednisone, and concomitant administration of adrenocorticotropic hormone by I.V. drip to help control new blistering. In the acute stage, patients may require I.V. therapy to replace tissue fluid and electrolyte losses. Less severe conditions may be controlled with low-dose corticosteroids, sometimes given on alternate days, which are also suitable for maintenance therapy. Long-term management may also include immunosuppressives (such as methotrexate, cyclophosphamide, and azathioprine) or, possibly, gold therapy with or without concomitant corticosteroids.

Topical application of fluorinated corticosteroids and open wet dressings may also be beneficial.

Additional considerations
• The patient on corticosteroids and immunosuppressives must be observed closely for signs of secondary infection and possible complications of drug therapy, especially hepatotoxicity and bone marrow depression with immunosuppressives. Infection can be prevented by washing hands thoroughly and wearing gloves before touching lesions. The patient should be told that the reason for wearing gloves is to protect him from infection.

• Cool wet compresses and baths, and topical application of fluorinated topical corticosteroids may ease discomfort.

• In acute stages, the patient's weight and electrolytes should be monitored daily, since significant fluid loss may occur through the skin. I.V. replacement therapy may be required.

• The patient needs good nutrition with a diet high in protein and calories.

• Good mouth care is needed for the patient with oral lesions. He should follow a soft diet, and use a topical anesthetic mouthwash, such as lidocaine, to alleviate mouth pain. Special dental care may be necessary to maintain healthy gums.

Decubitus Ulcers
(Pressure sores, bedsores)

Decubitus ulcers are localized areas of cellular necrosis that occur most often in the skin and subcutaneous tissue overlying bony prominences. These ulcers may be superficial, caused by local irritation to the skin with subsequent maceration of the surface, or deep, originating in underlying tissue. Deep lesions often go undetected until they penetrate the skin surface, by which time they've usually caused extensive subcutaneous damage.

Causes

Pressure, particularly over bony prominences, interrupts normal circulatory function and causes most decubitus ulcers. The intensity and duration of such pressure governs the severity of the ulcer; pressure exerted over an area for a moderate period (1 to 2 hours) produces tissue ischemia and increased capillary pressure, leading to edema and multiple small-vessel thromboses. An inflammatory reaction gives way to ulceration and necrosis of ischemic cells. In turn, necrotic tissue predisposes to bacterial invasion and subsequent infection.

The patient's position determines the pressure exerted on the tissues. For example, if the head of the bed is elevated, or the patient assumes a slumped position, gravity pulls his weight downward and forward (toward the foot of the bed). This shearing force causes deep ulcers due to ischemic changes in the muscles and subcutaneous tissues, and occurs most often over the sacrum and ischial tuberosities.

Predisposing conditions for decubitus ulcers include altered mobility (due to immobilization and prolonged bed rest, impaired neurologic function, altered sensorium, or chronic illness), inadequate nutrition (leading to weight loss and subsequent reduction of subcutaneous tissue and muscle bulk), and a breakdown in skin or subcutaneous tissue (as a result of edema, incontinence, fever, pathologic conditions, or obesity).

Signs and symptoms

Decubitus ulcers commonly develop over bony prominences. Early features of superficial lesions are shiny, erythematous changes over the compressed area, caused by reactive hyperemia (vasodilation in the affected area when pressure is relieved). Superficial erythema progresses to small blisters or erosions and, ultimately, to necrosis and ulceration.

An inflamed area on the surface of the skin may be the first sign of underlying damage when pressure is exerted between deep tissue and bone. Bacteria, localized in a compressed site, cause inflammation and, eventually, infection, which leads to further necrosis of the surrounding tissue. A foul-smelling, purulent discharge may seep from a lesion that penetrates the skin from beneath. Infected, necrotic tissue prevents healthy granulation of scar tissue; a black eschar may develop around the edges and over the lesion.

Diagnosis

Decubitus ulcers are obvious on physical examination. Wound culture and sensitivity testing of the exudate in the ulcer identify infecting organisms. Based on these findings, antibiotics may be necessary. If severe hypoproteinemia is suspected, due to disease or severe protein loss through serous exudate in the lesion, total serum protein values and serum albumin studies may be appropriate.

Treatment and additional considerations

Successful treatment must relieve pressure on the affected area, keep the area clean and dry, and promote healing. Frequent repositioning is the most effective way to both prevent and heal decubitus ulcers. The hospital staff member should:

• check the skin of bedridden patients during each shift for possible changes in color, turgor, temperature, and sensation; examine an existing ulcer for any change in size or degree of damage; use, if necessary, pressure relief aids and topical agents as adjuncts to treatment. The function of such equipment should be explained to the patient.

• prevent pressure sores by repositioning the bedridden patient at least every 2 hours around the clock; minimize the effects of a shearing force by using a footboard and by not raising the head of the bed to an angle that exceeds 60°; keep the patient's knees slightly flexed for

SPECIAL AIDS FOR PREVENTING AND TREATING DECUBITUS ULCERS

Pressure relief aids:
- *Gel flotation pads* disperse pressure over a greater skin surface area, and are relatively convenient and adaptable for home and wheelchair use.
- *Water mattress* distributes body weight equally but is heavy and awkward; "mini" water beds (partially filled rubber gloves or plastic bags) may be used for small areas, such as heels and feet.
- *Alternating pressure mattress* contains tubelike sections, running lengthwise, that deflate and reinflate, changing areas of pressure; however, this mattress is noisy and its effectiveness remains unproven. It should be used with a single untucked sheet, since multiple layers of linen decrease its effectiveness. All connections have to be secure and the air hoses must be free of kinks.
- *Egg crate mattress* minimizes area of skin pressure with its alternating areas of depression and elevation: soft, elevated foam areas cushion skin; depressed areas relieve pressure. This mattress should be used with a single, loosely tucked sheet and is adaptable for home and wheelchair use. If the patient is incontinent, the mattress should be covered with a plastic sleeve.
- *Sheepskin* is soft, dry, absorbent, and easy to clean. It should be in direct contact with the patient's skin. Sheepskin is available in sizes to fit elbows and heels and is easily adaptable to home use.

- *Turning bed* is available in various makes and models (Stryker or Foster frame, Circ-Olectric bed, Roto-Rest). A turning bed is ineffective without adjuvant therapy. It also limits free movement, and is expensive and impractical for general use.

Topical agents:
- Gentle soap
- Zinc oxide cream
- Absorbable gelatin sponge
- Granulated sugar (mechanical irritant to enhance granulation)
- Dextranomer (inert, absorbing beads)
- Karaya gum patches
- Topical antibiotics (*only* when infection is confirmed by culture and sensitivity tests)
- Silver sulfadiazine cream (antimicrobial agent)
- Oxychlorosene calcium (antiseptic used for irrigations and wet-to-dry packs, in 0.4% solution)
- Povidone-iodine packs (remain in place until dry)

Skin-damaging agents which should be avoided:
- Harsh alkali soaps
- Alcohol-based products (witch hazel and astringents), which can cause vasoconstriction
- Tincture of benzoin (can cause painful erosions)
- Hexachlorophene (can irritate the central nervous system)

short periods (prolonged flexion may result in severe contractures); perform passive range-of-motion exercises, or encourage the patient to do active exercises, if possible.
- give meticulous skin care; keep the skin clean and dry without the use of harsh soaps; gently massage the skin around the affected area—not on it—to improve circulation and prevent damage to the skin and capillaries around the affected area (this will promote healing); rub moisturizing lotions into the skin thoroughly to prevent maceration of the skin surface; change bed linens frequently for patients who are diaphoretic or incontinent.
- clean open lesions with a 3% solution of hydrogen peroxide or normal saline solution; use dressings, if needed, that are porous and tape that is hypoallergenic; debride necrotic tissue, if necessary, to allow healing. (One method is to apply open wet dressings and allow

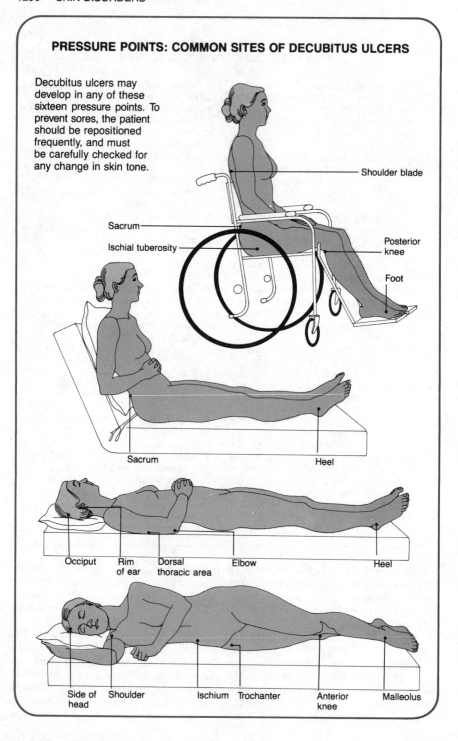

PRESSURE POINTS: COMMON SITES OF DECUBITUS ULCERS

Decubitus ulcers may develop in any of these sixteen pressure points. To prevent sores, the patient should be repositioned frequently, and must be carefully checked for any change in skin tone.

Shoulder blade

Sacrum

Ischial tuberosity

Posterior knee

Foot

Sacrum

Heel

Occiput

Rim of ear

Dorsal thoracic area

Elbow

Heel

Side of head

Shoulder

Ischium

Trochanter

Anterior knee

Malleolus

them to dry on the ulcer. Removal of the dressings mechanically debrides exudate and necrotic tissue. Other methods include surgical debridement with a fine scalpel blade, and chemical debridement through application of proteolytic enzyme agents.)
• encourage adequate intake of food and fluids to maintain body weight and promote healing; consult with the dietary department to provide a diet high in protein, calories, vitamins, and iron—all essential for granulation of new tissue; encourage the debilitated patient to eat frequent, small meals that include protein- and calorie-rich supplements; assist weakened patients to eat their meals.

Benign Skin Lesions

Common benign skin lesions include moles (pigmented nevi), freckles (ephelides), café au lait spots, lentigines, and seborrheic keratoses. These lesions are generally benign and are not usually cosmetically disfiguring.

Causes and incidence

Moles are thought to be an inherited characteristic, but the causes of other benign skin lesions are unknown. Moles are relatively uncommon in young children; only 1% to 3% of such lesions are congenital. They occur most often in young adults and, generally, disappear with advancing age. *Freckles* appear in fair-skinned, genetically predisposed persons (usually around ages 5 to 7) who are exposed to ultraviolet light. *Café au lait spots* affect about 10% of the population and are present at birth or appear later in life. *Lentigines* occur in childhood and are not sun-related, often appearing on nonexposed areas. They're associated with inherited disorders, such as multiple lentigines and both Moynahan's and Peutz-Jegher syndromes. Senile lentigines (liver spots) develop on sun-damaged skin in older persons. *Seborrheic keratoses* appear equally in older men and women, often in those with familial tendencies.

Signs and symptoms

Moles may be junctional, compound, or dermal, and range in color from yellow to brown or black. Their color and shape generally remain consistent, except during pregnancy, when they may darken.

Freckles are small (2 to 5 mm), flat, transient, circumscribed, brown macules that are irregularly scattered; they're most conspicuous during the summer because of more exposure to sunlight.

Café au lait spots are pale brown, uni-

COMMON MOLES

• *Junctional:* flat to slightly raised lesion, usually light to dark brown; found anywhere on body

• *Compound:* generally slightly raised and tan to dark brown, with melanocytes present in both dermis and epidermis; found anywhere on body

• *Dermal:* elevated, 2 to 10 mm in diameter, fleshtone to brown; most common on upper body; may contain hairs

• *Blue:* slightly elevated, less than 5 mm in diameter; color results from pigment deep within dermis and overlying collagen, reflecting blue light while absorbing other wavelengths; most common in women on head, neck, and arms

• *Lentigo maligna* (melanotic freckle of Hutchinson): initially flat, irregularly pigmented, tanned spot that gradually enlarges and darkens; most common on the face, and in persons over age 50; about one third progress to lentigo maligna melanoma.

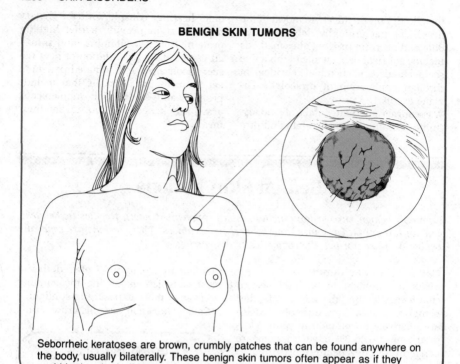

BENIGN SKIN TUMORS

Seborrheic keratoses are brown, crumbly patches that can be found anywhere on the body, usually bilaterally. These benign skin tumors often appear as if they could be brushed off but are actually difficult to remove.

form patches, more variably shaped than freckles. One to three spots are considered normal, but more than six may be characteristic of neurofibromatosis or Albright's syndrome.

Lentigines are round or oval, circumscribed macules, less than 3/8″ (1 cm) in diameter; they're generally darker than freckles but don't darken when exposed to sunlight, as freckles do. They commonly develop at sites of severe sunburn and on palms, soles, and mucous membranes.

Seborrheic keratoses are usually bilateral, symmetric, and less than 3/8″ (1 cm); they're located in areas that have an increased number of sebaceous glands, such as the chest, back, abdomen, and face. These lesions are usually yellow to brown, with velvety or waxy verrucal surfaces.

Diagnosis
Typical appearance usually confirms

benign skin lesions. Incisional (punch) or excisional biopsy may be necessary to rule out suspected malignancy. (Shave biopsy is contraindicated.)

Treatment and additional considerations
Generally, benign skin lesions don't require treatment. However, lesions that are cosmetically disfiguring or suspected of malignant transformation may require excision. When moles change in color, size, shape, or texture, or begin to ulcerate, bleed, or itch, malignant transformation is possible and must be considered. Seborrheic keratoses that are cosmetically undesirable (such as on the face) require simple curettage with pressure for hemostasis.

Because freckles become darker and more conspicuous after exposure to sunlight, fair-skinned, freckled persons may want to avoid excessive exposure and use sunscreens.

Selected References

Arndt, Kenneth A. MANUAL OF DERMATOLOGIC THERAPEUTICS. Boston: Little, Brown & Co., 1978.

Braverman, Irwin M. SKIN SIGNS OF SYSTEMIC DISEASE. Philadelphia: W.B. Saunders Co., 1970.

Cameron, Geraldine. *Pressure Sores: What to do when Prevention Fails*, NURSING79. 9:1:42-47, January 1979.

Fitzpatrick, Thomas B., et al. DERMATOLOGY IN GENERAL MEDICINE, 2nd ed. New York: McGraw-Hill Book Co., 1979.

Moschella, Samuel L., et al. DERMATOLOGY, Vols. 1 and 2. Philadelphia: W.B. Saunders Co., 1975.

Rook, Arthur, et al, eds. TEXTBOOK OF DERMATOLOGY, Vols. 1 and 2, 2nd ed. Philadelphia: J.B. Lippincott Co., 1972.

Sauer, Gordon C. MANUAL OF SKIN DISEASES, 4th ed. Philadelphia: J.B. Lippincott Co., 1980.

Stewart, William D., et al. DERMATOLOGY: DIAGNOSIS AND TREATMENT OF CUTANEOUS DISORDERS, 4th ed. St. Louis: C.V. Mosby Co., 1978.

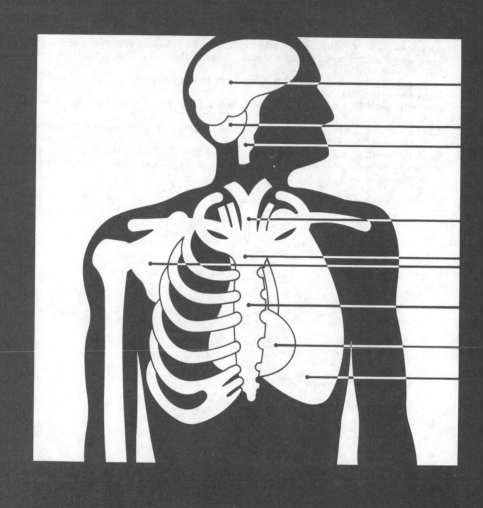

Appendices and Index

RARE DISEASES

DISEASE	DEFINITION AND CHARACTERISTICS
Akureyri disease: benign myalgic encephalomyelitis	Acute encephalitic/myelitic process marked by symptoms of damage to the white matter of the brain or spinal cord
Albarrán's disease: colibacilluria	Presence of *Escherichia coli* in the urine; may be associated with cystitis, pyelonephritis, and asymptomatic bacteremia; symptoms may include frequency, with burning and bladder pain.
Albers-Schönberg disease: osteopetrosis	Rare bone disorder marked by disorganization of bone structure that causes dense sclerotic bones vulnerable to recurrent fractures. Malignant variant begins in utero and progresses rapidly to cause marked anemia, hydrocephalus, cranial nerve involvement, hepatosplenomegaly, and fatal infection. Benign variant causes milder anemia and fewer neurologic abnormalities.
Arc-welders' disease: siderosis	Benign pneumoconiosis that can occur in iron ore miners, welders, metal grinders, and polishers from the inhalation and retention of iron
Armstrong's disease: lymphocytic choriomeningitis (LCM)	Central nervous system and influenzalike illness that may be associated with rash, arthritis, or orchitis. A zoonotic virus that causes meningitis and encephalitis. (Incidence rises in winter, when mice move indoors.) Probable port of entry is through the respiratory tract. Viremia occurs and LCM virus crosses the blood-brain barrier.
Baló's disease: leukoencephalitis periaxialis concentrica	Atypical form of Schilder's disease (see also Schilder's disease) causing concentric demyelination; most common in immunodeficient persons
Barometer-maker's disease: chronic mercurial poisoning	Soreness of gums, loosening of teeth, salivation, fetid breath, griping diarrhea, weakness, death
Basel disease: keratosis follicularis, Darier's disease	Any skin condition marked by formation of horny growths
Bateman's disease: molluscum contagiosum	Mildly contagious skin disease marked by formation of small waxy globular epithelial tumors containing semifluid caseous matter, or solid masses on the face, eyelids, breasts, and inner surfaces of thighs and genitalia
Bauxite workers' disease: bauxite pneumoconiosis, Shaver's disease	Occupational disorder causing rapid and progressive pneumoconiosis and leading to empyema; may be accompanied by pneumothorax
Behr's disease: degeneration of the macula retinae	Familial spastic paraplegia with or without optic atrophy; hyperactive tendon reflexes and sensory disturbances in adolescents and adults
Black disease	Rare infectious necrotic hepatitis
Blinding filarial disease: onchocerciasis, "river blindness"	Invasion of eye tissues by the filarial worm, which is enclosed in fibrous cysts or nodules

CAUSE	TREATMENT
Damage chiefly to white matter of brain or spinal cord secondary to perivascular cellular infiltration and perivenous myelination that may follow measles and smallpox, or vaccination against smallpox and rabies	Discontinuation of smallpox vaccine, use of measles vaccine to eliminate postinfectious encephalomyelitis, use of killed duck embryo vaccine for postrabies vaccination to decrease encephalomyelitis
Usually transmitted by fecal contamination, but airborne and fomes contamination are possible. Can be prevented by limited use of Foley catheters associated with rigorous aseptic technique; isolation of infectious patients; appropriate use of antibiotics, steroids, and cytotoxics in infection-prone patients; and increased fluid intake to flush urinary tract	Antibiotic treatment selected according to results of in vitro sensitivity tests. *E. coli* is sensitive to gentamycin (90%), ampicillin (85% to 90%), tetracycline (75%); streptomycin (50%); and high concentrations of penicillin (50%)
Malignant variant transmitted as autosomal recessive trait; benign variant transmitted as autosomal dominant trait. Increased bone mass secondary to defect in remodeling bone, resulting in thickened cortices (increased density). Bone is mechanically abnormal and fractures easily.	Transfusion of nucleated marrow cells from a healthy, clinically normal donor (almost always a sibling); associated splenectomy may decrease erythrocyte destruction and increase erythrocytic life span and effectiveness
Inhalation and retention of iron after exposure to iron oxide fumes and dust	Limiting or preventing exposure to iron dust or fumes prevents progression of this disease.
Viral infection that follows exposure to food or dust contaminated by rodents. Can be prevented by careful handwashing (although mode of transmission may be airborne).	Supportive and symptomatic management
Viral infection from the papovaviruses (JC virus).	Supportive and symptomatic management; invariably fatal
Mercury poisoning resulting from chronic exposure to mercury or its vapors	Evacuate stomach, lavage with milk or sodium bicarbonate but treat with BAL (dimercaprol) as soon as possible to prevent fatal progression
Unknown	No specific therapy, but keratolytic lotions and moistening skin to prevent cracking, drying, and skin breakdown may be useful.
A large virus of the pox group	Incision and drainage of tumor contents, followed by cleansing with iodine base solution
Inhalation of dust particles of alumina and silica (bauxite)	Elimination of exposure to bauxite
Hereditary form of cerebellar ataxia	No confirmed treatment; vitamin B therapy sometimes indicated
Clostridium novyi	Immediate surgical debridement and antibiotic therapy (usually 20 mU/day of penicillin by continuous IV infusion)
Onchocerca volvulus transmitted by the blackfly *(Simulium* and *Eusimulium)*	Diethylcarbamazine to destroy microfilarial but has little effect on the adult worm. Antihistamines treat possible allergic reactions. This condition leads to blindness despite treatment.

RARE DISEASES (continued)

DISEASE	DEFINITION AND CHARACTERISTICS
Bouillaud's disease: endocarditis	Rheumatic endocarditis
Breisky's disease: kraurosis vulvae	Vulval atrophy and dryness of skin and mucous membranes
Brown-Symmers disease	Acute serous encephalitis in children
Bruck's disease	Condition marked by deformity of the bones, multiple fractures, ankylosis of joints, atrophy of muscles
Bulimia	Obsessive eating associated with ritualistic vomiting and purging to maintain a desired weight level. Leads to electrolyte imbalance and may impair hepatic and renal function.
Castellani's disease: bronchospirochetosis	Hemorrhagic bronchitis, bronchopulmonary inflammation of the bronchial mucous membrane; usually follows the common cold
Central core disease of muscle	Rare muscle disease in which severe hypotonia causes weakness and arrests motor development in infancy. A central core in each muscle fiber is diagnostic.
Charrin's disease	Pyogenic infections causing formation of blue pus; may cause urinary tract infections or otitis externa
Chester's disease: xanthomatosis	Excessive accumulation of lipids in the long bones, marked by the formation of foam cells in skin lesions
Chiari-Frommel disease: Frommel's disease	Postpartum condition marked by uterine atrophy, persistent lactation, galactorrhea, prolonged amenorrhea, and low levels of urinary estrogen and gonadotropin
Cockayne's syndrome	Hereditary syndrome consisting of dwarfism, with retinal atrophy and deafness, associated with progeria, prognathism, mental retardation, and photosensitivity
Concato's disease	Progressive malignant polyserositis, with large effusions into the pericardium, pleura, and peritoneum
Conradi's disease: dysplasia epiphysealis punctata	Abnormal development of the secondary bone-forming center; marked by depressions or pinpoint structures
Creutzfeldt-Jakob syndrome: spastic pseudoparalysis, Jakob-Creutzfeldt disease	Rapidly progressive dementia developing between ages 40 and 65; accompanied by neurologic symptoms, such as myoclonic jerking, ataxia, aphasia, visual disturbances, and paralysis. EEG is abnormal early, with a distinct pattern useful for diagnosis.
Crocq's disease: acrocyanosis	Symmetrical cyanosis of the hands and feet; distinguished from Raynaud's disease by persistent discoloration.
Csillag's disease: lichen sclerosis et atrophicus	Acute inflammatory dermatitis, such as heat rash, prickly heat, miliaria rubra; chronic atrophic and lichenoid dermatitis
Czerny's disease	Joint pain, with swelling
Darier's disease: keratosis follicularis	Skin condition marked by excessive formation of horny growths, usually on the trunk, face, ears, nasolabial furrows, and scalp
Deutschländer's disease	Tumor of the metatarsal bones

CAUSE	TREATMENT
Delayed sequel to pharyngeal infection of group B streptococci	No specific cure; supportive therapy to reduce mortality/morbidity
Probable hypoestrinism	Surgery
Viral pathogens (rabies, measles, mumps, rubella, influenza)	Supportive care; control of intracranial pressure; correction of metabolic problems, disseminated in travascular coagulation, bleeding, renal failure, pulmonary emboli, and pneumonia; invariably fata
Unknown	Symptomatic and supportive management
Abnormal mental state marked by overwhelming obsession with food. Compulsion to eat may be related to low blood glucose levels.	Treatment difficult but successful at special clinics. Hypnotherapy used occasionally.
Spirochete infection	Bed rest and fluid intake; antipyretics, analgesics, and antibiotics; nebulization; humidified therapy
Transmitted as autosomal dominant trait	Symptomatic and supportive management
Pseudomonas aeruginosa	Increased fluid intake to flush urinary tract; appropriate antibiotics; vitamin C to increase glomerular filtration rate
Disturbances of lipid metabolism	Unknown
Possibly pituitary dysfunction or tumor	Treatment of underlying illness
Transmitted as autosomal recessive trait	Effective treatment unknown; symptomatic management; establishment of protective environment
Mycobacterium tuberculosis	Thoracentesis and parenteral or oral antitubercular antibiotics, such as apreomycin, para-aminosalicylic acid, and ethionamide
Hereditary	Supportive management, ensuring adequate calcium intake
Probably related to a latent virus; may be dependent on genetically determined susceptibility to a common agent, common environment, or familial dietary habits	Effective treatment unknown; symptomatic and supportive management that establishes a protective environment. Invariably fatal.
Vasospastic disturbance of smaller arterioles of the skin of unknown cause	Reassurance and protection from exposure to cold; vasodilators may be prescribed for cosmetic reasons
Keratin obstruction of sweat ducts	Symptomatic management, including cool environment, application of calamine lotion, and desquamation by ultraviolet rays
Serous effusion in a joint space or cavity	Treatment of inflammation; aspiration of joint space
Unknown	Systemic antibiotics can induce temporary amelioration.
Unknown	Surgery

RARE DISEASES (continued)

DISEASE	DEFINITION AND CHARACTERISTICS
Diamond-skin disease: swine erysipelas	Acute febrile vascular disease, causing localized swelling and inflammation of the skin and subcutaneous tissue
Dubois' disease: congenital syphilis	Multiple thymic abscesses in congenital syphilis
Duhring's disease: dermatitis herpetiformis	Chronic inflammatory disease marked by erythematous, papular, vesicular, bullous, or pustular lesions, with tendency to grouping and associated with itching and burning
Dukes' disease: fourth disease	Marked by myalgia, headache, fever, pharyngitis, conjunctivitis, generalized adenopathy, desquamation following confluent raised erythema
Dupré's disease: meningism	Noninflammatory irritation of the brain and spinal cord, with symptoms simulating meningitis
Durand's disease	Marked by headache, with upper respiratory tract, meningeal, and gastrointestinal tract symptoms
Duroziez's disease: congenital mitral stenosis	Narrowing orifice of the mitral valve that obstructs blood flow from atrium to ventricle
Eales's disease	Condition marked by recurrent hemorrhages into the retina and vitreous, mainly affecting males in the second and third decades of life
Economo's disease: lethargic encephalitis, Vienna encephalitis, sleeping sickness	Epidemic encephalitis marked by increasing languor, apathy, and drowsiness, progressing to lethargy; usually occurs in winter
Elevator disease	Respiratory distress affecting persons who work in grain elevators; a form of occupational pneumoconiosis
Engel-Recklinghausen disease: hyperparathyroidism, osteitis fibrosa cystica generatisata	Fibrous degeneration of bone, with the formation of cysts and fibrous nodules on bone affected
Engman's disease	Infectious eczematoid dermatitis
Eosinophilic endomyocardial disease: Löffler's endocarditis, Löffler's syndrome	Benign self-limiting pneumonitis marked by transient eosinophilic infiltration of the lungs and associated with marked eosinophilia in the blood and sputum, involving endocardium and myocardium
Epstein's disease: pseudodiphtheria, mononucleosis	Classic heterophil-positive infectious mononucleosis, occasionally complicated by neurologic diseases, i.e., encephalitis or transverse myelitis
Eulenburg's disease: myotonia congenita, Thomsen's disease	Slowly progressive disease of the skeletal muscles; similar to muscular dystrophy
Fifth disease: erythema infectiosum	Contagious form of macula, showing rose-colored eruptions diffused over the skin
File-cutters' disease	Lead poisoning from inhalation of particles of lead that arise during file-cutting
Fish-skin disease	Condition of dry and scaly skin resembling fish skin; two forms: hystrix and vulgaris
Fish-slime disease	Rapidly progressive septicemia following a puncture wound by the spine of a fish

CAUSE	TREATMENT
Streptococcus pyogenes; capillary congestion follows dilatation of superficial capillaries resulting from stress, inflammation, or external heat stimulation	Penicillin or erythromycin; application of cool magnesium sulfate compresses; aspirin for pain; and fluid replacement, as needed
Treponema pallidum, a spirochete transmitted by venereal contact	Penicillin, or in allergic patients, oxytetracycline, chlortetracycline, or erythromycin
Cause unknown; most prevalent in males	Removal of sources of reflex irritation; application of antiseptic to excoriated areas
Most likely a viral exanthema of Coxsackie-ECHO group	Symptomatic and supportive management
Unknown	Symptomatic and supportive management
Viral infection	Symptomatic and supportive management
Congenital	Surgical management, if possible; otherwise, supportive management
Possible causes include sickle cell anemia, tuberculosis, obscure vasculitis	Treatment of underlying causes
Arthropod-borne virus or sequela of influenza, rubella, varicella, or vaccinia	Symptomatic management, including appropriate antibiotics for secondary infection
Inhalation of dust particles, causing irritation and inflammation of respiratory tract	Elimination of exposure to dust
Marked osteoclastic activity secondary to parathyroid hyperfunction, with calcium/phosphorus metabolic disturbances	Control of parathyroid hyperactivity
Endogenous and exogenous agents	Topical application of corticosteroids, bath oils, lubricants, and topical antibiotics for secondary infections
Tubercle bacillus, privet pollen, *Ascaris, Trichinella*	Antibiotics for secondary endocarditis or myocarditis
Epstein-Barr virus	Symptomatic management, including appropriate antibiotics; generally benign course
Transmitted as autosomal dominant trait	Treatment comparable to that for muscular dystrophy
Capillary congestion from dilatation of superficial capillaries caused by nerves, heat, sunburn, general inflammation	Symptomatic treatment
Inhalation of lead particles	Avoidance of exposure to lead
Congenital	Effective treatment unknown
Septic substances introduced into blood through puncture wound	Supportive and symptomatic management of septicemia and secondary infections

RARE DISEASES (continued)

DISEASE	DEFINITION AND CHARACTERISTICS
Flax-dresser's disease	Pulmonary disorder of flax-dressers
Flecked retina disease	Group of retinal disorders, including fundus flavimaculatus, fundus albipunctatus, drusen, and congenital macular degeneration; all may be primary abnormalities at retinal pigment epithelium
Fleischner's disease	Inflammation of bone and cartilage affecting the middle phalanges of the hand
Fourth venereal disease: balanoposthitis	Specific gangrenous and ulcerative inflammation of the glans penis and prepuce; granuloma inguinale
Frankl-Hochwart's disease: polyneuritis cerebralis meniformis	Recurrent, progressive symptoms, including progressive deafness, ringing in the ears, dizziness, and a sensation of fullness/pressure in the ears; vertigo
Friedländer's disease: endarteritis obliterans	Chronic, progressive thickening of the intima, leading to stenosis or obstruction of the lumen
Friedreich's disease: paramyoclonus multiplex, Friedreich's ataxia	Tremors resembling those in multiple sclerosis, with evidence of cerebellar involvement of its pathways
Fürstner's disease; pseudospastic paralysis	Excessive tone and spasticity of muscles; exaggeration of tendon reflexes but loss of superficial reflexes; positive Babinski response
Gensoul's disease: Ludwig's angina	Infection of the sublingual and submandibular spaces, characterized by brawny induration of the submaxillary region, edema of the sublingual floor of the mouth, and elevation of the tongue
Gerlier's disease: endemic paralytic vertigo, paralyzing vertigo	Nervous system disorder in farmworkers and stableworkers, marked by pain, vertigo, paresis, and muscle contractions
Graefe's disease: ophthalmoplegia progressiva	Gradual paralysis of the eye, affecting first one eye muscle then the other
Grinder's disease: pneumoconiosis	Permanent deposition of particles in the lungs
Habermann's disease	Sudden onset of a polymorphous skin eruption of macules, papules, and occasionally vesicles, with hemorrhage
Haff disease	Condition affecting fishermen of the Haff lagoon, which joins the Baltic Sea; characterized by severe pain in the extremities, with accompanying weakness and weariness with myoglobinuria
Hagner's disease	Obscure bone disease resembling acromegaly, associated with increased soft-tissue growth after puberty; increased metabolic rate, with increased sweating and sebaceous activity
Heerfordt's disease: uveoparotid fever	Variant of sarcoidosis
Hemoglobin C–thalassemia disease	Simultaneous heterozygosity from hemoglobin C and thalassemia; characterized by mild hemolytic anemia and persistent splenomegaly
Henderson-Jones disease: osteochondromatosis	Presence of numerous benign cartilaginous tumors in the joint cavity or in the bursa of a tendon sheath
Heubner's disease	Syphilitic inflammation of tunica intima of cerebral arteries
Hodgson's disease	Aneurysmal dilatation of the proximal aorta, resulting in cardiac hypertrophy

CAUSE	TREATMENT
Inhalation of flax particles	Avoidance of exposure to flax
Congenital	Supportive and symptomatic management
Unknown	Anti-inflammatory agents (including steroids in severe cases) and analgesics
Sexual transmission of *Candida albicans*	Topical application of amphotericin B or nystatin and treatment of underlying causes, such as diabetes mellitus or malnutrition
Inflammation of the nerves (of the membranous labyrinth)	Bed rest, antihistamines
Trauma, pyogenic bacterial infection, infective thrombi, syphilis	Endarterectomy
CNS damage secondary to trauma, or infection	Treatment of underlying disease
Lesions of upper motor neurons or cerebrum	Treatment of underlying disease
Usually abscesses of the second and third mandibular molars	Large doses of penicillin; significant airway obstruction may require tracheotomy.
Disease of the internal ear from pressure of cerumen on the drum membrane	Symptomatic management; scopolamine for combatting nausea
Usually secondary to brain lesions	Treatment of underlying disease, corrective lenses
Inhalation of dust particles	Irreversible pulmonary disease; eliminating exposure to dust particles can prevent further irritation of tissues
Virus resembling smallpox	Supportive management; isolation may be necessary
Arsenic poisoning from waste water of cellulose factories; by direct contact with or ingestion of fish that have been exposed to toxins	Supportive and symptomatic management
Growth hormone—secreting tumors that develop after puberty	Management of cardiovascular complications; surgery for large tumors and irradiation (proton beam or heavy particle treatment and supravoltage)
Impaired regulation of thymus-derived lymphocytes (T cells) and bone marrow-derived lymphocytes (B cells)	Adrenal corticosteroids to suppress inflammation and control symptoms
Hereditary and congenital	Supportive management, including transfusions for severe anemia, and folate therapy
Irritation and trauma	Resection of tumor, with curettage and bone grafts
Treponema pallidum	Supportive management, including antibiotic therapy
Degenerative process involving the elastic and muscular components of the medial layer; hypertension, aortic dissection, trauma	Surgery

RARE DISEASES (continued)

DISEASE	DEFINITION AND CHARACTERISTICS
Hoffa's disease	Proliferation of fatty tissue (solitary lipoma) in the knee joint
Huchard's disease	Chronic arterial hypertension
Hünermann's disease: dysplasia epiphysealis punctata	Failure of ossification of center in bone formation
Hutchinson-Gilford disease: progeria	Premature old age marked by small stature, wrinkled skin, and gray hair, with attitude and appearance of old age in very young children
Hutinel's disease	Tuberculous pericarditis, with cirrhosis of the liver in children
Hydatid disease	Hepatic infection marked by development of expanding cysts (hydatid cysts); cysticerosis by *Taenia solium*
Hydatid disease, alveolar	Invasion and destruction of tissue as endogenous budding of cysts form an aggregate over the affected organ—usually the liver—and may metastasize
Hydatid disease, unilocular	Infection causing marked formation of single or multiple unilocular cysts
Iceland disease: epidemic neuromyasthenia, benign myalgic encephalomyelitis	Marked by headaches, muscle pain, low-grade fever, lymphadenopathy, fatigue, paresthesia; outbreaks occur in summer, usually in young women
Isambert's disease	Acute miliary tuberculosis of the larynx and pharynx
Jaffe-Lichtenstein disease: cystic osteofibromatosis	Form of polyostotic fibrous dysplasia marked by an enlarged medullary cavity with a thin cortex, which is filled with fibrous tissue (fibroma)
Jaksch's disease: anemia pseudoleukemica infantum	Syndrome of anisocytosis, peripheral red blood cell immaturity, leukocytosis, and hepatosplenomegaly that usually occurs in children under age 3
Jansen's disease: metaphyseal dysostosis	Skeletal abnormality with nearly normal epiphyses in which the metaphyseal tissues are replaced by masses of cartilage
Jensen's disease: retinochoroiditis juxtapapillaris	Inflammation of the retina and choroid marked by small inflammatory areas on the fundus close to the papilla
Kawasaki disease: mucocutaneous lymph node syndrome	High fever for 5 or more days, associated with conjunctivitis, generalized lymphadenopathy, palmar desquamation, swollen tongue and pharyngitis, body rash; most prevalent in preschool children, but age ranges from infancy to adolescence
Kienbock's disease: (1) lunatomalacia, (2) traumatic syringomyelia	(1) Slowly progressive osteochondrosis of the semilunar (carpal lunate) bone from avascular necrosis; (2) cavity formation in the spinal cord
Kirkland's disease	Acute throat infection, with regional lymphadenitis
Knight's disease	Perianal infection following skin abrasion (so called because of prevalence in equestrians)
Köhler's bone disease: tarsal scaphoiditis, epiphysitis juvenilis	Osteochondrosis of the tarsal navicular bone in children; onset about age 5
Krabbe's disease: globoid cell leukodystrophy	Rapidly progressive cerebral demyelination, with large globoid bodies in the white matter, associated with irritability, rigidity, tonic seizures, convulsions, blindness, deafness, and progressive mental deterioration

CAUSE	TREATMENT
Tissue trauma	Aspiration or surgery
Arteriosclerosis	Supportive management, including reduction of arterial pressure
Unknown	Supportive and symptomatic management
Acquired immunodeficiency; sarcoma meningiomas	No known treatment
Mycobacterium tuberculosis	Tuberculostatic agents
Ingestion of fish or meat contaminated by larvae of tapeworms of the genus *Echinococcus* or fecal-oral route of *T. solium*	Antilarval treatment with thiobendazole steroids
Infection by *Echinococcus multilocularis* (larvae)	Symptomatic management and surgery; usually fatal
Infestation by *Echinococcus granulosus* (larvae); hydatid tapeworm in dogs and cats	Symptomatic management; surgery
Infection probable but possibly psychosocial phenomenon	Symptomatic management
Mycobacterium tuberuclosis	Tuberculostatic agents
May be a lipoid granuloma	Symptomatic and supportive management; surgery
Malnutrition, chronic infection, malabsorption hemoglobinopathies	Treatment of underlying causes
Unknown	Surgery
Unknown; probably an autoimmune process	Steroids may induce improvements.
Unknown	Symptomatic management to avoid arterial damage that has caused ruptured aneurysms and fatal heart damage
(1) Degenerative process, precipitated by trauma; (2) trauma	(1) Immobilization of wrist for several months; if ineffective, surgery; (2) possibly surgery
Unknown	Appropriate antibiotics and symptomatic management
Trauma	Symptomatic management
Unknown but trauma suspected	Protection of foot from excessive use of trauma. If pain is severe, plaster cast may be required for 6 to 8 weeks. Complete spontaneous recovery may occur.
Familial	Symptomatic management; death by age 2

DISEASE	DEFINITION AND CHARACTERISTICS
Kugelberg-Welander disease: juvenile progressive muscular atrophy	Slowly progressive muscular atrophy resulting from lesions of the anterior horns of the spinal cord; usual onset in preschool or adolescent years
Kümmell's disease: posttraumatic spondylitis	Intercostal neuralgia, with spinal pain and motor disturbances in the legs
Kuru	Chronic, progressive, and fatal neurologic disease found only in New Guinea
Kyrle's disease	Form of follicular disease marked by keratotic pegs in the hair follicles and eccrine ducts, penetrating the epidermis and extending into the corium, causing foreign-body reaction and pain
Larsen's disease: Larsen-Johansson disease	Accessory center of ossification within the patella, associated with flat facies and short metacarpals
Leiner's disease: erythroderma desquamativum	Generalized exfoliative dermatitis and erythroderma, chiefly affecting newborn breast-fed infants; probably identical to severe seborrheic dermatitis
Lenegre's disease	Acquired complete heart block
Lesch-Nyhan syndrome	Disorder of purine metabolism marked by mental and physical retardation, spastic cerebral palsy, compulsive self-mutilation of fingers and lips by biting; hyperuricemia and excessive uricaciduria
Letterer-Siwe disease: nonlipid reticuloendotheliosis	Hemorrhagic tendency, with eczematoid skin eruptions, lymph node enlargement, hepatosplenomegaly, progressive anemia
Lewandowsky-Lutz disease	Widespread red or red-violet lesions resembling verruca plana, having a tendency to become malignant
Lichtheim's disease	Subacute degeneration of the spinal cord, associated with pernicious anemia
Little's disease	Form of cerebral spastic paralysis and stiffness of the limbs, associated with muscle weakness, convulsions, bilateral athetosis, and mental deficiencies
Lung fluke disease: *Paragonimus westermanii, Paragonimus heterotrema*	Parasitic hemoptysis, or oriental hemoptysis from pulmonary cysts
MacLean-Maxwell disease	Chronic condition of the calcaneus, marked by enlargement of the posterior third and by sensitivity to pressure
Magitot's disease	Osteoperiostitis of the alveoli of the teeth
Malibu disease: surfers' nodules	Hyperplastic, fibrosing granulomas occurring over bony prominences of the feet and legs of surfers
Maple syrup urine disease	Enzyme defect in the metabolism of the branched chain amino acids, resulting in mental and physical retardation, feeding difficulties, and a characteristic odor of urine
Marburg disease: Marburg virus disease	Severe viral disease, characterized by skin lesions, conjunctivitis, enteritis, hepatitis, encephalitis, and renal failure
Marie-Strümpell disease: von Bechterew's syndrome, rheumatoid spondylitis	Progressive immobility of sacroiliac joints, paravertebral soft tissues, and spinal articulations; most prevalent in males, ages 10 to 30
Marie-Tooth disease	Progressive neuropathic (peroneal) muscular atrophy
Marion's disease	Obstruction of the posterior urethra resulting from muscular hypertrophy of the bladder neck or absence of the flexiform dilator fibers

CAUSE	TREATMENT
Transmitted as autosomal recessive or dominant trait	Supportive management; normal life span probable
Compression fracture of the vertebrae	Management of fracture; extension of spine
Slow virus thought to be associated with cannibalism	No effective treatment; invariably fatal
Unknown	Symptomatic management
Unknown	Supportive management; surgery
Allergic, hereditary, and psychogenic causes suspected	Symptomatic management
Primary degeneration of the conduction system	Artificial pacemaker; supportive management
Defective enzyme transmitted by female carriers as sex-linked recessive trait	Symptomatic and supportive management, including protective restraints; usually fatal in childhood
Probably transmitted as autosomal recessive trait	Symptomatic and supportive treatment of anemia
Virus identical to or closely related to the virus of common warts	No effective treatment
Vitamin B_{12} deficiency	Correction of vitamin B_{12} deficiency
Congenital; birth trauma, fetal anoxia, or maternal illness during pregnancy	Preventive measures and symptomatic management
Infestation by trematodes or flukes	Parasitotropic agents; symptomatic and supportive management of hemoptysis
Trauma	Supportive shoes; avoidance of prolonged standing; surgery
Usually secondary to gingivitis	Steroid therapy for extreme inflammation; antibiotics for secondary infection
Repeated trauma from surfboard	Supportive shoes; avoidance of prolonged standing
Transmitted as autosomal recessive trait	Supportive management
Exposure to African green monkeys	Symptomatic and supportive management; usually fatal
Unknown; hereditary predisposition possible	Management to suppress pain and inflammation; supportive maintenance of a functional posture
Unknown	Surgery
Congenital	Surgery

DISEASE	DEFINITION AND CHARACTERISTICS
Martin's disease	Periosteoarthritis of the foot
Maxcy's disease	Rickettsial infection endemic in southeastern United States
Meyer-Betz disease: idiopathic, spontaneous, or familial myoglobinuria	Myoglobinuria, which may be precipitated by strenuous exertion or possibly by infection, and marked by tenderness, swelling, and muscle weakness
Microdrepanocytic disease	Sickle cell thalassemia; anemia involving simultaneous heterozygosity for hemoglobin and thalassemia
Milroy's disease	Chronic lymphatic obstruction, causing lymphedema of the legs sometimes associated with edema of the arms, trunk, and face
Minamata disease	Severe neurologic disorder characterized by peripheral and circumoral paresthesia, ataxia, mental disabilities, and loss of peripheral vision
Minor's disease	Hematomyelia, involving the central parts of the spinal cord; marked by sudden onset of flaccid paralysis, with sensory disturbances
Minot's disease	Self-limiting hemorrhagic disease of the newborn
Morton's toe: metatarsalgia	Metatarsal pain
Mozer's disease: myelosclerosis	Sclerosis of the spinal cord; obliteration of the normal marrow cavity by the formation of small spicules of bone
Mule spinner's disease	Warts or ulcers, especially on the scrotum, that tend to become malignant; common among operators of spinning mules in cotton mills
Mushroom picker's disease	Allergic respiratory disease of persons working with moldy compost prepared for growing mushrooms
Norrie's disease: atrophia bulborum hereditaria	Bilateral blindness resulting from retinal malformation, with mental retardation and deafness
Olivopontocerebellar atrophy	Progressively deteriorating neurologic disease marked by ataxia, dysarthria, action tremor that develops late in middle life; often mistaken for mental illness; usually normal deep tendon reflexes, associated with occasional rigidity and other extrapyramidal signs
Opitz's disease	Thrombophlebitic splenomegaly
Otto's disease: arthrokatadysis	Osteoarthritic protrusion of the acetabulum
Owren's disease: parahemophilia	Rare hemorrhagic tendency resulting from deficiency of coagulation Factor V
Paas's disease	Familial disorder marked by skeletal deformities, such as coxa valga, shortening of phalanges, scoliosis, spondylitis
Patella's disease	Pyloric stenosis, following fibrous stenosis in patients with tuberculosis
Pearl-worker's disease	Recurrent inflammation of bone, with hypertrophy
Pelizaeus-Merzbacher disease: sudanophilic leukodystrophy	Hyperplastic centrolobar sclerosis marked by nystagmus, ataxia, tremors, choreoathetotic movements, parkinsonian facies, mental deterioration; begins early in life, predominantly in males
Pellegrini's disease: Pellegrini-Stieda disease, Köhler-Pellegrini-Stieda disease	Semilunar bony formation in the upper portion of the medial lateral ligament of the knee
Perrin-Ferraton disease	Snapping hip

CAUSE	TREATMENT
Trauma, excessive walking	Supportive shoes; avoidance of prolonged standing
Rickettsieae	Treatment of underlying disease
Unknown; familial tendencies possible	Bed rest; anti-inflammatory agents; steroids in extreme cases; analgesics for pain
Hereditary transmission	Management of anemia
Congenital and hereditary	Surgery
Alkyl mercury poisoning	Avoidance of causative agents; supportive and symptomatic management; usually fatal
Unknown	Treatment of underlying disease; supportive management
Unknown	Supportive management
Abnormality of the foot, or osteochondrosis	Supportive shoes; analgesics
Unknown	Surgery
Unknown	Surgery
Airborne irritant, usually mold	Supportive and symptomatic management
Transmitted as X-linked trait	Unknown
Transmitted as autosomal or recessive trait	No effective treatment; death usually follows pneumonia secondary to loss of cough reflex
Thrombosis of the splenic vein	Symptomatic and supportive management, including anticoagulation
Degenerative changes, probably hereditary	Surgery, if night traction and rest ineffective
Transmitted as autosomal recessive trait	Supportive management
Hereditary	Unknown
Secondary to tuberculosis	Surgery
Inhalation of pearl dust	Avoidance of exposure to pearl dust
Familial transmission as a sex-linked recessive trait	No effective treatment; invariably fatal in several years
Trauma	Surgical correction; supportive management
Unknown	No effective treatment

RARE DISEASES *(continued)*

DISEASE	DEFINITION AND CHARACTERISTICS
Plaster-of-Paris disease	Limb atrophy after prolonged enclosure in a plaster splint
Pneumatic hammer disease	Vasospastic disease of the hands
Poncet's disease	Rheumatic symptoms associated with tuberculosis
Pulseless disease	Progressive obliteration of the brachiocephalic trunk and the left subclavian and left common carotid arteries above their origin on the aortic arch (loss of pulse in both arms)
Purtscher's disease	Retinal angiopathy, with edema, hemorrhage, and exudation
Recklinghausen's disease of bone: osteitis fibrosa cystica	Presence of fibrous nodules on affected bones
Refsum's disease	Defect in metabolism of phytanic acid, marked by chronic polyneuritis, retinitis pigmentosa, and cerebellar signs (mild ataxia) with persistent elevation of protein in cerebrospinal fluid
Ritter's disease	Dermatitis exfoliativa neonatorum
Robles' disease	Onchocerciasis of the fibroid nodules, lymph, subcutaneous connective tissue, and eyes
Roger's disease	Presence of small asymptomatic ventricular septal defects
Rummo's disease	Downward displacement of the heart (cardioptosis); also known as Wenckebach's disease
Rust's disease	Tuberculous spondylitis of the cervical vertebrae
Sacroiliac disease	Chronic inflammation of the sacroiliac joint, associated with tuberculosis
Schanz's disease	Inflammation of the Achilles tendon
Schilder's disease: leukoencephalopathy	Diffuse degeneration of the brain in infancy or adolescence, characterized by loss of myelin and progressive loss of cerebral function, leading to spasticity, optic neuritis, blindness, and dementia
Scholz's disease: leukoencephalopathy	Demyelination of the white substance of the brain, producing sensory aphasia, cortical blindness, deafness, weakness, spasticity of the limbs, and eventually complete paralysis and dementia
Schridde's disease	Generalized edema; abnormal accumulation of serous fluid in the cellular tissue or in a body cavity
Sever's disease	Epiphysitis of the calcaneus
Shuttlemaker's disease	Faintness, shortness of breath, headaches, nausea
Silo-filler's disease	Pulmonary inflammation, often associated with acute pulmonary edema
Smith-Strang disease	Defective methionine absorption, resulting in white hair, mental retardation, convulsions, attacks of hyperpnea, and characteristic odor of urine
Sponge-diver's disease	Burning, itching, erythema, necrosis, and ulceration of skin common in Mediterranean divers
Stargardt's disease	Degeneration of the macula lutea, marked by rapid loss of visual activity and abnormal appearance and pigmentation of the macular area
Strümpell-Leichtenstern disease: hemorrhagic encephalitis	Lateral sclerosis, in which spasticity is limited to the legs

CAUSE	TREATMENT
Prolonged immobilization	Removal of cast; use or exercise of the affected limb
Prolonged trauma from use of pneumatic hammer	Avoidance of trauma
Mycobacterium tuberculosis	Tuberculostatic agents
Arteriosclerosis; loss of pulse in both arms	Surgery
Trauma—usually a crushing injury to the chest	Treatment of underlying injury and supportive management
Marked osteoclastic activity secondary to parathyroid hyperfunction	Control of parathyroid hyperfunction
Hereditary transmission as autosomal recessive trait	Symptomatic and supportive management
Unknown	Unknown
Onchocerca volvulus	Parasitotropic agents
Congenital	Surgery, if defects become symptomatic
Probably congenital	Unknown
Mycobacterium tuberculosis	Tuberculostatic agents
Mycobacterium tuberculosis	Tuberculostatic agents
Trauma	Symptomatic management with anti-inflammatory agents, steroids, analgesics
Unknown; possibly familial	Symptomatic and supportive management; invariably fatal
Transmitted as X-linked recessive trait	Symptomatic and supportive management
Congenital	Management of fluid and electrolyte balance; symptomatic and supportive management
Inflammation secondary to trauma, irritation	Treatment of underlying cause
Inhalation of wood dust	Supportive respiratory management; avoidance of exposure to wood dust
Inhalation of oxides of nitrogen and other gases that collect in silos	Supportive respiratory management; avoidance of exposure to silo gases
Transmitted as autosomal recessive trait	Unknown
Irritation by toxins of sea anemones of the *Sagartia* and *Actinia* genera	Symptomatic management, with local application of calamine lotion and treatment with antihistamines for hives and itching
Hereditary transmission	Corrective lenses as symptomatic treatment; supportive management
Hereditary transmission	Supportive management

RARE DISEASES (continued)

DISEASE	DEFINITION AND CHARACTERISTICS
Swediaur's disease: Schwediauer's disease	Inflammation of the calcaneal bursa
Tangier disease	Deficiency of high-density lipoprotein in the serum, with storage of cholesterol esters in the tonsils and other tissues
Tarabagan disease	Plague in humans
Thiemann's disease	Vascular necrosis of the phalangeal epiphysis, resulting in deformity of the interphalangeal joints
Thomson's disease: Rothmund-Thomson syndrome	Developmental hyperkeratotic lesions and xerodermatous changes
Tommaselli's disease	Pyrexia and hematuria
Trevor's disease	Dysplasia epiphysealis hemimelica
Tyrosinemia	*Hereditary form:* results in liver failure and renal tubular failure, hypoglycemia, rickets, darkening of the skin, and mild mental retardation; occasionally causes liver cancer *Transient form:* usually in premature newborns, marked by elevation of blood tyrosine
Tyzzer's disease	Necrotic lesions of liver and intestine
Vaisuani's disease	Progressive pernicious anemia in puerperal and lactating women, with malabsorption of vitamin B_{12}
Verneuil's disease	Syphilitic disease of the bursae
Vidal's disease	Lichen simplex chronicus; pruritic, discrete, confluent, lichenoid, papular eruptions
Volkmann's disease	Tibiotarsal dislocation, causing deformity of the foot
Von Hippel-Lindau disease	Phakomatosis angiomatosis of the retina, cerebellum, spinal cord, and less commonly cysts of the pancreas, kidneys, and other viscera; onset usually in third decade and marked by symptoms of retina or cerebral tumors
Wegner's disease	Osteochondritic separation of the epiphyses
Werdnig-Hoffmann paralysis: progressive muscular atrophy of infancy	Progressive degeneration of anterior horn cells and bulbar motor nuclei in a fetus or infant. Onset marked by hypotonia, with abducted and externally rotated hips and flexed knees; reflexes absent. Later marked by accessory use of respiratory muscles.
White-spot disease: lichen sclerosus et atrophicus	Characterized by irregular flat-topped papules with keratotic plugging. Often asymptomatic but may cause itching, soreness, atrophy, especially in genital areas.
Witkop's disease: Witkop-Von Sallmann disease	Benign intraepithelial dyskeratosis affecting the oral mucosa and bulbar conjunctiva
Wolman's disease	Xanthomatosis in infants; associated with calcification of the adrenal glands, failure to thrive, vomiting, diarrhea, hepatomegaly, splenomegaly, and foam cells in skin lesions and bone marrow.

CAUSE	TREATMENT
Irritation of bursa	Symptomatic management, with application of warm moist heat, anti-inflammatory agents, and analgesics
Excessive cholesterol intake	Reduction of serum cholesterol levels
Bite of an ectoparasite of the Mongolian marmot (tarabagan)	Parasitotropic agent
Familial tendency	Unknown
Hereditary transmission	Unknown
Quinine toxicity	Discontinue quinine; symptomatic and supportive management
Unknown	Unknown
Autosomal recessive trait, resulting in excess of tyrosine in blood and urine	Tyrosine restriction; liver transplant may be successful; otherwise, fatal early in childhood
Bacillus piliformis transmitted through contact with rodents or dogs	Symptomatic management and appropriate antibiotics
Inadequate secretion of intrinsic factor from gastric mucosa	Correction of vitamin B_{12} deficiency
Treponema pallidum	Early treatment of syphilis
Psychogenic origin suspected	Unknown
Congenital	Surgery
Transmitted as autosomal dominant trait	Early surgical intervention
Congenital syphilis	Effective treatment of syphilis during pregnancy
Transmitted as autosomal recessive trait	Symptomatic and supportive management; no effective treatment. Death usually occurs in a year, but if disease limited to legs, progression is slower.
Unknown but often associated with Caucasian females; some familial incidence	Symptomatic management
Hereditary	No effective treatment; symptomatic management depending on severity
Transmitted as autosomal recessive trait	No known treatment; invariably fatal

Acknowledgments

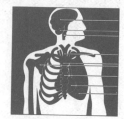

p. 12   © Martin Green, MD, 1979
p. 17   (upper right) © Carroll H. Weiss, RBP, 1980
p. 17   (lower right) © Carroll H. Weiss, RBP, 1980
p. 45   Ashley Montagu, *The Elephant Man, A Study in Human Dignity.* New York: E.P. Dutton, 1979.
p. 46   © Carroll H. Weiss, RBP, 1980
p. 57   (upper right) © Carroll H. Weiss, RBP, 1973
p. 63   Thomas Staudenmayer
p. 140 © Camera MD Studios, Inc., 1980
p. 150 Photo courtesy: *Consultant Magazine,* Greenwich, Conn.: Cliggott Publishing Co., 1972.
p. 157 © Carroll H. Weiss, RBP, 1980
p. 164 Tom McHugh/Photo Researchers
p. 165 Photo courtesy: *Consultant Magazine.* Greenwich, Conn.: Cliggott Publishing Co., 1971.
p. 167 © Carroll H. Weiss, RBP, 1980
P. 201 Paul A. Cohen
p. 216 © Carroll H. Weiss, RBP, 1980
p. 247 Photo courtesy: Roswell Park Memorial Institute, Department of Urologic Oncology, Buffalo, N.Y.
p. 271 Photo courtesy: Roswell Park Memorial Institute, Department of Urologic Oncology, Buffalo, N.Y.
p. 273 © Carroll H. Weiss, RBP, 1980
p. 274 © Carroll H. Weiss, RBP, 1980
p. 279 (upper right) © Carroll H. Weiss, RBP, 1980
p. 279 (lower right) © Carroll H. Weiss, RBP, 1980
p. 309 Photo courtesy: Ivan L. Roth, University of Georgia, Athens.
p. 313 Photo courtesy: Ivan L. Roth, University of Georgia, Atlanta.
p. 324B © Charles Gardner
p. 324D The Gram Stain Library, © Schering Corporation, Kenilworth, N.J. 07033

p. 342 Photo courtesy: Center for Disease Control, Atlanta, Ga.
p. 344 © Alfred T. Lamme, 1973
p. 361 © Carroll H. Weiss, RBP, 1978
p. 374 © Carroll H. Weiss, RBP, 1980
p. 389 © Carroll H. Weiss, RBP, 1980
p. 403 Photo courtesy: Center for Disease Control, Atlanta, Ga.
p. 407 © Carroll H. Weiss, RBP, 1976
p. 523 © Carroll H. Weiss, RBP, 1980
p. 529 © Carroll H. Weiss, RBP, 1980
p. 537 Photo courtesy: Marc S. Lapayowker, MD, Temple University Hospital, Philadelphia.
p. 539 © Carroll H. Weiss, RBP, 1980
p. 558 Photo courtesy: Eleanor M. Brower, RN, and Clyde L. Nash, Jr., MD, University Spine Center, Cleveland, Ohio .
p. 563 © Carroll H. Weiss, RBP, 1980
p. 570 © Carroll H. Weiss, RBP, 1980
p. 589 © Robert Ford, RBP, 1976
p. 601 Photo courtesy: Lucy Rorke, MD, Children's Hospital, Philadelphia.
p. 654 © Carroll H. Weiss, RBP, 1980
p. 678 Photo courtesy: Marc S. Lapayowker, MD, Temple University Hospital, Philadelphia.
p. 696 Photo courtesy: Marc S. Lapayowker, MD, Temple University Hospital, Philadelphia.
p. 744 © Carroll H. Weiss, RBP, 1973
p. 819 Photo courtesy: *Consultant Magazine.* Greenwich, Conn.: Cliggott Publishing Co., 1977.
p. 824 Photo courtesy: *Consultant Magazine.* Greenwich, Conn.: Cliggott Publishing Co., 1974.
p. 862 Photo courtesy: *Consultant Magazine.* Greenwich, Conn.: Cliggott Publishing Co., 1974.
p. 865 Photos courtesy: *Consultant Magazine.* Greenwich, Conn.: Cliggott Publishing Co., 1975.

p. 867   © Robert Ford, RBP, 1976
p. 882   © Carroll H. Weiss, RBP, 1980
p. 896   Photo courtesy: Majorie Beyers and Susan Dudas, *The Clinical Practice of Medical-Surgical Nursing.* Boston: Little, Brown & Co., 1977. Ron Hurst, Photographer.
p. 897   Photo courtesy: Majorie Beyers and Susan Dudas, *The Clinical Practice of Medical-Surgical Nursing.* Boston: Little, Brown & Co., 1977. Ron Hurst, Photographer.
p. 928   Photo courtesy: Dr. Edward Foord, Burlington County Memorial Hospital, Mount Holly, N.J.
p. 950   Photo courtesy: Sharon R. Reeder, et al., *Maternity Nursing.* Philadelphia: J.B. Lippincott Co., 1976.
p. 952   Photo courtesy: Dr. Edward Foord, Burlington County Memorial Hospital, Mount Holly, N.J.
p. 991   Photo courtesy: Center for Disease Control, Atlanta, Ga.
p. 994   Photo courtesy: Center for Disease Control, Atlanta, Ga.
p. 1055 © Carroll H. Weiss, RBP, 1980
p. 1056 © Carroll H. Weiss, RBP, 1980
p. 1108 Photo courtesy: Peter G. Lavine, MD, Crozer-Chester Medical Center, Chester, Pa.
p. 1144 Paul A. Cohen
p. 1175 © Muriel Laban Nussbaum, 1977
p. 1178 © Carroll H. Weiss, RBP, 1980
p. 1182 © Carroll H. Weiss, RBP, 1980
p. 1183 Photo courtesy: Heather Boyd-Monk, RN, Wills Eye Hospital, Philadelphia, Pa.
p. 1185 Photo courtesy: Wills Eye Hospital, Philadelphia, Pa.

p. 1202 © Tom Merrill, 1977
p. 1206 © Muriel Laban Nussbaum, 1977
p. 1232 Photo courtesy: *Consultant Magazine.* Greenwich, Conn.: Cliggott Publishing Co., 1978.
p. 1257 © Carroll H. Weiss, RBP, 1980
p. 1262 © Carroll H. Weiss, RBP, 1980
p. 1264 Photo courtesy: Evelina A. Bernardino, M.D., Dermatology, St. Mary Hospital, Langhorne, Pa.
p. 1265 © Christopher Papa, MD, 1978
p. 1266 © Carroll H. Weiss, RBP, 1980
p. 1267 (lower right) Photo courtesy: Reed and Carnrick, Pharmaceuticals, Kenilworth, N.J.
p. 1267 (upper right) © Carroll H. Weiss, RBP, 1980
p. 1268 Photo courtesy: Reed and Carnrick, Pharmaceuticals, Kenilworth, N.J.
p. 1268 Photo courtesy: Reed and Carnrick, Pharmaceuticals, Kenilworth, N.J.
p. 1275 © Carroll H. Weiss, RBP, 1980
p. 1278 (top to bottom) © Carroll H. Weiss, RBP, 1977
p. 1278 © Carroll H. Weiss, RBP, 1980
p. 1280 (top to bottom) © Carroll H. Weiss, RBP, 1980
p. 1280 © Carroll H. Weiss, RBP, 1980
p. 1280 © Carroll H. Weiss, RBP, 1978
p. 1284A-D Photos courtesy: Edward Glifort, Department of Dermatology, University of Pennsylvania, Philadelphia; and Gerald Pearlman, Skin and Cancer Hospital, Temple University Health Sciences Center, Philadelphia.
p. 1286 © Carroll H. Weiss, RBP, 1980

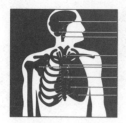

Sources of Additional Information

Al-Anon Family Group Headquarters
1 Park Ave.
New York, N.Y. 10016

Alateen World Service Headquarters
1 Park Ave.
New York, N.Y. 10016

Alcoholics Anonymous (AA)
General Service Board of Alcoholics
Anonymous
468 Park Ave., S.
New York, N.Y. 10016

American Association of Diabetes Educators
(AADE)
Box 56
North Woodbury Rd.
Pitman, N.J. 08071

American Association of Sex Educators,
Counselors and Therapists (AASECT)
5010 Wisconsin Ave., N.W.
Washington, D.C. 20016

American Cancer Society (ACS)
777 3rd Ave.
New York, N.Y. 10017

Association for Children with Retarded Mental
Development (A/CRMD)
902 Broadway
New York, N.Y. 10010

American Diabetes Association (ADA)
600 5th Ave.
New York, N.Y. 10020

American Foundation for the Blind (AFB)
15 W. 16th St.
New York, N.Y. 10011

American Red Cross (ARC)
17th and D Sts., N.W.
Washington, D.C. 20006

American Rheumatism Association (ARA)
% Arthritis Foundation
3400 Peachtree Rd., N.E.
Atlanta, Ga. 30326

American Speech-Language-Hearing
Association
10801 Rockville Pike
Rockville, Md. 20852

Anorexia Nervosa and Associated Disorders
(ANAD)
550 Frontage Rd., Suite 2020
Northfield, Ill. 60093

Arthritis Foundation (AF)
3400 Peachtree Rd., N.E.
Atlanta, Ga. 30326

Center for Disease Control
1600 Clifton Rd., N.E.
Atlanta, Ga. 30333

Committee to Combat Huntington's Disease
(CCHD)
250 W. 57th St., Suite 2016
New York, N.Y. 10019

Cystic Fibrosis Foundation
6000 Executive Blvd., Suite 309
Rockville, Md. 20852

Epilepsy Foundation of America (EFA)
1828 L St., N.W., Suite 406
Washington, D.C. 20036

Herpetics Engaged in Living Productively
(HELP)
260 Sheridan Ave.
Palo Alto, Calif. 94306

International Association of Laryngectomees
(IAL)
% American Cancer Society
777 3rd Ave.
New York, N.Y. 10017

Juvenile Diabetes Foundation (JDF)
23 E. 26th St.
New York, N.Y. 10010

Muscular Dystrophy Association, Inc.
810 7th Ave.
New York, N.Y. 10019

Myasthenia Gravis Foundation
15 E. 26th St.
New York, N.Y. 10010

National Foundation—March of Dimes
1275 Mamaroneck Ave.
White Plains, N.Y. 10605

National Hemophilia Foundation (NHF)
25 W. 39th St.
New York, N.Y. 10018

National Huntington's Disease Association
(NHDA)
1441 Broadway, Suite 501
New York, N.Y. 10018

National Lupus Erythematosus Foundation
(NLEF)
5430 Van Nuys Blvd., Suite 206
Van Nuys, Calif. 91401

National Multiple Sclerosis Society (NMSS)
205 E. 42nd St.
New York, N.Y. 10017

National Neurofibromatosis Foundation
340 E. 80th St.
New York, N.Y. 10021

National Parkinson Foundation (NPF)
1501 N.W. 9th Ave.
Miami, Fla. 33136

National Retinitis Pigmentosa Foundation
(NRPF)
Rolling Park Bldg.
8331 Mindale Circle
Baltimore, Md. 21207

National Psoriasis Foundation
6415 Southwest Canyon Court, Suite 200
Portland, Oreg. 97221

National Reye's Syndrome Foundation (NRSF)
509 Rosemont
Bryan, Ohio 43506

National Society for Autistic Children (NSAC)
1234 Massachusetts Ave., N.W., Suite 1017
Washington, D.C. 20005

National Sudden Infant Death Syndrome
Foundation (NSIDSF)
310 S. Michigan Ave., Suite 1904
Chicago, Ill. 60604

National Tay-Sachs and Allied Diseases
Association (NTSAD)
122 E. 42nd St.
New York, N.Y. 10017

President's Committee on Mental Retardation
Regional Office Bldg. #3
7th & D Sts., S.W.
Washington, D.C. 20201

Reach to Recovery Foundation
% American Cancer Society (ACS)
777 3rd Ave.
New York, N.Y. 10017

Smokenders
37 N. 3rd St.
Easton, Pa. 18042

Spina Bifida Association of America (SBAA)
343 S. Dearborn Ave., Suite 319
Chicago, Ill. 60604

United Cerebral Palsy Associations (UCPA)
66 E. 34th St.
New York, N.Y. 10016

United Ostomy Association
1111 Wilshire Blvd.
Los Angeles, Calif. 90017

United Parkinson Foundation (UPF)
220 S. State St.
Chicago, Ill. 60604

U.S. Committee for the World Health
Organization (USC-WHO)
777 United Nations Plaza, 9A
New York, N.Y. 10017

Women Organized Against Rape
P.O. Box 64
Harrisburg, Pa. 17108

Index

Page numbers in boldface refer to major entries.

Gomori's stains, histoplasmosis and, 368
Gonadotropin
human chorionic, 917, 918
hypothyroidism in children and, 821
testicular cancer and, 244
Gonioscopy, 1176
Gonorrhea, **989-992**
epididymitis and, 801
statistics for, 990t
Goose bumps (gooseflesh), 1253
Gorging, self-imposed, 107-109
Gout, **522-525**
Sydenham's description of, 524t
Gouty arthritis, **522-525**
Grading of malignant diseases, 182-183
Graefe's disease, 1308
Graft-versus-host (GVH) reactions, 35
Gram-negative infections
bacilli, **329-350**
cocci, **316-317**
See also names of infections
Gram-positive infections
bacilli, **317-329**
cocci, **308-315**
See also names of infections
Gram's stains, 1256
anthrax and, 328
bronchiectasis and, 494
candidiasis and, 362
gas gangrene and, 324
septic arthritis and, 521
Grand mal seizures
alcoholism and, 101
epilepsy and, 606
Granulocytopenia, **1068-1070**
chronic lymphocytic leukemia and, 294
dengue and, 398
epidemic typhus and, 411
Granuloma fungoides, **286-288**
Granuloma inguinale, **1001-1002**
Granulomatosis, lipophagia, **683-684**
Granulomatous colitis, **677-678**
Granulosa-lutein cysts, 925-926
Graves' disease, **825-829**
pernicious anemia and, 1028
simple goiter and, 824
thyroiditis and, 822
Grawitz's tumor, **233-234**
Gray scale ultrasonography, ectopic pregnancy and, 947
Great vessels (great arteries), transposition of, **1093-1095**
Grinder's disease, 1308
Grippe, **381-382**
Grotton's papules, 568
Growth hormone (GH), 855
pituitary tumors and, 194
G 6-PD deficiency, pattern of transmission, 39t
Guillain-Barré syndrome, **624-**

627
botulism and, 322
mononucleosis and, 402
neurogenic bladder and, 794
peripheral neuritis and, 644
respiratory acidosis and, 471
syndrome of inappropriate antidiuretic hormone and, 905
testing for thoracic sensation and, 626t
Gunshot wounds, 134-136
Günther's disease, 889, 890t
Guthrie screening test, 53
Gynecologic disorders, **911-938**
external structures, 912-914, 913t
follicular cycle, 916t
internal structures, 913t, 914
pelvic examination, 920
sources of pathology, 920
See also names of disorders
Gynecomastia
Klinefelter's syndrome and, 64, 65
lung cancer and, 211
testicular cancer and, 244
Gyri, 580

H

Habermann's disease, 1308
Haff disease, 1308
Hager's sign, 918
Hagner's disease, 1308
Hair, 1253-1254
Hager's sign, 918
Hallucinations
chronic brain syndrome and, 100
schizophrenia and, 94-95
Hallucinogens, abuse of, 105t
Hallux valgus, **551-552**
Haloperidol
Huntington's disease and, 619
manic-depressive illness and, 94
schizophrenia and, 97
Halothane, nonviral hepatitis and, 730
Hamartoma, 1164
Hammer toe, 552t
Hand, postoperative care of 218t
Hansen's disease, **358-360**
Hartnup disease, pattern of transmission, 39t
Hashimoto's thyroiditis, 822
hypothyroidism in adults and, 818
simple goiter and, 824
Hay fever, **11-33**
HB$_s$Ag, 728
Headache, **603-605**
cluster, 603
hyperpituitarism and, 815
migraine, 603, 604, 605

clinical features of, 604t
Head injuries, **120-129**
See also types of injuries
Hearing, **1210-1213**
audiometric testing, 1211-1213
Hearing loss, 1211-1213, **1227-1229**
medullary cystic disease and, 758
Paget's disease and, 549
perforated eardrum and, 128
scrub typhus and, 413
Heart, **1076-1083**
amyloidosis of, 887t
the cardiac cycle, 1077-1079
common anomalies, 1092b,c
conduction, 1079
normal, 1145t
normal anatomy, 1092a
transport system and, 1076
See also Cardiovascular disorders; names of disorders
Heart attack, see Myocardial infarction
Heart block, 1141t
Heartburn
esophageal diverticula and, 663
gastroesophageal reflux and, 655
peptic ulcers and, 671
Heart disease
acquired inflammatory, **1096-1104**
esophageal atresia and, 657
pattern of transmission, 39t
tracheoesophageal fistula and, 657
valvular, **1104-1108**
forms of, 1105t-1107t
See also Cardiovascular disorders; names of disorders
Heart failure
congestive, 1116t, **1118-1120**
cor pulmonale and, 466
Paget's disease and, 548
Heart sounds, 1077-1079, 1080, 1081
Heart syndrome, athletic, **1166-1167**
Heart valves, 1076-1077
Heat cramps, **151-153**, 152t
Heat exhaustion, **151-153**, 152t
Heatstroke, **151-153**, 152t
Heat syndrome, **151-153**
managing, 152t
Heavy chain diseases, **1067-1068**
Hebephrenic schizophrenia, **95**
Heberden's nodes, 538
Heerfordt's disease, 1308
Helminth infections, **426-438**
See also names of infections
Hemangiomas, 206-207
Hemangiosarcoma, 270
Hematologic disorders, **1019-1073**

Page numbers in boldface refer to major entries.

Page numbers in boldface refer to major entries.

Page numbers in boldface refer to major entries.